Handbook of Fathers an
Development

Hiram E. Fitzgerald
Kai von Klitzing
Natasha J. Cabrera
Júlia Scarano de Mendonça
Thomas Skjøthaug
Editors

Handbook of Fathers and Child Development

Prenatal to Preschool

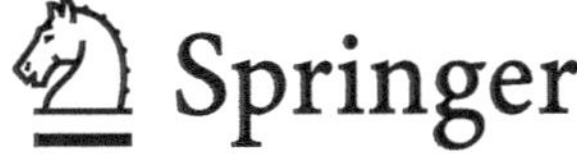

Editors
Hiram E. Fitzgerald
Michigan State University
East Lansing, MI, USA

Natasha J. Cabrera
University of Maryland
College Park, MD, USA

Thomas Skjøthaug
Division of Mental Health
Akershus University Hospital HF
Lørenskog, Norway

Kai von Klitzing
Department of Child and Adolescent Psychiatry
University of Leipzig
Leipzig, Sachsen, Germany

Júlia Scarano de Mendonça
Graduate Program in Educational Psychology
Centro Universitário FIEO
Osasco, São Paulo, Brazil

ISBN 978-3-030-51029-9 ISBN 978-3-030-51027-5 (eBook)
https://doi.org/10.1007/978-3-030-51027-5

This Springer imprint is published by the registered company Springer Nature Switzerland AG
The registered company address is: Gewerbestrasse 11, 6330 Cham, Switzerland

Foreword

Some Reflections on the Last 50 Years of Fatherhood Research: Progress, Promises, and Challenges

As this volume illustrates so well, as a field we have come a long way in both overcoming the idea that fathers are the forgotten parents and in unveiling the curtain that shrouded fathers in mystery. They are neither forgotten nor a mystery any longer but have assumed their rightful place along with mothers as central agents in the socialization of children. It was not always the case and with few exceptions such as early studies of wartime absent fathers, it was not until the 1960s and 1970s when the modern study of fathers began.

The Early Descriptive Phase

In the beginning, the goal was a descriptive one with the aim being to discover how men acted with infants and young children. These early efforts by Lamb (1976, 1981), Pederson and Robson (1969), and Parke (1979; Parke & Sawin, 1976) suggested that fathers as well as mothers were more capable as caregivers than previously imagined. In their role as fathers, men were competent feeding agents and expressed warmth and nurturance just as well as mothers even with newborn babies. They were able to read infant signals as well as mothers and adjusted their speech when addressing infants just as mothers did. And the infants responded accordingly. Infants developed attachments not just to mothers but to fathers as well and even used fathers as social referencing agents in stressful situations. These early studies not only confirmed that fathers were competent but in many ways were comparable to mothers in their ability to be engaged, nurturant, and competent caregivers. Consistent with evolutionary design, infants and young children were protected by a family social system in which redundancy and interchangeability between mothers and fathers were key components.

Other work in this early period underscored that a complete portrait of the emergence of fathering begins well before birth as studies of fathers during pregnancy and childbirth so well documented. Early studies of the couvade syndrome (Trethowan & Conolon, 1965) suggested that father's as well as mother's behaviors and emotions shift across the prenatal period. Moreover, the presence or absence of fathers during childbirth (Entwisle & Doering,

1981) was identified as a worthwhile topic of investigation – a reminder that fathering from the onset of pregnancy is embedded in a family system of couple and developing fetus (see Dayton, Malone, & Brown, 2020; Tolman & Walsh, 2020).

At the same time, as the overlapping aspects of paternal and maternal parenting style were being discovered, the unique features of opposite sex parents' interactive styles were being documented and described. Mothers and fathers differed in several ways. First, as consistent with cultural gender norms that guided maternal and paternal roles and responsibilities in this earlier era of the 1960s and 1970s, men in spite of their competence as caregivers were largely breadwinners while the major caregiving role fell to mothers. Even when adjusting for time available with infants and children, mothers spent a larger portion of their time in caregiving than fathers. Fathers, in turn, spent a larger proportion of their time with their offspring in playful interactions. Of course, mothers engaged in playful exchanges with their infants and young children just as fathers changed diapers and fed their infants but they each had specialized parts in the socialization story with mothers as caregivers and fathers as playmates.

Even the style of play differed across mothers and fathers. Fathers emerged as the physical play experts who routinely engage in touch and tickle routines and rough and tumble sequences. In contrast, mothers are less physical and more verbal and talkative when engaging their infants and are more likely to use toys as props in their play bouts, while fathers are less likely to engage in toy-mediated play. Mothers are more didactic and more likely to engage in teaching the infant and toddler during their playful exchanges. Finally, fathers' physical play is more arousing, stimulating, and exciting as well as more unpredictable and erratic. In contrast, maternal play is smoother and more predictable and modulated with gradual rather than abrupt changes in tempo and excitability. These stylistic differences between parents continue to be evident across the preschool period, and some would argue that paternal humor and sarcasm replaces physical play style as the child develops (See Vallotton, Foster, Harewood, Cook, & Adekoya, 2020).

The looming issue, however, was whether or not fathers make a difference in children's development. Abundant evidence has clearly documented that father involvement clearly matters for social as well as cognitive and language development. Studies in the decades of the 1980s and 1990s found that play and other forms of paternal involvement as well as aspects of interactive style such as contingent responsiveness were linked with enhanced social development (i.e., higher social acceptance by peers) (see Hennigar, Cabrera, & Chan, 2020), less deviant behavior (see Godleski & Eiden, 2020; McMahon, 2020), as well as academic achievement and linguistic and cognitive competence (see Panecsofar, 2020; Duursma, Ho, Grenyer, & Herbert, 2020; Meuwissen, 2020).

A related issue that was identified early and is of continuing interest is not only the effects of fathers on children but the impact of becoming a father on men's own psychological development including their mental health, their self-identity, and their occupational success (See Paulson, 2020; Skjøthaug, 2020; von Klitzing & White, 2020). Early work by Snarey (1993) guided by

Erikson's (1975) concept of generativity was particularly significant in guiding this line of inquiry. Involved fathering was, in turn, linked to societal generativity as indicated by caring for other younger adults such as serving as a mentor, providing leadership, and contributing to generational continuity. As both this work and Bradley (2020) remind us, fathering is best understood through an intergenerational and life span lens in which earlier childhood alters later adjustment as an adult, including the enactment of the father role which, in turn, alters subsequent cohorts of children.

Finally, the effects of the onset of fatherhood on maternal well-being and the marital relationship was the focus of studies of the transition to parenthood from the 1960s onward (see Palkovitz, 2020; Shears, 2020). Another important focus of inquiry from the earliest days of this descriptive era of fatherhood research was the documentation of the variability across fathers in their enactment of the paternal role. Often cast as the search for the determinants of fathering, this search focused on a variety of factors at several levels of analysis including individual characteristics such as paternal attitudes, motivation and skills, their quality of relationship with their family of origin, men's mental and physical health, and their age at the time of the onset of parenthood (in early adolescence vs on time vs late timed onset). The gender and birth order of the child with whom the father was involved were further determinants (see Volling, Steinberg, & Kuo, 2020). At the family level, the quality of the couple relationship and maternal gatekeeping were discovered as determinants of father involvement (see Frascarolo, Favez, Tissot, & Fivaz-Despeuringe, 2020). Finally, changing societal trends such as the shifts in maternal employment and the work schedules and job characteristics (degree of autonomy vs highly controlled; level of stress) of fathers emerged as important determinants of both father involvement and the quality of fathering behaviors. In sum, in this early descriptive phase, the main outlines of the fatherhood agenda were established, but only in the form of preliminary sketches and outlines of the contours of the issues. As this volume underscores, major advances over the ensuing decades have been made in flushing out the details and providing a clearer and more complete picture of the father's role. Moreover, as noted below, in the early stages, less attention was devoted to the explanatory processes that account for the effects of fathering on children and other players. We turn to the search for processes next.

From Description to Process

While progress in describing the father's role in the family was a necessary first step, identification of the underlying process that either accounted for paternal behavior or for the effects of fathers on their children is a needed next step. Several significant process advances are noteworthy. Following the work on father as a physical play partner, researchers discovered that infants and young children were learning important lessons in the context of play that, in turn, could, in part, account for the father's impact on children's social behavior with peers. First, when fathers were more democratic and less coercive and controlling in their father–child exchanges, children were more popular with their peers, in part, due to their ability to initiate activities and their capacity to respond appropriately to the social bids of their partners. Second, children learn to read and respond to their father's emotional signals or cues in the course of play bouts. The skill of being able to decipher a play partner's emotional messages is a critical one for maintaining a successful social exchange. Third, in the context of play, children learn to use their own emotional signals to regulate the interactions of their father playmate. Again, this skill of being able to accurately and clearly communicate one's emotions to an interactive partner is valuable and accounts, in part, for children's success in their peer interactions.

In sum, several emotion-related processes are acquired in the context of father-child play, which, in turn, transfers to other non-parental social contexts. Play between father and child is indeed not idle but a context for learning transferable skills about how to send and read other people's emotions in the course of social exchanges (see Bergmann & Klein, 2020; Paquette, Gagnon, & de Medeiros, 2020).

Closely related to emotional regulatory processes are a distinct but important additional mediator between fathering and child outcomes, namely attention regulatory abilities. These processes include the ability to attend to relevant cues, sustain attention, to refocus attention through such processes as cognitive distraction and cognitive restructuring, and other efforts to purposely reduce the level of emotional arousal in stressful situations. Attentional processes organize experience and play a central role in cognitive and social development beginning in early childhood. In summary, the ability to regulate attention is a further important mediator through which parental behavior, including paternal behavior, may influence children's social competence. In addition to learning to manage emotions in social encounters, children also develop cognitive representations or cognitive scripts that serve as guides to social exchanges with other social partners. Attachment theorists offer cognitive working models, whereas social and cognitive psychologists have suggested scripts or cognitive maps as guides for social action. Research within the attachment tradition have found support for Bowlby's argument that representations vary as a function of child-parent attachment history (see Brown & Aytuglu, 2020).

For example, children who had been securely attached infants were more likely to represent their family in their drawings in a coherent manner, with a balance between individuality and connection, than children who had been insecurely attached. In turn, securely attached children have better peer relationships. Research in the social interactional tradition as well as the attachment perspective reveals links between parent and child cognitive representations of social relationships and, in turn, their peer relationships. These include cognitive representations as well as scripts for dealing successfully with social partners. Other work suggests that father–child interaction is related to children's "theory of mind" competence, a clear asset for achieving social skills.

In addition, a variety of other process avenues have been identified, including the father as a manager of children's social contacts and a coach and guide in novel social situations. Clearly significant progress has been made in documenting not only the father's significant role in children's development but also in delineating a myriad of process pathways through which these effects are achieved.

Finally and of major significance as evidence of theoretical progress, there have emerged in the last several decades major theoretical models that aim at the integration of current knowledge and serve as guides for future work on fathering (see Fitzgerald, von Klitzing, Cabrera, Mendonça, & Skjethaug, 2020). These theoretical models are ambitious in scope and underscore the multiple social, demographic, cognitive, and biological/neurological factors which function as determinants of father involvement and, in turn, outline the processes and pathways which account for the effects of variations in fathering on child outcomes. Although single studies seldom encompass the array of factors outlined in these models, they serve as valuable heuristic devices for organizing current and guiding future work in this area.

Some Caveats and Challenges

Several more recent advances have challenged this relatively neat package of findings and progress and have opened up new avenues of inquiry. Many of these new directions are captured in this volume. The first challenge is based on the fact that much of the pioneering work was carried out in Western cultures or more accurately with Euro-American and middle class fathers. It was assumed that these findings would be universally valid across other cultures and generalizable to non-European American groups in North America and in Europe (see Rabie, Skeen, & Tomlinson, 2020; de Mendonca & Bussab, 2020). In the past several decades, these assumptions have been questioned on several fronts and have forced us to confront the variability in father behaviors across cultures and subcultures but also challenged some of our assumptions about the central features of the father role. For example, the well-established finding that the physical play style is the hallmark of the father's role has been questioned. Findings from a variety of non-Western cultures (Taiwan, India, Africa, Thailand) suggest that fathers rarely engage in physical play and few mother–father differences in play style are found (Roopnarine, Hooper, Ahmeduzzaman, & Pollack, 1993). These cross-cultural observations may lead to a reevaluation of the pathways through which fathers influence their children's development and lead to a rethinking of the father's role in fostering emotional regulation in children at least in some cultures (Lamb, 1987; Shwalb, Shwalb, & Lamb, 2013).

A related challenge to the centrality of physical play for fathers not only in other cultures but in Western cultures comes from the monitoring of secular changes in male and female roles. The movement of women into the workforce is well documented and the resulting increase in father involvement in caregiving is well established. Men and women are becoming increasingly similar in their distribution of caregiving responsibilities and their level of involvement, although women still engage in more childcare than men. However, at the same time there are notable shifts in styles of interaction that warrant more attention. The gender-of-parent differences, on average, are relatively small, and there is a good deal of overlap between mothers and fathers in both the style of play as well as in the absolute amount of time devoted to playful interactions. Fathers do not own the physical play franchise; mothers have a mixed play repertoire too, and can and do bounce and tickle as well as read and converse with their children. In the same vein, fathers, like mothers, play with toys, read books, and engage in pretend play in addition to their supposedly signature style of arousing and stimulating physical play. Both mothers and fathers contribute to their children's development in a myriad of playful ways. The stylistic differences in play between fathers and mothers became enshrined in our views of mothers and fathers based on work conducted 20–30 years ago when traditional conceptions of fathers' role predominated, maternal employment was still relatively uncommon and viewed negatively, and fathers were much less involved in the day-to-day care of their infants. As men in contemporary society have expanded their range of involvement to include more caregiving and managerial parenting activities, the predominance of play as the distinctive feature of the father role has diminished in importance. Play has become merely one of a variety of ways that fathers (and mothers) are involved with their children. Some leading father scholars (Lamb & Lewis, 2010) have revised their earlier views of the uniqueness of father play.

Moreover, demographic shifts in North America away from a predominantly white Euro-American profile to a more diverse culturally and racially complex picture are well documented. These changes have led to an increased interest in a range of ethnic and racial groups of fathers, which, in turn, has led to a reevaluation of our prior conclusions about paternal roles and behavior. Recent work has not only been devoted to a wide range of racial/ethnic groups, including African American, Latino, Asian American, and to a lesser extent native American fathers, but this evidence questions many stereotypes about the role of these fathers in the lives of their children (see Gadsden & Iruka, 2020; Mogro-Wilson, 2020; Allison-Burbank & Collins, 2020). These efforts have challenged stereotypes concerning both levels of involvement as well as bringing into question assumptions about the hierarchical and authoritarian nature of the fathering styles of these men in these racial groups. For example, comparisons across ethnic groups (African and European American) revealed either few differences in level of father involvement or in some studies African American fathers are higher in their levels of caregiving and play than European American fathers.

Along with a renewed focus on a range of racial and ethnic groups, there is increasing recognition that the cultural trends of involved fathers apply most clearly to economically and educationally advantaged families and to intact two-parent families while they apply less readily to less economically well-off and less-educated fathers and families (see Keizer, 2020). Especially as economic inequality has increased, it is important to recognize that income disparities between fathers have yielded more variability across social classes in the patterns of fathering. Most attention in the research literature has been devoted to the study of fathers in two-parent intact families. According to a recent survey of journal articles from 1930 to 2006, 76% of the fathers were from two-parent families and the rest were focused on divorced, single, or nonresident father families (Goldberg, Tan, & Thorsen, 2009). However, many fathers cohabit with their partners (rather than marry) while others may be divorced or not in residence with their partner but remain involved in the lives of their children. There is a renewed interest in documenting patterns of fathering among economically disadvantaged fathers who are often not residing with their offspring. Although these fathers may not be physically present, recent work has found these nonresidential fathers often rely on contact at a distance and communicate via phone or social media rather than face-to-face. Moreover, disadvantaged fathers provide input such as nurturance, play and leisure activities, safety, moral guidance, discipline, as well as contact through connections with the extended family and community. Studies reveal complex patterns of involvement while showing that these alternative involvement strategies are important for children's development.

It is not merely the disadvantaged, nonresident fathers who have received increased attention but other men who "father at a distance" and have limited face-to-face contact with their children due to incarceration, military deployment, or migration patterns (see Bocknek, 2020). Although divorced fathers have received plenty of research attention, these other men have remained in the research shadows, yet their circumstances are deserving of further scrutiny if we wish to understand the full range of fathering. Recent work has begun to examine the ways in which these men who are separated from their children are able to maintain contact and father from afar and in doing so impact their children's development and adjustment. While the issue of father military deployment has a long history, more sophisticated measurement and more fully developed theoretical frameworks have given new prominence to this topic (see Walsh & Rosenblum, 2020). In view of the high rates of incarceration among men, especially minorities in the USA, the focus on the effects of incarceration on men's fathering roles is a welcome advance. Similarly, the current concern about immigration policies and patterns has led to a heightened interest in the study of transnational fathering. Together, these alternative fathering arrangements across space and time have underscored the high degree of variability in fathering profiles and seriously challenged our traditional focus on residential fathering.

At the other extreme and in recognition of the plethora of family forms and caregiving arrangements in contemporary families there has been increased attention given to highly involved fathers such as those in reverse role families. In these families, fathers take on major caregiving roles while mothers assume the breadwinning role. Although relatively rare several decades ago (Russell, 1983), there has been a significant increase in these types of family arrangements in recent years (see Lee & Lee, 2020). These arrangements not only underscore the malleability of parental roles but provide unique opportunities to assess the effects of heightened father involvement on children's development and the relative importance of mothers and fathers in the socialization process.

Another challenge is the recent work on gay and lesbian families which has raised provocative issues for the field of fatherhood research. As the evidence suggests, children in families of same-sex parents develop adequately in terms of social-emotional adjustment (Golombok, 2015; Miller, Kors, &

Macfie, 2017; Patterson, 2016). These data help us address the uniqueness of fathers' and mothers' roles in the family. Moreover, they help provide clarity on the important issue of how essential fathers (Silverstein & Auerbach, 1999) and mothers (Parke, 2002, 2013) are for the successful socialization of their children. Moreover, these insights raise the possibility that our focus on the gender of the parent may be too narrow. Instead, it could be helpful to recast the issue and ask whether it is the extent to which exposure to males and/or females is critical or whether it is exposure to the interactive style typically associated with either mother or father that matters. Perhaps the style of parenting and gender of the parent who enacts the style can be viewed as partially independent. More attention to the kinds of parenting styles evident in same-gendered parental households will help us address the uniqueness of father and mother roles in the family and help provide needed clarity on the important issue of how essential fathers or mothers are for children's development.

A further challenge/opportunity is the re-biologization of fatherhood. In the early years of fatherhood research, much attention was devoted to the social, economic, and demographic determinants of fathering. Less emphasis was devoted to the biological underpinning of fathering behaviors, in part, due to the assumption that the lack of biological preparedness accounted for fathers' limited involvement in caregiving of children. Moreover, direct social experience of contact with infants was assumed to be sufficient for the activation of fathering behaviors as demonstrated in studies of adoption. Fortunately, recent evidence has challenged the assumption that fathers are biologically unprepared for fatherhood. Studies suggest that fathers experience hormonal changes accompanying the birth of an infant, which, in turn, makes them more ready for social interaction and more sensitive to infant social signals (Storey, Walsh, Quinton, & Wynne-Edwards, 2000; see Gettler, 2020). Moreover, some of the most striking evidence that fathers are biologically prepared for caregiving come from recent studies of how our brains react when we are exposed to babies. From the earliest days of life, fathers (as well as mothers) are neurologically primed to respond to infants. Using brain imaging techniques such as fMRI, they show more neural activation when shown pictures of babies than pictures of animate objects. Fathers and mothers show higher levels of activity in emotional processing areas of the brain when exposed to infant cries than nonparents. Other brain imaging studies found that men respond neurologically more to the cries of their own infants than to the distress signals of unrelated infants (see Grande, Tribble, & Kim, 2020). In sum, our brains as well as our hormones prepare not just mothers but fathers too for the challenges of caregiving. Including biological markers in our studies of fathering, along with our more established social and cognitive indices, will yield a fuller understanding of the multiple levels that determine fathering.

Another significant trend is the increasing interdisciplinarity of fathering research. In many ways, a psychological approach to fathering has a unique identity with its focus on intra-familial processes, such as actor attitudes, cognitions and beliefs, and the dynamic interchanges between and among family members. However, it is unlikely that we can fully understand fathers without recognizing the contributions of other disciplines. Sociologists inform us about issues of ethnicity, class, inequality, and demographic shifts while anthropologists alert us to cross-cultural variations. Economists document shifts in economic opportunities and struggles. Medical professionals provide insights about family illness, disease, and wellness-promoting strategies while evolutionary theorists clarify the trade-offs between the costs and benefits of father involvement for men. Additionally, legal scholars offer glimpses into how families are helped or hindered by laws and social policies that directly affect families. Historians remind us that cross time shifts in family forms, beliefs, and practices are constantly under revision. Beyond these traditional contributors to the study of fathers, some disciplines such as architecture and urban design have not received sufficient attention. The effects of living in multi-family households or in intergenerational housing on father roles are poorly understood. Our challenge is to examine how these innovations in housing arrangements alter various aspects of family life. As scholars of fathering, we need to understand better how these cross- disciplinary insights modify our process-oriented explanations of father functioning. A fuller understanding of fathering requires an interdisciplinary perspective.

Finally, the field has recognized that fathering research has important implications for the guidance of social and public policy. In part due to the acceptance of fathers as critical socializing agents in the healthy development of children, policy makers have increasingly undertaken the development of programs and policy guidelines aimed at supporting the father's role in the family (see Osborne, 2020). Public agencies such as state and federal governments have become active promoters of father involvement through awareness and educational campaigns as well as by recognizing the importance of such initiatives as family leave. While these policy efforts lag behind the policies of many European countries, especially Scandinavian countries, clear awareness and some progress is evident. Moreover, government support of father-directed intervention programs which are aimed at increasing father involvement is a welcome advance. These intervention efforts should be lauded not only as policies to strengthen father involvement but as valuable opportunities for theory evaluation. For example, these efforts can help establish direction of causality effects and provide some further evidence that the direction of effects flow in part from father to child. (see Pruett & Pruett, 2020; Fletcher, Macdonald, & St George, 2020; DeGarmo, 2020). Relatedly, private organizations such as the National Fatherhood Initiative, the National Centre on Fathering, the National At-Home Dad Network, Dad Central Canada and Polimundo, represent international efforts on behalf of fathers. In summary, policy makers are becoming significant partners in the fatherhood enterprise by aiding in translating scholarly advances into social action on behalf of fathers.

Final Thoughts

We have come a long way in the past half century not only in recognizing fathers as central players in family life and in the lives of our children but in beginning to understand the range of ways in which they alter children's development. We have made significant progress in outlining the pathways and processes through which these effects are achieved. Finally, we have attracted the attention of policy makers who have joined as active partners in promotion of father involvement. At the same time, significant challenges await, including broadening our definition of fathering to include a wider range of fathers who operate outside the traditional nuclear family model. Significant challenges await us about the necessity of fathers in light of the emerging work on lesbian parent families. This volume suggests that we are making advances on all of these issues, but as is always the case in scientific endeavors, this remains a progress report with much future work to be accomplished.

University of California, Riverside
Riverside, CA, USA
Ross D. Parke

References

Allison-Burbank, J. D., & Collins, T. (2020). Native American fathers and their sacred children. In H. E. Fitzgerald, K. von Klitzing, N. Cabrera, J. S. de Mendonça, & T. Skjøthaug (Eds.), *Handbook of fathers and child development: Prenatal to preschool*. New York: Springer.

Bergmann, S., & Klein, A. M. (2020). Fathers' emotional availability with their children: Determinants and consequences. In H. E. Fitzgerald, K. von Klitzing, N. Cabrera, J. S. de Mendonça, & T. Skjøthaug (Eds.), *Handbook of fathers and child development: Prenatal to preschool*. New York: Springer.

Bocknek, E. (2020). A family systems perspective on paternal absence, presence, and engagement. In H. E. Fitzgerald, K. von Klitzing, N. Cabrera, J. S. de Mendonça, & T. Skjøthaug (Eds.), *Handbook of fathers and child development: Prenatal to preschool*. New York: Springer.

Bradley, R. H. (2020). Fathers and their very young children: Future directions. In H. E. Fitzgerald, K. von Klitzing, N. Cabrera, J. S. de Mendonça, & T. Skjøthaug (Eds.), *Handbook of fathers and child development: Prenatal to preschool*. New York: Springer.

Brown, G. L., & Aytuglu, A. (2020). Father-child attachment relationships. In H. E. Fitzgerald, K. von Klitzing, N. Cabrera, J. S. de Mendonça, & T. Skjøthaug (Eds.), *Handbook of fathers and child development: Prenatal to preschool*. New York: Springer.

Dayton, C., Malone, J., & Brown, S. (2020). Pathways to parenting: The emotional journeys of fathers as they prepare to parent a new infant. In H. E. Fitzgerald, K. von Klitzing, N. Cabrera, J. S. de Mendonça, & T. Skjøthaug (Eds.), *Handbook of fathers and child development: Prenatal to preschool*. New York: Springer.

de Mendonca, J. S., & Bussab, V. S. R. (2020). Father-child interactional synchrony as a function of maternal and paternal depression in low-income Brazilian families. In H. E. Fitzgerald, K. von Klitzing, N. Cabrera, J. S.

de Mendonça, & T. Skjøthaug (Eds.), *Handbook of fathers and child development: Prenatal to preschool.* New York: Springer.

DeGarmo, D. S. (2020). Designing and tailoring preventive interventions for fathers' parenting. In H. E. Fitzgerald, K. von Klitzing, N. Cabrera, J. S. de Mendonça, & T. Skjøthaug (Eds.), *Handbook of fathers and child development: Prenatal to preschool.* New York: Springer.

Duursma, E., Ho, C. J., Grenyer, B. F., & Herbert, J. S. (2020). Fathers talking and reading with their 3-year-olds during shared bookreading. In H. E. Fitzgerald, K. von Klitzing, N. Cabrera, J. S. de Mendonça, & T. Skjøthaug (Eds.), *Handbook of fathers and child development: Prenatal to preschool.* New York: Springer.

Entwisle, D., & Doering, S. G. (1981). *The first birth.* Baltimore: Johns Hopkins University Press.

Erikson, E. (1975). *Life history and the historical moment.* New York: W. W. Norton.

Fitzgerald, H. E., von Klitzing, K., Cabrera, N., Mendonça, d., & Skjethaug, T. (2020). Fathers and their very young children: A developmental systems perspective. In H. E. Fitzgerald, K. von Klitzing, N. Cabrera, J. S. de Mendonça, & T. Skjøthaug (Eds.), *Handbook of fathers and child development: Prenatal to preschool.* New York: Springer.

Fletcher, R., Macdonald, J. A., & St George, J. M. (2020). Connection, IT and identity: SMS4dads as health promotion for new fathers. In H. E. Fitzgerald, K. von Klitzing, N. Cabrera, J. S. de Mendonça, & T. Skjøthaug (Eds.), *Handbook of fathers and child development: Prenatal to preschool.* New York: Springer.

Frascarolo, F., Favez, N., Tissot, H., & Fivaz-Despeuringe, E. (2020). Fathers' place and role in family relationships. In H. E. Fitzgerald, K. von Klitzing, N. Cabrera, J. S. de Mendonça, & T. Skjøthaug (Eds.), *Handbook of fathers and child development: Prenatal to preschool.* New York: Springer.

Gadsden, V. L., & Iruka, I. (2020). African American fathers and their young children: Lessons from the field. In H. E. Fitzgerald, K. von Klitzing, N. Cabrera, J. S. de Mendonça, & T. Skjøthaug (Eds.), *Handbook of fathers and child development: Prenatal to preschool.* New York: Springer.

Gettler, L. (2020). Biological Influences on fathers. In H. E. Fitzgerald, K. von Klitzing, N. Cabrera, J. S. de Mendonça, & T. Skjøhaug (Eds.), *Handbook of fathers and child development: Prenatal to preschool.* New York: Springer.

Godleski, S., & Eiden, R. D. (2020). Fathers' antisocial behavior and early childhood. In H. E. Fitzgerald, K. von Klitzing, N. Cabrera, J. S. de Mendonça, & T. Skjøthaug (Eds.), *Handbook of fathers and child development: Prenatal to preschool.* New York: Springer.

Goldberg, W. A., Tan, E. T., & Thorsen, K. (2009). Trends in academic attention to fathers, 1930-2006. *Fathering: A Journal of Research, Theory, and Practice, 7*, 159–179.

Golombok, S. (2015). *Modern families.* Cambridge, UK: Cambridge University Press.

Grande, L., Tribble, R., & Kim, P. (2020). Neural plasticity in human fathers. In H. E. Fitzgerald, K. von Klitzing, N. Cabrera, J. S. de Mendonça, &

T. Skjøthaug (Eds.), *Handbook of fathers and child development: Prenatal to preschool*. New York: Springer.

Hennigar, A., Cabrera, N., & Chan, Y. (2020). Fathers and social development. In H. E. Fitzgerald, K. von Klitzing, N. Cabrera, J. S. de Mendonça, & T. Skjøthaug (Eds.), *Handbook of fathers and child development: Prenatal to preschool*. New York: Springer.

Keizer, R. (2020). The role of fathers in the intergenerational transmission of (dis)advantages: Linking sociological stratification questions to developmental psychology research. In H. E. Fitzgerald, K. von Klitzing, N. Cabrera, J. S. de Mendonça, & T. Skjøthaug (Eds.), *Handbook of fathers and child development: Prenatal to preschool*. New York: Springer.

Lamb, M. E. (Ed.). (1976). *The role of the father in child development*. New York: Wiley.

Lamb, M. E. (1981). The development of father-infant relationships. In M. E. Lamb (Ed.), *The role of the father in child development* (Rev. ed.). New York: Wiley.

Lamb, M. E. (Ed.). (1987). *The father's role: Cross-cultural perspectives*. Mahwah, NJ: Lawrence Erlbaum Associations, Inc.

Lamb, M. E., & Lewis, C. (2010). The development and significance of father-child relationships in two-parent families. In M. E. Lamb (Ed.), *The role of the father in child development* (5th ed., pp. 94–153). New York: Wiley.

Lee, S. J., & Lee, J. Y. (2020). Stay at home fathers. In H. E. Fitzgerald, K. von Klitzing, N. Cabrera, J. S. de Mendonça, & T. Skjøhaug (Eds.), *Handbook of fathers and child development: Prenatal to preschool*. New York: Springer.

McMahon, T. J. (2020). Fatherhood, substance use, and early child development. In H. E. Fitzgerald, K. von Klitzing, N. Cabrera, J. S. de Mendonça, & T. Skjøthaug (Eds.), *Handbook of fathers and child development: Prenatal to preschool*. New York: Springer.

Meuwissen, A. S. (2020). Fathers and children's executive functions. In H. E. Fitzgerald, K. von Klitzing, N. Cabrera, J. S. de Mendonça, & T. Skjøthaug (Eds.), *Handbook of fathers and child development: Prenatal to preschool*. New York: Springer.

Miller, B. G., Kors, S., & Macfie, J. (2017). No differences? Meta-analytic comparisons of psychological adjustment in children of gay fathers and heterosexual parents. *Psychology of Sexual Orientation and Gender Diversity, 4*, 14–22.

Mogro-Wilson, C. (2020). Latino American fathers and their preschool children. In H. E. Fitzgerald, K. von Klitzing, N. Cabrera, J. S. de Mendonça, & T. Skjøthaug (Eds.), *Handbook of fathers and child development: Prenatal to preschool*. New York: Springer.

Osborne, C. (2020). Fathers and public policy. In H. E. Fitzgerald, K. von Klitzing, N. Cabrera, J. S. de Mendonça, & T. Skjøthaug (Eds.), *Handbook of fathers and child development: Prenatal to preschool*. New York: Springer.

Palkovitz, R. (2020). Fathering and being fathered: Developmental interdependence. In H. E. Fitzgerald, K. von Klitzing, N. Cabrera, J. S. de Mendonça, & T. Skjøthaug (Eds.), *Handbook of fathers and child development: Prenatal to preschool*. New York: Springer.

Panecsofar, N. (2020). Father's contributions to children's language development. In H. E. Fitzgerald, K. von Klitzing, N. Cabrera, J. S. de Mendonça, & T. Skjøthaug (Eds.), *Handbook of fathers and child development: Prenatal to preschool*. New York: Springer.

Paquette, D., Gagnon, C., & de Medeiros, M. (2020). Fathers and the activation relationship. In H. E. Fitzgerald, K. von Klitzing, N. Cabrera, J. S. de Mendonça, & T. Skjøthaug (Eds.), *Handbook of fathers and child development: Prenatal to preschool*. New York: Springer.

Parke, R. D. (1979). Perspectives on father-infant interaction. In J. D. Osofsky (Ed.), *Handbook of infant development* (pp. 549–590). New York: Wiley.

Parke, R. D. (2002). Fathers and families. In M. H. Bornstein (Ed.), *Handbook of parenting. Volume 3: Being and becoming a parent* (2nd ed., pp. 27–73). Mahwah, NJ: Erlbaum.

Parke, R. D. (2013). *Future families: Diverse forms, rich possibilities*. Malden, MA/Oxford, UK: Wiley Blackwell.

Parke, R. D., & Sawin, D. B. (1976). The fathers role in infancy: A reevaluation. *The Family Coordinator, 25*, 365–371.

Patterson, C. J. (2016). Parents' sexual orientation and children's development. *Child Development Perspectives, 11*, 45–49.

Paulson, J. (2020). Prenatal and postnatal depression. In H. E. Fitzgerald, K. von Klitzing, N. Cabrera, J. S. de Mendonça, & T. Skjøthaug (Eds.), *Handbook of fathers and child development: Prenatal to preschool*. New York: Springer.

Pederson, F. A., & Robson, K. S. (1969). Father participation in infancy. *American Journal of Orthopsychiatry, 39*, 466–472.

Pruett, K., & Pruett, M. K. (2020). Engaging fathers of young children in low income families to improve child and family outcomes: A preventive intervention perspective. In H. E. Fitzgerald, K. von Klitzing, N. Cabrera, J. S. de Mendonça, & T. Skjøthaug (Eds.), *Handbook of fathers and child development: Prenatal to preschool*. New York: Springer.

Rabie, S., Skeen, S., & Tomlinson, M. (2020). Fatherhood and early childhood development in sub-Saharan Africa. In H. E. Fitzgerald, K. von Klitzing, N. Cabrera, J. S. de Mendonça, & T. Skjøthaug (Eds.), *Handbook of fathers and child development: Prenatal to preschool*. New York: Springer.

Roopnarine, J. L., Hooper, F., Ahmeduzzaman, M., & Pollack, B. (1993). Gentle play partners: Mother-child and father-child play in New Delhi, India. In K. Macdonald (Ed.), *Parent-child play*. Albany, NY: State University of New York Press.

Russell, G. (1983). *The changing role of fathers*. St. Lucia, QLD: Queensland University Press.

Shears, J. K. (2020). Fathers reflections of their fathers: The use of text mining to find meaning in narratives. In H. E. Fitzgerald, K. von Klitzing, N. Cabrera, J. S. de Mendonça, & T. Skjøthaug (Eds.), *Handbook of fathers and child development: Prenatal to preschool*. New York: Springer.

Shwalb, D. W., Shwalb, B. J., & Lamb, M. E. (Eds.). (2013). *Fathers in cultural context*. New York: Routledge.

Silverstein, L. B., & Auerbach, C. F. (1999). Deconstructing the essential fathers. *American Psychologist, 54*, 397–407.

Skjøthaug, T. (2020). Antecedents of fathers' stress in fatherhood. In H. E. Fitzgerald, K. von Klitzing, N. Cabrera, J. S. de Mendonça, & T. Skjøthaug (Eds.), *Handbook of fathers and child development: Prenatal to preschool*. New York: Springer.

Snarey, J. (1993). *How fathers care for the next generation*. Cambridge, MA: Harvard University Press.

Storey, A. E., Walsh, C. J., Quinton, R. L., & Wynne-Edwards, K. E. (2000). Hormonal correlates of paternal responsiveness in new and expectant fathers. *Evolution and Human Behavior, 21*, 79–95.

Tolman, R. M., & Walsh, T. B. (2020). Ghosts in the ultrasound: Expectant fathers' experience of trauma. In H. E. Fitzgerald, K. von Klitzing, N. Cabrera, J. S. de Mendonça, & T. Skjøthaug (Eds.), *Handbook of fathers and child development: Prenatal to preschool*. New York: Springer.

Trethowan, W. H., & Conolon, M. F. (1965). The couvade syndrome. *British Journal of Psychiatry, 111*, 57–66.

Vallotton, C., Foster, T. W., Harewood, T., Cook, J., & Adekoya, A. (2020). Fathers and young children at play: A scoping review of studies of father figures play with sons and daughters from birth to preschool. In H. E. Fitzgerald, K. von Klitzing, N. Cabrera, J. S. de Mendonça, & T. Skjøthaug (Eds.), *Handbook of fathers and child development: Prenatal to preschool*. New York: Springer.

Volling, B. L., Steinberg, E. J., & Kuo, P. X. (2020). Is it easier the second time around? Fathers' roles across the transition from one child to two. In H. E. Fitzgerald, K. von Klitzing, N. Cabrera, J. S. de Mendonça, & T. Skjøthaug (Eds.), *Handbook of fathers and child development: Prenatal to preschool*. New York: Springer.

von Klitzing, K., & White, L. (2020). Fathers in psychotherapy. In H. E. Fitzgerald, K. von Klitzing, N. Cabrera, J. S. de Mendonça, & T. Skjøthaug (Eds.), *Handbook of fathers and child development: Prenatal to preschool*. New York: Springer.

Walsh, T. B., & Rosenblum, K. (2020). Fathering across military deployment and reintegration. In H. E. Fitzgerald, K. von Klitzing, N. Cabrera, J. S. de Mendonça, & T. Skjøthaug (Eds.), *Handbook of fathers and child development: Prenatal to preschool*. New York: Springer.

Foreword

The Global Fatherhood Charter

I have a word of caution for all those researching fatherhood: be prepared to be frustrated at how your research is ignored. Your time will come, but this time is measured in generations, not years! Communicating fatherhood research does not just face all the normal barriers that new research faces. It challenges deeply held emotions among practitioners and policy makers, emotions that cannot easily be admitted by those trading in objectivity. Over the last 20 years of trying to communicate fatherhood research into policy and practice in order to improve child development, I have had plenty of time to reflect on why it is so relentlessly difficult.

Nothing about fatherhood can match the deep emotional appeal of the loving mother. When resources are tight – as they are everywhere all the time – the priority will always be supporting the mother-child bond, even when engaging with fathers also improves outcomes. Policies, services, workplaces and cultures will favour the mother-child bond for the foreseeable future almost everywhere in the world.

Meanwhile, the male provider model still holds tight, however much the aspirations of men to be caring grow. In every country in the world, men do less care than women, even in the Nordic countries (van der Gaag, Heilman, Gupta, Nembhard & Backet (2019)). To this we must add the idea that the role of the male is to be strong and to provide support, not to receive support and not to be seen as weak and needy. In this world view, fathers should focus on self-reliance, not on being helped by services or policy makers. The best research on this phenomenon comes from neonatal care, where fathers face enormous pressures and fears and are most in need of help. Nowhere is the demand to be "the strong one" stronger than in such extremities (Fisher et al., 2018).

Closely linked to this is the idea that fathers are powerful and have agency. If they are not doing the "right things", the solution is not help but for them to man-up and take responsibility. The entire narrative in UK around parental leave, for example, is "why don't fathers take leave?" rather than focusing on policy and institutional barriers that might be limiting their ability to take it.

Finally, all the research about the value of collaborative parenting for child development faces the challenge of the idea that men and women live in fundamental competition with each other. Won't men use co-parenting to "take over"? In my early years of advocacy, I was described as a "wolf in sheep's clothing" by a senior UK politician: all talk of love and care on the outside, but with a hidden agenda to dominate.

This is a gloomy outlook, to be sure, but for researchers who are patient, there is an end in sight. Human parenting has been shown by anthropologists to be enormously flexible in response to context (Hrdy, 2009) and the modern economy is driving change towards much more sharing of roles. Millennial parents have a very different outlook from the older generations that still hold the power to shape policy and practice. If you want to see this, just take a trip into the social media world, where the celebration of loving fatherhood is in full swing. I recently assembled 11 viral videos about father-child bonding, with 0.4 billion views between them (familyincluded.com/viral-videos-fathers-bonding). When this generation are decision-makers in the global field of child development, the time for fatherhood research to become mainstream will come. In the meantime, our job is to lay foundations and hasten the progress of the incoming tide.

The traditional approach to fatherhood support is to work with services to deliver programs to support fathers. But these are proving to be remarkably unsustainable – in most cases, the programs fizzle out as soon as the designated pilot funding runs out – however good the child outcomes prove to be – or as soon as the sole advocate within the service moves on. The prevailing culture reasserts itself, focusing exclusively on mother-child bond. And yet, in every community in the world there are fathers discovering the joy of loving care of their infants, succumbing to human biology and psychology, and acting as early adopters of changing gender roles. These people are the future and the foundation for change. In my view, the focus should be on supporting fathers and their partners as advocates in their communities to support other parents. The appeal is to the most basic instinct of all: "experience the love of your child". And this is where the research comes in.

Throughout the time I was involved in raising my children, I had privileged access to the research on fathers and child development, which was entirely unavailable to any of my peers through "parenting" channels. I devoured the findings about the benefits to children of co-parenting. I followed and still follow every new discovery about the biology and neurobiology of fatherhood. Since 2015, I have charted all new developments in the field of fathers and maternal and newborn health – nearly 300 reports since 2015 on FamilyIncluded.com. I edit ChildandFamilyBlog.com, working closely with Michael Lamb (1987, 2004; Shwalb, Shwalb, & Lamb, 2013; Lewis & Lamb, 2007), and this is a platform that reports on important fatherhood research when it emerges. Earlier this year, I called on leading fatherhood researchers to define the fatherhood agenda on the basis of accumulated knowledge to date, which resulted in the Fatherhood Charter, reproduced below.

This knowledge is immensely empowering. It makes sense of something that contradicts prevailing culture. It supports the transition from private experience to public engagement. And yet, hardly any fathers (or mothers) see it.

So what can fatherhood researchers do now, beyond doing more research and advancing knowledge? My invitation is to organize to communicate research globally to fathers and to the mothers who are their partners and co-parents. I am inviting fatherhood researchers and advocates to come together globally to support particularly those fathers who are taking the additional step of publicly advocating change towards more support for father-child relationships in society. These fathers need inspiration, they need evidence and they need strength. Knowledge is power and we can give this to them.

The Global Fatherhood Charter

1. The loving care of a father is a foundation for his child's wellbeing and creates a life-long relationship.
2. The loving care of father can be as powerful and important as that of a mother.
3. All fathers, both biological and non-biological, have an innate ability to bond with their babies from the first days. A father's brain changes when he actively cares for his child, generating enhanced capacity for care and empathy.
4. Loving care takes many forms. Each family and each father-child relationship is unique.
5. Fathers are family, and family caregivers are among the most important influences on children's development, wellbeing and health. This is so even when fathers do not live permanently with their children.
6. A harmonious community of care around a child, with parents and caregivers supporting each other, is a foundation for the child's healthy development.
7. Fatherhood, like motherhood, is a journey. Fathers need time and practice – to care for, nurture, play with, and teach their children.
8. Loving fatherhood means respect for and collaboration with the mother and the absence of violence.
9. To provide the care and form the relationships that children need, fathers need support and validation from their partners, families, communities and society.
10. Maternal and newborn health services, early years services, and economic self-sufficiency services should offer, and encourage the use of, support for fathers and other family caregivers in ways that engage creatively with the local culture and socioeconomic conditions. They should provide information and help about how to support maternal and child health and child development. They should support family caregivers' relationships with their children and a harmonious community of care for children within families. They should offer support for all caregivers to meet their children's financial needs. This support should be accessible to fathers even if they live apart from the mother.
11. Workplaces and employment laws should honour and support the caring responsibilities of both fathers and mothers.
12. Fathers' involvement in the first 1000 days of their children's life should be a focus of international early childhood development strategies.

13. Promotion of gender equality needs to include support for fatherhood. Equal economic opportunities for women and men must include the opportunity to share the care of their children.
14. Men are inherently loving and caring beings. Men's caring instincts and emotional life should be celebrated as part of what it is to be a man in today's cultures.
15. Loving fatherhood and men's caregiving of all kinds should be recognised and celebrated as an inspiration to other fathers, mothers, grandparents and caregivers, in this generation and the next.

Relevant Web Pages

Child and Family Blog, ChildandFamilyBlog.com
Family Included, FamilyIncluded.com

Child and Family Blog Duncan Fisher, OBE
Crickhowell, UK

References

Fisher, D., Khashu, M., Adama, E. A., Feeley, N., Garfield, C. F., Ireland, J., et al. (2018). Fathers in neonatal units: Improving infant health by supporting the baby-father bond and mother-father coparenting. *Journal of Neonatal Nursing, 24*(6), 306–312.

Hrdy, S. B. (2009). *Mothers and others*. Cambridge, MA: Harvard University Press.

Lamb, M. E. (Ed.). (1987). *The fathers' role: Cross cultural perspectives*. Hillsdale, NJ: Lawrence Erlbaum Associates.

Lamb, M. E. (Ed.). (2004). *The role of the father in child development* (4th ed.). New York: Wiley.

Lewis, C., & Lamb, M. E. (2007). *Understanding fatherhood*. York, UK: Joseph Rowntree Foundation.

Shwalb, D. W., Shwalb, B. J., & Lamb, M. E. (Eds.). (2013). *Fathers in cultural context*. New York: Routledge.

Van der Gaag, N., Heilman, B., Gupta, T., Nembhard, C., & Barket, G. (2019). *State of the world's fathers: Unlocking the power of men's care*. Washington, DC: Promundo.

Preface

Thirty-eight years ago, the senior editor for this volume published a revision of his book on infancy and early childhood. Seven pages in the chapter on socialization were devoted to the father's role as caregiver. That may not sound like much today, but back then that much attention given to father as caregiver was relatively unique, especially with respect to the period of human development spanning conception to preschool. The theoretical framework throughout the book stressed that a baby is a system embedded in a more complex family system that, in turn, is part of an increasing number of adjunctive systems that directly and/or indirectly influence the family, and therefore the infant. Unfortunately, at the time, the developmental sciences did not reflect well the role of the father in the infant's emergent world beyond his sperm-producing role in conception. That was soon to change.

General research on infant development literally exploded during the second half of the twentieth century spurred on by Bowlby's attachment theory, Piaget's theory of genetic epistemology, and various forms of evolutionary theory. Researchers such as Ross Parke, Michael Lamb, and countless others tackled a wide variety of issues related to the role of the father in early child development, including capturing the diversity of fathering across many of the world's cultures.

In the early part of this century, a team of investigators led by Natasha Cabrera began to focus on efforts to create a conceptual model to give an organizational framework to guide research on fathers and assess their influence on early child development. This volume is a continuation of the early conception of father as part of a dynamic family system, combined with a more contemporary bio-ecological view of father within a dynamic systems framework.

We chose to focus on the prenatal to preschool age period specifically to capture the father's influence on child development within the concept of a family as a dynamic system of interacting personalities, which collectively affect the biopsychosocial organization of the infant and young child. Fortunately, we found many colleagues who share the same interest and the book dreamed about so long ago is now a reality.

According to the U. S. Census Bureau, there were 6,475,000 single parent father families in the USA in 2018, 86.6% of whom worked full- or part-time. Many infants and young children in father-only household families receive supplemental care from someone else and/or at some other place. We believe these numbers alone support a more active and robust research agenda focused on fathers as caregivers and the father caregiving environment.

We deeply appreciate the commitment of the authors who contributed to this volume. They have played a key role in helping us bring attention to contemporary knowledge of the diverse ways that fathers influence early development and how they are influenced themselves by the dynamics of family life and the adjunctive systems that they encounter.

Not surprisingly, we have used the Cabrera team's most recent model to guide the organization of this volume, address core areas of early development, and provide diverse theoretical perspectives and ecological contexts. An underlying theme is that early human development is the time when each individual's biopsychosocial organization is shaping the foundation of a life course pathway that is positioned somewhere on the risk to resilience continuum, but which continues to change over the life course.

From a philosophical frame, this is a book about becoming, replete with what Overton might refer to as moments (being) in the life-course. Some moments have a profound negative effect (trauma, adverse childhood experiences) and others have positive effects (secure attachment, nurturing father), but the individual is always floating in a sea of potential change driven by the fluctuating balance of risk and resilience.

All chapters were peer reviewed (anonymously) by two of the editors. In addition, Laurie Van Egeren, Goeff Twitchell, Andren-Ann SDeneault, and Avery Henniger provided additional assistance. Every chapter was revised at least once during the production process, consistent with our effort to have a peer-reviewed orientation to the volume. We extend our deep thanks to Judy Jones and Michelle Tam at Springer for their assistance throughout the two-year production process and are ever thankful to Kamaraj Shanthini, Mario Gabriele and their teams of copy and production editors and staff who play an unseen yet vital role in the Springer Nature publication process.

East Lansing, MI, USA Hiram E. Fitzgerald
Leipzig, Germany Kai von Klitzing
College Park, MD, USA Natasha J. Cabrera
Osasco, São-Paulo, Brazil Júlia Scarano de Mendonça
Lørenskog, Norway Thomas Skjøthaug

Contents

Part II Prenatal and Perinatal Influences

Part III Father-Child Transaction in Early Development

Contributors

Anike R. Adekoya, MS, LLMFT Human Development and Family Studies, Michigan State University, East Lansing, MI, USA

Regina L. Alexander, MS Virginia Consortium Program in Clinical Psychology, Old Dominion University, Norfolk, VA, USA

Joshuaa D. Allison-Burbank, MA, CCC-SLP University of Kansas Center on Developmental Disabilities, Lawrence, KS, USA

Alp Aytuglu Department of Human Development and Family Science, University of Georgia, Athens, GA, USA

Sarah Bergmann, PhD Department of Child and Adolescent Psychiatry, Psychotherapy and Psychosomatics, University of Leipzig, Leipzig, Germany

International Psychoanalytic University Berlin, Berlin, Germany

Erika London Bocknek, PhD, LMFT Department of Educational Psychology, Wayne State University, Detroit, MI, USA

Robert H. Bradley, PhD Center for Child and Family Success, Arizona State University, Tempe, AZ, USA

Geoffrey L. Brown, PhD Department of Human Development and Family Science, University of Georgia, Athens, GA, USA

Suzanne Brown, Ph.D., MSW School of Social Work, Wayne State University, Detroit, MI, USA

Vera Sílvia Raad Bussab, PhD Department of Experimental Psychology, Institute of Psychology, University of São Paulo, São Paulo, Brazil

Natasha J. Cabrera, PhD Department of Human Development and Quantitative Methodology, University of Maryland, College Park, MD, USA

Olivia D. Chang School of Social Work, University of Michigan, Ann Arbor, MI, USA

Yu Chen, BA Department of Human Development and Computational Methodology, University of Maryland, College Park, MD, USA

Tanya Coakley, PhD, MSW Department of Social Work, University of North Carolina at Greensboro, Greensboro, NC, USA

Anthony (Thosh) Collins Well For Culture, Miami, FL, USA

Jody Cook, MPH Human Development and Family Studies, Michigan State University, East Lansing, MI, USA

Carolyn Joy Dayton, PhD, LP, LMSW, IMH-E IV® School of Social Work & Merrill Palmer Skillman Institute for Child & Family Development, Wayne State University, Detroit, MI, USA

David S. DeGarmo, PhD Department of Counseling Psychology and Human Services, Prevention Science Institute, University of Oregon, Eugene, OR, USA

Julio Macario de Medeíros École de psychoéducation, University of Montreal, Montreal, QC, Canada

Júlia Scarano de Mendonça, PhD Graduate Program in Educational Psychology, Centro Universitário FIEO, Osasco, São Paulo, Brazil

Elisabeth Duursma, EdD School of Education, University of Wollongong, Wollongong, NSW, Australia

Rina D. Eiden, PhD Department of Psychology, Consortium for Combating Substance Abuse, Pennsylvania State University, State College, PA, USA

Kelsey T. Ellis, MS Virginia Consortium Program in Clinical Psychology, Old Dominion University, Norfolk, VA, USA

Nicolas Favez, PhD FPSE, Uni Mail, University of Geneva, Geneva, Switzerland

Duncan Fisher, OBE Child and Family Blog, Crickhowell, UK

Hiram E. Fitzgerald, PhD, IMH-E IV® Department of Psychology, Michigan State University, East Lansing, MI, USA

Elisabeth Fivaz-Depeursinge, PhD Lausanne University, Grandvaux, Switzerland

Richard Fletcher, PhD Fathers and Families Research Program – Faculty of Health and Medicine, The University of Newcastle, Callaghan, NSW, Australia

Tricia Foster, PhD Occupational Therapy Program, School of Health Sciences, Eastern Michigan University, Ypsilanti, MI, USA

France Frascarolo-Moutinot, PhD Lausanne University, Lausanne, Switzerland

Vivian L. Gadsden, EdD Graduate School of Education, University of Pennsylvania, Philadelphia, PA, USA

Carole Gagnon École de psychoéducation, Université de Montréal, Montréal, QC, Canada

Lee T. Gettler, PhD Department of Anthropology, Eck Institute for Global Health, University of Notre Dame, Notre Dame, IN, USA

Stephanie Godleski, PhD College of Liberal Arts, Department of Psychology, Rochester Institute of Technology, Rochester, NY, USA

Leah Grande, MA Department of Psychology, University of Denver, Denver, CO, USA

Brin F. Grenyer, PhD Illawarra Health and Medical Research Institute and School of Psychology, Wollongong, NSW, Australia

Tamesha Harewood, MS, MA, PhD Human Development and Family Studies, Michigan State University, East Lansing, MI, USA

Avery Hennigar, MPH Department of Human Development and Computational Methodology, University of Maryland, College Park, MD, USA

Jane S. Herbert, PhD School of Psychology and Early Start, University of Wollongong, Wollongong, NSW, Australia

Cheryl Jialing Ho School of Psychology and Early Start, University of Wollongong, Wollongong, NSW, Australia

Iheoma U. Iruka, PhD Center for Early Education Research & Evaluation, HighScope Educational Research Foundation, Ypsilanti, MI, USA

Renske Keizer, PhD Erasmus School of Social and Behavioral Sciences, Erasmus University Rotterdam, Rotterdam, The Netherlands

Pilyoung Kim, PhD Department of Psychology, University of Denver, Denver, CO, USA

Seongtae Kim, PhD Statistics and Analytics Consulting Center, Department of Mathematics & Statistics, North Carolina A&T State University, Greensboro, NC, USA

Joshua Kirven, MSW PhD Department of Social Work, Winthrop University, Rock Hill, SC, USA

Annette M. Klein, PhD International Psychoanalytic University Berlin, Berlin, Germany

Patty X. Kuo, PhD Department of Child, Youth and Family Studies, University of Nebraska-Lincoln, Lincoln, NE, USA

Joyce Y. Lee, MSW School of Social Work, University of Michigan, Ann Arbor, MI, USA

Shawna J. Lee, PhD, MSW School of Social Work, University of Michigan, Ann Arbor, MI, USA

Jacqui A. Macdonald, PhD School of Psychology, Deakin University, Burwood, VIC, Australia

Johanna C. Malone, PhD Harvard Medical School and Cambridge Health Alliance, Cambridge, MA, USA

Thomas J. McMahon, PhD Yale University School of Medicine, Connecticut Mental Health Center, New Haven, CT, USA

Alyssa S. Meuwissen, PhD Center for Early Education and Development, University of Minnesota, St. Paul, MN, USA

Cristina Mogro-Wilson, PhD, MSW School of Social Work, University of Connecticut, Hartford, CT, USA

Cynthia Osborne, PhD LBJ School of Public Affairs, University of Texas at Austin, Austin, TX, USA

Rob Palkovitz, PhD University of Delaware, Newark, DE, USA

Nadya Pancsofar, PhD Department of Special Education, Language, and Literacy, The College of New Jersey, Ewing, NJ, USA

Daniel Paquette, PhD École de psychoéducation, Université de Montréal, Montréal, QC, Canada

Ross D. Parke, PhD Department of Psychology and Center for Family Studies, University of California, Riverside, Riverside, CA, USA

James F. Paulson, PhD Department of Psychology, Old Dominion University, Norfolk, VA, USA

Kyle Dean Pruett, MD Yale Study Center, Northampton, MA, USA

Marsha Kline Pruett, PhD School for Social Work, Smith College, Northampton, MA, USA

Stephan Rabie, PhD Institute for Life Course Health Research, Department of Global Health, Stellenbosch University, Stellenbosch, South Africa

Katherine L. Rosenblum, PhD Departments of Psychiatry and Obstetrics & Gynecology, University of Michigan, Ann Arbor, MI, USA

Jeffrey Shears, PhD, MSW The JMSW Program, University of North Carolina at Greensboro & NC A&T State University, Greensboro, NC, USA

Sarah Skeen, PhD Institute for Child and Adolescent Health Research, Masiphulisane Research Centre, Stellenbosch University, Khayelitsha, South Africa

Thomas Skjøthaug, PhD Division of Mental Health, Grorud DPS, Akershus University Hospital, Lørenskog, Norway

Emily J. Steinberg, BA Department of Psychology, Fordham University, Bronx, NY, USA

Jennifer Mary StGeorge, PhD Family Action Centre, Faculty of Medicine & Health, University of Newcastle, Callaghan, NSW, Australia

Hervé Tissot, PhD FPSE, University of Geneva, Geneva, Switzerland

Centre d'Etuide de la Famille, CHUV Site de Cery, Prilly, Switzerland

Richard M. Tolman, PhD School of Social Work, University of Michigan, Ann Arbor, MI, USA

Mark Tomlinson, PhD Department of Psychology, Stellenbosch University, Matieland, Stellenbosch, South Africa

Michelle L. Townsend, PhD Illawarra Health and Medical Research Institute and School of Psychology, University of Wollongong, Wollongong, NSW, Australia

Rebekah Tribble Department of Psychology, University of Denver, Denver, CO, USA

Claire D. Vallotton, PhD Human Development and Family Studies, Michigan State University, East Lansing, MI, USA

Brenda L. Volling, PhD Department of Psychology, University of Michigan, Ann Arbor, MI, USA

Kai von Klitzing, MD Department of Child and Adolescent Psychiatry, University of Leipzig, Leipzig, Germany

Tova B. Walsh, PhD, MSW Sandra Rosenbaum School of Social Work, University of Wisconsin, Madison, WI, USA

Lars O. White, PhD Department of Child and Adolescent Psychiatry, University of Leipzig, Leipzig, Germany

About the Editors

Hiram E. Fitzgerald, Ph.D., is University Distinguished Professor in the Department of Psychology at Michigan State University. His major areas of research include the study of infant and family development in community contexts, the impact of fathers on early child development, the etiology of alcohol use disorders, and the scholarship of university-community engagement. He is a Fellow of the American Psychological Association and the Association of Psychological Science. He is a recipient of the Zero to Three Dolley Madison Award for Outstanding Lifetime Contribution to the Development and Well-Being of Very Young Children and the WAIMH designation as Honorary President.

Kai von Klitzing, M.D., Professor of Child and Adolescent Psychiatry, University of Leipzig, Germany; Psychoanalyst for adults, adolescents, and children, Swiss Psychoanalytical Society and German Psychoanalytical Association/IPA; Training Analyst; Editor of the journal *Kinderanalyse* (Child Analysis); Associate-Editor of the *Infant Mental Health Journal*, President of the World Association for Infant Mental Health. Scientific interests: developmental psychopathology, early triadic relationships (mother–father–infant), children's narratives, psychotherapy (individual and family), childhood maltreatment, and neurobiology.

Natasha J. Cabrera, Ph.D., is Professor of Human Development at the University of Maryland. Her research focuses on father involvement and children's social and cognitive development, adaptive and maladaptive factors related to parenting, ethnic and cultural variations in fathering and mothering behaviors, family processes in a social and cultural context and children's development, and the mechanisms that link early experiences to children's school readiness. She is the Co-editor of the *Handbook of Father Involvement: Multidisciplinary Perspectives, Second Edition* (Taylor & Francis, 2013)

Júlia Scarano de Mendonça, Ph.D., is Professor in the Graduate Program in Educational Psychology at Centro Universitário FIEO, Osasco, São Paulo, Brazil. Her research focuses on family functioning and fathers' role in Brazilian low-income families in the context of post-partum depression, family influences on the child's emotion regulation skills and empathy, and on the development of mental health prevention programs in risky families for post-partum depression and in the school setting in low-income Brazilian contexts.

Thomas Skjøthaug, Ph.D., is a Specialist in Clinical Psychology at Akershus University Hospital, Division of Mental Health, Grorud, Norway. Skjøthaug's research involves investigation of fathers' adverse childhood experiences and fathers' mental health during pregnancy, pathways from pregnancy to experienced stress postpartum, and fathers' prenatal attachment patterns with interactional quality postpartum. He is also interested in how political arrangements affect fathers' involvement, i.e., parental and paternal leave.

About the Contributors

Anike R. Adekoya, M.S., LLMFT, is a doctoral student of Human Development and Family Studies at Michigan State University focusing on Couple and Family Therapy. She brings a womanist/feminist relational perspective to her clinical and academic work. Her research interests highlight the role of context, focusing on interpersonal relationships, including parent-child dynamics, intersectionalities, historical and ongoing transgenerational trauma, and culturally informed mental health interventions, especially within communities of color.

Regina L. Alexander, M.S., is currently a doctoral student in the Virginia Consortium Program in Clinical Psychology. Her research interests include the impact of parental relationships on child development, specifically in underrepresented and understudied populations. Her previous work has examined the impact of compassionate love and maternal gatekeeping on the co-parenting relationship. Ms. Alexander looks forward to continuing to contribute to the literature related to family relationships and interactions.

Joshuaa D. Allison-Burbank, M.A., CCC-SLP(Diné/Acoma Pueblo), is a speech-language pathologist at the University of Kansas. His research interests include community capacity building, parent training and advocacy, and epidemiologic surveillance of neurodevelopmental disabilities. Joshuaa is currently pursuing his doctoral degree with an emphasis on neurodevelopmental disabilities and public health. Joshuaa is a Lecturer in the KU Speech-Language-Hearing Department and an Adjunct Lecturer in the Communication Sciences and Disorders Program at the University of Vermont

Alp Aytuglu is a doctoral student in the Department of Human Development and Family Science at the University of Georgia. He received his master's degree in applied developmental psychology after studying in Ozyegin University, Istanbul. His research interests include first-time fathers' readiness and preparedness for parenting, fathers' experiences of their transition to fatherhood, maternal gatekeeping, and fathers' influence on their children's social-emotional and cognitive development.

Sarah Bergmann, Ph.D., is a Psychologist and Research Associate in the Department of Child and Adolescent Psychiatry, Psychotherapy and Psychosomatics, University of Leipzig, and at the International Psychoanalytic University Berlin. For the past few years, her main topic of research has been the relationship quality between parents and their young children including a specific focus on gender differences in and predictors as well as child outcomes of the quality of parent-child interactions.

Erika London Bocknek, Ph.D., LMFT, is Assistant Professor of Educational Psychology at Wayne State University in Detroit, MI. She studies social emotional development in young children in the context of parenting and family relationships. Her research and clinical practice emphasize resilience promotion in populations at risk by highlighting routines, rituals, and strategies that strengthen family bonds. Dr. Bocknek currently serves as Associate Editor of the *Infant Mental Health Journal.*

Robert H. Bradley, Ph.D., is Director of the Center for Child and Family Success at Arizona State University. He has served on research panels for federal agencies such as the NIH, CDC, NSF, IES, HRSA, and Head Start. Dr. Bradley was associate editor for *Child Development* and *Early Childhood Research Quarterly*. He has more than 350 publications dealing with parenting, family environment, early education, fathers, and childcare. Dr. Bradley is co-developer of the HOME Inventory.

Geoffrey L. Brown, Ph.D., is an Assistant Professor in the Department of Human Development and Family Science at the University of Georgia. His research has focused on family relationships and social-emotional development in infancy and early childhood, with an emphasis on the development of early father-child relationships. His work has documented the correlates and consequences of father involvement and father-child attachment security as well as the development of early parent-child relationships in rural African American populations.

Suzanne Brown, Ph.D., MSW, is an Associate Professor of Social Work at Wayne State University. Her research program examines risk and resilience in the lives of women affected by substance abuse. Her work is grounded in developmental and attachment theory and focuses on the influence of social networks on substance abuse recovery and on early parenting competence.

Vera Sílvia Raad Bussab, Ph.D., is a Full Professor in the Department of Experimental Psychology at the University of São Paulo since 1975. Bussab is a member of the commission of the Brazilian Society of Ethology, a member of the research group on Evolutionary Psychology of the National Association of Graduate Research in Psychology, and a member of the research group on Behavior and Evolution from the National Council of Scientific and Technological Development in Brazil. She has been working mainly on the following topics: ethological approach, development, attachment, day care, animal behavior, sexual and reproductive strategies, and psychopathology.

Olivia D. Chang is an undergraduate student at the University of Michigan studying psychology. Broadly, her research interests focus on the significance of intersecting identities (e.g., race, ethnicity, gender) in physical and mental well-being. She has published in *Eating and Weight Disorders* and *Personality and Individual Differences*. In the future, she hopes to continue to study the impact of intersecting identities (e.g., multiethnoraciality) in relation to family dynamics and child well-being.

Yu Chen, B.A., is a first-year doctoral student working with Dr. Natasha Cabrera at University of Maryland. Yu earned her Bachelor of Arts degree in Psychology and Economics from Grinnell College and worked as a Lab Manager at Temple University after graduation. Her research focuses on how parent-child interactions and home environment shape child outcomes. She is particularly interested in low-income mothers and fathers' language input and the quality of their interactions with infants and young children.

Tanya Coakley, Ph.D., M.S.W., is a Professor and Associate Chair for Research in Social Work at the University of North Carolina at Greensboro. Her expertise is in quality foster care, effective transcultural parenting, fathers' involvement, minority health disparities, risky sexual behavior in youth, and quantitative assessment. She earned a Ph.D. in Social Work and a Minor in Statistics from the University of Tennessee-Knoxville. Her work promotes children's psychological and social functioning, such as good coping and behavior skills. She also focuses on health and development through effective interventions and resources for parents and families, typically minority and poor.

Anthony (Thosh) Collins was born and raised in the Salt River Reservation in Arizona where he is now a family man, community organizer, and an active participant in cultural and ceremonial gatherings. He is a board member and senior trainer for the Native Wellness Institute. Thosh, along with his wife Chelsey Luger, co-founded WELL FOR CULTURE, an Indigenous wellness initiative that promotes holistic wellness and ancestral teachings to optimize contemporary Indigenous lifestyles. Thosh and Chelsey travel to indigenous communities all over the USA and Canada to teach workshops about their indigenous wellness model the "7 Circles of Wellness." Thosh has dedicated his life to helping shift the collective consciousness of indigenous communities and people in regards to prioritizing holistic health for the benefit of future generations.

Jody Cook, M.P.H., is a graduate student in Human Development and Family Studies at Michigan State University. She applies her public health knowledge to the implementation of parent- and teacher-focused interventions to enhance caregiver practices and ultimately the caregiver-child relationship. Jody is interested in parenting and caregiving in the context of stressors, such as poverty and military deployment, and studies the impacts of stress on caregiver-child relationships, especially for fathers and their young children.

Carolyn Joy Dayton, Ph.D., is the Associate Director of the Infant Mental Health Program at the Merrill Palmer Skillman Institute for Child and Family Development at Wayne State University. Her research focuses on early parenting processes with an emphasis on fathering in urban settings. Dr. Dayton's program of research informs her clinical work with families and aims to identify biological and psychosocial risk and resilience factors that influence parenting processes and early child development.

David S. DeGarmo, Ph.D., is a prevention science methodologist interested in family stress models and program evaluation of preventive interventions for families at risk for compromised parenting. His active research in the University of Oregon Prevention Science Institute involves a blended group and online intervention for single fathers and comparison of multi-model interventions for military mothers and fathers. A major focus of his work is on independent and interactive effects of fathering. Dave teaches methodology in the College of Education and the Department of Educational Methodology, Policy, and Leadership (EMPL) at the University of Oregon and is a former postdoctoral fellow of the NIMH Family Research Consortium.

Julio Macario de Medeiros has a master's degree in psychology (Universidade Federal de Pernambuco, Brazil). His research main interest is children's social-emotional development. In Brazil, he worked 6 years as adult and child psychotherapist, including children with special needs (deafness and ELA). Currently, he's enrolled as a Ph.D. student at Université de Montréal, where he studies the father-child relationship in order to identify and prevent problems on the children's socio-emotional development.

Elisabeth Duursma, Ph.D., is a Senior Lecturer in Education at the University of Wollongong, Australia. She received her doctorate in Human Development and Psychology from the Harvard University Graduate School of Education in Cambridge, USA. Previously she worked at Reach Out and Read (ROR) in Boston as Director of Research Initiatives and at the University of Groningen (the Netherlands). Elisabeth's research focuses on father involvement, particularly in young children's language and literacy development.

Rina D. Eiden, Ph.D., is a Developmental Psychologist and Professor in the Department of Psychology, Pennsylvania State University, University Park, PA. She is interested in understanding developmental trajectories of risk and resilience among children of substance using parents from the prenatal period to adolescence. She is an APA Division 50 Fellow and has published extensively in this area.

Kelsey T. Ellis, M.S., is a doctoral candidate in the Virginia Consortium Program in Clinical Psychology. Her work is focused on the contextual factors of parent psychopathology and how these factors influence parent-child interactions, specifically related to child maltreatment. Her previous work has spanned from experimental research looking at inhibitory processes in parent decision-making to examining the role of paternal and maternal attachment patterns on adult child outcomes.

Nicolas Favez, Ph.D., is Full Professor of Clinical Psychology specialized in family and interpersonal relationships at the University of Geneva, Switzerland, and is Co-Director of the Research Unit of the Center for Family Study (IUP, Lausanne University Hospital). His research activities and teaching relate to family and couples relations, observation and assessment methodology, and therapeutic work with couples and families. He has carried out several research projects focused on the influence of early family relationships on child cognitive and affective development. He has published a variety of books and papers on family interactions.

Duncan Fisher, OBE has championed the communication of fatherhood research into public policy and practice since 1996. He co-founded the Fatherhood Institute in UK, which engaged with maternal health and early years services. Fisher became a leading advocate for leave entitlements in UK that encourage early co-parenting. He received an Order of the British Empire (OBE) by the Queen in 2008 for his "services to children." In 2014, he co-founded the Child and Family Blog, a project of Cambridge University, Princeton University, and the Jacobs Foundation (Switzerland) that is developing new ways of communicating child development research into policy and practice. He is now working in developing countries and developing a "Global Fatherhood Academy."

Elisabeth Fivaz-Depeursinge earned a Ph.D., in Child Development from Geneva University, Switzerland, in 1965 and has taught at Lausanne Medical School of Medicine until retirement. Her research focus was on non-verbal communication in family triads, couple therapy, and medical consultations. She has published a variety of articles on three-way communication between infant and parents, including two books, *The Primary Triangle* (Basic Books, 1999) and *The Baby and the Couple* (2014).

Richard Fletcher, Ph.D., is Associate Professor in the Family Action Centre, Faculty of Health and Medicine, the University of Newcastle, NSW, Australia. Richard's expertise includes the design and conduct of research into fathers' role in families across diverse settings: new fathers, antenatal support, rough and tumble play, Aboriginal fathers, and fathers using the Web. He is Principal Investigator on a range of projects delivering SMS4dads. He is editor of the *Fatherhood Research Bulletin*.

Tricia Foster, Ph.D., OTR/L, is an Assistant Professor in the Occupational Therapy Program at Eastern Michigan University. She studies young children's early experiences and environments for both typically developing children as well as children with special needs. Tricia's teaching and research include a strong focus on how to support parents in the early intervention process through family-centered services. Tricia is also a pediatric occupational therapist, with experience in both early intervention and school-based practice.

France Frascarolo-Moutinot, Ph.D., received a doctoral degree for research on links between father's involvement and infant sociability from Geneva University (Switzerland) in 1994 and was Co-director of the Research Unit of the Center for Family Study (IUP, Lausanne University Hospital) until retirement. Her research focus was on non-verbal communication in family triads. She has published a variety of articles and book chapters on fathers, family communication, and assessment of family interaction.

Vivian L. Gadsden, Ed.D., is the William T. Carter Professor of Child Development and Education at the University of Pennsylvania and Director of the National Center on Fathers and Families. Dr. Gadsden's research and scholarly interests focus on children and families across the life-course, from early childhood through the aging process, particularly children, parents, and communities at the greatest risk for academic and social vulnerability by virtue of race, gender, ethnicity, poverty, and immigrant status.

Carole Gagnon is a doctoral candidate at Université de Montréal, École de psychoéducation. She holds a DESS in Community Health from Université de Montréal. Her research main interest is child attachment relationship with parents. Her work focuses on fathering and mothering behaviors associated with infant and young child attachment security. The results of this work could have implications for the development of interventions targeting the unique contributions of fathers and mothers to child attachment security.

Lee T. Gettler, Ph.D., is an Assistant Professor in Anthropology at the University of Notre Dame and directs the Hormones, Health, and Human Behavior Laboratory. Much of his past research focused on the way in which men's hormonal physiology responds to major life transitions, such as marriage and fatherhood. He currently researches the psychobiology of motherhood and fatherhood, parents' physical and mental health, and child growth and development in the USA, the Philippines, and Congo-Brazzaville.

Stephanie Godleski, Ph.D., is a Clinical Psychologist and an Assistant Professor in the Department of Psychology at the Rochester Institute of Technology. The primary focus of her research is pathways of risk and resilience in predicting social competence across the lifespan. Specifically, she has focused on protective (e.g., parenting) and maladaptive (e.g., prenatal exposure) processes that predict and maintain negative social-emotional developmental and health outcomes.

Leah Grande is a third-year student in the Clinical Child Psychology Ph.D. program at the University of Denver, working with Dr. Pilyoung Kim. Leah received her bachelor's degree in psychology and cognitive science from the University of Virginia and then worked as a project coordinator for Dr. Joseph Allen. Leah is interested in the intergenerational transmission of parenting as well as the long-term health and brain development consequences of early life experience.

Brin F. Grenyer, Ph.D., is a practicing Clinical Psychologist and Senior Professor of Psychology at the University of Wollongong. He is Scientific Director and Principal Investigator for the Illawarra Born Cross-Generation Health Study. Major publications and scientific discoveries from this work have included the role of parental psychological factors prior to birth on infant developmental milestones. At the University he serves as Director of Professional and Clinical Psychology Training.

Tamesha Harewood, Ph.D., is Assistant Professor of Human Development and Family Studies at Michigan State University. She brings her background in human resources to her study of adult learners as they develop knowledge and skills about early child development, care, and education. Her scholarly interests focus on professional development of the pre-service early childhood workforce and parental influences on children's early development. Contributions include research indicating effects of early father-child relationships on children's later cognitive and language development.

Avery Hennigar, M.P.H., is a third-year doctoral student in Human Development and Quantitative Methodology at the University of Maryland, College Park. Her research explores how characteristics of low-income and ethnic minority families are related to the early home environment and the cognitive and social development of young children through parenting practices. She is also interested in how interventions can be most effective for at-risk families and the application of research to policy.

Jane S. Herbert, Ph.D., is an Associate Professor at the University of Wollongong, Australia. She is an expert in infant cognition and development based in the School of Psychology at the University of Wollongong. She is the director of the Wollongong Infant Learning Lab (WILL) and leads the Family, Learning and Interaction (FLINT) research theme at Early Start at the University of Wollongong. Her research considers how maturation and environmental experiences impact the child's developing brain and cognitive abilities and on parent-child interactions.

Cheryl Jialing Ho is currently pursuing her Ph.D. in Psychology at University of Wollongong. Her research interests include the study of cognitive abilities and interaction during infancy, and parent-child book-reading interactions. Her doctoral dissertation will explore how parent's book-reading practices change as babies become increasingly mobile and verbal.

Iheoma U. Iruka, Ph.D., is the Chief Research Innovation Officer and Director of The Center for Early Education Research and Evaluation at HighScope, providing strategic direction and leading national and local projects. Iheoma is engaged in projects and initiatives focused on how evidence-informed policies and systems in early education can support the optimal development and experiences of children of color. She has been engaged in addressing the excellence and well being of young diverse learners, especially Black Children. Prior to returning to the University of North Carolina,

Chapel Hill, she was at High Scope and the Buffett Institute at the University of Nebraska.

Renske Keizer, Ph.D., is Full Professor in Family Sociology at the Erasmus University Rotterdam, the Netherlands. Keizer's primary research interest is the role that families, and in particular fathers, play in strengthening, maintaining, or weakening social inequalities. Her research straddles sociology, pedagogical sciences, demography, and developmental psychology. In 2016, she was selected as one of the 25 most talented young scholars of all Dutch and Flemish universities. Since 2019, Professor Keizer is member of the Young Academy, the Royal Netherlands Academy of Sciences.

Pilyoung Kim, Ph.D., is an Associate Professor of Psychology and Director of the Family and Child Neuroscience Lab at the University of Denver, Denver, Colorado. She received her B.A. from Korea University in South Korea, her Ph.D. in Developmental Psychology from Cornell University, and completed her postdoctoral training at NIMH. Her areas of expertise include developmental affective/social neuroscience, intergenerational transmission of poverty and parenting, and neural plasticity of the parental brain.

Seongtae Kim, Ph.D., is Associate Professor in the Department of Mathematics and Statistics at North Carolina A&T State University, where he has been teaching and doing research in the area of statistics and data science since 2013. Dr. Kim's research areas include data science, time series analysis, statistical genomics, and STEM education. His research focuses on boosting the impact of data science on behavioral and social science and public health. He has published more than 40 articles in scholarly journals including *Nature Genetics* and *Proceedings of the National Academy of Sciences*. Prior to joining North Carolina A&T State University, he worked as Biostatistician at the Center for Cancer Genomics at Wake Forest School of Medicine. He received his Ph.D. in Statistics from North Carolina State University in 2007.

Joshua Kirven, Ph.D., M.S.W., is an Associate Professor in the Department of Social Work at Winthrop University and Part-Time Instructor at North Carolina A&T State University in Greensboro, NC. He is a research-practitioner with over 20 years of experience as an educator. Dr. Kirven's research areas are fatherhood, neighborhood leadership and safety, public health, and social conscious capitalism. He has an array of practice experience with micro solution-oriented, evidence-based interventions and macro programming across communities and public-private sectors. He is a Fulbright Scholar and graduate of Hampton University, University of South Carolina, and The Ohio State University, respectively.

Annette M. Klein, Ph.D., is Professor of Developmental Psychology at the International Psychoanalytic University Berlin. Her research focuses on the following topics: parent-child interactions (emotional availability, attachment), their determinants and associations with children's symptoms and social competences; internalizing symptoms and disorders from preschool to school age and their relation to psychosocial and biological risk factors; and development under risk conditions (e.g., severe life events, experiences of abuse/neglect).

Patty X. Kuo, Ph.D., is a Visiting Assistant Professor in the Department of Psychology and Faculty Affiliate of the William J. Shaw Center for Children and Families at the University of Notre Dame. She received her Ph.D. in Developmental Psychology from the University of Michigan. Her research focuses on understanding the interplay between family relationship functioning and biopsychosocial processes within individual development.

Joyce Y. Lee is a doctoral student in the Joint Ph.D. Program in Social Work and Developmental Psychology, University of Michigan. Ms. Lee has three broad research interests: (1) studying the role of father involvement and father engagement in child development; (2) developing, implementing, and evaluating technology-based parent education programs that are inclusive of fathers; and (3) examining ways to incorporate fathers in preventing child maltreatment and treating its effects on children early on.

Shawna J. Lee, Ph.D., is Associate Professor at the University of Michigan School of Social Work, where she is Director of the Parenting in Context Research Lab. Her main area of research is fathers' parenting behaviors and father-child relations, child maltreatment prevention, and the effects of parental corporal punishment on child well-being. She currently leads a multi-site study to implement and evaluate a program for low-income fathers, in collaboration with home visitation programs in Michigan.

Jacqui A. Macdonald, Ph.D., is a Senior Lecturer and Research Fellow in Developmental Psychology at Deakin University, Australia. She leads Deakin's Men and Parenting Pathways program of research and co-leads the Lifecourse Sciences Theme within Deakin's Centre for Social and Early Emotional Development (SEED). She is on the Scientific Advisory Group of Australia's longitudinal study of men's health, "Ten to Men," and she is co-convener of the Australian Fatherhood Research Consortium. @JacquiMacd

Johanna C. Malone, Ph.D., is a Lecturer in Psychiatry (part-time) at Harvard Medical School. She serves as faculty at the Massachusetts Institute for Psychoanalysis and a Clinical Supervisor at Cambridge Health Alliance. She is the Associate Editor of *Psychoanalytic Psychology* and a Co-editor for child and adolescent personality sections of the *Psychodynamic Diagnostic Manual (PDM-2).* Her writing focuses on the centrality of developmental processes to experience. Her private practice is in Cambridge, Massachusetts.

Thomas J. McMahon, Ph.D., is a Professor in the Departments of Psychiatry and Child Study at the Yale University School of Medicine. He is interested in ways the principles of developmental psychopathology can be used to understand the impact parental addiction has on family process and the well-being of fathers, mothers, and children. He is particularly interested in parenting as a treatment issue for men in systems of care and the development of parent intervention for men.

Alyssa S. Meuwissen, Ph.D., is a Research Associate in the Center for Early Education and Development (CEED) at the University of Minnesota-Twin Cities. Her work is focused on evidence-based interventions to support positive interactions between young children and the adults in their lives, with much of her research focused on fathers as an understudied population. She is passionate about promoting strong child cognitive and social development by getting research findings to the adults who can use them.

Cristina Mogro-Wilson, Ph.D., is a recognized scholar and expert in health disparities with Latino families. Her research has made substantial contributions to improving Latino families by identifying modifiable factors associated with substance use and parenting in Latino populations. Dr. Mogro-Wilson's work focuses on how culture informs parenting practices, and how to better engage and retain fathers in substance abuse treatment. Dr. Mogro-Wilson has added to the knowledge on what makes individuals and family units more effective at prevention of substance use, and what protects individuals and families that are in at-risk situations. Dr. Mogro-Wilson's work informs culturally responsive practice and education regarding understudied ethnic and racial minority populations.

Cynthia Osborne, Ph.D., is the Associate Dean for Academic Strategies at The University of Texas at Austin LBJ School of Public Affairs and Director of both the Child and Family Research Partnership and the Center for Health and Social Policy. She is a child and family policy expert and program evaluator. Osborne holds a Ph.D. in Demography and Public Affairs from Princeton University and a Master's degree in Public Policy from Harvard's Kennedy School of Government.

Rob Palkovitz, Ph.D., is Professor of Human Development and Family Sciences at the University of Delaware. His research focuses on father-child relationship quality and developmental outcomes for men and their children. He has studied factors influencing father involvement, diverse patterns of transitions to and within fatherhood, fathers' birth attendance and bonding, fathers' attitudinal and personality factors, the effects of timing on fathering, coparenting, fathering and religious faith, fathers' midlife development, and executive function in fathers' resource management.

Nadya Pancsofar, Ph.D., is an Associate Professor at The College of New Jersey where she coordinates programs in Early Childhood Special Education and Early Childhood Deaf Education. Her work focuses on fathers' contributions to early development and learning, fathers' school involvement, and home-school partnerships for children with and without disabilities. Her previous research has specifically considered contextual influences on fathering and the roles of fathers in children's early language development.

Daniel Paquette, Ph.D., earned a master's degree in biology (ethology) and a Ph.D. in anthropology (primatology) from Université de Montréal. He studied play and dominance relationships during the development of captive chimpanzees. Postdoctoral studies led him to do researches on the development of attachment and aggression in children of teenage mothers in youth protection services. His research at the School of psychoeducation now focuses on the father-child relationship, rough-and-tumble play, and peer competition.

Ross D. Parke, Ph.D., is Distinguished Professor of Psychology Emeritus and past Director of the Center for Family Studies at the University of California, Riverside. Parke was educated at the Universities of Toronto and Waterloo and was previously affiliated with the Universities of Wisconsin and Illinois and the Fels Research Institute. His is a past President of both SRCD, from which he received the Distinguished Scientific Contribution to Child development award, and the Developmental Psychology Division of the American Psychological Association, who awarded him the G. Stanley Hall award for his research contributions. He served as an editor of *Developmental Psychology* and the *Journal of Family Psychology.* Parke is author of *Fathers, Fatherhood*, and *Future Families:Diverse Forms, Rich Possibilities*; co-author of *Child Psychology*, *Social Development*, and *Throwaway Dads*; and most recently co-edited with Glen Elder *Children in a Changing World:Socio-cultural and Temporal Perspectives* (2019). He has studied fathering since the late 1960s.

James F. Paulson, Ph.D. Paulson's research program focuses on early family development with an emphasis on parents' characteristics and their impact. His work specifically seeks to further clarify fathers' impact during this time period, with an eye for parallels between paternal and maternal psychopathology in their impact on the family and developing children. Dr. Paulson completed a Ph.D. in Clinical Psychology, with a postdoctoral fellowship in Pediatric Psychology. He maintains a practice working with children and families.

Kyle Dean Pruett, M.D., Clinical Professor of Child Psychiatry and Nursing, served as Director of Medical Studies at the Yale School of Medicine's Child Study Center, where he received both the Lifetime Distinguished Teaching and Lifetime Achievement awards. He co-directed the 1100+ family "Supporting Father Involvement" project funded by the California Office of Child Abuse and Neglect and has published more than hundred original scientific articles as well as numerous books including the classic *Nurturing Father* (American Health Book Award). He is a member of the PBS National Advisory Board and Sesame Workshop Board of Directors and was co-host of the "Children's Town Meeting" for ABC News the Saturday after 9/11.

Marsha Kline Pruett, Ph.D., ABPP, is the Maconda Brown O'Connor Chair at the Smith School of Social Work and a Clinical/Community

Psychologist. She maintains a clinical practice focused on parenting issues, groups, couples, and families. A prolific writer for scholarly and lay audiences, Dr. Kline Pruett specializes in family issues pertaining to father involvement, life transitions, early development, conflict, and family law – particularly parenting plans for very young children among separated or divorced families.

Stephan Rabie, Ph.D., is a Junior Researcher with the Institute for the Life Course Health Research in the Department of Global Health at Stellenbosch University, South Africa. His work focuses on the development and implementation of community-based interventions in resource-constrained settings. His research interests include child and family health, male-specific health improvement strategies, and cross-cultural assessment. He has worked on a number of projects in South Africa, Lesotho, and Ghana.

Katherine L. Rosenblum, Ph.D., IMH-E, is a clinical and developmental psychologist with expertise in early emotional development. Her research and clinical work at the University of Michigan focuses on trauma and relationship disruptions in early childhood, parent mental health, interventions to enhance parent-child relationships, the special needs of young children in the context of military families, adoption, and foster care. Dr. Rosenblum also leads the Strong Families initiative that is part of the University of Michigan's M-SPAN initiative, focused on building effective outreach and support for military families with young children during and following deployment.

Jeffrey Shears, Ph.D., is a jointly appointed Professor in the Social Work Departments at North Carolina A&T State University and University of North Carolina – Greensboro, where he is also the Director of the Joint Master of Social Work Program (JMSW). Dr. Shears earned his BSW and Masters in Education Administration from North Carolina A&T State University and his Ph.D. in Social Work from the University of Denver. His research interests are fathering, multicultural issues, and quantitative research with an emphasis on data sharing among social service agencies. Dr. Shears has an extensive list of academic publications on fathering featured in national and internationally refereed journals.

Sarah Skeen, Ph.D., is Co-Director of the Institute for Life Course Health Research and a Senior Researcher in the Department of Global Health at Stellenbosch University in South Africa. She has extensive experience working in child and family research, with a focus on community-based interventions in low resource settings. Her work focuses on developing, implementing, and/or evaluating early child development, adolescent, and parenting programs. She has worked on a number of projects in South Africa, Lesotho, Kenya, Malawi, and Zambia.

Emily J. Steinberg is a doctoral student in Clinical Psychology at Fordham University. Her research focuses on the relationship between family factors, youth psychopathology, and treatment outcome for children and adolescents with internalizing disorders.

Jennifer Mary StGeorge, Ph.D., is Senior Lecturer in Family Studies in the Family Action Centre, Faculty of Health and Medicine, at the University of Newcastle, Australia. Her current research investigates father-child stimulating play and its effects on children's social and emotional development. Jennifer is a member of the Ten to Men Scientific Advisory Group. She has a particular interest in using observational and qualitative methodologies to explore behavioral and psychological aspects of child development and parenting.

Hervé Tissot, Ph.D., is Director of the Research Unit of the Center for Family Study (IUP, Lausanne University Hospital) and is also Researcher and Lecturer at the University of Geneva. He is a specialist of observation and assessment of interactions in families with young children. His research interests are the interplay between individuals and group-level dynamics, the impact of marital and co-parenting relationships on child development, and the impact of family-level relationships on child emotion regulation. Some of his recent work focused on the impact of postpartum depression on the development of mother-father-infant relationships.

Richard M. Tolman, M.S.W., is the Sheldon D. Rose Collegiate Professor of Social Work at the University of Michigan. He received his doctorate in social welfare from the University of Wisconsin-Madison and MSW from University of Michigan. His research on fathers grows from his extensive work with prevention of abuse by men towards their partners and children. Current projects include prevention of abuse during pregnancy and involvement of men as allies to end violence against women.

Mark Tomlinson, Ph.D., works at the Department of Psychology at Stellenbosch University and studies factors that contribute to compromised maternal health, infant and child development in contexts of high adversity, the impact of maternal depression on infant and child health and development, and community-based home visiting intervention programs. He has completed five RCTs aimed at improving maternal and child health and infant development and is currently implementing three other trials (including in Lesotho). He is on the Editorial Board of *PLoS Medicine*, is an Associate Editor of *Infant Mental Health Journal*, and is also on the Editorial Boards of *Psychology, Health and Medicine* and *Mental Health and Prevention*.

Michelle L. Townsend, Ph.D., is a Research Fellow at the Illawarra Health and Medical Research Institute and the School of Psychology at the University of Wollongong. Her career encompasses child protection, out-of-home care, and early intervention positions. Dr. Townsend's research interests include developmental origins of adult health and disease, parenting, long-term outcomes from adverse childhood experiences, and child and adolescent development and well-being.

Rebekah Tribble is a Research Coordinator in the Family and Neuroscience Lab in the Department of Psychology at the University of Denver. She earned her Master's degree in Integrative Physiology from fNIRS at the University of Colorado Boulder in 2013. Her research interests include intergenerational parenting, resilience, discrimination, coping strategies, functional near-infrared spectroscopy () with infants and mothers, and infant neuroimaging.

Claire D. Vallotton, Ph.D., is Associate Professor of Human Development and Family Studies at Michigan State University. Her research and teaching focus on the first 3 years of life in the context of important relationships with parents and other caregivers. Her scholarly contributions include research showing long-term effects of early father-child relationships on children's cognitive, language, and social development. Her scholarship is applied in early care and education, infant mental health, and social work.

Brenda L. Volling, Ph.D., is Lois Wladis Hoffman Collegiate Professor of Psychology at the University of Michigan. She received her Ph.D. in Human Development and Family Studies from Penn State University. Her research focuses on family relationship functioning and young children's social and emotional development. She is the Principal Investigator of the Family Transitions Study, a longitudinal investigation of changes in children's adjustment and family adaptation after the birth of an infant sibling.

Tova B. Walsh, MSW, Ph.D., is an Assistant Professor of Social Work and affiliate of the Center for Child & Family Well-Being and the Institute for Research on Poverty at University of Wisconsin–Madison. Through her research, she aims to better understand and meet parenting support needs through parenting interventions in early childhood. She focuses in particular on the support needs of expectant and new fathers and of parents in military-connected families.

Lars O. White, Ph.D., M.Sc., is a Research Team Leader at the Department of Child and Adolescent Psychiatry, University of Leipzig. He received his doctorate from the University of Leipzig in collaboration with the Max Planck Institute for Evolutionary Anthropology on social exclusion and mentalizing in young children. The present focus of his research is on the long-term effects of child maltreatment and neglect as well as child psychotherapy. He completed postgraduate studies at the University College London, the Anna Freud Centre, and the Yale Child Study Center as well as the International Psychoanalytic University.

Part I

Fathers, Developmental Systems, and Relationships

1 Overview to Part I: Fathers, Developmental Systems, and Relationships

Hiram E. Fitzgerald

> Before there were humans there were no fathers.
> (Kraemer, 1991, p. 377)

In his fascinating historical account on the "Origins of Fatherhood," Kraemer (1991, p. 377) asserts that "Fatherhood is a human social invention and patriarchy, the rule of the father" emerged from recognition that males played an essential role in procreation. While patriarchy rapidly, in historical time, replaced matriarchy and men created male gods to rule over all of the dominions, child rearing during infancy and early childhood became the sole responsibility of women. Therefore, in a more contemporary world it should not be surprising that most theories of early human development were developed by men, they gave special importance to the quality of the mother-child relationship with respect to child outcomes, particularly the negative ones as implied by the concept of "mother blame." Kraemer references Goodall's work with Chimpanzee's, with whom humans share about 99% of their DNA, to illustrate that for non-human primates there is no such concept as "father." What a difference 1% makes for human primates, who socially constructed the concept of father. Alas, the social construction of fatherhood that humans (men) created did not include having males play any major role in child rearing during the early years of their life. As Kraemer notes, "within a space of a few thousand years, the idea of male parent became the divine leader who could do his own creating by inventing things and controlling people" (p. 390).

Today there is a different story evolving, one that evolutionary psychologists may or may not be able to count as an adaptation, but clearly it reflects a change in relationships, a key component of adaptation (Tooby & Cosmides, 2005). The change concerns the role of fathers in child development, beyond economic provider and power-broker, to one involving his contribution to child development through caregiving and his relationships with his children. The central theme of the opening section of the volume, then, is relationships. Infant research over the past 50 years has documented the extraordinary early organization and development of neurobiological brain networks; hormonal, emotional, and behavioral regulatory systems; and the systemic embodiment of experience into the child's mental representations of self, others, and self-other relationships. How fathers contribute to the development of the children they conceive is partially determined at conception. The conceptus incorporates the evolutionary history contained in the ovum and sperm that create the new cell. How that cell evolves when interacting with its environments will depend on a host of factors, not the least of which is the environment it expe-

H. E. Fitzgerald (✉)
Department of Psychology, Michigan State University, East Lansing, MI, USA
e-mail: fitzger9@msu.edu

H. E. Fitzgerald et al. (eds.), *Handbook of Fathers and Child Development*,
https://doi.org/10.1007/978-3-030-51027-5_1

riences prenatally and throughout its postnatal life. This volume attends to questions related to how fathers (social or biological) contribute to the systemic organization of the newly conceived and developing conceptus through birth and the first 5 postnatal years.

In Chap. 2 the editors focus on two core themes to provide a foundational framework for the volume. The first theme is that fathers' contributions to child development are best informed by systems theories. System theories are not specific to fathers, they are specific to examining how the component parts of organized systems are related to one another and are expressed within the dynamic processes that regulate system functions. Second, those processes critical to system components are relationships. In a family system, they are the reciprocal relationships among family members, broader kinships, and all of the adjunctive systems that influence the family.

In Chap. 3, Palkovitz discusses the interdependent relational aspects of fathering and of being fathered that have life-altering, developmental consequences for both fathers and their children. He focuses on how father-child relationships bring developmental benefits and outcomes of interdependent meanings and processes in the context of everyday intergenerational father-child relationships. A key aspect of intergenerational transmission of fathering involves a broader ecological scan of adjunctive system influences on family dynamics and parenting. In Chap. 4, Keizer asserts that much about fathers' role in the intergenerational transmission of (dis) advantages can be revealed by linking sociological stratification questions to developmental psychology research on father involvement. In Chap. 5, Shears and his colleagues focus specifically on the father-child relationship. There is a growing research literature examining the father-child relationship, specifically within the context of low-income communities. Using narratives generated by men discussing their remembrances of their fathers, Sears et al. explore through text mining how these retrospective stories provide insight into how becoming a father has influenced their lives across generations.

One of the family relationships that affect children are those between parents. In Chap. 6, Frascarola and colleagues focus on the quality of the co-parenting, the quality of the marital relationship, the father's interest in being involved, and maternal gatekeeping with respect to parenting and child care. The diversity of families is enormous, and the concept of a nuclear family no longer captures the contexts within which many children are reared. Bocknek follows, in Chap. 7, with a review of the effects of father presence and absence in the family on child development outcomes. She refers to literature indicating that fathers contribute in consistent and meaningful ways to their children's development across residential patterns. The discussion derives conceptual meaning based on boundary clarity/ambiguity in families, especially within families dealing with psychological/sociological issues that impact family separation including mental health problems, substance use, trauma, and incarceration.

Studying the early influences of parenting practices advances understanding of critical factors that influence the biopsychosocial development of children. When translated into non-scientific language, it also can inform parents about successful ways to raise their children. But unless scientific knowledge leads to positive social policies, the weight of factors external to the family often create barriers to effective parenting practices. In the final chapter in Part I, Osborne describes current policies designed to support fathers and evidence indicating whether such policies lead to positive outcomes, relative to those designed to support mother and child well-being. She offers recommendations for enhancing policy practices in support of fathers and child well-being.

References

Kraemer, S. (1991). The origins of fatherhood: An ancient family process. *Family Process, 30*, 377–392.

Tooby, J., & Cosmides, L. (2005). Conceptual foundations of evolutionary psychology. In D. M. Buss (Ed.), *The handbook of evolutionary psychology* (pp. 5–67). Hoboken, NJ: John Wiley & Sons.

2 Fathers and Very Young Children: A Developmental Systems Perspective

Hiram E. Fitzgerald, Kai von Klitzing, Natasha J. Cabrera, Júlia Scarano de Mendonça, and Thomas Skjøthaug

Research in human development has expanded knowledge about the period of infancy and early childhood. The majority of this work related to parenting has focused on the importance of the mother-infant attachment relationship for positive social-emotional development. In 1965, Nash challenged researchers to go beyond the mother-child dyad by directing more attention to the role of the father in child development. Nash posited that the "relative lack of the father [in child development research] may have distorted our understanding of the dynamics of development, and …adversely affected the rearing of males" (p. 261). Within a decade, responses to Nash's challenge were evident as researchers demonstrated fathers' competence in performing routine caregiving tasks (Parke, 1979; Parke & Sawin, 1976), and generated theories about fathers' role and/or involvement in child development (Biller, 1971; Lamb, 1976; Lamb & Lamb, 1976; Pleck, 1981), including mother-father-newborn interactions (Parke & O'Leary, 1976), and attachment relationships (Clarke-Stewart, 1978; Cohen & Campos, 1974). Ten years after Nash's article, Lamb (1975) followed with a catalyzing article about "forgotten fathers" shortly followed by Hagstad and Speicher (1981) who referred to grandfathers as "forgotten men" (McGreal, 1994). The race to discover what role and/or impact fathers have on child development was officially launched! Literature reviews spanning 1964–1980 evidence at least 1292 published articles on fathers, with the primary foci on fathers and their children (172 articles), father absence (154), fathers and pregnancy (146), and fathers and sons (118) (Price-Bonham, 1976; Price-Bonham, Pittman, & Welch, 1981). Based on Lewis' (2012) estimate of the annual rate of publications concerning fathers and child development since 1965, there would be nearly 32,000 studies in the literature (Fitzgerald, 2014). Yet, Lewis queried, "Why do we know so little about fathers, when there is so much research on them" (Lewis, 2012, p. 229).

H. E. Fitzgerald (✉)
Department of Psychology, Michigan State University, East Lansing, MI, USA
e-mail: fitzger9@msu.edu

K. von Klitzing
Department of Child and Adolescent Psychiatry, University of Leipzig, Leipzig, Germany

N. J. Cabrera
Department of Human Development and Quantitative Methodology, University of Maryland, College Park, MD, USA

J. S. de Mendonça
Graduate Program in Educational Psychology, Centro Universitário FIEO, Osasco, Sao Paulo, Brazil

T. Skjøthaug
Division of Mental Health, Grorud DPS, Akershus University Hospital, Lørenskog, Norway

H. E. Fitzgerald et al. (eds.), *Handbook of Fathers and Child Development*,
https://doi.org/10.1007/978-3-030-51027-5_2

Fathers

While it may be the case that "Before there were humans there were no fathers (Kraemer, 1991, p. 377)," and that "Fatherhood is a human social invention and patriarchy, the rule of the father," it is not true that paternal (male) caring behavior is unique to human primates (Huck & Fernandez-Duque, 2013; Snowdon & Suomi, 1982). Geary (2005) posits that adult primate males benefit from participating in infant care, including assisting in the infant's survival, sharing the female's reproductive burden, and enhancing chances of future mating. However, the extent to which non-human primate males are involved in infant care varies greatly. For example, Huck and Fernandez-Duque (2013) summarize evidence indicating that Strepsirrhine males (lemurs, tarsiers, langurs) are rarely involved, but black-and-white snub-nosed monkeys are moderately so. Cercopithecine (Old World Monkeys) monkeys range from low to moderate involvement, whereas Platyrrhines (New World Monkeys, titi monkeys, and owl monkeys) have high levels of involvement, primarily involving carrying behavior. Snowdon and Suomi's (1982) review of paternal behavior in non-human primates suggests the variation of male involvement depends on the extent to which adult males have early experiences with infants, or when infants achieve an older age and emit behaviors that trigger adult male involvement. For example, they note that marmost and golden lion tamarin mothers carry their newborns more than fathers do, but after several postnatal weeks, father and brothers become principal caretakers of golden lion tamarin infants. Cotton tamain and pygmy marmoset males, however, engage in carrying behavior from birth. Interestingly, although rhesus monkey males rarely interact with infants, they engage in some caretaking behaviors when the mother becomes impaired, similar to some human fathers (de Mendonça, Vera, Bussab, Rodriguez, & Cossette, 2013; Hops et al., 1987).

At the beginning of the 1970s decade of the discovery of father, Barry and Paxton (1971) published findings about father involvement from their survey of 186 societies. They listed 10 predictors of increased paternal involvement:

1. The line of descent is bilateral or matrilineal rather than patrilineal.
2. Monogamy or limited polygyny is practiced.
3. A high male god does not rule.
4. Males are not circumcised.
5. Games of physical skill, rather than games of strategy are played.
6. Birds or small animals, rather than large game, are hunted.
7. Animal husbandry is nonexistent or unimportant.
8. Land transport is human rather than by pack animals.
9. Adolescent males are not segregated.
10. The training of children is responsibility and obedient is relatively lenient.

Studies reported in Shwalb, Shwalb, and Lamb (2013) evidence considerable within culture and cross-cultural variation in father involvement in countries spanning six continents, somewhat mirroring the variation among nonhuman primates, with cultural practices playing a major role in such variation. On the other hand, some paternal behaviors seem more alike than different across cultures. For example, MacKey's (1996) multicultural study indicated when father, mother, and infant are together, fathers typically yield caregiving to the mother, even though they competently provide such care when she is absent.

In the United States, there are 70 million fathers, nearly 25 million of whom are in a marital relationship that includes children under 18 years of age. According to Livingston (2013), there are at least 2.6 million single father households, a nine-fold increase since 1960 (see Table 2.1). In addition, there are 214,000 stay-at-home fathers, and fathers caring for 18% of all preschoolers during times when the mother is at work. Research on fathers since Nash's challenge and Lamb's lament clearly indicates that fathers contribute broadly to child development (Cabrera, Fitzgerald & Shannon, 2007; Diamond, 2007;

Table 2.1 Children in Single-Parent Families by Race. National Kids Count data

Location	Race	Date Type	2010	2011	2012	2013	2014
United States							
	American Indian	Number	350,000	355,000	345,000	329,000	341,000
		Percent	52%	53%	53%	52%	53%
	Asian & Pacific Islander	Number	539,000	559,000	579,000	557,000	578,000
		Percent	16%	17%	17%	16%	17%
	Black or African American	Number	6,533,000	6,509,000	6,493,000	6,427,000	6,382,000
		Percent	66%	67%	67%	67%	66%
	Hispanic or Latino	Number	6,674,000	6,890,000	7,008,000	7,044,000	7,190,000
		Percent	41%	42%	42%	42%	42%
	Non-Hispanic White	Number	9,329,000	9,466,000	9,358,000	9,289,000	9,181,000
		Percent	24%	25%	25%	25%	25%
	Two or more Races	Number	1,586,000	1,655,000	1,703,000	1,758,000	1,797,000
		Percent	42%	42%	43%	43%	42%
	Total	Number	24,297,000	24,718,000	24,725,000	24,647,000	24,689,000
		Percent	34%	35%	35%	35%	35%

Definitions: Children under age 18 who live with their own single parent either in a family or subfamily. In this definition, single-parent families may include cohabitating couples but do not include children living with married stepparents. Children who live in group quarters (e.g., institutions, dormitories, or group homes) are not included in this calculation. © 2016 The Annie E. Casey Foundation. With permission according to web-based use description

Fitzgerald, Mann, Cabrera, Sarche, & Qin, 2010; Fitzgerald, & Bradley, 2012; Palkovitz, 1980; Tamis-LaMonda & Cabrera, 2002). Indeed, as von Klitzing (2011) observed, there is a sense that "Fathers *have* to be different from mothers, to help children orient themselves in multi-dimensional developmental space" (p. 157). Although there are direct effects, fathers also influence children indirectly via mediation through the child's mother, or by influences that are exogenous to the family. Yet, there are many unanswered questions related to what fathers do that contribute to their influence on child development.

Their visibility as unique contributors to child development continues to be questioned, especially with respect to the earliest years of human development. In this volume, we set the stage for a comprehensive review of fathers' involvement in child development from the prenatal years to preschool, a period of human development marked by the early organization of neurobiological networks, hormonal, emotional, and behavioral regulatory systems, and the systemic embodiment of experience into the child's mental models of self, others, and self-other relationships.

Although fathers are no longer forgotten or invisible parents (Saracho & Spokek, 2008).

Fathers and Early Childhood Development

Developmental scientists have long viewed infant care as an outgrowth of the mother's biological relationship to her conceptus and newborn. At the extreme was Margaret Mead's comment that the father is "a biological necessity but a social accident." Thus, the father's role was conceptualized as that of family provider and companion to his wife, rather than as caregiver to his infant and young child. Moreover, fathers have generally been perceived as being uninterested and less nurturant toward infants, less competent to care for them, and more interested in non-caregiving roles. Parke and Sawin (1976) dispelled these views in their observational studies of fathers and their newborns that demonstrated precisely the opposite of these erroneous perceptions of fathers' interests and competencies. Fathers apparently already agreed with their findings. In 1943, Gardner asked fathers to describe their roles with respect to child rearing. They talked about providing guidance related to economic, social, and educational issues and noted they spent time disciplining, teaching words, answering questions, and playing with children under six. Pederson and Robson (1969) found similar descriptions 26 years later, albeit from mothers reporting about their husband's involvement with infants and toddlers. Regardless of the source or when the data were collected, by the 1970s researchers began to think differently about the ecological validity of parenting research (Bronfenbrenner, 1974; McGreal, 1981), noting that few infants and young children are socialized within the bounded context of a mother-child dyad. Infants and very young children interact with a considerable number of socializing influences, not just those provided by father and mother, and not just in the home.

The strongest evidence of father effects involves negative outcomes, particularly with respect to fathers and sons. Much of this evidence derives from studies of father absence. Although the father presence does not assure that he will be a positive influence on child development any more than mother presence does, it is highly correlated with positive child outcomes (Table 2.1). Unfortunately, we know more about fathers in the context of child abuse (Lee, Bellamy, & Guteman, 2019; Guterman and Lee (2005), substance use disorders (Fitzgerald & Bockneck, 2013; Zucker, Wong, Puttler, & Fitzgerald, 2003), neighborhood violence (Fitzgerald, McKelvey, Schiffman, & Montanez, 2006), marital conflict (Cummings, Goeke-Morey, & Raymond, 2004), and divorce (Amato & Sobolewski, 2004), than we know about their positive influences on very young children's cognitive development (Cabrera, Fitzgerald, Bradley, & Roggman, 2007; Cook, Roggman & Boyce, 2011), social competence (Colonnesi, Zeegers, Majdandzic, van Steensel, & Bogels, 2019), self-efficacy, self-identity, behavior and emotion regulation, and positive peer relationships (Bockneck, Brophy-Herb, Fitzgerald, Schiffman, & Vogel, 2014; Bocknek, Dayton, Brophy-Herb, Raveau, & Fitzgerald, 2017; Cabrera & Tamis-LaMonda, 2013; Volling & Cabrera, 2019). In addition, we need to learn more about cultural influences that affect father-child relationships (Lamb, 1987; Mackay, 1996; Shwalb et al., 2013), as well as their relationships within single families (Brott, 1999), biracial families and families of color (Fitzgerald, Johnson, Qin, Villarruel, & Norder, 2019), families with same-sex caregivers (Bos, Knox, vanRijn-van Gelderen, & Gartrell, 2016; Crowl, Ahn, & Baker, 2007), or any other type of family (Parke, 2013).

Cabrera and Tamis-LeMonda (2013) emphasized two core themes to guide efforts to understand father involvement in child development; identifying positive and negative factors that influence involvement, and assessing within and between culture variations. Other investigators suggest that the study of paternal parenting needs to focus on (1) the direct assessment of fathers, (2) assessing their presence rather than their absence, (3) recognizing that father effects on child development and presence in the home are not necessarily the same, (4) determining his influence on children's gender role differentiation, (5) involving him in family interventions, and (6) understanding father and mother as components of a dynamic system of interacting personalities (Fitzgerald, Mann, & Barrett, 1999; Loukas, Twitchell, Piejak, Fitzgerald, & Zucker, 1998). More recently, Cabrera and Volling (2019) recommended that researchers explicitly attune to four core issues related to future research on fathers and child development (Table 2.2).

Core Issue 1: Emphasize that fathers are important to children's development and researchers need to know they matter to children.

Core Issue 2: Use an ecological systems approach and family focus for understanding fathering, mothering, and co-parenting.

Core Issue 3: Understand that fathers (and mothers) are part of diverse family and social systems.

Core Issue 4: Consider that the study of fathers may uncover "new" parenting constructs that predict children's development (pp. 112–113).

Table 2.2 Correlates of Negative and Positive Involvement on Child Development

Negative Father Involvement with Child Development (includes father absence)
Cognitive Development
Lower: scores on intelligence tests, grade point averages, advanced education attainment
Trouble with mathematical and puzzle tasks
Difficulty paying attention
Higher likelihood of being expelled or dropping out of school
Poor school achievement
Social, Emotional, and Moral Development
Poor social and emotional regulation
Difficulty delaying gratification
More impulsive
A weaker sense of right and wrong
Developmental Psychopathology
Higher rates of suicide, aggression, bullying, antisocial behavior, physical and sexual abuse, alcohol use disorders, illicit drug use, possession of weapons, conduct and anxiety disorders, involvement with crimination justice system
Deviant peer group selections
Earlier onset of sexual intercourse, smoking, alcohol abuse
Positive Father Involvement with their Children
Cognitive and Language Development
More use of 5-W questions in language interactions
Higher school attendance and less problems
More likely to enjoy school
Higher academic achievement, GPA, test scores
Better problem solving skills
More self-direction and initiative
Social, Emotional & Moral Development
High life satisfaction
More playful, socially competent, socially mature, tolerant, and understanding
Better capacity for relatedness, sibling relationships
Stronger moral values
Developmental Psychopathology
Less depression, stress, frustration, antisocial behavior, bullying, involvement with criminal justice system
Fewer behavior problems

Adapted from Fitzgerald (2017)

The direction of effects for these recommended guidelines focuses on explanatory and predictive approaches to study fathers and child development (Barlas & Carpenter, 1990), perhaps because there is no overarching theory driving research involving father-infant/child relationships (Kotelchuck, 1976, Pederson, 2002, Yogman, 1982) such as there is with attachment-driven studies of mother-child relationships. For fathers, investigators have used social relational theory (Kuczynski & Parkin, 2007) and self-determination theory (LaGuardia & Patrick, 2008; Ryan & Deci, 2000), and others draw attention to social capital theories, ecological models, and essential father theory (Pleck, 2007) as well as attachment theory, particularly with respect to infancy and early childhood (Brown, Mangelsdorf, Shigeto, & Wong, 2018). Paquette's activation relationship theory shows promise for understanding fathers' influence on the organization of children's behavioral regulation skills, especially for boys (Paquette, 2004). Using the risky situation procedure, Paquette and his colleagues found that fathers' activation relationships with their sons were different than their attachment relationships and provided their sons with support for risk taking and behavioral control (Paquette & Bigras, 2010; Paquette & Dumont, 2013). Fletcher, StGeorge, & Freeman, 2013) proposed that rough and tumble play provides another context wherein fathers facilitate organization of self-control and reduction of aggressive behavior in boys.

While there is no agreement on one overarching theory driving research on father's parenting behaviors, there is consensus that father research must address a wide range of methodological issues to augment measurement tools and research methods primarily developed for research with mothers rather than research with fathers (Roggman, Fitzgerald, Bradley, & Raikes, 2002; Volling & Cabrera, 2019).

Father Roles

The shift from emphasis on mother-child relationships to one that stresses broader influences on child development especially affected research with fathers (Pleck, 2007; Roggman, Bradley, & Raikes, 2013). While there is no single definition of father involvement, studies of fathers now span diverse ways that societies or cultures define family and assign roles and responsibilities, oftentimes regardless of their biological connection to the child (Lamb, 1987; Shwalb et al., 2013). Even with the rapidly changing family configurations, including diminution of the nuclear family, most children are reared in a context that includes an adult male, who may or may not be in residence, or who may or may not be their biological parent. These conditions, and others like them, suggest evolving roles for men in children's lives and the likelihood of diverse, rather than single, pathways through which they influence children's development.

Atran, Medin, and Ross (2005) view culture as consisting of networks or patterns of publicly shared mental representations, and behaviors in ecological context. Thus, culture attitudes and stereotypes are social constructions expressed in the scripts and social mores that define parents and other caregivers. "Beliefs are constructed through the exchange of social meanings among peoples as individuals integrate personal experiences with their participating in the parenting role suggested by the culture at a particular point in history" (McGillicuddy-DeLisi & Subramanian, 1996, p. 147). Lamb et al. (1987) identified four historical set points that augured changes in cultural stereotypes about the role of fathers in family life and child rearing. According to Lamb et al. (1987), during Colonial Times, fathers were perceived to be disciplinarians. When the Industrial Revolution moved fathers' work space outside of the home, his role shifted to greater involvement in active play. Following World War II his role shifted again to parenting that focused on sex-role differentiation, particularly with respect to gender stereotypes (see Biller, 1971). Finally, in contemporary Western societies the father's role expectations now focus more on being an active caregiver and sharing parenting with his partner (Cabrera, Tamis-LeMonda, Bradley, Hofferth, & Lamb, 2000).

Cultural mental representations and broad categorizations of father's role are useful in historical context, but in reality, fathers have always been involved with more activities that affect children than might be implied by such broad cultural characterizations. As indicated in Table 2.3, Lamb concluded that fathers perhaps should be studied by what they actually do to engage children, be available to them, and responsible for the provision of resources to them. Palkovitz (2002b) identified 14 activities that could influence fathers' involvement in children's cognitive, affective, and behavioral development. Snarey's (1993) study of fathers' parental generativity involved interviews when the fathers were 25, 31, and 47 years of age. Fathers reported the extent to which they supported their children (birth to age 10) and then their adolescents (11–21 years old) in social-emotional development, intellectual-academic development, and physical-athletic development. There were 12 activities in each content domain at each age level. The average number of activities was 9.3, although there was considerable variation when fathers were divided into three groups: low (35%, 0 to 6 activities), average (41%, 7–12 activities), and high involvement (24%, 13–24 activities). The mean number of activities they participated in during childhood (5.04) was significantly greater than during adolescence. (4.24). Fathers were more involved with more social-emotional and physical athletic activities during childhood, and more intellectual-achievement activities during adolescence. There was more continuity for engaging in social-emotional activities across age periods than was the case for the other two content domains. Interestingly, the three types of activities were not significantly correlated in childhood.

In Bretherton, Lambert, and Golby's (2006) study of fathers of preschool children, fathers commented on the lack of affection, support, and engaged relationships, and degree of authoritarian parenting they received from their own fathers. The number of fathers who perceived themselves as similar to their own fathers was considerable, but many fathers also worked to change the paternal role to one that reworked the role they remembered from their own past. Sharabany, Seher, and Gal-Kraaz (2006) noted that fathers who perceived that their fathers were more accepting tended to have a strong interest in behavioral regulation, which mothers reported as contributing to their children's better positive behaviors. Shears, Robinson, and Emde (2002)

Table 2.3 Dimensions of father involvement in child development

Source			
Lamb, Pleck, Charnov, and Levine (1987)	Dimensions		
	Engagement Availability Responsibility	Direct contact & shared interactions Presence and accessibility Resource availability to child	
Palkovitz (2002a)	Domains	Simultaneously occurring continua	Possible actions
	Cognitive Affective Behavioral	Time invested Degree of involvement Observability Salience of involvement Directedness Proximity	Communicating Teaching Monitoring Engaging in thought processes Providing Showing affection Protecting Supporting emotionally Running errands Caregiving Engaging in child-related maintenance Sharing interests Being available Planning Sharing activities

Adapted from Cabrera et al. (2007)

found that low-income fathers who reported a positive relationship with their own fathers viewed themselves as better fathers than fathers who did not report positive relationships with their fathers.

Atran et al.'s (2005) concept of cultural practices as mindsets within ecological context demands that research on fathers' role in child rearing must extend beyond parenting research in Western cultures. Valaiquette-Trssier, Vosselin, Young, and Thomassin (2019) conducted a systematic review of studies published between 2005 and 2016 that focused on parenting stereotypes in cultures/countries outside of North America. Five stereotypes were identified, with considerable variation within and across groups. All groups seemed to agree that financial provider was a father role. All groups also agreed that fathers should be role models, guides, and moral teachers, with the exception of nonresidential fathers in Russia. Fathers in Ethiopia, Kenya, and Mexico did not agree that being an educator was part of fathers' role. Nearly all studies agreed with fathers as protectors, but there was the least support for fathers as disciplinarians. Descriptions of fathers' roles in countries around the world document considerable variation (Bornstein, 2010; Lamb, 1987; Shwalb et al., 2013). Indeed, Werner (1988) pointed out that Western theories of socialization fail to recognize that the exclusive care of infants by their mothers is the exception rather than the rule when considered from cross-cultural perspectives.

Clearly, gaining a deeper understanding of the father's role within family systems will enable a broad range of researchers, practitioners, and policy makers to address family systems perspectives, but only if they avoid decoupling fathers from the multiple relationships and sets of conditions that define family and within which children develop (Loukas et al., 1998). Kaplan and Garner's (2017) Dynamic Systems Model of Role Identity, developed to re-conceptualize identity formation during adolescence, has relevance for re-conceptualizing father's role identity as well. From a dynamic systems perspective, fathers' role identity becomes more contextually diverse, encompassing multiple actions that may vary as a function of culture, family dynamics, marital quality, child gender, child age, and the impact of exogenous systems on the father and/or the family system. Currently, we know little about these processes, particularly from the father's point of view.

Infancy and early childhood provide numerous occasions for children to model sex-role behavior and to construct their initial working models of what it is to be a father, mother, spouse, or parent. These mental representations incorporate adult behavior and interpersonal dynamics, including such behaviors as drinking and smoking, and such dynamics as marital conflict. Children remember events that are consistent with gender-role stereotypes better than events that are inconsistent, and, remarkably, when events are not consistent with stereotypes, preschool age children distort the information to make it consistent (Davidson, 1996). Like father, like son is driven by the son's identification processes as it is by the father's modeled behavior, although father's differential interactions with sons and daughters play a key role in the son's identification with the father (Lytton & Romney, 1991), although his behavior may vary as a function of child age. For example, Cannon, Schoppe-Sullivan, Mangelsdorf, Brown, and Sokolowski (2008) observed that middle-class American mothers' behaviors were more influential in triadic interactions with 3-month-old infants than were fathers, whereas de Mendonça, Bussab, and Kärtner (2019) found that Brazilian fathers were more influential in triadic interactions with 3-year-old children especially positive interactions involving daughters. de Mendonca et al. suggest that less interactional synchrony between father-son dyadic interactions and father-mother-son triadic interactions may reflect the father's stronger adherence to traditional gender role behavior with its emphasis on autonomy and independence for boys, and compliance and dependence for girls.

According to Lorber and Egeland (2009, p. 912), "Infancy is characterized by rapid development of emotion regulatory capacity, patterns of relating to others, and internal representations of relationships; each is surmised to be important to the development of externalizing problems. Maladaptive infancy parenting may negatively impact these capacities and behaviors during a period in which they are thought to be highly sensitive to environmental input, thus setting the stage for the development of persistent externalizing psychopathology."

Diamond (2007) notes that fathers play a key role in helping their preschool sons to establish a sense of their categorical self (What am I), but their role changes when helping their adolescent sons to develop a sense of identity that spans the boundaries of "me" and "not me" as they strive to understand their identity and answer the question, "Who am I?" (also see, Fitzgerald, Wong, & Zucker, 2013).

Fathers, Family Systems, and Relational Developmental Science

In 2006, researchers gathered at the University of Maryland to discuss a proposed heuristic model to guide research on father influences on child development. The discussions were intensive and lead to a special journal issue focused on modeling approaches to research on fathers and child development (Cabrera et al., 2007). Six years later Cabrera and her colleagues offered a revised model, incorporating the complexity and extent to which that literature had grown. They shifted their focus from questions related to how fathers are involved in child development, to more pointed questions concerning what it is that fathers do that contributes to child development across the broad issues that comprise development (Cabrera, Fitzgerald, Bradley, & Roggman, 2014a). In one sense, they needed a model that would represent "the link between the *culture of fatherhood*, the norms, values and beliefs surrounding men's behavior, and the *conduct of fatherhood*, what fathers do, their parental behavior" (LaRossa, 1997, p. 117).

Cabrera et al. shifted to a systems approach to guide research on fathers, focusing on organismic explanatory/predictive models of father involvement rather than mechanistic models (Barlas &

Carpenter, 1990; Yu, 2006). They aligned with developmental history theory with its roots in Schneirla's (1957) emphasis on the study of "....progressive changes in the organization of an individual considered as a functional adaptive systems through its life history" (p. 79), and Werner's (1957) orthogenetic principle, which asserted that development "proceeds from a state of relative globality and lack of differentiation to a state of increasing differentiation, articulation, and hierarchic integration." (p. 126). Today developmental science focuses on organizational models of development (Yates, Egeland, & Sroufe, 2003) that adaptive behavior and function are emergent, epigenetic, relational, systemic, organized, constructive, and hierarchically integrated (Ford & Lerner, 1992; Laszlo, 1972, 1996; Miller, 1976; Sameroff, 1983; von Bertalanffly, 1968) and sometimes chaotic (Levine & Fitzgerald, 1992). Furthermore, these dynamic and organizing processes begin at conception and affect "the emergence of new structural and functional properties and competences at all levels of analysis...as a consequence of horizontal and vertical coactions among the organism's parts including organism-environmental coaction" (Gottlieb, 1991, p. 7) (Table 2.4).

Table 2.4 Contrasting Paradigms of Science

Mechanistic Paradigm	Organismic Paradigm
Reactive organism	Active organism
Basic metaphor: Machine	Basic metaphor: Living organism
Elementaristic: The whole is predictable from the parts	Holistic: Parts derive their meaning from the whole
Mechanistic	Teleological (purposive)
Behavioral change: Determined by efficient and material causes	Behavioral change: Structures and functions change during development (epigenetic)
Continuity: Present behavior is predictable from early behavior in an additive sense	Discontinuity: Changes in the parts or in the organization of the parts result in a whole with new systemic properties; properties are emergent in the sense that they cannot be predicted from the sum of the parts.
Causation: Material, efficient	Causation: Material, efficient, final, formal
Unidirectional, sequential	Reciprocal, transactional, synergistic

Adapted from Fitzgerald, Strommen, and McKinney (1982), p. 19

The purpose of heuristic models is to generate a map or flow-chart to guide examination of pathways in space and time that may explain or predict the effect of prior occurring events on some outcome of interest. With heuristic models in hand, one can generate research models designed to assess the influence of specific aspects of the model that may explain or predict positive or negative correlates on the outcome. The model developed by Cabrera et al. was intended to:

(a) Organize systematically the study of fathers in relation to their children's well-being and development within a transactional dynamic systems framework,
(b) To take into account the factors that affect fathers' involvement with their children,
(c) To consider the factors that mediate or moderate the pathways from father involvement to child outcomes, and
(d) To consider fathers' characteristics and parenting as mediators and moderators of other influences on their children's development (p. 348).

From a dynamic relational perspective, the individual is always contextually embedded in subsystems (biological, intraindividual, interindividual, social, emotional, cognitive, and cultural) that may or may not have meaningful influences at the moment (proximal), or over the life course. Because individual development is unique, probabilistic, and changing through life course transitions, determinants predicting outcomes can change over time. Such changes are captured by the developmental principles of multifinality (there are multiple ways to reach the same outcome) and equifinality (the same developmental pathway can predict different outcomes) (Cicchetti & Rogosch, 1996), which describe the diversity of developmental pathways within open systems (Fig. 2.1).

Diverse developmental pathways are produced in part by genetic and epigenetic (gene–environment interplay) factors and by the host of life course experiences that impact the individual

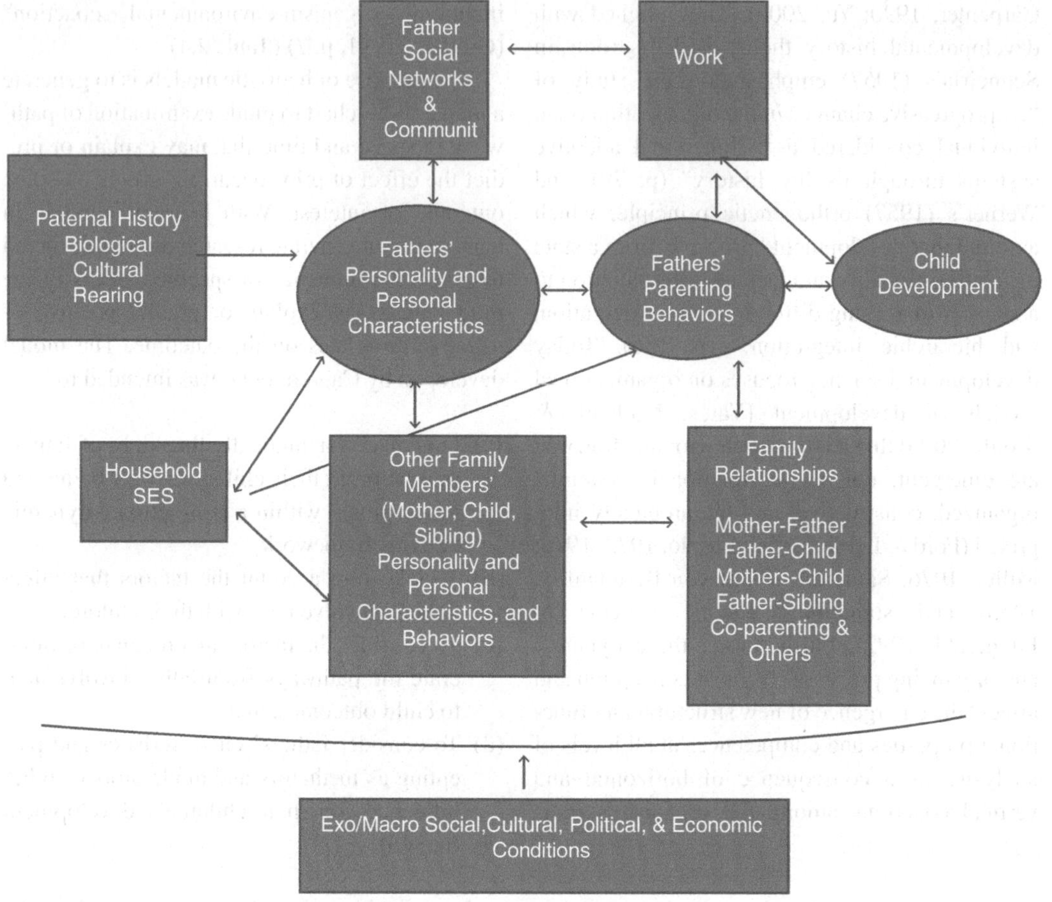

Fig. 2.1 Heuristic model to guide research on fathers and child development. (Reprinted from: Cabrera, Fitzgerald, Bradley, and Roggman (2014b). With permission: © John Wiley & Sons)

through family and broader system transactions. Both risk and resilience factors can accumulate or change over the life course, and with respect to the infancy and early childhood period, greater attention has been given to risk factors than to those that promote resilience. For example, the concept of cumulative risk through adverse childhood experience has drawn considerably more attention (Felitti et al., 1998; Rutter, 1979; Sameroff, Seifer, Zax, & Barocas, 1987) than has literature on cumulative resilience (Masten, 2014; Hays-Grudo & Morris, 2020), particularly with respect to mother-child transactions and bioecological variables that affect the family (Bronfenbrenner & Morris, 2006). Little attention has been given to father effects within either the risk or resilience literatures, with the exceptions of paternal substance abuse (Fitzgerald & Eiden, 2007), antisocial behavior and violence (Golding & Fitzgerald, 2019), marital conflict (Cummings et al., 2004), and absence from the home. Cummings et al. suggest that study of father effects on child development would be enhanced by emphasizing three research pathways focused on (a) parenting and father-child relationships, (b) children's exposure to father marital conflict, and (c) father's overall and specific psychological functioning (Feinberg et al. 2011). For example, questions of interest may concern the effects of fathers' antisocial behavior (Loukas, Fitzgerald, Zucker, & Von Eye, 2001) or depression (de Mendonça et al., 2013) on father-child relationships or marital conflict. Figure 2.2 illustrates major transitional periods during the

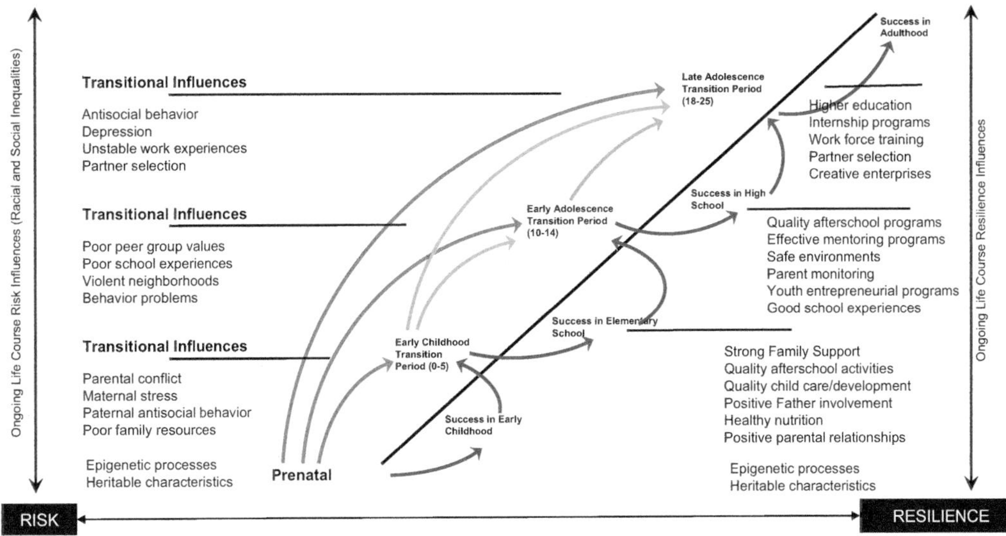

Fig. 2.2 Transactional periods: Dynamic factors affecting positioning on the risk-resilience continuum from conception to adulthood. Source: Fitzgerald (2010). (Reprinted with permission © Michigan State University Board of Trustees)

first 25 years of life and known sources of risk and resilience promoting experiences (Fitzgerald et al. 2013). The following are descriptive of major aspects of each of these transitional periods:

- Prenatal through Early Childhood (Conception to 5 years)
  - Rapid physical, cognitive, and social emotional development
  - Organization of neurobiological, behavioral, and mental networks
  - Foundation established for transition from home school
- Middle Childhood/Early Adolescence (6–15 years)
  - More autonomy and skill development but increased exposure to risk
  - Cultural and family identity sets trajectory for success in school
  - Increased exposure to peers and broader community networks
  - Rapid neurobiological and psychological changes through puberty
- Late Adolescence/Early Adulthood (16–25 years)
  - Establishing identity as knower and fostering a growth mindset
  - Transitioning from home and school to post-secondary education/training, employment, and self-sufficiency
  - Acquiring skills and attitudes to be successful in a rapidly changing workplace (adapted from Fitzgerald et al. (2019), pp. 4–5.

The statistical risk for psychopathology or life-course outcomes does not indicate a general vulnerability for psychopathology (Richters & Weintraub, 1990). Because contextual events play a pivotal role in the organization, disorganization, and reorganization of developmental pathways, neither resilience nor vulnerability is a fixed attribute of the individual (Rutter, 1990). The challenge is to identify the critical variables that guide individuals onto developmental pathways, that shift them to other pathways, and that predict the life course at various time periods over the life span considering both distal and proximal events.

In the study of human development, the shift to an expanded view of the child's multidimensional space occurred when investigators brought fathers, father-mother relationships, gene-environment interplay, and co-parenting into their efforts to understand child development (Cabrera et al., 2014a). From a developmental systems perspective, the search for causal determinants of behavior must consider intraindividual (within the individual), interindividual (between individuals), contextual (social-historical-temporal events or situations), and organismic-environmental transactional (ecological, bidirectional) sources of variance, rather than relying on simple main effects models (Fitzgerald, Davies, Zucker, & Klinger, 1994; Fitzgerald, Zucker, & Yang, 1995). Because development is dynamic and transactional, things are always subject to change as family dynamics shift, children and caregivers become older, adjunctive systems influencing individuals and families change, and developmental transitions are negotiated. For example, during the prenatal period many expectant fathers provide positive support to their partner and think about their future interactions with the child to be (Dayton et al., 2016), in ways that are reminiscent of Lebovici's (1988) concepts of the imaginary and fantasized infant that are aspects of the pregnant women's perceptions of her infant and motherhood. However, other expectant fathers show increases in psychological distress, alcohol use and abuse, sexually deviant behaviors, extramarital affairs, spousal interpersonal violence, neuroticism, and immature ego defenses (Boyce, Condon, Barton & Corkindale, 2007; Curtis, Blume, & Blume, 1997). Others may gain weight, have sleep difficulties, increased restlessness, and minor health problems (Connor & Denson, 1990), characteristic of couvade syndrome (Trethowan & Conlon, 1965). First time parents often doubt their abilities to be adequate parents, with feelings of inadequacy tied to conscious or unconscious negative experiences in their own childhoods. Such "ghosts in the nursery" have been described for mothers (Fraiberg, Adelson, & Shapiro, 1975) and fathers (Barrows, 2004) and can challenge parental relations with infants as well as behavioral interactions. For example, typical maternal left side-holding preferences are disrupted resulting in more right-side holding for mothers who are stressed or otherwise troubled by events characterized their own early childhood relations with their parents (deChateau, 1991). Trevathan (1987) found that mothers who held their newborns on the left side immediately after birth initiated breastfeeding earlier than did mothers who had a right-side holding preference, perhaps because newborns tend to more quickly turn to the right when in a left-side hold, than to turn to the left when in a right-side hold. Thus, they more quickly contact the breast for feeding. In addition, feeding on the left breast positions the infant to see the left side of the mother's face, the more emotionally expressive side. The organizational dynamics of these initial dyadic transactions are disrupted by maternal depression, the infant's delivery position, and other organizers related to the development of lateralized behaviors during infancy and early childhood (Fitzgerald, et al., 1991). Fathers in contrast do not have strong left-side holding preferences, nor do they tend to hold infants as much as mothers do, but no equivalent research has been conducted to determine whether or how father behavior relates to the early organization of the infant's neurobiological networks. Studies of neurobiological and hormonal influences in infant-parent interactions show similarities and differences in mothers and fathers (Atzil, Henaler, Sagoory-Sharon, Weintroub, & Feldman, 2012; Feldman, Gordon, Schneiderman, Weisman, & Zaggory-Sharon, 2010; Swain et al., 2014), and it is reasonable to hypothesize that male and female infants respond differentially as well.

Much more needs to be learned about the extent to which fathers' own childhood experiences impact his parenting attitudes, beliefs, and attitudes. Curtis et al. (1997) found that fathers' prenatal perceptions of the marital relationship, and his postnatal perceptions of his partners' ability to put herself in his place were related to his problem behaviors. Snarey's (1993) study of the extent of father involvement in childhood and adolescence also examined aspects of fathers' own childhoods in relation to their involvement with their own children. Fathers reported on 10 characteristics of their own parenting: father's and mother's relationship quality, unsuitable supervisory styles, use of physical punishment, education level, and occupational levels. In addition, they reported on a variety of family characteristics: child age and sex, number of children, generativity chill (a measure of the extent to which there was ever a threat to children's death or illness), the wife's work outside the home and her education, the father's education, and the father's marital affinity (whether he ever considered divorce). Predictors of the fathers' total quantity of parental generativity from his past were their fathers' IQ and their mothers' education (5% of variance). Concurrent predictors of their parental generativity were in order: their own marital affinity, wife's employment, generativity chill, and wife's education, which combined accounted for an additional 22% of the variance related to parental generativity.

Table 2.5 summarizes which variable for the fathers' boyhood and current family were predictive of content domains at each age level. Note that concurrent factors explain more of the variance in predicting relationships than do boyhood factors.

Heuristic models conceptualizing causal pathways can capture explanatory events in the moment (Overton, 2013, 2015), but when applied to longitudinal designs with person-oriented analyses, they can also describe changes in life-course trajectories. Cabrera et al.'s (2014a) heuristic model begins with the father's biological, cultural, and rearing history as the set points for the study of his involvement in child rearing. They then entered various adjunctive influences that may mediate or moderate father's parenting behaviors over time, including all of the dynamics of his relationships with family members as well as influences from other exogenous adjunctive systems. In infancy, influences begin with the transition to fatherhood. Greenberg and Morris (1974) captured fathers' reactions at the birth of their firstborn child, labeling their sense of absorption, preoccupation, and interest in all facets of the newborn as engrossment. If the birth is not of a firstborn, the pressures on daily activities, family conflicts, and routines are not just additive, but involve adjustments for all relational dynamics within the family system (Volling et al., 2019; Volling & Elins, 1998). Using a person-centered approach, Volling et al. (2019) studied maternal and paternal depressive symptoms during the pregnancy of a second child and at 1, 4, 8, and 12 postnatal months. They identified four types of families distinguished by the level of parental depressive symptoms [high (H) and low (L)]: mother and father H, mother H and

Table 2.5 Predictors of Fathers Childrearing Support with Assessment Domains: Significant findings only. S (social-emotional), I-A (intellectual-achievement, P-A (physical-athletic)

	Father Involvement Childhood			Father Involvement Adolescence			Fathers Global
Fathers Boyhood & Home	S-E	I-A	P-A	S-E	I-A	P-A	
Father IQ	X		X	X			X
Father-son relation quality							
Unsuitable supervision style				X			
Use of physical punishment				X			
Father education	X						
Father occupation				X			
Mother unsuitable supervision	X					X	
Mother education		X	X		X	X	
Fathers Current Family							
Child age	X	X		X	X	X	X
Generativity chill			X	X		X	X
Wife's working			X			X	X
Wife's education				X	X	X	X
Father's education					X		
Father's marital affinity	X			X	X		X

Adapted from Snarey (1993)

father L, mother L and father H, and mother and father L. In families where mothers and fathers were high in depressive symptoms, there was high marital negativity, parenting stress, and low parental efficacy. Their children scored high on both externalizing and internalizing behavior problems. Family and child problems were higher when fathers had more depressive symptoms than mothers.

Zucker et al. (2003) also used a person-centered approach to track the effect of family adversity on child externalizing behavior over four waves of the Michigan Longitudinal Study (MLS), from ages 3 to 14. Families in the MLS were recruited to the study based on father characteristics (alcoholism and antisocial behavior), family presence of a 3–5 year old son, and two biological parents. All other family members were also recruited but their characteristics were not part of the selection process. Community comparison families were recruited with the same criteria, with the exception that fathers did not have a diagnosis of alcoholism (Zucker et al., 2000). Family adversity (FA) was defined as high or low on the basis of family psychopathology. Child (boys) psychopathology (CP) was classified based on ratings of externalizing and internalizing behavior (high or low). Assessment during the preschool period revealed four developmental pathways which were labeled nonchallenged (FA and CP low), troubled (FA low, CP high), resilient (FA high, CP low), and vulnerable (FA and CP high). Parents in the high FA group had high rating in marital negativity and parenting stress and low rating in parental efficacy. Their preschool age children (vulnerable group) scored highest in both externalizing and internalizing behavior, a pattern that continued across the 4 waves of the study, closely followed by children in the troubled group. Parents of the preschool boys who were reactive, hyperactive, and had short attention spans were more likely to be spanked and treated negatively and to score higher on externalizing behaviors (Wong, Zucker, Puttler, & Fitzgerald, 1999). Resilience and nonchallenged children scored lower in externalizing and internalizing behavior, and higher in measures of achievement skills. However, in early adolescence (12–14) resilient children scored higher in internalizing problems than nonchallenged children. Each of these longitudinal studies provides evidence that negative aspects of father behavior influence family and child functioning, whereas positive father behavior is associated with less family stress and child behavior problems.

A family changes when additional siblings come into the system, or when any change affects the initial composition of the family unit (e.g., death or divorce of a parent, presence of a grandparent or a partner, loss of family income). But individuals from conception onward are increasingly embedded in more complex systems. The infant's primary system includes the caregiving setting and the individual(s) involved in providing care. The primary system could consist of the home environment and include parents, siblings, grandparents, or other kin. Or, the primary system could consist of non-biological parents, a single parent, or an institution (orphanage, supplemental child care setting). All other systems affecting the primary system are adjunctive to the primary system. Adjunctive systems include the work environment, supplementary care settings, religious institutions, or neighborhood peer groups. Insofar as biological fathers are concerned, their connection to the family system ranges from core, to various degrees of connectivity ranging from membership in a nuclear family, to various forms of distal connectivity, or none at all (Fig. 2.3).

Thus to understand father effects on child development one must also understand the degree to which he is physically present in the family system, or, if not, the extent to which he has access to his children or to their mother (Schermerhorn & Cummings, 2008). This multifactorial approach suggests five major sources of analyses relevant to the structure and function of any family system. First, the subsystems or individual components of the system must be identified and described, e.g., accessing the presenting state characteristics of individual family members, including genetic differences that may ultimately trigger different behavioral propensities or sensitivities (Belsky, 1984). Second,

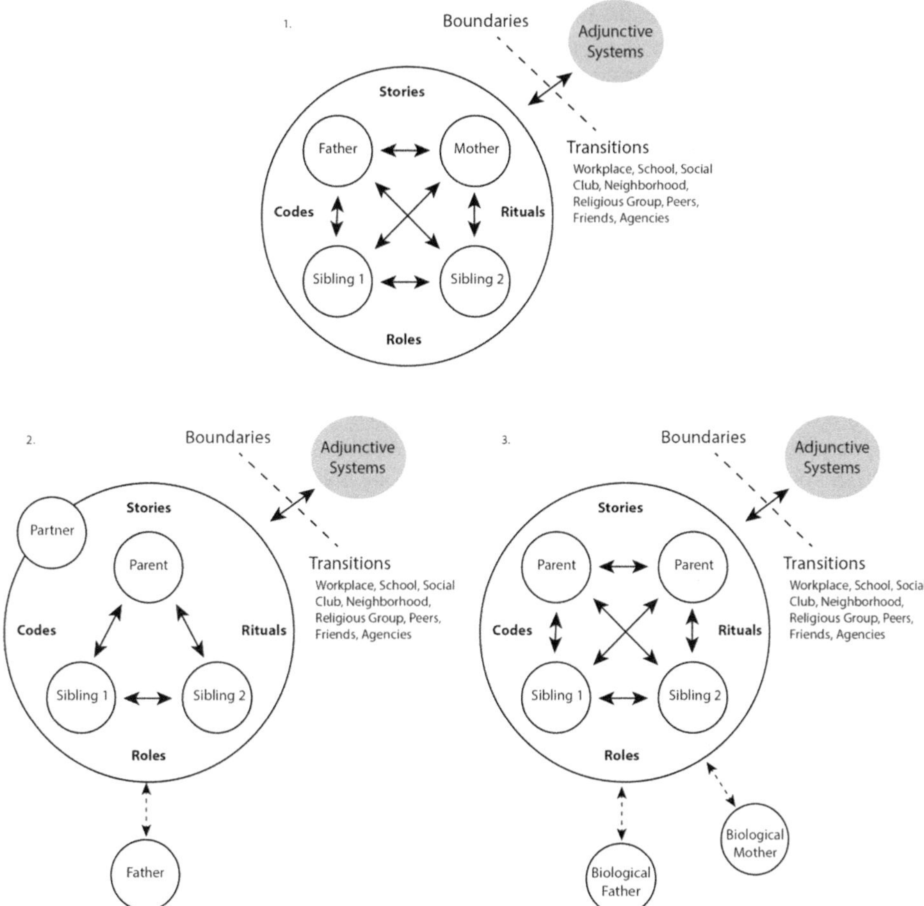

Fig. 2.3 Possible transactional linkages in a primary family system (1) consisting of or mother, father, and their children, (2) in which there is a single parent, with or without contact with an adult partner, and (3) or two same-sex parents with or without contact with children's biological father. Other configurations are possible depending upon the structure of the primary family system and the exogenous adjective systems that interact with the family system

the structural and functional connections of subunits must be identified and described (e.g., assessing spousal, parent-child, sibling, and kin relationships). Third, one must identify and describe the properties that emerge when this collection of components is joined together into a specific dynamic structure (e.g., assessing family traditions, values, beliefs, resources, and cohesiveness) (Sameroff, 2003). Fourth, one must identify adjunctive systems that may have direct effects on the family unit or that affect the family indirectly via individual members, that is, describing and assessing the impact of adjunctive systems or environtype (Sameroff, 2003) that affect individual and family functioning. This includes evaluating the well-being of the community and neighborhood, and the social-historical events that contribute to cultural values. Finally, one must describe, and eventually test, predictive models of change in the individual, the family, and the ecosystem over time (e.g., assessing models of system organization, as well as bifurcations that lead to system disorganization and reorganization) (Fitzgerald et al., 1995).

The Cabrera et al. model is informed by Bronfenbrenner's bioecological model, which views the individual as embedded within a family system (microsystem), which in turn is embedded in increasingly broader exogenous mesosystems (school, work, religious institutions, organizations), which in turn are nested in exosystems (to which the individual child is not directly connected), nested in macrosystems (cultural, political, economic and geographic), all of which are embedded in time, space, and place (chronosystems) (Bronfenbrenner, 1974; Bronfenbrenner & Morris, 2006). However, the model goes beyond nested sources of variance, positing a fully recursive dynamic relational approach, wherein parts and wholes are always dialectic, synergistic, and transactional (Overton, 2013, 2015; Sameroff, 1982, 1995; Whitherington, 2015). Note that even within the family microsystem and its myriad dyadic, triadic, and more complex transactions, children are exposed to the family histories that mother and father recount through what Sameroff (2003) refers to as family codes, rituals, stories, myths, and roles, which provide varying degrees of regulation that define the family system. Codes provide the glue that forms a family system or unit, relative to broader society. Rituals refer to family activities that assign roles and meaning to family practices, such as the way that families celebrate occasions (birthdays, anniversaries, successes) that provide children with a sense of regularity and connectivity. Stories are about inter-generativity: parents repeating stories about their parents and relatives, their lives prior to having children, and other family issues that give children a sense of continuity and family meaning. Myths are those beliefs within families that are not totally believed in, not fully contested, but form part of the intergenerational glue, whether they are true or not. All of these form aspects of what Sameroff (1995) asserts when he notes that an individual "cannot exist separated from its environment and an environment cannot exist separated from the perspectives of an organism [individual]" (p. 677). Studies of the influence of such family dynamics have not been sufficiently studied with respect to such issues as intergenerational transmission of either fathers or mothers' individual personal histories.

Fathers and Policy

Fein (1978) viewed parenting as an androgynous activity equally performed by men and women, with the exceptions of gestation and lactation. He recommended active research on fathering in several key areas, including (a) prenatal and perinatal experiences, (b) father-infant interactions, including the development of social-emotional relationships, (c) fathers in non-traditional care settings, and (d) the effects of parenting on fathers themselves. Equally important to his self-described "emergent perspective" was a focus on changes in social policy to enable implementation of greater father involvement in child rearing, including provision for parental leave for both mothers and fathers. His proposed inclusion of fathers is as relevant today as it was four decades ago. When Hellman, Levtov, van der Gaag, Hassick, and Barker (2017) published the *State of the World's Fathers*, 92 of the world's 195 countries recognized by the United Nations offered some form of paternal leave. A follow-up study focused specifically on changes in social and economic policies needed to enhance father involvement in childcare, including policies to change social and gender norms across all sectors of society, to increase the economic and physical security of families, to assist couples and parents abilities to thrive together, and to put individual father's care activities into action (Van de Gaag, Helman, Gupta, Normbhard & Barker, 2019). These will not be easy tasks. For example, studies continue to indicate that most men define their social roles and role identities as family providers. Conversely, other studies indicate that nearly 85% of fathers agree that they should participate in childcare, including with their infants and very young children.

Drawing upon developmental systems theory, Yoshikawa and Hsuch (2001) suggest approaches to policy change may be more effective if they were based on the actual realities of human development, rather than politically expedient non-science informed perspectives. Relational dynamic systems theory in all of its forms aligns with the importance of transitional periods in human development and the rich diversity in life course pathways. Constructing policy issues related to such diversity may lead to more efficient and effective support for families than broad-based infusion of resources that are not linked to the developmental needs of families at the moment. McKinney, Fitzgerald, Winn, and Babcock (2017) note that "Just as children, families, schools, neighborhoods, and communities change over time, so too, must policies change to assure the provision of services that were intended when the policies were first established." This would include policies aligned with the risk to resilience concept, so that fathers were able to secure work and reconnect with their families following incarceration, military service, or severe economic downturns. Or, qualify for paternal leave following the birth of their baby in order to develop a relationship with the baby, and to provide relief and support for the mother. Research with fathers and families guided by Bronfenbrenner's model positing the interaction of multiple levels of adjunctive influences on the family is well suited for assessing the impact of macrosystem laws and policies on family functioning as well as monitoring changes in such policies to assess whether they achieve their intended outcomes. As Huston (2005) notes, "Any research may generate information that informs policy." However, "Researchers and practitioners are trained in their respective fields, usually not social policy" (McKinney et al. p. 173) and are not especially skilled at translating their research findings to practice or to policy. Clearly, stronger transdisciplinary bridges must link behavioral and life science research with policy makers in order to translate research into effective practice guided by the sciences of diffusion and dissemination, and on-going program evaluation. Evidence points to the importance of father involvement in the lives of children, in their own personal growth, and in enhanced quality of relationships with their parent partners. Tracking these changes over time and determining, "What works, under when circumstances, and how?" (Office of Planning Research and Evaluation, 2016, p. 1) should inform social policies and assure efficient and effective resources are allocated to strengthen successful programs to enhance fathers' involvement in the lives of their children.

Summary and Key Points

Sixty years of intensive scientific study of infancy and early childhood across broad developmental disciplines have produced, arguably, more information about the earliest period of human development than any other period. The origins of human development at the individual level begin at conception, as the conceptus starts on its unique life course pathway organizing, developing, and adapting to experience. The interplay of genetic, epigenetic processes, and lived experience positions each individual along the risk to resilience continuum throughout the life course. During the conception to age five years of human development all of the individual's component neurobiological, hormonal, behavioral, and mental subsystems organize and integrate to prepare the individual for adapting to increasingly complex systemic influences over the life course. Most parents play a key role during the earliest years providing nearly all of the ingredients needed for infants to transition through the earliest years secure, nourished, safe, supported, and positioned on the resilience side of the risk to resilience continuum. Other parents do not or cannot provide such support and infants proceed through development adapting to or negotiating a variety of risks.

The vast amount of behavioral and social science studies of early development have focused on maternal contributions to infant development, guided by attachment theory and its focus on the provision of security and emotional development. In the 1960s and 70s, researchers began to turn attention to the role that fathers play in child development, focusing first on their competence to perform routine caregiving tasks. Gradually, broader questions within the context of a disciplinary shift from the emphasis on cause-effect and dyadic relationships to one emphasizing the dynamic reciprocal relationships among family members were asked. At the beginning of the current century, the Zeitgeist was set and theories and models specific to fathers and child development began to emerge and guide broad inquiry regarding what fathers do, and how they influence child development. In addition, by embracing systems approaches to research, father researchers focused on relational dynamics in an effort to identify direct, indirect or no effect of father contributions to children's development. Their efforts provide ample qualitative and quantitative evidence that fathers contribute independently as well as indirectly to the quality of children's development during infancy and early childhood. As cultural mores change and family structures and functions continue to diversity, researchers are now well-positioned to advance substantive inquiry concerning the role that men play in the early development of children.

Fathers are part of a family system that traditionally has been studied within the context of nuclear families, or families where the father is physically absent. The increase in single parent father families, gay families, and adoptive families and families where the father may be psychologically present, though physically absent has received a commensurate increase in research interest with respect to fathers and child development.

Fathers influence children's cognitive development and behavioral regulation in ways that are not yet clearly understood, although evidence suggests that encouragement of rough and tumble play and risk taking is related to decreases in son's aggression and externalizing behaviors. Evidence suggests that fathers play a key role in sex role differentiation, emphasizing social and emotional support and protection of their daughters and encouraging risk taking and autonomy in their sons.

Role expectations for fathers as parents vary greatly across cultures and within multi-cultural societies. Moreover, across cultures and societies, overarching descriptors of father's roles within families do not reflect the diverse activities they engage in, nor the transitions in activities over the life span.

Fathers' involvement in parenting is influenced by their perceptions of the quality of the marital relationship; the poorer the perceived (or actual) quality, the less they are involved in childcare, or engage in more harsh parenting. Little is known about the impact of the quality of partner relationship among gay parents with respect to caregiving behaviors.

Cultural context influences father involvement in caregiving particularly during infancy and very early childhood. In most cultures, mothers are perceived to be the lead parent with respect to very early childcare, although fathers express interest in being more involved in childcare and often do share in care for their infants and young children.

Social policies, developed primarily to support mother-led families and dual-parent heterosexual families, create barriers for alternative family structures and for fathers who are nonresidential. Parental leave policies specific to fathers promote active involvement in caregiving and shared parenting with mothers and/or partners. Policies related to providing more support for fathers as parents, including their involvement in parent improvement programs or caregiving skills development, are underfunded and/or under-utilized.

References

Amato, P. R., & Sobolewski, J. M. (2004). The effects of divorce on fathers and children: Nonresidential fathers and stepfathers. In M. E. Lamb (Ed.), *The role of the father in child development* (pp. 341–367). Hoboken, NJ: Wiley.

Atran, S., Medin, D. L., & Ross, N. O. (2005). The cultural mind: Environmental decision making and cultural modeling within and across populations. *Psychological Review, 112*, 744–776.

Atzil, S., Henaler, T., Sagoory-Sharon, O., Weintroub, Y., & Feldman, R. (2012). Synchrony and specificity in the maternal and paternal brain: Relation to oxytocin and vasopresson. *Journal of the American Association for Child and Adolescent Psychiatry, 51*, 789–811.

Barlas, Y., & Carpenter, S. (1990). Philosophical roots of model validation: Two paradigms. *Systems Dynamics Review, 6*, 148–166.

Barrows, P. (2004). Fathers and families: Locating the ghost in the nursery. *Infant Mental Health Journal, 25*, 408–428.

Barry, H. A., & Paxton, C. M. (1971). Infancy and early childhood: Cross-cultural codes. *Ethnology, 10*, 466–509.

Belsky, J. (1984). The determinants of parenting: A process model. *Child Development, 55*, 83–96.

Biller, H. B. (1971). *Father, child and sex role*. Lexington, MA: D. C. Heath.

Bockneck, E. L., Brophy-Herb, J. E., Fitzgerald, H. E., Schiffman, R. F., & Vogel, C. (2014). Stability of biological father presence as a proxy for family stability: Cross-racial associations with the longitudinal development of emotion regulation in toddlerhood. *Infant Mental Health Journal, 35*, 309–321.

Bocknek, E. L., Dayton, C., Brophy-Herb, H. E., Raveau, H., & Fitzgerald, H. E. (2017). Routine active playtime with fathers is associated with toddlers' emotion regulation competencies. *Merrill-Palmer Quarterly, 63*(1), 105–134.

Bornstein, M. H. (Ed.). (2010). *Handbook of cultural developmental science*. New York: Taylor & Francis.

Bos, H. M., Knox, J., vanRijn-van Gelderen, L., & Gartrell, N. K. (2016). Same-sex and different-sex parent households and child health outcomes: Findings from the National Survey of Children's Health. *Journal of Developmental and Behavioral Pediatrics, 37*, 179–187.

Boyce, P., Condon, J., Barton, J., & Corklindale, C. (2007). First time fathers' study: Psychological distress in expectant fathers during pregnancy. *Australia and New Zealand Journal of Psychiatry, 41*, 718–715.

Bretherton, I., Lambert, J. D., & Golby, B. (2006). Modeling and reworking childhood experiences : Involved father representations of being parented and parenting of a preschool child. In O. Mayseless (Ed.), *Parenting representation: Theory, research, and clinical implications* (pp. 177–207). New York: Cambridge University Press.

Bronfenbrenner, U. (1974). Developmental research, public policy, and the ecology of childhood. *Child Development, 45*, 1–5.

Bronfenbrenner, U., & Morris, P. A. (2006). The bioecological model of human development. In P. Mussen (Ed.), *Handbook of child psychology*. Hoboken, NJ: Wiley.

Brott, A. A. (1999). *The single father: A dad's guide to parenting without a partner*. New York: Abbeville Press.

Brown, G. L., Mangelsdorf, S. C., Shigeto, A., & Wong, M. S. (2018). Associations between father involvement and father-child attachment security: Variations based on timing and type of involvement. *Journal of Family Psychology, 32*, 1015–1024.

Cabrera, N., Fitzgerald, H. E., & Shannon, J. (Eds.) (2007). Special Issue. Fatherhood: Understanding the impact of fathers on child development. *Applied Developmental Science, 11*(4), 185–272.

Cabrera, N., Fitzgerald, H. E., Bradley, R. H., & Roggman, L. (2007). Modeling the dynamics of paternal influences on children over the life course. *Applied Developmental Science, 11*(4), 185–190.

Cabrera, N., Fitzgerald, H. E., Bradley, R. H., & Roggman, L. (2014a). The ecology of father-child relationships: An expanded model. *Journal of Family Theory and Review, 6*, 336–354.

Cabrera, N., Fitzgerald, H. E., Bradley, R. H., & Roggman, L. (2014b). The ecology of father- child relationships: An expanded model. *Journal of Family Theory and Review, 6*, 336–354.

Cabrera, N. J., & Tamis-LeMonda, C. S. (Eds.). (2013). *Handbook of father involvement: Multidisciplinary perspectives* (2nd ed.). New York: Rutledge.

Cabrera, N. J., Tamis-LeMonda, C. S., Bradley, R. H., Hofferth, S., & Lamb, M. E. (2000). Fatherhood in the twenty-first century. *Child Development, 71*, 127–136.

Cabrera, N., & Volling, B.L. (2019). Moving research on fathering and children's development forward: Priorities and recommendations for the future. *Monographs of the Society for Research in Child Development, 84*(1), 107–117.

Cannon, E., Schoppe-Sullivan, S. J., Mangelsdorf, S. C., Brown, G. I., & Sokolowski, M. S. (2008). Parent characteristics as antecedents of maternal gatekeeping and fathering behavior. *Family Process, 47*, 501–519.

Cicchetti, D., & Rogosch, F. A. (1996). Equifinality and multifinality in developmental psychopathology. *Development and Psychopathology, 8*(4), 597–600. https://doi.org/10.1017/S0954579400007318

Clarke-Stewart, K. A. (1978). And daddy makes three: The father's impact on mother and young child. *Child Development, 49*, 466–478.

Cook, G. A., Roggman, L. K., & Boyce, L. E. (2011). Fathers' and mothers' cognitive stimulation in early play with toddlers. Predictors of 5th grade reading and math. *Family Science, 3*, 131–145.

Cohen, L. B., & Campos, J. J. (1974). Father, mother, and stranger as elicitors of attachment behaviors in infancy. *Developmental Psychology, 10*, 146–154.

Colonnesi, C., Zeegers, M. A. J., Majdandzic, M., van Steensel, F., & Bogels, S. M. (2019). Fathers' and mothers' early mind-mindedness pedicts social competence and behavior problems in childhood. *Journal of Abnormal Child Psychology, 47*, 1421–1435.

Connor, G. K., & Denson, V. (1990). Expectant fathers' response to pregnancy: Review of literature and implications for research in high-risk pregnancy. *Journal of Perinatal and Neonatal Nursing, 4*, 33–42.

Crowl, A., Ahn, S., & Baker, J. (2007). A meta-analysis of developmental outcomes for children of same-sex and heterosexual parents. *Journal of GLBT Family Studies, 4*, 385–407.

Cummings, E. M., Goeke-Morey, M. C., & Raymond, J. (2004). Fathers in family context: Effects of marital quality and marital conflict. In M. E. Lamb (Ed.), *The role of the father in child development* (pp. 196–221). Hoboken, NJ: Wiley.

Curtis, J. A., Blume, L. B., & Blume, T. W. (1997). Becoming father: Marital perceptions and behavior of fathers during pregnancy. *Michigan Family Review, 3*, 31–44.

Davidson, D. (1996). The role of schemata in children's memory. In H. Reese (Ed.). *Advances in Child Development and Behavior, 26* (pp 35–58). New York: Academic Press.

Dayton, C. J., Buczkowski, R., Muzik, N., Goletz, J., Hicks, L., Walsh, T. B. et al. (2016). Expectant fathers' beliefs and expectations about fathering as they prepare to parent a new infant. *Social Work Research, 40*, 225–236

deChateau, P. (1991). Clinical applications of asymmetrical behavioral communication in parent-infant interaction. In H. E. Fitzgerald, B. M. Lester, & M. W. Yogman (Eds.). *Theory and research in behavioral pediatrics, Vol 5* (pp 185–208). New York: Plenum Press.

de Mendonça, J. S., Bussab, V. S., & Kärtner, J. (2019). Interactional synchrony and child gender differences in dyadic and triadic family interactions. *Journal of Family Issues, 40*, 959–981.

de Mendonça, J. S., Vera, S. R., Bussab, V. S. R., Rodriguez, A., & Cossette, L. (2013). Postpartum depression, father involvement, marital and co-parental relationship from mothers' and fathers' perspectives in a low-income Brazilian sample. *Family Science, 2*, 164–173.

Diamond, M. J. (2007). *My father before me: How fathers and sons influence each other throughout their lives*. New York: W. W. Norton.

Fein, R. A. (1978). Research on fathering: Social policies on and an emergent perspective. *The Journal of Social Issues, 34*, 122–135.

Feinberg, M. E., Jones, D. E., McDaniel, B. T., Liu, W., & Almeida, D. (2011). New fathers and mothers daily stressors and resources influence parent adjustment and family relationships. In B. L. Volling & N. J. Cabrera (Eds.), Advancing research and measurement on fathering and children's development. *Monographs of the society for research in child development*, 84(1), 18–34.

Feldman, R., Gordon, L., Schneiderman, I., Weisman, O., & Zaggory-Sharon, O. (2010). Natural variation in maternal and paternal care as associated with systematic changes in oxytocin folloing parent-infant contact. *Psychoneuroendocrinology, 35*, 1133–1141.

Felitti, V. J., Anda, R. F., Nordenberg, D., Williamson, D. F., Spitz, A. M., Edwards, V., et al. (1998). Relationship of childhood abuse and household dysfunction to many of the leading causes of death in adults: The Adverse Childhood Experiences (ACE) Study. *American Journal of Preventive Medicine, 14*(4), 245–258.

Fitzgerald, H. E. (2010). A community driven framework for systems change. *The Engaged Scholar, 5*, 20–21.

Fitzgerald, H. E. (2014). Wrapping up and moving on. *Infant Mental Health Journal, 35*, 527–528.

Fitzgerald, H. E. (2017). *Early origins of violence in males*. Chicago: Santa Fe Educational Boys Foundation.

Fitzgerald, H. E., & Bradley, R, (Eds.). (2012). Special Issue. Paternal family relationships, child risk, and child outcomes. *Family Science, 3*, 141–265.

Fitzgerald, H. E., & Bockneck, E. L. (2013). Fathers, children, and the risk-resilience continuum. In N. J. Cabrera & C. S. Tamis-LaMonda (Eds.), *Handbook of father involvement: Multidisciplinary perspectives* (2nd ed., pp. 168–185). New York: Routledge.

Fitzgerald, H. E., Davies, W. H., Zucker, R. A., & Klinger, M. (1994). Developmental systems theory and substance abuse. In L. L. L'Abate (Ed.), *Handbook of developmental family psychology and psychopathology* (pp. 350–372). New York: Wiley.

Fitzgerald, H. E., & Eiden, R. D. (2007). Paternal alcoholism, family functioning, and infant mental health. *Journal of ZERO TO THREE, 27*, 11–18.

Fitzgerald, H. E., Harris, L. J., Barnes, C. L., Wang, X., Cornwell, K. D., Kamptner, N. L., Dagenbach, D., & Carlson, D. (1991). The organization of lateralized behavior during infancy. In H. E. Fitzgerald, B. M. Lester, & M. W., Yogman (Eds). *Theory and research in behavioral pediatrics, Vol. 5* (pp 155–184). New York: Plenum Press.

Fitzgerald, H. E., Johnson, D. J., Qin, D. B., Villarruel, F. A., & Norder, J. (2019). Introduction: A developmental systems perspective on children and prejudice. In H. E. Fitzgerald et al. (Eds.), *Handbook of children and prejudice: Integrating research, practice, and policy* (pp. 3–22). Cham, Switzerland: Springer Nature.

Fitzgerald, H. E., Mann, T., & Barrett, M. (1999). Fathers and infants. *Infant Mental Health Journal, 20*, 213–345.

Fitzgerald, H. E., Mann, T., Cabrera, N., Sarche, M., & Qin, D. (2010). Tidlig barndom og identitet I multikulturelle miljoer (Infancy and identity in multicultural context). In V. Moe, K. Slinning, & M. B. Hansen (Eds.), *Handbook of infant and toddler psychology* (pp. 269–282). Oslo, Norway: Gyldendal Akademisk.

Fitzgerald, H. E., McKelvey, L. M., Schiffman, R. F., & Montanez, M. (2006). Exposure to neighborhood violence and paternal antisocial behavior on low-income families and their children. *Parenting: Research and Practice, 6*, 243–258.

Fitzgerald, H. E., Strommen, E. A., & McKinney, J. P. (1982). *Developmental psychology: The infant and young child*. Homewood, IL: The Dorsey Press.

Fitzgerald, H. E., Wong, M. M., & Zucker, R. A. (2013). Early origins of alcohol use and abuse: Mental representations, relationships, and the risk-resilience continuum. In N. Suchman, M. Pajulo, & L. C. Mayes (Eds.), *Parenting and substance addiction: Developmental approaches to intervention* (pp. 126–155). New York: Oxford University Press.

Fitzgerald, H. E., Zucker, R. A., & Yang, H.-Y. (1995). Developmental systems theory and alcoholism: Analyzing patterns of variation in high-risk families. *Psychology of Addictive Behaviors, 9*, 8–22.

Fletcher, R., StGeorge, J., & Freeman, E. (2013). Rough and tumble play quality: Theoretical foundations for a new measure of father-child interaction. *Early Child Development and Care, 178*, 746–759.

Ford, D. H., & Lerner, R. M. (1992). *Developmental systems theory: An integrative approach*. New York: Sage Publications.

Fraiberg, S., Adelson, E., & Shapiro, V. (1975). Ghosts in the nursery: A psychoanalytic approach to the problems of impaired infant-mother relationships. *Journal of the American Academy of Child Psychiatry, 14*, 387–421.

Geary, D. C. (2005). Evolution of paternal investment. In D. M. Buss (Ed.), *The evolutionary psychology handbook* (pp. 483–505). Hoboken, NJ: Wiley.

Glueck, S., & Glueck, E. (1968). *Delinquents and nondelinquents in perspective*. Cambridge, MA: Harvard University Press.

Golding, P., & Fitzgerald, H. E. (2019). The biopsychosocial development of prenatal, infant, and toddler boys and the origins of violence in males. *Infant Mental Health Journal, 22*(3), 393–415.

Gottlieb, G. (1991). The experiential canalization of behavioral developmental theory. *Developmental Psychology, 27*, 4–13.

Greenberg, M., & Morris, N. (1974). Engrossment: The newborn's impact upon the father. *American Journal of Orthopsychiatry, 44*, 520–531.

Guterman, N. B., & Lee, Y. (2005). The role of fathers in risk for physical abuse and neglect: Possible pathways and unanswered questions. *Child Maltreatment, 10*, 136–149.

Hagstad, G. O., & Speicher, J. L. (1981). *Grandparents and family influence. Views of three generations*. Paper presented at the meeting of the Society for Research on Child Development, Boston, MA.

Hays-Grudo, J., & Morris, A. S. (2020). *Adverse and protective childhood experiences: A developmental perspective*. Washington, D. C.: American Psychological Association.

Hellman, B., Levtov, R., van der Gaag, N., Hassick, A., & Barker, G. (2017). *State of the world's fathers: Time for action*. Washington, DC: Promundo.

Hops, H., Biglan, A., Sherman, L., Arthus, J., Friedman, L., & Osteen, V. (1987). Home observations of family interactions of depressed women. *Journal of Consulting and Clinical Psychology, 55*, 341–346.

Huck, M., & Fernandez-Duque, E. (2013). When dads help: Male behavioral care during primate infant development. In K. B. H. Clancy et al (Eds.), *Building babies: Primate development in proximate and ultimate perspective. Developments in primatology: Progress and prospects*, 37, 361–385.

Huston, A. C. (2005). Connecting the science of child development to public policy. *Society for Research in Child Development Social Policy Report, 19*(5), 1–20.

Kaplan, A., & Garner, J. K. (2017). A complex dynamic systems perspective on identity and its development: The dynamic systems model of role identity. *Developmental Psychology, 2017*, 53,2036–53,2051.

Kotelchuck, M. (1976). The infant's relationship to the father: Experimental evidence. In M. E. Lamb (Ed.), *The role of the father in child development* (p. 1976). New York: Wiley.

Kraemer, S. (1991). The origins of fatherhood: An ancient family process. *Family Processes, 30*, 377–392.

Kuczynski, L., & Parkin, C. M. (2007). Agency and bidirectionality in socialization: Interactions, transactions and relational dialectics. In J. E. Grusee & P. Hastings (Eds.), *Handbook of socialization: Theory and research* (pp. 259–283). New York: Guilford.

LaGuardia, J. G., & Patrick, H. (2008). Self-determination theory as a fundamental theory of close relationships. *Canadian Psychology, 49*, 201–209.

Lamb, M. E. (1975). Fathers: Forgotten contributors to child development. *Human Development, 18*, 245–266.

Lamb, M. E. (Ed.). (1976). *The role of the father in child development*. New York: Wiley.

Lamb, M. E. (Ed.). (1987). *The father's role: Cross-cultural perspectives*. New York: Routledge.

Lamb, M. E., & Lamb, J. E. (1976). The nature and importance of the father-infant relationship. *The Family Coordinator, 25*, 379–386.

Lamb, M. E., Pleck, J. H., Charnov, E. L., & Levine, J. A. (1987). A biosocial perspective on paternal behavior and involvement. In J. B. Lancaster, J. Altmann, A. S. Rossi, & L. R. Sherrod (Eds.), *Arent across the lifespan: Biosocial dimensions* (pp. 111–142). New York: Aldine de Gruyter.

LaRossa, P. (1997). *The modernization of fatherhood: A social and political history*. Chicago: The University of Chicago Press.

Laszlo, E. (1972). *Introduction to systems philosophy: Toward a new paradigm of contemporary thought*. New York: Harper & Row.

Laszlo, E. (1996). *The systems view of the world: A holistic vision for our time*. Cresskill, NJ: Hampton Press.

Lebovici, S. (1988). Fantasmatic interactions and intergenerational trauma. *Infant Mental Health Journal, 9*, 10–19.

Lee, S. L., Bellamy, J. L., & Guteman, N. B. (2019). Fathers physical child abuse and neglect: Advancing the knowledge base. *Child Maltreatment, 14*, 227–231.

Levine, R. L., & Fitzgerald, H. E. (Eds.). (1992). *Analysis of dynamic psychological systems: Vol. 1: Basic approaches to general systems, dynamic systems and cybernetics*. New York: Plenum.

Lewis, C. (2012). Commentary: What are the links between fathering, family relationships, risk and child outcomes? Methodological and theoretical issues. *Family Science, 3-4*, 229–232.

Livingston, G. (2013). *The rise of single fathers: A ninefold increase since 1960*. Pew Research Center. www.pewresearch.org.

Loeber, M. F., & Egeland, B. (2009). Infancy parenting and externalizing psychopathology from childhood through adulthood: Developmental trends. *Developmental Psychology, 45*, 909–912.

Loukas, A., Fitzgerald, H. E., Zucker, R. A., & Von Eye, A. (2001). Parental alcoholism and co-occurring antisocial behavior: Prospective relationships to externalizing behavior problems in their young sons. *Journal of Abnormal Child Psychology, 29*(2), 91–106.

Loukas, A., Twitchell, G. R., Piejak, L. A., Fitzgerald, H. E., & Zucker, R. A. (1998). The family as a unity of interacting personalities. In L. L'Abate (Ed.), *Handbook of family psychopathology* (pp. 35–59). New York: Guilford Publications.

Lytton, H., & Romney, D. (1991). Parents' differential socialization of boys and girls: A meta-analysis. *Psychological Bulletin, 109*, 267–296.

MacKey, W. C. (1996). *The American father: Biocultural and developmental aspects*. New York: Plenum Press.

Masten, A. S. (2014). Global perspectives on resilience in children and youth. *Child Development, 85*, 6–20.

McGillicuddy-DeLisi, A. V., & Subramanian, S. (1996). How do children develop knowledge? Beliefs of Tanzanian and American mothers. In S. Harkness & C. M. Super (Eds.), *Culture and human development* (pp. 143–168). New York: Guilford.

McGreal, C. E. (1981). The father's role in the socialization of his infant. *Infant Mental Health Journal, 2*, 216–225.

McGreal, C. E. (1994). The family across generations. In L. L'Abate (Ed.), *Handbook of developmental family psychology and psychopathology* (pp. 116–131). New York: Wiley.

McKinney, M., Fitzgerald, H. E., Winn, D.-M., & Babcock, P. (2017). Public policy, child development research and boys at risk: Challenging, enduring, and necessary partnership. *Infant Mental Health Journal, 38*, 166–176.

Miller, J. G. (1976). *Living systems*. New York: McGraw Hill.

Nash, J. (1965). The father in contemporary culture and current psychological literature. *Child Development, 36*, 261–297.

Office of Planning, Research & Evaluation, United States Department of Health and Human Services, Administration for Child and Families. (2016). *What works, under what circumstances, and how? Methods for unpacking the "black box" of programs and policies*. Office of Planning, Research and Evaluation, Report No. 2016-54. Washington, DC: Author.

Overton, W. F. (2013). A new paradigm for developmental science: Relationism and relational-developmental systems. *Applied Developmental Science, 2013*(17), 94–107.

Overton, W. F. (2015). Processes, relations, and relational-developmental-systems. In W. F. Overton & P. C. M. Molenaar (Eds.), *Handbook of child psychology and developmental science Vol. 1: Theory and method* (pp. 9–62). New York: Wiley.

Palkovitz, R. (1980). *Predictors of involvement in first time fathers*. Dissertation Abstracts International. University Microfilms order no. 705-801.

Palkovitz, R. (2002a). Involved fathering and child development: Advancing our understanding of good fathering. In C. S. Tamis-LeMonda & N. Cabrera (Eds.), *Handbook of father involvement* (pp. 33–64). Mahwah, NJ: Lawrence Earlbaum.

Palkovitz, R. (2002b). *Involved fathers and men's adult development: Provisional balances*. Mahwah, NJ: Lawrence Erlbaum.

Paquette, D. (2004). Theorizing the father-child : Mechanisms and developmental outcomes. *Human Development, 39*, 70–82.

Paquette, D., & Bigras, M. (2010). The risky situation: A procedure for assessing the father-child activation relationship. *Early Child Development and Care, 18*(2), 171–189.

Paquette, D., & Dumont, C. (2013). The father-child activation relationship, sex differences, and attachment disorganization in toddlerhood. *Child Development Research, 2013*, 102860.

Parke, R. D. (1979). Perspectives on father-infant interaction. In J. D. Osofsky (Ed.). *Handbook of infant development*. New York: John Wiley & Sons.

Parke, R. D. (2013). *Future families: Diverse forms, rich possibilities*. New York: Wiley Blackwell.

Parke, R. D., & Sawin, D. B. (1976). The fathers' role in infancy: A re-evaluation. *The Family Coordinator, 25*, 365–371.

Pederson, F. A. (Ed.). (2002). *The father-infant relationship: Observational studies in the family setting*. New York: Praeger Press.

Pederson, F. A., & Robson, K. S. (1969). Father participation in infancy. *American Journal of Orthopsychiatry, 39*, 466–472.

Pleck, J. H. (1981). *The myth of masculinity*. Cambridge, MA: MIT Press.

Pleck, J. H. (2007). Why could father involvement benefit children? Theoretical perspectives. *Applied Developmental Science, 11*, 196–202.

Price-Bonham, S. (1976). Bibliography of literature related to the role of fathers. *The Family Coordinator, 35*, 489512.

Price-Bonham, S., Pittman, J. F., & Welch, C. O. (1981). The father role: An update. *Infant Mental Health Journal, 2*, 264–289.

Richters, J., & Weintraub, S. (1990). Beyond diathesis: Toward an understanding of high-risk environments. In J. Rolf, A. S. Masten, D. Cicchetti, K. H. Nuechterlein, & S. Weintraub (Eds.), *Risk and protective factors in the development of psychopathology* (pp. 67–96). Cambridge, MA: Cambridge University Press.

Riegel, K. F. (1976). The dialectics of human development. *American Psychologist, 31*, 689–700.

Roggman, L., Fitzgerald, H. E., Bradley, R., & Raikes, H. (2002). Overview of methodological, measurement, and design issues in studying fathers: An interdisciplinary perspective. In C. Tamis-LeMonda & N. Cabrara (Eds.), *Handbook of father involvement: Multidisciplinary perspectives* (pp. 1–30). Mahwah, NJ: Lawrence Erlbaum.

Roggman, L. A., Bradley, R. H., & Raikes, H. H. (2013). Fathers in family contexts. In N. J. Cabrera & C. S. Tamis-LeMonda (Eds.), *Handbook of father involvement: Multidisciplary perspectives* (2nd ed., pp. 186–201). New York: NY: Routledge.

Rutter, M. (1979). Protective factors in children's responses to stress and disadvantage. In M. W. Kent &

J. E. Rolf (Eds.), *Primary prevention of psychopathology: Vol. 3. Social competence in children* (pp. 49–74). Hanover, NH: University Press of New England.

Rutter, M. (1990). Psychosocial resilience and protective mechanisms. In J. E. Rolf, A. L. Masten, D. Cicchtti, K. H. Nuechterlein, & S. Weintraum (Eds.), *Risk and protective factors in the development of psychopathology*. Cambridge, MA: Cambridge University Press.

Ryan, R. M., & Deci, E. L. (2000). Self-determination theory and the facilitation of intrinsic motivation, social development, and well-being. *American Psychologist, 55*, 68–78.

Sameroff, A. J. (1982). Development and the dialectic: The need for a systems approach. In W. A. Collins (Ed.), *Minnesota symposium on child psychology* (Vol. 15). Hillsdale, NJ: Lawrence Erlbaum Associates.

Sameroff, A. J. (1983). Developmental systems: Contexts and evolution. In W. Kessen (Ed.), *Handbook of child psychology: (4th Ed). Vol. 1. History, theory, and methods* (pp. 237–294). New York: Wiley.

Sameroff, A. J. (1995). General systems theories and developmental psychopathology. In D. Cicchetti & D. J. Cohen (Eds.), *Developmental psychopathology. Vol. 1. Theory and methods* (pp. 659–695). New York: Wiley.

Sameroff, A. J. (2003). Developmental systems: Contexts and evolution. In W. Kessen & P. H. Mussen (Eds.), *Handbook of child psychology. Vol. 1. History theories and methods* (pp. 237–294). New York: Wiley.

Sameroff, A. J., Seifer, R., Zax, M., & Barocas, H. (1987). Early indicators of developmental risk: The Rochester Longitudinal Study. *Schizophrenia Bulletin, 13*, 383–394.

Saracho, O. N., & Spokek, K. B. (2008). Fathers: The invisible parents. *Early Child Development and Care, 178*, 821–836.

Schermerhorn, A. C., & Cummings, E. M. (2008). Transactional family dynamics: A new framework for conceptualizing family influence processes. In R. V. Kail (Ed.), *Advances in child development and behavior* (pp. 187–250). Amsterdam: Elsevier.

Schneirla, T. C. (1957). The concept of development in comparative psychology. In D. B. Harris (Ed.), *The concept of development* (pp. 78–108). Minneapolis, MN: University of Minnesota Press.

Sharabany, R., Seher, A., & Gal-Kraaz, J. (2006). Life father, like son? Fathers attitudes to childrearing in light of their perceived relationships with own parents, and their attachment concerns. In O. Mayseless (Ed.), *Parenting representations: Theory, research, and clinical implications* (pp. 239–261). New York: Cambridge University Press.

Shears, J. K., Robinson, J., & Emde, R. N. (2002). Fathering relationships and their associations with juvenile delinquency. *Infant Mental Health Journal, 23*, 79–87.

Shwalb, D. W., Shwalb, B. J., & Lamb, M. E. (2013). *Fathers in cultural context*. New York: Routledge.

Snarey, J. (1993). *How fathers care for the next generation: A four-decade study*. Cambridge, MA: Harvard University Press.

Snowdon, C. T., & Suomi, S. J. (1982). Paternal behavior in primates. In H. E. Fitzgerald, J. A. Mullins, & P. Gage (Eds.), *Child nurturance: Vol. 3: Studies of development in nonhuman primates* (pp. 63–108). New York: Plenum Press.

Swain, J. E., Kim, R., Spicer, J., Ho, S. S., Dayton, C. J., Elmadih, A., et al. (2014). Approaching the biology of human parental attachment: Brain imaging, oxytocin, and coordinated assessments of mothers and fathers. *Brain Research, 1580*, 78–101.

Tamis-LaMonda, C. S., & Cabrera, N. (Eds.). (2002). *Handbook of father involvement: Multidisciplinary perspectives*. Mahwah, NJ: Lawrence Erlbaum.

Trethowan, W. H., & Conlon, M. R. (1965). The Couvade Syndrome. *British Journal of Psychiatry, 3*, 57–66.

Trevathan, W. R. (1987). *Human birth: An evolutionary perspective*. Hawthorne, NY: Aldine de Gruyter.

Valaiquette-Trssier, S.-L., Vosselin, J., Young, M., & Thomassin, K. (2019). A literature review of cultural stereotypes associated with motherhood and fatherhood. *Marriage & Family Review, 55*, 299–329.

Van der Gaag, N., Heilman, B., Gupta, T., Nembhard, C., & Barker, G. (2019). *State of the world's fathers: Unlocking the power of men's care*. Washington, DC: Promundo-US.

Volling, B. L., & Cabrera, N. J. (Eds.). (2019). Advancing research and measurement on fathering and children's development. *Monographs of the society for research in chill development*, Serial No 332. 84, No. 1.

Volling, B. L., & Elins, J. L. (1998). Family relationships and children's emotional adjustment as correlates of maternal and paternal differential treatment: A replication with toddler and preschool Siblings. *Child Development, 69*, 1640–1656.

Volling, B. L., Yu, T., Gonzalez, R., Tengelitsch, E., & Stevenson, M. M. (2019). Maternal and paternal trajectories of depressive symptoms predict family risk and children's emotional and behavioral problems after the birth of a sibling. *Development and Psychopathology, 31*, 1307–1324.

von Bertalanffly, L. (1968). *General systems theory*. New York: George Braziller.

Von Klitzing, K. (2011). Commentary on the special issue. *Family Science, 2*, 156–158.

Werner, H. (1957). The concept of development from a comparative and organismic point of view. In D. B. Harris (Ed.), *The concept of development* (pp. 125–148). Minneapolis, MN: University of Minnesota Press.

Werner, E. E. (1988). A cross-cultural perspective on infancy: Research and social issues. *Journal of Cross-Cultural Psychology, 19*, 96–113.

Whitherington, D. C. (2015). Dynamic systems in developmental science. In W. F. Overton & P. C. M. Molenaar (Eds.), *Handbook of child psychology and developmental science Vol. 1: Theory and method* (pp. 63–112). New York: Wiley.

Wong, M. M., Zucker, R. A., Puttler, L. I., & Fitzgerald, H. E. (1999). Heterogeneity of risk aggregation for alcohol problems between early and middle childhood. Nesting structure variations. *Development and Psychopathology, 11*, 727–744.

Yates, T. M., Egeland, B., & Sroufe, A. (2003). Rethinking resilience: A developmental process perspective. In S. S. Luthar (Ed.), *Resilience and vulnerability: Adaptation in the context of childhood adversities* (pp. 243–266). New York: Cambridge University Press.

Yogman, M. (1982). Development of the father-infant relationship. In H. E. Fitzgerald, B. M. Lester, & M. Yogman (Eds.), *Theory and research in behavioral pediatrics* (pp. 221 279). New York: Plenum.

Yoshikawa, H., & Hsueh, J. (2001). Child development and social policy: Toward a dynamic systems perspective. *Child Development, 72*, 1887–1903.

Yu, C. H. (2006). *Philosophical foundations of quantitative research methodology*. Laham, MD: University Press of America.

Zucker, R. A., Fitzgerald, H. E., Refior, S. K., Puttler, L. I., Pallas, D. M., & Ellis, D. A. (2000). The clinical and social ecology of childhood for children of alcoholics: Description of a study and implications for a differentiated social policy. In H. E. Fitzgerald, B. M. Lester, & B. S. Zuckerman (Eds.), *Children of alcoholics: Research, health and policy issues* (pp. 109–141). New York: Routeledge Falmer.

Zucker, R. A., Wong, M. M., Puttler, L. I., & Fitzgerald, H. E. (2003). Resilience and vulnerability among sons of alcoholics: Relationship to developmental outcomes between early childhood and adolescence. In S. S. Luthar (Ed.), *Resilience and vulnerability: Adaptation in the context of childhood adversities* (pp. 76–103). New York: Cambridge University Press.

Fathering and Being Fathered: Developmental Interdependence

3

Rob Palkovitz

Fathering entails relationships, and relationships are fundamentally important to the people engaged in them. Yet, this obvious truth is sometimes forgotten or obscured by efforts to objectively study and analyze the key components of father-child relationships and their developmental consequences for men and their children. When we focus on devising precise measures of fathering behaviors or developmental outcomes, we can lose sight of the fact that father-child relationships are a complex, interactive system that we are attempting to characterize with our precise measures. Both the scholarly literature and casual conversations with our friends indicate that it is no overstatement to declare that father-child relationships are truly life-transformative for men and their children. Specifically, fathering and being fathered have consequences that are long-lasting and have important and salient implications that provide an affective, behavioral, and cognitive overlay for all other aspects of life, both for fathers and for their children.

The goal of this chapter is to present a relational understanding of fathering and being fathered. The developmental and theoretical literature reviewed will establish that fathering and being fathered represent *inter*dependent experiences that have life-altering consequences for both fathers and their children. A central focus of the chapter is to elaborate *how* father-child relationships are conducted and experienced across life to bring developmental benefits and outcomes of the interdependent meanings and processes that occur in the context of intergenerational father-child relationships.

Considerations of Father Absence

It is important to recognize at the outset of this discussion that not all families are characterized by the existence of positive father-child relationships. And, in the overall view of family functioning, when it comes to consistent, positive father engagement, the unfortunate reality is that there truly are "haves" and "have nots." Further, although the focus of this chapter is on the mutual benefits of positive father engagement for both fathers and their children, the reality is that virtually all father-child relationships could be "better" in some regards. What the theoretical and empirical literature well establishes is that families benefit when they are characterized by primarily positive paternal engagement. Consistently positive father-child relationship quality is more likely to be associated with fathers and children who share attributes of developmental optimization, reaching their potential, and experiencing fulfilling contexts of life.

R. Palkovitz (✉)
University of Delaware, Newark, DE, USA
e-mail: robp@udel.edu

H. E. Fitzgerald et al. (eds.), *Handbook of Fathers and Child Development*,
https://doi.org/10.1007/978-3-030-51027-5_3

Father Absence in Contrast to Fatherlessness

The word, father, designates at least one biological relationship, and subsequently, one, or a small number of specific and unique persons who fill socially constructed roles in the life of their children. Despite widespread contemporary usage of the term, *there is, in fact, no such thing as a fatherless child.*

Children who do not perceive that a father is materially involved in a significant way in their lives, eventually come to know, in ways that are hurtful to their wellbeing, that though they may not currently experience the presence of a father in their lives, that their very existence depended on a father. That discrepancy denotes a loss and that loss is typically associated with uncomfortable realities. Their father may be negligent, absent, deceased, or incarcerated, but children are not fatherless.

Although there is immense variability in the level of ongoing engagement and relationship quality with their child across their lifetime, the fact remains that no children exist without the participation of a biological father to achieve their conception, even if his role is limited to a sperm donor. Their relationship to their biological father forms a foundational part of the child's emerging identity and gives anchor to their origin story. Recent general commercial availability of genetic analysis has resulted in people reporting the unsettling disruption of identity that occurs when their origin story is contradicted by genetic results that stand in contrast to their longstanding understanding of who their biological father is. Knowing your father is foundational to self-understanding, a basis for the way we conduct many aspects of our life and relationships.

The father absence literature has been rightfully criticized on the basis of numerous structural differences that tend to get overlooked in many of the simplistic correlational summaries of its findings. However, there is a basic truth that still permeates—father absence is often associated with a deficit in emotions and behavioral competence in children—issues that manifest in both internalizing and externalizing problems. Though not truly fatherless, father absent or father-deficient children suffer developmental consequences across all domains of development.

Fathering and Being Fathered

It is in the context of father-child relationships that some of the biggest issues of life get addressed. For involved fathers, by their own reports, fathering has been found to be among, if not *the* most, central determiner of life satisfaction, meaningfulness, or purpose (Palkovitz, 2002).

In various ways, father-child relationships address one's sense of origin, identity, trajectory, and possibilities and purposes in life. Both fathers and their children, in parallel, interdependent, yet unique manners consider questions such as, "where did I come from?", "why am I here?", "where am I going in life?" As elaborated in detail below, these identity and purpose issues are grounded in everyday components of father-child relationships and behavioral interactions. It is in commonplace encounters that the answers to these big questions of life get anticipated and adjusted offering both glimpses of hope and looming threats to fulfillment.

It is not the purpose of this chapter to present a comprehensive review of the fathering literature in regard to broad domains of developmental outcomes for fathers and their young children—rather, that is the focus of multiple content chapters that follow in subsequent sections in this volume. The primary focus of this chapter is to present an accessible understanding of *how* father-child relationships come to take on such central meanings through ongoing processes of relational interaction. In doing so, we will focus together on both theoretical underpinnings of development and relationships, and briefly summarize central conclusions of the selected empirical literature. This is done in an effort to establish a clear understanding of how father-child relationship quality shapes both fathers' and young children's wellbeing and developmental outcomes through the context of ordinary interactions, that, over time, constitute a relational history with associated meanings, expectations, and evaluations of self and other. In order to articulate how such meanings and processes yield outcomes, it is necessary to first think about the nature of close relationships and how they are experienced by their participants.

Framing the Characteristics of Close Relationships and Scientific Inquiry

Families are groups of people who have close interpersonal relationships that evolve across time. Amato and Gilbreth (1999, p. 558) summarize Berscheid and Peplau's (1983) characterization of close relationships as those involving a high degree of interdependence, reflected in four attributes: "(a) the individuals have frequent contact, (b) the relationship is of long duration, (c) the degree of mutual impact is strong, and (d) the relationship involves diverse kinds of activities." Although not all father-child relationships are characterized by all four of these elements, it is still the case that many father-child relationships are appropriately portrayed as close relationships.

Despite the fact that close interpersonal relationships are often numericized and quantitatively analyzed by social scientists, father-child relationships are not built on or experienced through numeric algorithms. Rather, fathers and children interact in contexts where their behaviors toward one another have associated affect and cognitions through which the quality of the relationship is perceived. Important qualities and components of relationships, such as emotional and cognitive features, are conceptualized and inferred from the events and behaviors that people share together. As such, relationships are multidimensional and challenging to objectively characterize.

Stated another way, interpersonal relationships are organic, moving, growing, and changing experiences shared by two or more people. As active co-participants, fathers and their children are characterized by agency, choices, discrepant developmental capacities, understandings, and motives. Clearly, father-child relationships have many subjective elements.

In contrast, research studies are intended to bring objective, standardized ways of observing, measuring, and analyzing phenomena. By nature, research brings a purposeful and reductionistic focus on particular elements of a relationship, unable to capture all components of relationships in real time, or to represent their multitudinous changes across time. As such, scientific studies offer a partial, incomplete lens to the experiences, processes, and meanings of father-child relationships.

In actuality, key elements of relationships cannot be directly observed; they consist of both cognitive and affective elements that defy overt recording, and they have characteristics that have multiple interactive layers of structure and function. They have many elusive qualities; qualities that matter to both fathers and their children, qualities that shape the affect, behaviors, and cognitions of everyday encounters. If that were not complex enough, the interdependent feelings, behaviors, and thoughts of relationships change rapidly and exert influence across the relational history of fathers and children. The net result is that it is challenging to adequately scientifically encompass, operationalize, and measure father-child relationships in a manner that captures anything beyond their most central, basic, or important elements.

It is also the case that father-child relationships do not exist in a social or environmental vacuum. They are situated in a complex array of diverse demographic, cultural, and environmental contexts that mediate and moderate their unfolding across time (see, e.g., Marsiglio, Roy, & Fox, 2005). Another significant challenge to studying and understanding patterns of father-child relationships lies in the increasing diversity of fathers across myriad dimensions beyond SES, ethnicity, age, and living arrangements, who are situated in seemingly countless contexts of fathering relationships across time (Marsiglio et al., 2005). Residential status, marital or relational status, health, mental health, employment status, and spirituality represent a limited sampling of factors that converge to contribute to fathering diversity. Each father's constellation of diversity factors positions him with different resources and challenges to bring to the contexts of father-child interactions (Palkovitz & Hull, 2018).

Father-Child Relationships Develop Asynchronously across Time

Scientific advancements in the field of human development and family sciences have yielded an expanding appreciation for the complexity of relationships between developing individuals whose maturational outcomes are multiply determined, dynamic, and systemically embedded (Baltes, Staudinger, & Lindenberger, 1999). A central understanding is that all individuals (including both fathers and children) continually develop. That is, they manifest changes that are functionally significant and relatively permanent across biological, psychological, social, and spiritual domains of development. Fathers and their children often are developing in different developmental domains in different ways, rates, and directions at the same time (Palkovitz, 2007).

The implication is that fathers and children have different developmental capacities to plan, engage in, represent, comprehend, and regulate relationships. As a result, every shared father-child interaction is perceived differently by each participant (Dyer, Day, & Harper, 2014). Although fathers and their children experience discrepant perceptions, and have asynchronous developmental abilities and life course trajectories, many father-child dyads maintain meaningful connections and relationship quality across the first 5 years of the child's life, and well beyond.

Juxtaposed with the conceptual richness and understanding held by developmentalists and family scientists regarding the complexity and dynamic contexts of father-child relationships and their development, the current empirical literature on fathering is characterized by relatively narrow and static assessments of father involvement in child rearing. It is common for researchers to record the frequency of selected father behaviors toward children, a thin proxy of father-child relationship quality. A focus on fathers' behavior typically ignores the bidirectional, conditional, and transactional nature of relationships. In fact, scholars have long been reporting that mere behavioral frequencies of fathers toward their children do not predict important characteristics of child wellbeing or of father-child relationship quality (see, e.g., Amato & Gilbreth, 1999).

Palkovitz (2019) suggests that if we want to better represent the meanings and processes of father-child relationships and how they change over time, it is crucial for fathering scholarship to move beyond reductionistic foci on behavioral components of father involvement *toward* children and to more fully embrace the multiple characterizations of fathers' relationships *with* their children (Palm, 2014). Specifically, broader conceptualizations of father-child relationships have the potential to simultaneously honor the substantive contributions of fathering research that has focused on father involvement with children, while expanding the empirical focus of fathering to include multifaceted *relational qualities* of father-child relationships rather than specific behavioral *quantities*.

The professional literature has begun to make the shift from a nearly singular focus on father involvement toward children to a broader conceptualization of father-child relationship quality. As early as 1997, I began to write concerning the limitations of focusing primarily on fathers' behaviors toward their children while failing to meaningfully measure fathers' affect and cognitions as well. Current understandings of father-child relationship quality have placed a focus on the interdependence of fathers' and children's affect, behavior, and cognitions to more fully represent the lived experiences of fathers and children (Palkovitz, 2019). While we have known for years that paternal warmth, positive attachments, positive father engagement, closeness, and a sense of care make positive contributions to children's wellbeing, it is only recently that studies of positive father engagement have been expanded to focus beyond behavior to a more encompassing sense of father-child relationship quality. The interdependent processes and meanings in the child are equally important to articulate and support.

View 1: Interpersonal Relationships Are Complex

From one vantage point, father-child relationships are very complex. They consist of a system of countless interdependent feelings, behaviors, and thoughts toward one another and in response to one another. Figure 3.1 presents a graphic representation of the systemic nature of fathers' and children's feelings, behaviors, and thoughts in any given interaction.

In essence, Fig. 3.1 represents what is a "snapshot" in time of a specific father-child relationship. In contrast, Sameroff (2009) has established that development takes place through an unfolding of sequentially interdependent transactional interactions between a person and their environment. Applying Sameroff's reasoning and extending his transactional model to father-child relationships, the implication is that the interdependent affect, behaviors, and emotions of fathers and their children sequentially influence one another across time. That is, subsequent interactions are causally altered by the history of key interactional elements in the father-child relationship. Any time we have the opportunity to observe a father and child interacting, the interaction we observe is dependent on previous thoughts, behaviors, and feelings that they each brought into their previous interactions. In addition, future relational interactions will be influenced by current interactions. Figure 3.2 presents an elaboration of Sameroff's (2009) transactional model as it applies to the systemic interactions of the affect, behavior, and cognitions of father-child relationships. Fathers' and children's relational history, the match or discrepancy between the expectations, experiences, and evaluations sets both fathers' and children's expectations for and appraisals of future interactions.

Figure 3.2 is an adaption of Sameroff's (2009) model of the transactional nature of development created to represent fathers' and children's affect, behavior, and cognitions at times 1, 2, 3, & 4. The figure is intended to illustrate that fathers' affect, behaviors, and cognitions at time 1 are simultaneously and interdependently linked to the child's affect, behaviors, and cognitions at time 1. In addition, the figure represents that fathers' and children's relational characteristics at time 1 influence their own attributes at time 2. Further, each participant's characteristics at time 1 influences the other's at time 2. The framed section of Fig. 3.2, focusing attention on relational qualities between time 1 and time 2, shows the time frame represented in Fig. 3.3, where interdependent

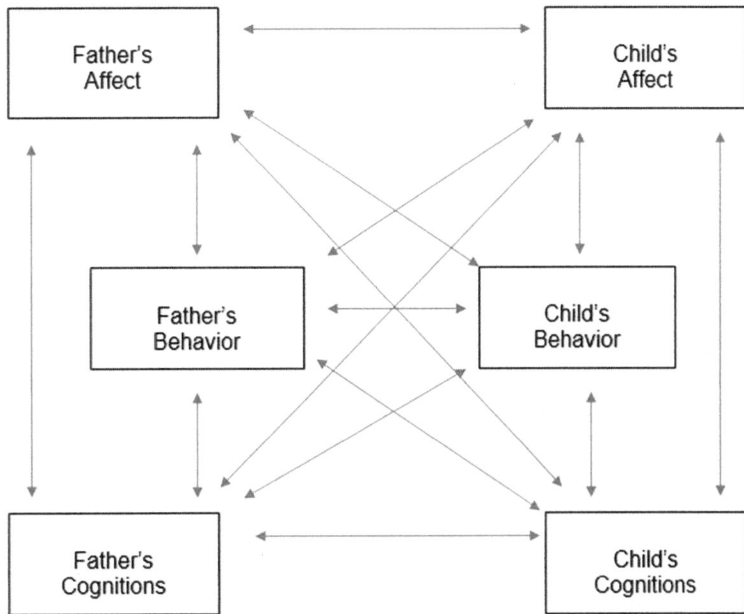

Fig. 3.1 Interdependence of fathers' and children's affect, behavior, and cognitions

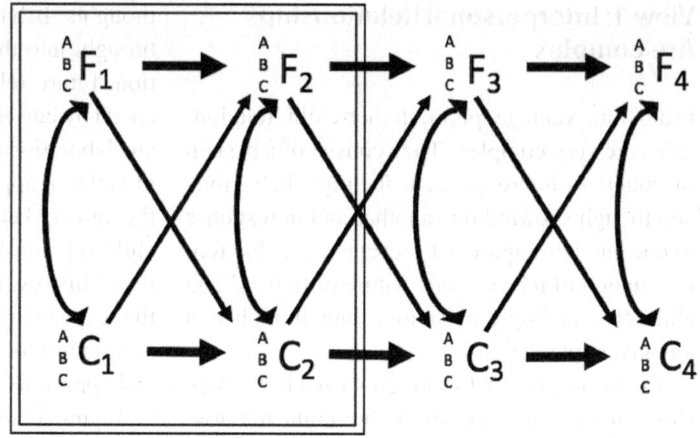

Fig. 3.2 The Transactional nature of father-child relationships across time. F father, C child, A affect, B behavior, C cognition. Numerals 1–4 represent time 1, time 2, time 3 & time 4

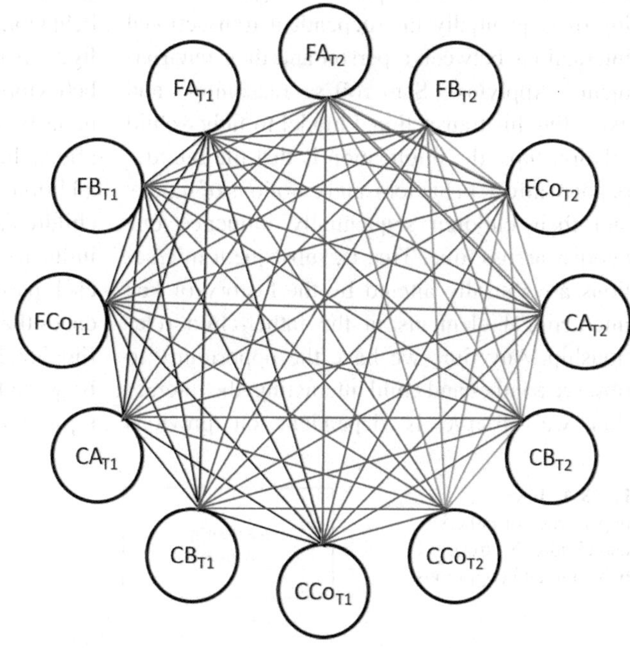

Fig. 3.3 Interdependence of fathers' and children's affect, behavior, and cognition from time 1 to time 2

relationships from each relational attribute in time 1 exert unidirectional influence on each relational attribute at time 2. In addition, at time 1 and at time 2, there is complete interdependence between fathers' and children's affect, behavior, and cognitions. The density of the represented relationships illustrates the complexity of father-child relationships either when snapshots of interactive qualities are represented in a single time or when they are viewed across an expanse of time.

The boxed area of Fig. 3.2 is, in reality, a simplification of the interdependent influences of fathers and their children in a number of regards. First, although the figure represents fathers' and children's feelings, behaviors, and thoughts, it does not represent other variables, factors, or contexts that influence father-child relationship quality. Specifically, it does not reflect variables such as physical and mental health, developmental abilities or disabilities, motivations, social support networks, or any other contextual elements demonstrated by a rich and varied literature to mediate and moderate father-child relationships (Palkovitz, 2019). Second, the highlighted area does not elaborate in detail the actual transactional nature of father's and children's affect, behavior, and cognitions. Specifically, each partner's feelings, behaviors, and thoughts reciprocally influence the other's at each time. Equally important, and missing from Fig. 3.2, is a representation of the unidirectional influences exerted by each factor (e.g., fathers' behavior at time 1) on all subsequent elements (father's affect, behavior, and cognitions, child's affect, behavior, and cognitions at time 2). Figure 3.3 provides a representation of both interdependent (within time) and unidirectional (across time) influences of fathers' and children's feelings, behaviors, and thoughts. Clearly, there are many interdependent forces at work in each father-child interaction, and their influences persist in complex relationships across time.

A further limitation of Figs. 3.2 and 3.3 in representing the lived experience of fathers' and children's relationship quality has to do with the representation of time in the figures. Specifically, the lapse from time one (T_1) to time two (T_2) could represent the minimal elapsed time, as in observing the interdependent nature of parents' and children's behavior within moments of a brief interaction (see, e.g., Tronick et al., 1998). Alternatively, the lapse between T_1 and T_2 could represent months, years, or decades, as is often the case in between waves of data collected in longitudinal studies.

A final observation in regard to the complexity of father-child relationships is that even limiting variables of interest to affect, behavior and cognitions, attempting to gather data in a manner that is representative of the myriad interactive transactions that children experience with their engaged fathers over the period of an hour, day, week, or year, presents extreme challenges to researchers. Having a sample large enough to allow analyses of even a handful of variables over time represents a significant challenge to researchers who want to capture meaningful elements of father-child relationship quality and to conduct robust statistical analyses.

View 2: Interpersonal Relationships Are Simple

From an alternative perspective, father-child relationships are fairly simple. If we can disregard mediating and moderating influences of other pertinent variables (e.g., hormones, neural networks, representations, social scripts), and focus on just the feelings, behaviors, and thoughts that fathers and their children direct toward each other, those are the main components that determine both father-child relationship quality and the developmental outcomes for both fathers and their children (Palkovitz, 1997). In essence, those three foci, affect, behavior, and cognition are the three things that always matter in father-child-relationship quality. These are the characteristics that influence fathers' and children's experiences and expectations of one another as well as their appraisals of their relationship quality and their individual roles in contributing toward relational quality.

Further, expanding to simultaneously and interactively consider just those three factors, affect, behavior, and cognitions, represents a conceptually rich advancement over studies with a singular focus on fathers' behavior toward children (i.e., involvement). Detailed interviews with fathers indicate that they are aware of and able to articulate their feelings, behaviors, and thoughts toward their children during open-ended conversations (Palkovitz, 2002). In fact, these are components that are frequently represented in the lived experiences of everyday dads and their children.

Reconciling the Two Views

Though we know that the development of father-child relationships is interdependent, multidirectional, multiply determined, asynchronous, contextually embedded, and transactionally dynamic, it is possible to identify a few central components that explain large degrees of variability in perceived relationship quality. In conversations with fathers and children concerning their daily experiences, both fathers and their children find ways to discuss or represent the affect, behaviors, and cognitions that characterize the quality of their relationships. Simply stated, fathers and children are aware of these components of their relationship and focus on them when representing their interactions with others. The implication is that, as fathers or their children improve the affect, behavior, or cognitions that they contribute to the father-child relationship, they have the realistic potential to precipitate subsequent positive developmental cascades (Masten, 2014) into the system of father-child relationship quality.

Theoretical Foundations of Father-Child Relationship Quality

Numerous theoretical approaches and their associated empirical bases establish the importance of different components of father-child relationships in influencing the lived experiences and developmental outcomes of fathers and their children. Specifically, attachment, father-child closeness, parenting styles, identity theory, father presence, mutual regulation models, resource theory, and paternal sensitivity and relational synchrony have each been elaborated, to varying degrees, to bring important understandings to the experiences and outcomes of fathering and being fathered.

Attachment

When considering the developmental components of children's experiences of father-child relational quality, a logical place to begin is with children's attachment toward their fathers. Bowlby's attachment theory (1969) advances that parent-child relationships are the foundation for children's social relationships and sense of self. Specifically, it is the nature and quality of interactions an infant has with parents and others that help them to learn about themselves, others, and how to relate. As early as 1964, Schaffer and Emerson conducted ground-breaking work in father-infant attachment, finding that most of infants formed an attachment to their fathers by the second year of life. Subsequent systematic analyses of empirical studies have identified paternal warmth and sensitivity as formative features father-infant attachment (Cox, Owen, Henderson, & Margand, 1992; Van Ijzendoorn & De Wolff, 1997).

Bowlby (1969) elaborated attachment theory to explain that infants construct internal working models (IWMs), expectations about relationships, based on their ongoing history of experience with attachment figures, and reflecting the quality of relationship with those figures (Peluso, Peluso, White, & Kern, 2004). As such, IWMs can be thought of as a child's cognitive frameworks for understanding the self, the world, and relationships with others. Solomon and George (1996) write about IWMs serving as the source of the child's self-appraisal and confidence regarding their acceptableness and worthiness of care and protection, and of the attachment figure's availability, desire, and capability to provide care and protection. Clearly, IWMs reflect father-child relationship quality to influence children's sense of self-worth and their sense of trustworthiness of others and their circumstances in life. Bretherton and Munholland (1999) articulated that, throughout life, a person's interactions with others are shaped by components of their IWMs; memories, expectations, and representations of others as trustworthy (or not), the self as valuable (or not), and the self as effective when interacting with others (or not). As such, internal working models can be understood as a cognitive prototype that helps one to formulate sense of self, expectations of, and responses to others. As articulated, and consistent with Figs. 3.1 and 3.2, IWMs have affective, behavioral, and cognitive components and implications for approaching, experiencing, and evaluating all future interpersonal interactions.

Father-Child Closeness

Bronfenbrenner (1994) articulated that parents' mental representations of attachment are formed in proximal processes, which require direct contact between parents and children. In a manner similar to children's formation of IWMs, parental IWMs would include associated affective components. The implication is that proximal processes, direct behavioral interactions, can yield feelings of emotional closeness (or distance). In elaborating key attributes of father presence (see below) Krampe (2009, p. 883) states,

> The core of the offspring's feelings about the father is whether or not the child feels close to him. Conceptually, emotional closeness or distance represents the coming together of a number of other interpersonal elements: a sense of trust, the feeling of being accepted, favorably received, and welcomed; the experience of intimacy and sense of knowing and being known by the other; the recognition that one has a (psychological) place with the other (i.e., father), and is important to him. Despite the significance of each of these factors in adult relationships, there is relatively little work on this aspect of the parent–child bond, particularly between children and their fathers.

Parenting Styles

Baumrind's (1971) classic work identified parental warmth and control as central components of parenting style. Contemporary scholarship on paternal style continues to highlight paternal warmth and control, along with other relationship quality attributes. A wide variety of research studies have documented that parenting styles predict child well-being in the domains of academic performance, problem behaviors, prosocial development, and social competence (see, e.g., Adamsons & Johnson, 2013; Anderson, Kaplan, & Lancaster, 1999; Conger & Elder, 1994; Gavin et al., 2002; McBride & Rane, 1997).

It has been well established that paternal styles tend to systematically differ from mothers' (Palkovitz, Trask, & Adamsons, 2014), and various components of fathers' style have been linked to child wellbeing and developmental outcomes. A detailed body of literature verifies that fathers' play styles (see, e.g. Vollotton, Foster, Harewood, Cook, & Adekoya, 2020) can facilitate children's social and emotional regulation, provided that fathers are sensitively attentive to their children's signals during play.

The style of father-child interactions interdependently affects fathers' and children's cognitive functioning. Specifically, Slade (2005) detailed the relationships between parents' reflective functioning (RF), the capacity of a parent to hold their child's mental state in mind as it relates to affect regulation, and productive social relationships. Slade describes RF at the interface between psychoanalytic theories and attachment, current thinking in neuroscience, and social psychological understandings of self-regulation. Slade advances that it is parent's capacity to reflect upon the child's internal cognitive and affective experience that is key to the facilitation of a secure attachment and to an array of other developmental outcomes. Slade has further articulated that nonreflective and dysregulated caregiving profoundly disrupts self-development in children.

Fonagy et al. (2002, p. 6) describe RF as the ability of a person to give meaning and organization to internal states so that they can be "communicated to others and interpreted in others to guide collaboration in work, love, and play." This variety of mentalization integrates affective and cognitive ways of knowing to think about feeling and to feel about thinking. These functions have both been previously identified as metacognitive processes related to perspective taking and metacognitive monitoring (Main, 1991). These processes are held to be at the heart of sensitive caregiving, which, in turn, gives rise to children's capacity to develop mentalizing competence of their own. Viewed integratively, this body of literature indicates that incomplete perspectives of father-child relationship quality are afforded by looking at father-child relationships in isolation from parenting style.

Identity Theory

A vital construct of identity theory is that fathers have an internalized standard of performance (e.g., cognitive expectations) yoked with being a father, and that fathers regularly engage in reflected appraisals (Maurer, Pleck, & Rane, 2001) by utilizing their executive functions of monitoring and evaluating their performance against their role prescriptions (Dyer, Kauffman, Fagan, Pearson, & Cabrera, 2018). When there is a match between their cognitive standards and their perceived role performance, fathers tend to feel validated (Burke, 1991). In contrast, if they perceive that they fall short of their standard, feelings of inadequacy, accompanied by negative affect, result from the dissonance experienced. Fathers' personal identity is validated by father-child closeness because closeness indicates that the father is meeting his internalized standard. In contrast, father-child conflict more frequently yields feelings of inadequacy, because their standard is not being attained or surpassed.

Fathering role centrality, another aspect of paternal identity has been positively associated with levels of father involvement in both home-based observational studies (Palkovitz, 1984) and large longitudinal data sets (Adamsons & Pasley, 2016; Pasley, Futris, & Skinner, 2002). Additionally, role occupancy perspectives of father identity (Doherty, Kouneski, & Erickson, 1998) link paternal engagement in various fathering roles with changes in behavior and cognitions over time (Palkovitz, 2002). Data interpreted from the role occupancy perspective supports the contention that the effects of fatherhood roles on men's lives are moderated by the degree to which men affectively, behaviorally, and cognitively embrace and engage in fathering roles.

Father Presence

Krampe (2009) advanced the construct of father presence, expanding on Lamb's prior (e.g., 1997) ideas regarding father's accessibility to children. Father presence is conceptualized to have several components that represent affective, behavioral, and cognitive domains. Krampe (p. 875) describes the primary elements of father presence to include:

> (a) an inner sense of father in the child that orients him or her to the father; (b) the child's relationship with the personal father; (c) other family influences on father presence in the child; and (d) cultural and religious beliefs about the father found in the larger societal context, which are transmitted to the child in the family and other primary groups.

Krampe identifies emotional accessibility within father-child relationships as a central component of the expressive dimension. An additional, instrumental, dimension includes the child's perception of father involvement, principally represented through behavioral interactions and related components that foster the child's development.

Krampe and Newton (2006, p. 162) articulate that father presence encompasses "affective, behavioral, and cognitive/perceptual elements that we operationalize as the son's or daughter's feelings about the father, his/her physical relationship with the father, and the adult child's perception of the father's involvement with him/her."

Mutual Regulation Model and Dyadically Expanded States of Consciousness

Tronick (1989) and his colleagues (1998) advanced models of infant self-regulation where infants seek states of emotional connectedness with caregivers in order to achieve dyadic states of consciousness, or shared meaning. The basic idea is that infants observe the affect and behavior of caregivers, facilitated through processes of caregivers' emotional scaffolding, in order to enter into a dyadic state of organization with the caregiver. In essence, the infant seeks mutual regulation (i.e., to be "in synch") with the affect and behaviors of the caregiver to experience a joint state of consciousness. The processes, which are viewed to be inherent in humans, require a mutual mapping of elements of each partner's affective, behavioral, and cognitive states of consciousness into the other partner's brain. These assertions are consistent with the recent scholarly emphasis on shared perspective taking, theory of mind, and associated developmental outcomes (see, e.g., Decety & Sommerville, 2003).

In multiple experiments, researchers have had adults practice "still face" responses during interactions with infants, resulting in emotional distress, behavioral dysregulation, and general breakdown of behavioral organization (see, Adamson & Frick, 2003 for a historical review).

This scholarship establishes that in the first months of life, infants engage in interactions with others that require mutual regulation of affect, behavior, and cognitions. Achievement of mutual regulation and synchrony potentially leads to dyadic expanded states of consciousness and generally positive outcomes. Lack of mutual regulation leads to affective, cognitive, and behavioral dysregulation and general distress. In summary, very early in life, infants appear to be highly motivated and capable of processing and making meaning of complex dyadic interactions that reflect affective, behavioral, and cognitive components of relationship quality.

Resource Theory of Fathering

Palkovitz and Hull (2018) focus on the intersectionality of fathers' affect, behaviors, and cognitions in utilizing executive functions such as monitoring, planning, and evaluating their personal, interpersonal, and contextual resources to facilitate the quality of their relationships with their children. Resource theory is father-centric, and emphasizes the interdependence of fathers' affect, behavior, and cognitions in fathers' resource management, lived experiences, and father-child relationships. A limitation is that resource theory does not centrally articulate children's affect, behavior, and cognitions or the specifics of interdependent father-child interactions into the theory. Nonetheless, it offers an elaborated view of central aspects of fathers' affective, behavioral, and cognitive characteristics and how they intersectionally influence father-child relationship quality.

Paternal Sensitivity and Relational Synchrony

Lamb and Lewis (2013) affirm that paternal sensitivity is instrumentally shaped by fathers' experiences of their own childhood relationships. This view is consistent with the construct of internal working models, briefly discussed above. Several researchers have found that men who had loving and secure relationships with their caregivers are more sensitive, attentive, and involved than fathers who recounted poor caregiving relationships as children (Bretherton, Lambert, & Golby, 2006; Cowan, Cohn, Cowan, & Pearson, 1996; Shannon, Tamis-LeMonda, & Cabrera, 2006). Fathers' sensitivity to infant signals (Lamb, 2010) as well as their warmth, responsiveness, and consistency of responding to children (Carson & Parke, 1996; Fagan & Iglesias, 1999; Ninio & Rinott, 1988) have been documented as important factors in influencing father-child relationship quality.

Brown et al. (2007, p. 213) analyzed various empirical studies conducted across different ages of children and focusing on different domains of child outcomes, concluding that it appears that fathers' positive affect, warmth, and emotional support "load onto the same dimension," best described as positive emotions. Multiple studies support the importance of positive emotional expression between fathers and their children (see, e.g., Cox et al., 1992; Frosch, Cox, & Goldman, 2001; Volling, McElwain, Notaro, & Herrera, 2002).

Creating Interdependent Understandings of Fathering and Being Fathered

When considering the convergence of these theoretical and empirical findings, it has been widely recognized that "the amount of time that fathers and children spend together is probably much less important than what they do with that time" (Lamb & Tamis-LeMonda, 2004, p. 10). Brown et al. (2007, p. 215) conclude that their results "speak to the importance of considering qualitative dimensions of fathers' parenting—in addition to father involvement—in research on fathering and child outcomes in general, and father-child attachment security in particular."

ABCs of Father-Child Relationship Quality

Macon, Tamis-LeMonda, Cabrera, and McFadden (2017) elaborate that psychology entails the study of persons' affect, behaviors, and cognitions, concluding that the work of applied researchers and interventionists should address fathers' "affective values (parenting beliefs), their behaviors (teaching targeted skills, such as how to read to children), and their cognitions (knowledge about child development and best practices in parenting)" (Macon et al., 2017, p. 2658).

Viewed as a whole, the reviewed scholarship supports the conviction that father-child relationship quality hinges on the interdependence of both fathers' and children's affective, behavioral and cognitive processes as opposed to placing primary focus on fathers' behavior toward children. As clearly supported by theoretical and empirical literature, father-child relationships consist of a series of behavioral interactions that have associated thoughts and feelings. The processes and meanings of relationships as well as the quality of those relationships are manifested in the transactionally unfolding behaviors, thoughts, and feelings of father-child interactions over time. The way that we come to represent our relationship with our father is that we call to mind (i.e., bring into consciousness or think about) a sense of who he is toward us—our representation of our interaction history with him, and those cognitions have associated feelings. In describing father presence, Krampe (2009, p. 882) concurs:

> Analytically, there appears to be three broad dimensions where individuals may directly bond or connect with their male parent. One is affective, based on feelings for him. The second is cognitive or perceptual, and includes the child's view of the father's involvement with him or her. The third is physical, and consists of direct body-based encounters and interaction with the father.

Palkovitz (2007, 2018) has reviewed and summarized these considerations by stating that in terms of father-child relationship quality, three things always matter: the affective climate of the relationship, the behavioral style, and relational synchrony (connection). He designated these factors as the ABCs of father-child relationship quality, and articulated that the ABCs work together systemically. Positive attributes in each factor transactionally result in positive developmental cascades into the larger system of father-child relationship quality, and negativity or deficits are associated with decrements in father-child relationship quality and well-being for both fathers and children.

Briefly summarized, Palkovitz (2018) posits that the affective (A) factor is the foundational lynchpin of fathering and being fathered. It comprises the sense of closeness, love, warmth, caring, and attachment. Across the life of father-child relationships, it is expressed in "being there" for one another, relational security, or having one another's back. It yields a sense of relational security, an abiding sense that things are good between fathers and children. The B factor refers to the behavioral components of father-child interaction, encompassing the mutuality of behavioral engagement and behavioral style. The B factor is manifested in countless everyday encounters, engaging in the behaviors associated with doing things together. As stated previously, the vast majority of fathering research has focused on the behavioral involvement of fathers toward their children. The third element of central importance, C, represents the connections between fathers and their children's affective, behavioral, and cognitive components of relating to one another. It is manifested in constructs such as goodness of fit, relational synchrony, mutual regulation, and sensitivity to one another's signals. Father-child connections are facilitated by behaving (B) in a manner that builds the sense of closeness and love (A) by doing the right things, in the right time, in the right way to facilitate the mutuality of the relationship.

In the absence of an adequate base in the affective foundations of the relationship, both fathers and children tend to manifest internalizing problems along with low self-esteem, confidence, and competence. Conversely, when the A factor is primarily positive and consistently manifested over time, fathers and children are characterized by well-being in their sense of self, including self-worth, self-confidence, self-competence, and a sense of belonging.

When father-child relationship quality is characterized by positive behavioral qualities associated with the B factor, both fathers and children tend to manifest fewer externalizing problems. In addition, they are characterized by positive developmental outcomes in both cognitive skills such as executive function and theory of mind, with spillover into positive social development, such as positive peer relationships and social cognition. Positive B factors in father-child relationship quality are associated with greater educational attainment, better outcomes in substance use, and delayed sexual initiation and pregnancy outcomes in children.

Interdependence in Processes and Meanings of Fathering and Being Fathered

It is a challenge to present father-child relational interdependence in a manner that captures the simultaneous richness of factors and experiences of both fathers and their children. We will begin by individually describing their simultaneous experiences, processes, and meanings of fathers and children separately, and later to attempt an integrative narrative to bring them together.

Relational Processes and Meanings in Children

Early in infancy, children have the capacity to respond to the affect and behavior of adults, and appear to be motivated to enter into synchrony with them through processes of mutual regulation (Tronick, 1989). A child's sense of his or her relationship with their father is grounded in bouts of mutual regulation as well as in the context of their developing attachment relationships and the associated formation of internal working models. Each subsequent encounter contributes more data to the child's experiential understanding of the nature and quality of the relationship he or she has with their father—resulting in either more positive affect and appraisal (e.g., closeness, positivity), or greater distance and emotional hurt (e.g., mistrust, disappointment).

Their perceived relationship to their father forms a foundational part of the child's emerging identity and gives anchor to their origin story. Knowing your father is foundational to self-understanding, a basis for the way we conduct many aspects of our life and relationships.

In summary, for infants, the primary processes of importance are grounded in mutual regulation, the formation of attachments and associated internal working models, yielding a sense of trust versus mistrust (Erikson, 1993) along with an emergent sense of identity. According to Bronfenbrenner (1991, p. 2), in order to develop "intellectually emotionally, socially and morally a child requires participation in progressively more complex reciprocal activity on a regular basis over an extended period in the child's life, with one or more persons with whom the child develops a strong, mutual, irrational, emotional attachment and who is committed to the child's well-being and development, preferably for life." This principle has frequently been simply translated and stated as: "every child needs at least one adult who is irrationally crazy about him or her."

Sabey, Rauer, Haselschwerdt, and Volling (2018) conducted the only known study to collect data from both parents and their children to document how parents demonstrate love toward their children. They found that parents most often express love to their children by playing or doing things together, followed by demonstrating affection, helping or supporting, and giving gifts or treats. It is the repeated engagement in these everyday experiences that shape young children's understanding of the self, others, and how to relate.

Relational Processes and Meanings in Fathers

The poet, William Wadsworth stated that "the child is father to the man." Perhaps he was reflecting on the continuity of development from early childhood experiences to developmental outcomes later in life. Alternatively, he may have been observing the profound and life-changing pathways of men who give themselves over to engaging in fathering roles across time in their child's life.

Men's reports of their lived experience of fathering document the centrality that relational components hold for them. A man's identity is indelibly changed when he assumes the role of father. Fathering identity is a central component of the developmental meanings and processes that causes fathering to exert a developmental pull on committed fathers (Palkovitz, 2002).

As Cowan (1991) has eloquently elaborated, a developmental transition entails an interdependent, long-lasting, and functionally significant change in both a sense of self and in subsequent behaviors of the person experiencing the transition. As such, transitions to fatherhood are not merely demarcated by the birth of a child, and in fact, may occur asynchronously with the event of birth or adoption. Fathers may experience the transition to fatherhood prior to trying to conceive a child or long after a child's birth, for example when assuming a fictive kin, step father, or adoptive father role. Specifically, the transition to fathering is experienced by men who cognitively and behaviorally embrace the role of father, experience the "fatherhood click" (Daniels & Weingarten, 1988) or decide to assume responsibility as a father in a child's life. Both role centrality and role occupancy—designating self as father and engaging in the role—brings life-changing differences that define fathers' lived experiences, self-concepts, sense of efficacy, and meaning in life in addition to dictating much of their daily expenditure of time, emotional capital, and money (Palkovitz, 2002).

Simply stated, engaged fathering occupies much of a man's focus and time, providing countless opportunities for shaping his developmental outcomes. Because fathering is a common context of life for men's adult development, it may be overlooked as a primary contributor to manifested developmental status. But, as my own research has documented (Palkovitz, 2002) engaged fathers tend to see fathering as the primary shaper of who they have become. In fact, fathering relationships are cited by fathers to be a primary source of emotional experience, and the emotions of fathering run the gamut from the most positive, joyous, and exhilarating to the most negative. In open-ended interviews, fathers recount that the emotions of fathering include love, joy (fun), pride, self-gratification (purpose), as well as fear, anger, frustration, disappointment, and even futility.

For fathers, the centrally important processes and meanings of father-child relationships have to do with fathering identity, self-appraisal, purpose & meanings, sense of closeness (influenced by their adult IWMs), and a sense of fun/enjoyment. Men who are committed to fathering as a central role in their lives engage in frequent self-appraisal. They think about their performance in the role of fathering, and the quality of their relationship with their children (closeness). They plan for and monitor many components of their relationship with their children. The skills of fathering simultaneously integrate with and differentiate from other aspects of life and transfer to other contexts and relationships (Palkovitz, 2002). There are positive developmental cascades that ripple into positive outcomes in relationships with their partners and in the community. The lived experience of fathering consumes much of involved fathers' time, energy, emotions, and focus.

Engaged, committed fathering has been demonstrated to exert a developmental pull on men, which they report to "make them better persons" than they would have otherwise been if they did not invest their time and effort into building a relationship with their children (Palkovitz, 2002). Specifically, involved fathers report making changes that they would not have otherwise made for the sake of their children.

Integrating Fathers' and Children's Relational Experiences into a Developmental Understanding

Palkovitz (2002) conducted a qualitative study with a diverse group of involved fathers who recounted that the affective, behavioral, and cognitive connections they have with their children are central to their lived experiences as fathers and the way they see themselves as men. At the same time that fathers have integrated feelings, behaviors, and thoughts with their children, their children concurrently have affective, behavioral, and cognitive experiences in interacting with their fathers. Consequently, a more inclusive model of father-child relationship quality needs to simultaneously consider the interdependence of fathers' and children's affect, behavior, and cognitions, as depicted in Fig. 3.1. Repeated opportunities for interaction across both brief and lengthy spans of time transactionally influence the developing history of father-child relationship quality across time (Figs. 3.2 and 3.3). Each new father-child interaction is grounded in past experiences of characteristics such as perceptions of mutuality, closeness, care, or disappointments, hurts, and lack of mutuality. Across time, and grounded in an ongoing history of fathering and being fathered, men and their children come to interdependently constructed understandings of self and others. Lasting developmental outcomes and senses of well-being (or their lack) are forged in the everyday relational interactions of fathers and their children.

Importance of the Early Years for Fathers and Children

The first years of life have been repeatedly identified by developmentalists as foundational in setting the stage for wellbeing and the attainment of milestones and achievement. The story that has emerged regarding fathering and being fathered is, in some ways, very nuanced, complicated, and infinitely difficult to capture because of the multiple layers of interacting factors across real time. On the other hand, these are things that my immigrant grandmother, a sensitive caregiver who did not complete high school, could have articulated in conversations about intergenerational relationships. In fact, when you question sensitive caregivers about how to best care for young children, they focus on and express elements centrally related to the ABCs of fathering. Fathers who are mindful of and regularly practice these principles have children who are characterized by positive developmental outcomes. In turn, children use their emerging relational skills to invest back into their social relationships, including their relationships with their fathers. Fathers who regularly ignore the ABCs contribute to deficits in the manifold of skills commonly termed theory of mind and executive function, and consequently, their children have challenges in peer relationships, school readiness, and meeting subsequent developmental milestones and indicators of wellbeing or success. This is particularly true when extreme deficits persist across time or exposure to adverse childhood experiences occur (Masten, 2014).

Summary and Key Points

Creating scholarly representations of interpersonal relationships is a perilous enterprise. Attempting to faithfully represent the central aspects, meanings, and processes of dynamic and important relationships is particularly challenging. At any time, fathers and children are developing (i.e., making functionally significant, relatively permanent changes across bio-psycho-social-spiritual domains) by engaging in processes with meanings that are not uniform across developmental eras and social addresses. That is, fathers and their children often are developing in different developmental domains in different ways, rates, and directions at the same time. Fathers and their children have different developmental capacities to represent, understand, and regulate relationships. As a result, every shared father-child interaction is perceived differently by each participant. What may be perceived to be primarily a positive interaction by either the child or the father may be experienced, processed, and remembered quite differently by the other. Yet, the shared interactions are characterized by *inter*dependent feelings, behaviors, and thoughts, and the central processes of development are the same for fathering and being fathered. In their everyday interactions, fathers' and children's feelings (affect) behaviors and cognitions (ABCs) combine to shape the quality of their relationships.

This chapter has articulated the everyday processes that allow fathers and children maintain meaningful connections and relationship quality across the life span while experiencing discrepant perceptions, asynchronous developmental abilities, and life course trajectories.

References

Adamson, L. B., & Frick, J. E. (2003). The still face: A history of a shared experimental paradigm. *Infancy, 4*(4), 451–473.

Adamsons, K., & Johnson, S. (2013). An updated and expanded meta-analysis of nonresident fathering and child well-being. *Journal of Family Psychology, 27*, 589–599. https://doi.org/10.1037/a0033786

Adamsons, K., & Pasley, K. (2016). Parents' fathering identity standards and later father involvement. *Journal of Family Issues, 37*(2), 221–244.

Amato, P. R., & Gilbreth, J. G. (1999). Nonresident fathers and children's well-being: A meta-analysis. *Journal of Marriage and the Family, 61*(3), 557–573.

Anderson, K., Kaplan, H., & Lancaster, J. (1999). Paternal care by genetic fathers and stepfathers I: Reports from Albuquerque men. *Evolution and Human Behavior, 20*, 405–431. https://doi.org/10.1016/S1090-5138(99)00023-9

Baltes, P. B., Staudinger, U. M., & Lindenberger, U. (1999). Lifespan psychology: Theory and application to intellectual functioning. *Annual Review of Psychology, 50*(1), 471–507.

Baumrind, D. (1971). Current patterns of parental authority. *Developmental Psychology, 4*(1p2), 1.

Berscheid, E., & Peplau, L. A. (1983). The emerging science of relationships. In H. H. Kelly, E. Berscheid, A. Christensen, J. H. Harvey, T. L. Huston, G. Levinger, E. McClintock, L. A. Peplau, & D. R. Peterson (Eds.), *Close relationships* (pp. 1–19). New York: W. H. Freeman.

Bowlby, J. (1969). *Attachment. Attachment and loss: Vol. 1. Loss*. New York: Basic Books.

Bretherton, I., Lambert, J. D., & Golby, B. (2006). Involved fathers of preschool children as seen by themselves and their wives: Accounts of attachment, socialization, and companionship. *Attachment & Human Development, 7*, 229–251.

Bretherton, I., & Munholland, K. A. (1999). Internal working models in attachment relationships: A construct revisited. In J. Cassidy & P. R. Shaver (Eds.), *Handbook of attachment: Theory, research, and clinical applications* (pp. 89–111). New York: The Guilford Press.

Bronfenbrenner, U. (1991). What do families do? *Institute for American Values, Winter/Spring*, 2.

Bronfenbrenner, U. (1994). Ecological models of human development. *Readings on the Development of Children, 2*(1), 37–43.

Brown, G. L., McBride, B. A., Shin, N., & Bost, K. K. (2007). Parenting predictors of father-child attachment security: Interactive effects of father involvement and fathering quality. *Fathering, 5*(3), 197.

Burke, P. J. (1991). Identity processes and social stress. *American Sociological Review, 56*(6), 836–849.

Carson, J. L., & Parke, R. D. (1996). Reciprocal negative affect in parent child interactions and children's peer competency. *Child Development, 67*(5), 2217–2226.

Conger, R. D., & Elder, G. H. (1994). *Families in troubled times: Adapting to change in rural America. Social institutions and social change*. Hawthorne, NY: Aldine de Gruyter.

Cowan, P. A. (1991). Individual and family life transitions: A proposal for a new definition. In P. A. Cowan & M. Hetherington (Eds.), *Family transitions* (pp. 3–30). Hillsdale, NJ: Lawrence Erlbaum Associates.

Cowan, P. A., Cohn, D. A., Cowan, C. P., & Pearson, J. L. (1996). Parents'attachment histories and children's externalizing and internalizing behaviors: Exploring family systems models of linkage. *Journal of Consulting and Clinical Psychology, 64*(1), 53.

Cox, M. J., Owen, M. T., Henderson, V. K., & Margand, N. A. (1992). Prediction of infant-father and infant-mother attachment. *Developmental Psychology, 28*(3), 474.

Daniels, P., & Weingarten, K. (1988). *The fatherhood click: The timing of parenthood in men's lives*.

Decety, J., & Sommerville, J. A. (2003). Shared representations between self and other: A social cognitive neuroscience view. *Trends in Cognitive Sciences, 7*(12), 527–533.

Doherty, W. J., Kouneski, E. F., & Erickson, M. F. (1998). Responsible fathering: An overview and conceptual framework. *Journal of Marriage and the Family, 60*(2), 277–292.

Dyer, W. J., Day, R. D., & Harper, J. M. (2014). Father involvement: Identifying and predicting family members' shared and unique perceptions. *Journal of Family Psychology, 28*(4), 516.

Dyer, W. J., Kauffman, R., Fagan, J., Pearson, J., & Cabrera, N. (2018). Measures of father engagement for nonresident fathers. *Family Relations, 67*(3), 381–398.

Erikson, E. H. (1993). *Childhood and society*. London: WW Norton & Company.

Fagan, J., & Iglesias, A. (1999). Father involvement program effects on fathers, father figures, and their Head Start children: A quasi-experimental study. *Early Childhood Research Quarterly, 14*(2), 243–269.

Fonagy, P., Steele, M., Steele, H., Leigh, T., Kennedy, R., Mattoon, G., et al. (2002). Attachment, the reflective self, and borderline states: The predictive specificity of the Adult Attachment Interview and pathological emotional development. In S. Goldberg, R. Muir, & J. Kerr (Eds.), *Attachment theory: Social, developmental and clinical perspectives* (pp. 223–279). Hillsdale, NJ: Analytic Press.

Frosch, C. A., Cox, M. J., & Goldman, B. D. (2001). Infant-parent attachment and parental and child behavior during parent-toddler storybook interaction. *Merrill-Palmer Quarterly, 1982*, 445–474.

Gavin, L. E., Black, M. M., Minor, S., Abel, Y., Papas, M., & Bentley, M. (2002). Young, disadvantaged fathers' involvement with their infants: An ecological perspective. *Journal of Adolescent Health, 31*, 266–276. https://doi.org/10.1016/S1054-139X(02)00366-X

Krampe, E. M. (2009). When is the father really there? A conceptual reformulation of father presence. *Journal of Family Issues, 30*(7), 875–897.

Krampe, E. M., & Newton, R. R. (2006). The father presence questionnaire: A new measure of the subjective experience of being fathered. *Fathering: A Journal of Theory, Research & Practice about Men as Fathers, 4*(2), 159–190.

Lamb, M. E. (1997). The development of father–infant relationships. In M. E. Lamb (Ed.), *The role of the father in child development* (pp. 104–120). Hoboken, NJ: Wiley.

Lamb, M. E. (2010). The development and significance of father-child relationships in two-parent families. In *The role of the father in child development* (5th ed., pp. 94–153). Hoboken, NI: Wiley.

Lamb, M. E., & Lewis, C. (2013). Father-child relationships. *Handbook of Father Involvement: Multidisciplinary Perspectives, 2*, 119–135.

Lamb, M. E., & Tamis-LeMonda, C. E. (2004). The role of the father: An introduction. In M. E. Lamb (Ed.), *The role of the father in child development* (pp. 1–31). Hoboken, NJ: Wiley.

Macon, T. A., Tamis-LeMonda, C. S., Cabrera, N. J., & McFadden, K. E. (2017). Predictors of father investment of time and finances: The specificity of resources, relationships, and parenting beliefs. *Journal of Family Issues, 38*(18), 2642–2662.

Main, M. (1991). Metacognitive knowledge, metacognitive monitoring, and singular (coherent) vs. multiple (incoherent) models of attachment: Findings and directions for future research. In C. M. Parkes, J. Stevenson-Hinde, & P. Marris (Eds.), *Attachment across the life cycle* (pp. 127–159). London: Tavistock-Routledge.

Marsiglio, W., Roy, K., & Fox, G. L. (2005). *Situated fathering: A focus on physical and social spaces*. Lanham: Rowman & Littlefield Publishers.

Masten, A. S. (2014). *Ordinary magic: Resilience in development*. New York: Guilford Publications.

Maurer, T. W., Pleck, J. H., & Rane, T. R. (2001). Parental identity and reflected appraisals: Measurement and gender dynamics. *Journal of Marriage and Family, 63*(2), 309–321.

McBride, B., & Rane, T. (1997). Role identity, role investment, and paternal involvement: Implications for parenting programs for me. *Early Childhood Research Quarterly, 12*, 173–197. https://doi.org/10.1016/S0885-2006(97)90013-2

Ninio, A., & Rinott, N. (1988). Fathers' involvement in the care of their infants and their attributions of cognitive competence to infants. *Child Development, 59*(3), 652–663.

Palkovitz, R. (1984). Parental attitudes and fathers' interactions with their five-month-old infants. *Developmental Psychology, 20*, 1054–1060.

Palkovitz, R. (1997). Reconstructing "involvement": Expanding conceptualizations of men's caring in contemporary families. In A. Hawkins & D. Dollahite, (Eds.), Generative Fathering: Beyond Deficit Perspectives. Thousand Oaks, CA: Sage, pp. 200–216.

Palkovitz, R. (2002). *Involved fathering and men's adult development: Provisional balances*. Mahwah, NJ: Lawrence Erlbaum Associates, Inc.

Palkovitz, R. (2007). Challenges to modeling dynamics in a developmental understanding of father-child relationships. *Journal of Applied Developmental Science, 11*, 190–195.

Palkovitz, R. (2018). *Fathering for life: The importance of fathering for child development*. Keynote address at the Taiwan Family Policy Conference, Taipei, Taiwan (October).

Palkovitz, R. (2019). Expanding our focus from father involvement to father-child relationship quality. *Journal of Family Theory & Review, 11*(4), 576–591.

Palkovitz, R., & Hull, J. (2018). Toward a resource theory of fathering. *Journal of Family Theory & Review, 10*(1), 181–198.

Palkovitz, R., Trask, B. S., & Adamsons, K. (2014). Essential differences in the meaning and processes of mothering and fathering: Family systems, feminist and qualitative perspectives. *Journal of Family Theory and Review, 6*, 406–420.

Palm, G. (2014). Attachment theory and fathers: Moving from "being there" to "being with". *Journal of Family Theory & Review, 6*(4), 282–297.

Pasley, K., Futris, T. G., & Skinner, M. L. (2002). Effects of commitment and psychological centrality on fathering. *Journal of Marriage and Family, 64*(1), 130–138.

Peluso, P. R., Peluso, J. P., White, J. F., & Kern, R. M. (2004). A comparison of attachment theory and individual psychology: A review of the literature. *Journal of Counseling & Development, 82*(2), 139–145.

Sabey, A. K., Rauer, A. J., Haselschwerdt, M. L., & Volling, B. (2018). Beyond "lots of hugs and kisses": Expressions of parental love from parents and their young children in two parent, financially stable families. *Family Process, 57*(3), 737–751.

Sameroff, A. (2009). *The transactional model*. New York: American Psychological Association.

Shannon, J. D., Tamis-LeMonda, C. S., & Cabrera, N. J. (2006). Fathering in infancy: Mutuality and stability between 8 and 16 months. *Parenting, 6*(2–3), 167–188.

Slade, A. (2005). Parental reflective functioning: An introduction. *Attachment & Human Development, 7*(3), 269–281.

Solomon, J., & George, C. (1996). Defining the caregiving system: Toward a theory of caregiving. *Infant Mental Health Journal: Official Publication of the World Association for Infant Mental Health, 17*(3), 183–197.

Tronick, E. Z. (1989). Emotions and emotional communication in infants. *American Psychologist, 44*, 112–119.

Tronick, E. Z., Bruschweiler Stern, N., Harrison, A. M., Lyons Ruth, K., Morgan, A. C., Nahum, J. P., et al. (1998). Dyadically expanded states of consciousness and the process of therapeutic change. *Infant Mental Health Journal: Official Publication of the World Association for Infant Mental Health, 19*(3), 290–299.

Van IJzendoorn, M. H., & De Wolff, M. S. (1997). In search of the absent father—Meta analyses of infant father attachment: A rejoinder to our discussants. *Child Development, 68*(4), 604–609.

Volling, B. L., McElwain, N. L., Notaro, P. C., & Herrera, C. (2002). Parents' emotional availability and infant emotional competence: Predictors of parent-infant attachment and emerging self-regulation. *Journal of Family Psychology, 16*(4), 447.

Vollotton, C., Foster, T., Harewood, T., Cook, J., & Adekoya, A. (2020). Fathers and young children at play: A scoping review of studies of father figures play with sons and daughters from birth to preschool. In H. E. Fitzgerald, K. von Klitzing, N. Cabrera, J. S. de Mendonca, & T. Skjothaug (Eds.), *Handbook of fathers and child development: Prenatal to preschool.* Springer Nature: Gham, Switzerland.

4 The Role of Fathers in the Intergenerational Transmission of (Dis)advantages: Linking Sociological Stratification Questions to Developmental Psychology Research

Renske Keizer

The target deadline of the Millennium Declaration, and the Millennium Developmental Goals (MDG) as its practical and measurable articulation, was reached in 2015. Evaluations show that progress has been made in improving child outcomes worldwide (Hulme, 2009), although readers have to be aware that the picture is most likely too rosy, given that mental and emotional disorders among young children often go undetected (Lyons-Ruth et al., 2017). Despite progress, the MDGs have also left some major issues on the table. Some of the most important, and challenging ones, are SES inequalities, i.e., inequalities in (children's) social, behavioral, emotional, cognitive, psychological, and financial outcomes by socioeconomic status. The MDGs focus on average progress measured at the country and global level has masked inequalities that lie behind these averages (Kabeer, 2010): studies show that even in countries where there has been progress toward the MDGs, inequalities in child outcomes have grown. Realizing that the issue of inequality has been neglected, the post-2015 development agenda has prioritized combating inequality (UN, 2012; Save the Children, 2012). Scholarly attention for the issue of inequality, in the last decade, has been directed toward obtaining a better understanding of how social (dis)advantages are transmitted intergenerationally to children. There is now consensus in the literature that the intergenerational transmission of (dis)advantages from parents onto their children is often filtered through intra-familial dynamics, in particular parenting (Conger, Conger, & Martin, 2010; Ermisch, Jantti, & Smeeding, 2012; Kalil, 2014; Lareau, 2000; McLanahan, 2004; Putnam, 2015). Parenting creates a largely unseen but distinct division line between families, leading to widening gaps in social mobility and inequality that may last for generations (Kalil & Mayer, 2016; McLanahan, 2004; Putnam, 2015).

Historically, studies that have examined the impact of parenting on inequality in child outcomes have mainly focused on mothers (Augustine, Cavanagh, & Crosnoe, 2009; Augustine, Prickett, & Kimbro, 2016; Hsin & Felfe, 2014; Kalil, Ryan, & Corey, 2012; Milkie, Nomaguchi, & Denny, 2015). We know comparatively little about how inequalities develop through father's parenting. This is startling, given that current demographic trends

R. Keizer (✉)
Erasmus School of Social and Behavioral Sciences, Erasmus University Rotterdam, Rotterdam, The Netherland
e-mail: keizer@essb.eur.nl

H. E. Fitzgerald et al. (eds.), *Handbook of Fathers and Child Development*,
https://doi.org/10.1007/978-3-030-51027-5_4

may exacerbate in particular fathers' role in the intergenerational transmission of (dis)advantages. Father involvement has become, and much more so than maternal involvement, increasingly polarized (Edin, Tach, & Nelson, 2014; Furstenberg Jr., 1988; Settersten & Cancel-Tirado, 2010). Specifically, higher educated fathers, who have significant skills and resources, flexible jobs, and stable families, are increasingly able to expand their fathering roles beyond breadwinning, and these men are also more likely to adhere to norms of intensive parenting. Lower educated men, on the other hand, have been retreating from their roles as fathers altogether (Perelli-Harris et al., 2011; Roy, 2014). This suggests that deriving benefits from fathers' parenting might have increasingly become a higher social class privilege (Settersten & Cancel-Tirado, 2010) and, therefore, fathers' parenting may play a pivotal role in the intergenerational transmission of (dis) advantages.

In this chapter, I argue that much can be learned about the influence fathers have on their children's development and, more specifically, about how inequalities in child outcomes develop through fathers' parenting, by linking sociological stratification questions to developmental psychology research on father involvement. The chapter will start with a review of the sociological literature on fathers' role in the intergenerational transmission of (dis)advantages. Then, I review developmental psychological/pedagogical literature on the role of father-child interactions in child development. Subsequently, I will briefly discuss two existing theories that have integrated sociological and developmental psychological insights on the role of parents in the intergenerational transmission of (dis)advantages, and I will show what these theories have taught us so far about fathers' role in the intergenerational transmission of (dis)advantages. Finally, I will elaborate on the limitations of these existing theories and provide suggestions for future theoretical developments on fathers' role in the intergenerational transmission of (dis) advantages.

The Role of Fathers in the Sociological Stratification Literature

Theory

A sociological perspective on fathers' roles in children's lives assumes that fathers influence their children's development primarily via the intergenerational transmission of economic, social, and cultural resources. These resources are unequally generated and distributed across families, and differ by socioeconomic status. Socioeconomic status (SES) is a combined economic and sociological measure of a person's economic and social position in relation to that of others, based on income, education, and occupational status. Traditionally, scholars have solely used fathers' SES as indicator of family SES, given that many mothers, until the 1960s, were not active on the labor market or had to leave the labor force once they entered marriage and/or became pregnant.

Prevailing sociological theories on how parental SES may contribute to inequalities in child outcomes rely either on a parental investment model (i.e., parental investment of time and money) and/or on a socialization/social reproduction model (i.e., parental or school socialization through modeling or teaching). When investigating the influence of parents' SES, scholars often, based on the work of Bourdieu (1986), differentiate between the economic, social, and cultural aspects of SES. Bourdieu argued that positions in the social world can best be ordered according to differences in the amount and composition of economic, social, and cultural capital. Economic capital refers to the benefits that individuals or families have accumulated by virtue of having money, property, and/or wealth. With respect to economic capital, fathers with higher SES can advance their children's outcomes by providing them with financial resources (i.e., being able to pay tuition for private schooling, being able to pay for piano lessons or sport memberships). Social capital refers to the benefits accruing to individuals or families by virtue of their ties with others. With respect to social capital, fathers with higher SES can be involved in clubs or are members of certain associations that help their children move higher up the socioeconomic ladder. Finally, cultural capital refers to people's knowledge, intellectual skills, social abilities, norms, and values that provide advantages in achieving a higher social status in society. With respect to cultural capital, fathers with higher SES status can help their children do well in school by familiarizing them with those actions and content (i.e., museums, books, and digital media) that are valued in the educational system. In particular, with respect to differences in cultural capital, scholars have argued and shown that parents with different levels of SES hold different values related to childrearing (e.g., Kohn, 1963) and differ in how they parent their children (Lareau, 2002).

Kohn showed that parents transfer values that are appreciated in the workforce to their children. In middle- and higher-class jobs, skills such as intellectual stimulation and independent decision-making are desired. As a consequence, middle and higher social class parents internalize "self-direction" in their behavior, and, albeit consciously or unconsciously, socialize their children in these skills. Lower class jobs often require skills such as conformity to rules and requirements; skills that are subsequently internalized and passed on to their children. Lareau (2000) showed that parents from higher social classes are more aware of the importance of time investments in cultivating children's human and social capital. Using data collected from extensive fieldwork among 88 white and black children from middle class, working class, and poor families, Lareau (2002) argued that middle and higher class families engage in *concerted cultivation:* engaging in deliberate efforts to facilitate their children's development by enrolling them in several leisure activities, by engaging in active parenting that includes intervening and advocating on their child's behalf in social institutions, and by creating a cognitive stimulating home environment using language games and educational material (i.e., books). An important advantage of this form of parenting is that children learn how to get along with both adults and same-age peers through organized activities. In addition, children develop a "sense of entitlement": they have experiences in which their opinions matter and are taken into consideration. Lower class families, on the other hand, rely to a greater extent on *natural growth*: They perceive children's development as more spontaneous, and thus create a relatively less orchestrated environment. Lower class children participate less in organized activities and spend more of their free time with other children in the neighborhood. They learn how to get along with each other on the street, often outside the realm of parental supervision. The desired attitude with respect to adults and parents is that of obedience. Whereas both approaches to parenting have their advantages, Lareau argues that schools' expectations of the parental role are more in line with *concerted cultivation*. The parenting practices of middle/higher social class parents thus generate behaviors, beliefs, and attitudes that are relatively more beneficial for their children's developmental and life outcomes.

In sum, a sociological perspective on fathers' role in the intergenerational transmission of (dis) advantages assumes that fathers influence their children's development primarily via the intergenerational transmission of economic, social, and cultural capital. This capital is unequally generated and distributed across families, and differs by SES. As such, from a sociological perspective, fathers can play a key role in stratification processes, as fathers socialize their children into their class positions. Below I will provide a short overview of recent findings on linkages between fathers' SES, fathers' parental involvement, and child outcomes.

Empirical Findings for Linkages Between Fathers' SES, Fathers' Parental Involvement, and Child Outcomes

SES is a construct that captures various dimensions of a person's economic and social position, including prestige, power, and economic well-being. There is consensus among scholars that income, education, and occupational status provide adequate coverage of these dimensions (Bradley & Corwyn, 2002). Scholars have argued that each of these dimensions demonstrates different levels of stability across time and differentially predicts family processes and child adjustment (Duncan & Magnuson, 2003).

When scholars use the theoretical framework in which parenting practices are conceptualized as class-specific cultural practices, most attention has been devoted to parents' educational attainment. Given that in most societies mothers still shoulder childcare responsibilities and are often the primary caretaker (e.g., Dermott, 2015; Doucet, 2013, most of these studies have investigated how mothers' educational attainment socializes children into their class positions. There are relatively fewer studies that have investigated the role that fathers' educational attainment plays. Nevertheless, there is empirical evidence that fathers' educational attainment is related to fathers' parental involvement. Several studies have shown that highly educated fathers are more involved in both developmental and routine childcare activities than their lower-educated counterparts (Bianchi, Robinson, & Milkie, 2006; Hook & Wolfe, 2012; Marsiglio, 1991). A recent study by Altintas (2016) showed that higher-educated fathers spend significantly more time in developmental childcare activities, and that the gap between high- and low-educated parents' time investment in developmental childcare activities has widened over the years. In line with these findings, Gracia (2014) showed that father's education had a significant positive effect on his physical care when the youngest child was aged 0–5 and a significant positive effect in his interactive care, especially in teaching activities, when the youngest child was aged 3–5 years. Studies also show that higher educated fathers are more likely to read to their children (Cabrera, Hofferth, & Chae, 2011; Duursma, Pan, & Raikes, 2008; Malin et al., 2012) and have more frequent interactions than can be characterized as playful (e.g., Grossmann et al., 2002). Although most of these studies have been conducted in high-income countries, similar findings are found in low- and middle-income countries. Using data from 98,464 three- and four-year-old children in 44 low- and middle-income countries, Jeong, McCoy, and Fink (2017) found robust associations between both fathers' education levels and children's development scores. Controlling for the impact of mothers' education and mothers' provision of support for learning, they found that fathers' provision of support for learning (i.e., books, stimulating interactions) was a key mechanism through which parental education relates to children's development. Finally, although most of the abovementioned findings pertain to young children, studies have also revealed that higher-educated fathers are more engaged in their adolescent children's academic activities than lower-educated ones (e.g., Yeung, Sandberg, Davis-Kean, & Hofferth, 2001). When scholars use the theoretical framework in which SES is linked with time investments in children, scholars have often turned to employment status and employment hours. Again, most of the literature has focused on mothers. The literature on linkages between fathers' employment and father involvement is inconclusive. There are studies that find a negative association between employment and father involvement (Roeters, Lippe, & Kluwer, 2009), but others find no or only very weak associations between fathers' employment and time spent with children (Hook & Wolfe, 2012; Pleck & Masciadrelli, 2004). McGill (2014) showed in her study that fathers' work hours were negatively related to father involvement, albeit only with respect to physical care for children. Fathers' work hours did not have an impact on the level of responsibility the father took for caring for his child, nor did it impact the amount of time farther spent in play or activity-related activities with his child. The sparse literature on linkages between paternal employment and child outcomes is also inconclusive (Parcel & Menaghan, 1994; Harvey, 1999). However, moderation effects are found. For example, Harvey showed that for low-income families, fathers' working more hours tended to be associated with higher language scores for children, whereas the opposite was true for high-income families. These somewhat counterintuitive findings suggest that fathers' work hours imply different things for families with different levels of income. When families have difficulties making ends meet, fathers' increased work hours may benefit their children's outcomes as increased work hours implies more (much needed) income, whereas for families that have no difficulties making ends meet, increased work hours may be detrimental for children's outcomes, as increased work hours implies that fathers can spend less time with their children. Given the lack of direct effects for paternal employment, scholars are turning to other occupational measures for fathers. A recent study by Gracia (2012) showed that fathers employed in post-industrial occupations are more involved in childcare and sociocultural activities with children than those employed in industrial occupations.

When scholars use the theoretical framework in which SES is associated with financial resources, they have used measures of family income or combined measures of educational attainment and occupational status with income to construct an overall SES index. Only rarely do studies investigate the individual contribution of fathers' income to paternal involvement or child outcomes across the entire spectrum of the income distribution. However, scholars have investigated paternal involvement among low-income fathers (e.g., Bocknek, Brophy-Herb, Fitzgerald, Schiffman, & Vogel, 2014; Cabrera, Ryan, Mitchell, Shannon, & Tamis-LeMonda, 2008; Duursma et al., 2008). With notable exceptions, these studies on low-income fathers often pertain to non-resident fathers, making it difficult to assess differences in the impact of low- versus high-income fathers, given that the nature of their involvement often differs substantially (daily interactions of resident fathers versus child support payment and face to face contact of non-resident fathers). Nevertheless, there is consensus in the literature that fathers' financial resources enable families, among others, to afford houses in safer neighborhoods and to buy nutritious food, which in turn predict desirable childhood outcomes, including cognitive skills (Cabrera & Peters, 2000).

Limitations of a Sociological Perspective on Fathers' Role in the Intergenerational Transmission of Inequality

Although the abovementioned sociological perspectives underscore that fathers with higher SES status have more resources to invest in their children's developmental outcomes and that their socialization practices prepare their children better for positions higher on the societal ladder, neither of the two sociological perspectives engages with the emotional and/or relational aspects of parenting. This limits our understanding of the processes through which inequalities are transmitted across generations (see for similar criticism Moulin, Waldfogel, & Washbrook, 2017).

In contrast, developmental psychologists argue that fathers influence their children's development exactly through those characteristics that sociologists have neglected: via the quality of the interactions fathers have with their children. For a full and comprehensive understanding of the processes through which fathers transmit (dis) advantages onto the next generation, we need to complement the ones that we have derived from the sociological literature with those from the developmental psychological/pedagogical literature.

The Role of the Father in the Developmental Psychology/Pedagogical Literature

Theory

Although fathers have always played a central role in the sociological stratification literature, the role of fathers in their children's lives has only relatively recently gained ground in the developmental psychology/pedagogical literature. In these fields, parenting research has typically focused on questions regarding what mothers do with, and for, their children, and what influence maternal involvement has on children's development. The importance of father involvement only came into focus in the early 1970s

(Lamb & Lewis, 2013). At that time, paternal involvement was operationalized most frequently in terms of co-residence: fathers' presence in the child's household. The next generation of scholars refined the definition of father involvement, defining it in terms of time spent with the child, regardless of the type of activities undertaken. Little evidence was found, however, for a significant link between fathers' total amount of time spent with children and child development. Subsequently, fathering research gradually shifted toward conceptualizing father involvement as father's direct engagement with the child, through caretaking and other shared activities that might potentially promote child development (Pleck, 2007). Over time, the notion of the father as a co-parent gained ground (Pleck & Pleck, 1997), according to which fathers share the responsibilities of childrearing with mothers. To keep pace with flouring conceptualizations of fatherhood, research on father involvement evolved to encompass qualitative dimensions as well, including warmth and control (or: demandingness; Maccoby & Martin, 1983; Pleck, 2004). As readers might be able to tell from this brief description of historical developments in the field, the literature on fathers' role in child development has mainly been guided by societal questions, demographic developments, and empirical findings. Empirical studies on fathers' role in child development are abundant, but there are not many overarching theoretical perspectives to specifically "frame the conceptualization of fathering as an activity and of fatherhood as a status" (Lewis & Lamb, 2007, page 3), but see Pleck (2007) for a short overview of theoretical perspectives on fathers' influences on child development. I will therefore discuss more general frameworks on the quality of parent-child interactions below to understand the processes that underlie the influence of fathers on their children's lives.

Bronfenbrenner's (1979, 1986) ecological perspective on human development is one of the most commonly used frameworks to understand child development. In his model, different systems are identified that are nested within each other and that each has, by themselves, but also in interaction, an influence on children's development. Bronfenbrenner's ecological theory describes that children first and foremost develop through interactions with their immediate environment in the microsystem (i.e., proximal processes). As such, the quality of caregiver-child interactions is of the utmost importance in defining children's everyday experiences and in explaining developmental outcomes. In general, it is argued that high-quality parent-child interactions—characterized by sensitive and supportive parents who provide security and confidence—help children flourish, regardless of parents' gender. Sensitive parents are those parents who are able to perceive and to interpret accurately the signals and communications implicit in their infant's behavior, and given this understanding, to respond to them appropriately and promptly (Ainsworth, Blehar, Waters, & Wall, 2015). In contrast, parent-child interactions that are characterized as harsh, intrusive, or neglectful (rather than warm, and responsive) are considered to be detrimental for children's development.

Sensitivity is not only a central concept in the proximal processes described in Bronfenbrenner's ecological model. It also plays a key role in attachment theory. Attachment theory (Bowlby, 1982) is one of the most commonly used frameworks to understand how children's (socio-emotional and behavioral) skills develop through the parent-child relationship in the first years of life. Attachment theory centralizes the "affectionate bond" between a caregiver and a child. This bond is activated in times of distress and becomes visible in the child's preferential desire for proximity and/or contact with the caregiver. Attachment theory indicates that secure parent-child attachment relationships promote positive feelings of self-worth and importance (Sroufe, 2002; Thompson, 2006). More specifically, the trustworthy warmth of parents provides a foundation for children in infancy to develop mental representations of themselves (internal working model) as loveable and worthy of care. The trust generated by a supportive parent–child attachment relationship provides children with the confidence to explore and engage in new experiences while knowing that the parents' assistance is available. The positive internal working model gained from this fosters cognitive development and skills acquisition as well as social and emotional development. At the core of attachment theory is the claim that infants not only become attached to their biological mother but also to other caregivers who interact regularly with them, including fathers.

There are scholars who have argued that mothers and fathers have distinct and complementary attachment roles; the mother-child attachment relationship is posited to primarily provide warmth and security, whereas exploration is posited to be more central to the father-child attachment relationship. For this reason, the father-child attachment relationship has been coined an "activation relationship" (Dumont & Paquette, 2013). Paquette (2004) states that while mothers play an important role in children's need to be calmed and secured, the father-activation relationship satisfies the children's need to be stimulated, to overcome limits, and to learn to take chances. According to this theory, fathers represent the outside world, and tend to encourage their children to take risks more often than mothers do. Fathers, more than mothers, may demand their children to express and think over their ideas, encourage them to take initiative, and teach them that it is okay to disagree with each other. By promoting their autonomy, fathers are argued to facilitate the process of becoming more agentic.

In sum, these developmental psychological/pedagogical theories assume that fathers influence their children's development primarily via paternal sensitivity (the quality of father-child interactions) and (subsequently) via the nature and the quality of the father-child attachment and activation relationship.

Empirical Findings

There is general consensus in the literature that sensitive and supportive fathers have children who have fewer behavioral and emotional problems (for reviews see Cabrera, Tamis-LeMonda, Bradley, Hofferth, & Lamb, 2000; Lamb & Lewis, 2013). Furthermore, fathers' sensitive and supportive interactions have been linked to higher cognitive and language development and school achievement of children (Cabrera, Shannon, & Tamis-Le-Monda, 2007; Malin, Cabrera, & Rowe, 2014; Pancsofar & Vernon-Feagans, 2010; Tamis-LeMonda, Baumwell, & Cabrera, 2013). In addition, multiple studies have shown that the quality of fathers' interactions with their children is important for the development of empathy and social development in both sons and daughters (Leidy, Schofield, & Parke, 2013). In addition, research shows that the security of children's attachments to both their mother and to their father impact children's development, although there has been much less research on the impact of father-child than of mother-child attachment (Cowan & Cowan, 2019; see for a review Lamb & Lewis, 2013; Ranson & Urichuk, 2008). Some studies show that infant-mother attachments have more consistent predictive power than infant-father attachment, especially in two-parent families. Nevertheless, there is evidence that father-child and mother-child attachment both have independent and non-overlapping effects on children's development (e.g., Buttitta et al., 2019; Cowan, Cowan, Pruett, & Pruett, 2019; Grossmann et al., 2002; see for a review Lamb & Lewis, 2013).

Other studies find evidence for the importance of the father-child activation relationship for child outcomes (e.g., Dumont & Paquette, 2013; Gaumon & Paquette, 2013; Paquette & Dumont, 2013). Gaumon and Paquette, for example, find that the more positively activated children were in their relationship with their father, the fewer internalizing disorders they displayed. Although these studies highlight the importance of the father-child activation relationship for children's development, it is too preliminary to draw the conclusion that the activation relationship is unique to the father-child relationship, as the scholars involved in this line of work have not (yet) tested the importance of an equivalent mother-activation relationship for child outcomes.

Limitations of a Developmental Psychological/Pedagogical Perspective on Fathers' Role in the Intergenerational Transmission of Inequality

Although the abovementioned theories had close detail for the qualitative aspects of fathers' parenting and parent-child relationships, and offer a model of the micro-level processes that connect fathers' parenting processes to children's developmental outcomes, it generally does not take structural opportunities and constraints into account. It therefore often underestimates the degree to which social forces shape psychological states (Settersten Jr., 2009). Attachment theory, for example, even though one of its aims is to explain intergenerational continuities in human development, neglects the social and economic contexts in which parent-child bonds are embedded (see Mesman, van Ijzendoorn, & Sagi-Schwarz, 2016; Moulin et al., 2017).

Nevertheless, there is an increasing awareness in the developmental psychological/pedagogical literature that socioeconomic circumstances should be taken into account (e.g., Mesman et al., 2016 in Handbook of Attachment, p. 869). This might especially be important for fathers, as previous studies have shown that fathering is influenced to a greater extent than mothering, by contextual factors in the family (e.g., Bureau et al., 2017). Recent studies indeed suggest that socioeconomic characteristics are in particular important for fathers' quality of parenting. Teufl, Deichmann, Supper, and Ahnert (2019) showed that fathers' education was related to father-child attachment security, whereas the same was not observed for mothers.Although scholars in the field of psychology have proposed insightful ecological models of human development (such as the abovementioned model by Bronfenbrenner) and father involvement in particular (e.g., Cabrera, Fitzgerald, Bradley, & Roggman, 2014), such models are frequently misused in empirical work, overlooking the complex interplay between proximal processes and context (Tudge, Mokrova, Hatfield, & Karnik, 2009). We need to more closely integrate insights from sociological stratification studies into the developmental psychology literature on fathers' role in child outcomes, to be able to understand how inequalities in children's developmental outcomes develop through fathers' parenting. Below I will briefly discuss two existing theories that have integrated sociological and developmental psychological insights on the role of parents in the intergenerational transmission of (dis)advantages, and I will show what these theories have taught us so far about fathers' role in the intergenerational transmission of (dis)advantages. Finally, I will elaborate on the limitations of these existing theories and provide suggestions for future theoretical developments on fathers' role in the intergenerational transmission of (dis)advantages.

Existing theories that link SES to qualitative dimensions of fathers' parenting and child development

In this section, I describe two existing theoretical models that have integrated sociological and developmental psychological insights on the role of parents in the intergenerational transmission of (dis)advantages: the Family Stress Model (FSM) and the Interactionist Model of Socioeconomic Influence (IMSI). The Family Stress Model (e.g., Conger et al., 1992, 1993; Conger & Conger, 2002) posits that parenting reflects the influence of economic hardship. Stress and anxieties related to economic and financial struggles negatively affect the well-being of parents and strain the relationship between them. This heightened level of stress is then predicted to disrupt parenting, namely leading to harsher forms of parenting and hampering parental warmth and support. As such, economic hardship obstacles children's development through disrupting parenting. Numerous studies have investigated each arrow in the causal model of the FSM (for reviews see Conger & Donnellan, 2007; Masarik & Conger, 2017). Scholars have shown that economic hardship increases depressive symptoms among parents, which leads to harsher parenting as well as lower parental warmth (Guo & Harris, 2000; Gershoff, Aber, Raver, & Lennon, 2007; Kiernan & Huerta, 2008; Turney, 2012; Rijlaarsdam et al., 2013; Treanor, 2016; Sosu & Schmidt, 2017). Harsh parenting and lower parental warmth, subsequently, are related to more detrimental developmental outcomes for children (e.g., Pinquart, 2017).

Most of these studies, however, have been restricted to mothers. This is quite unfortunate, as the studies that include both mothers and fathers suggest that fathers' parenting practices may play a different role than mothers' in the intergenerational transmission of (dis)advantages. For example, Karras (2015) showed that material hardship only had a direct impact on fathers' symptoms of depression, while it had direct effects on both mothers' symptoms of anxiety and depression. Furthermore, she showed that fathers' parenting stress was related to his spanking behavior but not to his engagement with his child, while mothers' parenting stress was related to both. Wadsworth et al. (2013) also found differential processes for fathers and mothers in testing the Adaptation to Poverty-related Stress Model. They showed that economic strain reductions were uniquely associated with increased positive father–child relationships only, where secondary control coping was uniquely associated with decreases in negative mother–child relationships only. Furthermore, they found an indirect effect of reduced economic strain on child symptoms via positive parent–child interactions for fathers only. This suggests that the processes through which SES, in particular economic hardship, influences parenting and subsequently child outcomes differ by parent's gender. These findings underscore the importance of paying attention to the role that fathers, above and beyond mothers, play in the intergenerational transmission of (dis) advantages.

One of the big advantages of the FSM is that it provides a theoretical model for how SES (here: economic hardship) influences mothers' and fathers' parenting quality and subsequently child outcomes. As such, it integrates sociological insights on stratification with the developmental psychology literature on causal linkages between SES, parenting, and child outcomes. Nevertheless, the focus of the FSM is quite restricted from the perspective of Bourdieu's notion of economic, social, and cultural capital, as the focus is only put on the influence of a lack of economic capital. It is just as important and interesting to investigate to what extent the presence of economic, social, and cultural capital has on parenting quality and parent-child interactions and subsequently child outcomes.

This limitation is overcome in the Interactionist Model of Socioeconomic Influence (IMSI; Conger & Dogan, 2007 and Conger & Donnellan, 2007). The IMSI utilizes a broader lens on the influence of SES, and combines insights derived from both the parental involvement model and the family stress model to understand how SES through family processes influences child development. In addition to these two causal perspectives, it also incorporates a social selection perspective. The argument being that establishing a causal link that goes from SES to parenting to child outcomes requires accounting for selection effects as well. The model stresses the importance of controlling for characteristics of parents and children (e.g., parents' own genes, personality traits, childhood experiences, children's cognitive and non-cognitive skills) that may influence both the adaptation of different parenting practices as well as the experience of economic hardship. A big advantage of this model is that it allows for interplays between individual attributes and socioeconomic conditions across time and across multiple generations (Martin et al., 2010).

Compared to the FSM, the IMSI is relatively more new. Nevertheless, several studies have unfolded demonstrating how social selection and causation both play a role in linkages between SES, parenting, and child outcomes (e.g., Martin et al., 2010; Schofeld et al., 2011; Conger, Martin, Masarik, Widaman, & Donnellan, 2015). These studies revealed that personality (Schofeld) and behavior characteristics (Conger; Martin) of first-generation family members influenced their own SES as an adult, their levels of family stress and parental emotional investments, and also the behavioral characteristics of their child. In addition, the study by Martin et al. (2010) showed that SES was related to family stress of the member of the first generation. The family stress of this person subsequently influenced his/her child's behavioral outcomes. Furthermore, the adult SES of the first-generation family member influenced both material and emotional investments in his/her child. These material and emotional investments, in turn, predicted the behavioral outcomes of the child.

Accounting for selection effects, findings from studies applying the IMSI suggest that fathers play an important role in the intergenerational transmission of (dis)advantages, and they suggest that the processes differ between fathers and mothers. For example, the study by Martin et al. (2010) showed that the relationship between the first-generation family member's behavioral characteristics and their own parental emotional investments was only there for fathers. The relationship between family stress experienced by the first-generation family member and behavioral characteristics of their child was only there for mothers. Finally, the association between material investments of the first-generation's family member and their child's behavioral characteristics was only there for fathers. Again, these findings hint to an important role played by fathers in the intergenerational transmission of (dis)advantages and suggest that the processes that underlie the intergenerational transmission of (dis)advantages differ by fathers and mothers.

In sum, integrating insights from the sociological and the developmental psychology/pedagogical literature, both the FSM and the IMSI models highlight, although based on a relatively limited number of studies, that fathers play an important and sometimes different role compared to mothers, in the intergenerational transmission of (dis)advantages. More research that includes both mothers and fathers is needed to be able to draw a firm conclusion concerning the role that fathers play in the intergenerational transmission of (dis)advantages.

The Complex Interplay Between Proximal Processes and Context: Limitations of Existing Models and Suggestions for Future Theoretical Developments

Although the FSM and the IMSI help us advance our understanding of the role that fathers play in the intergenerational transmission of (dis)advantages, their conceptual models somewhat restrict us in the questions that we are able to answer about fathers' role. Below I will mention these limitations and formulate five suggestions for future theoretical developments.

Moving Beyond Mediation: Interactions between Fathers' SES and Parenting on Child Outcomes

The theoretical models mentioned above assume that the impact of the key characteristics in the model (personal characteristics, SES, family processes, child development) is unconditional. However, individuals (here: fathers) are active agents who not only mediate the effect of social structure but also make decisions and set goals that shape social structure. The ability to make specific choices or adapt to life events varies with people's resources or supports in the form of economic, cultural, and social capital. Thus, even though in theory all individuals and families can construct, negotiate, and traverse life course events, experiences, and outcomes, some are more successful in doing so than others. This suggests that a mediational model (from SES to father's parenting practices to child outcomes) may not suffice, as the effects of father involvement on child outcomes among low SES fathers are likely different from those among higher SES fathers, which implies moderation.

One the one hand, in line with the work of McLanahan's (2004) and Kalil et al. (2012) notion of a "developmental gradient", it can be argued that children from higher SES fathers benefit more from their fathers' parental involvement and parenting practices compared to children from lower SES fathers. By means of their social, economic, and cultural capital, fathers with higher SES might be better able to adjust the activities and the arrangements they make for their children to the needs of their child (Kalil et al., 2012). Or, arguing from the perspective of lower SES fathers, poverty and lower levels of education, which are associated with parental stress and harsh parenting, may limit the benefits of low-SES fathers' parental involvement and parenting practices for their children. Both ways of reasoning suggest that the same levels of parental involvement would yield greater returns for higher SES fathers in terms of their children's development. In line with these ideas, several studies have revealed that the impact of personal characteristics and parenting practices on child outcomes may depend on the level of SES. For example, the study by Reeb, Conger, and Martin (2013) revealed that the level of perceived economic strain that fathers perceive exacerbates the effect of paternal depressed mood on their hostile parenting behaviors. The study by Cabus and Ariës (2017) showed that even though parents with low SES are as much involved in the education of their children as the average Dutch family, their involvement is less effective in terms of children's learning outcomes.

On the other hand, fathers' involvement among low SES families may be more beneficial than for those in higher-SES families, since children in higher SES families have numerous other advantages and resources to fall back on. In their bioecological model of human development, Bronfenbrenner and Ceci (1994) posit that proximal processes in a child's immediate environment—such as parental involvement—promote child development more strongly in disadvantaged environments because the children in them have the most to gain. In this light, recent studies have revealed that fathers' parenting practices could offset the effects of socioeconomic disadvantage on children's cognitive outcomes (Hango, 2005). Future studies should follow up on this observation and investigate to what extent fathers' parenting practices might actually mitigate or strengthen the intergenerational transmission of (dis)advantages.

Moving Beyond Mothers' and Fathers' Independent Contributions

In the developmental and pedagogical literature, there is consensus that father-child relationships do not exist in a vacuum, but are instead contingent on other family relationships (e.g., Cabrera et al., 2014) and that the impact of father-child relationships on child development should be investigated while taking the larger family system into account (e.g., Cabrera, Fitzgerald, Bradley, & Roggman, 2007; Cabrera et al., 2014; Malmberg & Flouri, 2011; Sameroff & MacKenzie, 2003; Schacht, Cummings, & Davies, 2009). However, when investigating the role of parents in the intergenerational transmission of (dis)advantage, this insight has unfortunately not yet been fully incorporated. But please see the branch of literature that focuses on the intergenerational transmission of aggression and more broadly psychopathology for a notable exception (e.g., Ellis, Zucker, & Fitzgerald, 1997; Fitzgerald & Eiden, 2007).

First, scholars often take the SES of the parent with the highest SES as the indicator of the entire family or use family-level indicators of poverty, overlooking what these characteristics for each of the two parents look like. Because of increased educational homogamy (Cherlin, 2010; Komter, Keizer, & Dykstra, 2012), socioeconomic inequalities are more likely to be compounded within households, concentrating all maternal and paternal (dis)advantages on the same children. These trends have led to increased inequality in the availability, and quality of the investments, of (extended) family members (Mare, 2011), which is posed to be a major factor in the widening inequality among children (Esping-Andersen, 2015; Heckman, 2006). For a clear understanding of the role fathers play in passing on (dis)advantages, it is therefore not only important to know the socioeconomic background of fathers themselves, but also to take these characteristics of mothers into account.

Second, when investigating the role of fathers in child development from a family system perspective, scholars often merely control for the influence of mothers or take co-parental characteristics into account (see for a review, Cabrera, Volling, & Barr, 2018). As others have also stressed (Dagan & Sagi-Schwartz, 2018), and in light of our quest to better understand how parents transmit (dis)advantages onto their children, it would be more informative to see the integrative effect of mother-child attachment and father-child attachment on child development. Furthermore, a family system perspective would allow scholars to ascertain how fathers and mothers via dynamics such as marital conflict transmit inequality onto their children.

Moving Beyond Unidimensional or Aggregated Measures of SES

In order to fully understand how inequalities develop via fathers' parenting practices, it is crucial to disaggregate the different indicators of SES. As mentioned earlier, SES is a multidimensional construct capturing prestige, power, and economic well-being. There is consensus among scholars that income, education, and occupational status provide adequate coverage of these dimensions (Bradley & Corwyn, 2002). Unfortunately, scholars have often restricted themselves to using only one indicator of SES or compiling an aggregate measure. Only by disaggregating income, educational attainment, and occupational prestige, are we able to examine whether and through which pathways (i.e., parental investment versus family stress model) fathers' parenting practices mediate the link between SES and child outcomes.

Moving Beyond Infancy and Early Childhood

As children grow up and develop, behaviors within the parent-child relationship also require change in order to meet the new needs of the child. Parenting practices that might have been beneficial in infancy could be inappropriate or counter-effective in middle childhood and/or adolescence. The extent to which parents are able to adjust their involvement and monitor the child is largely based on parents' social, economic, and cultural capital (Kalil et al., 2012). Parents from lower social classes might have fewer abilities to monitor their children and to adjust their involvement accordingly. These findings suggest that, over time, a Matthew effect might occur (Merton, 1968), with better-off fathers, being able to remain a positive influence on their children by adequately monitoring their children, and adjusting the quantity and quality of their parenting to the changing needs of the child. Studies so far have often focused on early childhood. We need to incorporate a wider time span in order to be able to understand whether fathers' role in the intergenerational transmission of inequality actually becomes stronger over the years.

Moving Beyond Micro-level Processes: The Importance of Country Context

Theoretical models such as the FSM and the IMSI leave little room for the influence of macro contextual variables. This is unfortunate, as the extent to which inequalities in child outcomes produced by differences in fathers' parenting practices are mitigated might also strongly depend on the country context, in particular the extent to which policies address inequity in the resources families have to properly develop their children's potential (Cooke & Baxter, 2010; Esping-Andersen, 2015; Saraceno & Keck, 2010). Policies create conditions which may mitigate or strengthen social inequality (Garbarino, Governale, & Kostelny, 2019; Javornik, 2014). It is essential to know whether policies involve payments for care, (paid) leave, or the provision of care services, as the specific combinations of the items that make up policy packages create different options for parents, different possible experiences for children, and they define different responsibilities between mothers and fathers, and between families and society (Saraceno, 2011). When public support is offered in money rather than in kind, families use it to buy help or to augment the family budget while providing care directly. This tradeoff is likely different in families with different socioeconomic circumstances (e.g., Gornick & Meyers, 2008; Leitner, 2003). For example, the less compensated parental leave, the more it produces polarized behaviors among parents, mostly based on social class/education (Korpi, 2000; Saraceno, 2011). In the absence of generous paid paternity leave, mainly high SES fathers are capable to take short periods of (part-time) leave (Korpi, 2000). In line with this idea, research has shown that throughout developed countries, higher educated fathers are more involved in childcare and are more likely to take up paternity leave (Boll, Leppin, & Reich, 2013; Geisler & Kreyenfeld, 2018). It is important to take national context into account when investigating the role of fathers in the intergenerational transmission of (dis)advantages, as effective national polices (e.g., a child-related leave that is accompanied by generous financial benefits could) have the potential to equalize the leave uptake among fathers with different socioeconomic background and consequently lead to fewer social class disparities in children's resources and development. In this light, studies are encouraged to investigate to what extent and how country context buffers or strengthens fathers' role in the intergenerational transmission of (dis)advantages.

Summary and Key Points

Fathers play an important role in children's lives—that is something that all researchers, regardless of their disciplinary background, agree on. However, the perspective on the roles that fathers play differs between disciplines. A sociological perspective on fathers' role assumes that fathers influence their children's development primarily via the intergenerational transmission of economic, social, and cultural resources. These resources are unequally generated and distributed across families, and differ by SES. From a sociological perspective, fathers play a key role in stratification processes, as fathers socialize their children into their class positions. In contrast to the emphasis on investment and socialization, developmental psychological/pedagogical studies focus on fathers' role in the emotional and/or relational aspects of parenting assuming that fathers influence their children's development primarily via paternal sensitivity (the quality of father-child interactions) and via the nature and the quality of the father-child attachment and activation relationship. In this chapter, I have argued that we need both perspectives to obtain a comprehensive understanding of the role that fathers play in the intergenerational transmission of (dis)advantages. I have showed that theoretical models of FSM and IMSI have successfully integrated both perspectives, albeit with limited success when it comes to the understanding of the role that fathers play in the intergenerational transmission of (dis)advantages. This is partly related to the fact that most empirical studies are still restricted to mothers. When studies do take the roles of both mothers and fathers into account, there is suggestive evidence that the processes that underlie the intergenerational transmission of (dis)advantages differ between fathers and mothers. However, more research is needed to obtain a more accurate understanding of fathers' role in the intergenerational transmission of (dis)advantages. In this chapter, I have suggested five research avenues that may help us in accomplishing just that.

We need to:

- Move beyond mediation and assess interactions between fathers' SES and parenting on child outcomes
- Move beyond mothers' and fathers' independent contributions and truly take a family system perspective
- Move beyond unidimensional or aggregated measures of SES
- Move beyond infancy and early childhood
- Move beyond micro-level processes and assess the importance of country context

Obtaining a comprehensive understanding of the role that fathers play in the intergenerational transmission of (dis)advantages is not only important from a scientific perspective, but also from a societal one, in particular given that studies have revealed that it is easier to improve the average level of child outcomes, rather than reduce inequality between social groups in a given society (e.g., Kabeer, 2010). Understanding how inequalities in child outcomes are developed through fathers' parenting practices, and the extent to which micro-, meso-, and macro-level characteristics influence this development, will provide novel input for better-tailored policies to reduce inequality in child outcomes.

Acknowledgements I would like to thank Nicole Lucassen for her helpful comments on a previous version of this chapter. The present study was supported by a grant from the Netherlands Organization for Scientific Research (NWO MaGW VIDI; grant no. 452-17-005) and by a grant from the European Research Council (ERC StG; grant no. 757210).

References

Ainsworth, M. D. S., Blehar, M. C., Waters, E., & Wall, S. N. (2015). *Patterns of attachment: A psychological study of the strange situation*. Psychology Press.

Altintas, E. (2016). The widening education gap in developmental child care activities in the United States, 1965-2013. *Journal of Marriage and Family, 78*, 26–42.

Augustine, J. M., Cavanagh, S. E., & Crosnoe, R. (2009). Maternal education, early child care and the reproduction of advantage. *Social Forces, 88*(1), 1–29.

Augustine, J.M., Prickett, K.C., & Kimbro, R.T. (2016). Health-related parenting among U.S. Families and young children's physical health. *Journal of Marriage and Family*.

Bianchi, S. M., Robinson, J. P., & Milkie, M. A. (2006). *Changing Rhythms of American Family Life*. New York: Russell Sage Foundation.

Bocknek, E. L., Brophy-Herb, H. E., Fitzgerald, H. E., Schiffman, R. F., & Vogel, C. (2014). Stability of biological father presence as a proxy for family stability: Cross-racial associations with the longitudinal development of emotion regulation in toddlerhood. *Journal of Infant Mental Health, 35*, 309–321.

Boll, C., Leppin, J., & Reich, N. (2013). Paternal Childcare and Parental Leave Policies: Evidence from Industrialized Countries. *Review of Economics of the Household, 12*(1), 129–158.

Bourdieu, P. (1986). *The forms of capital*. In *Readings in Economic Sociology*. Oxford: Blackwell Publishers.

Bowlby, J. (1982). Attachment and loss: retrospect and prospect. *American Journal of Orthopsychiatry, 52*(4), 664.

Bradley, R. H., & Corwyn, R. F. (2002). Socioeconomic status and child development. *Annual Review of Psychology, 53*, 371–399.

Bronfenbrenner, U. (1979). *The ecology of human development*. Harvard University Press.

Bronfenbrenner, U. (1986). Ecology of the family as a context for human development: Research perspectives. *Developmental Psychology, 22*(6), 723.

Bronfenbrenner, U., & Ceci, S. J. (1994). Nature-nuture reconceptualized in developmental perspective: A bioecological model. *Psychological Review, 101*(4), 568.

Bureau, J.-F., Martin, J., Yurkowski, K., Schmiedel, S., Quan, J., Moss, E., et al. (2017). Correlates of child–father and child–mother attachment in the preschool years. *Attachment & Human Development, 19*(2), 130–150.

Buttitta, K. V., Smiley, P. A., Kerr, M. L., Rasmussen, H. F., Querdasi, F. R., & Borelli, J. L. (2019). In a father's mind: paternal reflective functioning, sensitive parenting, and protection against socioeconomic risk. *Attachment & Human Development, 21*(5), 445–466.

Cabrera, N., Fitzgerald, H. E., Bradley, R. H., & Roggman, L. (2007). Modeling the dynamics of paternal influences on children over the life course. *Applied Developmental Science, 11*(4), 185–189.

Cabrera, N., Fitzgerald, H. E., Bradley, R. H., & Roggman, L. (2014). The ecology of father-child relationships: An expanded model. *Journal of Family Theory & Review, 6*, 336–354.

Cabrera, N., & Peters, H. E. (2000). Public policies and father involvement. *Marriage & Family Review, 29*(4), 295–314.

Cabrera, N. J., Hofferth, S. L., & Chae, S. (2011). Patterns and predictors of father–infant engagement across race/ethnic groups. *Early Childhood Research Quarterly, 26*, 365–375.

Cabrera, N. J., Ryan, R. M., Mitchell, S. J., Shannon, J. D., & Tamis-LeMonda, C. S. (2008). Low-income, nonresident father involvement with their toddlers: Variation by fathers' race and ethnicity. *Journal of Family Psychology, 22*(4), 643.

Cabrera, N. J., Shannon, J. D., & Tamis-Le-Monda, C. (2007). Fathers' influence on their children's cognitive and emotional development: from toddlers to pre-K. *Applied Developmental Science, 11*(4), 208–213.

Cabrera, N. J., Tamis-LeMonda, C. S., Bradley, R. H., Hofferth, S., & Lamb, M. E. (2000). Fatherhood in the Twenty-First Century. *Child Development, 71*(1), 127–136.

Cabrera, N. J., Volling, B. L., & Barr, R. (2018). Fathers are parents, too! Widening the lens on parenting for children's development. *Child Development Perspectives, 12*(3), 152–157.

Cabus, S. J., & Ariës, R. J. (2017). What do parents teach their children? The effects of parental involvement on student performance in Dutch compulsory education. *Educational Review, 69*(3), 285–302.

Cherlin, A. J. (2010). Demographic trends in the United States: A review of research in the 2000s. *Journal of Marriage and Family, 72*(3), 403–419.

Conger, R. D., & Conger, K. J. (2002). Resilience in Midwestern families: Selected findings from the first decade of a prospective, longitudinal study. *Journal of Marriage and Family, 64*(2), 361–373.

Conger, R. D., Conger, K. J., Elder, G. H., Lorenz, F. O., Simons, R. L., & Whitbeck, L. B. (1993). Family economic stress and adjustment of early adolescent girls. *Developmental Psychology, 29*(2), 206.

Conger, R. D., Conger, K. J., Elder Jr., G. H., Lorenz, F. O., Simons, R. L., & Whitbeck, L. B. (1992). A family process model of economic hardship and adjustment of early adolescent boys. *Child Development, 63*(3), 526–541.

Conger, R. D., Conger, K. J., & Martin, M. J. (2010). Socioeconomic status, family processes, and individual development. *Journal of Marriage and Family, 72*(3), 685–704.

Conger, R. D., & Dogan, S. J. (2007). Social Class and Socialization in Families. In J. E. Grusec & P. D. Hastings (Eds.), *Handbook of Socialization: Theory and Research* (pp. 433–460). New York, NY: Guilford Press.

Conger, R. D., & Donnellan, M. B. (2007). An interactionist perspective on the socioeconomic context of human development. *Annual Review of Psychology, 58*, 175–199.

Conger, R. D., Martin, M. J., Masarik, A. S., Widaman, K. F., & Donnellan, M. B. (2015). Social and economic antecedents and consequences of adolescent aggressive personality: Predictions from the interactionist model. *Development and Psychopathology, 27*(4pt1), 1111–1127.

Cooke, L. P., & Baxter, J. (2010). 'Families' in international context: Comparing institutional effects across western societies. *Journal of Marriage and Family, 72*(3), 516–536.

Cowan, P. A., & Cowan, C. P. (2019). Introduction: bringing dads back into the family. *Attachment & Human Development, 21*(5), 419–425.

Cowan, P. A., Cowan, C. P., Pruett, M. K., & Pruett, K. (2019). Fathers' and mothers' attachment styles, couple conflict, parenting quality, and children's behavior problems: an intervention test of mediation. *Attachment & Human Development, 21*(5), 532–550.

Dagan, O., & Sagi-Schwartz, A. (2018). Early attachment network with mother and father: An unsettled issue. *Child Development Perspectives, 12*(2), 115–121.

Dermott, E., & Miller, T (2015). "More than the sum of its parts? contemporary fatherhood policy, practice and discourse." *Families, Relationships and Societies* 4(2):183–195.

Doucet, A. (2013). Gender roles and fathering. In N. J. Cabrera & C. S. Tamis-LeMonda (Eds.), *Handbook of father involvement* (pp. 297–319). Taylor & Francis: New York, NY.

Dumont, C., & Paquette, D. (2013). What about the child's tie to the father? A new insight into fathering, father-child attachment, children's socio-emotional development and the activation relationship theory. *Early Child Development and Care, 18*(3-4), 430–446.

Duncan, G. J., & Magnuson, K. A. (2003). Off with Hollingshead: socioeconomic resources, parenting, and child development. In M. H. Bornstein & R. H. Bradley (Eds.), *Socioeconomic status, parenting, and child development* (pp. 83–10). Mahwah, NJ: Erlbaum.

Duursma, E., Pan, B. A., & Raikes, H. (2008). Predictors and outcomes of low-income fathers' reading with their toddlers. *Early Childhood Research Quarterly, 23*, 351–365.

Edin, K., Tach, L., & Nelson, T. J. (2014). The diverging destinies of fathers and what it means for children's lives. In P. Amato, S. M. McHale, & A. Booth (Eds.), *Diverging Destinies: Families in an era of increasing inequality*. New York, NY: Springer.

Ellis, D. A., Zucker, R. A., & Fitzgerald, H. E. (1997). The role of family influences in development and risk. *Alcohol Health and Research World, 21*, 218–226.

Ermisch, J., Jantti, M., & Smeeding, T. M. (2012). *From parents to children: The intergenerational transmission of advantage*. New York, NY: Russell Sage.

Esping-Andersen, G. (2015). Welfare regimes and social stratification. *Journal of European Social Policy, 25*(1), 124–134.

Fitzgerald, H. E., & Eiden, R. D. (2007). Paternal alcoholism, family functioning, and infant mental health. *Zero to Three, 27*(4), 11–18.

Furstenberg, F.F., Jr. (1988). Good dads - bad dads: Two faces of fatherhood. In A.J. Cherlin (E.d.), *The Changing American Family and Public Policy* (pp.193-218). Washington, DC: Urban Institute

Garbarino, J., Governale, A., & Kostelny, K. (2019). Parenting and public policy. In M. H. Bornstein (Ed.), *Handbook of parenting. The practice of parenting* (Vol. 5, 3rd ed., pp. 491–514). Routledge: New York.

Gaumon, S., & Paquette, D. (2013). The father–child activation relationship and internalising disorders at preschool age. *Early Child Development and Care, 183*(3-4), 447–463.

Geisler, E., & Kreyenfeld, M. (2018). Policy reform and fathers' use of parental leave in Germany: The role of education and workplace characteristics. *Journal of European Social Policy, 29*(2), 273–291.

Gershoff, E. T., Aber, J. L., Raver, C. C., & Lennon, M. C. (2007). Income is not enough: Incorporating material hardship into models of income associations with parenting and child development. *Child Development, 78*(1), 70–95.

Gornick, J. C., & Meyers, M. K. (2008). Creating gender egalitarian societies: an agenda for reform. *Politics & Society, 36*(3), 313–349.

Gracia, P. (2012). *Diverging Parenting Behavior: Education, Gender, Class, and Institutions*. Dissertation. Universitat Pompeu Fabra.

Gracia, P. (2014). Fathers' child care involvement and children's age in Spain: A time use study on differences by education and mothers' employment. *European Sociological Review, 30*(2), 137–150.

Grossmann, K., Grossmann, K. E., Fremmer-Bombik, E., Kindler, H., Scheuerer-Englisch, H., & Zimmerman, P. (2002). The uniqueness of the child-father attachment relationship: Fathers' sensitive and challenging play as the pivotal variable in a 16-year longitudinal study. *Social Development, 11*(3), 307–331.

Guo, G., & Harris, K. M. (2000). The mechanisms mediating the effects of poverty on children's intellectual development. *Demography, 37*(4), 431–447.

Hango, D. (2005). Parental investment in childhood and educational qualifications: Can greater parental involvement mediate the effects of socioeconomic disadvantage? *Social Science Research, 36*(4), 1371–1390.

Harvey, E. (1999). Short-term and long-term effects of early parental employment on children of the National Longitudinal Survey of Youth. *Developmental Psychology, 35*(2), 445.

Heckman, J. J. (2006). Skill formation and the economics of investing in disadvantaged children. *Science, 312*(5782), 1900–1902.

Hook, J. L., & Wolfe, C. (2012). New fathers? Residential fathers' time with children in four countries. *Journal of Family Issues, 33*(4), 415–450.

Hsin, A., & Felfe, C. (2014). When does time matter? Maternal employment, children's time with parents, and child development. *Demography, 51*(5), 1867–1894.

Hulme, D. (2009). *The Millennium Development Goals (MDGs): A short history of the world's Biggest promise*, BWPI Working Paper, University of Manchester.

Javornik, J. (2014). Measuring state de-familialism: Contesting post-socialist exceptionalism. *Journal of European Social Policy, 24*(3), 240–257.

Jeong, J., McCoy, D. C., & Fink, G. (2017). Pathways between paternal and maternal education, caregivers' support for learning, and early child development in 44 low- and middle-income countries. *Early Childhood Research Quarterly, 41*, 136–148.

Kabeer, N. (2010). *Can the MDGs provide a pathway to social justice? The challenge of Intersecting inequalities*. New York, NY: UN Millennium Achievement Fund.

Kalil, A. (2014). Inequality begins at home: The role of parenting in the diverging destinies of rich and poor children. In P. Amato, S. M. McHale, & A. Booth (Eds.), *Diverging Destinies: Families in an era of increasing inequality*. New York, NY: Springer.

Kalil, A., & Mayer, S. E. (2016). Understanding the importance of parental time with children: Comment on Milkie, Nomaguchi, and Denny (2015). *Journal of Marriage and Family.*

Kalil, A., Ryan, R., & Corey, M. (2012). Diverging destinies: Maternal education and the developmental gradient in time with children. *Demography, 49*(4), 1361–1383.

Karras, C. A. (2015). *Material hardship and children's behavior across early childhood: examining the differential associations of maternal versus paternal parenting behaviors as mediators of material hardship on children's social and behavioral outcomes*. Doctoral dissertation. University of Texas.

Kiernan, K. E., & Huerta, M. C. (2008). Economic deprivation, maternal depression, parenting and children's cognitive and emotional development in early childhood. *The British Journal of Sociology, 59*(4), 783–806.

Kohn, M. L. (1963). Social class and parent-child relationships: An interpretation. *American Journal of Sociology, 68*, 471–480.

Komter, A. E., Keizer, R., & Dykstra, P. A. (2012). The men behind economically successful women: A focus on Dutch dual-earner couples. *Géneros, Multidisciplinary Journal of Gender Studies, 1*(2), 156–187.

Korpi, W. (2000). Faces of inequality: Gender, class and patterns of inequality in different Welfare states. *Social Politics Summer*, 127–191.

Korpi, W., Ferrarini, T., & Englund, S. (2013). Women's opportunities under different family policy constellations: Gender, class, and inequality tradeoffs in western countries re-examined. *Social Politics, 20*(1), 1–40.

Lamb, M., & Lewis, C. (2013). *Father–Child Relationships. In: Cabrera, N.J., Tamis-Le-Monda, C.S. Handbook of Father Involvement: Multidisciplinary perspectives (pp.119-134)* (2nd ed.). New York, NY: Routledge.

Lareau, A. (2000). *Home advantage: Social class and parental intervention in elementary education.* Rowman & Littlefield Publishers.

Lareau, A. (2002). Invisible inequality: Social class and childrearing in black families and white families. *American Sociological Review*, 747–776.

Leidy, M. S., Schofield, T. J., & Parke, R. D. (2013). Father's contributions to children's social development. In N. J. Cabrera & C. S. Tamis-LeMonda (Eds.), *Handbook of Father Involvement: Multidisciplinary perspectives* (pp. 151–167). New York, NY: Routledge.

Leitner, S. (2003). Varieties of Familialism. The caring function of the family in comparative perspective. *European Societies, 5*(4), 353–375.

Lewis, C., & Lamb, M. E. (2007). *Understanding fatherhood: A review of recent research.* Joseph Rowntree Foundation.

Lyons-Ruth, K., Todd Manly, J., Von Klitzing, K., Tamminen, T., Emde, R., Fitzgerald, H., et al. (2017). The worldwide burden of infant mental and emotional disorder. *Report of the taskforce of the world association for infant mental health, 38*, 695–705.

Maccoby, E. E., & Martin, J. A. (1983). Socialization in the context of the family: Parent-child interaction. In P. H. Mussen (Ed.), *Handbook of Child Psychology: Formerly Carmichael's Manual of child psychology.* Wiley.

Malin, J. L., Cabrera, N. J., & Rowe, M. L. (2014). Low-income minority mothers' and fathers' reading and children's interest: Longitudinal contributions to children's receptive vocabulary skills. *Early Childhood Research Quarterly, 29*, 425–432.

Malin, J. L., Karberg, E., Cabrera, N. J., Rowe, M., Cristaforo, T., & Tamis-LeMonda, C. S. (2012). Father–toddler communication in low-income families: The role of paternal education and depressive symptoms. *Family Science, 3*, 155–163.

Malmberg, L.-E., & Flouri, E. (2011). The comparison and interdependence of maternal and Paternal influences on young children's behavior and resilience. *Journal of Clinical Child & Adolescent Psychology, 40*(3), 434–444.

Mare, R. D. (2011). A multigenerational view of inequality. *Demography, 48*(1), 1–23.

Marsiglio, W. (1991). Paternal engagement activities with minor children. *Journal of Marriage and the Family, 53*, 973–986.

Martin, M. J., Conger, R. D., Schofield, T. J., Dogan, S. J., Widaman, K. F., Donnellan, M. B., et al. (2010). Evaluation of the interactionist model of socioeconomic status and problem behavior: A developmental cascade across generations. *Development and Psychopathology, 22*(3), 695–713.

Masarik, A. S., & Conger, R. D. (2017). Stress and child development: A review of the Family Stress Model. *Current Opinion in Psychology, 13*, 85–90.

McGill, B. S. (2014). Navigating new norms of involved fatherhood: Employment, fathering attitudes, and father involvement. *Journal of Family Issues, 35*(8), 1089–1106.

McLanahan, S. (2004). Diverging destinies: How children are faring under the second demographic transition. *Demography, 41*(4), 607–627.

Merton, R. K. (1968). *Social theory and social structure*. New York, NY: The Free Press.

Mesman, J., van Ijzendoorn, M. H., & Sagi-Schwarz, A. (2016). Cross-cultural patterns of attachment. In J. Cassidy & P. R. Shaver (Eds.), *Handbook of Attachment: Theory, research, and clinical applications* (pp. 852–877). New York: Guilford Press.

Milkie, M. A., Nomaguchi, K. M., & Denny, K. E. (2015). Does the amount of time mothers spend with children or adolescents matter? *Journal of Marriage and Family, 77*, 355–372.

Moulin, S., Waldfogel, J., & Washbrook, E. (2017). Parent-child attachment as a mechanism of intergenerational (dis)advantage. Families, Relationships and Societies.

Pancsofar, N., & Vernon-Feagans, L. (2010). Fathers' early contributions to children's language development in families from low-income rural communities. *Early Childhood Research Quarterly, 25*(4), 450–463.

Paquette, D. (2004). Theorizing the father-child relationship: Mechanisms and developmental outcomes. *Human Development, 47*, 193–219.

Paquette, D., & Dumont, C. (2013). Is father–child rough-and-tumble play associated with attachment or activation relationships? *Early Child Development and Care, 183*(6), 760–773.

Parcel, T. L., & Menaghan, E. G. (1994). Early parental work, family social capital, and early childhood outcomes. *American Journal of Sociology, 99*(4), 972–1009.

Perelli-Harris, B., Sigle-Rushton, W., Lappegård, T., Kreyenfeld, M., Berghammer, C., & Keizer, R. (2011). The educational gradient of nonmarital childbearing in Europe: emergence of a pattern of disadvantage? *Population and Development Review, 36*(4), 775–801.

Pinquart, M. (2017). Associations of parenting dimensions and styles with externalizing problems of children and adolescents: An updated meta-analysis. *Developmental Psychology, 53*(5), 873.

Pleck, E. H., & Pleck, J. H. (1997). Fatherhood ideals in the United States: Historical dimensions. In M. E. Lamb (Ed.), *The Role of the Father in Child Development* (pp. 33–48). New York, NY: John Wiley & Sons, Inc..

Pleck, J. H., & Masciadrelli, B. (2004). Paternal involvement in U.S. residential fathers: Levels, sources, and consequences. In M. E. Lamb (Ed.), *The Role of the Father in Child Development* (pp. 222–271). Hoboken, NJ: Wiley.

Pleck, J. H. (2007). Why could father involvement benefit children? Theoretical perspectives. *Applied Development Science, 11*(4), 196–202.

Pleck, J. (2004). Paternal involvement: Revised conceptualization and theoretical linkages with child outcomes. In M. E. Lamb (Ed.), *The Role of the Father in Child Development*. Hoboken, NJ: John Wiley & Sons.

Pleck, E. H., & Pleck, J. H. (1997). Fatherhood ideals in the United States: Historical dimensions. In M. E. Lamb (Ed.), *The Role of the Father in Child Development* (pp. 33–48). New York, NY: John Wiley & Sons, Inc..

Putnam, R. D. (2015). *Our Kids. The American Dream in Crisis*. New York, NY: Simon & Schuster.

Ranson, K. E., & Urichuk, L. J. (2008). The effect of parent–child attachment relationships on child biopsychosocial outcomes: a review. *Early Child Development and Care, 178*(2), 129–152.

Reeb, B. T., Conger, K. J., & Martin, M. J. (2013). Perceived economic strain exacerbates the effect of paternal depressed mood on hostility. *Journal of Family Psychology, 27*(2), 263–270.

Roeters, A., Lippe, T. V. D., & Kluwer, E. S. (2009). Parental work demands and the frequency of child-related routine and interactive activities. *Journal of Marriage and Family, 71*, 1193–1204.

Roy, K. (2014). Fathering from the long view: Framing personal and social change through life course theory. *Journal of Family Theory & Review, 6*(4), 319–335.

Rijlaarsdam, J., Stevens, G. W., Van Der Ende, J., Hofman, A., Jaddoe, V. W., Mackenbach, J. P., et al. (2013). Economic disadvantage and young children's emotional and behavioral problems: Mechanisms of risk. *Journal of Abnormal Child Psychology, 41*(1), 125–137.

Sameroff, A. J., & MacKenzie, M. J. (2003). Research strategies for capturing transactional models of development: The limits of the possible. *Development and Psychopathology, 15*(3), 613–640.

Saraceno, C. (2011). Childcare needs and childcare policies: A multidimensional issue. *Current Sociology, 59*(1), 78–96.

Saraceno, C., & Keck, W. (2010). Can we identify intergenerational policy regimes in Europe? *European Societies, 12*(5), 675–696.

Save the Children. (2012). *Born Equal. How reducing inequality could give our children a better future.* Save the Children, UK.

Schacht, P. M., Cummings, E. M., & Davies, P. T. (2009). Fathering in family context and child adjustment: A longitudinal analysis. *Journal of Family Psychology, 23*, 790–797.

Schofeld, T., Martin, M. J., Conger, K. J., Donnellan, M. B., Neppl, T., & Conger, R. D. (2011). Intergenerational transmission of adaptive functioning: A test of the interactionist model of SES and human development. *Child Development, 82*, 33–47.

Sroufe, L. A. (2002). From infant attachment to promotion of adolescent autonomy: Prospective, longitudinal data on the role of parents in development. In J. G. Borkowski, S. L. Ramey, & M. Bristol-Power (Eds.), *Monographs in parenting. Parenting and the child's world: Influences on academic, intellectual, and social-emotional development* (pp. 187–202). Mahwah, NJ: Lawrence Erlbaum Associates Publishers.

Settersten, R., & Cancel-Tirado, D. (2010). Fatherhood as a hidden variable in men's development and life courses.*Research in. Human Development, 7*(2), 83–102.

Sosu, E. M., & Schmidt, P. (2017). Economic deprivation and its effects on childhood conduct problems: The mediating role of family stress and investment factors. *Frontiers in Psychology, 8*, 1580.

Settersten Jr., R. (2009). It takes two to tango: the (un) easy dance between life-course sociology and life-span psychology. *Advances in Life Course Research, 14*, 74–81.

Tamis-LeMonda, C. S., Baumwell, L., & Cabrera, N. J. (2013). Fathers' role in children's language development. In N. J. Cabrera & C. S. Tamis-LeMonda (Eds.), *Handbook of father involvement: Multidisciplinary perspectives* (pp. 135–150). New York, NY: Routledge.

Teufl, L., Deichmann, F., Supper, B., & Ahnert, L. (2019). How fathers' attachment security and education contribute to early child language skills above and beyond mothers: parent-child conversation under scrutiny. *Attachment & Human Development*. https://doi.org/10.1080/14616734.2019.1589063

Thompson, R. A. (2006). The development of the person: Social understanding, relationships, conscience, self. In N. Eisenberg, W. Damon, & R. M. Lerner (Eds.), *Handbook of Child Psychology* (pp. 65–69). New York: Wiley.

Treanor, M. (2016). The effects of financial vulnerability and mothers' emotional distress on child social, emotional and behavioural well-being: A structural equation model. *Sociology, 50*(4), 673–694.

Tudge, J. R. H., Mokrova, I., Hatfield, B. E., & Karnik, R. B. (2009). Uses and misuses of Bronfenbrenner's bioecological theory of human development. *Journal of Family Theory & Review, 1*, 198–210.

Turney, K. (2012). Pathways of disadvantage: Explaining the relationship between maternal depression and children's problem behaviors. *Social Science Research, 41*(6), 1546–1564.

UN. (2012). *Addressing inequalities: The heart of the post-2015 agenda and the future we want for all.* Thematic Think Piece. ECE, ESCAP, UNDESA, UNICEF, UNRISD, UN Women.

Wadsworth, M. E., Rindlaub, L., Hurwich-Reiss, E., Rienks, S., Bianco, H., & Markman, H. J. (2013). A longitudinal examination of the adaptation to poverty-related stress model: Predicting child and adolescent adjustment over time. *Journal of Clinical Child & Adolescent Psychology, 42*(5), 713–725.

Yeung, W. J., Sandberg, J. F., Davis-Kean, P. S., & Hofferth, S. L. (2001). Children's time with fathers in intact families. *Journal of Marriage and the Family, 63*(1), 136–154.

5 Fathers' Reflections of their Fathers: The Use of Text Mining to Find Meaning in Narratives

Jeffrey Shears, Seongtae Kim, Joshua Kirven, and Tanya Coakley

Historical parent-child research has typically focused on the mother-child dyad when investigating early childhood development, effects of parenting, parent-child attachment, and many other child development topics. However, over the last forty years an increased focus has been placed on understanding the role of fathers, the impact they have on child development, and how to increase, expand, and support positive father involvement. Traditionally, fathers when compared to mothers have taken a less interactive role with children, often serving as a protector, financial provider, and disciplinarian (Shears, Summers, Boller, & Barclay-McLaughlin, 2006). However, more contemporary roles have emerged as fathers are becoming more likely to engage in caregiving responsibilities, serve as a partner to the child's mother, and act as another source of emotional support for their child. A father's involvement with his children can have important positive impacts on child development, particularly with respect to academic achievement, cognitive functioning, and emotional regulation (Popenoe, 1996). In addition to research on fathering roles and the impacts of father involvement on children, another area that has emerged in the fatherhood literature is the motivation of men to be involved with their children (Furstenberg & Weiss, 2000).

J. Shears (✉)
The JMSW Program, University of North Carolina at Greensboro & NC A&T State University, Greensboro, NC, USA
e-mail: jkshears@ncat.edu

S. Kim
Statistics and Analytics Consulting Center, Department of Mathematics & Statistics, North Carolina A&T State University, Greensboro, NC, USA

J. Kirven
Department of Social Work, Winthrop University, Rock Hill, SC, USA

T. Coakley
Department of Social Work, University of North Carolina at Greensboro, Greensboro, NC, USA

Predictors of Father Involvement

The understanding of what motivates fathers and predicts their involvement could serve as a foundation for increased father presence. Bolstering the factors that foster engagement and working to combat those that inhibit healthy father-child relationships can have a positive impact on families. Extensive research has been conducted to further understand what makes fathers more likely to be involved. Researchers have identified some factors that tend to predict the amount of positive involvement fathers have with their child. For example, studies have found that fathers who have higher levels of education are likely to be more involved (Roggman, Boyce, Cook, & Cook, 2002; Waanders, Mendez, & Downer, 2007; Cabrera, Ryan, Mitchell,

H. E. Fitzgerald et al. (eds.), *Handbook of Fathers and Child Development*,
https://doi.org/10.1007/978-3-030-51027-5_5

Shannon, & Tamis-LeMonda, 2008; Van Holland De Graaf, Hoogenboom, De Roos, & Bucx, 2018). Lamb (1997) identified determinants of father involvement as motivation, skills, and confidence regarding the role of the father, the availability of social supports, and supportive policies. Other external factors can also be predictive of father involvement. For example, fathers who are in a relationship with the child's mother are more likely to be involved with their child (Shears et al., 2006; Shears, Robinson, & Emde, 2002; Tach, Mincy, & Edin, 2010; Cabrera et al., 2008; Jessee & Adamsons, 2018). Shears and colleagues (2006) found that fathers expressed that a main way to "be there" for their children was to stay with the child's mother, endorsing a two-parent household as most beneficial for child development.

Theoretical explanations have been advanced to explain what motivates and predicts whether or not a father is involved with his children. Identity theory (Burke, 1980; Burke & Tully, 1977), especially the concept of roles, can be used to explain father's involvement with their children by examining the significance placed on the parental and paternal role (Ihinger-Tallman, Pasley, & Buehler, 1993; Maurer, Pleck, & Rane, 2001; Pasley, Petren, & Fish, 2014). A more positive self-identity and identity as a father can lead to higher levels of involvement with children (Beitel & Parke, 1998; Paisley, et al., 2014). A major contributor to the development and valuation of paternal identity is the partner's appraisal of the father's competence and importance in child-rearing duties (Maurer et al., 2001; Paisley, et al., 2014).

Self-determination theory (SDT) also has been used to understand father involvement. SDT explains behavior in terms of differing motivations either related to intrinsic (the self) or to extrinsic factors influences on parenting behaviors. Motivation related to intrinsic factors fosters a greater sense of autonomy and commitment (Bouchard, Lee, Asgary, & Pelletier, 2007). Hence, fathers who are more intrinsically motivated, as opposed to extrinsically motivated, are more likely to engage with their children in order to gain personal pleasure rather than to gain some sort of external reward. SDT also posits that intrinsically motivated father involvement would tend to be longer-lasting and more fulfilling than extrinsically motivated fathers (Bouchard et al., 2007).

Another researched area of predictive elements of father involvement focuses on how a father's experience impacts his parenting practices. Some suggest that how a man was fathered can predict how much and in what ways he will be involved with his own children (Baruch & Barnett, 1986; Cowan & Cowan, 1987, 1992; Russell, 1986; Sagi, 1982; Brown, Kogan, & Kim, 2017). Evidence suggests that patterns of fathering are reproduced across generations (Gerson, 1993; Popenoe, 1996); studies indicate that men who had more warm and nurturing experiences with their own fathers are more likely to continue those behaviors when they became fathers (Shears et al., 2002; Reuter & Biller, 1973; Hofferth, Pieck, & Vesely, 2012).

Intergenerational Transmission of Parenting

Evidence supportive of intergenerational parenting suggests that beliefs and behaviors related to parenting are passed from one generation to the next. Social learning theory (Bandura, 1977) and psychodynamic theory (Fraiberg, Adelson, & Shapiro, 1975) each address issues related to the intergenerational transmission of parenting.

Social learning theory posits that behaviors originate from those we have observed throughout life. Thus, children learn parenting behaviors by observing their own parents and apply those behaviors with their children. From another perspective, children do not only observe parenting practices, then incorporate or embed models as representations of parenting styles.

In her research with families, Fraiberg et al. (1975) asked the question, "what determines whether the conflicted past of the parent will be repeated with his child?" Guided by psychodynamic theory, she posited that repressed memories of one's childhood influence intergenerational parenting, a process that she referred to as having "ghosts in the nursery". Barrows (1999) argued that fathers can also "exert a powerful shaping influence on the infant's developing psyche" (p 335), influenced by their ghosts of childhood as well. Thus, intergenerational transmission of parenting practices appears to be guided both by observing parenting behaviors and forming representational models of parenting that would include both conscious and unconscious aspects of how one was parented, the neurobiological embodiment of memories of adversities experienced during childhood (Ammaniti and Gallese (2013)).

One might argue that much of what is learned from parents is not specifically just behaviors but relational dynamics. In short, parents can provide children with specific behaviors that might be learned and then internalized within the context of their environment. Relational developmental theory Lerner, Agans, DeSouza, and Hershberg (2014) draws attention to the contextual aspects that frame lived experiences. For example, Lerner et al. (2014) note:

> "In sum, embedded within a process-relational paradigm, models derived from relational developmental systems metatheory emphasize that all levels of organization within the ecology of human development are systemically integrated across life. As such, any variable from any level is embodied in, fused with, variables from all other levels; the structure and function of one variable is thus governed, or regulated, by the structure and function of other variables and, for the developing person, these developmental regulations mean that individual←→context relations are the basic unit of analysis within human development. Moreover, history (temporality) imbues in individual←→context relations the potential for relative plasticity in human development." (p 257).

Much of the research pertaining to the continuity of parenting behaviors derives from longitudinal studies using both prospective and retrospective self-report measures with first (G1), second (G2), and sometimes third generation (G3). Many studies have shown that harsh parenting in G1 is directly related to harsh parenting used by G2 (Simons, Whitbeck, Conger, & Wu, 1991; Neppl, Conger, Scaramella, & Ontai, 2009; Scaramella & Conger, 2003; Belsky, Conger, & Capaldi, 2009; Bailey, Hill, Oesterle, & Hawkins, 2009; Conger, Shofield, & Neppl, 2012). Hyoun, Capaldi, Pears, Kerr, and Owen (2009) found that G2 parents who had experienced neglect during childhood were 2.6 times as likely to report their own neglectful parenting behavior and twice as likely to report physically abusive parenting behavior; likewise, G2 parents who were physically abused were 5 times as likely to report physically abusive parenting behavior and 1.4 times as likely to report neglectful parenting with their own children.

Constructive, warm, and sensitive parenting have also been found to be transmitted across generations (Belsky, Jaffee, Sligo, Woodward, & Silva, 2005; Neppl et al., 2009; Kerr, Capaldi, Pears, & Owen, 2009; Simons, Beaman, Conger, & Chao, 1992). Simons et al. (1992) found that adolescents whose parents were supportive are more likely to believe that parenting impacts child development. Simons and colleagues found that supportive parenting was more strongly related to parenting beliefs related to female children than male children, whereas harsh discipline styles were more strongly related to discipline beliefs about male children.

As research supports the continuity of parenting behaviors between generations, it also supports mechanisms and mediating factors to explain the phenomenon such as interpersonal relations, social participation, role-specific modeling, social competence, and various child characteristics (Neppl et al., 2009; Shaffer, Burt, Obradović, Herbers, & Masten, 2009; Scaramella & Conger, 2003; Chen & Kaplan, 2001; Shears et al., 2002). Chen and Kaplan (2001) found that interaction styles and attachment patterns in the home can mediate the transmission of constructive parenting practices; they also found that the socialization of the child and social learning processes involving role-specific parenting practices mediate the transmission of parenting styles. Others support this as Shaffer et al. (2009) found that developing social competence with peers mediates the continuity of parenting behaviors between generations, and academic attainment has also been found to mediate the relationship of positive parenting between G1 and G2 (Neppl et al., 2009).

Research has also found evidence of mediating factors in the intergenerational transmission of harsh and abusive parenting. Scaramella and Conger (2003) found that observed hostile parenting in G1 predicted similar behaviors in G2 which were positively related to G3 behavior problems. However, the continuity in hostile parenting behaviors was only seen when the G3 child was rated as highly reactive and emotionally negative during an arm restraint task. Similarly, Neppl et al. (2009) found that externalizing behavior in G2 children mediated the transmission of harsh parenting from G1 to G2.

The theoretical underpinnings of SDT, psychodynamic, and RDS theories, combined with the evidence of directional impacts of both harsh and warm/sensitive parenting, along with support that these impacts are influenced by various covarying factors all suggest support for the idea that parental behaviors can potentially impact parenting attitudes and practices across generations.

Intergenerational Transmission of Parenting & Fatherhood

The intergenerational transmission of parenting has not been extensively researched relating specifically to fatherhood. The literature does suggest that the mechanisms of generational parenting apply to fathering behaviors and role transmission. Intergenerational transmission of parenting helps explain if and how fathers are involved with their children (Cowan & Cowan, 1987; Snarey, 1993; Sagi, 1982; Brown et al., 2017). Men's relationships with their own fathers during childhood are related to their perceptions of themselves as fathers and their attachment to their own children (Shears et al., 2002; Mallers, Charles, Neupert, & Almeida, 2010). Pleck (1997) posits that men either compensate for their father's lack of involvement or model their father's behavior, endorsing the strong influence of a father's relationship with his own father on his parenting behaviors (Baruch & Barnett, 1986; Russell, 1986; Sagi, 1982; Reuter & Biller, 1973; Guzzo, 2011). When men report a positive relationship with their own father, they are more likely to rate themselves as better fathers (Shears et al., 2002; Brown et al., 2017). The body of literature does not delineate specific fathering attitudes or behaviors that are transmitted; however, research suggests that a father's experiences with his own father influence the roles that he will adopt with his own children. Furstenberg and Weiss (2000) found that having a father present during childhood delayed the timing of family formation which suggests that early family formation is more likely to occur if a child did not grow up with an involved father. Additional research suggests that fathers are less likely to reside with their child if they did not live with their own father as a child (Furstenberg & Weiss, 2000; Sipsma, Biello, Cole-Lewis, & Kershaw, 2010).

The connection between intergenerational transmission of parenting and fatherhood is a new and growing body of literature. In contrast to most research concerning generational parenting, exploratory studies have found that men whose fathers were absent and uninvolved will sometimes work harder to be more available to their own children. These men may be attempting to compensate for the lack of a quality relationship with their father. Shears et al. (2006) found that fathers desired to have a more affectionate, involved relationship with their own child and expand their roles as father outside of those traditionally expected. Although some fathers expressed disappointment that the relationship with their father was not more positive, these fathers tended to participate with their child in many of the same activities they participated in with their father. Whether looking at a discontinuity or continuity in fathering behaviors, research has shown that experiences with one's father influences a man's attitudes toward fathering and parenting role.

Methodological Approaches to Examining Intergenerational Fathering

Although the intergenerational literature clearly documents and supports that behavioral and attitudinal continuities between generations, it is equally important to explore how this phenomenon has been explored and examine new ways to expand how we view intergenerational parenting. Much of this work has been explored utilizing traditional qualitative methods to collect data such as case studies and open-ended interviews as well as qualitative methods to analyze the data largely based on grounded theory.

Early intergenerational transmission of parenting work by Barrows and Barrows (2005) utilized clinical examples to show how fathers may impact future psychological development in their offspring. They highlight that father behaviors, personality, and psychopathology are sources of significant risk for their own child's psychopathology. Their research suggest that father's inability to deal with his own history of loss may impede his ability to provide emotional support to help his children.

Taylor and Behnke (2005) study explored the lived experiences of $n = 32$ Latino men who resided in Mexico and in rural and urban settings within the United States. Specifically, this study explored generative fathering in terms of immigration. Data were gathered through semi-structured interview instruments and contained mostly open-ended questions which allowed for in-depth interviewing. Researchers used a grounded theory approach to guide their analysis which used general themes and meanings related to father's experiences by utilizing NUD*IST. The researchers report that intergenerational influences seemed to impact fathering practices. Fathers reported being affected by their relationships with their fathers and agreed that this generative fathering impacted their current fathering role. Similarly to Shears et al. (2006) men often emulated their fathers or compensated while others reported more of a mixed model where they made a conscious decision to not participate in negative parental behaviors they witnessed from their father.

Wilkinson, Khurana, and Magora (2013) explored how, $n = 115$, young African American and Latino fathers described their relationships with their fathers and how it influenced their parenting. The study sought to examine how young fathers' experience with their fathers impacted the participants' involvement with their children using narrative data. Data were gathered using one-on-one in-depth open-ended interviews which included numerous probes to provide more in-depth data. The authors report utilizing a qualitative data analysis software NVIVO 7.0 and coded the responses using an interactive process. This allowed the researches to develop themes from the data and through multiple iterations of reading the transcripts a final coding structure emerged that conceptually fit the data into identified themes. The researchers concluded that some young fathers repeated similar patterns of being an absent father and negatively influencing their children and concluded that one's fathers can have a positive or negative impact on fathers' behaviors. The authors summarize that the intergenerational process is complex, and their study highlighted that although some fathers attempted to compensate for the negative influence of their fathers many fathers reported emulating their fathers' negative fathering behaviors.

Brannen, Parutis, Mooney, and Wigfall (2011) utilized two separate samples to study the intergenerational impacts of fathers in Britain and Poland. The study looked to explore what resources and practices do current fathers inherit from their own fathers by utilizing a biographic-narrative interview approach. The authors utilized this approach to better understand fathers' lives in relation to various cultural and historical context and includes various fathering perspectives to be compared across generations. This was a three-prong approach where respondents first provided an account of their childhood, secondly they were invited to elaborate on events or specific experiences. Lastly, using a more semi-structured approach, additional questions were asked related to the focus of the study. The authors suggested that this type of data collection provided rich narratives and interpretations of their experiences as fathers and sons. The researchers concluded that the types of resource provided were inherited by younger fathers and suggest that models of parenthood are passed on from older generations. It also suggests that access to cultural resources can assist or constrain fathering practices.

Utilizing data from a 30-year longitudinal study, Furstenberg & Weiss (2000) used a largely mixed-method approach utilizing descriptive analyses and open-ended qualitative data to understand how a father's early relationship with his father impacted his parenting. More specifically, the study looked to describe and explore how the long-term parental involvement patterns were sustained across generations specifically looking at responsible fathering behaviors. Utilizing n = 110 males the study findings suggested that early stable presence of father as a child was strongly linked to the timing of their own family formation. As a result, young fathers were less likely to be residing with their children if they also grew up with a non-residential father.

The Belsky et al. (2005) study examined whether childrearing and family climate experienced in early childhood, middle childhood, and early adolescence predicted parenting practices. More specifically the study examined if a positive childrearing history will predict a sensitive-stimulating fathering. The study utilized observational data, i.e., videotaped interactions between n = 99 fathers and their 36-month-old child. The study used a hierarchical regression to predict how childhood histories predicted observed parenting. The analyses failed to show that the father's parenting history predicted parenting practices with his three-year-old.

The Brown et al. (2017) study examined the intergenerational transmission of fathering among n = 132 young African American fathers in rural communities. The study examined if the quality of the relationship with their biological fathers influenced their own involvement with their young children. About 19.5% reported living with their biological dad as a child with 40.9% reporting that they never resided with their biological father. The study used several standard measures to assess father's involvement, relationship with birth father and social fathers. The study found that young fathers who reported close supportive relationships with their fathers were more likely to be involved with their children when compared to fathers who did not report a close supportive relationship with their dads.

The current study looks to add to this growing body of literature by utilizing the Early Head Start (EHS) Father Studies data to explore if parents' reflections about their parents, specifically fathers' reflections of their fathers, will provide necessary supplemental information regarding the intergenerational transmission of fathering. The present study will use a new technique to explore father's reflections on experiences with their own father by examining narrative responses. More specifically, we will look at the relationship between response length, response sentiment, and wordcloud using test mining, a new analytic method in the social sciences. There is little research examining whether the length of someone's response indicates anything about the sentiment of their words. By conducting this research study, we hope to add to the growing body of literature connecting intergenerational transmission of parenting to fatherhood, explore a new area of research regarding parents' reflections of their parents, as well as utilize text mining techniques within the social sciences.

Early Head Start Father Studies

Early Head Start (EHS) is a federally funded initiative that seeks to address the needs of low-income families who are expecting a child or who have infants or toddlers. The EHS program was established in 1994 with the main focal points of: promoting child development, furthering family development, and supporting community development (Love et al., 2005). The mission of EHS is to foster healthy outcomes for expectant mothers, enhance the development of young children, and encourage healthy functioning within families. The Early Head Start Research and Evaluation Project (EHSREP) was funded to evaluate the effectiveness of the EHS program. The EHSREP project utilized an experimental research design and recruited 3001 mothers and children who were 12 months or younger or the mothers were pregnant. Fathers were later recruited as a part of the EHS Father Studies when the child was two years old. Mothers identified the father-figure of the child and the EHS Father Studies consisted of biological fathers, father-figures, and grandfathers (Shears et al., 2006). Although all of the 3001 children involved in the EHSREP had a father, protocol required mothers to willingly identify their child's father or father-figure and then provided consent for him to be contacted. As a result, the EHS Father Studies' sample was well below $n = 3001$ EHSREP participants. The EHS Father Studies represents one of the early studies of fathering in low-income families. Boller et al. (2006) provide a detailed overview of the research design and data collection methods of the Early Head Start Research and Evaluation Project.

The EHS Father Studies sample included 727 fathers and father-figures of children at 24 months and 698 fathers and father-figures of children at 36 months who were identified by the mother involved in the EHSREP and agreed to participate in the EHS Father Studies. Approximately 64.2% at 24 months and 61.5% at 36 months were resident biological fathers; 16.4% at 24 months and 15% at 36 months were nonresident biological fathers; 15.6% at 24 months and 17.9% at 36 months were resident father-figures; and 4% at 24 months and 6% at 36 months were nonresident father-figures (Boller et al., 2006). Most fathers reported being employed 89% at 24 months and 92% at 36 months and the average level of education was less than 12 years. The average age of fathers was 27 years old when the EHSREP focus child was born.

Procedure & Interview Protocol

The EHS Father Studies involved both qualitative and quantitative data collection methods. Intensive semi-structured qualitative interviews were conducted and audiotaped with the participating fathers (Boller et al.,2006). The study utilized an embedded qualitative study to gain more exploratory information on fathers. When this study was conducted, it was decided that a qualitative component was necessary because there was so little information available about fathers—especially those from low-income backgrounds. Given the historical dearth of information on fathers, some basic exploratory data were needed to develop a sense of how fathers perceive and interpret the issues of parenting and program supports.

Standards of rigor for qualitative studies that are analogous to quantitative studies include the use of techniques to enhance credibility (analogous to validity), transferability (analogous to generalizability), and dependability (analogous to reliability) of the research process (Anfara Jr, Brown, & Mangione, 2002). The qualitative interview protocol included six primary or "grand tour" (Miles & Huberman, 1994) items: The interview protocol covered six major areas: (1) What does being a "good father" mean to you? (2) How has becoming a father impacted your life? (3) Talk about experiences with your own father. (4) What kinds of help or support do you get to do your job as a father? (5) What gets in the way of being a good father? (6) What are you proudest of about your child?

For each of these questions, a series of suggested probes was developed for use by interviewers. The probes were intended to elicit more elaborate responses to these questions. All EHS interviewers received the same training on the procedures of qualitative interviewing. Additionally, each interviewer participated in two project-wide conference calls to discuss and revise the probes throughout the data collection phase (Boller et al., 2006). This process is a type of peer debriefing intended to enhance the credibility of the study; an audit trail of the changes in protocols was also kept documenting the dependability of the study (Anfara Jr et al., 2002).

EHS Father Study Results

There have been numerous research studies utilizing both qualitative and quantitative data gathered from the EHSREP. These EHSREP studies represent a comprehensive view of fathering in the context of low-income families. One such study by Mckelvey et al. (2012) found that fathers teaching behaviors when the child was 24 and

36 months predicted children's math skills at ages 5, 7, & 10 years of age while also predicting language and literacy at age five. An early pilot study by Summers et al. (1999) explored how low-income fathers view the role of fathers in their families. The study utilized qualitative methods that included focus groups and open-ended interviews and data were analyzed using a traditional grounded theory approach to qualitative data. The results indicated that fathers talked about being there for their child and fathers described this role as being a caregiver, participating in play activities, being a role model, disciplinarian, and serving as a protector. Raikes, Summers, and Roggman (2005) examined fathers' participation in the Early Head Start Program utilizing both qualitative and quantitative data. The descriptive results indicated that a little less than half of the fathers reported participating in at least one program activity. These EHS program activities ranged from parent education programs, father only activities to transporting children to and from the Early Head Start Center. The study also reported fathers' responses to open-ended questions to support the quantitative descriptive data results. Another EHSREP study by Roggman et al. (2002) examined if father characteristics and psychosocial functioning predicted father involvement in the EHS program and with his child. The results indicate that fathers who had difficulty in being involved with their child were also less likely to be involved in the EHS program. The study also utilized case studies to share both successful and unsuccessful cases of father involvement in Early Head Start programming. In another study examining men who were reported to be biological fathers, Cabrera et al. (2004) found that EHS fathers were involved, engaged, and showed responsibility for their child. Their results indicate within this subsample of EHS fathers that 80% of two-year-old children have accessible fathers. Shears and Robinson (2005) found that EHS father's modern parental practices were highly correlated with mother's modern parenting and higher cognitive scores for children. Bradley, Shears, Roggman, and Tamis-LeMonda (2006) offer an extensive overview of many of the EHS Fatherhood Studies. It should be noted that this is not an exhaustive list of research conducted using the EHSREP data but provides an overview of various ways these data have been used to study fathering.

An early study by Shears et al. (2006) explored the meaning of fathering among fathers participating in the EHS Fatherhood Studies. The study explored how fathers talked about their experiences with their fathers and how this relationship influenced their own parenting. The study utilized 16 qualitative interviews of fathers in the two Denver EHS Fatherhood Studies sites. This qualitative study explored the open-ended questions "What does being a good father mean to you?" and "Talk about the experiences with your own father." The results indicated that fathering roles fall within two categories, traditional and contemporary fathering roles. In support of intergenerational parenting, men talked about how they often participated in similar activities with their children as their fathers had participated with them as a child.

The Current Study

To expand the previous work of Shears et al. (2006), the current study explores the EHS Fathers Studies qualitative data focusing on the audiotaped open-ended question embedded in the EHS Fatherhood Studies interviews when children were 24 and 36 months. Given that some tapes were inaudible or defective, there were a total of 575 available audiotaped interviews. Of these, there were 483 responses to the interview question "Talk about your experience with your father as a child." The final analysis used 370 fathers who also answered "Yes" to the question "Did you have father in life as a teen or child?" As a result, the 70 represents EHS Fatherhood Studies fathers who answered the research question when their child was at 24 months or 36 months, indicated that they had a father in their life as a teen or child, and there was an audible tape recording of the questions of interest. This current study sample includes biological residential fathers (66%), residential father-figures (15%), non-residential biological fathers (15%), and non-residential father -figures (4%). The present study seeks to analyze the answers given to the question "Talk about your experiences with your own father."

Data Analysis

Text mining as the main analytical method used to analyze the qualitative data in this study. The novel nature of this data analysis technique in the social sciences necessitates a more detailed explanation of text mining terminology and processes. Text mining is a subfield of the broader analytic method of data mining and is used to extract information and patterns from large sets of textual data via structuring them into a useful format. The survey and literature review regarding text mining is documented in Aggarwal and Zhai (2012), Berry (2004), and Hotho, Nürnberger, and PaaB (2005). This method enables us to quantitatively analyze textual data which have traditionally remained in the realm of qualitative analysis approaches. Text mining over qualitative research has some advantages such as fast processing of a large scale of data and utilization of emotion-free various quantitative methods to extract hidden information. At the same time, text mining has some disadvantages such as limited capabilities of quantitative methods to catch subtle nuances of text including negation (Hashimi, Hafez, & Mathkour, 2015; Feldman et al., 1998). Nonetheless, text mining is a complementary tool for qualitative analysis, and these two methods are often epistemically compatible (Yu, Jannasch-Pennell, & DiGangi, 2011).

To supplement the process of text mining, we used sentiment analysis (Agarwal, Xie, Vovsha, Rambow, & Passonneau, 2011; Pang & Lee, 2008) and topic modeling (Wang & Blei, 2011; Hu, Boyd-Graber, Satinoff, & Smith, 2014) which provides a computational way to identify and categorize the meaning of textual data. Sentiment analysis is sometimes called opinion mining or sentiment mining. Considering the large volume of interview participants, sentiment analysis is a useful tool to analyze the important qualitative data recorded in the interview responses and to understand interviewees' sentiment. Topic modeling is a type of unsupervised document classification technique. A common topic modeling method is latent Dirichlet allocation (LDA) proposed by Blei, Ng, and Jordan (2003), which has two principles: every document is a mixture of topics and every topic is a mixture of words (Silge & Robinson, 2017). Topic modeling helps identify hidden topics across a large number of individual interview responses. Both sentiment analysis and topic modeling depend on the bag-of-words model, a simple method in natural language processing. In the bag-of-words model, a textual document is converted to a bag of its words ignoring grammar, structure, and non-word characters (DiMaggio, 2015; Harris, 1954). The bag-of-words model is widely applied to many research areas including classification of documents (Erosheva, Fienberg, & Lafferty, 2004; Purpura & Hillard, 2006), text annotation in political science (Cardie & Wilkerson, 2008), and detecting textual cyberbullying (Dinakar, Reichart, & Lieberman, 2011).

The bag-of-words model and most other text mining methods require a series of data preprocessing. First, text sources are converted to a corpus, a collection of structured texts, to which various data cleaning techniques are applied. Second, the tokenization step removes punctuation, special characters, numbers, and excessive white spaces, and remove stop words such as "the", "a", "an", "of", tokenize a text to single words, and unify word cases. This step reduces the amount of word data. Third, the stemming step reduces inflected words to their word stem to amplify the information extraction. For example, "lov" is the word stem for "love", "loves", "loved", and "loving". The step clearly increases the frequencies of specific words. In a similar manner, upper cases are converted to lower cases. The result of this data preprocessing is a table (or matrix) of words that are used to extract the information of the text.

We used Text Mining to explore fathers' reflections of their fathers by looking at interview responses which are quantified into several variables such as *word count* and *sentiment score*. The interview responses given to the interview prompt, "Talk about experiences with your own father," were analyzed for the number of words in each response (word count) and the sum score of each response (sentiment score). A sentiment score is a function of the number of positive words and the number of negative words. There are two sentiment scores, Bing sentiment score and Afinn sentiment score. The Bing sentiment score is derived by a summation process of each word's ascribed score; words with a positive meaning were given the score of (+1) and words with a negative meaning were given the score of (−1). For example, if a participant's response recorded 17 positive words and 13 negative words, the response's sentiment score would be +4; from this score, we know that the participant used more positive words than negative words to describe his father. The sentiment score is quantified based on the lists of positive and negative words used in the English language (Hu & Liu, 2004; Liu, Hu, & Cheng, 2005), which is available in the tidytext package in R (Silge & Robinson, 2017). After feature extracting word count and sentiment score, a regression analysis was run on these two variables to see if word count has a linear relationship with the response's sentiment. The Afinn sentiment score is calculated as the sum of the word grades between −5 and 5 where the positive values indicate the positive sentiment (Nielsen, 2011). For the calculation of the Afinn score, we used the list of positive and negative words provided in the tidytext package in R.

In addition to the regression analysis, we used another analytic method, wordcloud, to create a visual representation of important themes found in the text. Wordcloud is based on the frequency of occurring words in a body of text (Meyer, Hornik, & Feinerer, 2008). The visual representation includes frequently occurring words with varying font sizes based on the number of times the word occurs. The more often the word occurs, the larger the font of that word in the wordcloud; therefore, larger words denote the higher frequency of that word in the body of text. In this study, we used a wordcloud with all combined responses to obtain a visual representation of important words and themes occurring in the participants' reflections about their fathers.

Fathers' Descriptions of their Fathers

Figure 5.1 represents the words fathers used in response to the open-ended question of "Talk about experiences with your own father." It should be noted that most participants were shown to use less than 200 words when talking about their own fathers when they were a child. The results show that the word "father" was the most frequently used response. Although "father" was the most frequently word used, one could hypothesize that men used the word "father" to discuss their fathers and the frequent use of the word may not have significant meaning in the context of the question. The words "time" and "lot" seem to be the most commonly used meaningful words and suggest that men associate their experiences with their father with time. This supports earlier work from the EHS research (Shears et al., 2006) study that identifies being a good father as spending time with their child. The word "lot" may have been used as an adjective to describe the amount of "time" for example "a lot". If this is the case, then both words (a) "lot" and "time" would have similar meanings. For example, fathers spent (a) "lot" of time or we did (a) "lot" of activities together which also infers spending time with their fathers when they were a child.

Another frequently used word was "child" and could be the case similarly to the word "father" and was more of a reflection of the time in his life (as a child) as he reflected on his relationship with his father. The next most frequently used word was the word "mother" which indicates that as fathers talked about their fathers they often reflected on and frequently mentioned their mothers. This is an interesting result as some research suggest that men tend to put fathering in a larger family context (Popenoe, 1996). The fathers included in this analysis all stated that they had a relationship with their fathers growing up. It is curious that so many fathers who had a

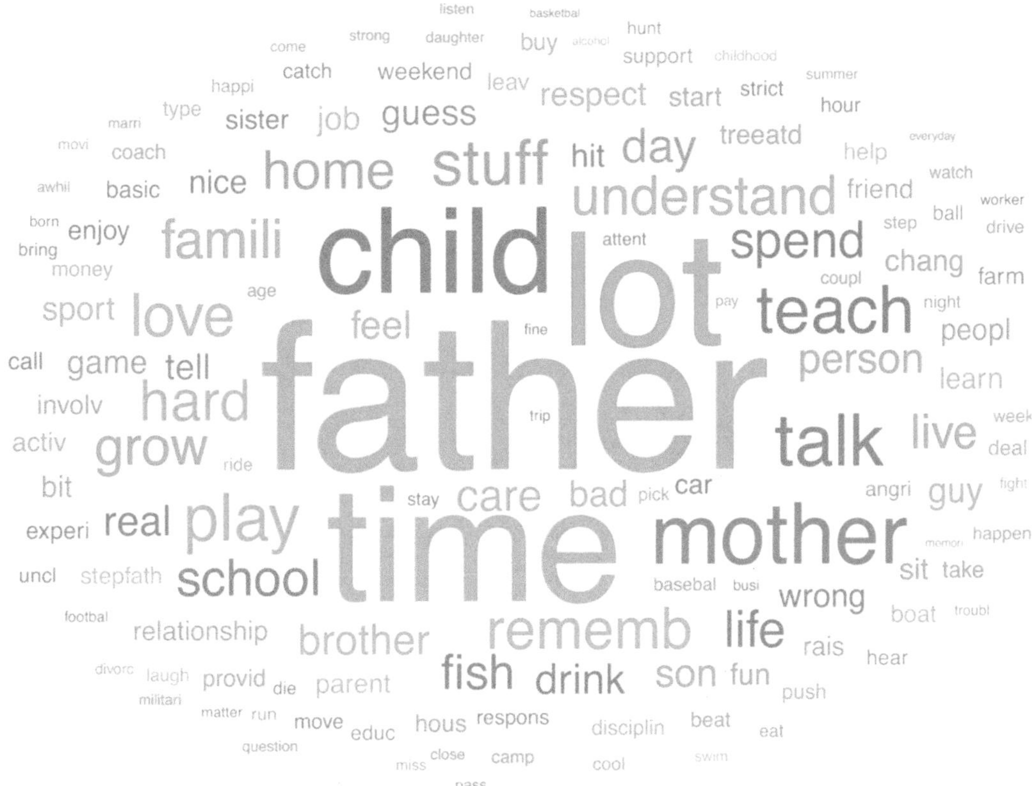

Fig. 5.1 Word cloud – childhood experiences with father

relationship with their fathers would mention their mothers when asked specifically to "Talk about experiences with your own father.".

The next set of frequently used words were "spend", "love", "talk", "teach", "understand", "play", "home", "stuff", "family", "grow", "hard", "school", and "rememb(ering)". With the exception of the word "hard" these words are viewed as both positive words and reflections of father-son interactions. As fathers reflected on their relationship as a child with their father they thought of doing things, i.e., "spend" (time, money, resources), "love", "talk", "teach", "understand", and "play" within the context of potentially positive institutions, i.e., "famili", "school", and "home".

There were several specific physical activities frequently mentioned by fathers such as "sport", "swim", "catch", "game", "active", and "fish", that suggest that reflections of their fathers as a child often involved their fathers sharing in physical father-son activities. Additionally, there were several descriptive words such as "learn", "care", "respect", "support", "relationship", "feel", and "change" that fathers often articulated as they reflected on their relationship with their father. These words tend to have a more emotional context to father's reflection of their fathers.

In Fig. 5.2a, b, two separate word clouds were generated using the Bing lexicon which classified words into positive and negative categories (Hu & Liu, 2004; Liu et al., 2005). The same color indicates the similar number of frequencies. The most frequent positive word is "love", which is followed by "respect", "nice", "fun", "enjoy", "support", and "help". The most frequent negative word is "hard", which is followed by "bad", "wrong", and "strict". The top 30 most frequently used words are presented in Table 5.1.

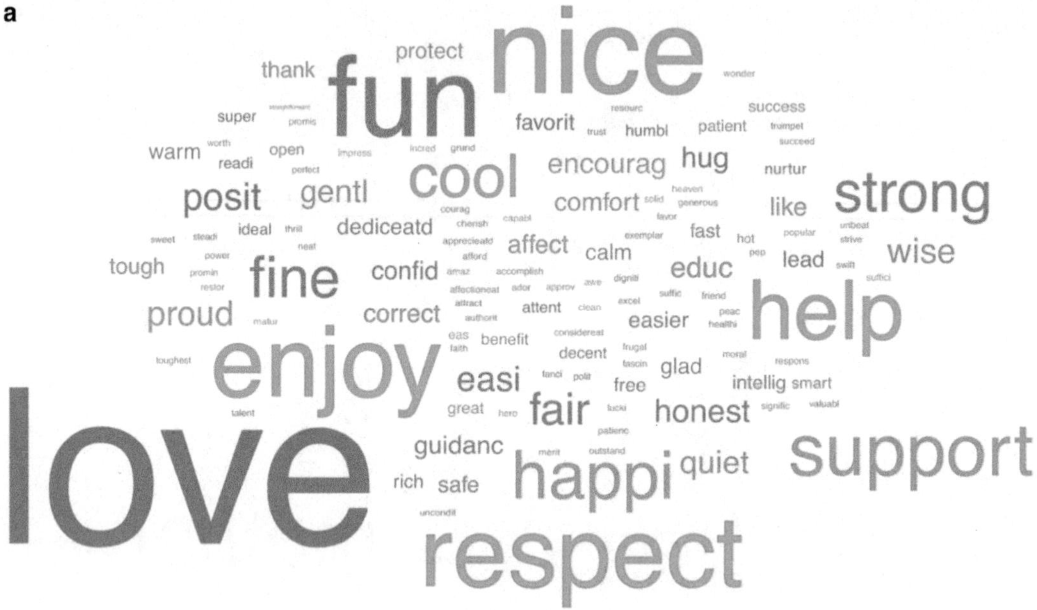

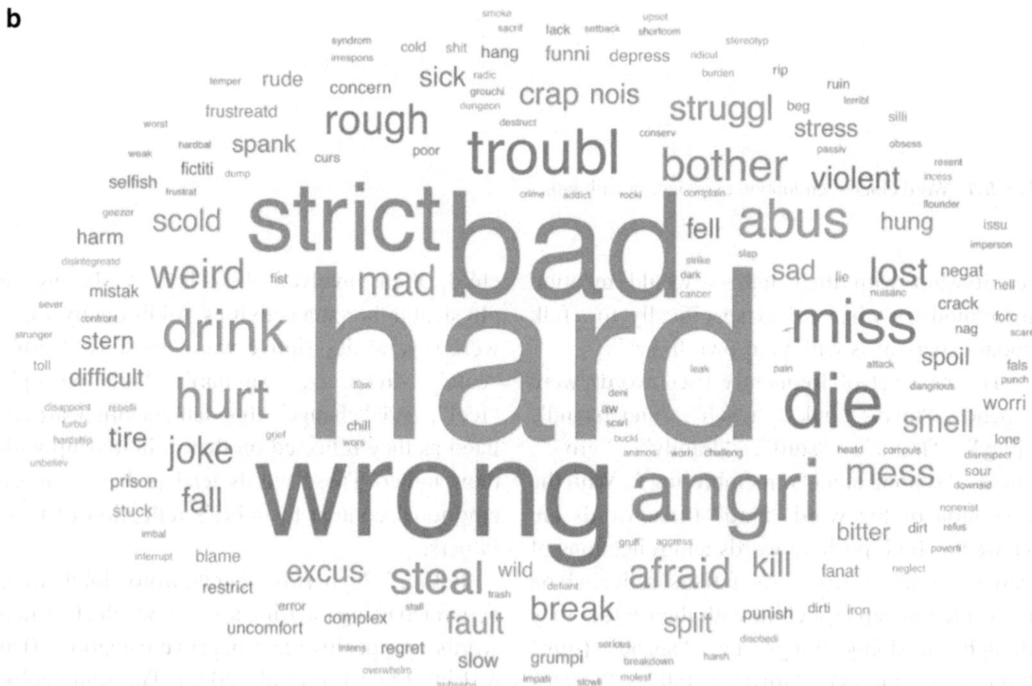

Fig. 5.2 (**a**). Word clouds of sentiment of positive words in the responses. (**b**). Word clouds of sentiment of negative words in the responses

Table 5.1 The 30 most frequently uses words in the response

	All		Positive		Negative	
Rank	Word	Count	Word	Count	Word	Count
1	Father	439	Love	65	Hard	66
2	Time	271	Nice	29	Wrong	33
3	Lot	223	Respect	27	Bad	32
4	Child	187	Enjoy	24	Strict	18
5	Mother	130	Fun	23	Angri	17
6	Talk	88	Help	18	Die	12
7	Teach	87	Support	18	Troubl	11
8	Understand	81	Happi	14	Drink	10
9	Play	80	Strong	12	Miss	10
10	Stuff	79	Cool	11	Abus	8
11	Rememb	78	Fine	10	Hurt	8
12	Hard	66	Fair	7	Bother	7
13	Famili	65	Posit	6	Steal	7
14	Love	65	Proud	6	Afraid	6
15	School	64	Easi	5	Mad	6
16	Home	63	Encourag	5	Rough	6
17	Grow	61	Gentl	5	Weird	6
18	Spend	61	Honest	5	Break	5
19	Brother	51	Quiet	5	Joke	5
20	Life	50	Wise	5	Lost	5
21	Person	48	Affect	4	Mess	5
22	Care	47	Comfort	4	Struggl	5
23	Day	47	Confid	4	Crap	4
24	Fish	47	Correct	4	Excus	4
25	Live	46	Dediceatd	4	Fall	4
26	Drink	42	Educ	4	Fault	4
27	Real	41	Guidanc	4	Kill	4
28	Feel	39	Hug	4	Scold	4
29	Guess	38	Calm	3	Smell	4
30	Game	35	Easier	3	Violent	4

The next step is to examine the positive and negative words fathers used as they discussed their experiences with their father as a child.

Positive Response Words when Talking about Fathers

The most positive word used when fathers reflected on their fathers as a child was "love" and is a powerful testament of how fathers reflected on their experiences with their fathers as a child. As the most frequently used word, "love" was used twice as much as the second most often used word "nice". This suggests fathers identified "love" as a term to best covey their reflections of their father.

Fathers also used words such as "nice" along with the words "respect", "enjoy", "fun", and "cool" most often as positive words when discussing their fathers. In the context of fatherhood, it could be that the words used either described their fathers or the father/son relationship. For example, being with my father was "fun" or "enjoy(ed)" time with my father or my dad was "cool", or the time spent with my dad was "cool". Fathers also used positive descriptive words in their response about their fathers such as "help", "support", "respect", "strong", and "happy". These descriptive words that fathers used reflected on their experience with their fathers, suggests that fathers were simply describing how they remembered their fathers, and/or how they felt as a son because of father's presence and interactions.

Negative Response Words when Talking about Fathers

Next, we wanted to explore the potentially negative words fathers used when talking about the experiences with their fathers as a child. The most common negative word used was "hard". The term makes one think of a father being a "hard" man or being "hard" to have a positive father-son relationship or could imply that their fathers were distant and/or aloof.

Fathers also used words such as "wrong", "bad", and "angry" when discussing their fathers. These negative words also support the most common negative word used by fathers, "hard". Fathers reflected on their fathers doing something wrong or feeling as if they had been wronged through the father-son relationship., Additionally, fathers using the word "bad", as in it was "bad" or a "bad" relationship, and "angry" as "angry" father or father was "angry". The use of these words clearly reflects negative aspects of their relationships with their fathers.

Another word commonly used that could have multiple connotations was the word "strict". Although we identified the word as negative, fathers could have used the word in a more positive or at least neutral context. Fathers also used the negative words "die", "drink", "hurt", "trouble", "abuse", and "bother". Particularly the words "bother" and "hurt" might all point to the emotional impact that the father-son relationship had on fathers. The word "miss" also has a negative connotation and may be fathers reflecting on how they "miss" (ed) out on not having a positive or nurturing relationship with their fathers. Remember that all these fathers responded that they had a "relationship" with their father as a child, but it is not clear whether the relationship was positive or negative.

The next step was to do a more in-depth analysis and explore fathers' responses using bigrams. Bigrams allow us to visualize words that are used in conjunction with other words. The bigrams show several clusters of words used with each other with two of the more complex clusters seemingly related to sports, with another on relationship with father and an additional one on "time". The word "time" is closely related to "spending", "found", "growing", and "hard" in conjunction with "worker" in affiliation with the word "time".

One of the more complex bigrams was the cluster of words used together that appear to be a focus on relationships. For example, such words were linked to the word "father" such as "typical father", "step-father", "biological father", "father-figure", "son father", "father teach", with "real cool" and "real close". This cluster of words suggest that the use of the word "father", "typical" "father" and "father" "figures" were used interchangeably and the words of "real" "close" or "real" "cool" were used to describe their father and or father-figure.

Another complex bigram was one with the words that were clearly associated with sports, i.e., "baseball team", "soccer coach", "coach baseball", "golf playing", "playing ball", "play catch", "play basketball", "play football", "basketball", "football games", and "video games". These words were often used together as fathers discussed their fathers. It is clear that fathers reflected on participating with their fathers in these activities or at the very least had wished their fathers had participated. Nevertheless, fathers tended to use these words together.

An additional complex bigram used the word "person" with "nice", "nice person", "nice guy", "responsible person", "sports person", "loved sports", "loved", "sports fanatic", and "nice guy". This bigram seems to suggest that fathers used words such as "nice", "person", or "nice" "guy" or "responsible" person along with "loved" "sports" or "sports" "fanatic" when discussing their relationship with their father. Unlike the previous bigram that revolved around participating in sports, this specific bigram

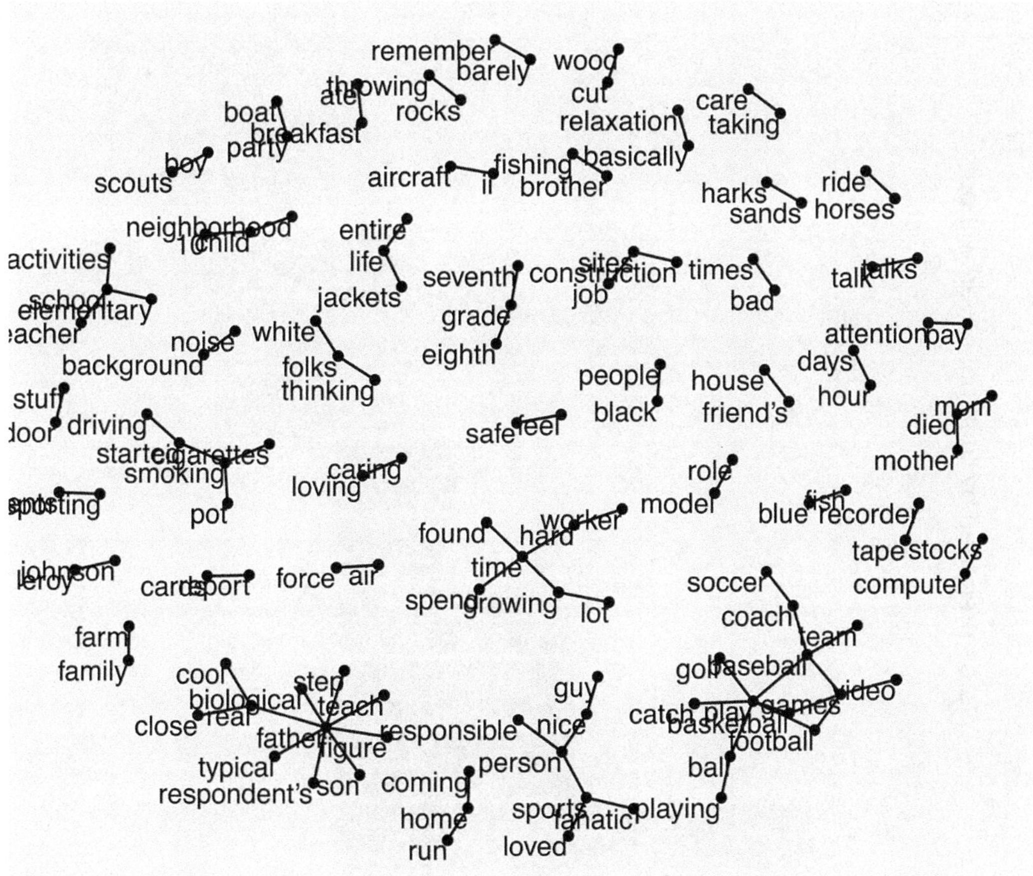

Fig. 5.3 Bigrams with at least two occurrences of the response

seems to be how fathers described their fathers (Fig. 5.3).

As we completed the sentiment analysis, we thought it was necessary to explore if there were a list of words that fathers used in describing their experiences with their father that were preceded by a negative word. We conducted an analysis on the words that followed "not", "no", "never", and "without". Figure 5.4 reveals that some of the words that could have been perceived as positive words changed when we analyzed these words being preceded by a negative word.

The most popular words preceded by a negative word was "work", "well", "respect", and "enough". For example, it could be that some fathers talked about their fathers with terms such as "never" "work", "not" "well", "no" "respect", or "not" "enough". Although this occurred at the most two times in the data file, it should be noted that understanding how fathers describe their experiences with their fathers necessitates understanding the words in context. It is important to note that fathers mostly used positive words in a positive way but there were some instances where these "positive" words in describing their fathers were used in a negative way to indicate a deficit or that fathers were expecting something from their fathers and used these words to show how their fathers failed to live up to their expectation when they were a child.

Similarly, we also explored negative words that were proceeded by a negative word. The most common word was "problem". As a standalone word, "problem" was seen as a negative word when describing the relationship with their father but the connotation changes when we add

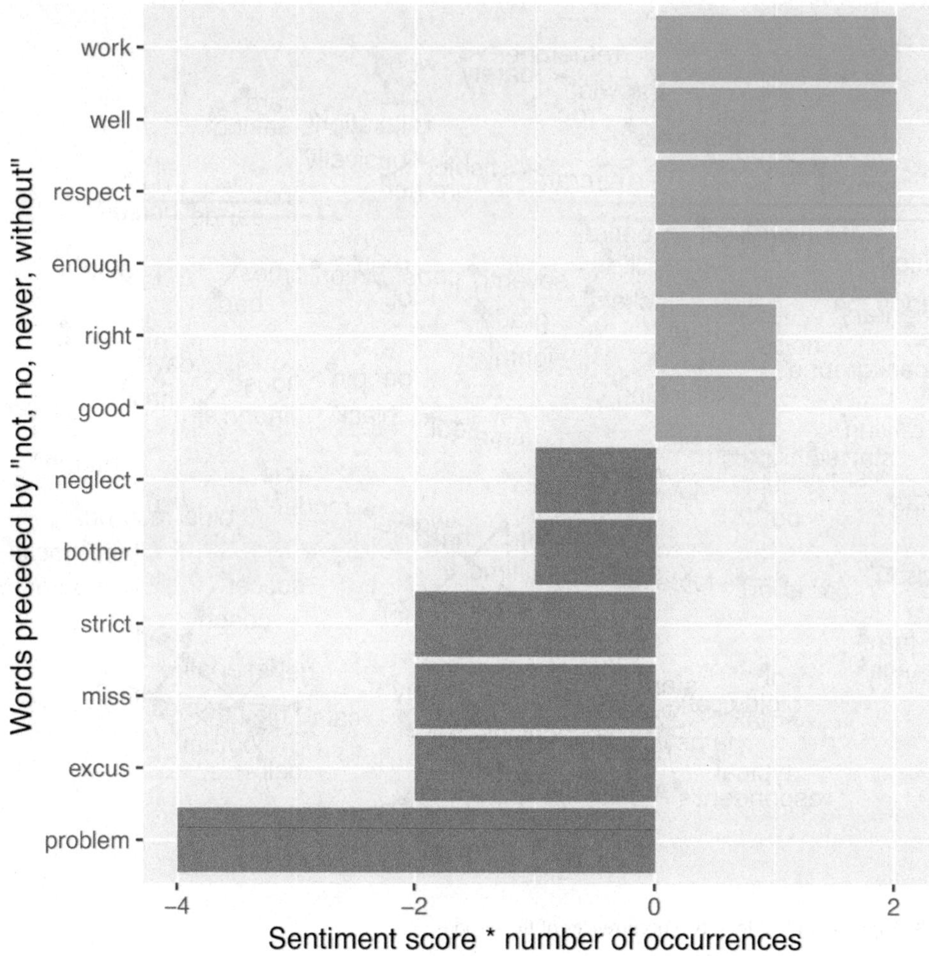

Fig. 5.4 Words preceded by negation words

the word "no" before it. This indicates that their father was "no" "problem" or maybe had "no" "problems".

Other negative words that might have had a more positive context were "abuse(ed)", "miss", and "strict". For example, "no" "abuse", "never" "miss(ed)", "not" "strict". In these instances, fathers used negative words preceded by a negative word seemingly to indicate more of what their fathers were not. He was "not" "abusive", or father was "not" "strict". Although these instances only occurred a few times, it reveals why this additional step in data analysis is very necessary to get a sense of how what fathers meant when discussing their fathers. However, in most instances, the positive and negative single words were indicative of the relationship that fathers described they had with their fathers. However, in a few instances, the meanings of these words were different when preceded by negative words. For negative words, fathers seem to validate that their fathers were good because they did not do certain negative things. When using positive words that were proceeded by a negative word describing their fathers seem to indicate that their father failed to do things that were expected of a father.

Figure 5.5 selected the top six topic models using the latent Dirichlet allocation (LDA) (Blei et al., 2003 method. The beta value in the x-axis

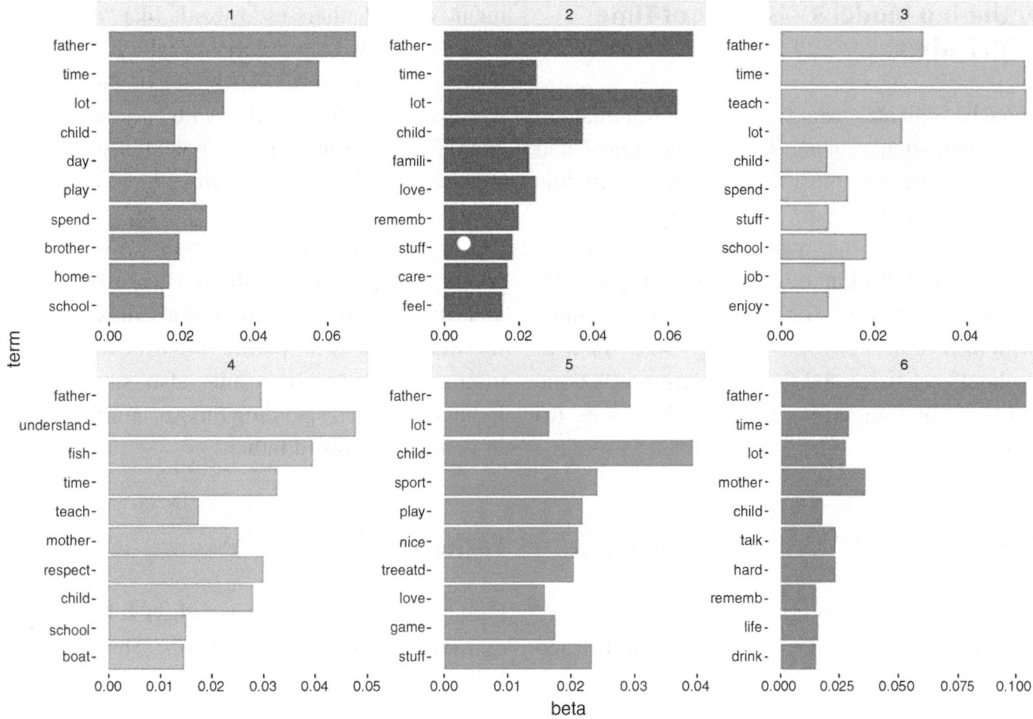

Fig. 5.5 The top 6 topic models of the responses

denotes the parameter of the Dirichlet prior on the per-topic word distribution, which is calculated using the tidytext package in R. The list of words on the y-axis, which were selected based on the beta values, allows the understanding of the topic modeled by the LDA. The interpretation of the word list often requires expert's knowledge in the application area (Silge & Robinson, 2017).

Models of Fathering

Fathering Model 1 – Spending Time with Father

Topic Model 1 indicates how time was spent with father. Here you can see from the mixture of words fathers discussed how they spent time with their fathers while growing up, with "fathers" being the most frequent word in the model followed by the word "time". The word (a) "lot" indicates the frequency of time spent participating in "play", with their "brother" at "home" or participating in "school" related activities. The words of "child" place these activities in context while the word "day" indicates activities that their fathers frequently participated in.

Fathering Model 2 – Emotional Connection

The words used in Topic 2 indicates what "fathers" typically did such as spent or shared "time" with the "child" and "fami" (ly) showing "love", "rememb" (ering), "care" taking and how this made them "feel" as a child. This model indicates how fathers' responses included words that suggested fathers did things that impacted their mutual emotional connection to their child and family.

Fathering Model 3 – Benefit of Time with Father

Model 3 indicates what was the benefit of having time with their fathers. The words "time" and "teach" were the most frequent words in this model. With "lot" and "spend" (ing) indicating this happened often with the outcome being "teach" (ing). Within the context of being a child, the fathers "enjoy" (ed) "spend" (ing) "time" with their fathers engage in doing "stuff" or with "school" activities and this interaction was done (a) "lot" or fathers would teach their sons (a) "lot".

Fathering Model 4 – Fathers Influence

Topic 4 model seems to be addressing "father" (s)' influence particularly with behavior, learned activities, and with child's "mother". Fathers used the word "understand" most frequently in this model and was often used with "fish" (ing), "teaching", showing "respect", "school" along with "boat" which probably is closely related to "fish" (ing). Another common word is "mother" which could indicate partnership with mother in that fathers influence many of these activities in partnership with mother.

Fathering Model 5 – Fathers' Active Experience with Father

This model seems to reflect on the "father" (s) active experiences with his father. As fathers reflected on their childhood, they discussed their experiences with their father. They used words like "sports", "play", "game" (s), and used words like "stuff" all the while being "nice" while doing it (a) "lot" and used words like "love" within this context.

Fathering Model 6 – Fathering Parenting Style

In this model "father" (s) was the most frequent word with "mother" (s) being the next most frequent word. Fathers used words like "time "and (a) "lot" with words such as "talk", "rememb" (ering), "life" there was also some potential negative words in this model with words such as "hard" and "drink". These potentially negative words further validate that this model addresses various fathers' parenting style. Fathers used words that might reflect his view of his father's parenting style. One of the positive role fathers identified in earlier EHSREP study in being there for their child was partnering with the child's mother. These early results also suggest that fathers identified spending time as another aspect of being an involved father.

Fathering Roles

Father descriptions of their fathers fell into several types of parenting behaviors. The parenting behaviors most associated with the words used by the fathers as they reflected on their fathers were "spending time", "relationship with mom", "emotional support", "play activities", "teaching children", and "physical activities".

Spending time – As fathers reflected on their fathers the results indicated that some of the most frequently used words were "time" and "a lot of time". With the frequency of these words, it can be deduced that men were describing a specific fathering behavior of spending time.

Relationship with mothers – In their reflection of their fathers, there was a high frequency of the word mother. One newer fathering behavior is to partner with the child's mother. The frequency of the use of the word mother maybe an indication of the fathering behavior of partnering with mom to raise their child.

Emotional support – fathers also used words such as love, care, respect, and support, which are identified with emotional support. Emotional support is one of the more contemporary roles that fathers have identified.

Playmate and Physical activities – The fatherhood research literature clearly articulates that being a child playmate is a vital role that fathers have adopted as their role.

Teacher – Early EHS work by Boller et al. (2006) talks about how being a teacher is a desirable role for young fathers. Fathers' reflection of their fathers also addressed this role as men frequently talked about teaching children.

Many of the fathering roles identified with this analysis support other research regarding how men view their own role as a father. It is an interesting finding that there are similar findings of fathering when these men were asked "talk about your experiences with your father" and a subset of fathers that were simply asked "What does being a good father mean to you?" We further explore these data by calculating sentiment scores from the father's narratives.

Sentiment Scores

The Bing sentiment score and the Afinn sentiment score were calculated as described above where the positive values indicate the positive sentiment. The number of words was calculated using the whole answer without any text mining cleaning. Table 5.2 presented the descriptive statistics of the sentiment scores and the number of words. Due to their definitions, the Afinn score has a higher variation than the Bing sentiment score. The Bing sentiment scores are closely centered at zero for both the mean and median while the median of the Afinn score is 2. The distribution of the number of words used in individuals is positively skewed, which is evident by the smaller median value of 45 compared to the mean of 73.8.

We hypothesized the relationship between the number of words and the sentiment score, that is, the interview participants with a negative sentiment score tend to talk more. The sentiment score was used as the dependent variable and the number of words as the independent variable in a simple linear regression. The residual of the simple linear regression showed severe symmetric heavy tails compared to the normal distribution. We addressed the heavy tail issue using the robust linear regression method in the heavy Lm package in R (Dempster, Laird, & Rubin, 1980; Lange & Sinsheimer, 1993). The results of the robust regression are summarized in Table 5.3.

The Bing sentiment score was calculated as the sum of the binary values (1 or −1) of positive and negative words. The Afinn sentiment score was calculated as the sum of the word grades between −5 and 5 where the positive values indicate the positive sentiment. The number of words was calculated using the whole answer without any text mining cleaning.

The two sentiment scores showed different results. The Bing sentiment score has a statistically significant relationship with the number of words (*P*-value =0.0036), whereas, the Afinn sentiment score was not statistically significant. In the Bing sentiment score analysis, the coefficient of −0.0038 for the number of words indicates that when an interviewer used one additional word, his sentiment scores decreased by 0.0038 on average. From this observation, it can be

Table 5.2 Descriptive Statistics of Sentiment Scores and Word Counts

	Min	Q1	Median	Q3	Max	Mean	SD
Sentiment score (Bing)	−10	−1	0	1	7	−0.07	2.18
Sentiment score (Afinn)	−19	−2	2	4	23	1.09	5.16
Number of words	1	25	45	86	1319	73.8	98.9

Table 5.3 Relationships between Word Counts and Sentiment Score

Dependent variable	Independent variable	Estimate	Std. Err	P-value
Sentiment score (Bing)	Intercept	0.275	0.1627	0.0964
	Word count	−0.0038	0.0013	0.0036
Sentiment score (Afinn)	Intercept	0.9536	0.3629	0.0086
	Word count	0.0002	0.0029	0.9569

inferred that fathers who spoke longer felt more negatively about their father.

Limitations

There were notable limitations in this study. First, because the interview was only semi-structured, some interviewees may have voiced their actual answer to the question in subsequent follow-up questions. Since only one question of the interview was analyzed in this study, the data in the follow-up questions were not included; this may have affected the study outcomes. Second, the text mining process was not able to account for phrases such as "don't like" that have a word score of 0 but have an actual negative sentiment. Similarly, the researchers in this study chose to denote the answers that had an overall score of 0 as negative since there was no neutral category. Lastly, all positive and negative words were given the same weight; therefore, words that connote a more negative or positive sentiment were scored the same as those with a less negative or positive connotation. For example, the words "abusive" and "didn't" were given the same score of −1. These limitations may have affected the results of this study. Although limitations exist, this study implemented a ground-breaking data analysis technique that could impact how we utilize qualitative data in fatherhood research. Qualitative research is a valuable aspect of research; however, qualitative research can be time-consuming and labor-intensive particularly with a large sample size. The use of text-mining could be beneficial in analyzing qualitative data by way of reducing time and labor needed to reach results.

Summary and Key Points

Fathers who do not carry positive reflections of being fathered may struggle with their parenting role. This challenge can be related to developmental regulations from how they navigated and adapted through exchanges during their upbringing, their relationship with their father and across their life span (Lerner et al., 2014). Fathers may rely on personal experiences and intuition compared to reaching out for assistance or support. Consideration to developmental science warrants attention toward understanding of intraindividual (within-person) change and interindividual (between-person) as it relates to human development and fathers parenting behavior (Lerner et al., 2014).

This study uses text mining, an innovative research approach to examine the power of words and experiential meaning in describing fatherhood in the context of being fathered. The text mining analyses offer initial inquiry to the question of how fathers reflected on being fathered. Intergenerational parenting suggests that how men were fathered may predict future parenting behaviors in men (Barrows, 1999). Future research is warranted to explore how men's reflections of their fathers might influence how they feel about themselves as a father and ultimately how they father their own children.

The results of this study also have some clinical applications in that it begins to examine how the relationship of current fathers with their own fathers impact their views and perceptions of child rearing. Initial findings of this research (Boller et al., 2006) showed that intergenerational transmission of parenting suggests that fathers tend to rely on old knowledge (past experiences, learned behaviors) compared to learning and seeking new knowledge on fathering.

The application of resiliency among fathers can be characterized as a strength across three factors: overcoming obstacles, sustained competence under stress, and recovery from trauma (Logan, 2018; Van Hook, 2019). Fathers need to know they matter and how their experiences with their own fathers may have impacted their parenting. Men who had positive experience with their fathers may emulate these with their own children while men who had less favorable experiences may overcome this and still be impactful fathers. Text-mining research may offer a new quantitative rigor toward future effective practice, policy, and research in working with fathers. With more quantitative rigor of text mining analyses, we can begin to examine if the frequency of words might predict fathers' parenting behaviors or if specific language models truly offer an insight on frequency and types of activities fathers have with their children. We can really begin to combine qualitative and quantitative research methodologies and ask research questions such as How does a father's reflection of his father predict the type and frequency of activities he participates in with his child? Do fathers who use negative words about their fathers also report lower levels of positive fathering behaviors and attitudes? Do sentiment scores impact childhood outcomes? Are there differences in fathers parenting attitudes and behaviors based on fathers' report of his father's latent Dirichlet allocation fathering method?

Our next step in this line of inquiry will be to examine men who fit specific models using text mining techniques and compare it with fathers' quantitative reports of their parenting styles and activities. We believe that we are just scratching the surface in exploring how text mining can be used to further understand the influences of father's parental behaviors.

References

Agarwal, A., Xie, B., Vovsha, I., Rambow, O., & Passonneau, R. (2011, June). Sentiment analysis of twitter data. In *Proceedings of the Workshop on Language in Social Media (LSM 2011)* (pp. 30–38).

Aggarwal, C. C., & Zhai, C. (Eds.). (2012). *Mining text data*. Boston, MA: Springer.

Ammaniti, M., & Gallese, V. (2013). *The birth on intersubjectivity. Psychodynamics, neurobiology and the self* (p. 236). W.W, Norton & Company.

Anfara Jr., V., Brown, K., & Mangione, T. (2002). Qualitative analysis on stage: Making the research process more public. *Educational Researcher, 31*(7), 28–38.

Bailey, J., Hill, K., Oesterle, S., & Hawkins, J. (2009). Parenting practices and problem behavior across three generations: Monitoring, harsh discipline, and drug use in the intergenerational transmission of externalizing behavior. *Developmental Psychology, 45*(5), 1214–1226.

Bandura, A. (1977). *Social learning theory*. Englewood Cliffs, NJ: Prentice Hall.

Barrows, P. (1999). Fathers in parent-infant psychotherapy. *Infant Mental Health Journal, 20*(3), 333–345.

Barrows, P., & Barrows, K. (2005). Fatherless sons: Psychoanalytic psychotherapy with bereaved boys. In A. Etchegoyen & J. Trowell (Eds.), *The importance of fathers: A psychoanalytic re-evaluation*. London: Routledge.

Baruch, G., & Barnett, R. (1986). Consequences of fathers' participation in family work: Parents' role strain and Well-being. *Journal of Personality and Social Psychology, 51*(5), 983–992.

Beitel, A., & Parke, R. (1998). Paternal involvement in infancy: The role of maternal and paternal attitudes. *Journal of Family Psychology, 12*(2), 268–288.

Belsky, J., Conger, R., & Capaldi, D. (2009). The intergenerational transmission of parenting: Introduction to the special section. *Developmental Psychology, 45*(5), 1201–1204.

Belsky, J., Jaffee, S., Sligo, J., Woodward, L., & Silva, P. (2005). Intergenerational transmission of warm-sensitive-stimulating parenting: A prospective study of mothers and fathers of 3-year-olds. *Child Development, 76*, 384–396.

Berry, M. W. (2004). Survey of text mining. *Computing Reviews, 45*(9), 548.

Blei, D., Ng, A., & Jordan, M. (2003). Latent dirichlet allocation. *Journal of Machine Learning Research, 3*, 993–1022.

Boller, K., Bradley, R., Cabrera, N., Raikes, H., Pan, B., Shears, J., et al. (2006). The early head start father studies: Design, Data Collection, and Summary of Father Presence in the Lives of Infants and Toddlers, Parenting., *6*(2–3), 117–143.

Bouchard, G., Lee, C. M., Asgary, V., & Pelletier, L. (2007). Fathers' motivation for involvement with their children: A self-determination theory perspective. *Fathering, 5*(1), 25–41.

Bradley, R., Shears, J., Roggman, L., & Tamis-LeMonda, C. (2006). Lessons learned from early head start for fatherhood research and program development. *Parenting, 6*(2–3), 259–271.

Brannen, J., Parutis, V., Mooney, A., & Wigfall, V. (2011). Fathers and intergenerational transmission in social context. *Ethics and Education, 6*(2), 155–170.

Brown, G. L., Kogan, S. M., & Kim, J. (2017). From fathers to sons: The intergenerational transmission of parenting behavior among African American young men. *Family Process, 57*, 165–180.

Burke, P. J. (1980). The self: Measurement requirements from an interactionist perspective. *Social Psychology Quarterly, 43*(1), 18–29.

Burke, P. J., & Tully, J. C. (1977). The measurement of role identity. *Social Forces, 55*(4), 881–897.

Cabrera, N. J., Ryan, R. M., Mitchell, S. J., Shannon, J. D., & Tamis-LeMonda, C. S. (2008). Low-income, nonresident father involvement with their toddlers: Variation by fathers' race and ethnicity. *Journal of Family Psychology, 22*(4), 643–647.

Cabrera, N., Ryan, R., Shannon, J., Brooks-Gunn, J., Vogel, C., Raikes, H., et al. (2004). Low-income fathers' involvement in their toddlers' lives: Biological fathers from the early head start research and evaluation study. *Fathering, 2*(1), 5–30.

Cardie, C., & Wilkerson, J. (2008). Text annotation for political science research. *Journal of Information Technology & Politics, 5*(1), 1–6.

Chen, Z.-Y., & Kaplan, H. B. (2001). Intergenerational transmission of constructive parenting. *Journal of Marriage and Family, 63*(1), 17–31.

Conger, R., Shofield, T., & Neppl, T. (2012). Intergenerational continuity and discontinuity in harsh parenting. *Parenting Science and Practice, 12*(2–3), 222–231.

Cowan, C. P., & Cowan, P. A. (1987). Men's involvement in parenthood: Identifying the antecedents and understanding the barriers. In P. W. Berman & F. A. Pedersen (Eds.), *Men's transitions to parenthood* (pp. 145–171). Hillsdale, NJ: Erlbaum.

Cowan, C. P., & Cowan, P. A. (1992). *When partners become parents: The big life change for couples*. New York, NY: Basic Books.

Dempster, A. Laird, N.M., & Rubin, D. B. (1980). Iterative reweighted least squares for linear regression when errors are normal/independent distributed. *Multivariate Analysis*, 35–57.

DiMaggio, P. (2015). Adapting computational text analysis to social science (and vice versa). *Big Data & Society, 2*(2), 2053951715602908; Adapting computational text analysis to social science (and vice versa). *Big Data & Society, 2*(2), 2053951715602908.

Dinakar, K., Reichart, R., & Lieberman, H. (2011). Modeling the detection of textual cyberbullying. In *fifth international AAAI conference on weblogs and* social *media*.

Erosheva, E., Fienberg, S., & Lafferty, J. (2004). Mixed-membership models of scientific publications. *Proceedings of the National Academy of Sciences, 101*(suppl 1), 5220–5227.

Feldman, R., Fresko, M., Kinar, Y., Lindell, Y., Liphstat, O., Rajman, M., ... & Zamir, O. (1998, September). Text mining at the term level. In *European Symposium on Principles of Data Mining and Knowledge Discovery* (pp. 65–73). Berlin, Heidelberg, Springer.

Furstenberg, F. F., & Weiss, C. C. (2000). Intergenerational transmission of fathering roles in at risk families. *Marriage & Family Review, 29*(2–3), 181–201.

Fraiberg, S., Adelson, E., & Shapiro, V. (1975). Ghosts in the nursery: A psychoanalytic approach to the problems of impaired infant-mother relationships. *Journal of the American Academy of Child Psychiatry, 14*(3), 387–421.

Gerson, K. (1993). *No Man's land: Men's changing commitments to family and work*. New York, NY: Basic Books.

Graaf, J., Hoogenboom, M., De Roos, S., & Bucx, F. (2018). Socio-demographic correlates of fathers' and mothers' parenting behaviors. *Journal of Child and Family Studies, 27*(7), 2315–2327.

Guzzo, K. (2011). New fathers' experiences with their own fathers and attitudes toward fathering. *Fathering: A Journal of Theory, Research, and Practice about Men as Fathers, 9*(3), 268–290. https://doi.org/10.3149/fth.0903.268

Harris, Z. S. (1954). Distributional structure. *Word, 10*(2–3), 146–162.

Hashimi, H., Hafez, A., & Mathkour, H. (2015). Selection criteria for text mining approaches. *Computers in Human Behavior, 51*, 729–733.

Hofferth, S. L., Pieck, J. H., & Vesely, C. K. (2012). The transmission of parenting from fathers to sons. *Parenting: Science and Practice, 12*(4), 282–305.

Hotho, A., Nürnberger, A., & PaaB, G. (2005). A brief survey of text mining. *Ldv Forum, 20*(1), 19–62.

Hu, M., & Liu, B. (2004, August). Mining and summarizing customer reviews. In *proceedings of the tenth ACM SIGKDD international conference on knowledge discovery and data mining* (pp. 168–177). ACM.

Hu, Y., Boyd-Graber, J., Satinoff, B., & Smith, A. (2014). Interactive topic modeling. *Machine Learning, 95*(3), 423–469.

Ihinger-Tallman, M., Pasley, K., & Buehler, C. (1993). Developing a middle-range theory of father involvement postdivorce. *Journal of Family Issues, 14*(4), 550–571.

Jessee, V., & Adamsons, K. (2018). Father involvement and father–child relationship quality: An intergenerational perspective. *Parenting: Science and Practice, 18*(1), 28–44.

Hyoun, K., Capaldi, D., Pears, K., Kerr, D., & Owen, L. (2009). Intergenerational transmission of internalizing ad externalizing behaviors across three generations; gender-specific pathways. *Criminal Behavior and Mental Health, 19*(2), 125–141.

Kerr, D. C. R., Capaldi, D. M., Pears, K. C., & Owen, L. D. (2009). A prospective three generational study of fathers' constructive parenting: Influences from family of origin, adolescent adjustment, and offspring temperament. *Developmental Psychology, 45*(5), 1257–1275.

Lamb, M. E. (1997). The development of father–infant relationships. In M. E. Lamb (Ed.), *The role of the father in child development* (pp. 104–120). Hoboken, NJ: John Wiley & Sons.

Lange, K., & Sinsheimer, J. S. (1993). Normal/independent distributions and their applications in robust regression. *Journal of Computational and Graphical Statistics, 2*(2), 175–198.

Lerner, R. M., Agans, J. P., DeSouza, L. M., & Hershberg, R. M. (2014). Developmental science in 2025: A predictive review. *Research in Human Development, 11*(4), 255–272.

Liu, B., Hu, M., & Cheng, J. (2005, May). Opinion observer: Analyzing and comparing opinions on the web. In *Proceedings of the 14th international conference on World Wide Web* (pp. 342-351). ACM.

Logan, S. (2018). *The black family: Strengths, self-help, and positive change*. Routledge Publishers.

Love, J. M., Kisker, E. E., Ross, C., Raikes, H., Constantine, J., Boller, K., et al. (2005). The effectiveness of early head start for 3-year-old children and their parents: Lessons for policy and programs. *Developmental Psychology, 41*(6), 885–901.

Mallers, M., Charles, S., Neupert, S., & Almeida, D. (2010). Perceptions of childhood relationships with mother and father: Daily emotional and stressor experiences in adulthood. *Developmental Psychology, 46*, 1651–1661.

Maurer, T. W., Pleck, J. H., & Rane, T. R. (2001). Parental identity and reflected-appraisals: Measurement and gender dynamics. *Journal of Marriage and Family, 63*(2), 309–321.

Mckelvey, L. M., Bokony, P. A., Swindle, T., Conners-Burow, N. A., Schiffman, R. F., & Fitzgerald, H. E. (2012). Father teaching interactions with toddlers at risk: Impacts on child cognitive outcomes. *Family Science, 2*(2), 146–155. https://doi.org/10.1080/19424620.2011.637710

Meyer, D., Hornik, K., & Feinerer, I. (2008). Text mining infrastructure in R. *Journal of Statistical Software, 25*(5), 1–54.

Miles, M., & Huberman, A. (1994). Miles and Huberman chapter 2. In *Qualitative Data Analysis: An expanded sourcebook*. Sage.

Neppl, T. K., Conger, R. D., Scaramella, L. V., & Ontai, L. L. (2009). Intergenerational continuity in parenting behavior: Mediating pathways and child effects. *Developmental Psychology, 45*(5), 1241–1256.

Nielsen, F. Å. (2011). A new ANEW: Evaluation of a word list for sentiment analysis in microblogs. *arXiv preprint arXiv:1103.2903*.

Pang, B., & Lee, L. (2008). Opinion mining and sentiment analysis. *Foundations and Trends® in Information Retrieval, 2*(1–2), 1–135.

Pasley, K., Petren, R., & Fish, J. (2014). Use of identity theory to inform fathering scholarship. *Journal of Family Theory and Review, 6*(4), 298–318.

Pleck, J. H. (1997). Paternal involvement: Levels, sources, and consequences. In M. E. Lamb (Ed.), *The role of the father in child development* (pp. 66–103). Hoboken, NJ: John Wiley & Sons.

Popenoe, D. (1996). *Life without father: Compelling new evidence that fatherhood and marriage are indispensable for the good of children and society*. Simon & Shuster.

Purpura, S., & Hillard, D. (2006, May). Automated classification of congressional legislation. In *Proceedings of the 2006 international* conference *on Digital government research* (pp. 219-225). Digital government Society of North America.

Raikes, H., Summers, J., & Roggman, L. (2005). Father involvement in early head start programs. *Fathering: A Journal of Theory, Research and Practice about men as fathers, 3*(1), 29–58.

Reuter, M. W., & Biller, H. B. (1973). Perceived paternal nurturance-availability and personality adjustment among college males. *Journal of Consulting and Clinical Psychology, 40*(3), 339–342.

Roggman, L. A., Boyce, L. K., Cook, G. A., & Cook, J. (2002). Getting dads involved: Predictors of father involvement in early head start and with their children. *Infant Mental Health Journal, 23*, 62–78.

Russell, G. (1986). Primary caretaking and role-sharing fathers. In M. E. Lamb (Ed.), *The father's role: Applied perspectives* (pp. 29–30). New York, NY: Wiley.

Sagi, A. (1982). Antecedents and consequences of various degrees of paternal involvement in child rearing: The Israeli project. In M. E. Lamb (Ed.), *Nontraditional families: Parenting and child development* (pp. 205–228). Hillsdale, NJ: Erlbaum.

Scaramella, L. V., & Conger, R. D. (2003). Intergenerational continuity of hostile parenting and its consequences: The moderating influence of children's negative emotional reactivity. *Social Development, 12*(3), 420–439.

Shaffer, A., Burt, K. B., Obradović, J., Herbers, J. E., & Masten, A. S. (2009). Intergenerational continuity in parenting quality: The mediating role of social competence. *Developmental Psychology, 45*(5), 1227–1240.

Shears, J., Robinson, J., & Emde, R. N. (2002). Fathering relationships and their associations with juvenile delinquency. *Infant Mental Health Journal, 23*(1–2), 79–87.

Shears, J., Summers, J., Boller, K., & Barclay-McLaughlin, G. (2006). Exploring fathering roles in low-income families: The influence of intergenerational transmission. *Families in Society: The Journal of Contemporary Social Services, 87*, 259–268.

Shears, J., & Robinson, J. (2005). Fathering attitudes and practices: Influences on children's development. *Child Care in Practice, 11*(1), 63–79.

Silge, J., & Robinson, D. (2017). *Text mining with R: A tidy approach*. O'Reilly Media, Inc..

Simons, R. L., Beaman, J., Conger, R. D., & Chao, W. (1992). Gender differences in the intergenerational transmission of parenting beliefs. *Journal of Marriage and the Family, 54*(4), 823–836.

Simons, R. L., Whitbeck, L. B., Conger, R. D., & Wu, C. (1991). Intergenerational transmission of harsh parenting. *Developmental Psychology, 27*(1), 159–171.

Sipsma, H., Biello, K., Cole-Lewis, H., & Kershaw, T. (2010). Like father, like son: The intergenerational cycle of adolescent fatherhood. *American Journal of Public Health, 100*(3), 517–524.

Snarey, J. R. (1993). *How fathers care for the next generation: A four-decade study*. Cambridge, MA: Harvard University Press.

Summers, J., Raikes, H., Butler, J., Spicer, P., Pan, B., Shaw, S., Langager, M., Mcallister, C., & Johnson, M. (1999). Low income fathers' and mothers' perceptions of the father role: A qualitative study in four early head start communities.

Tach, L., Mincy, R., & Edin, K. (2010). Parenting as a "package deal": Relationships, fertility, and nonresident father involvement among unmarried parents. *Demography, 47*(1), 181–204. https://doi.org/10.1353/dem.0.0096

Taylor, B., & Behnke, A. (2005). Fathering across the border: Latino fathers in Mexico and the U.S. *Fathering, 3*(2), 1–25.

Van Hook, M. P. (2019). *Social work practice with families. A resiliency-based approach* (3rd ed.). New York, NY: Oxford Press.

Waanders, C., Mendez, J. L., & Downer, J. T. (2007). Parent characteristics, economic stress and neighborhood context as predictors of parent involvement in preschool children's education. *Journal of School Psychology, 45*(6), 619–636.

Wilkinson, D., Khurana, A., & Magora, A. (2013). Intergenerational transmission of fathering among crime involved urban African American and Latino young men. *Spectrum: A Journal on Black Men, 2*(1), 19–45.

Wang, C., & Blei, D. M. (2011, August). Collaborative topic modeling for recommending scientific articles. In *Proceedings of the* 17th *ACM SIGKDD international conference on Knowledge discovery and data mining* (pp. 448–456). ACM.

Yu, C. H., Jannasch-Pennell, A., & DiGangi, S. (2011). Compatibility between text mining and qualitative research in the perspectives of grounded theory, content analysis, and reliability. *The Qualitative Report, 16*(3), 730–744.

A Family Systems Perspective on Father Absence, Presence, and Engagement

7

Erika London Bocknek

Across time, families, and communities, the definition of the fathering role in the United States has evolved and is nuanced (Fitzgerald, Mann, & Barratt, 1999). These definitions have been shaped by historical changes in society, like the industrial revolution, as well as the changing landscape of culturally relevant processes within American families (Cabrera, Fitzgerald, Bradley, & Roggman, 2007). While mothering remains a much more universal construct, the definition of fathering across groups is more heterogeneous (Cabrera, Fitzgerald, Bradley, & Roggman, 2014). This chapter describes methodological limitations in the measurement of absence and presence; discusses contemporary, population specific issues in the definition of father engagement; and, finally, presents a family systems perspective on the definition of father engagement in families. This chapter ends with implications for future research and practice that include nuanced and defined methods, a balance between culturally universal and culturally relative perspectives, and systemic approaches to research regarding fathering in families.

E. L. Bocknek (✉)
Department of Educational Psychology, Wayne State University, Detroit, MI, USA
e-mail: erika.bocknek@wayne.edu

Measurement of Father Presence and Absence

Research and policy alike have long decried the deleterious effects of father absence on outcomes for children. Research indicates that when fathers are present, children demonstrate better developmental (cognitive and social emotional), school-based, and behavioral (e.g., reduction in risk) outcomes across ages (e.g., Bocknek, Brophy-Herb, Fitzgerald, Schiffman, & Vogel, 2014; Dubowitz et al., 2001; East, Jackson, & O'Brien, 2006; Ellis et al., 2003). Other research has applied a more nuanced perspective on father presence. In one set of studies, researchers raise the question of whether or not presence is a positive contributor if fathers have mental health problems (Jaffee, Moffitt, Caspi, & Taylor, 2003) or if the relationship quality between parent and child is poor (Booth, Scott, & King, 2010). In yet another set of research, which is becoming the contemporary standard, researchers ask more fine-grained questions about the qualities of paternal involvement that make a difference in children's outcomes (Brown, Mangelsdorf, Shigeto, & Wong, 2018; Paquette & Dumont, 2013). Here, I review the historical binary definition of father presence and then discuss the evolving theoretical frameworks advanced by scholars to describe the complexities of father involvement.

H. E. Fitzgerald et al. (eds.), *Handbook of Fathers and Child Development*,
https://doi.org/10.1007/978-3-030-51027-5_7

Binary Measurement

Historically, father presence has been defined by residential status and/or marital status (Day & Lamb, 2003). Federal and local programs over the last 20 years have emphasized father presence as a measure of positive change: encouraging fathers to be in their children's lives was the programmatic goal. In fact, these initiatives emphasized increasing the marriage rates in order to improve father presence (Horn, 2003). If biological fathers did not live in the home where their children resided with a biological mother, the family is often determined to be "single mother headed," "father absent," or "disrupted," with two-parent married families considered "intact" (Bronte-Tinkew, Moore, & Carrano, 2006; Coley, 1998; Thomas, Farrell, & Barnes, 1996). Defining presence in this way presents two main problems. First, *father absence* as a function of divorce/non-romantic co-parenting overlaps with deficits in financial and social resources that contribute to positive outcomes (Tamis-Lemonda & McFadden, 2010). Second, contemporary research shows that the varying definition of fathering means that residential and/or romantic partnering status is not descriptive of the multitude of ways that fathers engage with their young children (Cabrera et al., 2004).

In a recent study (Bocknek, 2018), I invited 2-year-old children to participate with their biological mothers. Our research team asked mothers to identify their co-parents with secondary probes when necessary about the consistency of contact between biological father and child. Through that process, 75% of enrolled children participated with a biological mother and a biological father though only 16% of parents were married or cohabiting with each other. The families in this study were low-income families, residents of a large urban area, and mostly African American/Black. Moreover, observations in the lab demonstrated adaptive parenting engagement among these fathers (Richardson, Bocknek, McGoron, & Trentacosta, 2019). These data are consistent with large-scale studies in which nonresident fathers are reported by children's mothers to have regular contact with their children in a majority of cases. In the fathering substudy of the Early Head Start Research and Evaluation Project (EHSREP; Love et al., 2005), 70–80% of 2- to 3-year-olds maintained regular and consistent contact with their biological fathers despite varying patterns of residential statuses (Boller et al., 2006; Cabrera et al., 2004).

Theoretical Frameworks

To measure father absence/presence as a binary and an indicator of resilience for children is problematic in that it may be only a proxy for other variables including resources, family functioning, context, and fathering quality. It is also a low standard for influence. Mothers affect, language, microbehaviors, reflective functioning, mental health, and many other characteristics and behaviors have been analyzed in regard to their children's development for many decades (Beck, 1999; Lovejoy, Graczyk, O'Hare, & Neuman, 2000; Peck, 2003). Scholars cannot in good faith continue assessing good fatherhood as a question of showing up or not though historical perspectives paint fatherhood as more voluntary than motherhood (Piskernik & Ahnert, 2019). Thus, as the fatherhood literature has grown, so have nuanced theoretical definitions of father involvement. Seminal among them are the Lamb-Pleck tripartite model of father involvement (Lamb et al., 1987) and the Cabrera et al. (2007, 2014) heuristic model of the dynamics of paternal behavior and influence on children over time. The Lamb-Pleck tripartite model organized the most salient features of fathering behavior into three categories: engagement, accessibility, and responsibility. This model advanced thinking beyond presence/absence, adopting a more complex framework to describe unique contributions made by fathers to their families (for review, see Lamb, 2000). Cabrera and colleagues put forth another heuristic model that also made several important contributions to the study of fathers, children, and families. In this model, the authors discuss the context of fathering, emphasizing that the broader ecology and the mother-father relationship are critical in defining the quality and potential impact of father involvement. Similarly, Volling and Cabrera (2019) build upon Bronfenbrenner's ecological theory and emphasize the deep significance of relationships across system levels to the study of fathering. Still, scholars in the field have also suggested that science would be better served if definitions of parenting were gender inclusive and suggest there is little evidence for mother-specific and father-specific behaviors (Fagan, Day, Lamb, & Cabrera, 2014).

Research supports both perspectives. A significant body of literature has demonstrated that fatherhood is unique. Studies describe both specific behaviors that fathers engage in, such as rough-and-tumble play, that may be unique to male parents (Paquette & Dumont, 2013). In addition, studies also describe unique roles that fathers play supporting, buffering, and compensating for mothers who are posited as the normative primary caregivers to children (Martin, Ryan, & Brooks-Gunn, 2010). Roggman and colleagues defined fathers as the *primary playmate* in complement to mothers as the *primary caregiver*, emphasizing differential, gender-based behaviors and their unique role in the development of children's self-regulation (Roggman, Boyce, Cook, Christiansen, & Jones, 2007). Other research has focused on behaviors that fathers and mothers alike engage in that support optimal development among their children including sensitivity, cognitive stimulation, and racial socialization (Brown, Mangelsdorf, & Neff, 2012; Cooper, Smalls-Glover, Metzger, & Griffin, 2015; Lucassen et al., 2011; Shannon, Tamis-LeMonda, London, & Cabrera, 2002). This ongoing dialogue seeking to define the fathering role in the family is ultimately complex and in need of continued theoretical scaffolding.

Cultural Implications

This problem of measurement of father absence, presence, and engagement is not simply an esoteric scientific question but has significant policy and practice implications. Perhaps, the most significant among them is the way that values of the dominant culture become generalized across groups. The role of the father is uniquely sensitive to shifting historical, sociopolitical, and cultural forces. While mothers across groups and across time are likely to have established proximity to their children and engage in universal caregiving behaviors like feeding and soothing, fathers have been defined in heterogeneous ways across people, places, and time: breadwinner, teacher, disciplinarian, gender role socializer, playmate, and caregiver (Bocknek, Hossain, & Roggman, 2014; Fitzgerald et al., 1999). Thus, improving the scientific lens through which fathering is viewed is particularly critical from a position of cultural humility.

In White families who comprise the dominant culture in the United States, families are defined by adult-level relationships, and marriage and romantic partnering define who are the parents. However, in other communities, and in African American/Black families in particular, the family is defined by the relationships to the child. Research that seeks to define optimal father involvement from the perspectives of marriage, residence, and even co-parenting quality is likely applying a cultural standard that rigidifies African American/Black families in categories of risk. I highlight the experiences of African American/Black fathers here because they are at highest likelihood to be represented in categories of risk and to be the focus of racist perspectives and implicit bias in the scholarly literature. Despite lower marriage/cohabitation rates, African American/Black fathers are observed to be characteristically nurturant of their children and engage in egalitarian behaviors along with African American/Black mothers at higher rates compared to White and Latino fathers (Bocknek, Lewis, & Raveau, 2017; Boyd-Franklin, 2003). This example makes it clear that shifting definitions of father engagement is needed that incorporates the kind of systemic perspectives capable of balancing cultural relativism with cultural universalism.

Family Systems Theory

The scholarly dialogue regarding father engagement referenced above is evolving and discrepant in several ways. The earlier framing of fathers' contributions via binary absence and presence has largely evolved into finer-grained investigations of distinct behaviors. Efforts to adopt systemic perspectives have focused on subsystem functioning like co-parenting or examined circular patterns within systems including triadic interactions or father-child bidirectionality. This body of research has moved the field forward and demonstrated the unique and varied ways that fathers parent their children. Furthermore, increasingly complex research inquiries are compelling scholars to raise significant questions about whether or not fathers indeed occupy distinct parenting role attributes compared to mothers. Finally, culture and context are considered critical scientific constructs and are specifically relevant to the heterogeneous construction of fatherhood.

Efforts to define *father involvement* based on what many fathers *are* (e.g., married, residential) or *do* (e.g., teach, diaper, feed) is atheoretical and may be a cumbersome approach. Sophisticated models as described above have helped elucidate the critical tasks fathers may engage in to directly support the development of their children. In addition, these models support culturally universal definitions of fathering and allow culturally relevant adaptations to emerge. However, even with their application to theory and practice, questions remain about if and how fathers play central and critical roles in their children's lives and in what ways father presence matters. Bretherton (2009) noted that developmental psychology does not offer an explicit theory on family functioning but rather focuses on individual development in the context of specific subsystems and features like parenting and parent-child relationships. More recently, Volling and Cabrera (2019) note the lack of a broad theory to describe fatherhood and support research design. The intersection of a field like developmental psychology that focuses on children with a field like family therapy that has evolved theories on healthy families is imperative to the study of father involvement, a construct that can only be understood in the context of systems.

General Systems Theory

The field of family therapy has wrestled for 70 years with the question of family health and adaptation. A motivating force behind the once-emerging *general systems theory* (von Bertalanffy, 1969) was a response to *reductionism* that assumed that complex whole phenomena could be understood through analysis of individual parts of the system (Carr, 2016). General systems theory (GST) posits that systems are comprised of related parts that function in coordination and infuse information from the environment to move the system and its component parts toward unified goals. In the decades that have followed emergence of GST, the field of family therapy has answered the question of family health with defining system-level traits that contribute to optimal family functioning. Contemporary scholarship on fatherhood often adopts ecological perspectives that acknowledge intersecting variables across subsystems that influence father engagement like the co-parenting relationship, family stress, and child traits (Favez et al., 2012; McHale & Fivaz-Depeursinge, 2010; Parke & Cookston, 2019).

Family Stress Theory

Family stress theory (Boss, 1992; McCubbin, 1979; Patterson, 2002) defines maladaptation on multiple factors across multiple levels of a child's ecology that lead to outcomes beyond the nature of the stressor itself. *Stress* is created by change, often dramatic and characterized by hardship, but also as a function of normative transitions in the family life cycle. In response, families must reorganize and the ability to do so in ways that support the new and continuing needs of the system defines adaptation.

Fathers are absent from their families due to a multitude of stressors including divorce, incarceration, military deployment, and mental health and substance use problems. A body of research indicates that these stressors alone present risk to children (Arditti, Lambert-Shute, & Joest, 2003; Kelly & Emery, 2003; Ramchandani & Psychogiou, 2009). It is also clear that outcomes for children and for father engagement are heterogeneous with some families achieving resilience despite stress (Barnes, 1999). From a systems perspective, interpretation and resources to cope are additional factors leading to adaptation or maladaptation. The Family Adjustment and Adaptation Response Model (FAAR; Patterson, 1988, 2002) describes the ways in which the balance of family demands and family capabilities interacts with the meaning the family makes of the stressor (including acute stressors, transitions, or other events necessitating change) in order to shape family adaptation, or resilience of the family. When fathers are absent from families in any way, including a nonresidential father maintaining or evolving his own role, the family must effectively utilize resources to cope and make coherent sense of this transition in order to fully adapt.

The role of *perceptions* and *meaning* within the family regarding the fathering role and the impact of the absence are not well understood in the literature focused on fathers and their children, despite growing evidence that such variables play a significant role in defining father engagement (Fox & Bruce, 2001; Shears, Summers, Boller, & Barclay-McLaughlin, 2006). Family adaptation and reorganization in response to a stressor depend upon meaning at multiple levels: the meaning the family makes of the stressor itself, of each person's role in the family and continued role development through adaptive changes, and of future identity of the family system.

Role Boundaries

Patricia Minuchin (1985) synthesized important contributions from the field of family therapy to the study of child development in the following ways: components of a system (subsystems: individuals as well as relationships between individuals) are necessarily interdependent; processes are circular and not linear; thus, parenting patterns cannot be well understood based only on the parent's contributions in a vacuum; families seek homeostasis and even in the context of apparently maladaptive behaviors will seek familiar equilibrium; and a companion principle to homeostasis is that of dynamic change, and in families, this tends to be driving the rapidity of children's development. Finally, S. Minuchin (1974), P. Minuchin (1985), and others have written about the function of *boundaries* that indicate the edges of subsystems and are governed by rules and patterns of interactions.

Role boundaries define *who* is in a family and *what* each person does to define their role. Boundaries also define the repeated characteristics of subsystem relationships (e.g., father-child) in families. In families who achieve optimal levels of adaptation, boundaries must be consistent and clear but also flexible such that rare and special circumstances (e.g., short-term illness) allow role-typical behaviors to be shifted to another family member and shifted back without subsystem or system disruption post-stressor. A family role is defined by social norms perceived by the family from external cues and by internal rules and repeated experiences inside of the family. The fathering role may be particularly sensitive in periods of stress or change given its widely varying definition.

Role boundaries must be a positive contributor to the kind of balance between homeostasis and system evolution that support positive outcomes for the system and its component parts. This perspective is thus about process and furthermore is a concept that can be applied flexibly across groups who define fathering in different ways. The simple questions are as follows: Does father presence achieve flexible consistency such that other family members, children in particular, have predictable, positive expectations of their fathers? Does that role clarity support positive adaptation of the system and the family members within the system?

Boundary Ambiguity

Boundary ambiguity theory refers to the impact on the system when family members lack clarity on role definition and/or the rules governing particular roles (Boss & Greenberg, 1984). This theory is based on a symbolic-interactionist perspective and family stress theory (Boss, 2016). Role definition depends upon shared definitions of role attributes, or who does what and when within a family, and ambiguity of boundary occurs when there is incongruence in a shared definition such that it cannot be determined if a given family member is in or out of a family system and fully assuming his/her role.

Ambiguity of boundary caused by two types of ambiguous loss has been defined: physical presence in a family system with psychological absence (e.g., chronic illness, depression, complex grief) and physical absence with psychological presence (e.g., incarcerated parent, addiction, traumatic brain injury). In the context of psychological absence with physical presence, a family member is described as "here, but not here" creating a paradox of presence (Boss, 2016). Psychological presence with physical absence also creates a paradox. In these families, family members are physically missing, but often for unclear reasons. Confirming they are gone may be itself painful, and reorganizing family roles in ways that may conflict with social norms or internal processes may also be difficult. The central viewpoint in both types is that dysfunction in the family is created by the dissonance between psychological and physical forms of presence. This type of dissonance is particularly impactful on young children who lack abstract meaning-making skills and furthermore develop internal representations about self and self in relationship based on repeated and predictable interactions with important caregivers (Bowlby, 1969).

Boundary ambiguity theory advances the study of father absence, presence, and engagement. Within the rich set of fathering-related studies, conflicts arise if the broader question is to define a cohesive and universal framework underlying the effects of father absence, presence, and engagement on children's outcomes. Boundary ambiguity provides a theoretical basis for understanding complex phenomena.

Fathers may be physically absent from their families but remain psychologically present for a range of reasons. Ambiguous loss as a function of divorce, incarceration, or other physical losses that leave a psychological presence has the potential for dysfunction across a range of contexts. Likewise, psychological absence with physical presence is defined by a complex set of indicators in the family system, predicted by the loss but further defined by systemic and ecological traits. To examine father presence, absence, and engagement from this perspective confers risk and resilience across the rules, roles, and patterns of the family system.

Special Populations

Despite problems in measurement and definition, it is clear that paternal disengagement from children's lives affects millions of US children (Cabrera, 2010; Hairston, 1998). Here, I review specific special populations for whom role boundaries are diffuse and children's outcomes are at risk. As stated above, this theory may be relevant across a range of groups. Specific groups are chosen here where children are highly vulnerable due to related and cumulative patterns of risk. Also, these groups represent special populations for whom father absence as well as the impact of father absence on children and families is defined by intersystem coordination and incoherence as well as the primacy of perception and meaning.

Then, I discuss African American fathers from a perspective of role theory. This population requires special focus given a persistent though flawed narrative of absence, their overrepresentation in categories of risk below, and the lack of theoretical perspectives supporting strengths-based narratives.

Psychological Presence with Physical Absence

There are many situations in the life of a family when a family member may transition into or out of a family in an adaptive way. This loss may not always be marked with joy, including divorce and death, but clarity of role boundary following loss supports adaptation. Families are adaptive after loss where it is made clear if the person will return; if they do, what their role in the family will be; and if they will not, who else will take over their role. Furthermore, adaptation is supported by necessary resources to cope. In other situations, the loss is defined by ambiguity. For families for whom the loss itself is ambiguous or for whom the absent family member's role continuation has become unclear, intentionally shifting roles to adapt requires an affirmation of loss that may itself be painful or dysfunctional. In addition, because paternal physical absence may be viewed as more normative compared to maternal physical absence, families may struggle to apply coherent rules to new roles and patterns without a sense of urgency to do so. In other cases, families may struggle because role ideologies about gender-specific parenting are rigid and physically present caregivers feel unable to adopt new role attributes.

Divorce and Nonresidential Co-parenting Research suggests that 25% of children of divorced parents are at increased risk for poor outcomes, approximately double that of the general population (Greene, Anderson, Forgatch, Degarmo, & Hetherington, 2012). That means that 75% of children whose parents divorce are likely to adapt. Divorce creates increased risk but not in all circumstances. Divorce represents a family life cycle transition with increasing normativity: 40–50% of first marriages end in divorce (Center for Disease Control and Prevention, 2017). Adaptive transitions for families from single to multiple households are marked by coherent and clear revisions of family rules, roles, and patterns (Olmstead, Futris, & Pasley, 2009; Pilkington, Rominov, Brown, & Dennis, 2019). Egalitarian patterns often emerge in adaptive transitions as each household is now headed by a different parent, yet the main predictor of optimal health for children and their families is related to a sense of predictability about how each parent will conduct their role and when and how the child will engage with each parent. A coherent paternal role identity through this transition is a key correlate of positive adaptation, characterized by a father's satisfaction with his own parenting, supportive relationships between parents, and high-quality, patterned interactions between fathers and children (Madden-Derdich & Leonard, 2000).

Many families in the United States do not begin with marriage but rather with the birth of a shared child (Cabrera, 2010). This type of family is likely to earn low income, and economic adversity impacts paternal presence and engagement in multiple ways. This risk is particularly visible through common problems in child support provision. In addition, low-income fathers suffer from risks that impair consistent presence and engagement with their children including higher rates of underemployment, impaired mental and physical health, and incarceration. Studies with a systems focus emphasize patterns that support adaptivity: positive and clear fathering identity; strong co-parental communication, including among additional caregivers like extended family and new romantic partners; and higher resources (Jamison, Ganong, & Proulx, 2017; Sobolewski & King, 2005). In addition, research demonstrates that this family pattern may present in more adaptive ways among families of ethnoracial minority groups where processes circumscribing fathering identity based on residential status are more flexible (Boyd-Franklin, 2003; Cabrera, Ryan, Mitchell, Shannon, & Tamis-LeMonda, 2008).

Incarcerated Fathers Nearly three million children have an incarcerated parent in the United States, and 92% of those parents are fathers (Pew, 2010). At the present time, agencies typically tasked with monitoring and providing support to children affected by parental separation (e.g., departments of human services who oversee foster care and adoption services) are not comprehensively serving this population due to high rates of informal kinship care (Hanlon, Carswell, & Rose, 2007). The United States further lacks systematic programming for incarcerated parents to support parenting skills and the maintenance of relationships while incarcerated. It is also true that the justice system lends itself to ambiguity of boundary for families given that the system of bail is unclear and unfairly jails poor defendants, sentence lengths are approximate and shift based on system perceptions of inmate behavior and appeals, and the distance between jails and prisons varies widely from communities in which a given family may live making visitation often inconsistent or impossible. Finally, US jails and prisons lack appropriate spaces for parents to visit and connect with their children.

Families with an incarcerated family member are likely to be low-income families; incarcerated individuals are likely to be African American/Black with one in nine (11.4%) of African American/Black children impacted by parental incarceration (compared to 1.8% of White US children; Pew, 2010). Research shows that contact between fathers and their children is impacted by systemic risk factors as well as individual ones like a father's previous history of trauma (Galardi, Settersten Jr, Vuchinich, & Richards, 2017). Thus, adaptation is impaired by the lack of clarity of role maintenance as well as resources to cope with stress. The systemic issues related to nonresidential fathering intersect with this population as well including few resources and complex relationships with co-parents and families. Research demonstrates that the fathering role identity is particularly in peril among this group (Arditti, Smock, & Parkman, 2005). In addition, children of incarcerated parents are unlikely to have clear information about what happened to the incarcerated parent and if or when they will return (Bocknek, Sanderson, & Britner, 2009). Ambiguity of boundary for which many low-income families are at risk is amplified among families impacted by incarceration, and along with the typical lack of resources, this constellation of risk promotes maladaptation. However, at reentry, men with families to return to and fathering roles to resume demonstrate a more successful adaptation to society (Day, Acock, Bahr, & Arditti, 2005). This duality emphasizes the significance of clear role boundaries for development of fathers, families, and children alike.

Military Families These issues are surprisingly similar for military fathers whose deployment cycles may be indefinite and assigned with little notice to families to plan and cope. Huebner and colleagues (Huebner, Mancini, Wilcox, Grass, & Grass, 2007) write that the only certainty for military families is uncertainty, particularly in periods of war in a post-9/11 world. Ambiguity is present at immediate levels, through revisions in routines and goodbye rituals, and in emotional functioning where families may experience ongoing dissonance, for example, feeling both pride and guilt when coping with separation (Huebner et al., 2007). Military families have long been at the heart of the literature on ambiguous loss where families struggle to reorganize and confirm absence whereby fathering duties socially normed among many groups, like child discipline, become lost (Huebner et al., 2007). In fact, a recent study demonstrated that the stress caused children by paternal deployment was so significant that it did not differ for children whose fathers were combat versus non-combat deployed (Pexton, Farrants, & Yule, 2018).

Military fathers suffer from unique risk factors including the culture of the military that requires devotion and limits participation in other roles (MacDermid et al., 2005). There may also be unique sources of resilience for this group compared to other fathers with limited contact. Normative, positive narratives about military service (compared, for example, to incarceration) influence positive fathering role identity as well as maternal commitment to father-child contact (Yablonsky, Barbero, & Richardson, 2016). These protective factors are present despite similar rates of stress on both parents compared to other risk groups (Bello-Utu & DeSocio, 2015). Mental health problems among military fathers, as well as the families they leave, are significant and acute. These issues continue to impact presence and engagement among fathers after reunification (Knobloch & Knobloch-Fedders, 2017).

Physical Presence and Psychological Absence

Areas of the literature dealing with psychological absence may focus on subpopulations where the absent family member is ambiguously absent because physical presence is maintained, but the condition creating loss is degenerative or persistent (e.g., dementia; Boss, Caron, & Horbal, 1988; Boss, Caron, Horbal, & Mortimer, 1990). Here, I discuss two areas of paternal health and functioning that predicts ambiguity of boundary both because of the dissonance between physical and psychological presence and because the resolution and long-term course of role maintenance is unclear and often nonlinear.

Paternal Mental Health Problems Research shows that children's outcomes are impacted by paternal mental health problems with special scientific interest in paternal depression (Sethna, Murray, Netsi, Psychogiou, & Ramchandani, 2015), antisociality (LeMoine, Romirowsky, Woods, & Chronis-Tuscano, 2018), posttraumatic stress disorder (PTSD) (Parsons et al., 2018), and alcoholism (Fitzgerald & Bocknek, 2012).

Mental health disorders over the life span are persistent and include periods of functioning alongside periods of dysfunction. It is likely that the unpredictable manifestations of symptoms create ambiguity of boundary in families and underlie known associations between parental depression and family functioning and children's outcomes (Bocknek, Brophy-Herb, Fitzgerald, Burns-Jager, & Carolan, 2012). While mental health problems for parents can impact individuals across socioeconomic strata, low-income parents are at increased risk for poor mental health. Low-income families from ethnoracial minority groups face additional barriers to adequate diagnosis and treatment (Marrast, Himmelstein, & Woolhandler, 2016).

The impact of paternal depression appears to be predicted, buffered, and manifested in systemic patterns across the child's ecology. Bidirectional effects occur between paternal depression, co-parenting subsystem, and family stress and adaptation (Volling, Yu, Gonzalez, Tengelitsch, & Stevenson, 2018). Research demonstrates that fathers who have mental health problems are likely to co-parent with mothers who also are at greater risk for mental health problems (Anding, Röhrle, Grieshop, Schücking, & Christiansen, 2016). In fact, in the case of postpartum depression in particular, maternal postpartum depression is the most significant predictor of paternal postpartum depression (Paulson, Bazemore, Goodman, & Leiferman, 2016).

Paternal PTSD has been examined in relation to military deployment, traumatic birth, witnessing or experiencing violence, and persistent community violence (Bocknek et al., 2017; Hughes et al., 2019; Parsons et al., 2018). A common theme in this literature is that fathers attempt to cope with rigid internalizing patterns known to create emotional cutoff from present relationships. This distancing pattern is characteristic of a psychological absence despite physical presence and prevents open, flexible boundaries around role patterns needed for adaptation. Conversely, fathers impacted by PTSD have described their investment in the fathering role as a source of resilience for their own adaptation and resilience (Bocknek et al., 2017).

Antisocial behavior in fathers is a particular mental health problem that is less transient than a mood disorder. Fitzgerald, McKelvey, Schiffman, and Montañez (2006) demonstrated that the neighborhood moderates the relationship between paternal antisocial behavior and children's outcomes, further emphasizing the ways in which systemic perspectives can inform approaches to the study of and intervention with fathers and their children. In this study, fathers' meaning-making of their community experiences influences their own disciplinary approaches.

Paternal Substance Use Like mental health problems, problems related to parental substance use disorders impact individual functioning and family functioning (Stover & Kiselica, 2015). A substance abusing family member often ambiguously maintains their role, while patterns in subsystems become unclear and emotionally contracted (Boss & Greenberg, 1984). Research demonstrates that fathers with substance use disorders demonstrate ambiguity of boundary when under the influence of the substance, during withdrawal, and in periods when preoccupied with obtaining the substance (Mechling, Ahern, & Palumbo, 2018).

Substance abuse problems are co-mingled with mental health problems and affect varying levels of the child's ecology in similar ways. Research shows interrelationships between paternal substance use, maternal mental health problems and substance use, and child and youth maladaptation and risky behaviors (Das Eiden & Leonard, 2000). Substance use also represents a maladaptive pattern of coping with existing stress and thus blocks healthy patterns of system adaptation to emerge.

In particular, alcoholism impacts six million children in the United States and is the most significant substance abuse disorder worldwide (Das Eiden & Leonard, 2000; Fitzgerald & Bocknek, 2012). Paternal alcoholism predicts negative outcomes for young children in behavior, mental health, and cognitive functioning and is a strong predictor of children's later substance abuse (Leonard et al., 2000; Poon, Ellis, Fitzgerald, & Zucker, 2000). The research in this area demonstrates the multiple ways paternal alcoholism influences child functioning in nonlinear ways, reducing both paternal and maternal sensitivity (Das Eiden & Leonard, 2000). These emphases on nonlinear subsystem effects describe broader systemic characteristics that moderate risk-resilience pathways (Puttler, Fitzgerald, Heitzeg, & Zucker, 2017).

African American/Black Fathers

In general, non-White Americans including Latinx and American Indian/Alaskan Native fathers are overrepresented in the subgroups outlined above for whom mental health and sociopolitical risk are high. My work focuses on African American men and their families who are overrepresented across all categories of risk and whose resilience narratives have been persistently obscured.

African American fathers are specifically overrepresented in reports of *father absence* with African American/Black mothers overwhelmingly described as *single mothers* (Kim & Brody, 2005). These family patterns have unfolded through a history in which African American men were forcibly separated from their families; disproportionate minority confinement echoes this history of slavery today. Research demonstrates the significant and unique development of fathering role identity among African American/Black men (Roy, 2006). Presence, absence, and engagement are defined by intergenerational experiences of these constructs with a sense of role ideologies impacting fathering (Cooper, Ross, Dues, Golden, & Burnett, 2019). Social-systemic forces have restricted the capacity for African American/Black men to live with and parent their children across generations (Boyd-Franklin, 2003; Coley, 2001; McLoyd, 1990). This history defines father presence as anything but a binary; rather, father presence occurs on a continuum of levels of inadequate to adequate parenting and sometimes by multiple caregivers (Green, Chuang, Parke, & Este, 2019). Under stress of racism alongside and interrelated with the disproportionate risks to which African American families are exposed, patterns of resilience have emerged.

African American/Black families are resilient in culturally relevant ways that are informed by a long history of perseverance despite trauma and are also features of often close-knit and spiritually connected families and communities. Role patterns between African American/Black co-parents achieve greater fluidity, often termed *egalitarian*. The difference in phrasing here highlights the fact that these role pattern shifts do not occur as a feminist or postmodern approach to co-parenting and family life but rather represent adaptive behaviors in the context of external stressors. African American/Black women are likely to be breadwinners, and African American/Black men are just as likely to share in caregiving responsibilities like diaper changing and feeding (Cabrera, Hofferth, & Chae, 2011; McAdoo & Younge, 2009). African American/Black families may also be more likely than White families to incorporate kinship care providers and extended family members in definitions of parenting that represent resilience through transformed role coherence in the face of separation (Boyd-Franklin, 2003).

Summary and Key Points

This chapter discusses nuanced perspectives on paternal absence, presence, and engagement. Family systems theories advance trends in the fathering literature to incorporate subsystems in the family and consider broader sets of influences on father engagement. It is clear that among contemporary families, father presence is no longer a dichotomous construct with binary impact on children's outcomes. Fathers are present with their children in a multitude of ways, and there is a rich body of scholarship uncovering the many ways fathers engage with their children in a plurality of families (Cabrera, Hofferth, & Chae, 2001). Often, this type of research demonstrates bidirectional effects between the father-child relationship and other family subsystems (Feldman & Masalha, 2010). A systems perspective also elevates the theoretical framing to include wholly systemic features like fathering and family identity, role boundaries, and collective stress with systemic resources for coping and adaptation. In this chapter, I emphasize the ways that more complete systemic perspectives improve our collective understanding of father absence, presence, and engagement and how related definitions are context dependent.

Perspectives from family stress theory emphasize the role that *meaning* plays in adaptation (Patterson & Garwick, 1994). The family's definition of the stressor and of their own capacity to cope is a significant variable in how father presence or absence impacts child functioning. In the examples of the subpopulations described, ambiguity around the fathering role moderates the impact of the absence on the child and family. Intervention strategies with high-risk populations commonly seek to improve parenting skills with a focus on managing child behavior, buffering parental mental health problems, and improving communication between family members (Cowan, Cowan, Pruett, Pruett, & Wong, 2009; Pidano & Allen, 2015). Research is clear that fathers' cohesive role identities are highly significant to developmental outcomes for their own parenting as well as for their children (Cooper et al., 2019). This may be particularly true for ethnoracial minority fathers confronting stereotyped and biased definitions of fathering, thus reconciling external narratives with internal ideologies and complex levels of influence. Intervention can be improved to incorporate systemic perspectives regarding perception, and family narratives about role development include the ways that ethnoracial minority families define resilience.

Finally, a systems perspective places the role of cultural identity front and center in research conceptualization, design, and interpretation of findings. As described, the very definition of *presence* depends on social norms that are external to families as well as repeated experiences inside of families that define family rules. This may be complex for ethnoracial minority families who are managing expectations from the dominant culture, intergenerational perspectives, and current phenomena that underlie risk and resilience, including the role of racism in fathering identity and role development. Though a plethora of studies have defined culturally universal aspects of fathering that support theory development (e.g., McHale, Favez, & Fivaz-Depeursinge, 2018; Paquette & Bigras, 2010), this must be balanced with culturally relevant perspectives to ground translational science that can expertly support resilience promotion among families.

References

Anding, J. E., Röhrle, B., Grieshop, M., Schücking, B., & Christiansen, H. (2016). Couple comorbidity and correlates of postnatal depressive symptoms in mothers and fathers in the first two weeks following delivery. *Journal of Affective Disorders, 190*, 300–309.

Arditti, J. A., Lambert-Shute, J., & Joest, K. (2003). Saturday morning at the jail: Implications of incarceration for families and children. *Family Relations, 52*(3), 195–204.

Arditti, J. A., Smock, S. A., & Parkman, T. S. (2005). "It's been hard to be a father": A qualitative exploration of incarcerated fatherhood. *Fathering: A Journal of Theory, Research & Practice About Men as Fathers, 3*(3), 267–288.

Barnes, G. G. (1999). Divorce transitions: Identifying risk and promoting resilience for children and their parental relationships. *Journal of Marital and Family Therapy, 25*(4), 425–441.

Beck, C. T. (1999). Maternal depression and child behaviour problems: A meta-analysis. *Journal of Advanced Nursing, 29*(3), 623–629.

Bello-Utu, C. F., & DeSocio, J. E. (2015). Military deployment and reintegration: A systematic review of child coping. *Journal of Child and Adolescent Psychiatric Nursing, 28*(1), 23–34.

Bocknek, E. L. (2018). Family rituals in low-income African American families at risk for trauma exposure and associations with toddlers' regulation of distress. *Journal of Marital and Family Therapy, 44*(4), 702–715.

Bocknek, E. L., Brophy-Herb, H. E., Fitzgerald, H., Burns-Jager, K., & Carolan, M. T. (2012). Maternal psychological absence and toddlers' social-emotional development: Interpretations from the perspective of boundary ambiguity theory. *Family Process, 51*(4), 527–541.

Bocknek, E. L., Brophy-Herb, H. E., Fitzgerald, H. E., Schiffman, R. F., & Vogel, C. (2014). Stability of biological father presence as a proxy for family stability: Cross-racial associations with the longitudinal development of emotion regulation in toddlerhood. *Infant Mental Health Journal, 35*(4), 309–321.

Bocknek, E. L., Hossain, Z., & Roggman, L. (2014). Forward progress of scientific inquiry into the early father–child relationship: Introduction to the special issue on very young children and their fathers. *Infant Mental Health Journal, 35*(5), 389–393.

Bocknek, E. L., Lewis, M. L., & Raveau, H. A. (2017). African American fathers' mental health & child well-being: A cultural practices, strengths-based perspective. In *African American children in early childhood education: Making the case for policy investments in families, schools, and communities* (pp. 221–243). Bingley, UK: Emerald Publishing Limited.

Bocknek, E. L., Sanderson, J., & Britner, P. A. (2009). Ambiguous loss and posttraumatic stress in school-age children of prisoners. *Journal of Child and Family Studies, 18*(3), 323–333.

Booth, A., Scott, M. E., & King, V. (2010). Father residence and adolescent problem behavior: Are youth always better off in two-parent families? *Journal of Family Issues, 31*(5), 585–605.

Boss, P. (1992). Primacy of perception in family stress theory and measurement. *Journal of Family Psychology, 6*(2), 113.

Boss, P. (2016). The context and process of theory development: The story of ambiguous loss. *Journal of Family Theory & Review, 8*(3), 269–286.

Boss, P., Caron, W., & Horbal, J. (1988). Alzheimer's disease and ambiguous loss. In C. S. Chilman, E. W. Nunnally, & F. M. Cox (Eds.), *Families in trouble series, Vol. 2. Chronic illness and disability* (pp. 123–140). Thousand Oaks, CA: Sage Publications, Inc.

Boss, P., Caron, W., Horbal, J., & Mortimer, J. (1990). Predictors of depression in caregivers of dementia patients: Boundary ambiguity and mastery. *Family Process, 29*(3), 245–254.

Boss, P., & Greenberg, J. (1984). Family boundary ambiguity: A new variable in family stress theory. *Family Process, 23*(4), 535–546.

Bowlby, J. (1969). Attachment and loss: Volume I: Attachment. In *Attachment and loss: Volume I: Attachment* (pp. 1–401). London: The Hogarth Press and the Institute of Psycho-Analysis.

Boyd-Franklin, N. (2003). *Black families in therapy: Understanding the African American experience* (2nd ed.). New York: Guilford Press.

Boller, K., Bradley, R., Cabrera, N., Raikes, H., Pan, B., Shears, J., & Roggman, L. (2006). The early head start father studies: Design, data collection, and summary of father presence in the lives of infants and toddlers. *Parenting, 6*(2–3), 117–143.

Bretherton, I. (2009). Theoretical contributions from developmental psychology. In *Sourcebook of family theories and methods* (pp. 275–301). Boston: Springer.

Bronte-Tinkew, J., Moore, K. A., & Carrano, J. (2006). The father-child relationship, parenting styles, and adolescent risk behaviors in intact families. *Journal of Family Issues, 27*(6), 850–881.

Brown, G. L., Mangelsdorf, S. C., & Neff, C. (2012). Father involvement, paternal sensitivity, and father–child attachment security in the first 3 years. *Journal of Family Psychology, 26*(3), 421.

Brown, G. L., Mangelsdorf, S. C., Shigeto, A., & Wong, M. S. (2018). Associations between father involvement and father–child attachment security: Variations based on timing and type of involvement. *Journal of Family Psychology, 32*(8), 1015.

Cabrera, N. J. (2010). Father involvement and public policies. In M. E. Lamb (Ed.), *The role of the father in child development* (5th ed., pp. 517–550). Hoboken, NJ: Wiley.

Cabrera, N., Fitzgerald, H. E., Bradley, R. H., & Roggman, L. (2007). Modeling the dynamics of paternal influences on children over the life course. *Applied Development Science, 11*(4), 185–189.

Cabrera, N. J., Fitzgerald, H. E., Bradley, R. H., & Roggman, L. (2014). The ecology of father-child relationships: An expanded model. *Journal of Family Theory & Review, 6*(4), 336–354.

Cabrera, N. J., Hofferth, S. L., & Chae, S. (2011). Patterns and predictors of father–infant engagement across race/ethnic groups. *Early Childhood Research Quarterly, 26*(3), 365–375.

Cabrera, N. J., Ryan, R. M., Mitchell, S. J., Shannon, J. D., & Tamis-LeMonda, C. S. (2008). Low-income, nonresident father involvement with their toddlers: Variation by fathers' race and ethnicity. *Journal of Family Psychology, 22*(4), 643.

Cabrera, N. J., Shannon, J. D., Vogel, C., Tamis-LeMonda, C., Ryan, R. M., Brooks-Gunn, J., Raikes, H., & Cohen, R. (2004). Low-Income Fathers' Involvement in Their Toddlers' Lives: Biological Fathers From the Early Head Start Research and Evaluation Study. *Fathering: A journal of theory, research & practice about men as fathers, 2*(1).

Carr, A. (2016). The evolution of systems theory. In T. Sexton & J. Lebow (Eds.), Handbook of family therapy (pp. 27–43). New York: Routledge.

Center for Disease Control and Prevention. (2017). NVSS - Marriages and Divorces. Retrieved August 21, 2019, from https://www.cdc.gov/nchs/nvss/marriagedivorce.htm

Coley, R. L. (1998). Children's socialization experiences and functioning in single-mother households: The importance of fathers and other men. *Child Development, 69*(1), 219–230.

Coley, R. L. (2001). (In) visible men: Emerging research on low-income, unmarried, and minority fathers. *American Psychologist, 56*(9), 743.

Cooper, S. M., Ross, L., Dues, A., Golden, A. R., & Burnett, M. (2019). Intergenerational Factors, Fatherhood Beliefs, and African American Fathers' Involvement: Building the Case for a Mediated Pathway. *Journal of Family Issues, 40*(15), 2047–2075.

Cooper, S. M., Smalls-Glover, C., Metzger, I., & Griffin, C. (2015). African American fathers' racial socialization patterns: Associations with racial identity beliefs and discrimination experiences. *Family Relations, 64*(2), 278–290.

Cowan, P. A., Cowan, C. P., Pruett, M. K., Pruett, K., & Wong, J. J. (2009). Promoting fathers' engagement with children: Preventive interventions for low-income families. *Journal of Marriage and Family, 71*(3), 663–679.

Das Eiden, R., & Leonard, K. E. (2000). Paternal alcoholism, parental psychopathology, and aggravation with infants. *Journal of Substance Abuse, 11*(1), 17–29.

Day, R. D., Acock, A. C., Bahr, S. J., & Arditti, J. A. (2005). Incarcerated fathers returning home to children and families: Introduction to the special issue and a primer on doing research with men in prison. *Fathering: A Journal of Theory, Research & Practice About Men as Fathers, 3*(3), 183–200.

Day, R. D., & Lamb, M. E. (2003). Conceptualizing and measuring father involvement: Pathways, problems, and progress. In *Conceptualizing and measuring father involvement* (pp. 23–36). New York: Routledge.

Dubowitz, H., Black, M. M., Cox, C. E., Kerr, M. A., Litrownik, A. J., Radhakrishna, A., et al. (2001). Father involvement and children's functioning at age 6 years: A multisite study. *Child Maltreatment, 6*(4), 300–309.

East, L., Jackson, D., & O'Brien, L. (2006). Father absence and adolescent development: A review of the literature. *Journal of Child Health Care, 10*(4), 283–295.

Ellis, B. J., Bates, J. E., Dodge, K. A., Fergusson, D. M., John Horwood, L., Pettit, G. S., et al. (2003). Does father absence place daughters at special risk for early sexual activity and teenage pregnancy? *Child Development, 74*(3), 801–821.

Fagan, J., Day, R., Lamb, M. E., & Cabrera, N. J. (2014). Should researchers conceptualize differently the dimensions of parenting for fathers and mothers? *Journal of Family Theory & Review, 6*(4), 390–405.

Favez, N., Lopes, F., Bernard, M., Frascarolo, F., Lavanchy Scaiola, C., Corboz-Warnery, A., et al. (2012). The development of family alliance from pregnancy to toddlerhood and child outcomes at 5 years. *Family Process, 51*(4), 542–556.

Feldman, R., & Masalha, S. (2010). Parent–child and triadic antecedents of children's social competence: Cultural specificity, shared process. *Developmental Psychology, 46*(2), 455.

Fitzgerald, H. E., Mann, T., & Barratt, M. (1999). Fathers and infants. *Infant Mental Health Journal, 20*(3), 213–221.

Fitzgerald, H. E., McKelvey, L. M., Schiffman, R. F., & Montañez, M. (2006). Exposure of low-income families and their children to neighborhood violence and paternal antisocial behavior. *Parenting, 6*(2–3), 243–258.

Fitzgerald, H. E. & Bocknek, E. L. (2012). Fathers, children, and the risk-resilience continuum. In N. J. Cabrera & C. S. Tamis-LeMonda (Eds.), Handbook of fatherinvolvement: Multidisciplinary perspectives (2nd ed., pp. 168-185). New York: Routledge.

Fox, G. L., & Bruce, C. (2001). Conditional fatherhood: Identity theory and parental investment theory as alternative sources of explanation of fathering. *Journal of Marriage and Family, 63*(2), 394–403.

Galardi, T. R., Settersten Jr., R. A., Vuchinich, S., & Richards, L. (2017). Associations between incarcerated fathers' cumulative childhood risk and contact with their children. *Journal of Family Issues, 38*(5), 654–676.

Green, D. S., Chuang, S. S., Parke, R. D., & Este, D. C. (2019). Multidimensionality and complexities of fathering: A critical examination of Afro-Jamaican fathers'perspectives. *Sex Roles, 81*(9–10), 576–593.

Greene, S. M., Anderson, E. R., Forgatch, M. S., DeGarmo, D. S., & Hetherington, E. M. (2012). Risk and resilience after divorce. In F. Walsh (Ed.), Normal family processes: Growing diversity and complexity (p. 102–127). New York: The Guilford Press.

Hairston, C. F. (1998). The forgotten parent: Understanding the forces that influence incarcerated fathers' relationships with their children. *Child Welfare, 77*(5), 617.

Hanlon, T. E., Carswell, S. B., & Rose, M. (2007). Research on the caretaking of children of incarcerated parents: Findings and their service delivery implications. *Children and Youth Services Review, 29*(3), 348–362.

Horn, W. F. (2003). Is it working? Early evaluations of fatherhood-renewal programs. In *Black fathers in contemporary society: Strengths, weaknesses, and strategies for change* (pp. 138–152). New York: Russell Sage Foundation.

Huebner, A. J., Mancini, J. A., Wilcox, R. M., Grass, S. R., & Grass, G. A. (2007). Parental deployment and youth in military families: Exploring uncertainty and ambiguous loss. *Family Relations, 56*(2), 112–122.

Hughes, C., Foley, S., Devine, R. T., Ribner, A., Kyriakou, L., Boddington, L., & Holmes, E. A. (2019). Worrying in the wings? Negative emotional birth memories in mothers and fathers show similar associations with perinatal mood disturbance and delivery mode. *Archives of Women's Mental Health, 23*, 371–377.

Jaffee, S. R., Moffitt, T. E., Caspi, A., & Taylor, A. (2003). Life with (or without) father: The benefits of living with two biological parents depend on the father's antisocial behavior. *Child Development, 74*(1), 109–126.

Jamison, T. B., Ganong, L., & Proulx, C. M. (2017). Unmarried coparenting in the context of poverty: Understanding the relationship between stress, family resource management, and resilience. *Journal of Family and Economic Issues, 38*(3), 439–452.

Kelly, J. B., & Emery, R. E. (2003). Children's adjustment following divorce: Risk and resilience perspectives. *Family Relations, 52*(4), 352–362.

Kim, S., & Brody, G. H. (2005). Longitudinal pathways to psychological adjustment among Black youth living in single-parent households. *Journal of Family Psychology, 19*(2), 305.

Knobloch, L. K., & Knobloch-Fedders, L. M. (2017). *Reintegration difficulty of military couples following deployment*. University of Illinois Urbana United States.

Lamb, M. E., Pleck, J. H., Charnov, E. L., & Levine, J. A. (1987). A biosocial perspective on paternal behavior and involvement. *Parenting Across the Life Span: Biosocial Dimensions*, 111–142.

Lamb, M. E. (2000). The history of research on father involvement: An overview. *Marriage & Family Review, 29*(2–3), 23–42.

LeMoine, K. A., Romirowsky, A. M., Woods, K. E., & Chronis-Tuscano, A. (2018). Paternal antisocial behavior (but not paternal ADHD) is associated with negative parenting and child conduct problems. *Journal of Attention Disorders, 22*(13), 1187–1199.

Leonard, K. E., Eiden, R. D., Wong, M. M., Zucker, R. A., Puttler, L. I., Fitzgerald, H. E., et al. (2000). Developmental perspectives on risk and vulnerability in alcoholic families. *Alcoholism: Clinical and Experimental Research, 24*(2), 238–240.

Love, J. M., Kisker, E. E., Ross, C., Raikes, H., Constantine, J., Boller, K., et al. (2005). The effectiveness of early head start for 3-year-old children and their parents: Lessons for policy and programs. *Developmental Psychology, 41*(6), 885.

Lovejoy, M. C., Graczyk, P. A., O'Hare, E., & Neuman, G. (2000). Maternal depression and parenting behavior: A meta-analytic review. *Clinical Psychology Review, 20*(5), 561–592.

Lucassen, N., Tharner, A., Van IJzendoorn, M. H., Bakermans-Kranenburg, M. J., Volling, B. L., Verhulst, F. C., et al. (2011). The association between paternal sensitivity and infant–father attachment security: A meta-analysis of three decades of research. *Journal of Family Psychology, 25*(6), 986–992.

MacDermid, S., Schwarz, R., Faber, A., Adkins, J., Mishkind, M., & Weiss, H. (2005). Military fathers on the front lines. In *Situated fathering: A focus on physical and social spaces* (pp. 209–239). Lanham, MD: Rowman & Littlefield.

Madden-Derdich, D. A., & Leonard, S. A. (2000). Parental role identity and fathers' involvement in coparental interaction after divorce: Fathers' perspectives. *Family Relations, 49*(3), 311–318.

Marrast, L., Himmelstein, D. U., & Woolhandler, S. (2016). Racial and ethnic disparities in mental health care for children and young adults: A national study. *International Journal of Health Services, 46*(4), 810–824.

Martin, A., Ryan, R. M., & Brooks-Gunn, J. (2010). When fathers' supportiveness matters most: Maternal and paternal parenting and children's school readiness. *Journal of Family Psychology, 24*(2), 145.

McAdoo, H. P., & Younge, S. N. (2009). Black families. In *Handbook of African American psychology* (pp. 103–115). Thousand Oaks, CA: Sage.

McCubbin, H. I. (1979). Integrating coping behavior in family stress theory. *Journal of Marriage and the Family, 41*, 237–244.

McHale, J. P., Favez, N., & Fivaz-Depeursinge, E. (2018). The Lausanne Trilogue Play paradigm: Breaking discoveries in family process and therapy. *Journal of Child and Family Studies, 27*(10), 3063–3072.

McHale, J. P., & Fivaz-Depeursinge, E. (2010). Principles of effective co-parenting and its assessment in infancy and early childhood. In *Parenthood and mental health: A bridge between infant and adult psychiatry* (pp. 357–371). Chichester, West Sussex: Wiley-Blackwell.

McLoyd, V. C. (1990). The impact of economic hardship on Black families and children: Psychological distress, parenting, and socioemotional development. *Child Development, 61*(2), 311–346.

Mechling, B. M., Ahern, N. R., & Palumbo, R. (2018). Applying ambiguous loss theory to children of parents with an opioid use disorder. *Journal of Child and Adolescent Psychiatric Nursing, 31*(2–3), 53–60.

Minuchin, P. (1985). Families and individual development: Provocations from the field of family therapy. *Child Development, 56*, 289–302.

Minuchin, S. (1974). *Families and family therapy.* Cambridge, MA: Harvard University Press.

Olmstead, S. B., Futris, T. G., & Pasley, K. (2009). An exploration of married and divorced, nonresident men's perceptions and organization of their father role identity. *Fathering, 7*(3), 249.

Paquette, D., & Bigras, M. (2010). The risky situation: A procedure for assessing the father–child activation relationship. *Early Child Development and Care, 180*(1–2), 33–50.

Paquette, D., & Dumont, C. (2013). Is father–child rough-and-tumble play associated with attachment or activation relationships? *Early Child Development and Care, 183*(6), 760–773.

Parke, R. D., & Cookston, J. T. (2019). Commentary: Many types of fathers, many types of contexts: An agenda for future progress in fathering research. *Advancing Research and Measurement on Fathering and Children's Development, 84*(1), 132–146.

Parsons, A., Knopp, K., Rhoades, G. K., Allen, E. S., Markman, H. J., & Stanley, S. M. (2018). Associations of army fathers' PTSD symptoms and child functioning: Within-and between-family effects. *Family Process, 57*(4), 915–926.

Patterson, J. M. (1988). Families experiencing stress: I. The family adjustment and adaptation response model: II. Applying the FAAR model to health-related issues for intervention and research. *Family Systems Medicine, 6*(2), 202–237.

Patterson, J. M. (2002). Integrating family resilience and family stress theory. *Journal of Marriage and Family, 64*(2), 349–360.

Patterson, J. M., & Garwick, A. W. (1994). Levels of meaning in family stress theory. *Family Process, 33*(3), 287–304.

Paulson, J. F., Bazemore, S. D., Goodman, J. H., & Leiferman, J. A. (2016). The course and interrelationship of maternal and paternal perinatal depression. *Archives of Women's Mental Health, 19*(4), 655–663.

Peck, S. D. (2003). Measuring sensitivity moment-by-moment: A microanalytic look at the transmission of attachment. *Attachment & Human Development, 5*(1), 38–63.

Pexton, S., Farrants, J., & Yule, W. (2018). The impact of fathers' military deployment on child adjustment. The support needs of primary school children and their families separated during active military service: A pilot study. *Clinical Child Psychology and Psychiatry, 23*(1), 110–124.

Pidano, A. E., & Allen, A. R. (2015). The Incredible Years series: A review of the independent research base. *Journal of Child and Family Studies, 24*(7), 1898–1916.

Pilkington, P., Rominov, H., Brown, H. K., & Dennis, C. L. (2019). Systematic review of the impact of coparenting interventions on paternal coparenting behaviour. *Journal of Advanced Nursing, 75*(1), 17–29.

Piskernik, B., & Ahnert, L. (2019). What does it mean when fathers are involved in parenting? Advancing research and measurement on fathering and children's development. *Monographs of the Society of Research in Child Development, 84*(1), 64–78.

Poon, E., Ellis, D. A., Fitzgerald, H. E., & Zucker, R. A. (2000). Intellectual, cognitive, and academic performance among sons of alcoholics during the early school years: Differences related to subtypes of familial alcoholism. *Alcoholism: Clinical and Experimental Research, 24*(7), 1020–1027.

Puttler, L. I., Fitzgerald, H. E., Heitzeg, M. M., & Zucker, R. A. (2017). Boys, early risk factors for alcohol problems, and the development of the self: An interconnected matrix. *Infant Mental Health Journal, 38*(1), 83–96.

Ramchandani, P., & Psychogiou, L. (2009). Paternal psychiatric disorders and children's psychosocial development. *The Lancet, 374*(9690), 646–653.

Richardson, P., Bocknek, E. L., McGoron, L., & Trentacosta, C. (2019). Fathering across contexts: The moderating role of toddler respiratory sinus arrhythmia in predicting emotion regulation among African American families. *Developmental Psychobiology, 61*(6), 903–919.

Roggman, L. A., Boyce, L., Cook, G. A., Christiansen, K., & Jones, D. (2007). Playing with daddy: Social toy play, early head start, and developmental outcomes. *Fathering: A Journal of Theory, Research, and Practice About Men as Fathers, 2*(1), 83–108.

Roy, K. M. (2006). Father stories: A life course examination of paternal identity among low-income African American men. *Journal of Family Issues, 27*(1), 31–54.

Sethna, V., Murray, L., Netsi, E., Psychogiou, L., & Ramchandani, P. G. (2015). Paternal depression in the postnatal period and early father–infant interactions. *Parenting, 15*(1), 1–8.

Shears, J., Summers, J. A., Boller, K., & Barclay-McLaughlin, G. (2006). Exploring fathering roles in low-income families: The influence of intergenerational transmission. *Families in Society, 87*(2), 259–268.

Shannon, J. D., Tamis-LeMonda, C. S., London, K., & Cabrera, N. (2002). Beyond rough and tumble: Low-income fathers' interactions and children's cognitive development at 24 months. *Parenting: Science and Practice, 2*(2), 77–104.

Sobolewski, J. M., & King, V. (2005). The importance of the coparental relationship for nonresident fathers' ties to children. *Journal of Marriage and Family, 67*(5), 1196–1212.

Stover, C. S., & Kiselica, A. (2015). Hostility and substance use in relation to intimate partner violence and parenting among fathers. *Aggressive Behavior, 41*(3), 205–213.

Tamis-LeMonda, C. S., & McFadden, K. E. (2010). Fathers from low-income backgrounds: Myths and evidence. In M. E. Lamb (Ed.), *The role of the father in child development* (pp. 296–318). Hoboken, NJ: Wiley.

The Pew Charitable Trusts: Pew Center on the States. (2010). *Collateral costs: Incarceration's effect on economic mobility*. Washington, DC: Pew Charitable Trusts.

Thomas, G., Farrell, M. P., & Barnes, G. M. (1996). The effects of single-mother families and nonresident fathers on delinquency and substance abuse in Black and White adolescents. *Journal of Marriage and the Family, 58*(4), 884–894.

Volling, B. L., & Cabrera, N. J. (2019). Moving research on fathering and children's development forward: Priorities and recommendations for the future. *Advancing Research and Measurement on Fathering and Children's Development, 84*(1), 107–117.

Volling, B. L., Yu, T., Gonzalez, R., Tengelitsch, E., & Stevenson, M. M. (2018). Maternal and paternal trajectories of depressive symptoms predict family risk and children's emotional and behavioral problems after the birth of a sibling. *Development and Psychopathology, 31*(4), 1307–1324.

von Bertalanffy, L. (1969). *General system theory*. New York: George Braziller.

Yablonsky, A. M., Barbero, E. D., & Richardson, J. W. (2016). Hard is normal: Military families' transitions within the process of deployment. *Research in Nursing & Health, 39*(1), 42–56.

Fathers and Public Policy

8

Cynthia Osborne

Research is increasingly clear that fathers play an important and unique role in their children's development. Father involvement is associated with better outcomes on nearly every measure of child well-being, including academic achievement, emotional and physical health, and positive behaviors (Bronte-Tinkew, Carrano, Horowitz, & Kinukawa, 2008; Cabrera, Shannon, & Tamis-LeMonda, 2007; Carlson & Magnuson, 2011). Yet, more than half of children will spend some of their childhood living apart from their biological father, and many children have little involvement with their father from birth (Tach, 2014). These statistics are concerning because father absence is associated with an increased risk of a host of negative outcomes for children (McLanahan, Tach, & Schneider, 2013).

Today's families are increasingly complex and less stable, particularly families with lower levels of income and families of color. These family dynamics often fuel father absence, and family instability and complexity are associated with an increased risk of negative outcomes (Fomby & Cherlin, 2007; Fomby & Osborne, 2016; Osborne, Berger, & Magnuson, 2012; Osborne & McLanahan, 2007). Approximately two out of five children are born to unmarried parents, but approximately 70% of Black children, half of Latinx children, and the vast majority of children born to younger and less educated parents are born to unmarried parents (Martin, Hamilton, Osterman, & Driscoll, 2019; McLanahan, 2011). On average, unmarried relationships are less stable than marital relationships, such that the mother and father will separate and re-partner several times over the course of their child's young life (McLanahan & Beck, 2010; Osborne & McLanahan, 2007). Through re-partnering, children will acquire half- and stepsiblings as these new relationships form. Nearly 80% of children who are born to unmarried parents experience family instability (parental separation and re-partnering) or complexity (the introduction of half- or stepsiblings) by the time they are 5 years old (Edin, 2018). Fathers often have children across several households, such that the father will play multiple roles simultaneously (Edin & Nelson, 2013). For example, he might be a highly engaged resident stepfather to one child and an absent, nonresident father to his biological child. These multiple roles can lead to financial strain and difficulty in providing the emotional involvement that fathers idealize and children need to thrive.

Federal and state governments have come to recognize the important contributions that fathers make to their children's well-being and that these contributions extend beyond merely providing financial resources to the household. In the past 10 years, governments have increasingly

C. Osborne (✉)
LBJ School of Public Affairs, University of Texas at Austin, Austin, TX, USA
e-mail: cosborne@prc.utexas.edu

H. E. Fitzgerald et al. (eds.), *Handbook of Fathers and Child Development*,
https://doi.org/10.1007/978-3-030-51027-5_8

supported policies and programs to foster fathers' emotional and financial contributions, including through funding Responsible Fatherhood programs and enhancing the child support system to enable fathers to better meet their financial and emotional obligations (Tollestrup, 2018).

In this chapter, I discuss the policies and programs designed to support fathers' emotional and financial involvement with their children, and I compare these approaches with the policies and programs designed to support mothers of young children. Additionally, I discuss a broader set of policies that should be considered to ensure that fathers have the skills and resources necessary to be the fathers they aspire to be and that their children need.

The Role of the Father

Fathers vary considerably in the roles they play in their children's lives and in their level of needs that challenge their role as fathers. For example, some fathers are actively engaged in their children's lives and have a strong romantic and co-parenting relationship with their child's mother, whereas other fathers may have had very little contact with their child or their child's mother in several years, yet they strive to reconnect. Policies to support fathers should target the specific needs of fathers, because a one-size-fits-all approach will be ineffective.

In this chapter, I focus primarily on fathers with lower levels of education and income and who are not married to their child's biological mother. I focus on this group of fathers because, on average, these fathers struggle the most to provide for their children financially and to remain engaged in their child's life over the long term (Cabrera et al., 2007; Castillo, Welch, & Sarver, 2013; Coley & Chase-Lansdale, 1999). Yet, even among this narrowly defined group of lower-income, unmarried fathers, substantial variation exists. These fathers may be living with their child's mother; living separately but romantically involved with their child's mother; not in a romantic relationship with their child's mother, but actively co-parenting; or largely absent from their child's life. And, as stated earlier, fathers who have children with multiple partners may assume several of these roles simultaneously.

To be certain, most married fathers could benefit from programs that enhance their parenting skills, improve their relationship with their child's mother, or improve their job prospects. And all fathers could benefit from broader policies that support families, such as paid family leave. However, unmarried, lower-income fathers face considerable challenges in providing the emotional and financial resources their children need, and they are primarily the focus of the federal and state policies targeted toward fathers.

Focus of Fatherhood Policy

Traditionally, social policies were not targeted toward fathers, with the exception of child support policies. Arguably, policies that affect the criminal justice system or military have a disproportionate impact on men and therefore fathers, but those systems were not designed to increase child well-being. Policies, including fatherhood programs and child support policies, were originally designed to hold fathers accountable for financially supporting their children, and the policies paid little attention to the level of engagement or access the father had with his child. Policies were largely developed to replicate the breadwinner/homemaker stylized family of the 1950s, in which the father contributed financially to the household and the mother provided most of the child-rearing responsibilities (Huntington, 2015). In this stylized version of a family, upon separation, the courts assumed the father (the noncustodial parent) would continue working, and the court would determine the amount of money he needed to contribute to the household. The assumption was that the father would have a small role in the child-rearing responsibilities and the mother (the custodial parent) would have limited earnings (Murray & Hwang, 2014). Although today's policies and programs aimed at fathers have a larger focus on father involvement and parenting than they did in decades past, they are still largely based on encouraging the father to contribute financially to the household.

This policy emphasis on financial accountability for fathers is markedly different from the policies that are largely aimed at supporting mothers and their children, particularly mothers with lower levels of incomes. For mothers, the underlying assumption is that mothers are involved in their children's lives and policies, such as the Maternal, Infant, and Early Childhood Home Visiting (MIECHV) program, aim to give mothers the information and parenting skills they need to nurture their children (Congressional Research Service, 2018). Programs and policies also aim to identify needs that the mother may have (e.g., housing insecurity, depression, childcare instability) and connect mothers with necessary community resources to address these needs (Haskins & Sawhill, 2009; Osborne et al., 2014). If the mother does not have adequate resources to provide for her child independently, government policies provide aid through housing vouchers, food stamps, childcare subsidies, medical insurance, child support, and cash welfare, with some expectations that she will work to receive assistance.

These social policies apply to all custodial parents, regardless of whether the parent is a father or mother, but the overwhelming majority (80.4%) of custodial parents are mothers (Grall, 2020). Since 1960, the number of custodial fathers has increased substantially, and the rate of growth of single fathers is double that of single mothers (Livingston, 2013). However, custodial fathers are less disadvantaged than are custodial mothers. Compared to custodial mothers, custodial fathers are less likely to live in poverty, have higher levels of education and employment, and are more likely to be cohabiting with a partner who provides assistance in child-rearing activities. Despite their advantages over custodial mothers, custodial fathers still are worse relative to their married counterparts on all of the indicators mentioned above, and their children have similar outcomes as children raised by single mothers (Downey, Ainsworth-Darnell, & Dufur, 1998; Grall, 2020; Livingston, 2013).

Noncustodial parents may be eligible for some means-tested programs based on their personal needs to income, but the needs of providing for their children are not considered in the benefit levels provided, even if the noncustodial parent spends a great deal of time with their child. For example, parents may share physical custody of their child (e.g., the child spends every other weekend and rotating holidays with the noncustodial parent), and each parent may face food insecurity and qualify for SNAP benefits. The child's need for food will only be included within the allotment of benefits for the custodial parent, whereas the noncustodial parent will have to provide food for himself and the child without the additional benefit. This one-sided approach to supporting families may weaken the family system and discourage fathers from remaining engaged with their children.

Child Support

Perhaps, the policy that has the largest impact on fathers is the child support program. The reach of the federal child support program is immense, serving nearly 16 million children. More children are served by the child support program than by Social Security, Temporary Assistance for Needy Families (TANF), Child Care, and Supplemental Security Income (SSI) combined (Sorensen, 2016). One out of five children in the United States is in the child support system, and the program transfers over $30 billion dollars annually from the noncustodial parent (usually the father) to the custodial parent (usually the mother). The program is not means-tested, but families in the program are largely lower-income families, with more than half of families having incomes below 150% of the federal poverty line and over 80% having incomes below three times the poverty threshold. Of the families in the program who are poor and receive child support, the support accounts for over 40% of their monthly income (Sorensen, 2016).

The federal child support program was established in 1975 as Part D of Title IV of the Social Security Act. The program is administered at the state level, and the federal government reimburses the states for approximately two-thirds of their costs. Child support was established as a cost-recovery program for cash welfare. Child support payments collected from fathers were paid to the government to recoup payments made to mothers who received Aid to Families with Dependent Children (AFDC – now TANF) (Congressional Research Service, 2019). Child support remains a cost-recovery program, although the share of mothers on cash welfare (TANF) has dwindled substantially since the 1996 welfare reform, such that today only 5% of child support payments are retained by states (Sorensen, 2016).

The goals of the child support program are to establish and enforce the payment of child support orders to ensure that custodial parents (mothers) have the financial resources they need to provide for their child and to hold the noncustodial parents (fathers) financially accountable for their children. The program was established at a time when most children were born to married parents and the stylized family included a breadwinner father and a homemaker mother. As divorce rates rose substantially, child support payments from the father were intended to offset the loss of income that his leaving caused the household. The program was also established at a time of substantial increases in the cash welfare rolls (AFDC), and the goal was to hold fathers financially responsible for their children, rather than having mothers rely on the government for assistance (Cancian & Meyer, 2018).

Today, the program primarily serves families who have never been married and who are not on cash welfare (Sorensen, 2016). Because it was not designed with these families in mind, the program strains to meet the needs of today's complex families. The child support program works relatively well for families in which the father (noncustodial parent) has stable employment; the monthly child support payment is electronically withheld from his paycheck and transferred to the mother (custodial parent). However, for fathers whose employment patterns are erratic, the child support program is not flexible enough to serve these families well, and it is common for the father to amass substantial arrears and the mother and child to receive very little financial assistance (Cancian & Meyer, 2018; Miller & Mincy, 2012).

In recent years, the child support program has enhanced its goals to extend beyond the establishment and collection of child support payments, although these functions remain the primary measures that the federal government uses to determine and reward state performance. The Final Rule, issued in 2017 from the Office of Child Support Enforcement (OCSE), guided state child support offices to set "right-sized" orders that are based on the noncustodial parents' actual ability to pay, rather than imputed income, and the Rule ordered states to reduce their reliance on using civil contempt (jail) to enforce child support payments. The Rule also prohibited states from considering incarceration as voluntary unemployment, thus allowing fathers to modify their child support orders when they have lengthy prison stays (Office of Child Support Enforcement, n.d.).

Initially, the Rule proposed allowing states to use their funds to help noncustodial parents find employment and to establish parenting time orders alongside child support orders. These two elements were ultimately removed from the Final Rule, although these policy elements are top priorities for most fathers in the child support program.

Fathers often feel the child support program does not serve them well; it is a system that holds them financially accountable for their children, but does not support their emotional bond with their child (Edin & Nelson, 2013). Moreover, for fathers who have difficulty paying their required payment, the system can be punitive, leading to a loss of their driver's license or professional license or even to imprisonment. Families often prefer informal child support arrangements, either informal cash payments or in-kind contributions, to being involved in the formal child support system (Edin, 2018). These informal payments signal that the father is engaged and willing to take care of his child, without the enforcement of a formal system. Indeed, informal contributions, including cash and in-kind goods and services, are a stronger predictor of father involvement and healthier relationships than formal contributions through the child support system (Nepomnyaschy, 2007; Nepomnyaschy & Garfinkel, 2010).

Public policies have yet to strike the proper balance between holding fathers accountable for contributing to their child's financial well-being and recognizing the realities of the father's relationship with his child and co-parent and of the difficulties many fathers have in finding and maintaining steady employment that would allow them to support their child. Often, the formal child support system's punitive measures lead to lower levels of financial and emotional contributions to children, as fathers work in the underground economy or eschew their relationship with their child (Cancian, Heinrich, & Chung, 2013; Edin & Nelson, 2013).

In an effort to increase fathers' ability to pay child support, in 2012, the Office of Child Support Enforcement funded eight states to participate in a 5-year demonstration project to determine the impact that employment support programs have on improving child support payments among noncustodial parents who have difficulty making regular payments (Cancian, Meyer, & Wood, 2019). In addition to employment services, states provided a variety of services to fathers including enhanced child support services, parenting classes, and case management. The broad aim of the program was to increase the financial and emotional contributions of fathers to their children.

The demonstration project was rigorously evaluated using a randomized control trial design. The findings indicate that fathers who had access to the services earned more during the first year of the program (based on administrative records) and experienced greater economic stability with regard to housing and access to health and nutrition services. Participating fathers also reduced their child support obligations and payments during the first year substantially more than control fathers. A goal of the enhanced child support services was to set child support orders that were better aligned with what fathers could pay, which is what accounts for the lower child support orders of participating fathers. Unfortunately, despite the smaller order amounts, compliance with child support payments did not differ between the treatment and control groups (Cancian et al., 2019).

With regard to parenting, fathers in the programs reported a slightly greater sense of responsibility for their children compared to similar fathers who did not receive the parenting services, but the effects were very small. Participant fathers also reported spending an additional day with their child in the past 30 days (12.8 versus 11.8 days), compared to control fathers. Overall, the impacts of the demonstration project yielded relatively minimal impacts on improving participant fathers' emotional or financial contributions to his children (Cancian et al., 2019).

Responsible Fatherhood Programs

In an effort to increase fathers' involvement and support of their children, the federal government currently allocates $150 million annually to fund healthy marriage, responsible fatherhood, and prisoner reentry programs. The 1996 Personal Responsibility and Work Opportunity Reconciliation Act (PRWORA) emphasized marriage and father engagement, and the Clinton and Bush administrations supported demonstration projects and various efforts to promote relationship counseling and parenting skills. However, the Healthy Marriage and Responsible Fatherhood initiative authorized under the Deficit Reduction Act of 2005 and reauthorized in the Claims Resolution Act of 2010 expanded on these initial efforts by funding three types of programs: (1) the Healthy Marriage and Relationship Education (HMRE) programs offer marriage and relationship education, as well as services to promote economic stability; (2) the New Pathways for Fathers and Families (New Pathways) programs offer services focused on improving co-parenting relationships, enhancing parent-child engagement, and promoting economic mobility; and (3) the Responsible Fatherhood Opportunities for Reentry and Mobility (ReFORM) programs target fathers who will soon be released from incarceration or who were released within the prior 6 months. Not only are the services similar to the New Pathways services, but also they focus on connecting fathers with their communities (Fernandez, 2017; Office of Family Assistance, 2019).

The original impetus of the Responsible Fatherhood programs was to improve a father's economic stability in order to increase his child support payments. The programs have evolved to require a focus on co-parenting relationships and parenting skills, as well (Tollestrup, 2018). This expansion in focus was driven by research that shows that the parents' ability to co-parent, defined as the ability to make joint decisions about their child regardless of their romantic relationship, is a primary predictor of a father's financial contributions to his child. The co-parenting relationship and the father's financial contributions are also associated with the likelihood that the father will see his child more regularly (Hohmann-Marriott, 2011; Palkovitz, Fagan, & Hull, 2013; Ryan, Kalil, & Ziol-Guest, 2008).

The Responsible Fatherhood programs differ considerably in their aims, approach, and scope from the federal government's programs aimed largely at strengthening mothers' parenting skills. In 2010, Congress implemented the Maternal Infant Early Childhood Home Visiting (MIECHV) program, as part of the Affordable Care Act. The MIECHV legislation provides $400 million annually in formula and competitive grants to states to implement evidence-based home visiting programs targeted primarily to lower-income mothers. At least 75% of the MIECHV funds must be spent on programs that have been rigorously evaluated and meet the criteria established by the Home Visiting Evidence of Effectiveness (HOMVEE) clearinghouse. States are required to continuously evaluate their programs and to report on a common series of benchmark measures to demonstrate outputs of the program that are associated with child outcomes (Congressional Research Service, 2018).

By contrast, the Responsible Fatherhood programs are building an evidence base to identify programs that demonstrate a measurable impact on the stated goals of the programs, including co-parenting, father engagement, and economic stability. A large, federally funded, rigorous evaluation of four well-established Responsible Fatherhood programs found that the fathers who participated in the programs demonstrated more nurturing behaviors and engagement with their children, but the programs demonstrated no impact on co-parenting skills or economic mobility (Holcomb et al., 2019). Other evaluations with less rigorous designs have demonstrated similar modest to null impacts of the program models (Osborne, Michelsen, & Bobbitt, 2017).

The home visiting models also have relatively modest impacts on parenting behaviors and, with few exceptions, mostly null impacts on health and economic well-being (Filene, Kaminski, Valle, & Cachat, 2013; Nievar, Van Egeren, & Pollard, 2010; Sweet & Appelbaum, 2004), and no program model has a focus on improving co-parenting relationships. The home visiting field is attempting to identify the key or core elements of the program models and target services to the precise needs of a family (Supplee & Duggan, 2019). The hope is that a better alignment between program services and participant needs will improve the impacts of the program models.

The home visiting and Responsible Fatherhood programs differ in several other ways that may affect the impact the programs have on parents and children. Home visiting models frequently target new or expectant parents (mostly mothers) and provide services to the family in the family's home. The duration of the programs is quite long, often years, and most program models work jointly with the parent and child. The goals of the program models vary, but most aim to support the mother in her parenting role, identify any material needs or physical or mental health issues of the mother and child, and connect the family members to services in the community that can address these needs. The home visitors are trained professionals or paraprofessionals and have a caseload of approximately 20–25 families at a time.

By contrast, Responsible Fatherhood programs are typically short in duration (approximately 10–12 weeks) and meet in a group setting, with no children present. The group facilitator plays an important role in the success of the program by building a safe space for fathers to connect with one another. The facilitators seldom attend training sessions on the program model, and they have varied professional backgrounds. The programs target all fathers, not just new or expectant fathers, and the average age of fathers participating in the programs is 35 years old (Holcomb et al., 2019). Fathers typically enter the programs seeking job assistance or because they were strongly encouraged by a parole officer, child support caseworker, or judge. Fathers who enter the programs often have myriad problems, including low self-esteem, stress, and a sense of worthlessness, and therefore, the programs spend a substantial amount of time trying to build the father up and have him recognize the valuable role he can play in his child's life (Holcomb et al., 2019; Osborne et al., 2017).

One of the reasons for the small impacts of the Responsible Fatherhood programs may be that they are trying to do too much within one program. The home visiting programs focus on fewer outcomes (mostly parent-child interaction) over a substantially longer duration of time. Responsible Fatherhood programs, by contrast, attempt to cover many areas, including financial stability, co-parenting, father involvement, and improving the father's sense of self, over a short duration. These programs are also working with men who have a long history of unemployment, many of whom have not seen their child in months or years, who have children from several relationships, and have financial debts, including child support arrears that seem insurmountable. Fathers who complete the programs often comment that the programs were life affirming and helped them in many ways. But the programs have difficulty recruiting and retaining men in the programs (Holcomb et al., 2019; Osborne et al., 2017).

The evaluations of the child support demonstration project and of the Responsible Fatherhood programs reveal how difficult it is to meet the needs of fathers and their children. The child support demonstration project increased paternal employment and earnings but had very little impact on additional financial or emotional contributions to the child. The Responsible Fatherhood programs have not increased the financial stability of fathers nor the financial contributions fathers make to their children, and the programs have had only small impacts on father-child engagement. Neither the child support demonstration nor the Responsible Fatherhood program has improved the relationships between fathers and their children's other parent, which is essential for substantially increasing father involvement and child outcomes.

Parenting Time

The policy area most ripe for further development is in establishing and enforcing parenting time orders. Parenting time orders legally establish the minimum amount of time that a father (noncustodial parent) is entitled to see his child. Parents can jointly choose to modify the time each spends with the child informally, but the established order details the minimum amount of time that noncustodial fathers have to spend with their child. When married parents divorce, the judge will typically establish a child support order and a parenting time order when the divorce is finalized. However, most unmarried parents participate in the IV-D child support system, which typically only establishes child support orders, and if the parents want a parenting time order, they have to go through a separate court process (National Conference of State Legislatures, 2020). Most fathers (noncustodial parents) who participate in the federal child support program do not have a parenting time order, because the father would need to acquire the order in a family court, and the process may require representation and be costly (Lippold & Sorensen, 2013).

Texas is the only state that establishes a parenting time order with each child support order, and it has been following this approach for over three decades (Key, 2015). Written into the Family Code is the definition of a *standard possession order* that details the access and visitation arrangement, which for most families is the first, third, and fifth weekend of each month, rotating holidays, and longer periods of time during the summer. Exceptions are made for infants, especially those breastfeeding, and for families in which the father has not been present in the child's life for a substantial period of time (Texas Access, n.d.).

Specific attention is made to screen the families for issues of domestic or family violence, and in these instances, the amount of time allotted in the order may be zero. The zero-time parenting orders help to protect women in violent relationships, in which the father may try to use the child as a pawn. The parenting time order is enforceable, whereas without the order, if the father has established paternity, the father can legally access his children at any time and remove them from the mother.

In an attempt to increase father-child involvement, the federal government developed a small program called the Access and Visitation Mandatory Grants program, which provides a total of $10 million in annual funds to the states. The funds cannot be spent on establishing or enforcing legal parenting time orders, but the funds can be used for such things as providing mediation services to the co-parents that might lead to a negotiated parenting plan. The funds can also be used to provide supervised visitation or neutral spaces for parents in acrimonious or violent relationships to pick up or drop off their children (Office of Child Support Enforcement, 2007).

In 2012, the Office of Child Support Enforcement launched the Parenting Time Opportunities for Children pilot program to assist five state child support agencies in developing and implementing processes to establish parenting time orders alongside child support orders. The pilot program required each site to pay considerable attention to issues of family violence and to conduct an evaluation. The evaluation findings showed that state child support agencies developed innovative ways to incorporate parenting time orders with child support orders, although no state went as far as Texas and made it the default process. Noncustodial parents (fathers) appreciated the integration of parenting time with child support. The study also demonstrated that this issue needs to be addressed further at the federal and state level. If the goal of the system is to increase a father's financial and emotional connections to his child, then the allocation of resources and time must be decided in one process (Office of Child Support Enforcement, 2019).

Beyond establishing parenting time orders, states should also develop systems of enforcing parenting orders. Law enforcement and courts rarely enforce that noncustodial parents spend the time with their children that the parenting time orders allocate. This lack of enforcement is a concern for noncustodial parents (fathers) who are sometimes denied access to their child by the custodial mother, and it is a concern for custodial mothers associated with a father who fails to see his child. For noncustodial fathers kept from their children, the burden is emotional; for custodial mothers who do not have any support from their child's father, the burden is financial. And each instance may be harmful to the child's well-being. Several states are considering (and two have passed) legislation that includes a presumption that the parents will share (50–50) physical custody of their child (Fifield, 2016). This presumption only applies for divorcing families, and not for unmarried families who establish child support through the IV-D system. This new approach should be monitored to determine if it serves the best interest of the child and increases the overall financial and emotional well-being of the child.

Broader Social Policies

The child support program and Responsible Fatherhood programs are primarily aimed at serving fathers and increasing the financial and emotional involvement between the father and child. Fathers could benefit, however, from the range of other social programs that are primarily geared toward supporting custodial mothers and their resident children. Providing noncustodial fathers with greater access to resources, such as parenting programs, health care, housing vouchers, food stamps, paid family leave, and tax credits, may allow fathers to better provide for their children and improve father-child engagement (Berger, 2017). Currently, by design, our social policies provide substantially greater benefits to custodial parents (mostly mothers) than they do to noncustodial parents (mostly fathers) or childless adults (Wheaton & Sorensen, 2010). Even when benefits are offered to fathers in some states, such as paid family leave, the take-up rate of the benefits is quite small, or the benefit level is lower (Lenhart, Sweson, & Schulte, 2019; Smith, Duggan, Bair-Merritt, & Cox, 2012). In Europe, fathers are often extended the same benefits as mothers; however, take-up of the policies, such as paid leave, remains low among men (van Belle, 2016).

The federal earned income tax credit (EITC) is an effective policy at incentivizing labor force participation, supplementing income, and reducing child poverty. The federal EITC provides a very small benefit for childless adults, but the benefit for parents who have custody of their children for more than 6 months out of the year can be quite substantial. In the tax year 2019, the maximum benefit for a childless adult was $529, whereas a custodial parent with one dependent child could receive up to $3526 in a refundable credit, and a custodial parent with three dependent children could receive up to $6557 (Tax Policy Center, 2019). The benefit increases with higher levels of earnings until it plateaus and eventually fades out. Because the EITC is refundable, it provides income to families who have no tax burden. The federal EITC refund is an important source of income for many lower-income custodial mothers, but it provides limited support to noncustodial fathers.

Many states have their own version of the EITC that is offered as a percentage of the federal EITC. However, only one state provides an EITC to noncustodial parents. New York State has recently implemented a state earned income tax credit for noncustodial parents who are current on all of their child support payments. The benefit level is approximately 20% of what the father would receive if he filed for the federal EITC (for one child) or 2.5 times what the father would receive from the federal childless benefit (New York State, 2019). Although extending the EITC to noncustodial parents is a step toward stronger supports for fathers, the policy is still in its infancy and has not been used widely among eligible noncustodial fathers.

Summary and Key Points

The needs of fathers vary considerably based on their level of financial stability and their relationship with their child and their child's mother. Most of our social policies are designed to hold fathers financially accountable for providing for their children, and more recent policy approaches have recognized the importance of fathers' emotional support as well. To date, we have not been largely successful at improving the financial or emotional connections noncustodial fathers have with their children through policy. Most fathers are engaged with their children, and they provide financial support, albeit through informal rather than formal means. However, a substantial number of fathers are disengaged from their children and experience financial instability, and policies have not been very effective at improving their financial security or involvement with their children.

Our social policies have a different purpose for and approach toward supporting fathers than they do mothers. Financial accountability motivates most of the supports for fathers, whereas policies aimed at mothers focus on providing resources and skills to enhance child well-being. Each parent should be held accountable for ensuring that children's emotional and financial needs are met, but currently, fathers are largely held accountable for the child's financial needs, whereas mothers are held accountable for the child's emotional needs. A policy framework that recognizes and supports the importance of each parent's role in their children's lives would place the child at the center and ensure that each parent had the skills and resources necessary to provide for their child.

References

Berger, L. (2017). A safety net for 21-century families. *Pathways Magazine*. Retrieved from https://inequality.stanford.edu/sites/default/files/Pathways_Spring2017_Family-Safety-Net.pdf

Bronte-Tinkew, J., Carrano, J., Horowitz, A., & Kinukawa, A. (2008). Involvement among resident fathers and links to infant cognitive outcomes. *Journal of Family Issues, 29*(9), 1211–1244. Retrieved from http://online.sagepub.com/

Cabrera, N. J., Shannon, J. D., & Tamis-LeMonda, C. (2007). Fathers' influence on their children's cognitive and emotional development: From toddlers to pre-K. *Applied Developmental Science, 11*(4), 208–213. Retrieved from https://research.steinhardt.nyu.edu/scmsAdmin/uploads/006/903/Cabrera,%20N.%20J.,%20Shannon,%20J.%20D.,%20&%20Tamis-LeMonda,%20C.,%20Applied%20Dev.%20Sci.,%202007.pdf

Cancian, M., Heinrich, C., & Chung, Y. (2013). Discouraging disadvantaged fathers' employment: An unintended consequence of policies designed to support families. *Journal of Policy Analysis and Management, 32*(4), 758–784. Retrieved from https://doi.org/10.1002/pam.21707

Cancian, M., & Meyer, D. (2018). Reforming policy for single-parent families to reduce child poverty. *The Russell Sage Foundation Journal of the Social Sciences, 4*(2), 91–112.

Cancian, M., Meyer, D., & Wood, R. (2019). *Final impact findings from the child support parent employment demonstration (CSPED)*. Institute for Research on Poverty, University of Wisconsin–Madison. Retrieved from https://www.acf.hhs.gov/css/resource/final-impact-findings-from-csped

Carlson, M. J., & Magnuson, K. A. (2011). Low-income fathers' influence on children. *The Annals of the American Academy of Political and Social Science, 635*(95), 95–116. Retrieved from https://www.jstor.org/stable/29779412

Castillo, J. T., Welch, G. W., & Sarver, C. M. (2013). The relationship between disadvantaged fathers' employment stability, workplace flexibility, and involvement with their infant children. *Journal of Social Service Research, 39*(3), 380–396. Retrieved from https://doi.org/10.1080/01488376.2013.775089

Coley, R., & Chase-Lansdale, P. (1999). Stability and change in paternal involvement among urban African American fathers. *Journal of Family Psychology, 13*(3), 416–435. Retrieved from https://doi.org/10.1037/0893-3200.13

Congressional Research Service. (2018). *Maternal, Infant, and Early Childhood Home Visiting (MIECHV) Program: Background and Funding*. Retrieved from https://crsreports.congress.gov/product/pdf/R/R43930/18

Congressional Research Service. (2019). *Child Support Enforcement: Program Basics*. Retrieved from https://fas.org/sgp/crs/misc/RS22380.pdf

Downey, D. B., Ainsworth-Darnell, J. W., & Dufur, M. J. (1998). Sex of parent and children's well-being in single-parent households. *Journal of Marriage and Family, 60*(4), 878–893. Retrieved from https://www.jstor.org/stable/353631

Edin, K. (2018). Child support in the age of complex families: Government efforts to engage noncustodial fathers in supporting their children should take advantage of the reality that these dads care more about their offspring than is commonly assumed. *Issues in Science and Technology, 34*(2), 38(8). Retrieved from https://www.jstor.org/stable/44577405

Edin, K., & Nelson, T. (2013). *Doing the best I can: Fatherhood in the inner city*. Berkeley, CA: University of California Press.

Fernandez, M. A. (2017). National marriage initiative. In J. Carlson & S. B. Dermer (Eds.), *The SAGE encyclopedia of marriage, family, and couples counseling* (pp. 1137–1139). Thousand Oaks, CA: SAGE Publications, Inc.

Fifield, J. (2016). *More time for dads? States weigh changes to custody laws*. The Pew Charitable Trusts. Retrieved from https://www.pewtrusts.org/en/research-and-analysis/blogs/stateline/2016/03/15/more-time-for-dads-states-weigh-changes-to-custody-laws

Filene, J. H., Kaminski, J. W., Valle, L. A., & Cachat, P. (2013). Components associated with home visiting program outcomes: A Aeta-analysis. *Pediatrics, 132*(Supplement 2), S100–S109. Retrieved from https://doi.org/10.1542/peds.2013-1021H

Fomby, P., & Cherlin, A. J. (2007). Family instability and child well-being. *American Sociological Review, 72*(2), 181–204. Retrieved from https://www.jstor.org/stable/25472457

Fomby, P., & Osborne, C. (2016). Family instability, multipartner fertility, and children's externalizing behavior in middle childhood. *Journal of Marriage and Family, 79*, 75–93.

Grall, T. (2020). *Custodial mothers and fathers and their child support: 2015*. United States Census Bureau. Retrieved from https://www.census.gov/content/dam/Census/library/publications/2020/demo/p60-262.pdf

Haskins, R., & Sawhill, I. (2009). *Creating an opportunity society*. Brookings Institution Press, 191. Retrieved from https://www.jstor.org/stable/10.7864/j.ctt6wpgsh

Hohmann-Marriott, B. (2011). Coparenting and father involvement in married and unmarried coresident couples. *Journal of Marriage and Family, 73*(1), 296–309. Retrieved from https://doi.org/10.1111/j.1741-3737.2010.00805.x

Holcomb, P., Zaveri, H., Friend, D., Dion, R., Baumgartner, S., Clary, L., et al. (2019). *Supporting the fatherhood journey: Findings from the Parents and Children Together Evaluation (PACT)*. United States Department of Health and Human Services, Administration for Children and Families, Office of Planning, Research, and Evaluation. Retrieved from https://www.acf.hhs.gov/opre/resource/supporting-the-fatherhood-journey-findings-from-the-parents-and-children-together-evaluation-pact

Huntington, C. (2015). Family law and nonmarital families. *Family Court Review, 53*(2), 221–232.

Key, A. (2015). Parenting time in Texas child support cases. *Family Court Review, 53*(2), 258–266. Retrieved from https://doi.org/10.1111/fcre.12143

Lenhart, A., Sweson, H., & Schulte, B. (2019). *Lifting the barriers to paid family and medical leave for men in the United States*. Better Life Lab, New America. Retrieved from newamerica.org/better-life-lab/reports/lifting-barriers-paid-family-and-medical-leave-men-united-states/

Lippold, K., & Sorensen, E. (2013). *Characteristics of families served by the child support (IV-D) program: 2010 census survey results*. The Urban Institute. Retrieved from https://www.urban.org/research/publication/characteristics-families-served-child-support-iv-d-program-2010-census-survey-results

Livingston, G. (2013). *The rise of single fathers: A ninefold increase since 1960*. Pew Research Center. Retrieved from https://www.pewsocialtrends.org/2013/07/02/the-rise-of-single-fathers/#fn-17500-1

Martin, J. A., Hamilton, B. E., Osterman, M. J. K., & Driscoll, A. K. (2019). *Births: Final data for 2018*. United States Department of Health and Human Services, National Vital Statistics Report. Centers for Disease Control and Prevention. Retrieved from https://www.cdc.gov/nchs/data/nvsr/nvsr68/nvsr68_13-508.pdf

McLanahan, S. (2011). Family instability and complexity after a nonmarital birth: Outcomes for children in fragile families. In M. J. Carlson & P. England (Eds.), *Social class and changing families in an unequal America* (pp. 190–228). Stanford, CA: Stanford University Press.

McLanahan, S., & Beck, A. N. (2010). Parental relationships in fragile families. *The Future of Children, 20*(2), 17–37. Retrieved from https://www.jstor.org/stable/20773693

McLanahan, S., Tach, L., & Schneider, D. (2013). The causal effects of father absence. *Annual Review of Sociology, 39*, 399–427. Retrieved from https://www.jstor.org/stable/43049642

Miller, D. P., & Mincy, R. B. (2012). Falling further behind? Child support arrears and fathers' labor force participation. *Social Service Review, 86*(4), 604–635. Retrieved from https://doi.org/10.1086/668761

Murray, F. L., & Hwang, S. H. (2014). Fatherhood, responsible. In M. J. Coleman & L. H. Ganong (Eds.), *The social history of the American family: An encyclopedia* (pp. 522–526). Thousand Oaks, CA: SAGE Publications, Inc.

National Conference of State Legislatures. (2020). *Child support and parenting time orders*. Retrieved from https://www.ncsl.org/research/human-services/child-support-and-parenting-time-orders.aspx

Nepomnyaschy, L. (2007). Child support and father-child contact: Testing reciprocal pathways. *Demography, 44*(1), 93–112. Retrieved from https://doi.org/10.1353/dem.2007.0008

Nepomnyaschy, L., & Garfinkel, I. (2010). Child support enforcement and fathers' contributions to their non-marital children. *Social Service Review, 84*(3), 341–380. Retrieved from https://doi.org/10.1086/655392

New York State, Department of Taxation and Finance. (2019). *Noncustodial parent earned income credit*. Retrieved from https://www.tax.ny.gov/pit/credits/nceic.htm

Nievar, M. A., Van Egeren, L. A., & Pollard, S. (2010). A meta-analysis of home visiting programs: Moderators of improvements in maternal behavior. *Infant Mental Health Journal, 31*(5), 499–520. Retrieved from https://doi.org/10.1002/imhj.20269

Office of Child Support Enforcement. (2007). *A collaboration and strategic planning guide for states: Child access and visitation grant programs*. United States Department of Health and Human Services, Administration for Children and Families. Retrieved from https://www.acf.hhs.gov/css/resource/collaboration-and-strategic-planning-guide-access-and-visitation-grant

Office of Child Support Enforcement. (2019). *Parenting time opportunities for children research brief*. United States Department of Health and Human Services, Administration for Children and Families. Retrieved from https://www.acf.hhs.gov/css/resource/parenting-time-opportunities-for-children

Office of Child Support Enforcement. (n.d.). *Final rule summary*. United States Department of Health and Human Services, Administration for Children and Families. Retrieved from https://www.acf.hhs.gov/sites/default/files/programs/css/fem_final_rule_summary.pdf

Office of Family Assistance. (2019). *Healthy marriage & responsible fatherhood*. United States Department of Health and Human Services, Administration for Children and Families. Retrieved from https://www.acf.hhs.gov/ofa/programs/healthy-marriage

Osborne, C., Austin, J., Dion, M. R., Dyer, J., Fagan, J., Harris, K., et al. (2014). *Framing the future of responsible fatherhood evaluation research for the fatherhood research and practice network*. Responsible Fatherhood Workgroup. Retrieved from https://www.frpn.org/asset/framing-the-future-responsible-fatherhood-evaluation-research-the-fatherhood-research-and

Osborne, C., Berger, L., & Magnuson, K. A. (2012). Family structure transitions and changes in maternal resources and wellbeing. *Demography, 49*(1), 23–47.

Osborne, C., & McLanahan, S. (2007). Partnership instability and child wellbeing. *Journal of Marriage and Family, 69*, 1065–1083.

Osborne, C., Michelsen, A., & Bobbitt, K. (2017). *Fatherhood EFFECT evaluation final report: A comprehensive plan for supporting Texas fathers and families*. The University of Texas at Austin, Child and Family Research Partnership. Retrieved from https://childandfamilyresearch.utexas.edu/fatherhood-effect-evaluation-final-report-comprehensive-plan-supporting-texas-fathers-and-families

Palkovitz, R., Fagan, J., & Hull, J. (2013). Coparenting and children's well-being. In N. J. Cabrera & C. S.

Tamis-LeMonda (Eds.), *Handbook of father involvement* (2nd ed., pp. 202–219). New York: Routledge.

Ryan, R. M., Kalil, A., & Ziol-Guest, K. M. (2008). Longitudinal patterns of non-residential fathers' involvement: The role of resources and relations. *Journal of Marriage and Family, 70*(4), 962–977. Retrieved from https://doi.org/10.1111/j.1741-3737.2008.00539.x

Smith, T., Duggan, A., Bair-Merritt, M. H., & Cox, G. (2012). Systematic review of fathers' involvement in programs for the primary prevention of child maltreatment. *Child Abuse Review, 21*(4), 237–254. Retrieved from https://doi.org/10.1002/car.2195

Sorensen, E. (2016). *The child support program is a good investment*. United States Department of Health and Human Services, Administration for Children and Families, Office of Child Support Enforcement. Retrieved from https://www.acf.hhs.gov/css/resource/sbtn-child-support-program-is-a-good-investment

Supplee, L. H., & Duggan, A. (2019). Innovative research methods to advance precision in home visiting for more efficient and effective programs. *Child Development Perspectives, 13*(3), 173–179. Retrieved from https://doi.org/10.1111/cdep.12334

Sweet, M. A., & Appelbaum, M. I. (2004). Is home visiting an effective strategy? A meta-analytic review of home visiting programs for families with young children. *Child Development, 75*(5), 1435–1456. https://doi.org/10.1111/j.1467-8624.2004.00750.x

Tach, L. (2014). Social mobility in an era of family instability and complexity. *The Annals of the American Academy of Political and Social Science, 657*(1), 83–96. Retrieved from https://doi.org/10.1177/0002716214547854

Tax Policy Center. (2019). *EITC Parameters, 1975 to 2020*. Retrieved from https://www.taxpolicycenter.org/statistics/eitc-parameters

Texas Access. (n.d.). *Standard possession order and parenting time*. Retrieved from http://www.txaccess.org/standard-possession-order-and-parenting-time

Tollestrup, J. (2018). *Fatherhood initiatives: Connecting fathers to their children*. Congressional Research Services. Retrieved from https://fas.org/sgp/crs/misc/RL31025.pdf

van Belle, J. (2016). *Paternity and parental leave policies across the European Union*. Rand. Retrieved from https://www.rand.org/content/dam/rand/pubs/research_reports/RR1600/RR1666/RAND_RR1666.pdf

Wheaton, L., & Sorensen, E. (2010). Extending the EITC to noncustodial parents: Potential impacts and design considerations. *Journal of Policy Analysis and Management, 29*(4), 749–768. Retrieved from https://www.jstor.org/stable/40802190

Part II

Prenatal and Perinatal Influences

Overview to Part II: Prenatal and Perinatal Influences

9

Thomas Skjøthaug

Part II presents the early phases of fatherhood and emphasize updated research on men during their transition to becoming fathers. Despite current knowledge that fathers contribute importantly to their children's emotional, social, and cognitive development during pregnancy and infancy, emphasis has often been placed exclusively on the mothers' in research as well as in clinical practice. Fathers of today participate more actively in caregiving on early phases in their infants' lives than former generations of fathers did, and their influence is important for children's development. This underscores the importance of investigating paternal characteristics at an early point of time.

In Chap. 10, Gettler covers the evolutionary and comparative perspectives about human fathers' psychobiology. He covers the relevance of evolutionary perspectives to current understandings of contemporary men's biology and family system. Gettler reviews evidence related to the role that neuroendocrine, testosterone, plays in regulating fathers' parenting behaviors, illustrating the importance of understanding the relationship of biological mechanisms related to paternal parenting.

In Chap. 11, Grande, Tribble, and Kim provide current knowledge of how human fathers' brains support their relationship with their children. Fathers undergo processes of neural adaptations to parenthood that are similar, but also unique, when compared to the neural adaptations of mothers during parenthood. More specific, the chapter deals with fathers' neural responses to their own child, exemplified by the roles and impact of the neuroendocrine hormones vasopressin, oxytocin, and testosterone.

In Chap. 12, Dayton, Malone, and Brown review the various theories related to the emotional journeys during the prenatal period among fathers-to-be. Moreover, they cover literature related to fathering during the perinatal period as well as paternal thoughts and representations towards parenting an infant and they discuss risk and resilience factor when the father-infant relationship develops postnatally.

The following chapters address experiences of the unborn child in the ultrasound and how fathers' own adverse childhood experiences can induce stress postpartum. First, in Chap. 13, Tolman and Walsh recount how parents own past may influence their view of the child. For example, seeking connection, parents may speculate about family resemblances or suggest that a specific fetal movement indicates that the future child will one day become a soccer player due to their own soccer experiences. The authors discuss how such "ghosts from the past" make their presence already during pregnancy. Then in Chap. 14, Skjothaug discusses fathers' stress and

T. Skjøthaug (✉)
Division of Mental Health, Grorud DPS, Akershus University Hospital, Lørenskog, Norway
e-mail: tskjotha@getmail.no

H. E. Fitzgerald et al. (eds.), *Handbook of Fathers and Child Development*,
https://doi.org/10.1007/978-3-030-51027-5_9

how antecedents of such stress can be traced back to pregnancy, even before the child is born. Further, He addresses affiliated issues of stress research on father's pathways from conception towards fatherhood after the child is born and how to help understand and reduce such experience of stress.

In Chap. 15, Paulson, Ellis, and Alexander discuss how paternal depression arises through the lens of the family system and how this affects the developing family. They review fathers' adjustment during the early years of fatherhood (prenatal to postpartum) and the association with depression, risk, and protective factors, partner and family adjustment, and how such adjustment may predict important child development processes. They also suggest an integrative model in order to better understand paternal perinatal depression and how it may constitute risk to the family and developing children.

The final chapter in Part II, Chap. 16, reviews extant research of various reactions across the transition from one child to two, a relatively understudied aspect of family growth. Volling, Steinberg and Kuo suggest that fathers' engagement in child care during the family's increase in household members (another child) may help explain individual differences in children's adjustment across the transition to siblinghood. Further, they review how an increase in family size affects or changes parental competence and mental health.

Exploring Evolutionary Perspectives on Human Fatherhood and Paternal Biology: Testosterone as an Exemplar

10

Lee T. Gettler

In evolutionary terms, humans have a unique life history strategy compared to other primates, including our closest relatives, the Great Apes. In particular, we have highly vulnerable infants who grow and mature very slowly, often remaining reliant on investments from caregivers well into their second decade of life (Hrdy, 2009; Kaplan, Hill, Lancaster, & Hurtado, 2000; Kramer, 2010). This period of protracted and slow physical growth for our children is physiologically linked to the very high metabolic costs of our large brains (for body size), which is a distinguishing characteristic of our evolution as a species (Charnov & Berrigan, 1993; Kuzawa et al., 2014). Despite these elevated time- and resourced-based costs of raising our children to independence, humans often "stack" the dependency periods of offspring on top of one another, raising multiple costly offspring simultaneously, rather than waiting for each one to mature to independence before having another (as is common in almost all other primates) (Kaplan et al., 2000; Kramer, 2010). Consequently, in contemporary natural fertility populations, humans have substantially shorter spaces (inter-birth intervals) between children than is common in our closest primate relatives. Despite this "stacking" of the intensive costs of our vulnerable children, comparative demographic research in small-scale societies, such as foragers or hunter-gatherers, has shown that our offspring also survive to adulthood at much higher rates than do Great Ape young (Kaplan et al., 2000).

Hence, humans have evolved a suite of reproductive and developmental characteristics that cross-species comparative perspectives would suggest should come with trade-offs (e.g., producing more young in shorter periods of time would typically be traded off against offspring survival rates) (Kaplan et al., 2000; Kramer, 2010). In the evolutionary past, hominin mothers would not have been able to manage the energetic costs of raising multiple costly human/hominin offspring simultaneously. A female employing such a strategy (alone) would have experienced lower reproductive fitness (i.e., likely as a result of greater offspring mortality) relative to her peers who continued to engage in a reproductive strategy involving raising one offspring at a time, as is found among the Great Apes (Kaplan et al., 2000; Kramer, 2010). Consequently, in scholarship and frameworks focused on human evolution, it is virtually uniformly held that in ancestral human/hominin populations, mothers would have needed extensive help from cooperative caregivers (e.g., grandmothers, fathers, older siblings, non-parental kin, etc.) in order for the life history strategy I have just described to have

L. T. Gettler (✉)
Department of Anthropology, Eck Institute for Global Health, University of Notre Dame, Notre Dame, IN, USA
e-mail: Lee.T.Gettler@nd.edu

H. E. Fitzgerald et al. (eds.), *Handbook of Fathers and Child Development*,
https://doi.org/10.1007/978-3-030-51027-5_10

emerged evolutionarily in our lineage (Hawkes & Coxworth, 2013; Gettler, 2010; Gray & Crittenden, 2014; Kramer, 2010). Within this framework, often referred to as "cooperative breeding," humans have specifically evolved the capacity for committed, involved fathering (Gettler, 2014; Gray & Anderson, 2010). If this represents an adaptive suite of behavioral tendencies and capacities, then evolutionary theoretical perspectives, which I will describe below, posit that human males should have hormonal and neurobiological mechanisms that help facilitate the expression of that commitment (Gettler, 2014; Rosenbaum & Gettler, 2018). The study of those mechanisms has grown into an area of research that is sometimes referred to as "the biology of fatherhood," with a large body of literature on men's testosterone (T), a growing body of work on fathers' oxytocin, and comparatively less research on other pertinent psychobiological mechanisms such as prolactin, vasopressin, and cortisol (Abraham & Feldman, 2018; Gettler, 2014; Gray, McHale, & Carre, 2017; Rosenbaum & Gettler, 2018).

In this chapter, I first review evolutionary and (cross-species) comparative perspectives that serve as core foundations for making predictions about human fathers' psychobiology. Then, I review research on men's T, partnering/parenting status, and parenting behavior as an exemplar for the relevance of evolutionary perspectives to current understandings of contemporary men's biology and family systems. While T is only one neuroendocrine mechanism relevant to fathering (Abraham & Feldman, 2018; Gettler, 2014; Rosenbaum & Gettler, 2018), it is the most widely studied and thus a review the literature on this hormone can be considered illustrative of broader principles and questions that are relevant to "the biology of fatherhood" more broadly.

Evolutionary Theoretical Perspectives on Human Fathering

Evolutionary perspectives, particularly parental investment theory and life history theory (LHT), are commonly used as framing lenses for research on the physiological underpinnings of fathering among humans and other animals (Fernandez-Duque, Valeggia, & Mendoza, 2009; Gettler, 2014; Gray et al., 2017). Compared to parental investment theory, LHT is a more expansive theoretical framework and is extensively used in evolutionary biology and ecology. It focuses on the ways in which organisms must allocate limited resources, particularly energy, to mutually exclusive physiological demands related to growth, reproduction, and survival, and how species have evolved to "solve" these allocation trade-off challenges through a range of "LH strategies" (Hill & Kaplan, 1999; Stearns, 1992). Across species, variations in these LH strategies, which result from organisms exploiting different ecological niches and thus experiencing diverse selective pressures (e.g., predation; infectious disease) through (deep) evolutionary time, are often viewed on a fast-to-slow continuum and include a focus on the timing-length of key life events (e.g., age at reproductive maturity; length of the reproductive window; total life span) and related physical-behavioral characteristics (e.g., adult body size; number of lifetime reproductive events; number of offspring per reproductive event; time-energy devoted to parental investment) (Charnov & Berrigan, 1993; Promislow & Harvey, 1990).

Physiological signals (such as hormones and neurotransmitters) mechanistically mediate the trade-offs between these various time and energy demands. Thus, genetically underpinned physiological profiles that differ between individuals become more common in the population (i.e., positive selection within-species) across generations, as some organisms achieve higher fitness and pass along their genes at greater rates than others (Bribiescas & Ellison, 2008; Stearns, 1992). Although organisms are limited by phylogenetic inertia (meaning, in this case, that their ability to developmentally acclimate is constrained by the evolutionary history of their species), it is expected that organisms will have some adaptive capacity to flexibly adjust their individual allocation strategies in relation to their current circumstances, which is related to the biological concept of reaction norms (Stearns,

1992). For example, a developing (younger) organism will tend to grow faster and bigger under conditions of energetic abundance compared to contexts with nutritional constraints, while an adult might reduce energetic investments in reproduction when faced with an environment with high levels of infectious disease, enabling survival despite lower immediate reproductive prospects (Hill & Kaplan, 1999).

These facultative (environmentally sensitive) within-individual LH shifts and within-species ranges of variation in LH strategies manifest themselves through physiological pathways (e.g., hormonal axes and neurobiological systems). This multi-level perspective on variation serves as a foundation for considering individual-level differences in LH-relevant biological systems and their emergence or calibration across the life course in response to environmental conditions (Bribiescas & Ellison, 2008; Jasienska, 2013). In terms of fathering and its underlying biology, LHT provides a predictive framework for the ways in which adults (particularly male mammals, see below) face core trade-offs between mating and parenting in their allocations to reproductive effort when biparental care evolves (Fernandez-Duque et al., 2009; Gettler, 2014; Hill & Kaplan, 1999). While recent psychobiological models have provided a substantive, nuanced perspective challenging the applicability of a dichotomous breakdown of mating vs. parenting effort to human neuroendocrine physiology and behavior (van Anders, 2013; van Anders, Goldey, & Kuo, 2011), a substantial amount of work on the psychobiology of human fatherhood, particularly for T, has drawn from the LHT perspective to make predictions about the ways in which men's hormonal production will vary based on the transition to parenthood (and away from mating effort) or men's specific investments in parenting effort (e.g., direct caregiving) and cooperation with partners to raise children (Gettler, 2014; Gray, McHale, & Carre, 2017).

In that vein, a substantial amount of the existing research on the biology of fatherhood (across taxa) has focused on variability in testosterone (T) based on the Challenge Hypothesis, an evolutionary biological model that emerged from the study of birds and is used to explain LH trade-offs between mating and parenting (Gray, Straftis, Bird, McHale, & Zilioli, 2019; Wingfield, Hegner, Ball, & Duffy, 1990). In short, drawing on extensive ornithological behavioral physiological research, Wingfield et al. (1990) proposed that among species in which males invested time and energy in raising their young, their T would decline during the stages of the breeding season in which their offspring were dependent. This downregulation of T was argued to be a pathway that would facilitate males' focus on cooperative parenting demands and shift their devotion of time/energy away from mating opportunities with females and competition with males for territory while also allowing males to attenuate the physical and metabolic costs of long-term T upregulation. Meanwhile, among species in which males had not evolved to cooperate with mothers and/or to invest in their young, they would not show this characteristic T decline, on average, at the "investment" stage of the reproductive cycle and their T would remain elevated across the breeding season if they were continually engaging in extensive male-male competition. It is important to note that it is very common for bird fathers to invest in their young, with up to 90% of bird species showing biparental care, which is a much higher rate than in other vertebrate taxa, particularly mammals (see below) (Clutton-Brock, 1991). Thus, in birds exhibiting biparental care, this perspective suggests that in many species males have evolved (via natural selection) the capacity to reduce their T to help shift their behavioral and energetic allocations toward priorities that help to optimize their cooperation with females and the promotion of the survival, growth, and development of their offspring (Wingfield et al., 1990).

Compared to the patterns among birds, paternal investment is rare among mammals, occurring in only around 3–5% of mammalian species (Clutton-Brock, 1991; Gray & Anderson, 2010). This low prevalence of mammalian paternal care almost certainly reflects divergences in male and female reproductive strategies that emerged alongside the evolution of internal fertilization, internal gestation and viviparity, and lactation that characterize mammalian reproduction (Clutton-Brock, 1991). Collectively, these characteristics often reduce males' certainty of paternity and their ability to remain in proximity to their young between fertilization and eventual birth, contributing to the predominant mammalian pattern of males competing with one another for mating opportunities with multiple females, rather than partnering with a pregnant female and raising his (potential) offspring (Royle, Smiseth, & Kolliker, 2012). Because the hypothalamic-pituitary-gonadal axis that produces T is evolutionarily ancient and shared across vertebrates, the Challenge Hypothesis laid the groundwork for scientists to make predictions regarding shifts in T production based on mating and parenting effort in other vertebrate taxa in which biparental care evolved, including its rare occurrence in mammalian species, such as humans (Gray et al., 2019; Wingfield et al., 1990). Notably, any similarities in the physiology underlying paternal involvement among birds and mammals are the result of convergent evolution (rather than shared ancestry) and represent natural selection (or other evolutionary processes) repeatedly coopting similar neurobiological and hormonal pathways to promote paternal care, however diverse the ecological settings in which it evolves. This evolutionarily grounded approach to the study of the biology of vertebrate fathering has led to the observation that pair-bonded and/or invested vertebrate fathers commonly show similar physiological profiles, including particularly lower T during the periods in which they cooperate with mothers to raise vulnerable offspring (Fernandez-Duque et al., 2009; Gettler, 2014; Gray, McHale, & Carre, 2017).

Thus, this comparative perspective has served as a pillar for evolutionarily grounded biosocial or biocultural conceptual frameworks and empirical research aimed toward testing whether human fathers express psychobiological profiles similar to other invested vertebrate fathers and how those profiles might be shaped by the cultural and family system contexts in which they find expression (Abraham & Feldman, 2018; Gettler, 2014, 2016; Gray, McHale, & Carre, 2017; van Anders, 2013; van Anders et al., 2011). Human male capacities for intensive paternal care evolved alongside or downstream of the suite of life history characteristics I described at the outset of the chapter that distinguish humans from the Great Apes and other primates (Gray & Anderson, 2010; Kaplan et al., 2000). To briefly reiterate, human life history includes the birth of newborns who are relatively neurologically and physically underdeveloped, comparatively early weaning of those infants, the slow growth and development of our offspring through a unique "childhood" phase, and shortened inter-birth intervals (such that our hyper-dependent offspring are "stacked" on top of one another, under natural fertility conditions) (Kaplan et al., 2000; Kramer, 2010).

This suite of reproductive-fertility and developmental characteristics would have been too much of an energetic and time burden for a mother to successfully manage alone (in the evolutionary past), rendering it a maladaptive for reproductive fitness in the absence of the types of cooperative caregiving that we observe across contemporary societies (Kaplan et al., 2000; Kramer, 2010). From an evolutionary perspective, it is highly probable that fathers frequently made critical though variable contributions to the well-being of their children, along with mothers receiving assistance from other helpers, often referred to as allomaternal caregivers (their own older offspring, grandmothers, other female kin, etc.) (Gettler, 2010; Gray & Anderson, 2010; Hawkes & Coxworth, 2013; Kramer, 2010).

Conceptualizing Fathers' Roles in the Evolutionary Past

There is general (though not universal) agreement that fathers' provisioning of energetic resources was likely important to the evolution of human's life history strategy by helping to improve child health and survival (Gray & Anderson, 2010; Gurven & Hill, 2009; Kaplan et al., 2000). In that vein, fathers' contributions as providers have recently been linked to children's improved nutritional status and growth in small-scale societies in which the environmental conditions include evolutionarily relevant features (i.e., energetic constraint; infectious disease stress) (Boyette, Lew-Levy, & Gettler, 2018; Winking & Koster, 2015). Compared to the importance of paternal provisioning, there has been less of a focus in evolutionary frameworks and related research on the roles of fathers as direct, physical caregivers and as contributors via other pathways (e.g., cultivators of social capital or status within the community) to child well-being (Boyette et al., 2018; Gettler, 2010; Scelza, 2010; von Rueden, Gurven, & Kaplan, 2011). Relative to fathers' roles as providers, there are fewer lines of evidence available to reconstruct the potential roles fathers may have played as direct caregivers during our evolutionary past. In particular, in many contemporary societies, fathers' roles in such care are relatively modest (Gettler, 2010), despite the increasing recognition that sensitive, warm, and supportive fathering can benefit child's social and emotional development in settings such as the United States and Europe (Cabrera, 2020). Scholars working at the intersection of human psychobiology and social bonding have specifically argued that testing for physiological profiles that help facilitate nurturant, sensitive caregiving in contemporary fathers (and within other salient social relationships) can serve as one line of evidence to test whether such roles were evolutionarily adaptive, in light of cross-species comparative data and based on LHT (Gettler, 2014; van Anders, 2013).

In that vein, human fathers' psychobiology has been repeatedly linked to engagement in direct caregiving and nurturance, although these neuroendocrine-behavioral profiles are by no means canalized or fixed (Gettler, 2014; Gray, Reece, et al., 2017; van Anders, 2013). The evolutionary perspective lays the foundation for understanding why (ultimately) human fathers have these psychobiological capacities, and provides a useful framework for making predictions regarding the types of behaviors and social contexts that are most likely to elicit (potentially) evolutionarily advantageous profiles. Yet, importantly, relatively recent psychobiological frameworks (van Anders, 2013; van Anders et al., 2011) have made the observation that "parenting" represents a diffuse range of demands that might be most optimally met by varied levels of (for example) T, rather than a singular profile of invested fathers having low T. For a number of reasons (including phylogenetic inertia), evolutionary processes result in traits that are "good enough" and not perfect; thus, human psychobiological responses to partnering/parenting are flexible but cannot be expected to reflect unlimited plasticity to respond to all aspects of family life and demands outside the family and might be occasionally mismatched to contemporary demands (Gettler, 2016). This provides an opportunity to build from LHT tenets as well as newer psychobiological frameworks (van Anders, 2013; van Anders et al., 2011) by integrating culturally-grounded, family system perspectives and by emphasizing individual differences that may shape the expression of the biology of fatherhood (Gettler, 2016). To help illustrate these points, in the next section, I will briefly describe some of the physiological functions of T that are considered relevant to life history trade-offs across vertebrate species. I will then build from that foundation to review the human literature on men's T and partnering/parenting status. Finally, I will transition to a discussion of research exploring the relationships between men's T and their caregiving behavior.

Testosterone (T), Partnering, and Parenting Status

As I described above, both LHT and parental investment theory focus on trade-offs that occur between core fitness-relevant demands, such as reproduction versus maintenance of the body, as a consequence of time and energy being limited resources. In particular, both theoretical perspectives are consistent with the notion that mammalian males will face reproductive effort trade-offs between dedicating limited time and energetic resources toward mating effort versus toward the cooperative care of young in those rare species exhibiting biparental care. Indeed, aspects of the Challenge Hypothesis, outlined above, are likewise premised on similar ideas regarding the ways in which male birds in species with biparental care will seasonally shift away from mating effort and toward cooperative parenting of young, as the two (mating and parenting) are often incongruent as to their physiological underpinnings and behavioral demands (Gray et al., 2019; Wingfield et al., 1990). Across vertebrates, T is considered a key physiological mechanism helping to mediate these mating versus parenting trade-offs. In vertebrate males, elevated T often facilitates behaviors related to competition for resources, territory, and status. Similarly, higher T generally facilitates costly investment in physical attributes, such as larger body size, musculature, and ornamentation (such as colored plumage in certain birds) that facilitate attraction of mates and competition for resources and status (Bribiescas, 2001; Gray, Reece, et al., 2017; Hau, 2007). Based on these patterns, many of the early studies of the biology of human fatherhood focused on men's "life history status," with the prediction that, in some settings, partnered fathers would have lower T than single non-fathers, particularly (Gray, Kahlenberg, Barrett, Lipson, & Ellison, 2002).

Over the past two decades, many studies have documented that partnered fathers tend to have lower T than single non-fathers, although, as I will discuss, this does vary by cultural context. Moreover, multiple thorough synthetic reviews have been written on this topic, which give far greater coverage of the relevant literature than I am able to do here (reviewed in Gettler, 2014; Gray, Reece, et al., 2017; Roney & Gettler, 2015; van Anders et al., 2011; van Anders, 2013). Importantly, a recent meta-analysis showed that there is an overall pattern of partnered men, especially fathers, having lower T than other men, though the prevailing effect size is relatively modest (Grebe et al. 2019). A subsequent meta-analysis that used a somewhat different approach in trying to isolate the relationship between T and fathering (adjusting for partnering) found largely complementary supportive results, but again with a relatively modest effect size (Meijer, van IJzendoorn, & Bakermans-Kranenburg, 2019).

My primary purpose here is to discuss some of the early work in this area, especially as it relates to cross-cultural patterns, and to highlight some of the larger and longitudinal studies that have been conducted on this topic, as these are less subject to research design limitations pertinent to smaller, cross-sectional studies. Gray and colleagues conducted a number of foundational studies in this domain, including work on men in the Boston area, showing that married men (regardless of parenting status) had lower T than unmarried non-fathers. Married fathers and married non-fathers did not differ for T in either analysis (Gray et al., 2002; Gray, Campbell, Marlowe, Lipson, & Ellison, 2004). In a similar study among Chinese men in Beijing, Gray et al. later found that married fathers had lower T than both unmarried and married non-fathers, hinting at some cross-cultural differences compared to the earlier studies in the United States (Gray, Yang, & Pope, 2006). Around this same period, Gray and colleagues also tested related ideas in two Kenyan cultural groups in which polygyny is culturally sanctioned and thus the dynamics of T-competition and mating-partnering/parenting are potentially blurred, such that men could potentially look more similar for T across life history statuses. Among Kenyan Swahili men, unmarried and monogamously married men did not significantly differ for T, while polygynously married men (i.e., with multiple partners) had higher T than other males (Gray, 2003). In contrast, in a larger study of Ariaal pastoralists in Tanzania, unmarried men in their reproductive primes had higher T than their married peers, while polygynously married men did not have elevated T relative to other men (Gray, Ellison, & Campbell, 2007). In a complementary study of Senegalese men later conducted by a separate set of researchers, married fathers similarly had lower T than unmarried non-fathers (Alvergne, Faurie, & Raymond, 2009). However, among fathers, polygynous men had higher T than monogamously partnered fathers, which is consistent with the idea that men's mating effort and competition in the context of polygyny are correlated with elevated T (Alvergne et al., 2009).

These findings set helped to set the stage for a subsequent cross-cultural comparative study in Tanzania of two neighboring small-scale societies in which models of family life differ substantially (Muller, Marlowe, Bugumba, & Ellison, 2009). Among Hadza foragers, men and women generally partner monogamously and fathers frequently spend time in close proximity with their young children and are involved with hands-on care of them. In contrast, among the neighboring Datoga pastoralists, adult men spend much of their time away from women and young children, attending to responsibilities for herding and protecting livestock. Polygyny is also culturally sanctioned in this context (Muller et al., 2009). In their study, Muller et al. (2009) found that Hadza fathers had significantly lower T than non-fathers, whereas Datoga fathers and non-fathers had similar T. This was among the first studies to hint that father-child proximity and men's direct caregiving potentially had implications for the patterning of men's T based on parenting status, a theme I return to in the subsequent section on T and fathering behavior.

Subsequent longitudinal research built on these earlier studies to help address the "state" or "trait" question as it relates to T and men's partnering and parenting (e.g., Edelstein et al., 2017; Gettler, McDade, Feranil, & Kuzawa, 2011). That is, because prior studies were cross-sectional, they could not address the question of whether men with reduced T were more likely to become partnered fathers in some settings (trait) or whether the transition to committed partnering and parenting led to declines in T (state). In research from a large, multi-decade birth cohort study in Metropolitan Cebu in the Philippines, my colleagues and I demonstrated that men who had higher T as single non-fathers in young adulthood were more likely to become partnered fathers by their mid-20s. Meanwhile, those men who became newly partnered new fathers between the ages of 21 (baseline) and 26 (follow-up) experienced large biologically meaningful declines in their T, with fathers of newborns showing the steepest declines (Gettler et al., 2011). These patterns differed significantly from the relatively static T profiles of men who remained single non-fathers over the same time frame. Other longitudinal research likewise found that fathers' T was reduced in the first few months of parenthood, compared to non-parent controls (Perini, Ditzen, Hengartner, & Ehlert, 2012).

There are relatively few large, longitudinal studies of human psychobiology and partnering or parenting, but two such studies that focus solely on partnering complement our findings from the Philippines. In a large decade-long study of US military veterans, Mazur and Michalek (1998) showed that unwed men and men who changed marital status (married ↔ single) all had T that was consistently higher than men who remained married across the study period. Men who transitioned from being divorced to remarried showed significant declines in T during the decade of study. Meanwhile, married men who had elevated T at earlier time points in the study were more likely to become divorced by later time points. Drawing on the study in Cebu, our research team later showed a complementary finding showing that men with greater T functionality as young adults were more likely to experience relationship separation/dissolution by their mid-20s (Gettler et al., 2017). Additionally, in a recent, large, longitudinal study in Denmark, many of the core findings from Mazur and Michalek (1998) were replicated, as men who transitioned to marriage experienced declines in T and those that divorced/separated exhibited increases in T through time (Holmboe et al., 2017).

Finally, in addition to these longitudinal studies that help shed light on the bidirectional relationships between T and shifts in life history status, a small number of large cross-sectional studies have (in some cases) added clarity to these patterns, while also raising new questions. This is particularly important since it is known that studies with small sample sizes are prone to inflated effect sizes when they find statistically significant results (Button et al., 2013). In a US population representative study with over 1500 men ranging in age from 20 to 60 years old, my collaborator and I showed that partnered men residing with children had significantly lower T than men who were not residing with children and were either divorced or never married (Gettler & Oka, 2016). Men who were partnered but not residing with children tended to have modestly higher T than partnered men living with children but the effect size was small and did not reach statistical significance. These findings thus generally parallel the earlier foundation work on US men by Gray et al. (2002, 2004).

In contrast to these patterns that align with past work, data from a large study of military personnel (N = 4400+) found that for men in their early 30s, T increased based on the presence of children in their homes and increased as the number of children rose (Mazur, 2014). Based on the data reported in the study, it is not clear what explains the discrepancies between this study and other relevant work on US married fathers. However, contextualized within existing frameworks (Gettler, 2016; van Anders, 2013; van Anders et al., 2011), I discuss some possible explanations below in a subsequent section regarding the importance of models of fatherhood, cultural context, and individual differences. Finally, a recent work focusing on Jamaican fathers (n = 350) found that fathers' T did not vary according to relationship status (married, long-term partnered but unmarried, visiting [mothers and fathers live apart but jointly raise children) (Gray, Reece, et al., 2017). This contrasts somewhat with my team's earlier work from Cebuano men in the Philippines, which showed that residential fathers had lower T than non-residential fathers (Gettler, McDade, Agustin, Feranil, & Kuzawa, 2015). While over-interpreting non-significant findings is potentially fraught, these studies and the variation they point to within- and across-cultures points to the potential importance of local cultural models of fathering, partnering, and family life more broadly in influencing the expression of these psychobiological patterns (Gettler, 2016), which is a theme I focus on in the subsequent section.

Fathering Quantity in Relationship to T

As I have already noted, T is considered a key mechanism helping to facilitate trade-offs between mating and parenting effort. In terms of understanding how fathers' T might affect and be affected by the functioning of family systems, there are a number of key points that merit discussion before delving into the relevant literature. First, the majority of studies that have drawn on LHT to formulate hypotheses about paternal care have generally focused on the *quantity* of caregiving (e.g., time spent in direct care) rather than the *quality* of care. Likely, because of its focus on time and energy as limited resources that are allocated to competing demands, LHT has not generally been used to generate predictions about caregiving quality, to date (Kuo & Gettler, 2018). In addition, there is a long-standing recognition that behaviors that are commonly lumped under the headings of "mating" and "parenting" effort, which are often a core focus of LHT approaches to modeling the trade-offs men negotiate when the transition to parenthood, are not necessarily mutually exclusive or divisible (Smuts & Gubernick, 1992; van Anders, 2013). For example, in many societies, men's competition for resources and status could be considered relevant to both mating effort and parenting effort.

Nonetheless, a number of studies have found that when fathers are involved with direct care of their children and/or spend time in close proximity to them, they generally have lower T than fathers who are uninvolved in hands-on caregiving (Alvergne et al., 2009; Gettler et al., 2011; Gettler, McKenna, Agustin, McDade, & Kuzawa, 2012; Lawson et al., 2017; Mascaro, Hackett, & Rilling, 2013), although these findings are not ubiquitous, even in cultural settings in which they might be predicted to occur (e.g., Gray et al., 2002, 2004; see further relevant discussion below). A recent meta-analysis also found support for this pattern, but with a relatively small effect size, which (as the authors note) could potentially reflect limited attention to core contextual details regarding family systems and dynamics (Meijer, van IJzendoorn, & Bakermans-Kranenburg, 2019) as well as variability in study design (Kuo & Gettler, 2018). Nonetheless, a number of longitudinal studies have helped to shed some light on the direction of these effects. Research following US expectant fathers from the pre- to post-partum found that fathers whose T declined more across their partners' pregnancies were more engaged in infant care post-partum and their partners reported that the lower T fathers helped more with household tasks and were more supportive (Edelstein et al., 2017). In a separate larger study of US fathers, Kuo and colleagues found that fathers' whose T was lower the day after their babies were born reported participating in greater direct care and indirect parenting tasks related to the baby 2–4 months later (Kuo et al., 2018). Finally, my collaborators and I found that among Filipino men who were fathers at age 21–22 years, those who increased their time spent in childcare in the ensuing 4–5 years experienced declines in T over the same time frame, while fathers' T went up if they decreased their caregiving time during the follow-up period (Gettler et al., 2015).

Much of this work is consistent with T playing a role as a mechanism to help shift men's priorities as they transition to committed fatherhood, particularly in reference to a limited resource (i.e., time). This work is also broadly consistent with psychobiological frameworks pertaining to human social behavior and bonding that have helped to provide nuance to predictions regarding the ways in which men and women's T will correlate with various demands related to partnering and parenting. Specifically, van Anders (2013) and colleagues (2011) have proposed that lower T will tend to correlate with nurturing behavior in the formation and maintenance of social bonds (such as can occur between partners or between parents and children), whereas elevated T will tend to be correlated with behaviors related to competition, including for status and resources. To the extent that nurturing parental behaviors (e.g., sensitive, warm, supportive interactions) are widely recognized as benefitting child development outcomes in the United States, Europe, and similar societal settings, this framework offers predictions for the way in which reduced T among fathers could be linked to child well-being in certain contexts (e.g., Landry, Smith, & Swank, 2006).

Fathering Quality in Relationship to T

Relatively few studies have tested whether lower T is related to the *quality* of fathers' parenting and the findings in the existing literature are mixed (Kuo & Gettler, 2018). In studies of Israeli families, it was found that fathers who had lower T engaged in more affectionate touch and sensitive infant-directed speech (Weisman, Zagoory-Sharon, & Feldman, 2014) and were observed to be more behaviorally synchronized with their babies (Gordon, Pratt, Bergunde, Zagoory-Sharon, & Feldman, 2017). In an earlier work on Canadian men, fathers who had lower T expressed greater concern and sympathy toward a crying baby, when they were exposed to recorded infant distress (Fleming, Corter, Stallings, & Steiner, 2002). In the Netherlands, fathers' waking and evening T, respectively, were not significantly linked to their sensitivity or respect for their children's autonomy. However, fathers with steeper diurnal changes in T across the day were found to engage in higher quality parenting (as defined in the study) (Endendijk et al., 2016). The typical diurnal pattern reflects a peak around waking and nadir by early evening, which is reflected in the study (Endendijk et al., 2016). Thus, for the majority of men, the key finding of this research likely reflects that fathers with steeper diurnal declines in T across the day engaged in more sensitive, respectful parenting. Meanwhile, more recent work from the same research group has shown that fathers' levels of self-control moderated the relationship between T and parenting quality. Specifically, low-self-control fathers with higher T were less sensitive and less respectful of child autonomy, whereas lower T in such fathers correlated with higher quality parenting. The reverse pattern was found for higher T fathers (van der Pol et al., 2019). This most recent (2019) research from this team points to the importance of bringing individual differences into the study of human paternal psychobiology as is done in other related domains such as research on T and aggression or physiological responses to psychosocially stressful conditions (Carré et al., 2017; Oswald et al., 2006).

Notably, however, a number of studies have failed to find significant correlations between fathers' T and the quality of their parenting. For example, in a US-based sample, Kuo and colleagues (2015) did not find that fathers' basal T was predictive of various measures of observed parenting quality, including sensitivity, responsiveness, and intrusiveness, during a lab-based father-infant teaching task. In a separate, relatively large US-based study, Dorius et al. (2012) found no significant link between fathers' T and their children's reports of father-child closeness. It is important to note that this study did not have direct measures of fathering quality. Theoretically, father-child closeness is predicted to emerge (in part) via high-quality (sensitive, warm, authoritative) parenting in this setting, thus, conceptually, T could plausibly have been associated with father-child closeness as a mediator in the pathway linking fathering quality and T. As Kuo and Gettler (2018) have recently described, it is difficult to discern whether inconsistencies in this literature reflect distinct psychobiological processes in different settings or samples, lack of statistical power (in some cases), or research design differences that lead to variation in what family and individual fathering dynamics are found to be meaningfully correlated with men's T. For example, in the Dorius et al. (2012) study, the age range of children included was quite large (6–16 years old), and there are variable demands of parenting and emotionally connecting and bonding with children of those varying ages. Thus, "high-quality" parenting and "closeness" of parent-child bonds might well be correlated with differing psychobiological profiles in fathers as parenting demands shift with child age and development (Gettler, 2016; van Anders, 2013). In fact, the vast majority of the work I have reviewed above has been conducted with families with infants and toddlers in a relatively limited number of cultural settings. To better understand the bidirectional relationships between hormones such as T and men's roles in families, we need to explore these questions across a more diverse landscape of family systems and societal settings (Gettler, 2016).

The models from van Anders and colleagues likewise point to the importance of social and cultural context in the expression of psychobiological systems, which is a critical consideration for interpreting the biology of fatherhood across diverse settings (van Anders, 2013; van Anders et al., 2011). Complementing those frameworks, I proposed a culturally oriented evolutionary developmental model ("Becoming DADS"), with the DADS acronym standing for Duration, Attitude, Dedication, and Salience. In this framework, I posited that evolutionarily conserved but developmentally plastic physiological systems, such as the hypothalamic-pituitary-gonadal axis that produces T, are calibrated to respond to and facilitate culturally valued social and gender roles within societies, based on boys' childhood experiences within families and communities (Gettler, 2016). This model thus facilitates social neuroendocrine predictions based on locally valorized roles for and gender socialization of men as fathers and men's individual experiences as children while also emphasizing the importance of broader processes that influence those dynamics, such as political economy and local ecology.

For example, drawing on my prior work on T and fatherhood among Filipino men (e.g., Gettler et al., 2011, 2015), I discussed how political economic changes in the Philippines in the 1980s (especially via neoliberalization of the economy) led to many Filipino women traveling overseas to seek better paying work and also a feminization of labor opportunities in Cebu, the Philippines. I argued that these shifting labor and migration dynamics potentially helped to contribute to changing family roles regarding childcare, requiring some fathers to participate more intensively in childcare, running counter to prevailing cultural norms of masculinity and expectations of fathers. In families and communities transformed by these changes, the developmental experiences of children would have been shifted (i.e., boys receiving some care from their fathers and thereby internalizing gendered roles and identities and developing bio-behaviorally in tune with those culturally salient dimensions of family life) (Gettler, 2016). My colleagues and I recently published work on the multi-generational patterning of fathering behavior and parenting identity in Cebu (the Philippines) that align with the general predictions of this framework, as boys who had fathers who did some caregiving in the early 1980s and developed close relationships with them were, themselves, more involved as fathers ~25 years later and described caregiving as more central to their identities as parents (Gettler, Kuo, Bas, & Borja, 2019). However, in that study, our core findings were based on crossover statistical interactions, meaning that for boys who grew up with fathers who were uninvolved with childcare and nonetheless developed a close relationship with them, they (the second-generation men) grew up to recapitulate their fathers' parenting styles, with relatively less caregiving and less emphasis on it as a component of their parenting identities (Gettler et al., 2019).

Notably, our team observed these crossover effects for intergenerational patterning of paternal parenting styles in Cebu using data from the same sample on which we had previously shown that men becoming newly partnered new fathers had larger longitudinal declines in T than men remaining single non-fathers (Gettler et al., 2011). Our more recent (2019) results suggest that there was likely a meaningful subset of new fathers in that pool who did not see nurturant caregiving as a core part of their parental responsibilities or identities as fathers. Such individual-level insights might help to explain why, despite group-level aggregate findings such as declining T among newly partnered new fathers in Cebu (Gettler et al., 2011), we still see that ~25% of those new fathers exhibit relatively static or even increasing T across that same 4.5-year time period. A similar within-culture perspective on variation in models of fathering may help explain results I discussed previously from Mazur (2014) in which relatively young military fathers with more children had higher T, as opposed to lower levels that might be predicted based on increasing caregiving demands of more dependents as has been found in other research on non-military US fathers (Mascaro et al., 2013). In particular, there is a possibility that the orientation and engagement of military men in the sample to fathering were more consistent with competition (e.g., providing resources) and protection than nurturance, and those social neuroendocrine dynamics could explain the observed patterns (Mazur, 2014). While that interpretation is speculative, my colleagues and I recently published research on fathers' roles and psychobiology from a small-scale society in the Republic of the Congo that gives it credence and that helps to lay the groundwork for the importance of understanding local models of fathering and family life vis-à-vis men's neuroendocrine profiles.

This new research focuses on a small Bantu-speaking community of less than 200 who identify ethnically as Bondongo. They reside in a remote region of northern Republic of the Congo, far removed from major urban centers and with little market integration, and they subsist primarily via fishing and (non-mechanized) farming (Boyette et al., 2018). In this society, fathers' roles as providers of resources are culturally valued and those who are seen as better providers have children in better health (Boyette et al., 2018). Fathers' acquisition of resources often involves risky behaviors (e.g., scaling tall trees; fishing in dangerous waters) and men achieve higher status in the community through their abilities as providers. Meanwhile, the Bondongo do not culturally emphasize warm father-child relations or fathers' direct caregiving, including sensitive or nurturant involvement, and such behaviors are relatively uncommon (Boyette, Lew-Levy, Sarma, & Gettler, 2019; Gettler, Sarma, et al., 2019).

Thus, in contrast to prior research on paternal psychobiology in settings such as the United States/Europe, the Philippines, and Israel, "higher quality" paternal care among the Bondongo is unlikely to be linked to lower T. In contrast, a culturally situated and theoretically grounded hypothesis would be that committed Bondongo fathers would exhibit higher T (Gettler, 2016; Gray, McHale, & Carre, 2017; van Anders et al., 2011; van Anders, 2013). We found support for this prediction, as fathers who were seen as better providers had higher T than men seen as less effective providers, which we suggest is consistent with theorized links between risk taking, competition for status, and elevated T (Gray,

McHale, & Carre, 2017; van Anders et al., 2011; van Anders , 2013). To our knowledge, our findings were the first to correlate measures of fathers' roles as providers to elevated T; however, our results complement and build on prior anthropological research that has shown that the well-documented differences in T between married fathers vs. single men and non-fathers do not necessarily extend to societies in which cultural models of partnering differ (e.g., polygyny is practiced) and roles for fathers involve little contact with young children (Gray, 2003; Muller et al., 2009).

To sum up, I began this chapter with a brief overview of human life history and current thinking regarding evolutionary-oriented theoretical frameworks (LHT, parental investment theory) that are commonly used to frame predictions regarding human paternal psychobiology. A fundamental idea underlying those frameworks is that if humans/hominins experienced selection favoring increased levels of paternal care, it would have required proximate (i.e., underlying physiological) mechanisms to help facilitate those shifts in male priorities and behavioral patterns. Based on cross-species comparisons, T is a likely candidate to function in that specific mechanistic role and is among the most widely studied hormones in research on human partnering/parenting and psychobiology. However, as I have reviewed above, there is increasing evidence from studies of T and, to a lesser extent, oxytocin (Abraham & Feldman, 2018; Gettler, Sarma, et al., 2019) that the patterning of human paternal biology potentially varies based on intersections between local contexts and systems of meaning (e.g., cultural norms), environmental conditions (i.e., ecology), and individual-level characteristics. It is important to note that these perspectives are not at odds with one another; rather, a number of lines of evidence are typically used by evolutionary-focused scholars to argue for plastic and facultative aspects of fathers' involvement in our evolutionary past. Regardless of whether current variation in responses of fathers' physiology to diverse parenting demands reflects selection in our evolutionary past or is merely an example of contemporary bio-behavioral phenotypic plasticity (Gettler, 2014), I would argue that to the extent that we think modeling between-father differences in these biological patterns is potentially important to understanding fathers' effects on children and family systems, we need to continue to increase our attention to fathers' own developmental experiences and individual dispositions as well as the prevailing cultural values of their communities and societies (Gettler, 2016).

Summary and Key Points

Humans have a relatively "slow" life history in many respects, especially the prolonged and costly periods of growth and development that are characteristic of our children. Yet, compared to closely related species, the way we raise our children is differentiated by the fact that in many families, parents and other caregivers commonly raise multiple dependent children simultaneously, rather than focusing on ensuring that each child reaches maturity before having another. Evolutionary and comparative perspectives on the emergence of this LH strategy help provide a theoretically grounded foundation for considering the important roles that human fathers have likely played throughout the history of our species and how selection may have shaped men's psychobiology to help facilitate shifts toward committed partnering and parenting (Gettler, 2014; Gray & Anderson, 2010). In that vein, there are three key sets of points I would like to emphasize in closing this chapter.

First, evolutionary framing, including LHT, provides a critical foundation for proposing why men's neurobiological and hormonal systems would have the functional capacity to respond to certain forms of partnering and parenting (Gettler, 2014). While the current literature on the biology of fatherhood is increasingly consistent with the idea that there is plasticity in fathers' psychobiology based on social and ecological context, the neuroendocrine axis that produces T (for example) is evolutionarily ancient and highly conserved, being shared by all vertebrates, and is thus certainly not infinitely malleable (Gettler, 2016). Rather, evolutionary and comparative perspectives help us generate predictions about how hormones, such as T, may have been selected as mechanisms to mediate trade-offs between certain types of incongruent demands. In short, it is not theoretically appropriate to expect that fathers' neuroendocrine systems will have the functional capacities to respond adaptively to all the demands of daily life. For example, a US-based father who is committed to being a sensitive and nurturing parent may also work in a business occupation in which he will achieve success by behaving highly competitively and hierarchically. These day-to-day demands are likely to be best optimized through different psychobiological profiles, which cannot necessarily be concomitantly expressed because our biology has constraints in its plasticity. Evolutionary perspectives are critical to understanding and modeling the plausible range of possibilities for parental physiology in contemporary environments and family systems, including in the face of political economic and structural constraints and challenges (Gettler, 2016).

Second, a fairly cohesive picture has emerged regarding men having lower T as fathers in the context of committed romantic partnerships and when they are more involved with direct caregiving for their children. However, these patterns are not ubiquitous across cultures, including in settings in which polygynous marriage is culturally sanctioned and practiced and those in which fathers' roles generally do not include direct caregiving (Gettler, 2014; Gray, McHale, & Carre, 2017; van Anders, 2013). Moreover, recent research that my colleagues and I have published shows that in a society in which fathers' roles as providers require risky behavior and represent pathways to achieving social status in a hierarchical community "better" fathers (by local definitions) have higher T than other fathers (Boyette et al., 2019; Gettler, Sarma, et al., 2019). Thus, there is much that remains poorly understood about the manifestation of human fathers' biology (Abraham & Feldman, 2018; Gettler, 2014; Rosenbaum & Gettler, 2018), and researchers must be attentive to the importance of variation in cultural models of fatherhood and family life, including within subpopulations in large, diverse societies (Mazur, 2014), as this area of study continues to grow.

Finally, and on a related point, we need further insights on individual differences in men's neurobiological and endocrine responsiveness from parenting and to understand the sources of that variation. Psychobiological frameworks increasingly emphasize the importance of early-life social-family environments in shaping the physiological pathways through which parenting is later expressed in adulthood (Bos, 2017; Gettler, 2016), while a small number of studies have begun exploring individual-level traits (e.g., personality dimensions; genetics) that predict differential outcomes of higher vs. lower T in the context of family life (Gettler et al., 2017; Sarma, Kuo, Bechayda, Kuzawa, & Gettler, 2018; van der Pol et al., 2019). For those of us who are interested in questions of parental biology and child outcomes, these more nuanced observations may be critical to helping solve the "conundrum" of how or if fathers' psychobiological profiles are linked to the quality of their parenting and functioning within family systems.

References

Abraham, E., & Feldman, R. (2018). The neurobiology of human allomaternal care; implications for fathering, coparenting, and children's social development. *Physiology & Behavior, 193*, 25–34.

Alvergne, A., Faurie, C., & Raymond, M. (2009). Variation in testosterone levels and male reproductive effort: Insight from a polygynous human population. *Hormones and Behavior, 56*, 491–497.

Bos, P. A. (2017). The endocrinology of human caregiving and its intergenerational transmission. *Development and Psychopathology, 26*, 991–999.

Boyette, A. H., Lew-Levy, S., & Gettler, L. T. (2018). Dimensions of fatherhood in a Congo Basin village: A multimethod analysis of intracultural variation in men's parenting and its relevance for child health. *Current Anthropology, 59*(6), 1–9.

Boyette, A. H., Lew-Levy, S., Sarma, M. S., & Gettler, L. T. (2019). Testosterone, fathers as providers and caregivers, and child health: Evidence from fisher-farmers in the Republic of the Congo. *Hormones and Behavior, 107*, 35–45.

Bribiescas, R. G. (2001). Reproductive ecology and life history of the human male. *American Journal of Physical Anthropology, 116*, 148–176.

Bribiescas, R. G., & Ellison, P. T. (2008). How hormones mediate trade-offs in human health and disease. In S. C. Stearns & J. C. Koella (Eds.), *Evolution in health and disease* (2nd ed., pp. 77–93). Oxford, UK: Oxford University Press.

Button, K. S., Ioannidis, J. P., Mokrysz, C., Nosek, B. A., Flint, J., Robinson, E. S., et al. (2013). Power failure: Why small sample size undermines the reliability of neuroscience. *Nature Reviews Neuroscience, 14*(5), 365.

Cabrera, N. J. (2020). Father involvement, father-child relationship, and attachment in the early years. *Attachment & Human Development, 22*(1), 134–138.

Carré, J. M., Geniole, S. N., Ortiz, T. L., Bird, B. M., Videto, A., & Bonin, P. L. (2017). Exogenous testosterone rapidly increases aggressive behavior in dominant and impulsive men. *Biological Psychiatry, 82*(4), 249–256.

Charnov, E. L., & Berrigan, D. (1993). Why do female primates have such long lifespans and so few babies? Or life in the slow lane. *Evolutionary Anthropology, 1*, 191–194.

Clutton-Brock, T. H. (1991). *The evolution of parental care*. Princeton, NJ: Princeton University Press.

Dorius, C., Booth, A., Hibel, J., Granger, D. A., & Johnson, D. (2012). Parents' testosterone and children's perception of parent–child relationship quality. *Horm Behav, 60*(5), 512–519.

Edelstein, R. S., Chopik, W. J., Saxbe, D. E., Wardecker, B. M., Moors, A. C., & LaBelle, O. P. (2017). Prospective and dyadic associations between expectant parents' prenatal hormone changes and postpartum parenting outcomes. *Developmental Psychobiology, 59*, 77–90.

Endendijk, J. J., Hallers-Haalboom, E. T., Groeneveld, M. G., van Berkel, S. R., van der Pol, L. D., Bakermans-Kranenburg, M. J., et al. (2016). Diurnal testosterone variability is differentially associated with parenting quality in mothers and fathers. *Hormones and Behavior, 80*, 68–75.

Fernandez-Duque, E., Valeggia, C. R., & Mendoza, S. P. (2009). The biology of paternal care in human and nonhuman primates. *Annual Review of Anthropology, 38*, 115–130.

Fleming, A. S., Corter, C., Stallings, J., & Steiner, M. (2002). Testosterone and prolactin are associated with emotional responses to infant cries in new fathers. *Hormones and Behavior, 42*(4), 399–413.

Gettler, L. T. (2016). Becoming DADS: Considering the role of cultural context and developmental plasticity for paternal socioendocrinology. *Current Anthropology, 57*(S13), S38–S51.

Gettler, L. T., Kuo, P. X., Bas, A., & Borja, J. B. (2019). The roles of parents in shaping fathering across generations in Cebu, Philippines. *Journal of Marriage and Family, 81*(3), 662–678.

Gettler, L. T., & Oka, R. C. (2016). Are testosterone levels and depression risk linked based on partnering and parenting? Evidence from a large population-representative study of US men and women. *Social Science & Medicine, 163*, 157–167.

Gettler, L. T., Ryan, C. P., Eisenberg, D. T., Rzhetskaya, M., Hayes, M. G., Feranil, A. B., et al. (2017). The role of testosterone in coordinating male life history strategies: The moderating effects of the androgen receptor CAG repeat polymorphism. *Hormones and Behavior, 87*, 164–175.

Gettler, L. T., Sarma, M. S., Lew-Levy, S., Bond, A., Trumble, B. C., & Boyette, A. H. (2019). Mothers' and fathers' joint profiles for testosterone and oxytocin in a small-scale fishing-farming community: Variation based on marital conflict and paternal contributions. *Brain and Behavior, 9*, e01367.

Gettler, L. T. (2010). Direct male care and hominin evolution: Why male-child interaction is more than a nice social idea. *American Anthropologist, 112*(1), 7–21.

Gettler, L. T. (2014). Applying socioendocrinology to evolutionary models: Fatherhood and physiology. *Evolutionary Anthropology, 23*(4), 146–160.

Gettler, L. T., McDade, T. W., Agustin, S. S., Feranil, A. B., & Kuzawa, C. W. (2015). Longitudinal perspectives on fathers' residence status, time allocation, and testosterone in the Philippines. *Adaptive Human Behavior and Physiology, 1*(2), 124–149. https://doi.org/10.1007/s40750-014-0018-9

Gettler, L. T., McDade, T. W., Feranil, A. B., & Kuzawa, C. W. (2011). Longitudinal evidence that fatherhood decreases testosterone in human males. *PNAS, 108*(29), 16194–16199.

Gettler, L. T., McKenna, J. J., Agustin, S. S., McDade, T. W., & Kuzawa, C. W. (2012). Does cosleeping contribute to lower testosterone levels in fathers? Evidence from the Philippines. *PLoS One, 7*(9), e41559.

Gordon, I., Pratt, M., Bergunde, K., Zagoory-Sharon, O., & Feldman, R. (2017). Testosterone, oxytocin, and the development of human parental care. *Hormones and Behavior, 93*, 184–192.

Gray, P. B., McHale, T. S., & Carre, J. M. (2017). A review of human male field studies of hormones and behavioral reproductive effort. *Hormones and Behavior, 91*, 52–67. https://doi.org/10.1016/j.yhbeh.2016.07.004

Gray, P. B., & Crittenden, A. N. (2014). Father Darwin: Effects of children on men, viewed from an evolutionary perspective. *Fathering, 12*(2), 121–142.

Gray, P. B., Straftis, A. A., Bird, B. M., McHale, T. S., & Zilioli, S. (2019). Human reproductive behavior, life history, and the challenge hypothesis: A 30-year review, retrospective and future directions. *Hormones and Behavior*, S0018-506X(19)30003-0.

Gray, P. B. (2003). Marriage, parenting, and testosterone variation among kenyan swahili men. *American Journal of Physical Anthropology, 122*(3), 279–286.

Gray, P. B., & Anderson, K. G. (2010). *Fatherhood: Evolution and human paternal behavior*. Cambridge, MA: Harvard University Press.

Gray, P. B., Campbell, B. C., Marlowe, F. W., Lipson, S. F., & Ellison, P. T. (2004). Social variables predict between-subject but not day-to-day variation in the testosterone of US men. *Psychoneuroendocrinology, 29*(9), 1153–1162.

Gray, P. B., Ellison, P. T., & Campbell, B. C. (2007). Testosterone and marriage among Ariaal men of northern Kenya. *Current Anthropology, 48*(5), 750–755.

Gray, P. B., Kahlenberg, S. M., Barrett, E. S., Lipson, S. F., & Ellison, P. T. (2002). Marriage and fatherhood are associated with lower testosterone in males. *Evolution and Human Behavior, 23*(3), 193–201.

Gray, P. B., Yang, C. J., & Pope, H. G. (2006). Fathers have lower salivary testosterone levels than unmarried men and married non-fathers in Beijing, China. *Proceedings of the Royal Society B: Biological Sciences, 273*(1584), 333–339.

Gray, P. B., Reece, J., Coore Desai, C., Dinall, T., Pellington, S., & Samms Vaughan, M. (2017). Testosterone and Jamaican fathers: Exploring links to relationship dynamics and paternal care. *Human Nature: An Interdisciplinary Biosocial Perspective, 28*, 201–218. https://doi.org/10.1007/s12110-016-9283-6

Grebe, N. M., Sarafin, R. E., Strenth, C. R., & Zilioli, S. (2019). Pair-bonding, fatherhood, and the role of testosterone: A meta-analytic review. *Neuroscience & Biobehavioral Reviews, 98*, 221–233.

Gurven, M., & Hill, K. (2009). Why do men hunt? A reevaluation of "man the hunter" and the sexual division of labor. *Current Anthropology, 50*(1), 51–74.

Hau, M. (2007). Regulation of male life history traits by testosterone: Implications for the evolution of vertebrate life histories. *BioEssays, 29*, 133–144.

Hawkes, K., & Coxworth, J. E. (2013). Grandmothers and the evolution of human longevity: A review of findings and future directions. *Evolutionary Anthropology: Issues, News, and Reviews, 22*(6), 294–302.

Hill, K., & Kaplan, H. (1999). Life history traits in humans: Theory and empirical studies. *Annual Review of Anthropology, 28*, 397–430.

Holmboe, S. A., Priskorn, L., Jørgensen, N., Skakkebaek, N. E., Linneberg, A., Juul, A., et al. (2017). Influence of marital status on testosterone levels–A ten year follow-up of 1113 men. *Psychoneuroendocrinology, 80*, 155–161.

Hrdy, S. B. (2009). *Mothers and others: The evolutionary origins of mutual understanding*. Cambridge, MA: Belknap Press of Harvard University Press.

Jasienska, G. (2013). *The fragile wisdom: An evolutionary view on women's biology and health*. Cambridge, MA: Harvard University Press.

Kaplan, H., Hill, K., Lancaster, J., & Hurtado, M. (2000). A theory of human life history evolution: Diet, intelligence, and longevity. *Evolutionary Anthropology: Issues, News, and Reviews, 9*, 156–185.

Kramer, K. L. (2010). Cooperative breeding and its significance to the demographic success of humans. *Annual Review of Anthropology, 39*, 417–436.

Kuo, P. X., Braungart-Rieker, J. M., Lefever, J. E. B., Sarma, M. S., O'Neill, M., & Gettler, L. T. (2018). Fathers' cortisol and testosterone in the days around infants' births predict later paternal involvement. *Hormones and Behavior, 106*, 28–34.

Kuo, P. X., & Gettler, L. T. (2018). Theories relevant to hormones and parenting. In O. C. Schultheiss & P. H. Mehta (Eds.), *Routledge international handbook of social neuroendocrinology* (pp. 333–354). Abingdon, UK: Routledge.

Kuo, P. X., Saini, E. K., Thomason, E., Schultheiss, O. C., Gonzalez, R., & Volling, B. L. (2015). Individual variation in fathers' testosterone reactivity to infant distress predicts parenting behaviors with their 1-year-old infants. *Developmental Psychobiology*.

Kuzawa, C. W., Chugani, H. T., Grossman, L. I., Lipovich, L., Muzik, O., Hof, P. R., et al. (2014). Metabolic costs and evolutionary implications of human brain development. *Proceedings of the National Academy of Sciences of the United States of America, 111*(36), 13010–13015. https://doi.org/10.1073/pnas.1323099111

Landry, S. H., Smith, K. E., & Swank, P. R. (2006). Responsive parenting: Establishing early foundations for social, communication, and independent problem-solving skills. *Developmental Psychology, 42*(4), 627.

Lawson, D. W., Nuñez-de la Mora, A., Cooper, G. D., Prentice, A. M., Moore, S. E., & Sear, R. (2017). Marital status and sleeping arrangements predict salivary testosterone levels in rural Gambian men. *Adaptive Human Behavior and Physiology, 3*, 221–240.

Mascaro, J. S., Hackett, P. D., & Rilling, J. K. (2013). Testicular volume is inversely correlated with nurturing-related brain activity in human fathers. *Proceedings of the National Academy of Sciences, 110*(39), 15746–15751.

Mazur, A. (2014). Testosterone of young husbands rises with children in the home. *Andrology, 2*(1), 125–129.

Mazur, A., & Michalek, J. (1998). Marriage, divorce, and male testosterone. *Social Forces, 77*(1), 315–330.

Meijer, W. M., van IJzendoorn, M. H., & Bakermans-Kranenburg, M. J. (2019). Challenging the challenge hypothesis on testosterone in fathers: Limited meta-analytic support. *Psychoneuroendocrinology*, 104435.

Muller, M. N., Marlowe, F. W., Bugumba, R., & Ellison, P. T. (2009). Testosterone and paternal care in East African foragers and pastoralists. *Proceedings of the Royal Society B: Biological Sciences, 276*(1655), 347–354. https://doi.org/10.1098/rspb.2008.1028

Oswald, L. M., Zandi, P., Nestadt, G., Potash, J. B., Kalaydjian, A. E., & Wand, G. S. (2006). Relationship between cortisol responses to stress and personality. *Neuropsychopharmacology, 31*(7), 1583.

Perini, T., Ditzen, B., Hengartner, M., & Ehlert, U. (2012). Sensation seeking in fathers: The impact on testosterone and paternal investment. *Hormones and Behavior, 61*(2), 191–195.

Promislow, D. E. L., & Harvey, P. H. (1990). Living fast and dying young: A comparative analysis of life-history variation among mammals. *Journal of Zoology, 220*(3),

417–437. https://doi.org/10.1111/j.1469-7998.1990.tb04316.x

Roney, J. R., & Gettler, L. T. (2015). The role of testosterone in human romantic relationships. *Current Opinion in Psychology, 1*, 81–86.

Rosenbaum, S., & Gettler, L. T. (2018). With a little help from her friends (and family) part II: Non-maternal caregiving behavior and physiology in mammals. *Physiology & Behavior, 193*, 12–24.

Royle, N. J., Smiseth, P. T., & Kolliker, M. (2012). *The evolution of parental care*. Oxford, UK: Oxford University Press.

Sarma, M. S., Kuo, P. X., Bechayda, S. A., Kuzawa, C. W., & Gettler, L. T. (2018). Exploring the links between early life and young adulthood social experiences and men's later life psychobiology as fathers. *Physiology & Behavior, 193*(Pt A), 82–89.

Scelza, B. A. (2010). Fathers' presence speeds the social and reproductive careers of sons. *Current Anthropology, 51*(2), 295–303.

Smuts, B. B., & Gubernick, D. J. (1992). Male-infant relationships in nonhuman primates: Paternal investment or mating effort? In B. S. Hewlett (Ed.), *Father-child relations: Cultural and biosocial contexts* (pp. 1–30). New York: Aldine De Gruyter.

Stearns, S. C. (1992). *The evolution of life histories*. Oxford, UK: Oxford University Press.

van Anders, S. M., Goldey, K. L., & Kuo, P. X. (2011). The steroid/peptide theory of social bonds: Integrating testosterone and peptide responses for classifying social behavioral contexts. *Psychoneuroendocrinology, 36*(9), 1265–1275.

van Anders, S. M. (2013). Beyond masculinity: Testosterone, gender/sex, and human social behavior in a comparative context. *Frontiers in Neuroendocrinology, 34*(3), 198–210.

van der Pol, L. D., Groeneveld, M. G., van Berkel, S. R., Endendijk, J. J., Hallers-Haalboom, E. T., & Mesman, J. (2019). Fathers: The interplay between testosterone levels and self-control in relation to parenting quality. *Hormones and Behavior, 112*, 100–106.

von Rueden, C., Gurven, M., & Kaplan, H. (2011). Why do men seek status? Fitness payoffs to dominance and prestige. *Proceedings of the Royal Society B: Biological Sciences, 278*, 2223–2232. https://doi.org/10.1098/rspb.2010.2145

Weisman, O., Zagoory-Sharon, O., & Feldman, R. (2014). Oxytocin administration, salivary testosterone, and father–infant social behavior. *Progress in Neuro-Psychopharmacology and Biological Psychiatry, 49*, 47–52.

Wingfield, J. C., Hegner, R. E., Ball, G. F., & Duffy, A. M. (1990). The 'challenge hypothesis': Theoretical implications for patterns of testosterone secretion, mating systems, and breeding strategies. *The American Naturalist, 136*, 829–846.

Winking, J., & Koster, J. (2015). The fitness effects of men's family investments. *Human Nature, 26*(3), 292–312.

11 Neural Plasticity in Human Fathers

Leah Grande, Rebekah Tribble, and Pilyoung Kim

A well-established field of research that examines the neural adaptation to parenthood among mothers exists. Combined with a rich body of nonhuman animal research, the field of the human maternal brain has provided detailed understanding of the neurobiological basis of motherhood and neural risk markers for insensitive parenting (Feldman, 2015; Kim, Capistrano, & Congleton, 2016; Kim, Strathearn, & Swain, 2016; Lonstein, Lévy, & Fleming, 2015; Rutherford, Wallace, Laurent, & Mayes, 2015). In contrast, such understanding of the neurobiological basis of parenting for human fathers is limited. However, recent neuroimaging studies of human fathers provide insight to neural adaptation processes that fathers experience after they have their own children (Feldman, Braun, & Champagne, 2019).

In this chapter, we provide the current understanding of how human fathers' brains support their relationships with their children. First, we review available evidence that compares neural structure and functions among human mothers and fathers. When compared with mothers, fathers undergo similar but also unique processes of neural adaptation to parenthood. Second, as there are individual differences in parenting behaviors, there are individual differences in neural responses to children among fathers. We review several factors that are associated with these individual differences in the neural responses to their own child. Third, we review the role of hormones, specifically vasopressin, oxytocin, and testosterone, in the neural responses to their own child among human fathers. Finally, we discuss the implications of the empirical findings and suggest directions for future research.

L. Grande · R. Tribble · P. Kim (✉)
Department of Psychology, University of Denver, Denver, CO, USA
e-mail: pilyoung.kim@du.edu

Paternal Brain Circuitry

We start by introducing key brain regions that are involved in parenting. Research on the neural basis of fathering highlights several important brain networks, including subcortical regions important for parental motivation and reward, as well as cortical regions involved in emotional and cognitive empathy. Please see Fig. 11.1 for a visual representation of key brain networks implicated in human paternal behavior (Abraham et al., 2018; Feldman et al., 2019), including subcortical, mentalizing, embodied simulation, and "executive" networks.

Animal research has played an important role in mapping the paternal brain. Although paternal care is relatively common in birds and fish, only 3–5% of mammals exhibit paternal caregiving. Nonhuman animal research has focused on certain species that exhibit paternal care, such as the

H. E. Fitzgerald et al. (eds.), *Handbook of Fathers and Child Development*,
https://doi.org/10.1007/978-3-030-51027-5_11

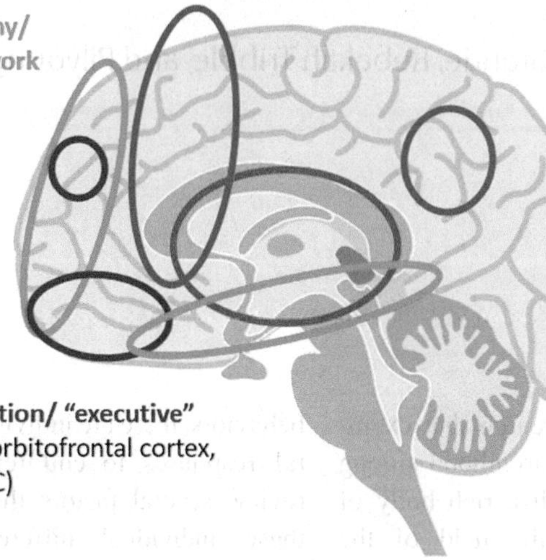

Emotional empathy/ embodied simulation network (e.g., insular-cingulate circuit, inferior parietal lobule)

Cognitive empathy/ mentalizing network (e.g., prefrontal-temporo-parietal circuit, superior temporal sulcus)

Emotion regulation/ "executive" network (e.g., orbitofrontal cortex, dorsolateral PFC)

Subcortical network (e.g., amygdala, hypothalamus, dopamine reward circuit)

Fig. 11.1 Paternal brain circuitry. This figure represents a number of brain networks involved in paternal caregiving, including the *subcortical network* (a conserved, limbic circuit shared with nonhuman animals), *mentalizing network* (implicated in cognitive empathy, the top-down understanding of others' mental states), *embodied simulation network* (implicated in emotional empathy, the bottom-up representation of others' emotions), and the *"executive" network* (important for emotion regulation and multitasking, thought to be the last to evolve). (Abraham, Raz, Zagoory-Sharon, & Feldman, 2018; Feldman et al., 2019) This is a schematic representation for descriptive purposes; circles do not accurately reflect the location of each brain region

biparental California mice, socially monogamous prairie voles, and nonhuman primates such as marmosets and tamarins (Snowden & Soumi, 1982). In some nonhuman primates such as the titi monkeys, infants are carried by fathers 90% of the time and demonstrate a preference for fathers over mothers (Fernandez-Duque, Valeggia, & Mendoza, 2009). Surprisingly, direct paternal care is absent in human's closest relatives; it is unclear how paternal care evolved in humans (Storey & Ziegler, 2016). However, studies of other animals suggest that consistent, high-quality paternal care tends to occur in the context of pair-bonding, and the neurobiological mechanisms underlying paternal care likely also support social behavior more generally (Fernandez-Duque et al., 2009).

Nonhuman animal research highlights the importance of subcortical and limbic structures in supporting paternal behavior. The medial preoptic area (MPOA) in the hypothalamus is well established as a critical area for parental care in both female and male rodents. MPOA lesions disrupt paternal care (Lee & Brown, 2002), optogenetic activation of the MPOA decreases infanticide (Tsuneoka et al., 2015), and exposure to pups increases c-Fos expression (a marker of neuronal activation) in the MPOA in species of male mice and prairie voles (Horrell, Saltzman, & Hickmott, 2019). During the transition to fatherhood, California mice show some plasticity in the MPOA, particularly decreased inhibition (Horrell et al., 2019). The basolateral and medial amygdala (Kirkpatrick, Kim, & Insel, 1994; Lee & Brown, 2002), bed nucleus of the stria terminalis (BNST) (de Jong, Chauke, Harris, & Saltzman, 2009; Kirkpatrick et al., 1994), and ventral pallidum (Akther, Fakhrul, & Higashida, 2014) are other subcortical structures implicated in paternal behavior in animal models. Lesions to the basolateral amygdala produce parenting impairments that are even more pronounced in male than female California mice, including reduced licking of pups and increased latency in retrieving, licking, and crouching over pups (Lee & Brown, 2002).

The subcortical, limbic circuit described in animal models is conserved in human fathers. Research demonstrates that regions such as the amygdala, the hypothalamus, and the dopamine reward circuit also play an important role in human paternal behavior (Abraham et al., 2014; Seifritz et al., 2003; see Fig. 11.1). The amygdala assists in the processing of biologically significant stimuli, emotion recognition, and salience (Adolphs, 2002; Dolan, 2002). More broadly, the amygdala is part of a set of limbic and cortical brain regions that assists in the regulation of caregiving behaviors, empathy, and perceptions of infant stimuli (Newman, 2007). By heightening parental anxiety and vigilance, this brain region enables parents to instinctively identify and instantly respond to infant distress, enhancing odds of infant survival. Additionally, the mesolimbic dopamine system promotes infant approach and enhances reward from the infant attachment relationship (Swain et al., 2014). Taken together, this subcortical circuit constitutes a phylogenetically early neural basis of paternal behavior with some shared structure and function across species.

The subcortical structures of the human paternal brain are connected to multiple, overlapping insular-cingulate and fronto-temporo-parietal networks (see Fig. 11.1). These networks can be differentiated as supporting both emotional and cognitive empathy in fathers (Feldman et al., 2019; Shamay-Tsoory, 2011). Bottom-up embodied simulation and insular-cingulate emotional empathy networks promote fathers' ability to identify with infant state, emotion, and behavior, including areas such as the anterior cingulate cortex (ACC), anterior insula, and inferior frontal gyrus (Abraham et al., 2018). By contrast, the mentalizing network involves more top-down cognitive processes, supporting the understanding of infant mental states, theory of mind, and attributions about child behavior (Abraham et al., 2018). This network consists of the prefrontal-temporo-parietal circuit, including areas such as the superior temporal sulcus (STS) and dorsomedial prefrontal cortex (dmPFC) (Feldman et al., 2019; Isik, Koldewyn, Beeler, & Kanwisher, 2017). Lastly, emotion regulation and "executive" networks support parental affect regulation, action selection, and multitasking, recruiting areas such as the orbitofrontal cortex (OFC) and dorsolateral prefrontal cortex (dlPFC) (Feldman et al., 2019). Cortical networks work in junction with one another and subcortical regions to promote paternal adaptation and parenting behaviors.

Structural Plasticity in Father Brains

Interest in paternal neural plasticity during the postpartum period has grown due to substantial evidence for maternal plasticity during this time. Fatherhood may increase the growth of new neurons. Marmoset fathers play an important role in caring for and feeding young and carry infants until they are 3 months old (Kozorovitskiy, Hughes, Lee, & Gould, 2006). First-time and experienced marmoset fathers have higher densities of dendritic spines on pyramidal cells in the prefrontal cortex (PFC) and an increased abundance of vasopressin receptors, a hormone important for paternal infant care and pair-bonding (Kozorovitskiy et al., 2006). Studies in the uniparental house mice demonstrate that interactions between a father and his pups stimulate neurogenesis in the olfactory bulb and hippocampus (Mak & Weiss, 2010). Some of these new cells mature into olfactory interneurons that facilitate recognition of his adult offspring's odors (Mak & Weiss, 2010). Growth of new neurons during the postpartum period may promote positive fathering behaviors, by potentially altering vasopressin signaling and supporting recognition of offspring odors.

Research has been mixed on whether fatherhood increases or inhibits neurogenesis and dendritic growth in the dentate gyrus of the hippocampus (Glasper et al., 2016; Glasper, Kozorovitskiy, Pavlic, & Gould, 2011; Lieberwirth, Wang, Jia, Liu, & Wang, 2013; Mak & Weiss, 2010). Among male prairie voles, fatherhood was found to decrease the survival of new cells in the dentate gyrus, as well as in the amygdala and ventromedial hypothalamus (Lieberwirth et al., 2013). Hyer and colleagues (2016) may help to explain these discrepant findings by demonstrating that fatherhood first reduced the survival of cells in the dentate gyrus, a part of the hippocampus, during the first week, and then maintained neurogenesis from 1 to 2 weeks postpartum among male California mice. Maintained neurogenesis from 1 to 2 weeks also coincided with a peak in fathers' pup retrieval and reduced anxiety-like behaviors, suggesting that pup exposure may relate to neural reorganization and affect postpartum (Hyer et al., 2016). Altered neuroplasticity and dendritic growth in the dentate gyrus, PFC, and other regions may help to facilitate paternal behavior during the postpartum period.

Few studies have examined structural changes among human fathers. Kim and colleagues (2014) measured 16 fathers' (*M* age = 36.31 years, SD = 4.92; US sample) anatomical changes from 2–4 weeks to 12–16 weeks postpartum. Gray matter volume increases were observed in the striatum/subgenual anterior cingulate cortex (including the hypothalamus and amygdala), lateral prefrontal cortex, and superior temporal gyrus (Kim, Rigo, et al., 2014). Gray matter volume decreases were observed in areas such as the orbitofrontal cortex (OFC), posterior cingulate cortex (PCC), insula, and fusiform gyrus (Kim, Rigo, et al., 2014). Although paternal gray matter increases were consistent with some research on maternal brain changes postpartum (Kim et al., 2010), observed gray matter decreases were unique to fathers. Decreases were observed in areas involved in the default mode network, such as the medial PFC and PCC. This may suggest that fathers are engaging less in the default mode network and instead directing attention toward parenting-relevant stimuli (Kim, Rigo, et al., 2014). Gray matter reductions were also observed in the OFC and insula, areas involved in processing emotion, as well as stress and uncertainty. Reductions in these areas may reflect decreased stress and ambiguity in the later postpartum period. Structural changes were also associated with fathers' mood and parenting behaviors. Gray matter increases in the striatum/subgenual ACC were associated with lower depressive symptoms; decreases in the OFC were associated with higher paternal intrusiveness, particularly during physical play with his infant (Kim, Rigo, et al., 2014). By contrast, in another study in Spain of 19 first-time fathers (*M* age = 35.21 years, SD = 4.30) and 17 control men without children (*M* age = 31.64 years, SD = 6.41), no gray matter changes were observed in fathers pre- and post-pregnancy (*M* weeks following parturition = 10.51, SD = 6.83), whereas pronounced gray matter decreases were observed among mothers (Hoekzema et al., 2017). These discrepant findings may be due to the time at which fathers' brains were assessed, as Hoekzema and colleagues (2017) assessed the paternal brain over a range of postpartum ages, as compared to prepregnancy, whereas Kim and colleagues (2014) assessed change within narrowly defined postpartum windows. It is possible that human paternal brain changes may wax and wane over the postpartum period, similar to patterns observed in animal studies (Hyer et al., 2016). Future research is needed to delineate normative structural changes among fathers during prenatal and postpartum periods, as well as how paternal mood and parenting are related to different neural trajectories.

Functional Adaptation in Father Brains: Comparison with Mother Brains

In addition to structural analyses, some researchers have examined neural network connectivity among mothers and fathers. Eighty-seven first-time parents in Israel (*M* age = 36.10 years, SD = 4.34), including 41 heterosexual parents (20 mothers, 21 fathers) and 48 homosexual fathers, viewed their interactions with their own and an unknown infant while in the MRI scanner (*M* infant age = 11 months, SD = 6.67) (Abraham et al., 2018). No differences were observed by gender or sexual orientation in the network connectivity of embodied simulation and mentalizing networks; this suggests that differences in neural parental empathy are due to individual differences and experience, rather than gender. Further, all parents showed greater connectivity within and between the two empathy networks when viewing their own, compared to an unknown, infant interaction (Abraham et al., 2018). This increased coherence to viewing one's own infant may be adaptive and an important marker of parental health and attachment. In an identical experimental paradigm, examining 45 primary caregiving parents in Israel (*M* age = 36.4 years, SD = 66.87), including 20 heterosexual biological mothers and 25 homosexual biological fathers, no connectivity differences were observed in core-limbic, embodied simulation, and mentalizing networks by gender (Abraham, Hendler, Zagoory-Sharon, & Feldman, 2016). Excitingly, greater parental integrity in these networks at 11 months predicted child development outcomes at age 3, such as increased positive emotionality, social engagement, and self-regulation, as well as child oxytocin and cortisol levels (Abraham et al., 2016, 2018). This finding highlights the potential importance of functional networks in the paternal brain for a father's long-term relationship with his child.

Functional changes in mothers and fathers with the birth of a child display both similarities and differences. One study observing biobehavioral synchrony conducted fMRI scans with 30 parents of 4–6-month-old infants (15 heterosexual, married couples; *M* age = 29.30 years, SD = 3.45; Israel sample); participants watched 2-minute segments of infant-related videos, some of their own infant and others of an unknown infant (Atzil, Hendler, Zagoory-Sharon, Winetraub, & Feldman, 2012). Videos consisted of mother-infant, father-infant, and infant solitary play. Researchers discovered that mother and father pairs displayed similar brain activations in social-cortical networks related to empathy and mentalizing including the dmPFC, inferior frontal gyrus, insula, and inferior parietal lobule when observing their own infant. Coordination of brain response within mother-father pairs may help to facilitate pair-bonding and co-parenting. In addition to synchrony, results also suggest specificity in maternal and paternal brain responses. Mothers displayed greater amygdala activation to their own infant cues compared with fathers. Additionally, plasma oxytocin, a key neurohormone underlying bond formation, was correlated with limbic activations only among mothers including the nucleus accumbens, amygdala, anterior insula, and ventral ACC. In contrast, oxytocin was correlated with higher activations in cognitive areas including the dorsolateral PFC, dorsal ACC, inferior parietal cortex, and precentral gyrus in fathers (Atzil et al., 2012). Fathering may rely more on socio-cognitive adaptation than mothering, whereas mothering demonstrates closer associations with phylogenetically ancient, limbic-motivational circuits. Plasma vasopressin levels were also associated with reductions in activation in the frontal and temporal gyrus in both mothers and fathers. Only among fathers, however, was vasopressin associated with inferior frontal gyrus and insula activation, areas important for emotional empathy and social cognition. Vasopressin is implicated in supporting defensive behaviors and male bonding in animal models (Bielsky, Hu, & Young, 2005). However, given the small sample size (*N* = 30) of this study, additional research is needed to tease out if oxytocin-limbic correlations are truly unique to mothers and vasopressin-brain connections unique to fathers.

Father Versus Mother Brains: Adaptations to Infant Cues

Fathers and mothers respond to infant vocalizations in differing ways. When rating infant cries, regardless of parenting status, women typically report feelings of sympathy and an urgency to care for the infant, whereas men often find the sounds aversive and even irritating in nature (Boukydis & Burgess, 1982; Zeifman, 2003). Pisapia and colleagues (2013) examined gender differences in response to infant hunger cries by gathering 18 healthy adults (9 females: *M* age = 31.50 years, SD = 4.27, and 9 males: *M* age = 35.38 years, SD = 4.63), half of whom were parents of children older than 4 years and half of whom were nonparents, and exposing them to infant cry sounds during rest and mind-wandering to investigate neural responses to infant cries. Participants were living in Italy and all of European descent. Researchers focused on the default-mode network given that deactivations are a reliable marker of an individual's engagement in their surroundings (De Pisapia, Turatto, Lin, Jovicich, & Caramazza, 2011). Women, regardless of if they were mothers themselves or not, displayed decreased activations in the dmPFC and PCC when compared to their male counterparts while listening to infant cries. Researchers concluded that the female brain interrupts ongoing mind-wandering, whereas the male brain continues in self-reflection typical of an awake resting state (De Pisapia et al., 2013), providing evidence for a stronger alloparental care tendency in females. Alloparental care is common in mammalian species in which adults other than the direct genetic parents act in a parental role.

Another study (Swain and colleagues 2003) used own baby cry stimuli at 2–4 weeks postpartum in 9 US mothers compared to an unknown baby cry and reported maternal activations in the midbrain, basal ganglia, cingulate, amygdala, and insula. By contrast, fathers showed less activation than mothers in the amygdala and basal ganglia in response to their own infant's cry (Swain et al., 2003; Swain et al., 2004). Participants were interviewed further regarding their experiences as parents; mothers reported being more preoccupied with their infant compared to fathers; thus, this lack of activation may be explained through fathers' reduced feelings of preoccupation. Together, the existing evidence suggests that mothers and fathers both show neural sensitivity to infant stimuli in some of the key neural regions involved in parenting. However, when compared, mothers' neural response to infant stimuli may be higher than fathers'. The difference between mothers and fathers may relate to their parenting experience and the amount of time they spend caregiving, as well as parental gender.

The Importance of Caregiving Experience

The human father's brain is thought to adapt to the parental role through active involvement in childcare, whereas some of the changes of a mothers' brain are driven by hormonal changes related to pregnancy and parturition. This emphasizes the importance of experience in developing functional changes in the paternal brain (Geary, 2000; Lamb, 2010). Studies demonstrate that the amount of childcare experience and involvement is associated with differences in fathers' parenting perceptions and hormonal responses during play (Gettler, McDade, Agustin, & Kuzawa, 2011; Hudson, Elek, & Fleck, 2001). The brains and biology of fathers are sensitive to childcare experiences, and their involvement in parenting impacts their children's development in turn. The role of caregiving experience in men has been examined primarily by comparing brain activation between fathers and non-fathers. In a small study of 20 men in Singapore, 10 fathers of children ages 3 years and younger (father *M* age = 33 years, SD = 3.2) and 10 non-fathers (*M* age = 32 years, SD = 4.5), participants underwent EEG and listened to a typically developing infant cry, a cry of an infant later diagnosed with autism spectrum disorder, infant laughter, and white noise (Truzzi, Islam, Valenzi, & Esposito, 2020). Researchers analyzed event-related potentials (ERP) focusing on well-known ERP waves. Specifically, a wave called P200 related to stimuli initial processing attentional levels and affective information (Carretié, Mercado, Tapia, & Hinojosa, 2001; Dennis & Chen, 2007; Singhal, Doerfling, & Fowler, 2002) resulted in a stronger response to white noise compared to infant laughter in fathers compared to non-fathers. Furthermore, fathers and non-fathers displayed opposite wave dynamics overall. Fathers' reaction to the white noise may be due to the importance of rapid reactions to unexpected threatening sounds in the environment to protect their child. By contrast, infant cry and laughter are familiar to fathers and therefore not threatening. In non-fathers, the atypical ASD cry and infant laughter exhibited a stronger P200 compared to fathers, suggesting the unfamiliarity and arousing nature of these sounds for non-fathers. Even in the very early stages of audio stimulus processing, fathers and non-fathers displayed differences in motor programming and language processing brain areas. This may underlie differential preparation of motor output in fathers and non-fathers, assisting fathers in their caregiving duties (Truzzi et al., 2020).

Another study looking at infant vocalizations further supports our understanding that the father's brain changes with experience. Seifrtiz and colleagues (2003) observed neural responses to infant crying and laughter in 10 mothers (*M* age = 31.6 years, SD = 4.5) and 10 fathers (*M* age = 36.2 years, SD = 4.7) with children younger than 3 years of age (*M* age = 1.3 years, SD = 0.8) living in Switzerland. Regardless of sex, parents displayed greater activations in the amygdala and interconnected limbic regions to infant crying than laughing, compared to 20 nonparents (10 women, *M* age = 27.6, SD = 3.7; 10 men, *M* age = 28.4, SD = 4.8) who displayed greater responses to infant laughing than crying (Seifritz et al., 2003). This suggests an experience-dependent modulation in brain responses regardless of the sex of the parent. Stimuli were collected from a standard international database with no age or reason for vocalizations reported of the infants recorded; therefore, additional studies should assess if similar findings occur in vocalizations that are age-matched to the parent's children. The infant cry response pattern in the amygdala found in fathers may occur from associative learning mechanisms, which is meaningful for adaptation to the demands associated with caring for a newborn.

Researchers have also examined how fathers and non-fathers respond differently to viewing child and adult stimuli. Eighty-eight US fathers of children aged 1–2 years old and 50 non-fathers (*M* age = 33.2 years, SD = 5.70) were instructed to share the emotion of an unknown child or adult while viewing their picture (Mascaro, Hackett, & Rilling, 2014). When viewing an unknown child, fathers showed greater activation in regions important for mentalizing, such as the temporoparietal junction; reward processing, such as the medial orbitofrontal cortex; and face emotion processing, such as the caudal middle frontal gyrus (Mascaro et al., 2014). By contrast, when presented with sexually provocative, adult images, fathers showed reduced activation in reward and motivation regions such as the dorsal caudate and nucleus accumbens (Mascaro et al., 2014). Neural adaptation to fatherhood may heighten reward and motivation circuits related to children while attenuating response to sexual stimuli. This may be associated with life history theory suggesting that fatherhood leads to the prioritization of own child caregiving over seeking another sexual mate (Figueredo et al., 2006; Gray & Crittenden, 2014).

Abraham and colleagues (2014) examined 89 first-time parents (*M* age = 36.1 years, SD = 4.34) raising their 4–17-month-old infants in Israel. We compared brain activations in 20 primary caregiving mothers, 21 secondary caregiving fathers, and 48 primary caregiving homosexual fathers while watching videotaped interactions between each parent and infant while undergoing functional brain imaging. Though primary caregiving mothers displayed greater activation in emotional processing networks including the bilateral amygdala, ventral anterior cingulate cortex, left IFG/insular cortex, and ventral tegmental area, secondary caregiving fathers displayed greater activation in socio-cognitive networks including the bilateral superior temporal sulcus (STS), ventromedial PFC, temporal poles, and lateral frontopolar cortex (Abraham et al., 2014). Activation in emotional processing networks has been linked with mammalian mothering (Kim et al., 2010; Toscano, Bauman, Mason, & Amaral, 2009). Specifically, the amygdala as part of this network undergoes structural changes during pregnancy and childbirth; therefore, greater activation in mothers is to be expected (Kim et al., 2010). Dissimilarly, socio-cognitive networks play a vital role in social cognition, biological motion, social goal interpretation, and prediction-making and updating regarding others' behavior. This pathway relates to paternal caregiving relying on later evolving structures impacted by the father's interactions with his infant once the infant is born (Allison, Puce, & McCarthy, 2000; Hein & Knight, 2008).

Interestingly, primary caregiving fathers exhibited greater parent-infant synchrony than secondary caregiving fathers, displayed by more parental repertoire in relation to infant social signals (Abraham et al., 2014). Additionally, primary caregiving fathers exhibited higher amygdala activation like mothers, higher superior temporal sulcus (STS) activity like secondary caregiving fathers, and functional connectivity between the amygdala and STS. Increased amygdala activations are related to parental vigilance and caregiving behaviors (Newman, 2007; Numan & Stolzenberg, 2009); thus, enhanced activations are adaptive in caring for one's infant and identifying infant cues to ensure infant survival. These primary caregiving fathers display, even without pregnancy, that adaptation to the parental role is possible in human fathers and that the amygdala is sensitive to the primary caregiving role. This also further suggests that differences in brain responses between mothers and fathers may in part be explained by the differences in the amount of parenting involvement between them. Among all fathers, the strength of amygdala-STS connectivity was greater when fathers spent more time in direct responsibility for childcare. The STS plays a key role in social perception, with projections to the amygdala establishing its role in mentalizing and social perception processes. Studies in biparental animals display this same integration of multiple brain networks (Allison et al., 2000; Hein & Knight, 2008; Lambert et al., 2011; Pelphrey, Morris, & Mccarthy, 2004). Stronger amygdala-STS connectivity has been linked with better social cue recognition; individuals with more complex social networks display greater amygdala-STS connectivity, suggesting greater ease in initiating and maintaining social bonds with others (Bickart, Hollenbeck, Barrett, & Dickerson, 2012). This finding suggests that amygdala-STS connectivity, a marker of the interconnected social perception network, may support growth and development that is independent of pregnancy and childbirth and dependent on caregiving experience.

Individual Differences in Father Brains

Although there are considerable differences between fathers and non-fathers' brain responses, there is also significant individual variability within fathers. Some researchers have explored how different characteristics, such as child gender and father age, emotional state, and parenting behaviors and attitudes contribute to differences in paternal brain response. First, a study examined differences in brain response between fathers of girls and fathers of boys (father M age = 33.0 years, SD = 5.67; US sample; 39.13% non-white) (Mascaro, Rentscher, Hackett, Mehl, & Rilling, 2017). Thirty-four fathers of 1–2-year-old girls showed greater neural responses when viewing their daughters' happy face, including enhanced activation in visual processing areas, the medial and lateral OFC, and the left middle frontal gyrus, compared to 35 fathers of 1–2-year-old boys (Mascaro et al., 2017). By contrast, fathers of boys showed heightened neural activation when viewing their sons' neutral face in the thalamus, medial OFC, and inferior temporal sulcus (Mascaro et al., 2017). These differences in brain response were associated with differences in how fathers play with daughters and sons. For example, fathers of daughters were more attentively engaged during play, sang more, and used more analytical language and language about sadness and the body (Mascaro et al., 2017). By contrast, fathers of sons engaged in more rough-and-tumble play and used more achievement language compared to the fathers of daughters. Greater medial and lateral OFC response to happy faces was associated with less rough-and-tumble play, whereas greater medial OFC response to neutral faces was associated with more rough-and-tumble play specifically for fathers of boys. Greater right lateral OFC was also associated with greater use of analytical language and singing during play.

Li and colleagues (2018) investigated how father's age influenced neural response to infant cries. Participants were 39 first-time US fathers, in age ranging from 23 to 40 years old (*M* age = 30.8 years, SD = 4.3; 44% non-white), with infants less than 4 months old (*M* infant age = 9.6 weeks, SD = 3.3). Many fathers could not distinguish between their own and unknown infant cries, and there was no significant difference between neural response to own and unknown cry stimuli. Older fathers found infant cries to be less aversive and also showed attenuated neural response in areas such as the dorsal ACC and anterior insula (Li et al., 2018). Heightened activation of these areas is thought to be related to emotional overarousal and has previously been associated with intrusive parenting (Musser, Kaiser-Laurent, & Ablow, 2012). Fathers who reported negative emotion (such as feeling annoyed or distressed) when listening to his own infant's cry showed increased activation in the right posterior middle temporal gyrus and right angular gyrus, which may suggest increased effort to process emotional information. On the other hand, fathers who reported negative emotion when listening to an unknown infant cry showed decreased activation in the thalamus and left caudate, areas important for parental motivation. Interestingly, Li and colleagues (2018) did not find differences in paternal brain activation related to fathers' depression, childhood abuse, stressful life events, or infant fussiness. This may have been due to limited sample variability (e.g., no participants reported moderate or severe depression), limited ecological validity due to listening to infant cries in the MRI scanner, and rigorous neuroimaging thresholds.

Kuo and colleagues (2012) and Mascaro and colleagues (2013) have examined the association between parenting attitudes and behavior and fathers' brain response. Among a sample of 10 fathers (*M* age = 33.9 years, range: 28–44 years; US sample; 40% non-white) of 2–4-month-old infants, greater paternal sensitivity and reciprocity were associated with less activation in the right orbitofrontal cortex (OFC) when viewing their own vs. unknown infant interactions (Kuo et al., 2012). This is somewhat surprising given the OFC's involvement in emotion, reward, and decision-making. Perhaps, sensitive fathers were highly responsive to both own and unknown infant stimuli, which influenced the contrast, or sensitive fathers had to engage the OFC more to understand unknown infants' emotional states, compared to his own infant. In another study, 36 US fathers (*M* age = 33.0 years, SD = 6.1; 41.7% non-white) of children aged 1–2 years listened to unknown infant cries; infant stimuli were obtained from an online database and consisted of two infants aged 3 and 5 months (Mascaro, Hackett, Gouzoules, et al., 2013). Fathers who endorsed high restrictiveness, such as being controlling of children's behavior and relying more on punishment, showed reduced anterior insula, ACC, and medial OFC activity when listening to unknown infant cries (Rickel & Biasatti, 1982), perhaps suggesting that decreased activity in these regions important for empathy results in the use of more controlling parenting and punishment. Alternatively, factors such as paternal mood, stress, and early experience could be associated with differences in both restrictiveness and paternal brain response. The different findings surrounding OFC activation (Kuo et al., 2012; Mascaro, Hackett, Gouzoules, et al., 2013) may be due to the nature of the task. The OFC has been consistently implicated in the regulation of negative affect. In a task involving aversive cry sounds (Mascaro, Hackett, Gouzoules, et al., 2013), OFC involvement could certainly support negative emotion regulation, whereas OFC involvement when viewing infant play interactions (Kuo et al., 2012) could reflect a variety of emotion and decision-making processes. The authors further examined this relation, as neither high nor low levels of restrictiveness were expected to be ideal. Research suggests that moderate levels of restrictiveness, characteristic of an authoritarian parenting style, are most predictive of positive child outcomes (Darling & Steinberg, 1993). In fact, the least restrictive fathers had the highest anterior insula activity, which is related to decreased paternal responsibility and involvement (Mascaro, Hackett, Gouzoules, et al., 2013). Fathers with a moderate level of anterior insula activity were the most involved in child caregiving, assessed by responsibility in remembering, planning, and scheduling tasks that revolve around their child's care. Overarousal in the anterior insula has been implicated in anxiety, as well as maternal intrusiveness and insecure/dismissing attachment styles (Musser et al., 2012; Simmons, Strigo, Matthews, Paulus, & Stein, 2006; Strathearn, Fonagy, Amico, & Montague, 2009). Likely, this suggests that there is an optimal level of empathy-related neural responding that supports effective parenting, a threshold beyond which leads to maladaptive parenting styles or withdrawal. Future research should continue to explore how paternal and infant characteristics alter fathers' brain response.

Associations Between Hormones and Father Brain

Vasopressin Research suggests that vasopressin may be highly influential particularly for fathers' bonding and parenting behaviors. In animal models, arginine vasopressin is associated with male bonding and territorial behaviors, such as mate-guarding (Carter, 1998). Fatherhood is associated with increases in vasopressin receptors and dendritic spines in the prefrontal cortex in marmosets, whose males help to raise the young (Kozorovitskiy et al., 2006). Vasopressin is also associated with enhanced social perception and face processing in humans (Guastella, Kenyon, Alvares, Carson, & Hickie, 2010), which may support parenting in fathers by heightening vigilance and social cognition networks. Fathers of young children exhibit higher vasopressin concentrations than fathers of older children (Gray, Parkin, & Samms-Vaughan, 2007). Administering vasopressin, but not oxytocin, intranasally increased implicit interest in infants among fathers-to-be compared to control men (Cohen-Bendahan, Beijers, van Doornen, & de Weerth, 2015). As discussed previously, plasma arginine vasopressin was associated with reduced inferior frontal gyrus and insula activation among fathers when viewing their own compared to unknown infant stimuli, suggesting its role in paternal social bonding (Atzil et al., 2012). Further, 41 fathers in Japan (*M* age = 33.6 years, SD = 4.2) with different genetic variants of the arginine-vasopressin receptor 1*A* show differential activation of the left inferior anterior PFC when viewing videos of their own child smiling (child *M* age = 1.6 months, SD = 0.7); by contrast, no differences are observed for 43 Japanese mothers (Nishitani et al., 2017). The reverse is true for oxytocin genetic variants, wherein differences are only observed among mothers (Nishitani et al., 2017). Vasopressin levels may hold significance for uniquely modulating paternal, rather than maternal, brain response to infant stimuli.

Oxytocin The neuropeptide oxytocin also plays an important role in social affiliative behaviors, particularly modulating parental behavior and neural response to infant stimuli. Vasopressin and oxytocin are structurally similar neuropeptides, differing from one another by only two amino acids (Carter, 1998). Oxytocin is closely linked to maternal-infant bonding, and increasing research suggests that higher oxytocin levels support paternal-infant bonding and positive fathering behaviors as well (Feldman, Gordon, Schneiderman, Weisman, & Zagoory-Sharon, 2010; Gordon, Zagoory-Sharon, Leckman, & Feldman, 2010a, 2010b; Weisman, Zagoory-Sharon, & Feldman, 2012). Oxytocin is synthesized in the paraventricular and supraoptic nuclei of the hypothalamus, is released by the posterior pituitary, projects to brain regions important for reward and attachment, and is released into peripheral circulation (Meyer-lindenberg, Domes, Kirsch, & Heinrichs, 2011; Wittfoth-Schardt et al., 2012). Oxytocin levels are higher among fathers than non-fathers (Mascaro et al., 2014), and oxytocin has been shown to increase during the first 6 months of fatherhood (Gordon et al., 2010a).

Oxytocin has been associated with both neural activations and reductions in social cognition, reward, and attention networks among fathers (Atzil et al., 2012; Li, Chen, Mascaro, Haroon, & Rilling, 2017; Wittfoth-Schardt et al., 2012).

Intranasal oxytocin administration, but not the administration of vasopressin, was associated with increased paternal activation in the caudate nucleus, dorsal ACC, and visual cortex in 30 US fathers (*M* age = 32.8 years, SD = 4.7) when viewing pictures of their 1–2-year-old toddler, which could reflect increased reward, empathy, and attention for their own child (Li et al., 2017). Paternal plasma oxytocin was also associated with increased hippocampal activation when viewing child pictures, which may have important implications for social memory (Mascaro et al., 2014). By contrast, other studies have found that oxytocin is associated with reduced neural responsivity. As discussed previously, plasma oxytocin levels were associated with increased limbic activation among mothers; however, among fathers, oxytocin level was correlated with reduced activation in socio-cognitive, cortical areas, such as the medial PFC, left inferior and superior frontal gyrus, and left ACC, when viewing own-infant interactions (Atzil et al., 2012). Additionally, Wittfoth-Schardt and colleagues (2012) demonstrated that intranasal oxytocin was associated with 19 German fathers' (*M* father age = 39.3 years, SD = 6.2; *M* child age = 4.6 years, SD = 1.0) reduced activations in the left globus pallidus when viewing their own and unfamiliar child pictures, as well as reduced connectivity between the globus pallidus and other reward and attachment regions (Wittfoth-Schardt et al., 2012). Oxytocin is involved in downregulating physiological responses to salient cues, both positive and negative, in order to reduce stress and pain perception. The authors hypothesized that reduced neural activation in socio-cognitive areas such as the globus pallidus may help to reduce social avoidance and facilitate approach behaviors in fathers (Wittfoth-Schardt et al., 2012).

Discrepant oxytocin findings may be due to the population, context, and method of oxytocin assessment or administration, as oxytocin is also released in times of stress in order to reduce anxiety (Tops, Peer, Korf, Wijers, & Tucker, 2007). Thus, in a highly stressed situation or population, higher oxytocin may indicate greater stress and cortisol response, and may not be associated with adaptive parenting outcomes. Whether via brain reductions or activations, neural modulation by oxytocin has important associations with paternal caregiving. In a previously described study, fathers' superior temporal sulcus activation when viewing an own-infant play interaction had a direct effect on observed father-infant synchrony during play, which was mediated by increases in oxytocin (Abraham et al., 2014). Oxytocin administration has also been shown to increase positive fathering behaviors by reducing testosterone levels (Weisman, Zagoory-Sharon, & Feldman, 2014).

The different patterns of oxytocin and vasopressin among mothers and fathers may further be associated with interaction style differences with children. Fathers engage in more rough-and-tumble play than mothers, which is thought to stimulate child risk-taking, exploration, and build confidence (Paquette, 2004). Some researchers have conceptualized fathers as the "primary playmate," helping to activate and arouse children (Paquette, 2004); this is in contrast to typical conceptualizations of high-quality maternal care, which involves more emphasis on soothing the child during times of distress. In observations of 71 Israeli mothers (*M* age = 28.9 years, SD = 5.22) and 48 fathers (*M* age = 29.3 years, SD = 4.26) interacting with their 4–6-month-old infants, fathers provided more stimulatory contact during play, whereas mothers engaged in more affectionate contact (Apter-Levi, Zagoory-Sharon, & Feldman, 2014). Interestingly, baseline vasopressin levels prior to the interaction were associated with more parental stimulatory contact, whereas oxytocin levels were associated with more affectionate contact (Apter-Levi et al., 2014). Feldman (2003) videotaped 100 Israeli mothers (*M* age = 27.7 years, SD = 3.93) and their partners, 100 fathers (*M* age = 30.37 years, SD = 4.99), playing with their first-born infants (*M* age = 4.72 months, SD = 0.72) and found that, although mother-infant and father-infant pairs show similar levels of synchrony (described as parental adaptation to the infant's state and signals), the type of synchrony differs. Mother-infant interactions typically involve low to moderate levels of arousal, which gradually increase in positive affect, as well as frequent affectionate touch and shared gaze and vocalizations. By contrast, father-infant interactions often contain sudden peaks in positive arousal, which increase in frequency during play. Paternal play is also characterized by stimulatory contact and a focus on the environment (Feldman, 2003). Stimulatory play with fathers has important implications for child development; in a study of 26 Australian fathers (*M* age = 37.4 years, SD = 3.7), high-quality paternal physical play with his 4-year-old child (*M* age = 51 months, SD = 3) was associated with fewer child emotional problems and fewer problems with peers (Fletcher, StGeorge, & Freeman, 2013). It is important to consider how paternal brain changes relate to fathers' parenting behaviors and experiences.

Testosterone Androgens play a large role in the reproductive axis and may also hold important implications for fathering and the paternal brain. In particular, testosterone is key to spermatogenesis, the maintenance of the genital tract, and the development of secondary sexual characteristics in males (Nelson, 2005). The state of being a father decreases testosterone levels over time (Gettler, McDade, Feranil, & Kuzawa, 2011), and overall, fathers have lower testosterone levels than non-fathers (Gray et al., 2007). This pattern is also observed among nonhuman primates; experienced marmoset fathers and fathers who frequently carry their young show lower testosterone concentrations (Nunes, Fite, & French, 2000; Nunes, Fite, Patera, & French, 2001). Testosterone is observed to influence and be modulated by human sexual interest, arousal, enjoyment, and not only fatherhood but also the anticipation of fatherhood (Dabbs Jr & Mohammed, 1992; Graham & Desjardins, 1980; Hellhammer, Hubert, & Schürmeyer, 1985; Hirschenhauser, Frigerio, Grammer, & Magnusson, 2002). Hirschenhauser and colleagues (2002) studied 27 Austrian and Italian male participants (*M* age = 33 years, SD = 1), observing testosterone levels over a 90-day period and discovered that men with partners who reported a current wish for children, thus prospective fathers, displayed a 28-day monthly interval that coincided with their partners' menstrual cycle, whereas single men or those who did not wish to have children did not exhibit this pattern of testosterone.

Testosterone levels in males are also modulated during his partner's pregnancy. Research (Storey, Walsh, Quinton, & Wynne-Edwards, 2000) reported that testosterone of 31 expectant Canadian fathers (age range: 25–40 years, all of European descent) was related to their partner's hormone levels; specifically, both prospective fathers and mothers had higher concentrations of prolactin and cortisol in the period just before the births of their children and lower postnatal concentrations of testosterone or estradiol, respectively. Additionally, expectant fathers reporting more couvade syndrome symptoms (such as weight gain and nausea, indicative of a "sympathetic pregnancy") had higher levels of prolactin and a significantly greater drop in testosterone following exposure to unknown infant stimuli, such as listening to recorded newborn cries from a neonate unit. This may suggest that prospective fathers respond and adapt to their partners' hormonal and fecundity phases. A similar pattern has been observed in marmoset and tamarin males, who show changes in testosterone and other hormones and weight gain starting in midgestation of their mate's pregnancy (Ziegler, Prudom, Schultz-Darken, Kurian, & Snowdon, 2006; Ziegler, Prudom, Zahed, Parlow, & Wegner, 2009; Ziegler, Washabaugh, & Snowdon, 2004). Weight gain among these nonhuman primates helps to prepare them for the high-energy demands of fathering, such as infant carrying (Ziegler et al., 2006).

Fathers display changes in testosterone as well in relation to infant cues. In a sample of 88 US fathers of children aged 1–2 years old and 50 non-fathers (*M* age = 33.2 years, SD = 5.70), lower levels of testosterone were associated with greater neural response to viewing happy child faces in the caudal middle frontal gyrus, an important area for facial emotion processing and empathy (Mascaro et al., 2014). It is hypothesized that reduced testosterone levels may function to enhance paternal empathy. As discussed previously, Mascaro and colleagues (2013) have also looked at relations between brain response, hormone levels, variations in the androgen receptor gene, and parental attitudes in association with unknown infant crying in 36 fathers of children aged 1–2. The study found that though levels of testosterone, prolactin, and oxytocin were not related to neutral responses to unknown baby cries, androgen receptor genes were. The number of CAG trinucleotide repeats in the first exon of the androgen receptor (AR) gene reflects the brain's sensitivity to testosterone and receptor density in the brain. Less sensitivity to testosterone in fathers was associated with increased neural responses in regions important for embodied simulation and empathy including the anterior insula and bilateral inferior frontal gyrus (IFG).

Parenting behaviors are related to testosterone levels, with fathers who spend at least 3 hours caregiving exhibiting lower testosterone (Gettler, McDade, Feranil, & Kuzawa, 2011). In one study, 10 US fathers (*M* age = 33.9 years; range: 28–44 years; 40% non-white) of infants 2–4 months old underwent neuroimaging while watching short video clips of their baby and then a sex-, age-, and ethnicity-matched baby they had not seen before (Kuo et al., 2012). Fathers with greater testosterone levels after interacting with their infant exhibited increased activation to their own infant compared to an unfamiliar infant in the left caudate (LC). The LC is associated with emotional and approach behaviors along with goal-directed action (Villablanca, 2010). This is somewhat surprising given prior research suggesting that high testosterone is associated with fewer paternal behaviors and fathers with high baseline testosterone tend to experience testosterone decreases as they interact more with their infants (Storey, Noseworthy, Delahunty, Halfyard, & McKay, 2011). However, experience-dependent elevations in testosterone in fathers could play a protective role; testosterone may increase in response to urgent infant vocalizations, potentially linking testosterone to parental protective behaviors (van Anders, Tolman, & Volling, 2012). Additional investigation into testosterone and its links to parenting behaviors and neural activations in fathers in response to their children is needed.

Mascaro and colleagues (2013) discovered testosterone and testicular volume as a predictor of parental caregiving among 70 US fathers (*M* age = 33.0 years, SD = 5.80) of children aged 1–2 years. Specifically, higher testicular volume and testosterone levels were associated with less paternal caregiving and fathers' reports of less desire for caregiving involvement. This was not related to extraneous factors like socioeconomic status that may interfere with the father's ability to be a more active and involved parent, such as hours fathers worked per week (Mascaro, Hackett, & Rilling, 2013). Fathers also underwent neuroimaging, and the effect of viewing their child's images resulted in activations in the fusiform gyrus, thalamocingulate, dorsolateral prefrontal cortex (dlPFC), and mesolimbic areas. Activations in the ventral tegmental area were correlated with more paternal caregiving. Further, brain activations when viewing their own infants' images decreased as testes volume increased. Fathers who display more activation in these reward areas of their brain may be more apt to care for their children and be involved as interactions with their child positively reinforce caregiving. Alternatively, fathers who spend more time with their children may come to find interactions with their children more rewarding, creating a stronger bond with them. Additional longitudinal research is needed to explore this association further. Testosterone appears to play an important role in facilitating partner hormonal synchrony and promoting paternal caregiving.

Summary and Key Points

In this chapter, we provided an overview of the current understanding of the neural adaptation to parenthood in human fathers. First, there are overlaps and differences between the maternal and paternal brain. Increased activations in the MPOA and striatum that are involved in parental motivation overlap between mothers and fathers. Increased activations in the amygdala, involved in detecting salience of infant cues, and in neural regions involved in empathy, mentalization, and emotion regulation are also observed in mothers and fathers. Similar to comparisons of mothers vs. non-mothers, fathers also exhibit increased neural responses to infant cues compared to non-fathers. This suggests that there are increased neural sensitivities to infant cues in parenthood.

Mothers and fathers also exhibit important differences, which suggest unique associations with hormones and parenting styles. Compared to mothers, fathers tend to exhibit more limited structural changes in the brain during the first few months postpartum. In response to infant stimuli, compared to mothers, fathers tend to show less neural activation in regions such as the amygdala and less deactivation in the default mode network. More limited changes among fathers compared to mothers may be associated with a number of biological and social factors, such as more limited hormonal changes that are associated with pregnancy and lactation, on average less time spent with children, and differences in parenting attitudes and societal expectations. Fathers tend to show greater activation in cortical regions involved in social cognition, rather than limbic regions. These differences may reflect fathering as deriving more from social and cultural processes, whereas the evolution of mothering is biologically embedded in reward and motivation processes. Observed differences also may be associated with the different interaction styles in mothers and fathers. Fathers have more physically stimulating interactive styles, whereas mothers have more emotionally sensitive interaction styles that may be supported by the amygdala and other limbic regions.

Next, as in mothers' brains, fathers' brains are sensitive to individual characteristics such as the amount of parenting experience, their own age, and child's gender. Primary caregiving fathers exhibited greater amygdala activations than secondary caregiving fathers. Older fathers perceived infant cry to be less aversive and exhibited attenuated activations in areas such as the dorsal ACC and anterior insula. Fathers exhibited different brain responses to daughters and sons. Moreover, several studies suggest associations between hormones and brain function among fathers. In fathers, vasopressin particularly plays an important role in parenting and pair-bonding. As in mothers, oxytocin was also associated with neural responses to child cues in fathers. Interestingly, in fathers, increased oxytocin levels can be associated with both increased and reduced neural activations in response to child cues; thus, more attention is needed to better understand the unique role of oxytocin vs. vasopressin in father brain activation. More uniquely in paternal care, fathers tend to have lower testosterone levels that are associated with altered neural sensitivity to own child cue and more sensitive parenting.

Our current understanding of human father brains provides insight into future directions of the research field. First, studies are limited that examine clinically at-risk fathers. Studies with mothers suggest that postpartum psychopathology, most commonly depression and anxiety, can influence maternal brain response to her children (Malak, Crowley, Mayes, & Rutherford, 2015; Wonch et al., 2016). Psychopathology in fathers also has significant impacts on parenting quality and child outcome; however, little is known about a neural risk marker for psychopathology or mechanism by which psychopathology influences parenting in fathers. Second, to further advance the understanding of the paternal brain, it would also be important to study environmental risk factors that may influence fathers' ability to parent and adjust to parenthood. The socioeconomic, racial, and ethnic diversity of fathers in many neuroimaging studies is limited. However, in studies with mothers, exposure to trauma and stressful environment (e.g., poverty) can negatively influence brain responses to children (Kim, Capistrano, & Congleton, 2016; Kim, Capistrano, Erhart, Gray-Schiff, & Xu, 2017; Kim, Fonagy, Allen, & Strathearn, 2014). Therefore, it would be important to understand the environmental conditions that support and do not support neural adaptation to parenthood in fathers. Third, although more limited compared to mothers, fathers exhibit hormonal changes during their partners' pregnancy (Saxbe et al., 2017). In studies with mothers, both hormonal and psychological adaptations such as increased oxytocin levels and increased attention to the infant's emotional cues (Feldman, Weller, Zagoory-Sharon, & Levine, 2007; Pearson, Lightman, & Evans, 2011) can predict more sensitive parenting after a child's birth. Therefore, studies that prospectively follow fathers from their partners' pregnancy to the postnatal period would provide insight into whether neural and psychological changes during pregnancy may predict their relationships with their children.

Last, an understanding of the psychopathology, environmental conditions, and prenatal biological adaptation of fathers can inform programs to support the successful adaptation to fatherhood. For example, fathers experiencing harsh environmental conditions such as poverty are less likely to stay involved in parenting, while their involvement is significant for supporting their children's positive development (Carlson & Magnuson, 2011). Understanding the unique neural and psychological processes of how fathers develop emotional bonds with their children would be critical to support fathers experiencing challenges to stay involved. Some fathers experience several unique challenges, such as the lack of a role model or parenting support from their own partners or others. Positive perceptions of parenting may be particularly important for fathers, compared to mothers, and may predict their involvement and the development of a positive relationship with their own child (Kim et al., 2015; Kim, Ho, Evans, Liberzon, & Swain, 2015). Therefore, neuroimaging work may provide insight into the unique aspects of fathering compared to mothering and ways to increase fathers' psychological well-being and support positive relationships between fathers and their children.

References

Abraham, E., Hendler, T., Shapira-Lichter, I., Kanat-Maymon, Y., Zagoory-Sharon, O., & Feldman, R. (2014). Father's brain is sensitive to childcare experiences. *Proceedings of the National Academy of Sciences, 111*(27), 9792–9797. https://doi.org/10.1073/pnas.1402569111

Abraham, E., Hendler, T., Zagoory-Sharon, O., & Feldman, R. (2016). Network integrity of the parental brain in infancy supports the development of children's social competencies. *Social Cognitive and Affective Neuroscience, 11*(11), 1707–1718. https://doi.org/10.1093/scan/nsw090

Abraham, E., Raz, G., Zagoory-Sharon, O., & Feldman, R. (2018). Empathy networks in the parental brain and their long-term effects on children's stress reactivity and behavior adaptation. *Neuropsychologia, 116*, 75–85. https://doi.org/10.1016/j.neuropsychologia.2017.04.015

Adolphs, R. (2002). Neural systems for recognizing emotion. *Current Opinion in Neurobiology, 12*(2), 169–177.

Akther, S., Fakhrul, A. A. K. M., & Higashida, H. (2014). Effects of electrical lesions of the medial preoptic area and the ventral pallidum on mate-dependent paternal behavior in mice. *Neuroscience Letters, 570*, 21–25. https://doi.org/10.1016/j.neulet.2014.03.078

Allison, T., Puce, A., & McCarthy, G. (2000). Social perception from visual cues: Role of the STS region. *Trends in Cognitive Sciences, 4*(7), 267–278.

Apter-Levi, Y., Zagoory-Sharon, O., & Feldman, R. (2014). Oxytocin and vasopressin support distinct configurations of social synchrony. *Brain Research, 1580*, 124–132. https://doi.org/10.1016/j.brainres.2013.10.052

Atzil, S., Hendler, T., Zagoory-Sharon, O., Winetraub, Y., & Feldman, R. (2012). Synchrony and specificity in the maternal and the paternal brain: Relations to oxytocin and vasopressin. *Journal of the American Academy of Child & Adolescent Psychiatry, 51*(8), 798–811. https://doi.org/10.1016/j.jaac.2012.06.008

Bickart, K. C., Hollenbeck, M. C., Barrett, L. F., & Dickerson, B. C. (2012). Intrinsic amygdala–cortical functional connectivity predicts social network size in humans. *Journal of Neuroscience, 32*(42), 14729–14741.

Bielsky, I. F., Hu, S.-B., & Young, L. J. (2005). Sexual dimorphism in the vasopressin system: Lack of an altered behavioral phenotype in female V1a receptor knockout mice. *Behavioural Brain Research, 164*(1), 132–136.

Boukydis, C. Z., & Burgess, R. L. (1982). Adult physiological response to infant cries: Effects of temperament of infant, parental status, and gender. *Child Development, 53*, 1291–1298.

Carlson, M. J., & Magnuson, K. A. (2011). Low-income fathers' influence on children. *The Annals of the American Academy of Political and Social Science, 635*(1), 95–116. https://doi.org/10.1177/0002716210393853

Carretié, L., Mercado, F., Tapia, M., & Hinojosa, J. A. (2001). Emotion, attention, and the 'negativity bias', studied through event-related potentials. *International Journal of Psychophysiology, 41*(1), 75–85.

Carter, C. S. (1998). Neuroendocrine perspectives on social attachment and love. *Psychoneuroendocrinology, 23*(8), 779–818.

Cohen-Bendahan, C. C. C., Beijers, R., van Doornen, L. J. P., & de Weerth, C. (2015). Explicit and implicit caregiving interests in expectant fathers: Do endogenous and exogenous oxytocin and vasopressin matter? *Infant Behavior and Development, 41*, 26–37. https://doi.org/10.1016/j.infbeh.2015.06.007

Dabbs Jr., J. M., & Mohammed, S. (1992). Male and female salivary testosterone concentrations before and after sexual activity. *Physiology & Behavior, 52*(1), 195–197.

Darling, N., & Steinberg, L. (1993). Parenting style as context: An integrative model. *Psychological Bulletin, 113*(3), 487–496. https://doi.org/10.1037/0033-2909.113.3.487

de Jong, T. R., Chauke, M., Harris, B. N., & Saltzman, W. (2009). From here to paternity: Neural correlates of the onset of paternal behavior in California mice (Peromyscus californicus). *Hormones and Behavior, 56*(2), 220–231. https://doi.org/10.1016/j.yhbeh.2009.05.001

De Pisapia, N., Bornstein, M. H., Rigo, P., Esposito, G., De Falco, S., & Venuti, P. (2013). Gender differences in directional brain responses to infant hunger cries. *Neuroreport, 24*(3), 142–146. https://doi.org/10.1097/WNR.0b013e32835df4fa

De Pisapia, N., Turatto, M., Lin, P., Jovicich, J., & Caramazza, A. (2011). Unconscious priming instructions modulate activity in default and executive networks of the human brain. *Cerebral Cortex, 22*(3), 639–649.

Dennis, T. A., & Chen, C.-C. (2007). Neurophysiological mechanisms in the emotional modulation of attention: The interplay between threat sensitivity and attentional control. *Biological Psychology, 76*(1–2), 1–10.

Dolan, R. J. (2002). Emotion, cognition, and behavior. *Science, 298*(5596), 1191–1194.

Feldman, R. (2003). Infant–mother and infant–father synchrony: The coregulation of positive arousal. *Infant Mental Health Journal, 24*(1), 1–23. https://doi.org/10.1002/imhj.10041

Feldman, R. (2015). The adaptive human parental brain: Implications for children's social development. *Trends in Neurosciences, 38*(6), 387–399. https://doi.org/10.1016/j.tins.2015.04.004

Feldman, R., Braun, K., & Champagne, F. A. (2019). The neural mechanisms and consequences of paternal caregiving. *Nature Reviews Neuroscience, 20*(4), 205–224. https://doi.org/10.1038/s41583-019-0124-6

Feldman, R., Gordon, I., Schneiderman, I., Weisman, O., & Zagoory-Sharon, O. (2010). Natural variations in maternal and paternal care are associated with systematic changes in oxytocin following parent–infant contact. *Psychoneuroendocrinology, 35*(8), 1133–1141. https://doi.org/10.1016/j.psyneuen.2010.01.013

Feldman, R., Weller, A., Zagoory-Sharon, O., & Levine, A. (2007). Evidence for a neuroendocrinological foundation of human affiliation: Plasma oxytocin levels across pregnancy and the postpartum period predict mother-infant bonding. *Psychological Science, 18*(11), 965–970. https://doi.org/10.1111/j.1467-9280.2007.02010.x

Fernandez-Duque, E., Valeggia, C. R., & Mendoza, S. P. (2009). The biology of paternal care in human and nonhuman primates. *Annual Review of Anthropology, 38*, 115–130.

Figueredo, A. J., Vásquez, G., Brumbach, B. H., Schneider, S. M., Sefcek, J. A., Tal, I. R., et al. (2006). Consilience and life history theory: From genes to brain to reproductive strategy. *Developmental Review, 26*(2), 243–275.

Fletcher, R., StGeorge, J., & Freeman, E. (2013). Rough and tumble play quality: Theoretical foundations for a new measure of father–child interaction. *Early Child Development and Care, 183*(6), 746–759. https://doi.org/10.1080/03004430.2012.723439

Geary, D. C. (2000). Evolution and proximate expression of human paternal investment. *Psychological Bulletin, 126*(1), 55.

Gettler, L. T., McDade, T. W., Agustin, S., & Kuzawa, C. W. (2011). Short-term changes in fathers' hormones during father–child play: Impacts of paternal attitudes and experience—ScienceDirect. *Hormones and Behavior, 60*(5), 599–606.

Gettler, L. T., McDade, T. W., Feranil, A. B., & Kuzawa, C. W. (2011). Longitudinal evidence that fatherhood decreases testosterone in human males. *Proceedings of the National Academy of Sciences, 108*(39), 16194–16199.

Glasper, E. R., Hyer, M. M., Katakam, J., Harper, R., Ameri, C., & Wolz, T. (2016). Fatherhood contributes to increased hippocampal spine density and anxiety regulation in California mice. *Brain and Behavior, 6*(1), n/a–n/a. https://doi.org/10.1002/brb3.416

Glasper, E. R., Kozorovitskiy, Y., Pavlic, A., & Gould, E. (2011). Paternal experience suppresses adult neurogenesis without altering hippocampal function in Peromyscus californicus. *The Journal of Comparative Neurology, 519*(11), 2271–2281. https://doi.org/10.1002/cne.22628

Gordon, I., Zagoory-Sharon, O., Leckman, J. F., & Feldman, R. (2010a). Oxytocin and the development of parenting in humans. *Biological Psychiatry, 68*(4), 377–382. https://doi.org/10.1016/j.biopsych.2010.02.005

Gordon, I., Zagoory-Sharon, O., Leckman, J. F., & Feldman, R. (2010b). Prolactin, oxytocin, and the development of paternal behavior across the first six months of fatherhood. *Hormones and Behavior, 58*(3), 513–518. https://doi.org/10.1016/j.yhbeh.2010.04.007

Graham, J., & Desjardins, C. (1980). Classical conditioning: Induction of luteinizing hormone and testosterone secretion in anticipation of sexual activity. *Science, 210*(4473), 1039–1041.

Gray, P. B., & Crittenden, A. N. (2014). Father Darwin: Effects of children on men, viewed from an evolutionary perspective. *Fathering: A Journal of Theory, Research & Practice about Men as Fathers, 12*(2), 121.

Gray, P. B., Parkin, J., & Samms-Vaughan, M. (2007). Hormonal correlates of human paternal interactions:

A hospital-based investigation in urban Jamaica. *Hormones and Behavior, 52*(4), 499–507.

Guastella, A. J., Kenyon, A. R., Alvares, G. A., Carson, D. S., & Hickie, I. B. (2010). Intranasal arginine vasopressin enhances the encoding of happy and angry faces in humans. *Biological Psychiatry, 67*(12), 1220–1222. https://doi.org/10.1016/j.biopsych.2010.03.014

Hein, G., & Knight, R. T. (2008). Superior temporal sulcus—It's my area: Or is it? *Journal of Cognitive Neuroscience, 20*(12), 2125–2136.

Hellhammer, D. H., Hubert, W., & Schürmeyer, T. (1985). Changes in saliva testosterone after psychological stimulation in men. *Psychoneuroendocrinology, 10*(1), 77–81.

Hirschenhauser, K., Frigerio, D., Grammer, K., & Magnusson, M. S. (2002). Monthly patterns of testosterone and behavior in prospective fathers. *Hormones and Behavior, 42*(2), 172–181.

Hoekzema, E., Barba-Müller, E., Pozzobon, C., Picado, M., Lucco, F., García-García, D., et al. (2017). Pregnancy leads to long-lasting changes in human brain structure. *Nature Neuroscience, 20*(2), 287–296. https://doi.org/10.1038/nn.4458

Horrell, N. D., Saltzman, W., & Hickmott, P. W. (2019). Plasticity of paternity: Effects of fatherhood on synaptic, intrinsic and morphological characteristics of neurons in the medial preoptic area of male California mice. *Behavioural Brain Research, 365*, 89–102. https://doi.org/10.1016/j.bbr.2019.02.029

Hudson, D. B., Elek, S. M., & Fleck, M. O. (2001). First-time mothers' and fathers' transition to parenthood: Infant care self-efficacy, parenting satisfaction, and infant sex. *Issues in Comprehensive Pediatric Nursing, 24*(1), 31–43.

Hyer, M. M., Hunter, T. J., Katakam, J., Wolz, T., & Glasper, E. R. (2016). Neurogenesis and anxiety-like behavior in male California mice during the mate's postpartum period. *European Journal of Neuroscience, 43*(5), 703–709. https://doi.org/10.1111/ejn.13168

Isik, L., Koldewyn, K., Beeler, D., & Kanwisher, N. (2017). Perceiving social interactions in the posterior superior temporal sulcus. *Proceedings of the National Academy of Sciences, 114*(43), E9145–E9152. https://doi.org/10.1073/pnas.1714471114

Kim, P., Capistrano, C., & Congleton, C. (2016). Socioeconomic disadvantages and neural sensitivity to infant cry: Role of maternal distress. *Social Cognitive and Affective Neuroscience, 11*(10), 1597–1607. https://doi.org/10.1093/scan/nsw063

Kim, P., Capistrano, C. G., Erhart, A., Gray-Schiff, R., & Xu, N. (2017). Socioeconomic disadvantage, neural responses to infant emotions, and emotional availability among first-time new mothers. *Behavioural Brain Research, 325*, 188–196. https://doi.org/10.1016/j.bbr.2017.02.001

Kim, P., Ho, S. S., Evans, G. W., Liberzon, I., & Swain, J. E. (2015). Childhood social inequalities influences neural processes in young adult caregiving. *Developmental Psychobiology, 57*(8), 948–960. https://doi.org/10.1002/dev.21325

Kim, P., Leckman, J. F., Mayes, L. C., Feldman, R., Wang, X., & Swain, J. E. (2010). The plasticity of human maternal brain: Longitudinal changes in brain anatomy during the early postpartum period. *Behavioral Neuroscience, 124*(5), 695–700. https://doi.org/10.1037/a0020884

Kim, P., Rigo, P., Leckman, J. F., Mayes, L., Cole, P., Feldman, R., & Swain, J. E. (2015). A prospective longitudinal study of perceived infant outcomes at 18-24 months: Neural and psychological correlates of parental thoughts and actions assessed during the first month postpartum. *Frontiers in Psychology, 6*. Retrieved from https://doaj.org

Kim, P., Rigo, P., Mayes, L. C., Feldman, R., Leckman, J. F., & Swain, J. E. (2014). Neural plasticity in fathers of human infants. *Social Neuroscience, 9*(5), 522–535. https://doi.org/10.1080/17470919.2014.933713

Kim, P., Strathearn, L., & Swain, J. E. (2016). The maternal brain and its plasticity in humans. *Hormones and Behavior, 77*, 113–123. https://doi.org/10.1016/j.yhbeh.2015.08.001

Kim, S., Fonagy, P., Allen, J., & Strathearn, L. (2014). Mothers' unresolved trauma blunts amygdala response to infant distress. *Social Neuroscience, 9*(4), 352–363. https://doi.org/10.1080/17470919.2014.896287

Kirkpatrick, B., Kim, J. W., & Insel, T. R. (1994). Limbic system fos expression associated with paternal behavior. *Brain Research, 658*(1–2), 112–118. https://doi.org/10.1016/S0006-8993(09)90016-6

Kozorovitskiy, Y., Hughes, M., Lee, K., & Gould, E. (2006). Fatherhood affects dendritic spines and vasopressin V1a receptors in the primate prefrontal cortex. *Nature Neuroscience, 9*(9), 1094–1095.

Kuo, P. X., Carp, J., Light, K. C., & Grewen, K. M. (2012). Neural responses to infants linked with behavioral interactions and testosterone in fathers. *Biological Psychology, 91*(2), 302–306.

Lamb, M. E. (2010). *The role of the father in child development* (5th ed.). John Wiley & Sons, Hoboken, New Jersey

Lambert, K. G., Franssen, C. L., Bardi, M., Hampton, J. E., Hainley, L., Karsner, S., et al. (2011). Characteristic neurobiological patterns differentiate paternal responsiveness in two Peromyscus species. *Brain, Behavior and Evolution, 77*(3), 159–175.

Lee, A. W., & Brown, R. E. (2002). Medial preoptic lesions disrupt parental behavior in both male and female California mice (Peromyscus californicus). *Behavioral Neuroscience, 116*(6), 968–975. https://doi.org/10.1037/0735-7044.116.6.968

Li, T., Chen, X., Mascaro, J., Haroon, E., & Rilling, J. K. (2017). Intranasal oxytocin, but not vasopressin, augments neural responses to toddlers in human fathers. *Hormones and Behavior, 93*, 193–202. https://doi.org/10.1016/j.yhbeh.2017.01.006

Li, T., Horta, M., Mascaro, J. S., Bijanki, K., Arnal, L. H., Adams, M., et al. (2018). Explaining individual variation in paternal brain responses to infant cries. *Physiology & Behavior, 193*, 43–54. https://doi.org/10.1016/j.physbeh.2017.12.033

Lieberwirth, C., Wang, Y., Jia, X., Liu, Y., & Wang, Z. (2013). Fatherhood reduces the survival of adult-generated cells and affects various types of behavior in the prairie vole (Microtus ochrogaster). *European Journal of Neuroscience, 38*(9), 3345–3355. https://doi.org/10.1111/ejn.12323

Lonstein, J. S., Lévy, F., & Fleming, A. S. (2015). Common and divergent psychobiological mechanisms underlying maternal behaviors in non-human and human mammals. *Hormones and Behavior, 73*, 156–185. https://doi.org/10.1016/j.yhbeh.2015.06.011

Mak, G. K., & Weiss, S. (2010). Paternal recognition of adult offspring mediated by newly generated CNS neurons. *Nature Neuroscience, 13*(6), 753–758. https://doi.org/10.1038/nn.2550

Malak, S. M., Crowley, M. J., Mayes, L. C., & Rutherford, H. J. V. (2015). Maternal anxiety and neural responses to infant faces. *Journal of Affective Disorders, 172*, 324–330. https://doi.org/10.1016/j.jad.2014.10.013

Mascaro, J. S., Hackett, P. D., Gouzoules, H., Lori, A., & Rilling, J. K. (2013). Behavioral and genetic correlates of the neural response to infant crying among human fathers. *Social Cognitive and Affective Neuroscience, 9*(11), 1704–1712.

Mascaro, J. S., Hackett, P. D., & Rilling, J. K. (2013). Testicular volume is inversely correlated with nurturing-related brain activity in human fathers. *Proceedings of the National Academy of Sciences, 110*(39), 15746–15751.

Mascaro, J. S., Hackett, P. D., & Rilling, J. K. (2014). Differential neural responses to child and sexual stimuli in human fathers and non-fathers and their hormonal correlates. *Psychoneuroendocrinology, 46*, 153–163. https://doi.org/10.1016/j.psyneuen.2014.04.014

Mascaro, J. S., Rentscher, K. E., Hackett, P. D., Mehl, M. R., & Rilling, J. K. (2017). Child gender influences paternal behavior, language, and brain function. *Behavioral Neuroscience, 131*(3), 262–273. https://doi.org/10.1037/bne0000199

Meyer-lindenberg, A., Domes, G., Kirsch, P., & Heinrichs, M. (2011). Oxytocin and vasopressin in the human brain: Social neuropeptides for translational medicine. *Nature Reviews Neuroscience; London, 12*(9), 524–538. http://dx.doi.org.du.idm.oclc.org/10.1038/nrn3044

Musser, E. D., Kaiser-Laurent, H., & Ablow, J. C. (2012). The neural correlates of maternal sensitivity: An fMRI study. *Developmental Cognitive Neuroscience, 2*(4), 428–436. https://doi.org/10.1016/j.dcn.2012.04.003

Nelson, R. J. (2005). *An introduction to behavioral endocrinology*. Sinauer Associates Inc. Sunderland, M.A.

Newman, J. D. (2007). Neural circuits underlying crying and cry responding in mammals. *Behavioural Brain Research, 182*(2), 155–165.

Nishitani, S., Ikematsu, K., Takamura, T., Honda, S., Yoshiura, K.-I., & Shinohara, K. (2017). Genetic variants in oxytocin receptor and arginine-vasopressin receptor 1A are associated with the neural correlates of maternal and paternal affection towards their child. *Hormones and Behavior, 87*, 47–56. https://doi.org/10.1016/j.yhbeh.2016.09.010

Numan, M., & Stolzenberg, D. S. (2009). Medial preoptic area interactions with dopamine neural systems in the control of the onset and maintenance of maternal behavior in rats. *Frontiers in Neuroendocrinology, 30*(1), 46–64.

Nunes, Fite, & French. (2000). Variation in steroid hormones associated with infant care behaviour and experience in male marmosets (Callithrix kuhlii). *Animal Behaviour, 60*(6), 857–865. https://doi.org/10.1006/anbe.2000.1524

Nunes, S., Fite, J. E., Patera, K. J., & French, J. A. (2001). Interactions among paternal behavior, steroid hormones, and parental experience in male marmosets (Callithrix kuhlii). *Hormones and Behavior, 39*(1), 70–82. https://doi.org/10.1006/hbeh.2000.1631

Paquette, D. (2004). Theorizing the father-child relationship: Mechanisms and developmental outcomes. *Human Development, 47*(4), 193–219. https://doi.org/10.1159/000078723

Pearson, R. M., Lightman, S. L., & Evans, J. (2011). Attentional processing of infant emotion during late pregnancy and mother–infant relations after birth. *Archives of Women's Mental Health, 14*(1), 23–31. https://doi.org/10.1007/s00737-010-0180-4

Pelphrey, K. A., Morris, J. P., & Mccarthy, G. (2004). Grasping the intentions of others: The perceived intentionality of an action influences activity in the superior temporal sulcus during social perception. *Journal of Cognitive Neuroscience, 16*(10), 1706–1716.

Rickel, A. U., & Biasatti, L. L. (1982). Modification of the block child rearing practices report. *Journal of Clinical Psychology, 38*(1), 129–134.

Rutherford, H. J. V., Wallace, N. S., Laurent, H. K., & Mayes, L. C. (2015). Emotion regulation in parenthood. *Developmental Review, 36*, 1–14. https://doi.org/10.1016/j.dr.2014.12.008

Saxbe, D. E., Edelstein, R. S., Lyden, H. M., Wardecker, B. M., Chopik, W. J., & Moors, A. C. (2017). Fathers' decline in testosterone and synchrony with partner testosterone during pregnancy predicts greater postpartum relationship investment. *Hormones and Behavior, 90*, 39–47. https://doi.org/10.1016/j.yhbeh.2016.07.005

Seifritz, E., Esposito, F., Neuhoff, J. G., Lüthi, A., Mustovic, H., Dammann, G., et al. (2003). Differential sex-independent amygdala response to infant crying and laughing in parents versus nonparents. *Biological Psychiatry, 54*(12), 1367–1375.

Shamay-Tsoory, S. G. (2011). The neural bases for empathy. *The Neuroscientist, 17*(1), 18–24. https://doi.org/10.1177/1073858410379268

Simmons, A., Strigo, I., Matthews, S. C., Paulus, M. P., & Stein, M. B. (2006). Anticipation of aversive visual stimuli is associated with increased insula activation in anxiety-prone subjects. *Biological Psychiatry, 60*(4), 402–409.

Singhal, A., Doerfling, P., & Fowler, B. (2002). Effects of a dual task on the N100–P200 complex and the early and late Nd attention waveforms. *Psychophysiology, 39*(2), 236–245.

Snowden, C. T., & Soumi, S. J. (1982). Paternal behavior in primates. In *Child nurturance Vol. 3: Studies of development in nonhuman primates* (Vol. 3, pp. 63–108). New York: Plenum Press.

Storey, A., Walsh, C. J., Quinton, R. L., & Wynne-Edwards, K. E. (2000). Hormonal correlates of paternal responsiveness in new and expectant fathers. *Evolution and Human Behavior, 21*(2), 79–95. https://doi.org/10.1016/S1090-5138(99)00042-2

Storey, A. E., Noseworthy, D. E., Delahunty, K. M., Halfyard, S. J., & McKay, D. W. (2011). The effects of social context on the hormonal and behavioral responsiveness of human fathers. *Hormones and Behavior, 60*(4), 353–361.

Storey, A. E., & Ziegler, T. E. (2016). Primate paternal care: Interactions between biology and social experience. *Hormones and Behavior, 77*, 260–271.

Strathearn, L., Fonagy, P., Amico, J., & Montague, P. R. (2009). Adult attachment predicts maternal brain and oxytocin response to infant cues. *Neuropsychopharmacology, 34*(13), 2655–2666. https://doi.org/10.1038/npp.2009.103

Swain, J., Leckman, J., Mayes, L., Feldman, R., Constable, R., & Schultz, R. (2003). *The neural circuitry of parent-infant attachment in the early postpartum*. Presented at the American College of Neuropsychopharmacology 42nd Annual Meeting.

Swain, J. E., Kim, P., Spicer, J., Ho, S. S., Dayton, C. J., Elmadih, A., et al. (2014). Approaching the biology of human parental attachment: Brain imaging, oxytocin and coordinated assessments of mothers and fathers. *Brain Research, 1580*, 78–101. https://doi.org/10.1016/j.brainres.2014.03.007

Swain, J. E., Leckman, J. F., Mayes, L. C., Feldman, R., Constable, R. T., & Schultz, R. T. (2004). Neural substrates of human parent-infant attachment in the postpartum. *Biological Psychiatry, 55*, 1S–242S.

Tops, M., Peer, J. M. V., Korf, J., Wijers, A. A., & Tucker, D. M. (2007). Anxiety, cortisol, and attachment predict plasma oxytocin. *Psychophysiology, 44*(3), 444–449. https://doi.org/10.1111/j.1469-8986.2007.00510.x

Toscano, J., Bauman, M. D., Mason, W., & Amaral, D. G. (2009). Interest in infants by female rhesus monkeys with neonatal lesions of the amygdala or hippocampus. *Neuroscience, 162*(4), 881–891.

Truzzi, A., Islam, T., Valenzi, S., & Esposito, G. (2020). Infant communicative signals elicit differential brain dynamics in fathers and non-fathers. *Early Child Development and Care, 190*(4), 549–557, https://doi.org/10.1080/03004430.2018.1482890

Tsuneoka, Y., Tokita, K., Yoshihara, C., Amano, T., Esposito, G., Huang, A. J., et al. (2015). Distinct preoptic-BST nuclei dissociate paternal and infanticidal behavior in mice. *The EMBO Journal, 34*(21), 2652–2670. https://doi.org/10.15252/embj.201591942

van Anders, S. M., Tolman, R. M., & Volling, B. L. (2012). Baby cries and nurturance affect testosterone in men. *Hormones and Behavior, 61*(1), 31–36.

Villablanca, J. R. (2010). Why do we have a caudate nucleus. *Acta Neurobiologiae Experimentalis (Wars), 70*(1), 95–105.

Weisman, O., Zagoory-Sharon, O., & Feldman, R. (2012). Oxytocin administration to parent enhances infant physiological and behavioral readiness for social engagement. *Biological Psychiatry, 72*(12), 982–989. https://doi.org/10.1016/j.biopsych.2012.06.011

Weisman, O., Zagoory-Sharon, O., & Feldman, R. (2014). Oxytocin administration, salivary testosterone, and father–infant social behavior. *Progress in Neuro-Psychopharmacology and Biological Psychiatry, 49*, 47–52. https://doi.org/10.1016/j.pnpbp.2013.11.006

Wittfoth-Schardt, D., Gründing, J., Wittfoth, M., Lanfermann, H., Heinrichs, M., Domes, G., et al. (2012). Oxytocin modulates neural reactivity to children's faces as a function of social salience. *Neuropsychopharmacology, 37*(8), 1799–1807. https://doi.org/10.1038/npp.2012.47

Wonch, K. E., de Medeiros, C. B., Barrett, J. A., Dudin, A., Cunningham, W. A., Hall, G. B., et al. (2016). Postpartum depression and brain response to infants: Differential amygdala response and connectivity. *Social Neuroscience, 11*(6), 600–617. https://doi.org/10.1080/17470919.2015.1131193

Zeifman, D. M. (2003). Predicting adult responses to infant distress: Adult characteristics associated with perceptions, emotional reactions, and timing of intervention. *Infant Mental Health Journal, 24*(6), 597–612.

Ziegler, T. E., Prudom, S. L., Schultz-Darken, N. J., Kurian, A. V., & Snowdon, C. T. (2006). Pregnancy weight gain: Marmoset and tamarin dads show it too. *Biology Letters, 2*(2), 181–183. https://doi.org/10.1098/rsbl.2005.0426

Ziegler, T. E., Prudom, S. L., Zahed, S. R., Parlow, A. F., & Wegner, F. (2009). Prolactin's mediative role in male parenting in parentally experienced marmosets (Callithrix jacchus). *Hormones and Behavior, 56*(4), 436–443. https://doi.org/10.1016/j.yhbeh.2009.07.012

Ziegler, T. E., Washabaugh, K. F., & Snowdon, C. T. (2004). Responsiveness of expectant male cotton-top tamarins, Saguinus oedipus, to mate's pregnancy. *Hormones and Behavior, 45*(2), 84–92. https://doi.org/10.1016/j.yhbeh.2003.09.003

Pathways to Parenting: The Emotional Journeys of Fathers as They Prepare to Parent a New Infant

12

Carolyn Joy Dayton, Johanna C. Malone, and Suzanne Brown

The role of the father in promoting children's healthy social-emotional development in childhood is well established. Fathers' active parenting of their young children is positively associated with a number of behavioral, cognitive, psychological, and social child outcomes (Cabrera & Tamis-LeMonda, 2013; Lamb, 2010). Further, fathers often play unique roles in the lives of their children, relative to mothers and other caregivers. For example, fathers tend to interact with their young children in physically active and engaged ways that promote the development of early child regulatory capacities (Anderson, St George, & Roggman, 2019; St George & Freeman, 2017). Very early in infancy however, the immediate postnatal work of newborn care is limited to a small number of observable parenting activities such as feeding, changing, bathing, and soothing the infant. Repeated engagement in these seemingly simple tasks forms the basis of the developing parent-infant relationship for both mothers and fathers. For instance, over time, a parent's capacity to effectively soothe the distressed newborn entrains self-regulatory capacities within the infant (Doi, Kato, Nishitani, & Shinohara, 2011; Zeman, Cassano, Perry-Parrish, & Stegall, 2006) and is associated with feelings of parenting competence in fathers (Dayton, Walsh, Oh, & Volling, 2015). Importantly, the roots of the father-child *postnatal* relationship begin even before the infant is born – they begin during pregnancy when the father's thoughts and feelings about his infant first evolve (Diamond, 2017; Leckman et al., 2004; Vreeswijk, Maas, Rijk, & van Bakel, 2014).

Fathering During Pregnancy and Early Infancy

For fathers who are present and involved with the mother of their infant, pregnancy is associated with biological, social, and psychological changes (Abraham & Feldman, 2018; Swain, Dayton, Kim, Tolman, & Volling, 2014), and these changes prepare him for parenting his newborn. For example, men undergo hormonal changes in the perinatal period (defined as pregnancy through the first 6 postnatal weeks; Milgrom & Gemmill, 2015), including decreases in testosterone (Saxbe et al., 2017) and increases in oxytocin (Gordon, Zagoory-Sharon, Leckman, & Feldman, 2010). In some cases, these biological

C. J. Dayton (✉)
School of Social Work & Merrill Palmer Skillman Institute for Child & Family Development, Wayne State University, Detroit, MI, USA
e-mail: carolyn.dayton@wayne.edu

J. C. Malone
Harvard Medical School and Cambridge Health Alliance, Cambridge, MA, USA

S. Brown
School of Social Work, Wayne State University, Detroit, MI, USA

H. E. Fitzgerald et al. (eds.), *Handbook of Fathers and Child Development*,
https://doi.org/10.1007/978-3-030-51027-5_12

changes may interact with sociocultural norms and contribute to the *Couvade syndrome*, an expectant father's biopsychosocial response to his partner's pregnancy that has been identified in many cultures and typically follows a culturally specific pattern including the experience of biological responses that mirror the woman's pregnancy experience (e.g., weight gain; Bogren, 1983, 1984; Brennan, Ayers, Ahmed, & Marshall-Lucette, 2007). While manifestations of the *Couvade syndrome* are relatively rare, the hormonal changes that most men experience during their partner's pregnancy are common, and they interact with psychosocial changes as fathers prepare psychologically to parent their new infant.

Although less is known about fathers who are experiencing contextual stress (e.g., poverty, racism, violence exposure), studies using community samples have demonstrated that the father's emotional connection with his infant emerges in pregnancy via the formation of internal representations of the infant and their relationship, and these representations develop as a father begins to imagine who his infant will be (Vreeswijk, Maas, Rijk, & van Bakel, 2014). A father might wonder, for example, who the infant will look like, what his or her personality will be like, and how difficult or easy it will be to care for the infant. This prenatal bonding process is critical for both the father and the infant because the quality of the father's prenatal bond is related to postnatal father-infant relationship qualities (Condon, Corkindale, Boyce, & Gamble, 2013; Luz, George, Vieux, & Spitz, 2017; Vreeswijk, Maas, Rijk, Braeken, & van Bakel, 2014) for at least two postnatal years (de Cock et al., 2016). Further, paternal prenatal bonding may also be related to the quality of the father's postnatal parenting behaviors (Dubber, Reck, Müller, & Gawlik, 2015; Foley & Hughes, 2018; Hjelmstedt & Collins, 2008), though in a recent meta-analysis, Foley and Hughes (2018) failed to find a significant relationship between prenatal thoughts and feelings about the infant and postnatal parenting. Finally, very preliminary data suggest that fathers' prenatal bonding may be related to child outcomes (de Cock et al., 2017). Importantly, and consistent with the ecological model of fathering put forth by Cabrera, Fitzgerald, Bradley, and Roggman (2007), the formation of this paternal-infant bond is influenced by the father's relational world including (but not limited to) the man's relationship with his partner in the present (Barrows, 2004; Condon et al., 2013) and his experience of being cared for in the past (Dayton, Brown, et al., 2019).

Because it involves the beginning of the parent-infant relationship, the perinatal period represents a critical developmental moment in the lives of parents and their infants. Historically, there was a focus on the physical care of the newborn with an assumption that mothers were better equipped to meet the newborn's basic needs. As our knowledge about the importance of very early parent-infant relationships to the later social-emotional development of young children has increased, an emphasis on the quality of early care and its influence on relationship development has emerged (Sroufe, 2005). Further, it has become clear that fathers, while not identical to mothers, are able and willing early caretakers of their infants (Dayton et al., 2015). Thus, understanding the emotional journeys of fathers during the perinatal period will allow us to better design and implement services that support the early father-infant relationship. To that end, this chapter will describe theories informing our understanding of fathering during the perinatal period and will review what is known about the risk and resilience factors that influence the father-infant relationship as it unfolds across the perinatal period. Specifically, this chapter will (1) review the extant literature on the meaning and importance of fathering in the perinatal period; (2) describe theoretical models that inform our understanding of early fathering; (3) discuss the emergence of paternal thoughts, feelings, and representations as they prepare to parent a new infant; (4) describe the development of the father-infant relationship in the perinatal period; and (5) discuss risk and resilience factors that affect the development of the father-infant relationship during the perinatal period. Finally, we will describe recent work from our own laboratory that informs our understanding of the pathways to parenting for risk-exposed fathers residing in an urban setting.

The Meaning and Importance of Fathering in the Perinatal Period

A father's role in the care of his children has changed dramatically over evolutionary and historical time (Zoja, 2018) and is diverse across cultures, largely based on prevailing parental ethnotheories within the family's primary cultural group (Harkness, Mavridis, Liu, & Super, 2015). Over the last few decades in the United States, fathers have become more actively involved in the direct care of their children (Bianchi, 2011). Although important differences exist across diverse cultural groups, the *meaning* of fatherhood in general in the United States has also changed in important ways over the past few decades (Lamb, 2010). Specifically, the importance of fathering to the social-emotional development of young children is more frequently acknowledged (Lamb, 2010). When fathers are involved very early in the lives of their children, they have the opportunity to form foundational and enduring relationships with them (Shannon, Cabrera, Tamis-LeMonda, & Lamb, 2009), and outcomes for mothers and children are improved (Giurgescu & Templin, 2015; Kroll, Carson, Redshaw, & Quigley, 2016; Sarkadi, Kristiansson, Oberklaid, & Bremberg, 2008).

The positive health effects that are associated with father involvement begin in pregnancy where improved prenatal, birth, and neonatal health outcomes and significantly lower per-infant healthcare costs have been identified (Alio, Salihu, Kornosky, Richman, & Marty, 2010; Salihu et al., 2014). In contrast, a lack of father involvement in pregnancy is associated with significantly higher infant mortality rates (Alio et al., 2011). Furthermore, in groups of fathers who are disadvantaged with respect to income and education, involvement during pregnancy is associated with a higher likelihood of continued involvement with their children across development (Cabrera, Fagan, & Farrie, 2008; Fagan & Palkovitz, 2007) and thereby has the potential to support resilience in young children who are exposed to poverty, violence, and other contextual risks (Jackson, Choi, & Preston, 2019).

Although less is known about the factors that are related to prenatal relationship development in fathers, relative to mothers, recent research has suggested that the pathways to parenting for fathers may be somewhat different than they are for mothers (Dayton, Brown, et al., 2019). These differences appear to continue during the postnatal period where parental sex differences in very early caregiving behaviors have been identified (Dayton et al., 2015). Given these findings, supporting the prenatal father-infant bond is an important target of intervention that has the potential to improve birth and relationship outcomes for fathers, mothers, and infants (Bond, 2010). To accomplish this, an understanding of the process of very early father-infant relationship development in the perinatal period is critical.

Understanding the Early Father-Infant Relationship: Theoretical Considerations

Family Systems Theory The childbearing years represent a significant developmental life stage for men and women who decide to become parents (Cowan & Cowan, 2012; McGoldrick & Shibusawa, 2012). As they move into this stage, parents prepare psychologically for birth. For first time parents, the transition to parenthood may be an especially significant milestone with the onset of a number of associated physical, emotional, and psychological changes (Nelson, Kushlev, & Lyubomirsky, 2014). From a family systems perspective, the move from a dyad to a family triad requires a reorganization of the romantic relationship as each parent develops a relationship with the infant and the co-parenting relationship becomes active within the parental subsystem (Shannon, Baumwell, & Tamis-LeMonda, 2013). The addition of subsequent children to the family also affects the overall functioning of the family system. The transition to siblinghood, for instance, when a second child is born into a family, influences the relationships within the family in important ways as parental roles shift to accommodate added childcare needs and the older sibling adjusts to changing family dynamics (Volling, 2005). As time goes on, for many families, the birth of additional children further increases the complexity of intrafamilial relationships. Moreover, diverse family arrangements, such as cohabitation versus independent living arrangements of the parents, blended family status, and multi-partner fertility, add additional complexity. The particular ways in which a family is organized influence the role of the father in that family system as well as the experience of the infant and the ways in which the father-infant relationship unfolds.

From an intergenerational systems perspective, Singley and Edwards (2015) have argued that young fathers of today are encountering a kind of "generation gap" wherein social norms are increasingly promoting early and engaged fathering, but their own experiences of being raised by "baby boomer" fathers provided a hands-off model of fathering. In heterosexual couples, fathers of today are also more likely than their own fathers were to have female partners who are working outside the home, leading to the need for shared parenting. Further, the tough, hands-off approach to fathering is consistent with hypermasculine identity development that then conflicts with contemporary expectations that compel men to sensitively parent their children (Cabrera, Tamis-LeMonda, Bradley, Hofferth, & Lamb, 2000; Diamond, 2017). The intersection of the tough, hands-off approach to fathering with contemporary expectations for father involvement may be especially powerful in early infancy, where parenting tasks that were previously considered "feminine" such as holding, rocking, and soothing their infants are required. As argued by Singley and Edwards (2015), men who experience this conflict as particularly stressful may develop feelings of anxiety, anger, and sadness that could ultimately influence their ability to bond with their infant during the perinatal period. An understanding of the ways in which a father's history of being parented and expectations about their own parenting unfold within the context of the father-infant relationship across the perinatal period is informed by attachment theory which we turn to next.

Attachment Theory Initially developed by John Bowlby (1982), attachment theory argues that individuals construct mental templates, or "working models," of their interpersonal environments that are first developed in infancy based on repeated interactions with one's caretakers and then revised over the life course based on interactions within other important relationships (i.e., friendships, romantic relationships, etc.). By adulthood, working models are presumed to be functioning in a stable, consistent, and unconscious manner and are therefore increasingly resistant to change (Collins & Read, 1994).

When an adult makes the transition to parenthood, a critical developmental shift becomes necessary – from activation of the attachment behavioral system in which the person seeks out trusted others (i.e., romantic partners, close friends) in times of distress to activation of the caregiving behavioral system in which the parent becomes the provider of care and protection to the child (Solomon & George, 1996). This transition typically begins during pregnancy, for both men and women, as they form internal working models of the infant by imagining who the infant will turn out to be (de Cock et al., 2016; Lebovici, 1988, 1993). Parents wonder, for example, what the infant will look and act like, who in the family the infant will "take after," and how the parent imagines he or she will care for this new infant. This experience of imagining the future infant ideally may be a joyful experience but, particularly in cases where parents have histories of developmental trauma, may also be haunted by intergenerational "ghosts" (Fraiberg, Adelson, & Shapiro, 1975; Malone & Dayton, 2015). In these cases, parents may experience the imagined infant (or themselves in relation to the infant) as having negative qualities taking after harsh, neglectful, or harmful individuals/experiences in the parents' past (Barrows, 2004).

For women, the prenatal period involves an intensely physical experience that unfolds across the weeks and months of pregnancy and coincides with a deepening of the maternal-fetal bond (Cohen & Slade, 2000; Yarcheski, Mahon, Yarcheski, Hanks, & Cannella, 2009). The unfolding of this process for men is less understood and is limited to social and psychological ways of bonding with the fetus. Efforts to more deeply understand the internal worlds of expectant fathers have been pursued within the psychoanalytic literature which we describe next.

Psychoanalytic Theory Within older psychoanalytic theory and practice, the father-child relationship was largely first conceptualized in the oedipal relationship and beyond (starting around age 3–5) (Freud, 1905/1953). It was at this phase of development that the child was thought to first grapple with the understanding of themselves in a world that was not just dyadically composed of mother and child but now also included an outside other (i.e., the father). This was thought to create a range of conflictual feelings around parental identifications, as well as intense experiences of competition, desire, and anxiety (Freud, 1905/1953; Klein, 1928; Fairbairn, 1952). In contrast, Burlingham (1973) encouraged psychoanalysts to take up the significance of the neglected *preoedipal* father-infant relationship (infancy and early childhood) rather than primarily focusing on the oedipal relationship and beyond. Burlingham also noted that in the early psychoanalytic literature, Freud regularly theorized about the *child's* fantasies about the father but gave little attention to the *father's* fantasies about his relationship with his child or infant. In particular, she wonders about Freud's absence of exploration of:

> —the father's fantasies in the period between impregnation and birth, and during the first weeks of the infant's life; the father's hopes and expectations concerning the child's growth and development; his jealousies of the mother's preoccupation with the infant; the arousal of his own feminine attitudes; the impact on all these attitudes of his own latent memories of his own father relationships. (Burlingham, 1973, p. 30)

It is as if Freud struggled to convey the unique richness of the father's hopes, fears, and experiences related to the expected baby and then to his first postnatal experiences in relation to the baby. Burlingham (1973) argued that the neglect of conceptualizing the early father-infant bond might actually distort our understanding of the mother-infant bond, for example, through inaccurately overemphasizing certain functions of the mother's role without taking into account the father's contributions. Similarly, Winnicott, who was prolific in his writing about the mother-child relationship, largely left the father untheorized or as Phillips (1988) states as a "relatively bland figure" (p. 28) (c.f. Formaini, 2004). The longstanding absence of this area of study has clear cultural parallels in the ways the father-infant bond is often inadequately supported or nurtured in contemporary society. In fact, Lamb (1976) has suggested that social scientists have unwittingly contributed to the devaluation of the father by almost exclusively focusing on mothers. And, at times, when fathers are considered in the literature, they are often undifferentiated from mothers (through references to "parents") in ways that imply that parents are interchangeable, rather than considering the complementary functions that one parent may have to the other (Diamond, 1986).

Further, when fathers have been considered directly, they are often treated as part of a triad (mother-father-infant) rather than focusing on the father's dyadic bond with the infant as significant in its own right. For example, Mahler (1971) and Abelin (1975) focused on the father's role in the separation and individuation process of the infant. Unlike the mother, Mahler theorized that the father enters into the infant's consciousness from the outside. This enables the father to provide a uniquely unambivalent role of support and accompaniment as the infant explores the world beyond the mother as part of the process of separation and individuation. This theoretical stance is consistent with contemporary work by Paquette (Gaumon & Paquette, 2013; Paquette, 2004) who has demonstrated that the early father-child relationship involves stimulating play in conjunction with limit setting that helps young children gain self-regulatory capacities and prepares them for life in the larger society.

Other theorists have emphasized the need to look beyond the triad of mother-father-infant to also consider directly the dyad of father and child (Benjamin, 1995; Blos, 1984; Diamond, 2017). Benjamin says,

> The function of the father … is dyadic, not triadic, that is to say, not rivalrous or forbidding, like the oedipal father. He does not so much represent the one who can exclusively love mother (as the child still imagines doing directly) as he embodies the desire for the exciting outside. What I wish to underscore is the importance of a second adult, not necessarily a male or a father, with whom a child can form a second dyad. (Benjamin, 1995, p. 57)

Benjamin's words bring us to the preoedipal period of father and baby together, a place and time where this relationship actually matters on its own terms. In this process of becoming a father, from a developmental perspective, Diamond (2017), like Singley and Edwards (2015), argues that the transition to fatherhood offers men a chance to take on (potentially) previously denounced or disavowed qualities such as being more empathic, vulnerable, and trusting. Fatherhood allows these qualities to be experienced directly as one's own – rather than solely belonging to the feminine domain. Further, Diamond posits that during pregnancy the father begins to see himself and his function as a guardian. This means "a watchful, protective presence for his infant, one who is ideally engaged in an intense mutual interaction with the mother." This developmental shift occurs as the father transitions from being the main character in the family story to the one standing close to the new center of the family's world, the infant.

In conceptualizing the internal experience of the father, Leckman and colleagues (Leckman et al., 2004) broaden the concept of the primary *maternal* preoccupation with the infant (first described by Winnicott, 1965) to consider the *paternal* preoccupation with the infant. In its original form, primary maternal preoccupation refers to an altered mental state that begins during the end of pregnancy and continues for the first months after birth in which the mother's attention and focus is centered almost completely on the infant's needs. The ability of the mother to enter this state is foundational to the infant's development of self. In broadening this concept to consider the "primary paternal preoccupation," Leckman and colleagues (Leckman et al., 1999) found that fathers went through a parallel experience that followed a similar time frame (later pregnancy to first postnatal months) but that the time devoted to thinking about the infant was approximately half of what they recorded in mothers (7 and 14 hours per day, respectively), yet still substantial.

Studies of early postnatal paternal parenting have found that fathers are actively engaged with their newborn infants. For example, Parke, Power, Tinsley, and Hymel (1980) observed fathers and mothers together with their infant 3 days after birth and found that (as a triad) there was no difference in the amount of time spent interacting with the infant, with the main difference being that mothers were more likely to hold the infant in their arms. In addition, when each parent was alone with the infant, Parke et al. (1980) found that fathers were as nurturing and involved with their infants as mothers, with a difference being that mothers were more likely to engage with their infants through smiling. In a more recent study, Dayton and colleagues (Dayton et al., 2015) examined early (1 month, 4 months, and 8 months of infant age) soothing behaviors of cohabitating mothers and fathers in a mainly Caucasian, middle-class sample and found that mothers and fathers spent similar amounts of time cuddling/rocking and carrying their infants to soothe them. Other soothing techniques (e.g., extra feedings, swaddling, singing) were used more frequently by mothers, however, and mothers reported the use of a wider variety of soothing techniques (7.7 on average) compared with fathers (5.9 on average). Taken as a whole, these findings point to both similarities and differences in the early parenting behaviors of mothers and fathers. Whether the internal experiences of parents vary by sex, and whether they are associated with early parenting behaviors, is a topic of great interest in contemporary research (Foley & Hughes, 2018).

In considering the expectant father's experience over the course of pregnancy, Diamond (1986), drawing heavily on the work of Herzog (1982), proposes seven stages of prospective fatherhood, which we briefly summarize:

1. *Getting Ready*: In this preconception stage, expectant fathers consciously think through aspects of timing, readiness, career issues, division of labor, and parent rearing beliefs. This stage is thought to be more rational and controlled than some of the later stages of expectant fatherhood. Experientially, unresolved developmental issues from a father's own history may emerge, including fears of surpassing his own father, fears of being abandoned by his partner, and even envy of women's creative capacities in pregnancy.
2. *Conception*: This stage includes both conception and the medical confirmation of pregnancy. While some men may feel conflicted about the anticipated life disruption, many will be more in touch with feelings of joy, including the wish to love another and be loved. Men in this stage often experience a sense of pride and a fuller positive sense of self.
3. *First Trimester*: In this stage, fathers begin to rework past and current relationships resulting in a shift in the sense of self. In doing this, expectant fathers may be thinking about the parenting they received as they begin to consider their own role as a paternal figure. This may bring up difficult feelings from the past and tensions between the sense of what they received and who they will become. Some men may also begin to struggle with feelings of loss regarding the changing relationship with their partner.
4. *Midpregnancy*: In midpregnancy, expectant fathers may become more in touch with the reality of the pregnancy. This is furthered through experiences such as seeing the baby in both still pictures and in motion through ultrasounds. The fetus is thus experienced as more alive. As a consequence of this, some men may begin to feel excluded from the relationship occurring between their partner and unborn infant. They may also be inspired in their own creative potentials within work or through other endeavors. Men may also feel more in touch with their own bodies and bodily symptoms as they attune and identify with their partner's experience and changing body.
5. *The Turn Toward One's Father and Fathering*: Expectant fathers may begin to experience an increasing pressure to sort out unresolved issues with their family of origin, particularly around concerns about how issues with their fathers may impact their own fathering. Diamond (1986) proposes that the working through of this stage enables men to feel more present throughout the remainder of pregnancy resulting in the emergence of sometimes previously suppressed tender and gentler feelings. Men who are less able to connect with a positive view of the past father are in what Herzog (1982, 2001) calls a state of "father hunger" and are expected to face more hurdles in being emotionally present in the remaining phases of pregnancy.
6. *Toward the End of the Second Trimester*: In this stage of pregnancy, expectant fathers may experience the fetus as separate not only from themselves but also from their partner. The experience of thirdness may lead to feelings of competition and jealousy. Herzog (1982) has speculated that this may be due to unconsciously re-experiencing old developmental feelings of recognizing that one is part of a particular triad (child-mother-father) as opposed to a more insular dyad (child-mother).
7. *The Last Trimester*: In this final stage of expectant fatherhood, Diamond (1986) describes a paradoxical experience in which the father both experiences an intensification of being oriented to the reality of the expected infant and also becomes imbued with a feeling of awe, with regard to a sense of there being "magical forces at work." This mixture of reality and magic may be an ideal state for the expectant father to be immersed in as he experiences the birth of his child.

In reflecting on Diamond's theorized stages for the expectant father, it is notable that they seem to be oriented to intact heterosexual father-mother couples in which the expectant father truly expected and was invested in the infant even prior to conception. Yet, we also see the universal struggle of the father trying to reconcile who he is and where he came from. Also evident is the father's anticipation not only of who he will be in a new relationship with an infant but also in a changed relationship with his partner, an experience of being part of a triad as well as separate dyads, and a new sense of an individual "self" as he sees and experiences himself as a father. Recent empirical work has examined fathers' shifting representations of themselves as fathers and of their emotional ties to their infant during the perinatal period, and we now turn to a review of that literature.

Paternal Thoughts, Feelings, and Representations of the Infant Across the Perinatal Period

Methodological Approaches

We begin this section with a description of the three methodological approaches that have been used to measure a father's internalized relationship with his infant across the perinatal period, namely, semi-structured qualitative interviews, self-report measures, and representational interviews. In reviewing this material, it is important to bear in mind that each of these approaches was initially developed and used with mothers. Indeed, as we have emphasized, within the parenting literature as a whole, mothers are typically considered the modal or default parent to which fathers are compared. Notable exceptions do exist, however, such as Paquette's activation theory, which argues for a unique role for fathers in parenting their young children (Paquette, 2004; Paquette & Bigras, 2010). As the fathering field moves forward, efforts to understand fathering using a father-centric approach will be important (Volling et al., 2019). In the meantime, we review the research that informs our current understanding of the emotional journeys of expectant fathers.

First, Semi-structured Qualitative Interviews The use of semi-structured, open-ended, qualitative interviews arguably provides the most room for a father-centric approach to data collection and analysis. Because they are exploratory in nature and use an inductive approach to data analysis, qualitative interviews allow the researcher to follow the father's lead in determining the manifest content of the interview. Qualitative interviews focus on a particular subgroup of the population to better understand their lived experiences. Within the perinatal fathering literature, this approach has been used with a number of father subgroups including, for example, first time fathers (Deave & Johnson, 2008), urban fathers (Dayton et al., 2016), adolescent fathers (Wilkes, Mannix, & Jackson, 2012), and fathers of preterm infants (Stefana, Padovani, Biban, & Lavelli, 2018). It has also been used to understand fathers' reactions to various fathering experiences such as attending the prenatal ultrasound (Walsh et al., 2014), engaging in infertility treatment (Herrera, 2013), and participating in genetic screening (Atkin, Berghs, & Dyson, 2015).

Second, Self-Report Measures Self-report measures capture the father's emotional connection or "bond" with the infant beginning during pregnancy. Examples include the Paternal Fetal Attachment Scale (PFA; Weaver & Cranley, 1983) and the Paternal Antenatal Attachment Scale (PAAS) (Condon, 1993). Each of these measures has a corresponding maternal version, and both versions assess the overall quality as well as specific components of the parental-fetal relationship. The most commonly used self-report measure of *paternal* prenatal bonding is the PAAS (Condon, 1993) which includes two subscales, quality of attachment and intensity of attachment. Self-report measures of prenatal bonding require considerably less time to administer and score than the more intensive interview assessments of prenatal relationship quality and have been found to be related to the more time-intensive and in-depth interview measures (Vreeswijk, Maas, Rijk, & van Bakel, 2014). For instance, Vreeswijk, Maas, Rijk, van Bakel, (2014) found that paternal prenatal bonding on the PAAS was highly correlated with a father's internal representation of his infant as measured by a semi-structured interview (WMCI, described below). Further, in a recent meta-analysis, Foley and Hughes (2018) found that, when combining data from mothers and fathers, self-report questionnaires assessing prenatal bonding were equally predictive of postnatal parenting as were representational interviews, which are described next.

Third, Representational Interviews A father's prenatal internal working model of his child, described by Vreeswijk and colleagues (Vreeswijk, Maas, Rijk, Braeken, & van Bakel, 2014) as the "meaning" of the child to the father, is measured using semi-structured interviews that are then transcribed and coded for narrative patterns within both content and process elements, leading to a categorization of the quality of his internalized relationship with his child, usually expressed as a typology. The most commonly used representational interview with fathers is the *Working Model of the Child Interview* (WMCI; Zeanah et al., 1993). Based on the father's narrative responses, a typology of *balanced*, *disengaged*, *distorted*, or *disrupted* representation is assigned. Each representational typology is related to a particular cognitive-affective regulatory stance the father has toward his infant (or fetus). Specifically, the narratives of fathers who hold *balanced* representations, the ideal, are well regulated with respect to the parent-child relationship. Fathers holding balanced representations are accepting of the infant's authentic self and describe warm and connected feelings toward their infants. In contrast, fathers holding *disengaged* representations of their infants are relatively emotionally "shut down" with respect to the father-infant relationship, and their interviews convey an emotional distance from the child. On the other end of the spectrum, fathers holding *distorted* representations of their child demonstrate over-activated affective ties to their infants that are characterized by expressions of strong emotions and emotional lability. Their interviews are often tangential and self-focused and convey a sense of distance from the child due to the intense and overwhelming feelings the father is experiencing. Finally, fathers holding *disrupted* working models of their child (Tooten, et al., 2014) tend to have histories of trauma and loss in their own backgrounds that manifest in their narratives as affective communication errors, role-boundary confusion, fearfulness, dissociation, disorientation, intrusiveness/negativity, and withdrawal (Crawford & Benoit, 2009).

There are pros and cons associated with each of these three methodological approaches to understanding the father's emotional tie to his infant. Taken together, they inform our understanding of the development of fathers' psychological, social, and emotional journeys across the perinatal period. Our current understanding of the development of the father-infant relationship during this period is described next.

Development of the Father-Infant Relationship in the Perinatal Period

Contemporary social norms in the United States compel fathers to "be involved" in the lives of their children beginning in pregnancy. In the prenatal period, for example, fathers are encouraged to attend birth and parenting classes with the mothers of their children and to be present during labor and delivery (Reed, 2005). Theoretically, feelings of connection to their infants during the prenatal period will increase the likelihood that men will, in fact, be involved (Cabrera et al., 2008). Indeed, paternal involvement during pregnancy is associated with later long-term father engagement in the lives of their children (Shannon et al., 2009). Further, the need for fathers to take on more childcare responsibilities has increased as more women have joined the workforce (Bianchi, Robinson, & Milke, 2006; Maume, 2011). However, expectant fathers encounter physical and social barriers that may diminish their feelings of connection with their infant during the prenatal period, potentially leaving them less emotionally prepared to care for their young children (Hanson, Hunter, Bormann, & Sobo, 2009).

At the most basic level, men do not physically carry their babies. This means, of course, that it is not physically obvious to others that they are expecting a baby and, therefore, they do not receive the volume of public responses – kind words, questions, and attention – that women do when their pregnancy begins to "show." The curiosity and kindness expressed by the larger society – strangers on the bus or at the grocery store – constitute a social acknowledgement of sorts, of the woman's status as a mother. If this is her first pregnancy, this new status represents a transition as she shifts to a new social category that carries with it (for good or bad) a set of social expectations and responsibilities. In this way, she is frequently reminded – by the outside social environment – that there is a change coming in her life. Although expectant fathers may have conversations with friends and family members who know of their expectant fatherhood status, they do not encounter the daily reactions from members of the larger society that women do. As a result, research has suggested that, during the transition to fatherhood, men's identities as fathers are often delayed with respect to mothers' and may undergo the most transformation during the postnatal period (Genesoni & Tallandini, 2009; Habib & Lancaster, 2010).

In addition to the lack of social reinforcement, men also do not have the physical connection with the infant that women do during pregnancy. Research using qualitative interview methodology suggests that this may influence the experiences of closeness to the infant that men feel during pregnancy. For example, in a qualitative study of expectant fathers in the United Kingdom, Ives (2014) found that first-time expectant fathers felt that they had a central role to play in the lives of their infants, but they also felt a sense of separation and distance. One father in Ives' study described this experience in the following way, "… I think she's [a] tiny bit more ahead because it's natural, she's physically feeling the changes… I think about myself as *preparing to become* a dad but you can see with her, she's *becoming* a mother, that's the difference [emphasis added]." In another qualitative investigation, Draper (2002) similarly found that men felt a distance from their infant during pregnancy. They described this distance in physical terms and sought out ways to connect to the infant in what Draper described as "body-mediated moments" such as watching and feeling (from the outside) the infant's movement in the womb, viewing the infant on the ultrasound scan, and, ultimately, being present during the labor and delivery process, which some fathers have described as the beginning of fatherhood (Poh, Koh, & He, 2014). It is important to note that fathers' reliance on body-mediated interactions with the infant places the mother in a gate-keeping role (Schoppe-Sullivan, Brown, Cannon, Mangelsdorf, & Sokolowski, 2008), such that she can inhibit or enable the father's engagement in the pregnancy- and infant-related events. Draper underscores the importance of the bodily experience of pregnancy for the woman that highlights the father's need to seek out body-mediated connections with their infant via the mother's body:

> Our experience of ourselves in the world is very much mediated by our bodies. The body is not merely a container for but, rather is our existence. Our experience of our bodies, our embodiment, is a social process located in social spaces with within a network of people. (Draper, 2002, p. 556)

Ives and others (Widarsson, Engström, Tydén, Lundberg, & Hammar, 2015) have also found that expectant fathers often feel ignored and even pushed away during prenatal medical appointments such as ultrasounds. In response to feeling unwelcome at the prenatal visit, one father in Ives' study reported wondering whether he should "wait outside" during the visits. Expectant mothers also witness the exclusion of their partners in healthcare settings. One expectant mother in Widarsson et al.'s (2015) qualitative study put it this way:

> The midwife hardly said hello to him [her partner], and then there was just a conversation between me and the midwife. So, he wondered afterwards, 'why was I there at all, the midwife treated me like air'… it was as if she didn't have a single question

for him, she never once spoke to him. (Widarsson et al., p. 1063)

These kinds of messages in healthcare settings, in particular, may reinforce a sense of distance from the infant for fathers who are seeking body-mediated connections with their infants and are especially concerning in the face of evidence that the prenatal ultrasound has the potential to increase fathers' feelings of connection with their infant (Rosich-Medina & Shetty, 2007; Walsh et al., 2014). Notably, however, some investigators have failed to find an increase in paternal bonding following attendance at a prenatal ultrasound (Righetti, Dell'Avanzo, Grigio, & Nicolini, 2005), raising the question of whether these disparate findings may be related to inconsistencies in the ways in which expectant fathers are treated during healthcare visits. Overall, the inherent contradiction of the contemporary societal narrative that men should be more involved in the lives of their children with experiences of being unwelcome at prenatal healthcare visits may leave men feeling uncertain about their role and is especially concerning given the importance of paternal prenatal involvement to maternal and infant health outcomes (Plantin & Olykoya, 2011) and to enduring father involvement in the lives of their children (Cabrera et al., 2008).

Taken as a whole, the lack of physical connection to the infant combined with the limited (relative to mothers) social reinforcement of the pregnancy could make it difficult for fathers to form stable and enduring prenatal emotional bonds with their infants. However, this does not appear to be the case for all, or even most, fathers (Habib & Lancaster, 2010; May, 1982). For instance, in a very early study of prenatal paternal-fetal bonding, May (1982) used qualitative methodology and found a pattern of increasing emotional investment in first time fathers across the course of the pregnancy. More recently, Habib and Lancaster (2010), using the PAAS, found small, but statistically significant, increases in paternal prenatal bonding from the first to the third trimester. These early studies suggest that fathers are, in fact, forming prenatal bonds with their infants over the course of the pregnancy. The quality of those bonds, however, may manifest differently in the prenatal period than they do for expectant mothers. For instance, in line with paternal feelings of distance that have been reported in the qualitative literature, Vreeswijk, Rijk, Maas, and Bakel (2015)) found that expectant fathers in a low-risk, community sample evinced higher rates of disengaged representations on the *Working Model of the Child Interview* (WMCI) (Zeanah et al., 1993) than mothers. Specifically, they reported that the distribution of WMCI typologies for mothers was 61% balanced, 27% disengaged, and 12% distorted, whereas the distribution for fathers was 44% balanced, 49% disengaged, and 7% distorted. These investigators interpreted the increased rate of disengaged representations in fathers (vs. mothers) as representative of fathers' overall emotional distance from the fetus and hypothesized that this may be due, in part, to the fathers' physical distance from his infant in the prenatal period. The results revealed that fathers' prenatal representations remained relatively stable across time: fathers' prenatal representations were significantly related to their postnatal representations when infants were 6 months of age (Vreeswijk, Maas, Rijk, Braeken, van Bakel, 2014). Specifically, 82.4% of fathers who had a balanced *prenatal* representation were also coded as balanced on the *postnatal* WMCI, and 49.6% with a non-balanced *prenatal* representation retained that category at the *postnatal* period. Despite this continuity, they also found that more fathers evinced balanced *postnatal* representations (64.4%) than balanced *prenatal* representations (43.6%). Their findings suggest that there is some continuity in representations across the perinatal period and also suggest that fathers may have an easier time bonding with their infants during the postnatal period.

The majority of the qualitative work that we have described in this section was conducted with fathers who were not burdened with exposure to contextual risk such as poverty and violence. For fathers who are exposed to these kinds of contextual risks, we might expect their pathways to parenting to be more challenging. In the following sections, we describe what is known about the risk factors influencing the father-infant relationship in fathers who are preparing to parent a new infant and the ways in which specific resilience factors may mitigate these risks.

Risk and Resilience Factors Affecting the Father-Infant Bond in the Perinatal Period

In this section, we review the risk and resilience factors affecting the development of the father-infant relationship that have been identified and replicated in the extant literature. Evidence suggests that once the father-infant relational bond has developed, it remains relatively stable across the perinatal period and at least the first 2 years of the child's life (de Cock et al., 2016; Luz et al., 2017). Therefore, understanding the risk and resilience factors affecting its development is critical to the establishment of father-friendly policies in the places and spaces that expectant fathers visit and, where necessary, the creation of interventions with expectant fathers.

In the last few years, there has been increased research in the area of paternal-infant perinatal relationship development (Julian, Muzik, Kees, Valenstein, & Rosenblum, 2018; Vreeswijk, Maas, Rijk, & van Bakel, 2014), including work from our own laboratory which is described below (Dayton, Brown, et al., 2019). Converging findings from a small, but growing, number of studies suggest two important factors that influence the development of the father-infant relationship during the perinatal period: (1) paternal symptoms of psychopathology (Cameron, Sedov, & Tomfohr-Madsen, 2016) and (2) the father's relationship with the mother of the infant (Ahlqvist-Björkroth et al., 2016).

Paternal Psychopathology The influence of perinatal psychopathology – including depression, anxiety, and post-traumatic stress – on *maternal* parenting and child outcomes has been well established (Falah-Hassani, Shiri, & Dennis, 2017; Furtado, Chow, Owais, Frey, & Van Lieshout, 2018; Woody, Ferrari, Siskind, Whiteford, & Harris, 2017; Yildiz, Ayers, & Phillips, 2017). More recently, a focus on psychopathology in early fatherhood has emerged in the clinical literature (Cameron et al., 2016; Kim & Swain, 2007; Sethna, Murray, Edmondson, Iles, & Ramchandani, 2018). A growing number of studies document the existence and effects of symptoms of psychopathology in men during the perinatal period, with a focus on depression (Underwood et al., 2017), some attention to anxiety (Korja et al., 2018), and very little attention to the influence of trauma on early fathering (for a notable exception see, Fredman et al., 2019). The fact that trauma has not been explored in the empirical perinatal fathering literature highlights a critical gap – the relative paucity of perinatal research focusing on fathers facing contextual risks such as poverty, racism, and chronic un/underemployment. Unlike their mainly Caucasian, middle-class counterparts (within the United States), expectant fathers who are living with these risk factors are much more likely to be exposed to higher rates of violence and trauma. Further, in the context of the established economic and racial health disparities in perinatal health outcomes for the mother and the infant, and the documented positive influence of father involvement on these outcomes, research that focuses on these populations is needed (Alhusen, Gross, Hayat, Rose, & Sharps, 2012; Bond, 2010).

To date, paternal perinatal depression has received the most empirical attention relative to other forms of psychopathology, leading to the possibility of determining trustworthy estimates of prevalence. For instance, in a recent meta-analysis of studies from multiple countries, Cameron et al. (2016) reported an overall random effect estimate of paternal perinatal depression of 8.4%, with little variation across the prenatal and postnatal periods and a notably higher rate of 13% for studies conducted in North America. Though the presence of anxiety in men in the perinatal period has received less empirical attention, a recent systematic review by Leach, Poyser,

Cooklin, and Giallo (2016) found that rates ranged from 4.1% to 16.0% in the prenatal period and 2.4% to 16.3% in the postnatal period.

Both depression and anxiety have been examined in relation to fathers' prenatal relationships with their infants. The results are mixed from these examinations but point to the possibility that prenatal paternal psychopathology poses a potential risk to the development of the relationship. Studies using the PAAS have generally found a negative relationship of bonding and psychopathology. For example, Brandão, Brites, Pires, Hipólito, and Nunes (2019) found that PAAS scores were negatively associated with paternal depression in a community sample of Portuguese parents. Interestingly, in this sample, anxiety was *positively* associated with paternal prenatal bonding in the regression model (standardized regression coefficient = 0.19; $p < 0.01$), though the correlation was not significant at the bivariate level ($r = -0.057$, ns). As described by the authors, mean levels of anxiety in this sample were within the normal range, and the authors wondered whether slight elevations in anxiety, at least for fathers, may result in a greater focus on the health and well-being of the fetus and motivation to care for the mother and infant. In a community sample of primarily Dutch fathers, Vreeswijk, Maas, Rijk, van Bakel, (2014) found that fathers' prenatal bonding as measured by the PAAS was negatively associated with symptoms of both depression and anxiety. However, the quality of their internal representations of the infant as measured by the WMCI was not associated with their symptoms of psychopathology. These findings differ from studies of maternal representations where psychopathology has been found to influence maternal working models (Korja et al., 2018). The authors speculate that one reason for the disparate findings may be that studies of maternal representations have utilized samples of mothers exposed to contextual risk, whereas Vreeswijk et al. (2015) utilized a low-risk, community sample of fathers, pointing, again, to the need for fathering studies that include diverse samples, especially samples of fathers exposed to contextual risk (e.g., poverty, racism, violence exposure).

The prevalence rates for depression and anxiety and their possible association with prenatal father-infant relationship development for men suggest that screening men for symptoms of psychopathology in the perinatal period is indicated (Kerstis et al., 2016). To date, however, most expectant and new fathers are not receiving routine mental health screenings (Musser, Ahmed, Foli, & Coddington, 2013). Complicating this picture is the fact that there are no diagnostic criteria for *paternal* perinatal depression included in the most frequently used diagnostic manual (DSM; American Psychiatric Association, 2013) and very few male-specific measures of perinatal depression (for a recent exception, see Stephen Matthey & Della Vedova, 2019). Instead, consistent with other approaches throughout the clinical and empirical literature, the DSM diagnostic criteria and measures of perinatal depression for women are often applied to men (Musser et al., 2013). For example, the most common measure used to assess perinatal depression in fathers is the Edinburgh Postnatal Depression Scale (EPDS; Da Costa et al., 2019) which was originally developed for use with mothers. Although the EPDS has been established as a valid measure for use with fathers (Matthey, Barnett, Kavanagh, & Howie, 2001), Singley and Edwards (2015) have argued that measures such as the EPDS that were originally designed for women may miss the mark when applied to men because their symptoms often manifest as anger and withdrawal such that the underlying depression is likely to be missed or misinterpreted. Further work is needed to determine whether perinatal depression may manifest differently for fathers and whether symptoms of psychopathology are robustly related to perinatal father-infant relationship development, especially in fathers exposed to contextual risk.

Couple Relationship Quality Prior work has demonstrated that the quality of the father's relationship with his romantic partner is consistently and robustly related to the quality of his parenting (Holland &

McElwain, 2013; Stroud, Durbin, Wilson, & Mendelsohn, 2011). This is also true for fathers within the perinatal period (Ahlqvist-Björkroth et al., 2016; Luz et al., 2017; Yu, Hung, Chan, Yeh, & Lai, 2012). For instance, in a low-risk sample of primarily well-educated and employed French couples, Luz et al. (2017) found that fathers' postnatal bonding (using the Paternal Antenatal Assessment Scale; Condon, 1993) was associated with self-reported marital quality and also with the quality of the parenting alliance. In addition, the strength of the *maternal* bond (using the Maternal Antenatal Assessment Scale; Condon, 1993) to the infant was related to the strength of the *paternal* bond. However, in this same study, maternal bonding was relatively independent from father- and couple-related variables. In other words, and consistent with some prior work, the maternal influence on the father-infant relationship was strong, whereas the opposite was not the case. In contrast, Ahlqvist-Bjorkroth and colleagues (2016) found that marital relationship quality for *both* mothers and fathers was associated with prenatal relationship quality as measured by the WMCI. In interpreting their results with regard to fathers, these investigators argue that a distressed marital relationship may decrease a mother's propensity to include the father in what Draper (2002) would call body-mediated experiences with the infant and thereby inhibit the healthy formation of the father-infant relationship through a process of prenatal gatekeeping. When parents are not married and not cohabitating, fathers may have an especially difficult time connecting with their infants in body-mediated ways during pregnancy. In the following section, we review data from a sample of urban-dwelling, expectant parents, the majority of whom were living apart and exposed to contextual risk during the pregnancy.

The Motown Family Relationships Laboratory: Early Fathering in an Urban Setting

We now turn to ongoing work in our own laboratory examining the process of prenatal bonding and relationship formation in a sample of poverty- and violence-exposed fathers and mothers ($n = 102$; for a sample description, see Dayton, Johnson, et al., 2019; Dayton, Matthews, Hicks, & Malone, 2017; Dayton et al., 2016). Investigations examining fathering in high-risk samples of men exposed to contextual risks have blossomed in the last few decades, generating a great deal of knowledge about the importance of father involvement in the lives of young children who, themselves, are risk exposed. However, as Volling and Cabrera (Volling et al., 2019) have recently pointed out, assessments of father "involvement," although they are critically important, do not offer a deep understanding of the process of early fathering. As they rightly highlight, we do not ask whether mothers are "involved" with their children. Instead, we try to understand, in nuanced and sophisticated ways, what they do, how they do it, and how, exactly, it matters for children. However, the majority of the studies examining the experiences of fathers in the perinatal period have focused on fathers who, although they may be struggling with perinatal psychopathology and relationship conflict, are otherwise facing very few contextual stressors such as poverty, racism, and the violence exposure that is associated with these circumstances. Our research at the Motown Family Relationships Laboratory is currently asking these how, where, what, and why questions related to father involvement in an urban sample of expectant fathers, many of whom are living in poverty and have been exposed to high levels of interpersonal and community violence. We have taken a biopsychosocial approach to understand the pathways to parenting these men travel in preparing to parent a new infant. We use the three types of measurement approaches described above – qualitative, self-report, and typological – and we additionally measure fathers' physiological responses to parenting stress (e.g., cortisol and testosterone production and heart rate variability). Here we briefly review some of our primary findings to date, including factors that influence prenatal bonding, fathers' views of early breastfeeding, and the importance of music in the lives of these fathers.

The Power of Relationships in the Lives of Expectant Fathers Experiencing Contextual Risk

As fathers prepared to parent a new baby, their self-report data and their answers to our interview questions made it clear that they were actively thinking about central relationships in their lives – past and current – and that these were primary contributors to the prenatal bonds they were forming with their infants. For example, in an examination of the association of risk and resilience factors with prenatal bonding using the PAAS (Dayton, Brown, et al., 2019), we found that a father's belief in the importance of early fathering to the healthy development of young children (Role of the Father Questionnaire; Palkovitz, 1984) was robustly ($r = 0.49, p < 0.01$) associated with his prenatal bonding. However, findings from the qualitative data (Dayton et al., 2016) suggest that fathers were primarily thinking about parenting their children when they were older – beyond the infancy and early childhood stage. Across interviews, fathers in this study described their intentions to parent their older children 281 times and described parenting their infants only 65 times. We argue that, taken together, these findings have important implications for intervening early with expectant fathers. Specifically, our results suggest that interventions that increase fathers' beliefs in their importance to the health and well-being of their infants and young children may improve their prenatal bonds with them.

Across the multiple methods used in this study, a father's history of relationships was found to be influential to his thoughts and feelings about his infant. On average, fathers in this sample reported high levels of childhood neglect and abuse in their own histories. Interestingly, in the quantitative analysis described above, a history of child neglect – but not abuse – was negatively associated with fathers' prenatal bonding scores. Data from the qualitative interviews help us understand the ways in which fathers were grappling with these feelings of father absence and neglect in their own lives (Dayton et al., 2016) as they prepared to parent a new baby. One father described the neglect of his father and went on to describe his intention to "be there" for his new baby in a way that his own father was not there for him:

> I wish [my father] would have been there more, and given more good advice instead of bad advice.... I have learned [about life] on my own... . Nothing that [my father] did I plan on doing with my child. (Dayton et al., 2016, p. 232)

> I will be there [for his own child], no matter what. No matter if I'm the brokest person in the world I will be there. And that was his [his father's] excuse, he said he wasn't there because he didn't have finances. But that ain't no excuse to me ... [so, the most important thing is] being there—me being there the whole time, and I'm gonna be there the whole time. And I'm proud of myself for actually coming to this. I've never done anything like this in my whole life. (Dayton et al., 2016, p. 229)

Another father described how other caretakers – all women – in his childhood helped to fill the gap of his father's absence and neglect:

> [My dad] didn't teach me nothing. My grandma was my dad and my mom [and] my aunt... . [My mom provided] help and support.... My mom straightened me out ... [and now] I know they are probably going to help support me when I need it [with the new baby]. (Dayton et al., 2016, p. 232)

Fathers' Views of Breastfeeding

Fathers reflected on their relationships as they prepared to parent across many domains. For example, in thinking about infant feeding decisions for their new infant, a father's very early relationship with his own mother was influential; fathers who had themselves been breastfed as infants were significantly more likely to say that they intended for their infant to be breastfed (Dayton, Johnson, et al., 2019). Further, they described the ways in which family relationships and norms influenced their feelings about breastfeeding. In the following case, a father who reported that he and his partner had not yet decided whether their baby would be breastfed describes a lack of knowledge about breastfeeding throughout his family system:

"Shoot don't nobody I know ever breastfed. My sister didn't breastfeed. My cousins didn't breastfeed. No one breastfed in my family that I know of." (Dayton, Johnson, et al., 2019)

Music in the Lives of Expectant Fathers

Many fathers in this study described that they planned to use music to calm and soothe their infants, and when asked about their memories of music from their childhoods, fathers described the relationships within which music was present in their lives (Dayton et al., 2017). More than two thirds of the participants explicitly referred to their mothers when thinking about their memories of music, and one third referred to their father (or a father figure). One father put it this way:

> [Music is] like the background music to your life. Like it [doesn't] matter what I'm feeling, I got a song for it. Whatever I'm going through in my life, I got a song for it. And you know whether it's good or bad as far as like the music I listen to … I just think it's a connection in some kind of way kinda like how smells and food and stuff … that can connect you to your memories and bring you back to that point. Like right now if I heard Bobby Brown playing I would just instantly think of my dad and the Friday night gatherings that he would have. (Dayton et al., 2017, p. 849)

Summary and Key Points

In closing, our understanding of the experience and roles of fathers during the perinatal period is in its very early stages. There have been significant changes in the societal expectations around father-infant interactions and involvement that are at times in conflict with ideas of masculinity. Yet a growing body of theory and research suggests that the father's participation and engagement in the prenatal phase and early infancy phase has benefits to the infant, mother, and father not only as individuals but also in relationship to one another. We hoped to emphasize the importance of assessing and learning about the father's internal experience of becoming a father, with particular attention to his representations of his infant and himself as a father. Given the need to consider the father-infant bond, we highlighted relevant risk and resilience factors particularly in the domains of paternal psychopathology and the quality of the couple's relationship. Finally, we closed the chapter by presenting a range of newly emerging qualitative and quantitative data about fathers and infants from the Motown Family Relationships Laboratory. The key points we wish to emphasize are as follows:

1. The father-infant relationship begins during pregnancy through the development of the father's internal representations of the infant. These paternal prenatal representations are predictive of qualities of the father-infant relationship, parenting, and child outcomes across early development.
2. Factors that influence the paternal perinatal bond include paternal mental health and the quality of the father's relationship with the mother. These areas deserve specific attention during prenatal care.
3. The growing body of literature addressing the perinatal paternal bond suggests that fathers would benefit from more inclusion and support during pregnancy and postpartum as they build a relationship with their baby, maintain and rework their relationship to their partners, and think about their own identity.

References

Abelin, E. L. (1975). Some further observations and comments on the earliest role of the father. *International Journal of Psychoanalysis, 56*, 293–302.

Abraham, E., & Feldman, R. (2018). The neurobiology of human allomaternal care; implications for fathering, coparenting, and children's social development. *Physiology & Behavior, 193*, 25–34. https://doi.org/10.1016/j.physbeh.2017.12.034

Ahlqvist-Björkroth, S., Korja, R., Junttila, N., Savonlahti, E., Pajulo, M., Räihä, H., et al. (2016). Mothers' and fathers' prenatal representations in relation to marital distress and depressive symptoms. *Infant Mental Health Journal, 37*(4), 388–400. https://doi.org/10.1002/imhj.21578

Alhusen, J. L., Gross, D., Hayat, M. J., Rose, L., & Sharps, P. (2012). The role of mental health on maternal-fetal attachment in low-income women. *Journal of Obstetric, Gynecologic, & Neonatal Nursing: Clinical Scholarship for the Care of Women, Childbearing Families, & Newborns, 41*(6), E71–E81. https://doi.org/10.1111/j.1552-6909.2012.01385.x

Alio, A. P., Mbah, A. K., Kornosky, J. L., Wathington, D., Marty, P. J., & Salihu, H. M. (2011). Assessing the impact of paternal involvement on racial/ethnic disparities in infant mortality rates. *Journal of Community Health, 36*(1), 63–68. https://doi.org/10.1007/s10900-010-9280-3

Alio, A. P., Salihu, H. M., Kornosky, J. L., Richman, A. M., & Marty, P. J. (2010). Feto-infant health and survival: Does paternal involvement matter? *Maternal and Child Health Journal, 14*(6), 931–937. https://doi.org/10.1007/s10995-009-0531-9

American Psychiatric Association. (2013). *Diagnostic and statistical manual of mental disorders* (5th ed.). Arlington, VA: American Psychiatric Association.

Anderson, S., St George, J., & Roggman, L. A. (2019). Measuring the quality of early father–child rough and tumble play: Tools for practice and research. *Child & Youth Care Forum*. https://doi.org/10.1007/s10566-019-09513-9

Atkin, K., Berghs, M., & Dyson, S. (2015). 'Who's the guy in the room?' Involving fathers in antenatal care screening for sickle cell disorders. *Social Science & Medicine, 128*, 212–219. https://doi.org/10.1016/j.socscimed.2015.01.039

Barrows, P. (2004). Fathers and families: Locating the ghost in the nursery. *Infant Mental Health Journal, 25*(5), 408–423.

Benjamin, J. (1995). *Like subjects, love objects: Essays on recognition and sexual difference*. New Haven, CT: Yale University Press.

Bianchi, S. M. (2011). Family change and time allocation in American families. *The Annals of the American Academy of Political and Social Science, 638*, 21–44. Retrieved from JSTOR.

Bianchi, S. M., Robinson, J. P., & Milke, M. A. (2006). *The changing rhythms of American family life*. New York: Russell Sage Foundation.

Blos, P. (1984). Son and father. *Journal of the American Psychoanalytic Association, 32*, 301–324.

Bogren, L. Y. (1983). Couvade. *Acta Psychiatric Scandinavia, 68*, 55–65.

Bogren, L. Y. (1984). The Couvade syndrome: Background variables. *Acta Psychiatrica Scandinavica, 70*, 316–320.

Bond, M. J. (2010). The missing link in MCH: Paternal involvement in pregnancy outcomes. *American Journal of Men's Health, 4*(4), 285–286. https://doi.org/10.1177/1557988310384842

Bowlby, J. (1980). *Attachment and loss*. Retrieved from http://proxy.lib.umich.edu/login?url=http://search.ebscohost.com/login.aspx?direct=true&db=psyh&AN=2003-00033-000&site=ehost-live&scope=site

Bowlby, J. (1982). Attachment and loss: Retrospect and prospect. *American Journal of Orthopsychiatry, 52*(4), 664–678. https://doi.org/10.1111/j.1939-0025.1982.tb01456.x

Brandão, T., Brites, R., Pires, M., Hipólito, J., & Nunes, O. (2019). Anxiety, depression, dyadic adjustment, and attachment to the fetus in pregnancy: Actor–partner interdependence mediation analysis. *Journal of Family Psychology, 33*(3), 294–303. https://doi.org/10.1037/fam0000513

Brennan, A., Ayers, S., Ahmed, H., & Marshall-Lucette, S. (2007). A critical review of the Couvade syndrome: The pregnant male. *Journal of Reproductive and Infant Psychology, 25*(3), 173–189.

Burlingham, D. (1973). The preoedipal infant-father relationship. *Psychoanalytic Study of the Child, 28*, 23–47.

Cabrera, N., Fagan, J., & Farrie, D. (2008). Explaining the long reach of fathers? Prenatal involvement on later paternal engagement. *Journal of Marriage and Family, 70*(5), 1094–1107. https://doi.org/10.1111/j.1741-3737.2008.00551.x

Cabrera, N., Fitzgerald, H. E., Bradley, R. H., & Roggman, L. (2007). Modeling the dynamics of paternal influences on children over the life course. *Applied Developmental Science, 11*(4), 185–189. https://doi.org/10.1080/10888690701762027

Cabrera, N., & Tamis-LeMonda, C. S. (2013). *Handbook of Father Involvement*. https://doi.org/10.4324/9780203101414

Cabrera, N., Tamis-LeMonda, C. S., Bradley, R. H., Hofferth, S., & Lamb, M. E. (2000). Fatherhood in the twenty-first century. *Child Development, 71*(1), 127–136. https://doi.org/10.1111/1467-8624.00126

Cameron, E. E., Sedov, I. D., & Tomfohr-Madsen, L. M. (2016). Prevalence of paternal depression in pregnancy and the postpartum: An updated meta-analysis. *Journal of Affective Disorders, 206*, 189–203. https://doi.org/10.1016/j.jad.2016.07.044

Cohen, L. J., & Slade, A. (2000). The psychology and psychopathology of pregnancy: Reorganization and transformation. In C. H. Zeanah Jr. & C. H. Zeanah Jr. (Eds.), *Handbook of infant mental health* (2nd ed., pp. 20–36). Retrieved from http://proxy.lib.umich.edu/login?url=http://search.ebscohost.com/login.aspx?direct=true&db=psyh&AN=2000-07057-002&site=ehost-live&scope=site

Collins, N. L., & Read, S. J. (1994). Cognitive representations of attachment: The structure and function of working models. In *Advances in personal relationships* (Attachment processes in adulthood) (Vol. 5, pp. 53–90). London, UK: Jessica Kingsley Publishers.

Condon, J., Corkindale, C., Boyce, P., & Gamble, E. (2013). A longitudinal study of father-to-infant attachment: Antecedents and correlates. *Journal of Reproductive and Infant Psychology, 31*(1), 15–30. https://doi.org/10.1080/02646838.2012.757694

Condon, J. T. (1993). The assessment of antenatal emotional attachment: Development of a questionnaire instrument. *British Journal of*

Medical Psychology, 66(2), 167–183. https://doi.org/10.1111/j.2044-8341.1993.tb01739.x

Cowan, P. A., & Cowan, C. P. (2012). Normative family transitions, couple relationship quality, and healthy child development. In *Normal family processes: Growing diversity and complexity* (4th ed., pp. 428–451). New York: The Guilford Press.

Crawford, A., & Benoit, D. (2009). Caregivers' disrupted representations of the unborn child predict later infant-caregiver disorganized attachment and disrupted interactions. *Infant Mental Halth Journal, 30*(2), 124-144.

Da Costa, D., Danieli, C., Abrahamowicz, M., Dasgupta, K., Sewitch, M., Lowensteyn, I., et al. (2019). A prospective study of postnatal depressive symptoms and associated risk factors in first-time fathers. *Journal of Affective Disorders, 249*, 371–377. https://doi.org/10.1016/j.jad.2019.02.033

Dayton, C. J., Johnson, A., Hicks, L. M., Goletz, J., Brown, S., Primuse, T., et al. (2019). Sex differences in the social ecology of breastfeeding: A mixed methods analysis of the breastfeeding views of expectant mothers and fathers in the U.S. exposed to adversity. *Journal of Biosocial Science, 51*(3), 374–393. https://doi.org/10.1017/S002193201800024X

Dayton, C. J., Matthews, W. K., Hicks, L. M., & Malone, J. C. (2017). The expression of music throughout the lives of expectant parents. *Psychology of Music, 45*(6), 839–854. https://doi.org/10.1177/0305735617692165

Dayton, C. J., Brown, S., Goletz, J., Hicks, L., Barron, C., Sperlich, M., et al. (2019). Pathways to parenting: Predictors of prenatal bonding in a sample of expectant mothers and fathers exposed to contextual risk. *Journal of Child and Family Studies*. https://doi.org/10.1007/s10826-019-01343-6

Dayton, C. J., Buczkowski, R., Muzik, M., Goletz, J., Hicks, L., Walsh, T. B., et al. (2016). Expectant fathers' beliefs and expectations about fathering as they prepare to parent a new infant. *Social Work Research, 40*(4), 225–236. https://doi.org/10.1093/swr/svw017

Dayton, C. J., Walsh, T. B., Oh, W., & Volling, B. (2015). Hush now baby: Mothers' and fathers' strategies for soothing their infants and associated parenting outcomes. *Journal of Pediatric Health Care, 29*(2), 145–155. https://doi.org/10.1016/j.pedhc.2014.09.001

de Cock, E. S. A., Henrichs, J., Klimstra, T. A., Maas, A. J. B. M., Vreeswijk, C. M. J. M., Meeus, W. H. J., et al. (2017). Longitudinal associations between parental bonding, parenting stress, and executive functioning in toddlerhood. *Journal of Child and Family Studies, 26*(6), 1723–1733. https://doi.org/10.1007/s10826-017-0679-7

de Cock, E. S. A., Henrichs, J., Vreeswijk, C. M. J. M., Maas, A. J. B. M., Rijk, C. H. A. M., & van Bakel, H. J. A. (2016). Continuous feelings of love? The parental bond from pregnancy to toddlerhood. *Journal of Family Psychology, 30*(1), 125–134. https://doi.org/10.1037/fam0000138

Deave, T., & Johnson, D. (2008). The transition to parenthood: What does it mean for fathers? *Journal of Advanced Nursing, 63*(6), 626–633. https://doi.org/10.1111/j.1365-2648.2008.04748.x

Diamond, M. J. (1986). Becoming a father: A psychoanalytic perspective on the forgotten parent. *Psychoanalytic Review, 73D*(4), 41–64.

Diamond, M. J. (2017). Recovering the father in mind and flesh: History, triadic functioning, and developmental implications. *The Psychoanalytic Quarterly, 86*(2), 297–334. https://doi.org/10.1002/psaq.12141

Doi, H., Kato, M., Nishitani, S., & Shinohara, K. (2011). Development of synchrony between activity patterns of mother-infant pair from 4 to 18 months after birth. *The Journal of Physiological Sciences, 61*(3), 211–216. https://doi.org/10.1007/s12576-011-0138-y

Draper, J. (2002). 'It's the first scientific evidence': Men's experience of pregnancy confirmation. *Issues and Innovations in Nursing Practice, 39*(6), 563–570. https://doi.org/10.1046/j.1365-2648.2002.02325.x

Dubber, S., Reck, C., Müller, M., & Gawlik, S. (2015). Postpartum bonding: The role of perinatal depression, anxiety and maternal–fetal bonding during pregnancy. *Archives of Women's Mental Health, 18*(2), 187–195. https://doi.org/10.1007/s00737-014-0445-4

Fagan, J., & Palkovitz, R. (2007). Unmarried, nonresident fathers' involvement with their infants: A risk and resilience perspective. *Journal of Family Psychology, 21*(3), 479–489. https://doi.org/10.1037/0893-3200.21.3.479

Falah-Hassani, K., Shiri, R., & Dennis, C.-L. (2017). The prevalence of antenatal and postnatal co-morbid anxiety and depression: A meta-analysis. *Psychological Medicine, 47*(12), 2041–2053. https://doi.org/10.1017/S0033291717000617

Fairbairn, W. R. D. (1952). *An object-relations theory of the personality*. New York: Basic Books.

Foley, S., & Hughes, C. (2018). Great expectations? Do mothers' and fathers' prenatal thoughts and feelings about the infant predict parent-infant interaction quality? A meta-analytic review. *Developmental Review, 48*, 40–54. https://doi.org/10.1016/j.dr.2018.03.007

Formaini, H. (2004). Peering into one of Winnicott's "Blank Spots". *American Imago, 61*(4), 527–538.

Fraiberg, S., Adelson, E., & Shapiro, V. (1975). Ghosts in the nursery: A psychoanalytic approach to the problems of impaired infant-mother relationships. *Journal of the American Academy of Child Psychiatry, 14*(3), 387–421.

Fredman, S. J., Le, Y., Marshall, A. D., Garcia Hernandez, W., Feinberg, M. E., & Ammerman, R. T. (2019). Parents' PTSD symptoms and child abuse potential during the perinatal period: Direct associations and mediation via relationship conflict. *Child Abuse & Neglect, 90*, 66–75. https://doi.org/10.1016/j.chiabu.2019.01.024

Freud, S. (1953). Three essays on the theory of sexuality. In J. Strachey (Ed. & Trans.), *The standard edition of the complete psychological works of Sigmund Freud* (Vol. 7, pp. 125–243). London, UK: Hogarth Press. (Original work published 1905).

Furtado, M., Chow, C. H. T., Owais, S., Frey, B. N., & Van Lieshout, R. J. (2018). Risk factors of new onset anxiety and anxiety exacerbation in the perinatal period: A systematic review and meta-analysis. *Journal of Affective Disorders, 238*, 626–635. https://doi.org/10.1016/j.jad.2018.05.073

Gaumon, S., & Paquette, D. (2013). The father–child activation relationship and internalizing disorders at preschool age. *Early Child Development and Care, 183*(3–4), 447–463. https://doi.org/10.1080/03004430.2012.711593

Genesoni, L., & Tallandini, M. A. (2009). Men's psychological transition to fatherhood: An analysis of the literature, 1989–2008. *Birth: Issues in Perinatal Care, 36*(4), 305–318. https://doi.org/10.1111/j.1523-536X.2009.00358.x

Giurgescu, C., & Templin, T. N. (2015). Father involvement and psychological well-being of pregnant women. *MCN: The American Journal of Maternal/Child Nursing, 40*(6), 381–387. https://doi.org/10.1097/NMC.0000000000000183

Gordon, I., Zagoory-Sharon, O., Leckman, J. F., & Feldman, R. (2010). Oxytocin and the development of parenting in humans. *Biological Psychiatry, 68*(4), 377–382. https://doi.org/10.1016/j.biopsych.2010.02.005

Habib, C., & Lancaster, S. (2010). Changes in identity and paternal-fetal attachment across a first pregnancy. *Journal of Reproductive and Infant Psychology, 28*(2), 128–142. https://doi.org/10.1080/02646830903298723

Hanson, S., Hunter, L., Bormann, J. R., & Sobo, E. J. (2009). Paternal fears of childbirth: A literature review. *The Journal of Perinatal Education, 18*(4), 12–20.

Harkness, S., Mavridis, C. J., Liu, J. J., & Super, C. M. (2015). Parental ethnotheories and the development of family relationships in early and middle childhood. *The Oxford Handbook of Human Development and Culture*. https://doi.org/10.1093/oxfordhb/9780199948550.013.17

Herrera, F. (2013). "Men always adopt": Infertility and reproduction from a male perspective. *Journal of Family Issues, 34*(8), 1059–1080. https://doi.org/10.1177/0192513X13484278

Herzog, J. M. (1982). On father hunger: The father's role in the modulation of aggressive drive and fantasy. In S. H. Cath, J. M. Gurwitt, & J. M. Ross (Eds.), *Father and child: Developmental and clinical perspectives*. Boston, MA: Little, Brown.

Herzog, J. M. (2001). Father hunger: Explorations with adults and children. Analytic Press.

Hjelmstedt, A., & Collins, A. (2008). Psychological functioning and predictors of father-infant relationship in IVF fathers and controls. *Scandinavian Journal of Caring Sciences, 22*(1), 72–78. https://doi.org/10.1111/j.1471-6712.2007.00537.x

Holland, A. S., & McElwain, N. L. (2013). Maternal and paternal perceptions of coparenting as a link between marital quality and the parent–toddler relationship. *Journal of Family Psychology, 27*(1), 117–126. https://doi.org/10.1037/a0031427

Ives, J. (2014). Men, maternity and moral residue: Negotiating the moral demands of the transition to first time fatherhood. *Sociology of Health and Illness, 36*(7), 1003–1019.

Jackson, A. P., Choi, J.-K., & Preston, K. S. J. (2019). Harsh parenting and Black boys' behavior problems: Single mothers' parenting stress and nonresident fathers' involvement. *Family Relations*, (0), 0. https://doi.org/10.1111/fare.12373

Julian, M. M., Muzik, M., Kees, M., Valenstein, M., & Rosenblum, K. L. (2018). Strong military families intervention enhances parenting reflectivity and representations in families with young children. *Infant Mental Health Journal, 39*(1), 106–118. https://doi.org/10.1002/imhj.21690

Kainz, G., Eliasson, M., & von Post, I. (2010). The child's father, an important person for the mother's well-being during the childbirth: A hermeneutic study. *Health Care for Women International, 31*(7), 621–635. https://doi.org/10.1080/07399331003725499

Kerstis, B., Aarts, C., Tillman, C., Persson, H., Engström, G., Edlund, B., et al. (2016). Association between parental depressive symptoms and impaired bonding with the infant. *Archives of Women's Mental Health, 19*(1), 87–94. https://doi.org/10.1007/s00737-015-0522-3

Kim, P., & Swain, J. E. (2007). Sad dads. *Psychiatry (Edgmont), 4*(2), 35–47.

Klein, M. (1928). Early states of the Oedipus complex. *International Journal of Psychoanalysis, 9*, 167–180.

Korja, R., Nolvi, S., Kataja, E.-L., Scheinin, N., Junttila, N., Lahtinen, H., et al. (2018). The courses of maternal and paternal depressive and anxiety symptoms during the prenatal period in the Finn Brain Birth Cohort study. *PLoS One, 13*(12). Retrieved from http://proxy.lib.umich.edu/login?url=http://search.ebscohost.com/login.aspx?direct=true&db=psyh&AN=2018-65485-001&site=ehost-live&scope=site

Kroll, M. E., Carson, C., Redshaw, M., & Quigley, M. A. (2016). Early father involvement and subsequent child behaviour at ages 3, 5 and 7 years: Prospective analysis of the UK Millennium Cohort Study. *PLoS One, 11*(9). Retrieved from http://proxy.lib.umich.edu/login?url=http://search.ebscohost.com/login.aspx?direct=true&db=psyh&AN=2016-47240-001&site=ehost-live&scope=site

Lamb, M. E. (1976). The role of the father: An overview. In J. E. Lamb (Ed.), *The role of the father in child development* (pp. 1–63). New York: Wiley.

Lamb, M. E. (2010). *The role of the father in child development* (5th ed.). (Michael E. Lamb, Ed.). Retrieved from http://proxy.lib.umich.edu/login?url=http://search.ebscohost.com/login.aspx?direct=true&db=psyh&AN=2010-04805-000&site=ehost-live&scope=site

Leach, L. S., Poyser, C., Cooklin, A. R., & Giallo, R. (2016). Prevalence and course of anxiety disorders (and symptom levels) in men across the perinatal period: A systematic review. *Journal of Affective*

Disorders, 190, 675–686. https://doi.org/10.1016/j.jad.2015.09.063

Lebovici, S. (1993). On intergenerational transmission: From filiation to affiliation. *Infant Mental Health Journal, 14*(4), 260–272.

Lebovici, S. (1988). Fantasmatic interaction and intergenerational transmission. *Infant Mental Health Journal, 9*(1), 10–19.

Leckman, J. F., Feldman, R., Swain, J. E., Eicher, V., Thompson, N., & Mayes, L. C. (2004). Primary parental preoccupation: Circuits, genes, and the crucial role of the environment. *Journal of Neural Transmission, 111*(7), 753–771.

Leckman, J. F., Mayes, L. C., Feldman, R., Evans, D. W., King, R. A., & Cohen, D. J. (1999). Early parental preoccupations and behaviors and their possible relationship to the symptoms of obsessive-compulsive disorder. *Acta Psychiatrica Scandinavica, 100*(S396), 1–26. https://doi.org/10.1111/j.1600-0447.1999.tb10951.x

Lee, S. J., Sanchez, D. T., Grogan-Kaylor, A., Lee, J. Y., & Albuja, A. (2018). Father early engagement behaviors and infant low birth weight. *Maternal and Child Health Journal*. https://doi.org/10.1007/s10995-018-2521-2

Luz, R., George, A., Vieux, R., & Spitz, E. (2017). Antenatal determinants of parental attachment and parenting alliance: How do mothers and fathers differ? *Infant Mental Health Journal, 38*(2), 183–197. https://doi.org/10.1002/imhj.21628

Mahler, M. S. (1971). A study of the separation-individuaton process and its possible application to borderline phenomena in the psychoanalytic situation. *Psychoanalytic Study of the Child*, 403–424.

Malone, J. C., & Dayton, C. J. (2015). What is the container/contained when there are ghosts in the nursery?: Joining Bion and Fraiberg in dyadic interventions with mother and infant. *Infant Mental Health Journal, 36*(3), 262–274. https://doi.org/10.1002/imhj.21509

Matthey, S., Barnett, B., Kavanagh, D. J., & Howie, P. (2001). Validation of the Edinburgh Postnatal Depression Scale for men, and comparison of item endorsement with their partners. *Journal of Affective Disorders, 64*(2–3), 175–184.

Matthey, S., & Della Vedova, A. M. (2019). Screening for mood difficulties in men in Italy and Australia using the Edinburgh Postnatal Depression Scale and the Matthey Generic Mood Questionnaire. *Psychology of Men & Masculinities*. https://doi.org/10.1037/men0000227

Maume, D. J. (2011). Reconsidering the temporal increase in fathers' time with children. *Journal of Family and Economic Issues, 32*(3), 411–423. https://doi.org/10.1007/s10834-010-9227-y

May, K. A. (1982). Three phases of father involvement in pregnancy. [Editorial]. *Nursing Research, 31*(6), 337–342.

McGoldrick, M., & Shibusawa, T. (2012). The family life cycle. In F. Walsh (Ed.), *Normal family processes: Growing diversity and complexity* (4th ed., pp. 375–398). New York: Guilford Press.

Milgrom, J., & Gemmill, A. (Eds.). (2015). *Identifying perinatal depression and anxiety: Evidence-based practice in screening, psychosocial assessment, and management*. Oxford, UK: Wiley.

Musser, A. K., Ahmed, A. H., Foli, K. J., & Coddington, J. A. (2013). Paternal postpartum depression: What health care providers should know. *Journal of Pediatric Health Care, 27*(6), 479–485. https://doi.org/10.1016/j.pedhc.2012.10.001

Nelson, S. K., Kushlev, K., & Lyubomirsky, S. (2014). The pains and pleasures of parenting: When, why, and how is parenthood associated with more or less well-being? *Psychological Bulletin, 140*(3), 846–895. https://doi.org/10.1037/a0035444

Palkovitz, R. (1984). Parental attitudes and fathers' interactions with their 5-month-old infants. *Developmental Psychology, 20*(6), 1054–1060. https://doi.org/10.1037/0012-1649.20.6.1054

Paquette, D. (2004). Theorizing the father-child relationship: Mechanisms and developmental outcomes. *Human Development, 47*(4), 193–219. https://doi.org/10.1159/000078723

Paquette, D., & Bigras, M. (2010). The risky situation: A procedure for assessing the father–child activation relationship. *Early Child Development and Care, 180*(1–2), 33–50. https://doi.org/10.1080/03004430903414687

Parke, R. D., Power, T. G., Tinsley, B. R., & Hymel, S. (1980). The father's role in the family system. *Parent-Infant Relationships*, 117–133.

Phillips, A. (1988). *Winnicott*. London, UK: Fontana.

Plantin, L., & Olykoya, A. (2011). Positive health outcomes of fathers' involvement in pregnancy and childbirth paternal support: A scope study literature review. *Fathering, 1*(9).

Poh, H. L., Koh, S. S. L., & He, H. G. (2014). An integrative review of fathers' experiences during pregnancy and childbirth. *International Nursing Review, 61*(4), 543–554. https://doi.org/10.1111/inr.12137

Reed, R. K. (2005). *Birthing fathers: The transformation of men in American rites of birth*. Piscataway, NJ: Rutgers University Press.

Righetti, P. L., Dell'Avanzo, M., Grigio, M., & Nicolini, U. (2005). Maternal/paternal antenatal attachment and fourth-dimensional ultrasound technique: A preliminary report. *British Journal of Psychology, 96*(1), 129–137. https://doi.org/10.1348/000712604X15518

Rosich-Medina, A., & Shetty, A. (2007). Paternal experiences of pregnancy and labour. *British Journal of Midwifery, 15*(2), 66–74.

Salihu, H. M., August, E. M., Mbah, A. K., Alio, A. P., Berry, E. L., & Aliyu, M. H. (2014). Impact of a federal healthy start program on feto-infant morbidity associated with absent fathers: A quasi-experimental study. *Maternal and Child Health Journal, 18*(9), 2054–2060. https://doi.org/10.1007/s10995-014-1451-x

Salihu, H. M., Salemi, J. L., Nash, M. C., Chandler, K., Mbah, A. K., & Alio, A. P. (2014). Assessing the economic impact of paternal involvement: A comparison of the generalized linear model versus decision analysis trees. *Maternal and Child Health*

Journal, 18(6), 1380–1390. https://doi.org/10.1007/s10995-013-1372-0

Sarkadi, A., Kristiansson, R., Oberklaid, F., & Bremberg, S. (2008). Fathers' involvement and children's developmental outcomes: A systematic review of longitudinal studies. *Acta Paediatrica, 97*, 153–158.

Saxbe, D. E., Edelstein, R. S., Lyden, H. M., Wardecker, B. M., Chopik, W. J., & Moors, A. C. (2017). Fathers' decline in testosterone and synchrony with partner testosterone during pregnancy predicts greater postpartum relationship investment. *Hormones and Behavior, 90*, 39–47. https://doi.org/10.1016/j.yhbeh.2016.07.005

Schoppe-Sullivan, S. J., Brown, G. L., Cannon, E. A., Mangelsdorf, S. C., & Sokolowski, M. S. (2008). Maternal gatekeeping, coparenting quality, and fathering behavior in families with infants. *Journal of Family Psychology, 22*(3), 389–398. https://doi.org/10.1037/0893-3200.22.3.389

Sethna, V., Murray, L., Edmondson, O., Iles, J., & Ramchandani, P. G. (2018). Depression and playfulness in fathers and young infants: A matched design comparison study. *Journal of Affective Disorders, 229*, 364–370. https://doi.org/10.1016/j.jad.2017.12.107

Shannon, J. D., Baumwell, L., & Tamis-LeMonda, C. (2013). Transition to parenting within context. In *Handbook of family theories: A content-based approach* (pp. 249–262). New York: Routledge.

Shannon, J. D., Cabrera, N., Tamis-LeMonda, C., & Lamb, M. E. (2009). Who stays and who leaves? Father accessibility across children's first 5 years. *Parenting: Science and Practice, 9*(1–2), 78–100. https://doi.org/10.1080/15295190802656786

Singley, D. B., & Edwards, L. M. (2015). Men's perinatal mental health in the transition to fatherhood. *Professional Psychology: Research and Practice, 46*(5), 309–316. https://doi.org/10.1037/pro0000032

Solomon, J., & George, C. (1996). Defining the caregiving system: Toward a theory of caregiving. *Infant Mental Health Journal, 17*(3), 183–197. https://doi.org/10.1002/(SICI)1097-0355(199623)17:3<183::AID-IMHJ1>3.0.CO;2-Q

Sroufe, L. A. (2005). Attachment and development: A prospective, longitudinal study from birth to adulthood. *Attachment & Human Development, 7*(4), 349–367. https://doi.org/10.1080/14616730500365928

St George, J., & Freeman, E. (2017). Measurement of father–child rough-and-tumble play and its relations to child behavior. *Infant Mental Health Journal, 38*(6), 709–725. https://doi.org/10.1002/imhj.21676

Stefana, A., Padovani, E. M., Biban, P., & Lavelli, M. (2018). Fathers' experiences with their preterm babies admitted to neonatal intensive care unit: A multi-method study. *Journal of Advanced Nursing, 74*(5), 1090–1098. https://doi.org/10.1111/jan.13527

Stroud, C. B., Durbin, C. E., Wilson, S., & Mendelsohn, K. A. (2011). Spillover to triadic and dyadic systems in families with young children. *Journal of Family Psychology, 25*(6), 919–930. https://doi.org/10.1037/a0025443

Swain, J. E., Dayton, C. J., Kim, P., Tolman, R. M., & Volling, B. L. (2014). Progress on the paternal brain: Theory, animal models, human brain research, and mental health implications. *Infant Mental Health Journal, 35*(5), 394–408. https://doi.org/10.1002/imhj.21471

Tooten, A., Hall, R. A. S., Hoffenkamp, H. N., Braeken, J., Vingerhoets, A. J. J. M., & van Bakel, H. J. A. (2014). Maternal and paternal infant representation: A comparison between parents of term and preterm infants. *Infant Behaviora nd Development, 37*, 366–379.

Underwood, L., Waldie, K. E., Peterson, E., D'Souza, S., Verbiest, M., McDaid, F., et al. (2017). Paternal depression symptoms during pregnancy and after childbirth among participants in the growing up in New Zealand study. *JAMA Psychiatry, 74*(4), 360–369. https://doi.org/10.1001/jamapsychiatry.2016.4234

Volling, B. L. (2005). The transition to siblinghood: A developmental ecological systems perspective and directions for future research. *Journal of Family Psychology, 19*(4), 542–549. https://doi.org/10.1037/0893-3200.19.4.542

Volling, B. L., Cabrera, N., Feinberg, M. E., Jones, D. E., McDaniel, B. T., Liu, S., ... Cookston, J. T. (2019, March 1). Advancing research and measurement on fathering and children's development. *Monographs of the Society for Research in Child Development, 84*(1). Serial No. 332. https://doi.org/10.1111/mono.12404

Vreeswijk, C. M. J. M., Maas, A. J. B. M., Rijk, C. H. A. M., Braeken, J., & van Bakel, H. J. A. (2014). Stability of fathers' representations of their infants during the transition to parenthood. *Attachment & Human Development, 16*(3), 292–306. https://doi.org/10.1080/14616734.2014.900095

Vreeswijk, C. M. J. M., Maas, A. J. B. M., Rijk, C. H. A. M., & van Bakel, H. J. A. (2014). Fathers' experiences during pregnancy: Paternal prenatal attachment and representations of the fetus. *Psychology of Men & Masculinity, 15*(2), 129–137. https://doi.org/10.1037/a0033070

Vreeswijk, C. M. J. M., Rijk, C. H. A. M., Maas, A. J. B. M., & Bakel, H. J. A. (2015). Fathers' and mothers' representations of the infant: Associations with prenatal risk factors. *Infant Mental Health Journal, 36*(6), 599–612. https://doi.org/10.1002/imhj.21541

Walsh, T. B., Tolman, R. M., Davis, R. N., Palladino, C. L., Romero, V. C., & Singh, V. (2014). Moving up the "magic moment": Fathers' experience of prenatal ultrasound. *Fathering: A Journal of Theory, Research, and Practice About Men as Fathers, 12*(1), 18–37. https://doi.org/10.3149/fth.1201.18

Weaver, R. H., & Cranley, M. S. (1983). An Exploration of paternal-fetal attachment behavior. [Editorial]. *Nursing Research, 32*(2), 68–72.

Widarsson, M., Engström, G., Tydén, T., Lundberg, P., & Hammar, L. M. (2015). 'Paddling upstream': Fathers' involvement during pregnancy as described by expectant fathers and mothers. *Journal of Clinical Nursing, 24*(7–8), 1059–1068. https://doi.org/10.1111/jocn.12784

Wilkes, L., Mannix, J., & Jackson, D. (2012). 'I am going to be a dad': Experiences and expectations of adolescent and young adult expectant fathers. *Journal of Clinical Nursing, 21*(1–2), 180–188. https://doi.org/10.1111/j.1365-2702.2011.03715.x

Winnicott, D. W. (1965). Primary maternal preoccupation. In *The maturational processes and the facilitating environment* (pp. 300–305). New York: Int. Univ. Press.

Woody, C. A., Ferrari, A. J., Siskind, D. J., Whiteford, H. A., & Harris, M. G. (2017). A systematic review and meta-regression of the prevalence and incidence of perinatal depression. *Journal of Affective Disorders, 219*, 86–92. https://doi.org/10.1016/j.jad.2017.05.003

Yarcheski, A., Mahon, N. E., Yarcheski, T. J., Hanks, M. M., & Cannella, B. L. (2009). A meta-analytic study of predictors of maternal-fetal attachment. *International Journal of Nursing Studies, 46*(5), 708–715. https://doi.org/10.1016/j.ijnurstu.2008.10.013

Yildiz, P. D., Ayers, S., & Phillips, L. (2017). The prevalence of posttraumatic stress disorder in pregnancy and after birth: A systematic review and meta-analysis. *Journal of Affective Disorders, 208*, 634–645. https://doi.org/10.1016/j.jad.2016.10.009

Yu, C., Hung, C., Chan, T., Yeh, C., & Lai, C. (2012). Prenatal predictors for father-infant attachment after childbirth. *Journal of Clinical Nursing, 21*(11–12), 1577–1583. https://doi.org/10.1111/j.1365-2702.2011.04003.x

Zeanah, C. H., Benoit, D., Barton, M., Regan, C., Hirshberg, L. M., & Lipsitt, L. P. (1993). Representations of attachment in mothers and their one-year-old infants. *Journal of the American Academy of Child & Adolescent Psychiatry, 32*(2), 278–286. https://doi.org/10.1097/00004583-199303000-00007

Zeman, J., Cassano, M., Perry-Parrish, C., & Stegall, S. (2006). Emotion regulation in children and adolescents. *Journal of Developmental and Behavioral Pediatrics, 27*(2), 155–168. Retrieved from psyh. (2006-07178-012).

Zoja, L. (2018). *The father: Historical, psychological and cultural perspectives*. Retrieved from http://proxy.lib.umich.edu/login?url=http://search.ebscohost.com/login.aspx?direct=true&db=psyh&AN=2002-11585-009&site=ehost-live&scope=site

Ghosts in the Ultrasound: Expectant Fathers' Experience of Trauma

13

Richard M. Tolman and Tova B. Walsh

An ultrasound provides a window into the womb, a somewhat disorienting fuzzy view of a life within a life. With organs and spine visible through transparent skin, these first images can appear ghostlike and otherworldly. These indistinct and confusing images seen on the screen are often subjected to parental (and sonographer) projections. For example, seeking connection, parents may speculate about family resemblances or suggest that a specific fetal movement indicates the future child will one day enjoy the same activities as the parent (e.g., a kick is interpreted to mean the child is a future soccer player) (Walsh, 2018). The ultrasound images collected, codified, and analyzed are intended, in the medical realm, to identify risk to the fetus. Whatever the medical value of the routine fetal ultrasound, it has become an almost universal ritual on the route to parenthood, often experienced as a social event and opportunity for connection with the baby. But if the internal experiences of the fathers who attend a prenatal ultrasound could be similarly displayed, one might also discern fuzzy transparent images: "ghosts" of traumas and adverse experiences that many fathers have lived through. In 1975, Selma Fraiberg, with colleagues Edna Adleson and Vivian Shapiro, published the groundbreaking paper "Ghosts in the Nursery: A Psychoanalytic Approach to the Problems of Impaired Infant-Mother Relationships." The paper introduced the concept of "ghosts in the nursery" to describe the intrusion of a parent's conflicted past on present-day parenting. The "ghosts" are metaphorical, representing maternal developmental experiences that then influence maternal-infant interactions. The "nursery" is also metaphorical, as the interactions of parents with their children of course exist across settings beyond a room the infant occupies. As Fraiberg described it, the conflicted past of a parent "may break through the magic circle in an unguarded moment," and parents and children "may find themselves reenacting a moment or a scene from another time…." These ghosts interfere in parental relationships with their children and "appear to do their mischief according to a historical or topical agenda, specializing in such areas as feeding, sleep toilet training or discipline…" (pp. 377–388).

While Fraiberg spoke of parents, she mainly considered maternal ghosts in her work. Barrows (2004) extended the metaphor of "ghosts in the nursery" to consideration of the developmental histories of fathers, challenging the infant mental health field's privileging of maternal "ghosts" over their paternal versions. Barrows makes a case for the importance of attending to the role of

R. M. Tolman (✉)
School of Social Work, University of Michigan, Ann Arbor, MI, USA
e-mail: rtolman@umich.edu

T. B. Walsh
School of Social Work, University of Wisconsin, Madison, WI, USA

H. E. Fitzgerald et al. (eds.), *Handbook of Fathers and Child Development*,
https://doi.org/10.1007/978-3-030-51027-5_13

fathers in child development, and he theorizes about the location of ghosts in the internal worlds of parents, concluding they are perhaps best considered as introjected objects. The therapeutic task becomes one of assisting parents to "assimilate" these objects into the ego, thus interrupting the transmission of parental experiences to their offspring.

Here we extend the "ghosts" metaphor beyond, or rather to before, an infant inhabits the nursery; we believe paternal "ghosts" begin to make their presence known during pregnancy.

These ghosts are present just below the surface of fathers' experience in the ultrasound, rarely if ever are they made evident in that setting or spoken about explicitly. However, in our interviews with fathers immediately after participating in an ultrasound appointment, these "ghosts of trauma past" emerge readily. Not ever directly bidden or specifically probed for, they emerge from conversation starters like "Tell me about your experience of the ultrasound today" or "What impact do you think the ultrasound today will have on your becoming a father?" That these questions elicit trauma narratives is in itself meaningful. These prenatal ghosts simultaneously influence the developing bond between expectant parent and child-to-be and also their relationship to their pregnant partner. (Note: the fathers we interviewed think and speak of the fetus as a "child" or "baby" "to-be," and we use these terms to be consistent with paternal representations.) The acknowledgement of the presence of these ghosts during the prenatal period presents an opportunity for preventive intervention to protect against a possible impairment of the parent-child relationship and the parent-child triad. There is extensive research to demonstrate that parents' own experiences as a child influence later parenting of their own children (Belsky, Conger, & Capaldi, 2009; Madden et al., 2015; Van IJzendoorn, 1992). More specifically, a parent's own early experience of adverse childhood experiences has been shown to influence their parenting stress and parenting practices (Lange, Callinan, & Smith, 2019; Lyons-Ruth & Block, 1996). Traumatic stress has been linked to decreased maternal ability to provide safe and sensitive parenting for children. Less is known about how trauma may impact upon fathering and upon paternal capacity to support their partners and co-parent effectively.

In this chapter, we will recount some of the paternal "ghosts" that emerge in the context of an interview after an ultrasound, at an important stage of the prenatal period. We explore not only the types of "ghosts" that emerge but also what it might mean that they surface at this particular moment in expectant fathers' lives. We will examine what implications this might have for how to best support men in their transition to fatherhood and how it might benefit them, their partners, and their children for us to heed these ghosts.

Transition to Fatherhood

Research demonstrates that fathers' active engagement with their children provides cognitive, behavioral, and social benefits that have lasting developmental benefits, from infancy to adolescence and beyond (Leidy, Schofield, & Parke, 2013; Pleck, 2010; Sarkadi, Kristiansson, Oberklaid, & Bremberg, 2008). This engagement can begin, or at least be shaped, during the prenatal period. Marsiglio (2008) conceptualized three domains of prenatal involvement—prenatal involvement with their pregnant partner, child (fetal)-focused prenatal activity, and the prospective construction of a father identity. Paternal involvement in the prenatal period can have profound influence on maternal and child health outcomes, including increasing mothers' health behaviors (Bloch et al., 2010; Teitler, 2001), earlier and increased prenatal care (Martin, McNamara, Milot, Haalle, & Hair, 2007; Singer, 2012), maternal well-being (Bloch et al., 2010), reduced smoking (Bloch et al., 2010; Martin et al., 2007), reduction of preterm births and low birth weight (Alio, Kornosky, Mbah, Marty, & Salihu, 2010; Bloch et al., 2010; Lee, Sanchez, Grogan-Kaylor, Lee, & Albuja, 2018), and lower infant mortality (Alio, Mbah, Koronosky, Wathington, Marty & Salihu, 2011) and prenatal paternal involvement is associated with later paternal engagement (Cabrera, Fagan & Farrie, 2008).

Paternal participation in prenatal care is increasing, and attendance at prenatal ultrasound examinations is rapidly becoming a norm in the United States. Expectant fathers are now playing an expanded role during pregnancy, labor, and delivery as compared to earlier eras. This raises issues for what men need to know about preparing themselves for fatherhood and to support their pregnant partner's health needs, which are altered and intensified during pregnancy.

Beyond knowledge needs, the transition to fatherhood raises many other concerns for men that can task their ability to adjust and cope. Yet, there are serious gaps in the availability of support for expectant fathers. In the prenatal healthcare system, expectant fathers recognize their role as "parent and partner" and yet experience treatment as "not-patient and not-visitor" (Steen, Downe, Bamford, & Edozien, 2012), which can lead to feelings of exclusion and alienation.

The prenatal period provides an opportunity to examine how paternal trauma may impact upon development of positive parenting and partnering. In our quantitative research, we have found that by both maternal report and paternal report, the great majority of men attend a prenatal ultrasound. In a nationally representative sample of households with children aged 10 and below, by maternal report (Walsh, Tolman, Singh, Davis, & Davis, 2017), we found that 80.3% of biological fathers attended a prenatal ultrasound visit. We replicated that study with a nationally representative study of men aged 18–35 and found that 88% of fathers of children aged 0–3 reported attending at least one ultrasound visit (Walsh et al., 2019). While disparities exist, e.g., fathers with less than high school education and low-income fathers are less likely to attend the ultrasound visit, even in these higher risk groups, the large majority of men report ultrasound attendance. Thus, in our view, prenatal visits serve as a convenient and meaningful site for engaging expectant fathers.

Qualitative Research with Expectant Fathers Attending Ultrasound

Initial Study

We have conducted a series of studies that have all included a one-on-one, semi-structured interview with expectant fathers who attended their partner's routine prenatal ultrasound. In our initial study, we recruited 22 men who attended a routine ultrasound with their pregnant partner at approximately 16–20 weeks' gestation. Our goal was to understand the experience of ultrasound attendance for expectant fathers and to explore the meaning and potential utility of engaging expectant fathers at this time of fatherhood. We interviewed fathers directly following the ultrasound examination, and in these interviews, we collected many accounts of the relief, exhilaration, and motivation that attending an ultrasound could produce. As one participant told us:

> You're just kind of like blown away… just kind of like wow, like a piece of you is just about to be here. That's really basically how I felt. I was just like so many emotions, I was just like happy, sad, excited, worried. It's just like all emotions just flash through your mind… It just felt like- the feeling's indescribable.

We were so struck by the power of these mainly positively valanced experiences that we characterized ultrasound as an opportunity for "moving up the magic moment" (Walsh et al., 2014). We noted that past literature focused on labor and delivery as a golden or magic moment for interventions to promote positive parent-child and partner relationships. But our interviews with fathers during pregnancy suggested that fathers' enchantment with the developing fetus and with the potential of what fatherhood might mean for them offered an earlier opportunity for engagement.

We identified a set of main themes from the interviews that reflect the significance of prenatal ultrasound attendance for fathers. These include (1) reassurance that the pregnancy is proceeding normally, (2) heightened reality of the pregnancy and child, (3) rapid expansion of thoughts and feelings about becoming a parent, (4) importance to partner relationship, (5) influence of the clinic setting, and (6) men's motivation to change as a result of pregnancy. We did not specifically probe for men's motivation to make changes—that theme emerged from participants who, unprompted, spoke about changes they wanted to make to enhance their health, relationships, finances, and work-life balance. This theme informed the design of our subsequent studies, which constitute most of this chapter. We set out in our subsequent work to learn more specifically how expectant fathers might be motivated by the ultrasound appointment and by the pregnancy overall to make changes in preparation for fatherhood.

Present Study In the second phase of our qualitative work, as in our initial study, we focused on recruitment of expectant fathers after attending a routine prenatal ultrasound appointment midway through pregnancy. We developed an interview protocol that we implemented across two settings, using recruitment methods and interview settings that diverged in some ways. Rather than creating a threat to comparability of the data, we believe these divergences give the common themes that emerged more credibility.

At one institution, we recruited as we did in the first study described. We approached expectant fathers who were present for a routine prenatal ultrasound and asked for their permission to interview them after the ultrasound. Both the expectant father and mother needed to give consent for this interview. When both members of the couple consented to be interviewed, we also asked for permission to sit unobtrusively in the ultrasound exam in order to monitor the expectant father's participation and responses during the exam. Twenty-five fathers participated in this study.

At the second institution, pregnant women and their partners were recruited from four obstetric and gynecology clinics. Flyers about the study included information that the study was open to expectant first-time parents, including both mothers and fathers, who attend a routine prenatal ultrasound examination at ~20 weeks' gestation. Ultimately, 22 expectant fathers from this site participated in the study. At this site, we met participants at the clinic prior to the ultrasound examination and conducted structured observation during the ultrasound, taking notes using an adaptation of the "Observation of Routine Screen Form" (Boukydis et al., 2006). The form was modified to record the engagement of fathers in addition to mothers and the nature as well as number of questions and comments during the exam, since this form has not previously been used in research with fathers. Following the exam, expectant fathers and mothers were interviewed individually.

Table 13.1 summarizes the demographic characteristics of the respondents in each setting. In both settings, we used the same interview protocol with expectant fathers. Interviews were semi-structured and audio-recorded and took approximately 30 minutes to complete. We kept

Table 13.1 Demographic characteristics of the sample

	Site 1 (N = 25)	Site 2 (N = 20)
Age in years		
≤ 24	6	2
25–34	11	17
≥ 35	7	1
Race/ethnicity		
White	9	14
Black	2	4
Asian	3	1
Latino	5	3
Native American	1	
Other (biracial or declined to answer)	5	
Education		
Some high school		–
High school	3	3
Some college	7	8
Completed college or more	15	9
Employment Full-time	23	18
Part-time Unemployed	1	–
	1	2
Household income per year		
<$25,000	4	1
$25,000–$49,999	9	8
$50,000–$74,999	2	4
>$75,000–	10	7

the time short to accommodate schedules as many of the fathers and mothers needed to return to work or childcare and to minimize interference with the couple's time together subsequent to the prenatal visit.

The broad domains of the interview included the following: (1) experience attending ultrasound and other prenatal visits, (2) thoughts and questions about father role during pregnancy, (3) personal goals in anticipation of fatherhood, and (4) perceived need for information and support in the transition to fatherhood.

Data Analysis

Each interview was professionally transcribed. We conducted thematic analysis of interview data, drawing on principles of grounded theory (Strauss & Corbin, 1998). We used an iterative process of review to develop codes for data interpretation, independently review transcripts and then discuss, repeat until we reached agreement on code definitions, and then apply final codes to the data. We conducted within-case and cross-case analyses and met regularly to discuss cases and identify emerging themes, which we verified by going back to the data. Transcripts were entered into Dedoose software 8.2 (Dedoose, 2019) and NVIVO 11 software (setting 2; QSR International, 2015) to assist with data analysis.

Results

A pattern emerged from our analysis of the interviews we conducted. Many fathers, as they reflected on their experience at the ultrasound and in prenatal care, their thoughts and feelings about becoming a father, and the changes they wished to make in preparation for fatherhood, spoke about their own past experience of traumas and adverse experiences. While we did not directly question fathers about the past, over time we began to anticipate that fathers might discuss these types of experiences. As interviewers, we were empathic toward fathers' accounts of their past experiences but did not probe them in detail or ask for additional description of what they had experienced. In the brief span of time available for the interviews and given that the exam and positive news about the health and normal development of the fetus was mainly a positively valenced event for fathers, we did not attempt to engage fathers in more detailed discussion of these emotionally charged topics. We listened and validated what fathers shared and then continued to prompt for the implications of their adverse experiences on their own readiness to be fathers.

Out of the accounts of past traumatic and adverse experiences, multiple categories emerged. We classified the experiences of *traumas* into several subcategories, including losses related to previous pregnancies, parental (both maternal and paternal) absence, abuse or neglect during childhood, and exposure to domestic violence and other violent environments. In the classification other *adverse childhood experiences*, subcategories included parental substance abuse, parental divorce or separation, and harsh discipline. In terms of other stressors or *adverse adult experiences*, the following subcategories emerged: pregnancy related, lack of support, and external stressors.

Traumas

Pregnancy Loss Discovered During Ultrasound

Some of the traumas that fathers raised concerned previous pregnancies. The salience of these traumas to the current interview situation seemed quite evident as the men had just attended a compelling prenatal visit focused on the current pregnancy. A traumatic loss discovered at a prior ultrasound could be triggered by a subsequent ultrasound, as one father described:

> …last time what happened was, I ended up fainting in one of these because it was during the miscarriage one and the lady just basically put the thing up, the, uh, ultra…what is it, the camera; she was going like this and she said, oh I'm sorry to let you know but, you know, this is … I was holding onto something and then I remember just hitting, I hit the floor….

This account may characterize the way fathers are largely unseen in prenatal care—no professional staff addressed this father's previous experience of passing out at an ultrasound with him in preparation for the current visit. The technician who conducted the current ultrasound most likely did not know this history and could not make adjustments in interacting with this father at a time of particular vulnerability.

Pregnancy Loss

The memory of a traumatic loss of a child during pregnancy, even when the memory was not directly linked to an ultrasound examination, could be triggered at important moments during a subsequent pregnancy. As one father with experience of a prior loss described, an ultrasound can prompt memories of how a prior ultrasound offered reassurance but ultimately the pregnancy was lost:

> We had this … where we're looking at [the ultrasound screen] and we're like, yeah, this looks good, you know and everything looked fine and, you know, then you find out that it's not… Obviously you want your kid to be fine, and you know to assume that it is and then all of a sudden found out it's not, is like devastating. That's what happened to us before so it … kind of shadows you… Right now that's kind of the only thing that I can think of….

Another respondent shows the complexity of the emotions regarding a pregnancy loss and the impact it may have on paternal-fetal attachment in a subsequent pregnancy. On the one hand, he wishes for more emotional preparation. On the other hand, he seems to deny the emotionality by noting that fathers are more logical than mothers. It seems he may be protecting himself from involvement with the fetus to manage the anxiety of the potential loss of the pregnancy:

> It's always scary for me; we had a miscarriage before…so there's, I feel like there's not really a lot of preparation emotionally going in there:… and what if it was a bad situation today? …So these are, these are kind of like mixed blessings for me to come and see that the heart is beating, but I feel like there's two lenses from the mother who's emotionally wrapped into it and looking at it from like; oh there's the heart and then the father who's more kind of, I don't know, I don't want to say logical or reasonable coming from a point of reason, but I think it's just a different view that a father has with looking at the ultrasound.

Parental Absence

The literature is replete with evidence of the negative impacts of father absence. Hence, many men are motivated to overcome such negative impacts as the absence of their own fathers to become good fathers themselves. The absence of their own fathers emerged as a key theme in our interviews:

> I just want things to be different. I didn't have a father I could go to and I want to be there for my son, want him to know he can come to me with anything. Just want to know what I need to know so I can get it right.

Of course, loss of a mother also resonates for a man as he prepares to become a parent himself. One respondent tied this preparation directly to his ability to be supportive to his partner and imagined an impact on his ability to co-parent:

> My mother was never in the picture so that's gonna be a hard part; is understanding what my wife is going through as a mom because there was never a mom in the picture.

Abusive/Neglectful Parent

While the loss or absence of a parent resonates deeply, the presence of an abusive parent looms large as well:

> I was beaten growing up you know so physical…I guess physical confrontation, gray area. Yeah, it damages you in ways that you really can't…you know you really can't imagine…You know I'm 27 years old now and I'm still dealing with nonsense from when I was 12 years old. You're like just…it's like hell, what are you gonna do? Just stay away from hitting them.

The expectant father who passed out upon learning about the pregnancy loss is one of the men in our sample who had experienced abuse in his own childhood. It's not hard to imagine the cumulative toll of loss and trauma that this man experienced creating an unbearable amount of anxiety in the context of becoming a father.

The interviews illuminated the salience of the intergenerational transmission process of childhood trauma during pregnancy:

> My father's been divorced twice so he doesn't…he doesn't want me being a father, he doesn't want me being a husband. He doesn't want me doing anything like that. He wants me to focus on myself and getting through this life alone because that's what he's doing… And I told him, I'm like, dad you are going to die a sad and lonely man. And both of my brothers have taken to…have taken to that lifestyle and I see what it does to people… and it sucks. … it's sad... I don't even call him dad anymore you know.

As this father exhibited, some expectant fathers have awareness of the risk of becoming such a father and strive to resist it and intentionally choose another way of being in relationships. Their accounts highlight the many forces at play in a man's transition to fatherhood and suggest the value of support for those who must not only resist repeating patterns of the past but identify new ways of going forward.

Exposure to Domestic Violence

Experiencing the abuse of one's parent by another can traumatize a child. Reflecting upon his own childhood experiences after attending an ultrasound for his future child, one father who was exposed to domestic violence as a child shared his relief upon learning that his expected child is male. Specifically, he was relieved to avoid the risk that a daughter would face from predatory men and how that might prompt his own violent response. This account also shows how some fathers recognize the risks of passing on their exposure to violence and work to resist its transmission:

> If it was a daughter I would have been at the police station right now like, save me a bed. …Cause it's crazy out here man and you don't know who to trust…And me having knowing that my momma and my sister got raped …I might be too protective now not knowing that I'm too protective because I know what's out here.

Exposure to Violent Environments

In addition to childhood exposure to family violence, some respondents also noted violent environments in discussing preparation for becoming a father. Here, the respondent recalls the extreme violence he experiences and suggests that the child he is expecting relates to his chance to reconcile his own traumatic history:

> I've been shot five times... just getting my son [is] a second chance, giving me a second chance through another body.

Interviewed immediately after attending an ultrasound, fathers regularly surfaced the greatest challenges they face and went on to discuss how that would impact their need to protect and care for their future child.

Other Adverse Childhood Experiences

Respondents also reported a host of other adverse childhood experiences, related to those we have classified as traumatic, but which, when we considered the overall context of what a father reported, did not warrant being classified as a trauma. As can be seen in the descriptions below, most of these were related to parenting, and these experiences were unsurprisingly on the minds of the expectant fathers as they looked ahead to becoming parents.

Parent with Problem Drinking/Drug Use

Many respondents discussed their own substance use and misuse as something they needed to change to be ready to parent their expected child. For several respondents, the history of substance misuse in their own family of origin was recalled as they discussed this:

> I want there to be laughter. There was never any laughter in the house and there still isn't. There's just, you know, two alcoholics and one want-to-be Christian. … And it's like okay what's the best way this can be avoided?

Whether reflecting on their own substance misuse or that of important people in their lives, fathers emphasized their wish to protect their children from exposure to substance misuse and the household environment of families struggling with substance misuse.

Harsh Parenting

Not all harsh parenting may be experienced as traumatic, though recent literature documents the negative developmental impact of physical punishment. Here again, we see the formulation of resistance to intergenerational patterns of discipline on the part of the expectant father:

> I come from a way more severe style of parenting and um, learning through [my partner] I was able to see, um, the part that I'm not that good about that... I just feel like no matter what happens I want to always be there to support my child, no matter how stupid thing they can possibly do, I'm gonna be there to love them and just make sure they always know that.

Fathers affirmed their wish to always "be there" for their child and often described a reliance of their partner to help them make needed adjustments to be the father they aspired to be.

Divorce and Parental Separation

Unsurprisingly, perhaps, even when not perceived as traumatic, parental separations found a place in the narratives of the expectant fathers, as they discussed their own readiness to parent their expected child:

> I had a really, I wouldn't say traumatic childhood, but some really messed-up family experiences that I'm still dealing with. But you know I buried my dad at 21, and my first memory is my parents divorcing when I was my son's age, my eldest son. So, and I got the whole wicked stepfather from whatever Disney film we picked....

Fathers referred to experiences of separation, reflected on the impact, and discussed how they want things to be different with their own child.

Sibling Health Crisis

Perhaps prompted by presence in a medical setting, with the aim of determining the health of the developing fetus, other threats to a child's health might be salient for expectant fathers:

> My younger sister, my only sister, has a, had two holes in her heart in the, I can't think of what it's called, in the walls of the heart. So she had like a heart murmur when she was born. ... I remember when they had to do open heart surgery on her. I remember even though I was so little because my parents and grandparents, everybody was really worried and I was scared too. So today I just really wanted to know about the heart.

Anxiety about the healthy development of the fetus is a prominent theme across our interviews. Fathers who had experience with health challenges among family members and close friends were particularly likely to invoke the possibility of health problems and highlight their relief following a reassuring ultrasound.

Major Stressors

Our interviews also unearthed accounts of numerous other stressful experiences and conditions that respondents linked to their readiness to be parents. We classified these in three subcategories: pregnancy related, lack of support, and external stressors.

Pregnancy Related

Some fathers described feeling initially ambivalent about the pregnancy and the stress and confusion that prompted:

> The test showed up positive and she was all ecstatic and I'm like; well I wasn't disappointed I'm just like uh, it's gonna be hard, it's gonna be exhausting. ... I don't not want the baby but maybe a little bit of I'm not ready or we're not going to be able to handle it with work and all that stuff.

Others described fears related to labor and delivery:

> When the day actually comes, well like I don't do well in situations where there's blood... I more than likely will probably pass out when my baby is born... I want to be there, I want to be a part of it obviously, but I don't...my wife doesn't need to just have a baby and then have her husband laying on the floor next to her.

For some fathers, worry about disconnection from their partner was foremost on their mind:

> The first few months [my girlfriend] was just, she was so sick it was hard to communicate about a lot of stuff because she would go to work all day and

> she'd come home... And she would just literally go to sleep on the couch or the bed at six, seven o'clock and that was it. You know we'd both get home from work by 5:30 or 6 o'clock. So, that was hard because I couldn't talk to her, couldn't do anything for her.

Across these examples of pregnancy-related stressors, fathers' worries all reflected a wish to be there for their partner and the baby, to be reliable, to know what needed to be done and do it to be effectively supportive, and to maintain connection.

Lack of Support

Fathers offered many examples of gaps in support available to them and recognized the absence of support as a barrier to their ability to find connection, empathy, and guidance for their parenting. The absence of family support was noted as a particular challenge. In some cases, the absence of support was attributed to family members' views about the pregnancy:

> My parents think we're too young, think we're making a mistake. Maybe money's tight but we'll make it work… That's the hardest part, that they're not happy about it.

In one instance, fresh grief and a parent's absence meant that support that would previously have been available was not currently available:

> My mom had a stroke not that long ago. So like there's just a lot of things that I'm thinking about and sometimes I just, some things fall by the wayside… Just I don't know, really wish we had a kid sooner because it would have made my mom so happy. Not sure how I'm gonna do it without her.

Fathers also described feeling isolated when support was not available from people who shared important aspects of their identity:

> I need to know more dads who know some of the struggles with the whole bi-racial thing. … you know not saying that only having a black family, only having a white family is a bad or good thing or whatever; it's just that they may, you may not fully understand the struggles or whatever, so it's nice to have people like you.

External Stressors

Fathers spoke of a number of stressors they face, which impact on their priorities as they anticipate their child's birth. Many fathers described significant financial stress and their recognition that their child would be depending on them:

> I need to get my own place, learn how to drive... I need to make sure I have a steady job because my child eating depends on me. If I don't work, he don't eat… I want to make sure that my child has every opportunity possible to do something great. So I'm gonna do whatever it takes….

Fathers also described work-related stress and concerns about balancing work and family:

> I have a fairly stressful job and so I'm worried about that. Like right now I don't have a ton of time so like when a kid comes … I don't know how it's all gonna fit.

In many ways, in discussing traumas, adverse childhood experiences, and other major past or current stressors that they face, fathers demonstrated their awareness that their behaviors and choices will shape their child's well-being and identified the opportunity to make choices to do differently in the future for the sake of their child and the father-child relationship they dream of.

Discussion

Men's openness and engagement in conversations following a prenatal ultrasound appointment demonstrate the promise of using that opportunity to reach out to expectant fathers in that setting. The pervasiveness of trauma and the potential pernicious impact it can have on partnering and parenting demonstrate the need to provide a gateway toward supportive services to address trauma and increase capacity to be effective fathers. Such services could help to address the risk that these traumatic and adverse events pose for effective parenting.

During pregnancy, both mothers and fathers develop a mental representation of the baby—they begin to imagine their future child and their relationship to that child. Their imagination is shaped by their own early experiences, including particularly attachment experiences. Pregnancy in general and prenatal ultrasound in particular present an opportunity to engage fathers and create space for them to reflect on their own relationship histories, the relationship they hope to build with their child, and the steps they will take to get there. Prenatal mental representations and parental-fetal (including maternal-fetal as well as paternal-fetal) attachment have been found to be associated with post-birth representations, parenting, and parent-child relationships (Benoit, Parker, & Zeanah, 1997; Condon & Corkindale, 1997; Siddiqui & Hägglöf, 2000). It is thus important to find ways to support all expectant parents during pregnancy. Given that most fathers attend an ultrasound exam or at least one prenatal visit, that engagement with the health-care system provides a prime opportunity for engaging, assessing, and supporting fathers in ways that will promote positive involvement, optimize attachment, and foster a supportive fathering trajectory.

Our research explored fathers' experiences in prenatal care and some of the traumas and sources of stress that emerged or became more salient during pregnancy, specifically at the ultrasound examination. Learning more about what fathers want and need from prenatal care and building understanding of potential opportunities to enhance father engagement in prenatal care settings hold promise for better supporting families at a critical moment for relationship development. In addition, in order to better engage and identify the needs of those fathers that do attend ultrasound, greater outreach is needed to welcome and encourage fathers' attendance and to connect with and support those fathers who do not attend.

In *Ghosts in the Nursery*, Fraiberg notes that many people experience pain or difficulty during childhood but that not all parents inflict that same pain on their children. She recognizes the motivation that parents bring, and we heard often in our interviews with fathers that they wanted to do better for their children and to resist the transmission of the painful past to the next generation. But Fraiberg also recognized that it is important to understand what can prevent the repetition. She emphasized the importance of remembering the pain. However, remembering alone is not enough to exorcise traumatic experiences. Fraiberg also noted although their parenting may be impacted, parents who have experienced adverse childhood experiences themselves may not seek or be receptive to support when offered:

> These parents may not come to us for professional guidance. Ghosts who have established their residence privileges for three or more generations may not, in fact, be identified as representatives of the parental past. There may be no readiness on the part of the parents to form an alliance with us to protect the baby. More likely we, and not the ghosts, will appear as the intruders. (pp. 388)

Our interviews hold some hope that some fathers could indeed welcome this help. Most fathers were eager participants in our interviews, and some acknowledged gratitude for the opportunity to focus on their own experiences in conversation with an empathic listener at the midpoint of a pregnancy. Fathers regularly referred back to their own history of adverse experiences, and some expressed active resistance to the potential that they would pass on these adverse experiences to their own children. Many seemed energized and motivated to exorcise these influences from their own parenting.

Given the salience of fathers' negative memories and experiences during this period, inviting fathers to reflect upon what is evoked during the pregnancy could be one component of prenatal care and support that might foster optimal developmental outcomes. Professionals can facilitate recognition that "ghosts" can influence the developing bond between parent and child-to-be and affirm the opportunity for fathers to reduce the power of such ghosts to intrude through conscious effort. This might include direct support or referrals for support, to remember, reflect upon, and avoid repeating the pain of the past.

Prompt Information for Couples with Prior Pregnancy Loss

Loss of a prior pregnancy and birth complications comprise one subset of traumatic experiences clearly and directly relevant in the prenatal care setting. One father who had experienced a prior pregnancy loss envisioned a way to address these issues, but he saw little chance of actual implementation:

> This is probably something that won't even be possible but…and the only reason I say it is because of what we went through before. Like when you're in there, just to have…and like I said, I don't know if it's possible, but to have someone in there that is like okay to tell you like that things are okay.

O'Leary (2009) describes the issues parents face in a subsequent pregnancy after a loss. She notes that fathers are frequently overlooked at the time of the loss and also during a subsequent pregnancy. Fathers' anxieties about the safety of the baby may be heightened, eliciting the need for more reassurance about the progress of the pregnancy and the viability of the fetus. Fathers' experiences of risk to the mother's life may also be activated, as we saw in our interviews. These feelings of anxiety and fear may result in paternal withdrawal or increased controlling behavior toward their pregnant partners Alternately, fathers may defer their own needs to the well-being of the expectant mother, to further protect her and the developing baby, at risk of neglecting their own well-being. Fathers' own well-being is important, and fathers influence the well-being of mothers and babies through positive and negative interactions before and after birth. Both in prenatal care and in the context of other services delivered during pregnancy (e.g., childbirth education, home visiting), attention to fathers' experiences and needs stands to benefit fathers and families.

Why Do these Traumas Emerge Openly?

Coates (2012) addressed the ways that a child might be a traumatic trigger for a parent. She notes that families are a "remembering context," that is, they are rich with situations that can readily evoke memories and affective schemas originating in parents' own childhood families. Clinically, this remembering context gains importance when the child becomes a reminder of earlier parental trauma experiences. She identifies several of the particular triggering contexts that have emerged in her practice, including medical examinations, delivery, baby's cries, baby's screams, defiance and temper tantrums, and physical resemblance. She emphasizes that such triggers are usually very specific.

We don't see this kind of specific triggering as the explanation for the emergence of trauma narratives in our interviews with expectant fathers, except in the examples where the previous trauma was clearly related to the prenatal setting, pregnancy, or labor and delivery itself. A more general mechanism would be needed to explain the broad range of both traumas and other adverse experiences that men spontaneously talked about in the context of preparing themselves for fatherhood. One underlying trigger would be the anxiety that is ambient during pregnancy. While an ultrasound examination that confirms the pregnancy is proceeding normally may quiet some of the immediate fears about the unborn child during pregnancy, it may leave deeper anxieties more accessible to men in the presence of a curious and empathic interviewer. We suspect the dispelling of the health concerns for the fetus and their partners, which would be the most readily available focus for the anxiety men feel, might leave room for the examination of other worries.

We also note that many men who re-experience these past traumatic and adverse events envision their ability to cope and manage these influences. Reestablishing a sense of control can help them contain the anxieties in the transition to fatherhood. When this control is directed toward healthful self-management (e.g., renouncing substance abuse), supportive behaviors toward their partners (e.g., supporting a pregnant partner's healthy eating), or toward preparation for the expected child (e.g., obtaining a crib or discussing names for the baby), this desire for control can be marshalled in service of positive developmental outcomes. If it takes the form of intrusive or coercive actions toward his partner, then the risk of adverse outcomes increases.

Not All Fathers Are Receptive to Support

Not all fathers were open about addressing their thoughts and feelings about emerging fatherhood midway through pregnancy. Some were reserved and gave primarily superficial answers. Some who named losses were reluctant to focus on them:

> Do you have any thoughts about how that might [the loss of your own father when you were two years old] impact your own being a dad? You said you already give yourself some slack and know that kids are resilient.
>
> Yeah, I think uh… Well I guess I haven't thought about that for a while... Um, no, I just think that um, I probably wouldn't be doing any favors to myself or the family by stressing out about, about anything you know. I'm already better relaxed and confident, so that's my tack for now.

A critical aspect of engaging fathers during pregnancy is taking the time to understand what each individual father is experiencing, what challenges he perceives, and what support he is open to. Unlike the context of our interviews, service providers have the opportunity to build a relationship over time and facilitate continued conversation and reflection that may lead to greater readiness to engage and to consider any actions that may be needed to achieve the desired father-child relationship.

Implications for Services

In order to meet the challenge of expectant fathers' needs of support, we note that changes in professional preparation and system changes are needed. Professionals that aid families during pregnancy should have the opportunity and the impetus as part of their training to reflect on their own beliefs and values about the role of a father. Identifying and attending personal beliefs and values that may contribute to a lack of father participation is important. Examples of such contributions may be that father participation is viewed as extra to the mothers, optional, or not important; that fathers represent more risk than positive value to their family; and that fathers are not suited to be caretakers during pregnancy and infancy. Enhancing father participation is a critical step toward enhancing professional capacity to recognize and respond to the needs of fathers. True engagement of fathers depends on individual and institutional commitment to communicate a clear and consistent message that fathers are welcome and valued and their needs matter. Prenatal care, maternal child health, and infant mental health home visiting are among the contexts in which professionals can leverage and create opportunities to include fathers in the provision of support to families surrounding the birth of a child. Our interviews suggest a potential for direct engagement with fathers that addresses their role in pregnancy, infancy, and beyond. Presuming high interest, listening and learning about fathers' own parenting motivation and goals, and offering resources to help fathers achieve their goals are strategies for establishing a foundation of trust to facilitate engagement. Attending to the way in which fathers wish to receive information and support is critical too. One father that we interviewed expressed a clear preference for verbal rather than written communication and opportunity to connect with peers:

> I tend to be more socially oriented, rather than book orientated, so [rather than read something] I want to talk to people about it. I want to have conversations with other men about having kids.

Eliciting and demonstrating sensitivity to fathers' individual needs and preferences for learning and support requires that professionals maintain awareness of the diversity among fathers and do not treat fathers as a monolithic group, and do not rely on gendered stereotypes to guide engagement strategies.

Some possible domains of intervention with both expectant fathers and mothers include prenatal support, diet and nutrition, smoking cessation, delivery involvement, breastfeeding allies, parenting preparation, parenting support, and relationship enhancement (Arora et al., 2000; Blackburn et al., 2005; Bottorff et al., 2006; Flouri & Buchanan, 2003; Singh & Newburn, 2000). The accounts of our interviewees demonstrate that at least some fathers perceive need of support in each of these areas. The period of pregnancy may present a window of heightened motivation to engage on the level necessary to establish behavior change. As one father told us,

> Having a kid is like the main encouragement [to quit]… I watched my parents grow up smoking and that's pretty much; I mean I'm not blaming them for it but, I never thought anything bad about it. I'm like, oh well my mom and dad did it… I think if parents smoke it has a big impact on if your kid takes up smoking at some point. And what it does to you is just horrible.

Supporting fathers toward this type of behavior change will benefit their partners and children.

Summary and Key Points

Across three qualitative studies, 69 expectant fathers were interviewed immediately after attending a prenatal ultrasound approximately midway through pregnancy. Fathers described powerful emotions evoked by attending the ultrasound and demonstrated interest and openness to reflecting on both where they have been and where they are going as they prepare for parenthood. Though our interviews were not designed to elicit "ghosts," in their reflections, fathers voluntarily spoke of many ghosts, i.e., unresolved traumas and painful early experiences that were (re-)emerging as salient in the context of the transition to parenthood.

Ghosts identified by fathers were many and varied. They included interpersonal traumas experienced in childhood (e.g., abuse and neglect, exposure to domestic violence) and adulthood (e.g., loss of a prior pregnancy), as well as adverse childhood experiences (e.g., parental separation or divorce, parental problem drinking or drug use) and ongoing stressors in adulthood (e.g., financial- or work-related stress). Many fathers, in naming their personal ghosts, described the ways they want things to be different for their own children.

Supporting fathers to recognize and exorcize ghosts holds promise for promoting healing, growth, and capacity to be a sensitive and responsive parent. Offered during the prenatal period, such support sets the stage for fathers to transmit a foundation of early love, unimpaired by pains of the past, that offers the best opportunity for their children to establish a core sense of security. Prenatal ultrasound and prenatal care more broadly offer a setting to encounter and engage expectant fathers and facilitate connections to care as needed. Care for expectant fathers stands to benefit mothers, children, and men themselves.

References

Alio, A. P., Kornosky, J. L., Mbah, A. K., Marty, P. J., & Salihu, H. M. (2010). The impact of paternal involvement on feto-infant morbidity among Whites, Blacks and Hispanics. *Maternal and Child Health Journal, 14*(5), 735–741.

Alio, A. P., Mbah, A. K., Kornosky, J. L., Wathington, D., Marty, P. J., & Salihu, H. M. (2011). Assessing the impact of paternal involvement on racial/ethnic disparities in infant mortality rates. *Journal of community health, 36*(1), 63–68.

Arora, S., McJunkin, C., Wehrer, J., & Kuhn, P. (2000). Major factors influencing breastfeeding rates: Mother's perception of father's attitude and milk supply. *Pediatrics, 106*(5), e67–e67.

Belsky, J., Conger, R., & Capaldi, D. M. (2009). The intergenerational transmission of parenting: Introduction to the special section. *Developmental Psychology, 45*, 1201.

Barrows, P. (2004). Fathers and families: Locating the ghost in the nursery. *Infant Mental Health Journal: Official Publication of The World Association for Infant Mental Health 25*(5), 408–423.

Benoit, D., Parker, K., & Zeanah, C. H. (1997). Mothers' representations of their infants assessed prenatally: Stability and association with infants' attachment classifications. *Journal of Child Psychology and Psychiatry, 38*, 307–313.

Bloch, J. R., Webb, D. A., Mathews, L., Dennis, E. F., Bennett, I. M., & Culhane, J. F. (2010). Beyond marital status: The quality of the mother–father relationship and its influence on reproductive health behaviors and outcomes among unmarried low income pregnant women. *Maternal and Child Health Journal, 14*(5), 726–734.

Boukydis, C. F. Z., Treadwell, M. C., Delaney-Black, V., Boyes, K., King, M., Robinson, T., et al. (2006). Women's responses to ultrasound examinations during routine screens in an obstetric clinic. *Journal of Ultrasound in Medicine, 25*, 721–728.

Blackburn, C. M., Bonas, S., Spencer, N. J., Coe, C. J., Dolan, A., & Moy, R. (2005). Parental smoking and passive smoking in infants: fathers matter too. *Health Education Research, 20*(2), 185–194.

Bottorff, J. L., Oliffe, J., Kalaw, C., Carey, J., & Mroz, L. (2006). Men's constructions of smoking in the context of women's tobacco reduction during pregnancy and postpartum. *Social Science & Medicine, 62*(12), 3096–3108.

Coates, S. (2012). The child as traumatic trigger: Commentary on paper by Laurel Moldawsky Silber. *Psychoanalytic Dialogues, 22*(1), 123–128.

Condon, J. T., & Corkindale, C. J. (1997). The correlates of antenatal attachment in pregnant women. *British Journal of Medical Psychology, 70*, 359–372.

Cabrera, N. J., Fagan, J., & Farrie, D. (2008). Explaining the long reach of fathers' prenatal involvement on later paternal engagement. *Journal of Marriage and Family, 70*(5), 1094–1107.

Dedoose. (2019). *Version 8.2, web application for managing, analyzing, and presenting qualitative and mixed method research data.* Los Angeles, CA: SocioCultural Research Consultants, LLC. https://www.dedoose.com

Flouri, E., & Buchanan, A. (2003). What predicts fathers' involvement with their children? A prospective study of intact families. *British Journal of Developmental Psychology, 21*(1), 81–97.

Lange, B. C. L., Callinan, L. S., & Smith, M. V. (2019). Adverse childhood experiences and their relation to parenting stress, and parenting practices. *Community Mental Health Journal, 55*(4), 651–662.

Leidy, M. S., Schofield, T. J., & Parke, R. D. (2013). Fathers' contributions to children's social development. *Handbook of Father Involvement: Multidisciplinary Perspectives, 2*, 151–167.

Lee, S. J., Sanchez, D. T., Grogan-Kaylor, A., Lee, J. Y., & Albuja, A. (2018). Father early engagement behaviors and infant low birth weight. *Maternal and Child Health Journal, 22*(10), 1407–1417.

Lyons-Ruth, K., & Block, D. (1996). The disturbed caregiving system: Relations among childhood trauma, maternal caregiving, and infant affect and attachment. *Infant Mental Health Journal, 17*(3), 257–275.

Madden, V., Domoney, J., Aumayer, K., Sethna, V., Iles, J., Hubbard, I., et al. (2015). Intergenerational transmission of parenting: Findings from a UK longitudinal study. *European Journal of Public Health, 25*(6), 1030–1035.

Marsiglio, W. (2008). Understanding men's prenatal experience and the father involvement connection: Assessing baby steps. *Journal of Marriage and Family, 70*(5), 1108–1113.

Martin, L. T., McNamara, M. J., Milot, A. S., Halle, T., & Hair, E. C. (2007). The effects of father involvement during pregnancy on receipt of prenatal care and maternal smoking. *Maternal and child health journal, 11*(6), 595–602.

NVivo qualitative data analysis software; QSR International Pty Ltd. Version 11, 2015.

O'Leary, J. (2009). Never a simple journey: Pregnancy following perinatal loss. *Bereavement Care, 28*(2), 12–17.

Pleck, J. H. (2010). Paternal involvement: Revised conceptualization and theoretical linkages with child outcomes. In M. E. Lamb (Ed.), *Role of the father in child development* (5th ed., pp. 58–93). Hoboken, NJ: Wiley.

Sarkadi, A., Kristiansson, R., Oberklaid, F., & Bremberg, S. (2008). Fathers' involvement and children's developmental outcomes: A systematic review of longitudinal studies. *Acta Paediatrica, 97*(2), 153–158.

Siddiqui, A., & Hägglöf, B. (2000). Does maternal prenatal attachment predict postnatal mother-infant interaction? *Early Human Development, 59*, 13–25.

Steen, M., Downe, S., Bamford, N., & Edozien, L. (2012). Not-patient and not-visitor: A metasynthesis of fathers' encounters with pregnancy, birth, and maternity care. *Midwifery, 28*(4), 362–371.

Strauss, A., & Corbin, J. (1998). *Basics of qualitative research: Techniques and procedures for developing grounded theory*. London, UK: Sage Publications.

Singer, B. J. (2012). The importance of unmarried residential fathers to maternal and child health: the association between prenatal involvement and birth outcomes (Doctoral dissertation).

Singh, D., & Newburn, M. (2000). Becoming a father: men's access to information and support about pregnancy, birth and life with a new baby. National Childbirth trust.

Teitler, J. O. (2001). Father involvement, child health and maternal health behavior. *Children and Youth Services Review, 23*(4–5), 403–425.

Van IJzendoorn, M. H. (1992). Intergenerational transmission of parenting: A review of studies in nonclinical populations. *Developmental Review, 12*, 76–99.

Walsh, T. (2018, June). Connecting while expecting: Prenatal ultrasound as a component of parental-fetal bonding. Paper presentation at the 2018 World Congress of the World Association for Infant Mental Health. Rome, Italy.

Walsh, T., Jones, M., Tolman, R., Lee, S. & Singh, V. (2019, Jan.). Early Service Experiences As a Barrier or Facilitator of Subsequent Service Engagement: An Examination of Father Engagement in Prenatal and Pediatric Care. Paper presentation at the 2019 Annual Conference of the Society for Social Work and Research. San Francisco, CA.

Walsh, T. B., Tolman, R. M., Palladino, C. L., Davis, R. N., Romero, V., & Singh, V. (2014). Moving up the 'magic moment': Fathers' experience of prenatal ultrasound. *Fathering, 12*(1), 18–37.

Walsh, T. B., Tolman, R. M., Singh, V., Davis, M. M., & Davis, R. N. (2017). Expectant fathers' presence at prenatal ultrasounds: An opportunity for social work engagement. *Social Work Research, 41*(3), 181–185.

Antecedents of Fathers' Stress in Fatherhood

14

Thomas Skjøthaug

Traditionally, the responsibility for rearing children has been largely left to mothers, and parents have had more differential roles in participation with their children than fathers of today (Cabrera, Tamis-LeMonda, Bradley, Hofferth, & Lamb, 2000). Social changes promote fathers as caregivers, and new social trends and ideals force a reconceptualizing of the traditional view of fathers as breadwinners and mothers as primary caregivers. Young fathers currently participate more actively in caregiving of their infants than former fathers have done, and the role of fathers as attachment figures for young children highlights the importance of employing fathers as participants and informants in research and caregiving. In some contemporary culture, fathers are more active in childcare and household work and go far beyond portrayals of men as "rough and tumble" playmates; they interact more as caregivers during their child's infancy (Shannon, Tamis-LeMonda, & Cabrera, 2006), and their influence in caregiving is commonly considered to be important for children's development in infancy and early childhood (Cabrera & Peters, 2000), even though it has sometimes been argued that fathers lack a "maternal instinct," understood as an inborn quality that supposedly makes mothers more sensitive to their babies than fathers (Solantus & Salo, 2005).

It is important to emphasize that fatherhood deserves more research and requires more knowledge: about the *transition* from man to father, *involvement* processes between father and child, obstacles *preventing* fathers' involvement, and evaluation of policy instruments and programs designed to include fathers in the care of their children (Tamis-LeMonda & Cabrera, 1999). Consequently, in line with the need of gaining more knowledge about these fatherhood issues are the experiences of *stress* in fatherhood.

The present chapter examines affiliated issues of stress research on father's pathways from conception toward fatherhood, such as childhood experiences, partner attachment, and fathers' mental health. Then the chapter sums up relevant issues to reduce the experience of stress, such as the transition from man to father, fatherhood involvement, autonomous ownership of the father's role, the importance of the couple relationship and the family triangle, and various aspects of how these measures are associated with fathers' experience of parenting stress postpartum.

Stress in Fatherhood

Becoming a father is a huge personal transition but unfortunately not exclusively a positive one. In this transition, we know that father's parenting

T. Skjøthaug (✉)
Division of Mental Health, Grorud DPS, Akershus University Hospital, Lørenskog, Norway
e-mail: tskjotha@getmail.no

H. E. Fitzgerald et al. (eds.), *Handbook of Fathers and Child Development*,
https://doi.org/10.1007/978-3-030-51027-5_14

is influenced by multiple intrafamilial and extrafamilial factors (Van Holland De Graaf, Hoogenboom, De Roos, & Bucx, 2014, Skjothaug, Smith, Wentzel-Larsen, Stänicke & Moe 2020). Previous research has shown that salient predictors of parental stress include negative life events; mental health problems, such as anxiety and depression; marital discord (Webster-Stratton, 1990); and parental developmental history (Belsky, 1984), and it is well known that parenthood can be experienced as stressful (Skjothaug, Smith, Wentzel-Larsen, & Moe, 2018). It has been found that stress influences parenting behavior and may be a determinant of dysfunctional parenting (Abidin, 1990, 1992, 1995; Belsky, 1984; Östberg & Hagekull, 2000).

Parenting stress can be defined as the discrepancy between the required resources of the parental role and the perceived resources available to meet those requests (Abidin, 1995). Further, Abidin specified various determinants of parenting stress, such as how parents *perceive* their child's behavioral characteristics, which tap into child temperamental characteristics of long-term predictive power (Abidin, 1982; Korn, 1984).

It has been found that parental developmental history and negative life events influence parental child perceptions and child behaviors, thereby resulting in experienced parental stress (Belsky, 1984; Webster-Stratton, 1990). Stress in the parent–child system during the first 3 years of life is especially important to consider in relation to the many facets of child–parent characteristics, family context, and life stress events. Even though we have some knowledge of parenting stress for both parents in child infancy, less is known concerning knowledge of the *antecedents* of fathers' stress and if stress expressed by their *child perception* can be traced back to their own characteristics and life experiences before the child is born (Barrows, 2004). Consequently, fathers' experiences measured before childbirth, such as father's own childhood experiences, attachment style, mental health, and spousal harmony, act in concert to shape child perceptions of their infants both directly and indirectly via other variables, which again may affect child development over time (Skjothaug et al., 2018; Skjothaug et al., 2020). Skjothaug and colleagues found that prospective fathers' mental health, as well as their own adverse childhood experiences, significantly predicted parenting stress, expressed as negatively perceived child behavior at 6 and 12 months postpartum. Even though there are many ways of expressing stress, this expression is an example of how one might express stress via child perception. So, how can such an effect arise? For example, fathers addressing their children's behavior negatively and throughout the first year of life may influence caregiving behavior negatively, which in turn may harm the children's development. And studies show that antecedents of such stress can be traced back to pregnancy, even before childbirth.

Some studies have focused upon *direct* associations, and an important goal of social science research is the analysis of causal processes. Further, studies have shown that multiple risks exceed the effect of the adverse developmental impacts of singular exposures (Trentacosta et al., 2008). During time, several variables may account for various effects and cooperate toward the outcome. Hence, the investigation of alternative causal mechanisms by examining the roles of *intermediate variables* situated in the path between predictors and outcome has been less studied, and most published mediation analyses have previously been based on the logic of the causal steps approach, inspired by an article published by Baron and Kenny (1986). According to their approach, in order for M to be considered to be a mediator of the effect of X on Y, one must first establish that there is a significant effect from X on Y. If there is such an effect, one might proceed to the next step (mediation analysis). If there is no such significant effect, according to Baron and Kenny's approach, one does not proceed with the analysis (Fig. 14.1).

As shown in the figure above, the total effect of X on Y is the direct one plus the sum of all the other effects. This means that there are multiple pathways that may exert effects on Y. If we suppose that X only exerts effect on Y via M and M', and they may have about equal magnitude but different signs, then the total effect may be close to zero, meaning about no net effect. In

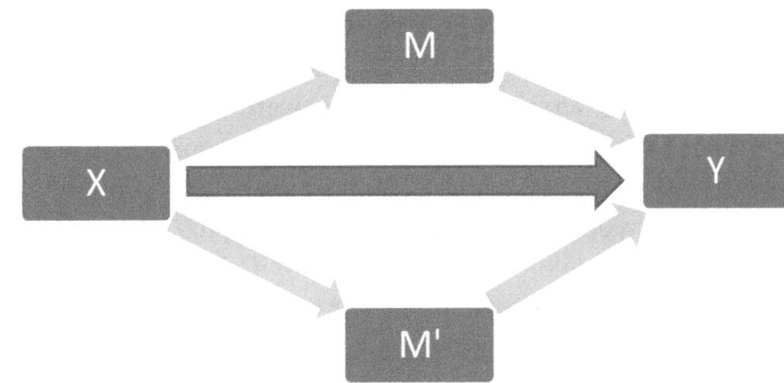

Fig. 14.1 X predicts Y directly. X also predicts Y via M and/or M'

such a case, this means that further analysis should stop, according to the causal steps approach. If so, we might end up underanalyzing data.

The estimation of causal effects has allowed researchers to explore whether a predictor affects outcome, while it cannot tell us *how* and *why* such an effect arises, which gives an excellent opportunity in future research. Hence, the estimation of causal relationships allows researchers to explore the degree to which predictors are related to outcomes. Such causal patterns are always possible outcomes within a dynamic systems framework because the predictors and estimated outcomes are contextual and may vary if contexts change. For example, a predicted set of father characteristics on child behavior will likely change if.the father's presence or "role" in the family changes.

According to such a mediator research view, is to explore how various antecedents of stress are influenced through time, not only by *directly* influencing stress but also *indirectly* via other variables. Such issues will be presented during the next parts of this chapter.

Adverse Childhood Experiences and Stress in Fatherhood

Adverse experiences in childhood are relatively common and are related to many public health problems later in life, such as heart problems (Anda, Butchart, Felitti, & Brown, 2010), autoimmune diseases (Dube et al., 2009), and depressive feelings (Chapman, Whitfield, Felitti, Edwards, & Anda, 2004). Such difficult experiences may include verbal and physical abuse, sexual abuse, substance abuse, mental illness, and divorce in the child's first 18 years of life. There is consensus that difficult childhood experiences pose a risk of developing health and social problems. There is also consensus that difficult childhood experiences increase the risk of social health problems (Anda et al., 2010), experienced stress in adolescence (Opacka-Juffry & Mohiyeddini, 2012), and depression (McEven & Gianaros, 2010) for many decades after exposure (Chapman et al., 2004).

However, most studies have looked at the contributions to isolated instances of abuse and the outcome of these, although we know that the cumulative effect of multiple instances of abuse and various forms of abuse increase the risk of developing poor health in adulthood (Chartier, Walker, & Naimark, 2010). Thus, the difference between children's outcome after exposure to isolated versus multiple instances of abuse may first become apparent many years after the events occurred (Anda et al., 2010). To understand how fathers affect children's development pathways from pregnancy, birth, and infancy, it is important to focus on the accumulation of risk and prevention factors, in addition to the child's individual constitution (Sameroff & Fiese, 2000a, b).

Difficult childhood experiences can also predict depression in fathers, but there are very few studies on the predictors of anxious and depressive feelings during pregnancy for expectant fathers. Skjothaug, Smith, Wentzel-Larsen, and Moe (2014) explored the question of how difficult childhood experiences reported retrospectively by expectant fathers were correlated with depressive and anxious feelings during pregnancy. The results showed the strongest correlation in the early stage of pregnancy (week 22) for both depressive and anxious feelings but were also correlated with the rest of the pregnancy (except for a lower level of anxious feelings toward the end of pregnancy). Other research has emphasized that the childhood experiences of fathers with their own parents, their current relationship with their mothers, and demographic factors can affect fathers' involvement during pregnancy and the childhood experiences of an expectant father and memories of his own childhood can affect how he views himself as a caregiver (Flykt et al., 2009) and infancy (Shannon et al., 2006).

Expectant fathers have had their own fathers as role models, and their cognitive understanding of "fatherhood" and "father" must be prepared and matured on a personal level. It is often the case that women identify with their own mothers and the mothers' child-rearing values when they themselves become mothers (Skjothaug et al., 2014). Thus, it is not so difficult to understand that expectant fathers also go through a similar process. As part of the process of becoming a father, it may be that many fathers have conflicting feelings about their own child-rearing values and the caregiving values they experienced from their parents. Such conflicts can also have consequences for how they view themselves as fathers and the feelings that this can generate. Fathers may therefore include and process their conscious and previous childhood experiences when they determine which values they will base their own fatherhood on. For example, healthcare providers may ask becoming fathers what they think about their anticipation of becoming a father, based on their own childhood memories.

Further, previous research has shown that negative life events may influence parental perceptions and behaviors (Webster-Stratton, 1990), thereby resulting in experienced stress. Longitudinal follow-up studies of adults whose childhood abuse was documented through records and interviews have consistently shown that their retrospective reports of childhood abuse were likely to underestimate, rather than to overestimate, the actual occurrence of abuse (Femina, Yeager, & Lewis, 1990; Williams, 1995) and may find it difficult to seek professional help when they experience mental health challenges (Addis & Mahalik, 2003).

It has further been demonstrated that adverse childhood experiences may influence later quality of life; the lasting effects of childhood abuse, neglect, and maltreatment are well recognized (Glaser, 2014).

Partner Attachment Style and Stress

Bowlby (1969) proposed that early experiences of care from attachment figures shape feelings, beliefs, and expectations of relationships across the life span, a phenomenon he described as "internal working models" (IWMs). He suggested that early attachment experiences prevail over time and influence later attachment relationships, such as the attachment relationships to romantic partners. Moreover, he thought that the adult's IWMs were related to the individual's own childhood experiences (Hazan & Shaver, 1987; Fox, Platz, & Bentley, 1995; Nelson-Coffey, Borelli, & River, 2017). In the same line of reasoning, it has been proposed that reported infant behavioral characteristics may be partly related to parental perceptions, rather than being true judgments of the child's character (Pauli-Pott, Mertesacker, Bade, Haverkock, & Beckmann, 2003). This implies that both parents' representations of their infant may be *present* even before the child is born and that such representations are related to parental interpretations of child characteristics and behavior after birth (Benoit, Zeanah, Parker, Nicholson, & Coolbear, 1997; Lebovici, 1994). This notion highlights that such perceptions may be rooted in and expressed via the father's own early exposures in childhood and his attachment experiences rather than purely expressing the child's actual behavior.

Bowlby (1969) further noted that parents yearn to be bonded to their baby during pregnancy and that this desire includes being psychologically close to their unborn child. He also proposed the concept of parenting alliance, which refers to the unique and specific component of the marital relationship that concerns parenting (Weissman & Cohen, 1985), a process that usually begins before birth (Luz, George, Vieux, & Spitz, 2007). Several studies suggest that a caregiver's own bonding experiences are associated with the quality of the child–caregiver attachment (Van IJzendoorn, 1995; Ward & Carlson, 1995). It is commonly assumed that the emotional relationship between parents and the child begins during pregnancy and that it continues into the postpartum period (Goulet, Bell, St-Cyr Tribble, Paul, & Lang, 1998). Consequently, in two-parent families, children simultaneously form attachment relationships with *both* their mother and their father (Easterbrooks & Goldberg, 1987). Newer studies, such as Dumont and Paquette (2013), offer new insights into father–child attachment. These workers compared two attachment procedures: the Ainsworth strange situation (Ainsworth, Blehar, Water, & Wall, 1978), which is the classic gold-standard method of assessing attachment quality, and a newer method, the risky situation (Dumont & Paquette, 2013). The strange situation measures a kind of parent–child attachment in which the parent takes on the role of comforting the child. Dumont and Paquette suggest that father–child attachment operates in a way that is different from merely comforting the children. According to Dumont and Paquette's activation theory, the child–father relationship consists of two dimensions: stimulation and discipline. Fathers encourage their children to *explore* the world as well as to be safe while doing so. They emphasize that the risky situation is a better predictor of children's socio-emotional development than the strange situation, even after controlling for paternal involvement. This view represents an alternative to classical attachment theory and conventional soothing practices.

When meeting first-time parents, it is especially important that the health services pay attention to both partners and their child bonding qualities and family interventions ought to take place during pregnancy in order to prevent later parenting stress. Research has shown that insecure adult attachment styles during pregnancy negatively predict parenting alliances 6 months postpartum (Bouchard, 2014). The parenting alliance has also been found to be associated with child adjustment (Belsky, Woodworth, & Crnic, 1996) and parental involvement (McBride & Rane, 1998).

Lastly, Skjothaug et al.'s (2020) research showed that more insecure partner attachment style among prospective fathers and their adverse childhood experiences strongly predicted paternal stress, mediated by mental health symptoms during pregnancy and spousal disharmony postpartum. This work shows that early predictors already measured before birth are associated with postpartum spousal disharmony, which in turn influences parenting stress and how fathers perceive their child's behavior in infancy and how elevated feelings of anxiety and depression lead to experiences of stress in fatherhood.

Mental Health of Fathers and Stress

Preparing for fatherhood includes going through a transformation of emotions (Finnbogadottir, Svalenius, & Persson, 2002). This process starts early in pregnancy with a mental preparation for fatherhood, and one process parents may experience is feelings of anxiety (Teixeira, Figueiredo, Conde, Pacheco, & Costa, 2009). Among prospective fathers, high levels of anxiety and depression are probably more prevalent in pregnancy than during the postpartum period (Teixeira et al., 2009). Heightened levels of anxiety among fathers-to-be seem to be associated with a lack of information about pregnancy, forthcoming childbirth, and poor social support (Condon, Boyce, & Corkindale, 2004). Early detection of depressive and anxious feelings in fathers during pregnancy is important because they are related to and predictors of depressive feelings in fathers after birth (Matthey, Barnett, Ungerer, & Waters, 2000). Both parents' personality traits, self-confidence, and depression during pregnancy can predict experienced stress after birth (Saisto, Salmela-Aro, Nurmi, & Halmesmäki, 2008).

Luoma et al. (2012) studied 194 fathers immediately after birth and found that 21 percent of the fathers and 24 percent of the mothers scored above the limit for depressive symptoms, indicating that depressive feelings can affect fathers immediately after birth, just the same as mothers. Additionally, high levels of anxiety and depression occur more frequently during pregnancy than after birth in both mothers (Andersson, Sundström-Poromaa, Wulff, Aström, & Bixo, 2006) and fathers (Condon et al., 2004). Some studies have shown increased anxiety levels as most prevalent during the first and third trimesters compared with the second trimester (Huizink, Mulder, Robles de Medina, Visser, & Buitelaar, 2004; Teixeira et al., 2009). It has also been shown that as many as 20% of fathers-to-be show high levels of anxiety during pregnancy, with a peak during the first and third trimester and higher levels in pregnancy, as compared to postpartum (Figueiredo & Conde, 2011). Similarly, Kim and Swain (2007) also found that more than 10% of fathers-to-be experienced some type of prenatal mood or anxiety disorder. Prevalence rates for "any" anxiety disorders are stable between the prenatal period (between 4.1% and 16%) and postpartum (between 2.4% and 18%) (Leach, Poyser, Cooklin, & Giallo, 2016). Other research reported that fathers' heightened levels of anxiety early in pregnancy predicted heightened levels of stress and depression later in pregnancy (Wee, Skouteris, Richardson, MacPhie, & Hill, 2015), thus highlighting the need for screening fathers-to-be for depression and anxiety in pregnancy. Surely, worries, preoccupations, generalized anxiety, and/or specific phobias can persist during pregnancy and into the postnatal period (Fenaroli & Saita, 2013). Ramchandani et al. (2008) reported that high prenatal symptom scores for depression and anxiety were the strongest predictors of paternal postnatal depression.

In addition, the research indicated that depression and depressive feelings in men are often associated with low satisfaction with their relationship with their partners and little social support (Wee et al., 2011), unemployment (Ballard & Davies, 1996), personal immaturity, and unplanned pregnancies (Schumacher, Zubaran, & White, 2008). The course of men's anxiety from the prenatal to the postnatal period tends to be stable, with a potential to decrease after birth (Leach et al., 2016). Also, there is an association between age and depressive symptoms among first-time fathers; younger fathers seem to be more vulnerable than older ones to develop depressive symptoms (Bergstrom, 2013).

Less research has focused upon the *predictors* of depressive and anxious feelings in fathers prenatally (Skjothaug et al., 2014), and there is also limited amount of research on the association between fathers' mental health and their perceptions of infant behavioral characteristics after birth (Parfitt, Ayers, Pike, Jessop, & Ford, 2014). The experiences of expectant fathers during pregnancy are described in some studies as more stressful than the postpartum period (Condon et al., 2004), while other studies indicate that the period from three to six months after birth is the most stressful for fathers (Paulson & Bazemore, 2010).

It has been found that parents with mental health problems in pregnancy experience stress elevation 12 months postpartum (Perren, Von Wyl, Bürgin, Simoni, & Von Klitzing, 2005), and comparable symptom scores have been found among depressed mothers and depressed fathers (Field et al., 2006; Figueiredo & Conde, 2011).

Even though there are fewer studies of the mental health of fathers as compared with mothers, it has been shown that during pregnancy depressed fathers may experience similar symptoms as reported by depressed mothers (Field et al., 2004; Field et al., 2006). In a 2010 meta-study with 28,000 participants (Paulson & Bazemore, 2010), researchers found that 10.4 percent of the fathers measured between the first trimester of pregnancy and the first year after birth had depression similar to a woman's postpartum depression. The level of depression in fathers was lower during the first 3 months (7.7 percent) and highest when measured later between 3 and 6 months (25.6 percent). This meta-study is important because it took many studies conducted in various locations around the world and compared the data. The study also points out the importance of focusing on the mental health of the depressed partner, as depression often occurs in both parents. Other studies report a higher rate of depression among women than in men, during pregnancy as well as 3 months after birth (Figueiredo & Conde, 2011).

Further, little attention has been given to the relations between fathers' depression and child development outcomes, and this is the case even though fathers' mental health in the postnatal period is associated with children's early behavioral and emotional development (Ramchandani et al. 2008).

For example, in a study of mediating factors, it was found that paternal depression and child outcomes were associated with and mediated through interparental conflict and maternal depression (Gutierrez-Galve, Stein, Hanington, Heron, & Ramchandani, 2015). It has also been shown that depression and anxiety mediate between parenting stress and parental dyadic adjustment at infant age 12 months (Rollè et al., 2017). More specifically and in the same line of research, Field et al. (2006) reported that fathers living with depressed mothers had significantly higher depression and anxiety scores than those living with nondepressed mothers. Hence, men with poor partner relationships are at risk for depression as much as women during the transition to parenthood (Matthey et al., 2000).

Recent research suggests that mothers' and fathers' depression may have differential effects on child development. Specifically, Fredriksen, von Soest, Smith, and Moe (2019) found that parenting stress plays a mediating role in the prediction of early child development from both parents' perinatal depressive symptoms. More specifically, Fredriksen et al. reported that fathers' (but not mothers') prenatal symptoms of depression were associated with child language development at 18 months (ibid). Another important issue concerns *who* should assess fathers' mental health during pregnancy and stress to provide reliable measures of fathers' mental health issues. As we know, men seldom attend mental health service, even when needed and warranted.

Assessment of Fathers' Depression

Massoudi, Hwang, and Wickberg (2013) found that about 90 percent of the public health nurses said that they seldom thought about the father's stress and less than one-fifth of the public health nurses had offered to have support conversations with fathers. Additionally, about 50 percent of public health nurses had an *ambivalent attitude* about the caregiving capacity of fathers as compared with mothers. In the assessment to detect fathers' symptoms of depressive feelings and depression, the Edinburgh Postnatal Depression Scale (EPDS) is currently used at many well-baby clinics. The questionnaire was originally created to measure depression in women after birth but is also thought to be a reliable, valid method of measuring depression in both parents during pregnancy (Matthey, Barnett, Kavanagh, & Howie, 2001; Cox & Holden, 2003; Skjothaug et al., 2014). The EPDS has proven to be a valuable, effective measurement tool for identifying depressive feelings after birth in women (Luoma et al., 2012) and men (Edmondson, Psychogion, Vlachos, Netsi, & Ramchandani, 2010). However, questionnaires and self-report measures of depression, specifically the use of the EPDS for men, have been criticized because men tend to use "externalizing" strategies when depressed; such strategies are not accounted for in the EPDS questionnaire. They rather include drug and alcohol abuse, road rage, aggression, suicide, risk-taking behaviors, cynicism, avoidance of social situations, and having affairs (Brownhill, Wilhelm, Barclay, & Schmied, 2005; Melrose, 2010; Matthey et al., 2001). Actually, it has been argued that the EPDS may be a general measure for assessing men's distress rather than depression (Matthey, 2008), since it picks up more worry, anxiety, and unhappiness than actual depression (Massoudi et al., 2013). Further research is encouraged where higher risk fathers participate and also other assessments than purely the EPDS alone, addressing depressive symptoms among fathers-to-be.

More knowledge about the mental health of fathers and the predictors of this are important so that the health services can provide the entire family with more and adequate assistance

(Fletcher, Matthey, & Marley, 2006). Depression in one of the parents should also trigger clinical awareness of the other parent; prevention and treatment should focus on the couple and the entire family rather than on the individual (Paulson & Bazemore, 2010).

It is also important to supplement the use of questionnaires with a clinical assessment, as most well-baby clinics are used to doing with the Edinburgh method. Knowledge about how fathers function as caregivers during the infancy period will increase the chance of prevention, detection, and treatment of mental illness and provide greater insight into intervention strategies for families at an early stage in the child's life. The kind of experiences fathers themselves have had as children with their own caregivers provides important knowledge about how they will be as fathers and what motivates them in their own fatherhood. Descriptions of fathers' experiences are often given by the mother as the informant. In clinical samples and research, there are also discrepancies and little correspondence between reporting based on fathers and mothers, respectively (Erlich, Cassidy & Dykas, 2011). Clearly, we need to address how to prevent stress both in research and in the clinics. The next part of the present chapter will reflect upon how to reduce stress among men in fatherhood.

Transition from Man to Father

Fathers are sometimes excluded from the infant's world, by the argument put forth that fathers lack the "mothering instinct," which is understood as an innate quality that supposedly makes mothers more sensitive to their children than fathers are (Solantus & Salo, 2005). The preparation from being a man to becoming a father includes going through a transformation of feelings (Finnbogadottir et al., 2002), and the first transition is preparing mentally to become a father during the pregnancy phase, which can result in anxiety (Teixeira et al., 2009). Men experience changes during their pathway to parenthood, and these changes are important in developing the relationship with their child (Musser, Ahmed, Foli, & Coddington, 2013). Therefore, fathers-to-be who experience a lack of information about pregnancy and childbirth, and who have little social support, also experience higher levels of anxiety (Condon et al., 2004). Furthermore, men experiencing a discrepancy between a more traditional male gender role and contemporary expectations of fathering behavior during pregnancy often experience distress (Singley & Edwards, 2015). Such distress may result in disconnection and withdrawal from the family and in some cases lead to mental health concerns, such as anxiety and depression. A consequence of being depressed may be that the father experiences his child's behavioral characteristics negatively and interacts with his child in a withdrawn way, thereby displaying less verbal and behavioral stimulation compared to nondepressed fathers. Hence, distressed fathers may initiate a compromised pattern of parenting which may potentially negatively affect their children's development (Sethna, Murray, Netsi, Psychogiou, & Ramchandani, 2015).

There is a relation between involvement in pregnancy and engagement with the child at ages 1 and 3 (Shannon et al., 2006; Cabrera, Fagan, & Farrie, 2008), suggesting stability of dedication over time. Studies have shown how highly engaged fathers contribute to more favorable outcomes; their children often have better cognitive development, better emotion regulation, better emphatic understanding toward peers (Radin, 1994), and score higher on intelligence tests (Gottfried, Gottfried, & Bathurst, 1988).

Increased levels of anxiety in expectant fathers appear to be related to a lack of information about pregnancy, the upcoming birth, and a low level of social support (Condon et al., 2004). Becoming a father necessarily implies a personal change from man to father. Children often encounter an expectation about the division of roles between the parents while they are young. It is often the case that boys mostly come in contact with women as role models in important social arenas, such as daycare, school, and the health services, because a majority of women are employed in these workplaces. The psychological preparation that boys undergo before they eventually become fathers may be somewhat different than it is for girls before they become mothers. This may be the case because today's fathers have not necessarily had their own fathers as role models, whereas the women of today have generally had their mothers as role models.

Finnbogadottir et al. (2002) studied seven expectant fathers to learn how the transition from man to father is experienced. The fathers said that the situation felt unreal, and they described feelings of inadequacy when they talked about the social and physical changes in light of their evolving feelings of responsibility during pregnancy.

Genesoni and Tallandini (2009) described the prenatal period as the most stressful for fathers because they experienced a psychological reorganization, a feeling of unreality, and a change in experienced partner contact and their own identity. The change in identity highlighted the values that manifest in the transition from man and partner to father and was most noticeable at the beginning of pregnancy. The transition in one's own self and the connection to role models and one's own identity, which is exemplified in concrete terms through the transformation from man to father, from two to three family members and the social change, were also described in the prenatal transition that fathers undergo. Such "transitions" are not so different from those found among women when they are expectant mothers. In the subsequent period, around birth, men say that they experience many feelings all at once and that they sometimes feel helpless, useless, worried, and vulnerable, in addition to great joy, of course. The final period described by Genesoni and Tallandini is the postpartum period in which the men's life situation was impacted by external circumstances such as social support and less time to establish good contact with the child, as well as a change in lifestyle and a sexual "down" period. Fathers may also feel that they have less free time and lack confidence in their own ability to handle their infant.

Interaction factors such as these are related to children's development. Although few studies have looked at the interaction of fathers with their children, some research has focused on the *behavior* of fathers during pregnancy and birth and how this behavior can predict the extent of their presence and involvement with their own children many years later (Shannon et al., 2006). This same study showed a correlation between the involvement of fathers in the pregnancy and their involvement with their child after birth. Other studies, such as the one conducted by Cabrera et al. (2008), found a stable correlation between prenatal involvement and involvement after birth, assessed when the children were 1 and 3 years old.

However, we know too little about other important factors, such as a man's motivation to become a father, the correlation between fathers' results orientation in fatherhood, and their long-term investment in their own children (Cabrera & Peters, 2000).

Smith (2010) shows how families can have an "attachment hierarchy," meaning that there is a distinction between which caregiving tasks are typically performed by the primary and secondary caregiver. He asserts that infants have a small network of caregivers and that cross-cultural studies suggest that infants choose one person as their "primary" caregiver (Van IJzendoorn & Sagi-Schwartz, 2008). However, children can have different qualities in their attachment to various caregivers, e.g., a child can be securely attached to her mother, while the child does not need to have the same quality in her attachment to her father (Howes & Spieker, 2008). In cases of divorce, focus is often placed on strengthening the bond between mother and child, which often has occurred at the expense of the relationship between father and child (Goldstein, Freud, & Solnit, 1979). More recent research has shown how infants have positive, meaningful attachments to both parents at about the same age, between six and eight months (Cabrera & Tamis-LeMonda, 2013). In order to ensure that relations between parents and children are maintained and strengthened, children need interactive experiences with both parents performing the same tasks, such as feeding, bathing, playing, boundary-setting, diaper changing, comforting (also at night), providing encouragement, and putting the child to bed. These are important, daily interactive tasks that promote children's psychosocial development and play a key role in the attachment between the caregiver and child. These tasks foster and maintain trust, security, and attachment to the parent (Lamb, 2002). It is crucial that fathers also have an opportunity to perform these tasks, both for their own sake and with regard to the child's development and attachment. By doing so, we might hope for less stress among men in their fatherhood role.

Paternal Involvement and Lack Thereof

Shannon and colleagues have shown how men's childhood experiences with their parents influence their involvement with their own child in infancy. They also showed that there is a relationship between prospective fathers' involvement in pregnancy and subsequent engagement with the child after birth (Shannon et al., 2006) and that a better partner relationship is likely to contribute to more involvement with the child (Shannon, Tamis-LeMonda, & Margolin, 2005). For example, Cabrera et al. (2008) found a stable association between fathers' prenatal involvement and their postnatal engagement with the children at ages 1 and 3. Thus, it is important to understand which factors are operating in fathers' capacity to be emotionally and practically involved with their children. One way of understanding involvement is to screen how many fathers attend and participate in the traditional health providers in the first-line services. Hence, it is mostly mothers who are seen at well-baby clinics, and less fathers are probably included in the clinics' activities because it is not assumed that they will accompany their children to various consultations. In spite of this, many well-baby clinics are trying to get more fathers to attend the various meetings at the clinics, which was not a matter of course for previous generations. Some public health nurses find that many fathers accompany their children to consultations from 8 to 12 months of age but that they attend fewer consultations during pregnancy. Some well-baby clinics have also established separate father groups and have put more focus on including fathers in various meetings. Of course, it is important that those of us who provide health services address the *mother's* challenges in the relevant childhood arenas, but we should also be aware of the *father's* challenges and take his experiences into account.

Previous generations of parents had a more traditional division of roles, and fathers from that time were not as visible during their child's infancy as they are now. Mothers had the main responsibility for the children, and mothers and fathers had different roles and responsibilities, with the father working mainly outside the home (Cabrera et al., 2000). Older research indicates a role division in which mothers talk and offer comfort, while fathers are more involved through physical play, especially with boys. The understanding of fathers' contribution to caregiving has been based primarily on the instrumental task in the family, such as finances, practical adaptations, and creating a protective sphere for the mother–child dyad (Lamb, 2010).

In general, fathers are now more active during their children's infancy, and they have responsibility for caregiving tasks that previously were reserved for mothers, such as changing diapers, providing comfort, looking after the children, and performing household tasks (Shannon et al., 2006). In most cases, therefore, the current generation of fathers during their child's infancy will not have their own fathers as role models because of the change in roles from an instrumental helper to a caregiver. This is generally not the case for today's mothers because they usually were raised by their mothers, who had responsibility for their infants (Fagerskiold, 2006).

How to Involve Fathers

Boys growing up without fathers seem especially prone to problems in the areas of sex-role and gender-identity development, school performance, psychosocial adjustment, and self-control (Hetherington & Stanley-Hagan, 1986). Girls are also affected by father absence; girls growing up without a father are at risk for early sexual activity and adolescent pregnancy (Ellis et al., 2003).

Cabrera has underscored the importance of encouraging researchers, educators, and practitioners to examine all aspects of fathering, including how men become fathers, the nature of father–child involvement, the barriers to involvement, and the design of effective policies and programs to include fathers (Tamis-LeMonda & Cabrera, 1999).The Clinton Administration launched a large-scale project called the Fatherhood Research Initiative as a result of what President Clinton described as a "fatherless America." The purpose was to promote research and policy instruments related to fathers' involvement with their children. The follow-up to this project was initiated by George W. Bush and was called the Healthy Marriage Initiative. The aim of this follow-up project was to avoid marriage dissolution and ensure that fathers remained with the family to counteract unhealthy development in children with an absent father.

Europe has launched a slightly different policy approach to affect the family constellation and involvement of fathers – namely, the father quota. Hence, Norway is in a unique position with regard to parental leave and the father quota, since the father quota was introduced already 20 years ago, in 1993, by Gro Harlem Brundtland's third government, and at that time it consisted of 4 weeks. Jens Stoltenberg's first government increased the quota to 5 weeks, and in 2010 it was extended to 14 weeks. Today (2019), Norwegian fathers have 15 dedicated father quota weeks (www.nav.no). This form of parental leave is one part of Norway's political effort to facilitate greater involvement by fathers with their children.

The notion of mandatory paternal leave, sometimes called "the daddy quota," is catching on in policymaking circles as a way to help women return to the workforce and encourage fathers to share in caregiving and bonding during a child's first year. Today, the "daddy quota means that 90% of fathers take parental leave" (https://apolitical.co/solution_article/norways-daddy-quota-means-90-of-fathers-take-parental-leave/). Nevertheless, some research, like Rege and Solli (2010), emphasizes in their study that the father quota actually increases the involvement of fathers with their children throughout their entire upbringing. Overall, the quota is regarded as an important instrument for increasing fathers' contact and involvement with their children. Generally, Cabrera and Peters (2000) underscore that there is little research that directly evaluates the effectiveness of existing social policies and programs targeted to increase father involvement, and in line with this view, the father quota as a policy instrument has undergone little evaluation. Few studies have looked at the efficacy of policy initiatives designed to encourage fathers to be more involved with their children. This illustrates the significance of studying more about how new social and policy initiatives can affect children's development. They emphasize the importance of mapping and tracking how new social trends influence children's development. The role of fathers as attachment figures for young children highlights the importance of employing fathers as autonomous participants and firsthand informants in research and caregiving.

As previously mentioned, there are very few studies on the involvement of fathers in the pregnancy, the psychological transition from man to expectant father, and how fathers function as caregivers. In addition, there is little research on the expectations that men have for their own fatherhood in the infancy period. There are also several reasons that it has been hard to obtain information from fathers. One reason is that it has been difficult to recruit fathers for research projects in this period of life (Cabrera & Peters, 2000; Flykt et al., 2009).

Previous research by Lamb, Pleck, Charnov, and Levine (1985) introduced the pillars that must be present in order for fathers to be involved with their children. He emphasized the importance of fathers' interest in direct interaction with their children during play and leisure activities when they were together, that they shared experiences, and that the fathers took responsibility for caregiving and played with the child. In order for this to be possible, the child must be accessible to the father, and the father must take responsibility for the child, with understanding and an accommodating attitude toward the child's needs and with participation in the planning and organization of the child's life.

In line with Lamb et al.'s (1985) thinking, Pleck (2010) has shown that fathers' involvement with their children should include three main components: (a) positive activities, (b) warmth and responsiveness, and (c) control. These are known "daily tasks" that are crucial for connection, involvement, and care in the contact between father and child. However, there are many ways to carry out these tasks, and there are different opinions about how this should be done.

Another indicator of engagement and involvement appears to be *couple satisfaction* and how parents interact with their children from an early age. Fathers interact more frequently with their children when both they and their partners have supportive attitudes about the father's involvement. Lundy (2002) described how disharmony in marriage negatively affected the quality of interaction with the child, as well as the level of security in the father–child connection. It is also the case that experienced couple satisfaction is strongly associated with depression in mothers (Beck, 1996), and depression in mothers may lead to depression in fathers (Goodman, 2004).

In order for fathers' involvement and knowledge to increase, it is important that hospitals and well-baby clinics take it seriously that mother, father, and child must be treated as a whole, rather than focusing only on the mother and child. When a midwife or pediatrician asks how the mother is doing – ask the father as well! Well-baby clinics should also ensure that the physical environment encourages an "equal" talk with both parents who are present and that all communication about the child and the child's development is conveyed to both parents, regardless of whether the midwife or public health nurse knows the mother best from previous interactions.

Relationship satisfaction with one's partner is one of the most important individual factors we must look at when we assess the parents' mental health, both during pregnancy and later. In order to develop an independent relationship to one's own fatherhood during the infancy period, the father must be included, and focus must be placed on him, both at clinics and in research, on an equal footing with the mother. The father's role as a caregiver should highlight fathers as independent participants and informants in research and at clinics and as caregivers for their children.

Autonomous Ownership of the father's Role

"Finance fathers" are often described in the Norwegian media as the type of father who prioritizes his job over spending time with his children, and they are more concerned with, than about, their children. If the general focus of the caregiving task is placed on performance, i.e., practical tasks with a clear "upkeep function" at the expense of attentive presence, security, and care, this will not necessarily help to build a good development pathway for the children. One might speculate that children who feel that their own needs do not get an independent space and who feel that their needs are secondary compared to their parents' needs may have difficulty developing their own identity and attachment, and they may lose contact with their own needs. Problems with balancing the needs of the father and his child affect not only the father but both parents, and there may be a tendency today for a larger share of women to work a lot and therefore have less time to spend with their children and home. Especially in Norway, this can be seen as a natural consequence of fathers assuming more responsibility on the home front than they did in the past due to Norway's welfare model where fathers have 15 weeks especially dedicated to paternal leave.

It is important that we view the father as an independent informant with regard to his own experiences, rather than focusing on the mother as the informant for the father's feelings. Ownership is motivated and adapted through mutual socialization with other fathers in the same situation. Socialization with other fathers helps to increase understanding of the father's role, increase mastery, and improve exchanges of knowledge and experiences, in the same way that postnatal gatherings do for mothers.

The Mother–Father–Child Triangle and Paternal Involvement in Childcare

Winnicott (1971) stated that a child's play and positive development presuppose *potential space,* which can be understood as the gradual separation between child and mother in an area between fantasy and reality. In this context, Green (2000) included fathers and how they may "break up" the dyadic relationship and form a triadic one, promoting the development of potential space.

Other researchers have also given due weight to the father's contribution to the family system, such as Chiland (1982), who emphasized the importance of including the father in the relationship. The importance of including fathers and focusing upon the triad, compared with the dyad only, has also been highlighted by more recent research than Winnicott and Chiland. Barrows (2004) described how the infant, already from birth, has to deal with numerous relationships. It is the characteristics of the parental couple that the child encounters which, above all else, will be of importance for the infant's future mental health. Barrows maintains that our internal representations (including ghosts from the past) may be reenacted within the current relationship in the heat of the moment (i.e., by *stress*), replaying scenarios from our own childhood that may have persisting influence across generations (Barrows, 2004). In the beginning of this chapter, it was reflected upon the importance of addressing mediating effects between predictor and outcome. In line with Barrows' thinking, Skjothaug et al. (2020) showed that fathers' perceived child behavior was highly stable during the second half-year of life, suggesting that their subjective perception and description of how the child behaves may be a lasting one. It is important to mention that the measure from this study was not an objective one, even though informative. The fathers' own opinion was surely colored by own experiences from the present and past. Further, the fathers' *adverse childhood experiences* and *partner attachment* were not significantly associated *directly* with stress, only *indirectly* when being mediated by spousal disharmony postpartum (which itself may be experienced as stressful). As described above, it is noteworthy that Barrows stated that it is not so much whose ghost it is that counts, whether it belongs to the father or the mother, but rather the nature of the interaction that ensues between the parents and how this interaction affects the infant. Barrows further stated that a united couple is deeply reassuring (and protective) for the infant and lays the foundation for its future emotional well-being, a notion that supports the importance of having fathers included in a mother–father–child triangle. He claims that more critical for the developing infant's future mental health than the father's individual role is the nature of the parental couple relationship, conveying the notion that the emotional climate within which the infant is born is of utmost importance (Barrows, 2004). This view is supported by previous research showing an association between unsatisfying marital relationships and parental stress (Grych & Clark, 1999; Saisto et al., 2008). Spousal disharmony has been found to have a mediating role; specifically, elevated anxious and depressive symptoms, more adverse childhood experiences, and less optimal partner attachment styles have been associated with more spousal disharmony postpartum and less positive perceived child behavior (more stress) postpartum (Skjothaug et al., 2018; Skjothaug et al., 2020).

Of course, we cannot be certain about how these fathers, based on their perceptions, actually interact with their children. But we may surmise that the caregivers' adverse experiences and mental health in childhood influence the interactional quality with their children. Other studies lend support to these findings concerning stress and spousal discord; reliable and active backing from one's partner seems to improve a parent's psychological and relational satisfaction, thus enhancing parenting ability (Vismara et al., 2016). Vismara's conclusion is also in line with one of Skjothaug et al.'s (2018, 2020) findings that depressive feelings predict negative perception of one's child, via the experience of spousal disharmony. Hence, fathers seem to be consistently more involved in interaction with their infants when both they and their partners have supportive attitudes to paternal involvement. Thus, Lundy (2002) reported that marital dissatisfaction adversely affected paternal synchrony and thus the security of infant–father attachment, underscoring the need of preventing spousal discord in order to prevent child misfortune.

The bond between the parents is vital to consider because a disharmonic spousal relationship negatively affects the quality of interaction with the child, as well as the level of security in the father–child connection (Lundy, 2002). Other research considering interactional quality between parents and their children, such as Parfitt, Pike, and Ayers (2013), found that parental *prenatal mental health*, especially anxiety, was associated with parent–infant interaction postpartum. The associations between prenatal mental health and parent–infant interaction were even stronger than those based on postnatal mental health scores (i.e., depression and posttraumatic stress). Specifically, fathers' prenatal symptoms were associated with higher unresponsiveness and infant passivity postpartum, whereas postnatal symptoms were associated with higher levels of infant difficulty in father–infant interaction. Insights from motherhood research show that during interaction with their children, depressed mothers often show less reciprocity and synchronicity and that they often fluctuate between being disengaged and intrusive (Luthar, D'Avanzo, & Hitches, 2003); these factors are related to the children's developmental outcome. This insight has transfer value to fathers interacting with their children, underscoring the need of treating couples and families, not only mothers, with their child individually, especially since mental health symptoms covariate between partners and influence their children.

Anxiety research on mothers has similarly shown that anxiety is associated with interactional quality; in a study of high-trait anxiety mothers, it was reported that these mothers were less sensitive and had reduced emotional tone during interaction with their toddlers (Nicol-Harper, Harvey, & Stein, 2007). This research has transfer value to fathers, and more recent research highlights fathers' prenatal mental health, especially anxiety, and its association with father–infant interaction at 3 months postpartum (Parfitt et al., 2013).

Summary and Key Points

Family interventions ought to be started early in order to prevent parenting stress in infancy, since predictors obtained during pregnancy are associated with postpartum spousal disharmony, which in turn influences parenting stress and how fathers perceive their child's behavior in infancy. Health providers should focus on treating the whole family, including the father, since we now realize that children's well-being is dependent on both parents and that they are better off with parents who communicate and cooperate. Knowledge of paternal attributes as caregivers is supposed to provide a basis for better understanding of prevention, detection, treatment, and intervention strategies for the children and their families at an early point of time. To understand how paternal attributes can impact on child development and mental health in the whole family, one should focus on the accumulation of risk and protective factors, in addition to taking the individual child's characteristics into consideration (Sameroff & Fiese, 2000a, b).

Healthcare providers need to motivate prospective fathers in their role as caregivers early in fatherhood. Fathers must be viewed as equal to mothers as caregivers, especially in child infancy. By providing qualified and updated information about the transition of a man to a father, by highlighting the importance of maintaining a harmonic spousal relationship, and by providing guidance of how fathers can evaluate their fatherhood on their own premises, one may improve the quality of life for developing children. Specifically, we must focus upon fathers' mental health in pregnancy, especially since fathers' adverse childhood experiences and partner attachment as well as symptoms of anxiety and depression during pregnancy predict paternal stress and a negative perception of child behavior at 6 and 12 months postpartum and men seldom attend mental health services when needed.

Surely, parenting stress and caretaking casualty (e.g., related to postpartum depression or high parenting stress) constitute environmental risks for developing socio-emotional problems in young children.

How can we impact the involvement of fathers with their children to reduce stress in a concrete way and view fathers as equal caregivers? Key aspects of achieving such an impact may be to motivate fathers and mothers to acknowledge the importance of fathers in the early stage of pregnancy (and of course on earlier points of time), inform them of what the transition from man to father may entail, increase their understanding that harmony in their relationship as a couple must be maintained, and ensure that fathers gain a sense of independent ownership on their own terms of their role as an important caregiver in the child's life. Well-baby clinics currently organize pre- and postnatal gatherings for the mothers at the clinics. Although fathers of today in Scandinavia are far more present in their children's early years than they were previously (cf. the father quota), no similar measures are arranged for men in Norway today. However, other measures, such as father groups, have been launched at well-baby clinics to include fathers and enhance the view of fathers as caregivers, but there is currently no systematic evaluation of such measures. Experience shows, though, that it is often easier for fathers to take part in arranged father groups when they are on parental leave and that fathers often do not participate to the same degree in the mother's consultations during pregnancy, perhaps because they are at work. In order to involve fathers early on in their fatherhood is to use them as independent informants in clinics, and research has most often reported fathers' experiences via mothers as the informant, especially since we know that there is usually a low correspondence between the experiences of fathers and what mothers report about those experiences. Adding the dimension of behavioral observation to parents' self-reports is needed as the correlations between behavioral observation and self-report measures are only weak to moderate (Alderfer et al., 2008). Another argument for using fathers as autonomous respondents instead of addressing fathers via mothers is that parents' subjective reports are not necessarily highly correlated. Lastly, future studies may address the child's gender in separate analyses, especially since research has shown that child gender may be related to parenting quality. As such, there is evidence that parents are more sensitive to their girls than to their boys (Lovas, 2005). It may be that fathers perceive more stress with girls than with boys; with same-gender child, it may be easier to recognize the needs of the child due to the parent's own experiences (Lam, McHale, & Crouter, 2013). Hallers-Haalboom et al. (2014) reported, however, that among 389 families with children between the ages of 1 and 3, the child's gender was not related to parenting in any of the analyses. They suggested that parent gender is more salient than child gender in the prediction of parenting practices in early childhood, a suggestion that is important to consider in future studies. In addition, future studies should strive to assess diverse methods to measure attachment security, not only by assessing soothing quality, as in the Ainsworth classic gold-standard method of evaluating child attachment quality, but also by employing newer methods, such as *the risky situation method* (Dumont & Paquette, 2013).

In addition to increase fathers' understanding of the father's role and to increase the involvement of fathers in their children's lives in order to reduce stress, it can be important to:

- Focus on the father's mental health and stress during fatherhood. Men seldom go to the doctor for mental health issues.
- Be aware of ethnic minority groups, low-income groups, and cultural differences, both at well-baby clinics and in research.
- Shed light on policy instruments designed to involve fathers; protect and support earmarking of the father quota. Men still find it is more

difficult to gain approval from their employers to take their father quota than women do with regard to maternity leave.

- Encourage fatherhood on its own terms and allow fathers to have ownership of their own fatherhood.
- Use more and different information methods and informants to increase specificity.
- Shed light on relationship satisfaction between the parents. Family interventions ought to take place already in pregnancy to prevent later parenting stress, especially since early predictors of paternal stress are associated with postpartum spousal disharmony, which in turn influences parenting stress and how fathers perceive their child's behavior in infancy.

References

Abidin, R. R. (1982). Parenting stress and the utilization of pediatric services. *Children's Health Care*, (2), 70–73. https://doi.org/10.1207/s15326888chc1102_5

Abidin, R. R. (1986). Parenting stress and the utilization of pediatric services. *Children's Health Care, 2*, 70–73. https://doi.org/10.1207/s15326888chc1102_5

Abidin, R. R. (1990). *Parenting stress index-manual* (2nd ed.). Charlottesville, VA: Pediatric Psychologists Press.

Abidin, R. R. (1992). The determinants of parenting behavior. *Journal of Clinical Child Psychology, 21*, 407–412. https://doi.org/10.1207/s15374424jccp2104_12

Abidin, R. R. (1995). *Parenting stress index: Professional manual* (3rd ed.). Odessa, FL: Psychological Assessment Resources, Inc.

Addis, M. E., & Mahalik, J. R. (2003). Men, masculinity, and the context of help seeking. *American Psychologist, 58*(1), 5–14.

Ainsworth, M. D. S., Blehar, M. C., Water, E., & Wall, S. (1978). *Patterns of attachment: A psychological study of the strange situation*. Hillsdale, NJ: Lawrence Erlbaum.

Alderfer, M. A., Fiese, B. H., Gold, J. I., Cutuli, J. J., Holmbeck, G. N., Goldbeck, L., et al. (2008). Evidence-based assessment in pediatric psychology: Family measures. *Journal of Pediatric Psychology, 33*(9), 1046–1061. https://doi.org/10.1093/jpepsy/jsm083

Anda, R. F., Butchart, A., Felitti, V. J., & Brown, D. W. (2010). Building a framework for global surveillance of the public health implications of adverse childhood experiences. *American Journal of Preventive Medisine, 39*, 93–98. https://doi.org/10.1016/j.amepre.2010.03.015

Andersson, L., Sundström-Poromaa, I., Wulff, M., Aström, M., & Bixo, M. (2006). Depression and anxiety during pregnancy and six months postpartum: A follow-up study. *Acta Obstetricia et Gynecologica Scandinavica, 85*, 937–944.

Ballard, C., & Davies, R. (1996). Postnatal depression in fathers, international depression in fathers. *International Review of Psychiatry, 8*, 65–71. *Based Approach*. The Guilford Press New York London.. https://doi.org/10.3109/09540269609037818

Baron, R. M., & Kenny, D. A. (1986). The moderator-mediator variable distinction in social psychological research: Conceptual, strategic, and statistical considerations. *Journal of Personality and Social Psychology, 51*(6), 1173–1182.

Barrows, P. (2004). Fathers and families: Locating the ghost in the nursery. *Infant Mental Health Journal, 25*(5), 408–432. https://doi.org/10.1002/imhj.20016

Beck, C. T. (1996). A meta-analysis of predictors of postpartum depression. *Nursing Research, 45*, 297–303.

Belsky, J. (1984). The determinants of parenting: A process model. *Child Development, 55*, 83–96. http://www.jstor.org/stable/1129836

Belsky, J., Woodworth, S., & Crnic, K. (1996). Trouble in the second year: Three questions about family interaction. *Child Development, 67*(2), 556–578.

Benoit, D., Zeanah, C. H., Parker, K. C. H., Nicholson, E., & Coolbear, J. (1997). "Working model of the child interview": Infant clinical status related to maternal perceptions. *Infant Mental Health Journal, 18*(1), 107–121. https://doi.org/10.1002/(SICI)1097-0355(199721)18:1<107::AID-IMHJ8>3.0.CO;2-N

Bergstrom, M. (2013). Depressive symptoms in new first-time fathers: Associations with age, Sociodemographic characteristics, and antenatal psychological Well-being. *Birth, 40*. https://doi.org/10.1111/birt.12026

Bouchard, G. (2014). The quality of the parenting alliance during the transition to parenthood. *Canadian Journal of Behavioral Science, 46*(1), 20–28. https://doi.org/10.1037/a0031259

Bowlby, J. (1969). *Attachment and loss: Vol. 1: Attachment*. New York: Basic Books.

Brennan, K. A., Clark, C. L., & Shaver, P. R. (1998). Self-report measurement of adult attachment. In J. A. Simpson & W. S. Rholes (Eds.), *Attachment theory and close relationships*. New York/London, UK: The Guilford Press.

Brownhill, S., Wilhelm, K., Barclay, L., & Schmied, V. (2005). 'Big build': Hidden depression in men. *Australian and New Zealand Journal of Psychiatry, 39*, 921–931. https://doi.org/10.1080/j.1440-1614.2005.01665.x

Cabrera, N., & Peters, H. E. (2000). Public policies and father involvement. *Marriage & Family Review, 29*, 295–314. https://doi.org/10.1300/J002v29n04_04

Cabrera, N. J., & Tamis-LeMonda, C. S. (2013). *In handbook of father involvement*. (2nd ed.). New York: Routledge Taylor & Francis Group.

Cabrera, N. J., Tamis-LeMonda, S. T., Bradley, R. H., Hofferth, S., & Lamb, M. E. (2000). Fatherhood in the twenty-first century. *Child Development, 71*, 127–136.

Cabrera, N. J., Fagan, J., & Farrie, D. (2008). Explaining the long reach of fathers' prenatal involvement on later paternal engagement. *Journal of Marriage and Family, 1, 70*(5). https://doi.org/10.1111/j.1741-3737.2008.00551.x

Chapman, D. P., Whitfield, C. L., Felitti, V. J., Dube, Shanta, R., Edwards, V. J., & Anda, R. (2004). Adverse childhood experiences and the risk of depressive disorders in adulthood. Journal of Affective Disorders. 82, 217–225. https://doi.org/10.1016/j.jad.2003.12.013.

Chartier, M. J., Walker, J. R., & Naimark, B. (2010). Separate and cumulative effects of adverse childhood experiences in predicting adult health and health care utilization. *Child Abuse & Neglect, 34*(6), 454–464.

Chiland, C. (1982). A new look at fathers. *The Psychoanalytic Study of the Child, 37*, 367–379.

Condon, J. T., Boyce, P., & Corkindale, C. J. (2004). The First-Time Fathers Study: A prospective study of the mental health and wellbeing of men during the transition to parenthood. *Australian and New Zealand Journal of Psychiatry, 38*, 56–64. https://doi.org/10.1111/j.1440-1614.2004.01298.x

Cox, J., & Holden, J. A. (2003). *A guide to the Edinburgh Postnatal Depression Scale (EPDS)*. London, UK: Gaskell.

Dube, S. R., Fairweather, D., Pearson, W. S., Felitti, V. J., Anda, R. F., & Croft, J. B. (2009). Cumulative childhood stress and autoimmune diseases in adults. *Psychosomatic Medicine, 71*(2), 243–250. https://doi.org/10.1097/PSY.0b013e3181907888

Dumont, C., & Paquette, D. (2013). What about the child's tie to the father? A new insight into fathering, father-child attachment, children's socio-emotional development and the activation relationship theory. *Early Child Development and Care, 183*, 430–446. https://doi.org/10.1080/03004430.2012.711592

Easterbrooks, M. A., & Goldberg, W. (1987). Toddler development in the family: Impact of father involvement and parenting characteristics. *Child Development, 55*, 770–752.

Edmondson, O. J., Psychogion, L., Vlachos, H., Netsi, E., & Ramchandani, P. G. (2010). Depression in fathers in the postnatal period: Assessment of the Edinburgh Postnatal Depression Scale as a screening measure. *Journal of Affective Disorders, 125*(1–3), 365–368. https://doi.org/10.1016/j.jad.2010.01.069

Ellis, B. J., Bates, J. E., Dodge, K. A., Fergusson, D. M., Horwood, L. J., Pettit, G. S., et al. (2003). Does father absence place daughters at special risk for early sexual activity? *Child Development, 74*, 801–822.

Erlich, K. B., Cassidy, J. & Dykas, M. J. (2011). Reporter discrepancies among parents, adolescents and peers: Adolescent attachment and informant depressive symptoms as explanatory factors. *Child Development, 82*, 999–1012. https://doi.org/10.1111/j.1467-8624.2010.01530.x

Fagerskiold, A. (2006). Support of fathers of infants by the child health nurse. *Scandinavian Journal of Caring, 20*, 79–85.

Femina, D. D., Yeager, C. A., & Lewis, D. O. (1990). Child abuse: Adolescent records vs. adult recall. *Child Abuse & Neglect, 14*(2), 227–231.

Fenaroli, V., & Saita, E. (2013). Fear of childbirth: A contribution to the validation of the Italian version of the Wijma Delivery Expectancy/Experience Questionnaire (WDEQ). *Testing, Psychometrics, Methodology in Applied Psychology, 20*, 1–24. https://doi.org/10.4473/TPM20.XXXXXX

Field, T., Diego, M., Hernandez-Reif, M., Schanberg, S., Kuhn, C., et al. (2004). Prenatal depression effects in the fetus and the newborn. *Infant Behavior and Development, 27*, 216–229. https://doi.org/10.1016/j.infbeh.2003.09.010

Field, T., Diego, M., Hernandez-Reif, M., Figueiredo, B., Deeds, O., Contogeorgos, J., et al. (2006). Antenatal paternal depression. *Infant Behavior and Development, 29*(4), 579–583. https://doi.org/10.1016/j.infbeh.2006.07.010

Figueiredo, B., & Conde, A. (2011). Anxiety and depression in woman and men from early pregnancy to 3-months postpartum. *Archives of Womens Mental Health, 14*, 247–255.

Finnbogadottir, H., Svalenius, E. C., & Persson, E. K. (2002). Expectant first-time fathers' experiences of pregnancy. *Midwifery, 19*, 96–105.

Fletcher, R. J., Matthey, S., & Marley, C. G. (2006). Addressing depression and anxiety among new fathers. *Medical Journal of Australia, 185*(8).

Flykt, M., Poikkeus, P., Sinkonen, J., Lindblom, J., Vilska, S., & Tiitinen, A. (2009). Prenatal expectations in transition to parenthood: Former infertility and family dynamic considerations. *Journal of Family Psychology, 23*, 779–789. https://doi.org/10.1037/a0016468

Fox, R. A., Platz, D. L., & Bentley, K. S. (1995). Maternal factors related to parenting practices, developmental expectations, and perceptions of child behavior problems. *Journal of Genetic Psychology, 156*, 431–441. https://doi.org/10.1080/00221325.1995.9914835

Fredriksen, E., von Soest, T., Smith, L., & Moe, V. (2019). Parenting stress plays a mediating role in the prediction of early child development from both parents' perinatal depressive symptoms. *Journal of Abnormal Child Psychology, 47*(1), 149–164.

Genesoni, L., & Tallandini, M. A. (2009). Men's psychological transition to fatherhood: An analysis of the literature, 1989–2008. *Birth, 36*(4), 305–318. https://doi.org/10.1111/j.1523-536X.2009.00358.x

Glaser, D. (2014). The effects of child maltreatment on the developing brain. Medico-Legal Journal, 2(3), 97–111. https//doi.org/10.1177/0025817214540395.

Goldstein, J., Freud, A., & Solnit, A. J. (1979). *Beyond the best interests of the child*. New York: The Free Press, MacMillan Publishing Co.

Goodman, J. H. (2004). Paternal postpartum depression, its relationship to maternal postpartum depression, and implications for family health. *Journal of Advanced Nursing, 45*, 26–25.

Gottfried, A. E., Gottfried, A. W., & Bathurst, K. (1988). Maternal employment, family environment, and children's development: Infancy through the school years). In A. E. Gottfried & A. W. Gottfried (Eds.), *Plenum studies in work and industry. Maternal employment and children's development: Longitudinal research* (pp. 11–58). New York: Plenum Press. https://doi.org/10.1007/978-1-4899-0830-8_2

Goulet, C., Bell, L., St-Cyr Tribble, D., Paul, D., & Lang, A. (1998). A concept analysis of parent-infant attachment. *Journal of Advanced Nursing, 28*(5), 1071–1081.

Green, A. (2000). On thirdness). In J. Abram (Ed.), *Andre Green at the squiggle foundation*. London, UK: Karnac Bookds.

Grych, J. H., & Clark, R. (1999). Maternal employment and development of the father-infant relationship in the first year. *Developmental Psychology, 35*, 893–903. https://doi.org/10.1037/0012-1649.35.4.893

Gutierrez-Galve, L., Stein, A., Hanington, L., Heron, J., & Ramchandani, P. (2015). Paternal depression in the postnatal period and child development: Mediators and moderators. *Pediatrics, 135*(2), 339–347. https://doi.org/10.1542/peds.2014-2411

Hallers-Haalboom, E. T., Mesman, J., Groeneveld, M. G., Endendijk, J. J., Van Berkel, S. R., Van der Pol, L. D., et al. (2014). Mothers, fathers, sons and daughters: Parental sensitivity in families with two .children. *Journal of Family Psychology, 28*(2), 138–147. https://doi.org/10.1037/a0036004

Hazan, C., & Shaver, P. (1987). Romantic love conceptualized as an attachment process. *Journal of Personality and Social Psychology, 52*, 511–524. https://doi.org/10.1016/j.jad.2013.09.038

Hetherington, E. M., & Stanley-Hagan, M. (1986). Divorced fathers: Stress, coping, and adjustment. In M. E. Lamb (Ed.), *The father's role: Applied perspectives* (pp. 103–134). New York: Wiley.

Howes, C., & Spieker, S. (2008). Attachment relationships in the context of multiple caregivers. In: J. Cassidy, & P. R. Shaver (red.), *Handbook of attachment: Theory, research, and clinical applications* (2nd ed. pp. 317–332). New York/London, UK: Guilford.

Huizink, A., Mulder, E. J. H., Robles de Medina, P. G., Visser, G. H. A., & Buitelaar, J. (2004). Is pregnancy anxiety a distinctive syndrome? *Early Human Development, 79*, 81–91. https://doi.org/10.1016/j.earlhumdev.2004.04.014

Kim, P., & Swain, J. E. (2007). Sad dads: Paternal postpartum depression. *Psychiatry, 4*, 35–47.

Korn, S. (1984). Continuities and discontinuities in difficult/easy temperament: Infancy to young adulthood. *Merrill-Palmer Quarterly, 30*, 189–199. http://www.jstor.org/stable/23086233

Lam, C. B., McHale, S. M., & Crouter, A. C. (2013). Parent-child shared time from middle childhood to late adolescence: Developmental course and adjustment correlates. *Child Development, 83*(2), 2089–2103. https://doi.org/10.1111/j.1467-8624.2012.01826.x

Lamb, M. E., Pleck, J. H., Charnov, E. L., & Levine, J. A. (1985). Paternal behavior in humans. *American Zoologist, 25*, 883–894.

Lamb, M. (2002). Placing children's interests first: Developmentally appropriate parenting plans. *Virginia Journal of Social Policy & the Law, 10*, 98–119.

Lamb, M. E. (2010). *The role of the fathers in child development*: fifth ed. John Wiley & Sons, Inc.

Leach, L. S., Poyser, C., Cooklin, A. R., & Giallo, R. (2016). Prevalence and course of anxiety disorders (and symptom levels) in men across the perinatal period: A systematic review. *Journal of Affective Disorder, 190*, 675–686. https://doi.org/10.1016/j.jad.2015.09.063

Lebovici, S. (1994). The way to subjectification. *Infant Mental Health Journal, 15*, 50–56.

Lovas, G. S. (2005). Gender and patterns of emotional availability in mother-toddler and father-toddler dyads. *Infant Mental Health Journal, 26*, 327–353. https://doi.org/10.1002/imhj.20056

Lundy, B. L. (2002). Father– And mother–infant face-to-face interactions: Differences in mind-related comments and infant attachment? *Infant Behavior and Development, 26*, 200–212.

Luoma, I., Puura, K. M., Äntymaa, M., Latve, R., Salmelin, R., & Tamminen, R. (2012). Fathers' postnatal depressive and anxiety symptoms: An exploration of links with paternal, maternal, infant and family factors. *Nordic Journal of Psychiatry*. *Advance online publication.* https://doi.org/10.3109/08039488.2012.752034

Luthar, S. S., D'Avanzo, K., & Hitches, S. (2003). Maternal drug abuse versus other psychological disturbances: Risks and resilience among children. In S. S. Luthar (Ed.), *Resilience and vulnerability. Adaptation in the context of childhood adversities* (pp. 105–129). Cambridge, UK: Cambridge University Press.

Luz, R., George, A., Vieux, R., & Spitz, E. (2007). Antenatal determinants of parental attachment and parenting alliance: How do mothers and fathers differ? *Intant Mental Health Journal, 38*(2), 183–197. https://doi.org/10.1002/imhj.21628

Massoudi, P., Hwang, C. P., & Wickberg, B. (2013). How well does the Edinburgh Postnatal Depression Scale identify depression and anxiety in fathers? A validation study in a population based Swedish sample. *Journal of Affective Disorders, 149*, 67–74. https://doi.org/10.1016/j.jad.2013.01.005

Matthey, S., Barnett, B., Ungerer, J., & Waters, B. (2000). Paternal and maternal depressed mood during the transition to parenthood. *Journal of Affective Disorders, 60*(2), 75–85. https://doi.org/10.1016/S0165-0327(00)00236-6

Matthey, S., Barnett, B., Kavanagh, D. J., & Howie, P. (2001). Validation of the Edinburgh Postnatal Depression Scale for men, and comparison of item endorsement with their partners. *Journal of Affective*

Disorders, 64(2–3), 175–184. https://doi.org/10.1016/S0165-0327(00)00236-6

Matthey, S. (2008). Using the Edinburgh Postnatal Depression Scale to screen for anxiety disorders. *Depression & Anxiety, 25*(11), 926–931. https://doi.org/10.1002/da.20415

McBride, B. A., & Rane, T. R. (1998). Parenting alliance as a predictor of fathers involvement: An exploratory study. *Family Relations, 47*(3), 229. https://doi.org/10.2307/584971

McEven, B. S., & Gianaros, P. J. (2010). Central role of the brain in stress and adaption: Links to socioeconomic status, health, and disease. *Annals of the New York Academy of Sciences, 1186*, 190–222. https://doi.org/10.1111/j.1749-6632.2009.05331.x

Melrose, S. (2010). Paternal postpartum depression: How can nurses begin to help? *Contemporary Nurse, 34*(2), 199–210. https://doi.org/10.5172/conu.2010.34.2.199

Musser, A. K., Ahmed, A. H., Foli, K. J., & Coddington, J. A. (2013). Paternal postpartum depression: What health care providers should know. *Journal of Pediatric Health Care, 27*(6), 479–485.

Nelson-Coffey, S. K., Borelli, J., & River, L. M. (2017). Attachment avoidance, but not anxiety, minimizes the joys of caregiving. *Attachment & Human Development, 19*(5), 504–531. https://doi.org/10.1080/14616734.2017.1326060

Nicol-Harper, R., Harvey, A. G., & Stein, A. (2007). Interactions between mothers and infants: Impact of maternal anxiety. *Infant Behavior & Development, 30*(1), 161–167.

Opacka-Juffry, J., & Mohiyeddini, C. (2012). Experience of stress in childhood negatively correlates with plasma oxytocin concentration in adult men. *Stress, 15*(1), 1–10.

Parfitt, Y., Ayers, S., Pike, A., Jessop, D. C., & Ford, E. (2014). A prospective study of the parent-baby bond in men and woman 15 months after birth. *Journal of Reproductive and Infant Psychology, 32*, 441–456. https://doi.org/10.1080/02646838.2014.956301

Parfitt, Y., Pike, A., & Ayers, S. (2013). The impact of parents' mental health on parent-baby interaction: A prospective study. *Infant Behavior & Development, 36*(4), 599–608.

Pauli-Pott, U., Mertesacker, B., Bade, U., Haverkock, A., & Beckmann, D. (2003). Parental perceptions and infant temperament development. *Infant Behavior and Development, 26*, 27–48. https://doi.org/10.1016/S0163-6383(02)00167-4

Paulson, J. F., & Bazemore, S. D. (2010). Prenatal and postpartum depression in fathers and its association with depression. A meta-analysis. *Journal of the American Medical Association, 303*, 19. https://doi.org/10.1001/jama.2010.605

Perren, S., Von Wyl, A., Bürgin, D., Simoni, H., & Von Klitzing, K. (2005). Depressive symptoms and psychosocial stress across the transition to parenthood: Associations with parental psychopathology and child difficulty. *Journal of Psychosomatic Obstetrics and Gynecology, 26*(3), 173–183.

Pleck, J. H. (2010). Paternal involvement: Revised conceptualization and theoretical linkages with child outcomes. In M. E. Lamb (Ed.), *The role of the father in child development* (5th ed., pp. 67–107). New York: Wiley.

Radin, N. (1994). Primary-caregiving fathers in intact families). In A. E. Gottfried & A. W. Gottfried (Eds.), *Redefining families: Implications for children's development* (pp. 11–54). New York: Plenum.

Ramchandani, P. G., Stein, A., O'Connor, T. G., & the ALSPAC team. (2005). Paternal depression in the postnatal period and child development: A prospective population study. *Lancet, 365*, 2201–2205. https://doi.org/10.1016/S0140-6736(05)66778-5

Ramchandani, P. G., Stein, A., O'Connor, T. G., Heron, J., Murray, L., & Evans, J. (2008). Depression in men in the postnatal period and later child psychopathology: A population cohort study. *Journal of the American Academy of Child & Adolescent Psychiatry, 47*, 390–398. https://doi.org/10.1097/CHI.0b013e31816429c2

Ramchandani, P. G., Domoney, J., Sethna, V., Psychogiou, L., Vlachos, H., & Murray, L. (2013). Do early father-infant interactions predict the onset of externalizing behaviours in young children? Finding from a longitudinal cohort study. *Journal of Child Psychology and Psychiatry, 54*(1), 56–64. https://doi.org/10.1111/j.1469-7610.2012.02583.x

Rege, M. & Solli, I. F. (2010). *The Impact of Paternity Leave on Long-Term Father Involvement.* CESifo Working Paper Series No. 3130. Cabrera, N. J. (2010). Father Involvement and Public Policies, In: Lamb, M. E (ed.) *The role of the Father in Child Development* (5th ed.). Wiley.

Rollè, L., Prino, L. E., Sechi, C., Vismara, L., Neri, E., Polizzi, C., et al. (2017). Parenting stress, mental health, dyadic adjustment: A structural equation model. *Frontiers in Psychology, 8*(839). https://doi.org/10.3389/fpsyg.2017.00839

Saisto, T., Salmela-Aro, K., Nurmi, J.-E., & Halmesmäki, E. (2008). Longitudinal study on the predictors of parental stress in mothers and fathers of toddlers. *Journal of Psychosomatic Obstetrics and Gynecology, 29*(3), 213–222. https://doi.org/10.1080/01674820802000467

Sameroff, A. J., & Fiese, B. H. (2000a). Transactional regulation: The developmental ecology of early intervention. In J. P. Shonkoff & S. J. Meisels (Eds.), *Handbook of early childhood intervention* (2nd ed., pp. 135–159). New York: Cambridge University Press.

Sameroff, A. J., & Fiese, B. H. (2000b). Models of development and developmental risk. In C. H. Zeanah (Ed.), *Handbook of infant mental health* (2nd ed., pp. 3–19). New York: Guilford Press.

Schore, A. N. (2009). Relational trauma and the developing right brain. An Interface of psychoanalytic self psychology and neuroscience. *Self and Systems: Annals of New York Academic Science, 1159*, 189–203.

Schumacher, M., Zubaran, C., & White, G. (2008). Bringing birth-reated paternal depression to the fore. *Women and Birth, 21*, 65–70.

Sethna, V., Murray, L., Netsi, E., Psychogiou, L., & Ramchandani, P. G. (2015). Paternal depression in the postnatal period and early father-infant interactions. *Parenting, Science and Practice, 15*(1), 1–8. https://doi.org/10.1080/15295192.2015.992732

Shannon, J. D., Tamis-LeMonda, C. S., & Margolin, A. (2005). Father involvement in infancy: Influences of past and current relationships. *Infancy, 8*, 21–414. https://doi.org/10.1207/s15327078in0801_2

Shannon, J. D., Tamis-LeMonda, C. S., & Cabrera, N. J. (2006). Fathering in infancy: Mutuality and stability between 8 and 16 months. *Parenting: Science and Practice, 6*, 167–188. https://doi.org/10.1080/15295192.2006.9681304

Singley, D. B., & Edwards, L. M. (2015). Men's perinatal mental health in the transition to fatherhood. *Professional Psychology: Research and Practice, 22*. https://doi.org/10.1037/pro0000032

Skjothaug, T., Smith, L., Wentzel-Larsen, T., & Moe, V. (2014). Prospective fathers' adverse childhood experiences, pregnancy-related anxiety, and depression during pregnancy. *Infant Mental Health Journal, 00*, 1–8. https://doi.org/10.1002/imhj.21485

Skjothaug, T., Smith, L., Wentzel-Larsen, T., & Moe, V. (2018). Does fathers' prenatal mental health bear a relationship to parenting stress at 6 months? *Infant Mental Health Journal, 39*, 537–551. https://doi.org/10.1002/imhj.21739

Skjothaug, T., Smith, L., Wentzel- Larsen, T., Stänicke, E. & Moe, V. (2020). Antecedents of fathers' perception of child behavior at child age 12 months. *Infant Mental Health Journal, 41:4*.

Smith, L. (2010). Tilknytning og omsorg for barn under tre år. *Tidsskrift for Norsk Psykologforening, 47*(9), 804–811.

Solantus, T., & Salo, S. (2005). Paternal postnatal depression: Fathers emerge from the wings. *The Lancet, 365*, 6.

Tamis-LeMonda, C. S., & Cabrera, N. (1999). Perspectives on father involvement: Research and policy. *Social Policy Report; Society for Research in Child Development., xiii*.

Teixeira, C., Figueiredo, B., Conde, A., Pacheco, A., & Costa, R. (2009). Anxiety and depression during pregnancy in women and men. *Journal of Affective Disorders, 119*, 142–148. https://doi.org/10.1016/j.jad.2009.03.005

Trentacosta, C. J., Hyde, L. W., Shaw, D. S., Dishion, T. S., Gardner, F., & Wilson (2008). *Journal of Child Psychology and Psychiatry, 49*(11), 1211–9. https://doi.org/10.1111/j.1469-7610.2008.01941.x

Van Holland De Graaf, J., Hoogenboom, M., De Roos, M., & Bucx, F. (2014). Socio-demographic correlates of fathers' and mothers' parenting behaviors. *Journal of Child and Family Studies, 27*, 2315–2327. https://doi.org/10.1007/s10826-018-1059-7

Van IJzendoorn, M. (1995). The association between adult attachment representation and infant attachment, parental responsiveness, and clinical status: A meta-analysis on the predictive quality of the adult attachment interview. *Psychological Bulletin, 113*, 404–410.

Van IJzendoorn, M. H., & Sagi-Schwartz, A. (2008). Cross cultural patterns of attachment: Universal and contextual dimensions. In: J. Cassidy, & P. R. Shaver (red.), *Handbook of attachment: Theory, research, and clinical applications* (2. utg., s. 880–905). New York/London: Guilford.

Wee, K. Y., Skouteris, H., Pier, C., Richardson, B., & Milgrom, J. (2011). Correlates of ante- and postnatal depression in fathers: A systematic review. *Journal of Affective Disorders, 130*, 358–377. https://doi.org/10.1016/j.jad.2010.06.019.

Weinfeld, N. S. (2002). Comments on Lamb's «Placing children's interests first». *Virginia Journal of Social Policy & the Law, 10*, 120–128.

Vismara, L., Rollè, L., Agostini, F., Sechi, C., Fenaroli, V., Molgara, S., et al. (2016). Perinatal parenting stress, anxiety, and first-time mothers and fathers: A 3-to 6-months postpartum follow-up study. *Frontiers in Psychology, 7*, 938. https://doi.org/10.3389/fpsyg.2016.00938

Ward, M., & Carlson, E. (1995). Associations among adult attachment representations, maternal sensitivity, and infant-mother attachment in a sample of adolescent mothers. *Child Development, 66*, 69–79.

Webster-Stratton, C. (1990). Stress: A potential disruptor of parent perceptions and family interactions. *Journal of Clinical Child Psychology, 19*, 302–312.

Wee, K. Y., Skouteris, H., Richardson, B., MacPhie, S., & Hill, B. (2015). The inter-relationship between depressive, anxiety and stress symptoms in fathers during the antenatal period. *Journal of Reproductive Infant Psychology., 33*, 359–373. https://doi.org/10.1080/02646838.2015.1048199

Weissman, S., & Cohen, R. S. (1985). The parenting alliance and adolescence. *Adolescent Psychiatry, 12*, 24–45.

Williams, L. M. (1995). Recovered memories of abuse in woman with documented child sexual victimization histories. *Journal of Traumatic Stress, 8*(4), 649–673.

Winnicott, D. W. (1971). *Playing and reality*. London, UK: Tavistock/Routledge.

Östberg, M., & Hagekull, B. (2000). A structural modeling approach to the understanding of parenting stress. *Journal of Clinical Child Psychology, 29*(4), 615–625. https://doi.org/10.1207/S15374424JCCP2904

15 Paternal Prenatal and Postpartum Depression

James F. Paulson, Kelsey T. Ellis, and Regina L. Alexander

To fully understand the factors that influence parents' functioning and its eventual effect on family and child development inevitably requires attention to expecting parents and their transition to the early family. Research in this tradition overwhelmingly emphasizes the mother's role in the family system, often positioning her characteristics as essential drivers of early child development (Cummings, Keller, & Davies, 2005). In particular, early maternal depression has been extensively documented as a predictor of negative child developmental, emotional, and behavioral outcomes (Bennett, Einarson, Taddio, Koren, & Einarson, 2004). Although a large body of research has accumulated around predictors and outcomes associated with maternal depression, research on paternal depression during this time is a newer and developing area. Recent studies of paternal depression have revealed that the incidence of depression is elevated prenatally in both mothers and fathers and remains elevated through the first year postpartum (Paulson & Bazemore, 2010). Moreover, depressive symptom severity is correlated between new parents, even when they do not cohabitate (Paulson, Dauber, & Leiferman, 2011).

In terms of paternal depression's implications for the family, this growing literature is providing evidence that bears similarity to established effects of maternal depression. Elevated paternal depression symptoms at 8 weeks postpartum were found to predict higher levels of child internalizing and externalizing behavior problems at child age 3.5 years. These same children of depressed fathers had higher rates of diagnosed psychopathology by age 7 years (Ramchandani et al., 2005; Ramchandani et al., 2011). Depression in fathers of infants has also been associated with reduced father-child activities, impaired bonding, increased parenting stress, and greater discord in the relationship with the child's mother (Bronte-Tinkew, Moore, Matthews, & Carrano, 2007; Edhborg, Matthiesen, Lundh, & Widstrom, 2005; Paulson, Dauber, & Leiferman, 2006).

Because of this growing literature, this chapter will address paternal depression through the lens of the family system in which it arises and the developing family that it affects. We will focus on evidence that suggests that fathers' adjustment during their partner's pregnancy and in the early period of new parenthood is (a) associated with an elevated risk of depression, (b) predicted by a range of risk and protective factors, (c) closely related to marital and family adjustment, (d) intertwined with maternal

J. F. Paulson (✉)
Department of Psychology, Old Dominion University, Norfolk, VA, USA
e-mail: jpaulson@odu.edu

K. T. Ellis · R. L. Alexander
Virginia Consortium Program in Clinical Psychology, Old Dominion University, Norfolk, VA, USA

H. E. Fitzgerald et al. (eds.), *Handbook of Fathers and Child Development*,
https://doi.org/10.1007/978-3-030-51027-5_15

adjustment, and (e) predictive of important child development processes. Using evidence from these findings, we will then suggest an integrative model of perinatal paternal depression family system for better understanding the emergence of paternal perinatal depression and how it conveys risk to the early family and developing children.

Definitions and Terminology

Various terms are used to refer to the period of time between conception to the end of the first year after delivery, with usage often following regional and national conventions. *Prenatal* is the term most often used to describe the pregnancy through delivery, whereas the duration and terminology for the period of time after delivery is much more variable, with times extending from 4 weeks to 1 year and terms that include *postnatal, postpartum, antenatal,* and *puerperium.* Other terms address the period from a midpregnancy to time 4-6 weeks after delivery as *perinatal* or *peripartum.* This mix of sometimes conflicting terminology is found in the literature describing depression that occurs during this time period (O'Hara, Wisner, Asher, & Asher, 2014), which is somewhat more consistent in characterizing a window of increased pregnancy, delivery, and postdelivery risk for depressive symptoms and other mental illness as stretching from early pregnancy to around 1 year after delivery, although this too varies. The Diagnostic and Statistical Manual of Mental Disorders (DSM-5) offers little clarity in its designation of a "peripartum onset" specifier under major depressive disorder, which can be coded when depression occurs sometime in pregnancy or within the first 6 postdelivery weeks (American Psychiatric Association (APA), 2013).

A far greater agreement can be found around the *nature* of depression during this time period, with most investigators agreeing that it is a manifestation of major depressive disorder. This aligns with current practice and DSM-5 criteria, which define major depressive disorder by the presence of one or more major depressive episodes in the absence of significant evidence of mania or hypomania (Uher, Payne, Pavlova, & Perlis, 2014). To meet the criteria for this disorder, five of nine symptoms must be present "nearly every day" during the same 2-week period. These symptoms include depressed mood, anhedonia, significant weight loss or gain, insomnia or hypersomnia, psychomotor agitation, fatigue, feelings of worthlessness, difficulties concentrating, and suicide ideation. Furthermore, these symptoms must cause clinically significant distress or impairment in daily functioning and must not be attributable to a substance or medical condition (APA, 2013). Based on this, classifying major depressive disorder during this time period separates it in severity and persistence from postpartum blues, or "baby blues," which has been common among mothers after delivery and which is now becoming increasingly adopted to address these same concerns in fathers (Hübner-Liebermann, Hausner, & Wittmann, 2012).

For the purposes of this chapter, we will use the terms *prenatal depression* and *postpartum depression* to refer to depression occurring before and after delivery (Falah-Hassani, Shiri, & Dennis, 2017). When reviewing research that measures depressive symptom severity, we will use the term *depressive symptoms* to differentiate this from clinical diagnosis.

History of Prenatal and Postpartum Depression in Fathers

A complete understanding of paternal prenatal depression must acknowledge the evolution of how researchers and developmentalists have historically approached fathers and their influence on child development. In 1976, Michael Lamb published the first edition of *The Role of the Father in Child Development.* It marked the first coherent effort to organize the then fragmentary research under one integrative summary that broke new ground in acknowledging fathers as meaningful developmental figures, both through their indirect impact on the family system and their direct engagement with the child. Lamb sought, in the first edition of this book, to provide an inclusive bibliography of research in the area, ending with a reference list of a few pages. By 1985, research in the fatherhood area had grown to the point that such a comprehensive bibliography was no longer feasible, and Lamb noted in his third edition introduction that such a bibliography would likely exceed the length of the written text in the book (Lamb et al., 1985).

Despite the growth in studying fathers as key developmental figures that can be observed in the late twentieth century, modern developmental research is still often faulted for including fathers only partially as a research or not at all. The reasons for this are likely multifactorial. First, because family structures often make mothers more available, they are more likely to be recruited as research participants. Many developmental theories, particularly those involving psychopathology, also tend to show a gender bias, centering influence (or blame) on mothers. Additionally, societal norms that have long been outpaced by our knowledge of fathers' role in development are still influential in investigators' conceptual and methodological approach to research, in particular, outdated norms that characterize fathers' primary, sometimes sole, role as breadwinning.

Building from this uncertain foundation in general developmental research on fathers' influence, work in specific subpopulations suffers from yet more disproportionate representation of fathers. In a 2010 meta-analysis of studies that document rates of depression among expecting and new fathers, we identified a total of 43 published peer-reviewed studies that documented rates of depression in fathers who were expecting a child or who had a child under age 1 year. Most of these articles documented studies that were not primarily focused on fathers, but collected their data as ancillary to main study purposes. Although the earliest study we were able to identify in this meta-analysis was published in 1984 (one of two studies published in the 1980s), about 75% were published after 2000. Much like in the broader child development literature, our understanding of fathers' experiences and their impact on the child and family system is new and rapidly evolving. As a corollary to the new and largely uncharted nature of paternal prenatal and postpartum depression, standardized practices for screening, identification, or treatment have yet to even be proposed.

Prevalence

A number of primary studies have sought to estimate the prevalence of depression in fathers during their partners' pregnancies and in their first postpartum year. This literature is international in scope, although most recent studies of prenatal and postpartum depression in fathers have been carried out largely in the developed world. For example, a study of 320 German fathers found that the prevalence of depression was 9.8% during their partners' pregnancy, falling to 7.8% during the postpartum period (Gawlik et al., 2014). A Hong Kong–based study of 320 fathers found that significant depressive symptomatology was present in 3.3% of expecting fathers during early pregnancy, rising to 4.1% in late pregnancy, and 5.2% at 6 weeks postpartum (Koh, Chui, Tang, & Lee, 2014). A study of 90 Mexican American fathers found that 9% of fathers met criteria for postpartum depression at both 15 and 21 weeks postpartum (Roubinov, Luecken, Crnic, & Gonzales, 2014). In a sample of 205 Iranian fathers, 11.7% evidenced significant depressive symptoms at 6–12 weeks postpartum (Kamalifard, Hasanpoor, Kheiroddin, Panahi, & Payan, 2014). In a sample of 885 Swedish fathers, 6.3% demonstrated significant depressive symptoms at 3 months postpartum (Massoudi, Hwang, & Wickberg, 2016).

These and many other studies have been synthesized in several recent meta-analyses. In 2010, an international meta-analysis synthesized 43 studies published between 1980 and 2009, finding that the average rate of paternal depression in pregnancy and the first postpartum year was 10.4% (Paulson & Bazemore, 2010). A more recent meta-analysis included 74 studies published between 1980 and 2015, reporting an average rate of paternal prenatal and postpartum depression of 8.4% (Cameron, Sedov, & Tomfohr-Madsen, 2016). Both of these meta-analyses note a number of common features among the research on paternal prenatal and postpartum depression: *First*, relatively few studies documenting this phenomenon were published prior to the year 2000, and the pace of publication has rapidly increased since that time. *Second*, there is significant heterogeneity of reported rates of depression that seems to covary with measurement method, location, year of publication, and maternal depression. *Last*, Cameron et al. (2016) points out significant gaps that exist in our knowledge of paternal depression during certain time periods during pregnancy and in the postpartum, particularly in the first trimester and 6–9 months postpartum.

Predictive, Risk, and Resilience Factors

Biological Factors

Recently, research has begun to examine the role that hormone changes during the prenatal and postpartum period may play in paternal depression. Some researchers have hypothesized that these hormone changes may lead to fathers' experience of depression during this time (Kim & Swain, 2007; Tuszyńska-Bogucka & Nawra, 2014), although the evidence for this hypothetical link is weak and correlational. Still, much of the thinking around causal biological mechanisms for prenatal and postpartum depression in women has been mirrored as a framework for proposing biological causes of fathers' depression.

One hypothesized predictor of paternal depression may be testosterone below baseline expected levels for age. Lower levels of testosterone have been associated with symptoms of depression in men (Seidman & Walsh, 1999). A systematic review and meta-analysis found support for this hypothesis and went on to describe relief in depressive symptoms with testosterone replacement therapy when compared to placebo (Zarrouf, Artz, Griffith, Sirbu, & Kommor, 2009). This effect has been extrapolated to suggest that some of the observed decreases in testosterone among men in the first few postpartum months (Berg & Wynne-Edwards, 2001) may play a causal role in paternal postpartum depression.

Another predictor of paternal prenatal and postpartum depression may be decreases in estrogens from baseline. Levels of estradiol, an estrogen that plays a key role in reproduction for both men and women, have been observed to increase in men during the last month of their partner's pregnancy and remain relatively high through the early postpartum period (Berg & Wynne-Edwards, 2001). Fleming and colleagues (2002) reported that higher levels of estrogen were associated with more father involvement in parenting. Taking these findings into consideration, Kim and Swain (2007) proposed that relative decreases in estrogens and potentially the lack of expected estradiol increase in expecting and new fatherhood may result in dysregulation of early parenting behaviors that may go on to impose a risk for depression. It should be noted that more work is needed to reconcile the proposition that lower levels of both estrogens and testosterone increase risk for depression, as estradiol typically inhibits testosterone production and availability (Schulster, Bernie, & Ramasamy, 2016).

Paternal depression may also be linked to lower cortisol levels (Kim & Swain, 2007; Tuszyńska-Bogucka & Nawra, 2014). Higher levels of cortisol, a hormone which regulates physiological reactions to stressful events, typically correlate with higher levels of stress. However, in the context of maternal perinatal depression, studies have reported that higher cortisol levels in mothers are generally associated with increased sensitivity to infant crying (Fleming, O'Day, & Kraemer, 1999) and lower level of depression (Fleming & Anderson, 1987). Thus, a lower level of cortisol among fathers may be related to difficulties in paternal bonding with the infant and in turn associated depressed mood (Kim & Swain, 2007).

Lower levels of vasopressin may be another predicting factor of paternal perinatal depression. Similar to oxytocin levels in mothers, vasopressin typically increases in fathers in the days and weeks after childbirth (Young, 1999). This increase in vasopressin is believed to ultimately enhance bonding between father and infant

(Wang, Ferris, & De Vries, 1994) by activating the prefrontal cortex and its associated increase in organizing and planning for the future (Kozorovitskiy, Hughes, Lee, & Gould, 2006). A number of investigators have proposed that because of this key role in early fatherhood, insufficient vasopressin production may disrupt early bonding and parenting engagement, which may also introduce vulnerability to depression (Kim & Swain, 2007; Tuszyńska-Bogucka & Nawra, 2014).

Finally, paternal prenatal and postpartum depression may be related to changes in prolactin levels, which is important for the onset and maintenance of parental behaviors. Prolactin levels in men typically increase during their partners' pregnancy and continue to increase during the first postpartum year. Higher levels of prolactin are associated with greater responsivity to infant stimuli among new fathers (Storey, Walsh, Quinton, & Wynne-Edwards, 2000). Thus, deficits in prolactin may impact fathers' ability to adapt to parenthood, thereby increasing risk for depression (Kim & Swain, 2007; Tuszyńska-Bogucka & Nawra, 2014).

Psychosocial Factors

Psychosocial predictors of maternal prenatal and postpartum depression have been studied and reported extensively, with robust findings suggesting that external stressful life events, parenting stress, problems in the partner relationship with the father, social support, economic strains, and many other factors increase the likelihood of expecting and new mothers' depression (Yim, Tanner Stapleton, Guardino, Hahn-Holbrook, & Dunkel Schetter, 2015). A newer and more limited effort has begun to characterize the role of these and similar factors in predicting fathers' depression. This growing literature points to several factors at the individual, social, and external stressor levels stress-related, as being predictive of the onset and persistence of paternal depression.

Individual Factors Individual factors such as sociodemographic background and underlying psychological processes have been identified as risk factors for paternal prenatal and postpartum depression. Sociodemographic factors such as age (e.g., <29 years; Bergström, 2013; Davé, Petersen, Sherr, & Nazareth, 2010), a low education level (Koh et al., 2014), unemployment status (Davé et al., 2010), and low social class and income (Davé et al., 2010; Koh et al., 2014) have been associated with paternal prenatal and postpartum depression. Furthermore, Bergström (2013) reported that first-time fathers, especially younger fathers, are at higher risk for depression and may experience the responsibilities associated with a new family as more troublesome. History of mental health concerns has also been linked to prenatal and postpartum depression in fathers. A longitudinal study looking at predisposing factors for postpartum depression in fathers reported that a history of severe depressive symptoms and having high anxiety after childbirth were its most significant predictors (Ramchandani et al., 2008).

Additionally, negative biases in processing information related to the self and life circumstances have been consistently linked to the onset and maintenance of depression (Baumeister, 2013; Kernis, 1993). Lower life satisfaction (Morse, Buist, & Durkin, 2000) as well as concerns about the future (Hall & Long, 2007; Morse et al., 2000) have also been linked to paternal prenatal and postpartum depression. Hall and Long (2007) suggested that fathers with lower life satisfaction are more likely to make negative appraisals of their circumstances, particularly their role as fathers. Fathers with low self-esteem (Koh et al., 2014) and poorer perceived parenting efficacy (deMontigny, Girard, Lacharité, Dubeau, & Devault, 2013) are also at a higher risk for prenatal and postpartum depression. Koh and colleagues (2014) suggested that poor self-esteem, in combination with work-family conflict, led to fathers experiencing a negative sense of control and in turn at greater risk of failing to meet their own parenting expectations.

Social Factors Social factors related to support, the partner relationship, and the parent-child relationship have been linked to paternal depression. Social support, defined broadly as an individual's available interpersonal resources, tends to be mobilized when the individual experiences life stress or psychological distress (Gao, Chan, & Mao, 2009). The extant literature suggests that fathers with lower social support are more likely to experience depression (Bielawska-Batorowicz & Kossakowska-Petrycka, 2006; Wee, Skouteris, Pier, Richardson, & Milgrom, 2011). Gao et al. (2009) found that when fathers perceived lower social support when compared to their partners, they were more likely to endorse more depressive symptoms. Moreover, a study examining gender differences among parents across various psychosocial risk factors for postpartum depression found that while lower social support was a significant predictor of postpartum depression in both mothers and fathers, mothers were impacted more strongly by stress and fathers experienced greater depression in the presence of lower self-esteem (Wang & Chen, 2006).

Additionally, individual relationships within the family play an important role in parent functioning. A meta-analysis of 30 studies found that one of the most common correlates of paternal prenatal and postpartum depression was having a partner with depression (Wee et al., 2011). Roberts and colleagues (2006) found that men with depressed partners were more likely to have three or more comorbidities, including depressive disorders, anxiety disorder, alcohol abuse, problem fatigue, and general affective problems. Additionally, multiple studies have reported that marital satisfaction has been negatively associated with paternal postpartum depression (Bielawska-Batorowicz & Kossakowska-Petrycka, 2006; deMontigny et al., 2013; Wee et al., 2011). Fathers describe communication, intimacy, and support from their spouse as being critical aspects of the partner relationship during the postpartum period (deMontigny & Lacharité, 2004); however, maintaining these supports, while also developing a co-parental alliance, is often challenging during this time (deMontigny et al., 2013). For example, a study of fathers' sense of exclusion from mother-infant bonding found that this posed a separate risk for their postpartum depression (Kim & Swain, 2007). Lower father-child engagement (Bronte-Tinkew et al., 2007), negative perceptions of their parental role (Zelkowitz & Milet, 1997), parenting stress (i.e., parenting distress, perceived difficult; deMontigny et al., 2013), and perception of a difficult infant temperament (Davé, Nazareth, Sherr, & Senior, 2005) have also been associated with paternal depression in pregnancy and the postpartum. Furthermore, because fathers may be slower to develop emotional bonds with their child, depression during this time period may be particularly disruptive (Anderson, 1996; Edhborg et al., 2005). Edhbord and colleagues (2005) reported that fathers who experience impaired bonding at 1 week postpartum also reported greater depressive symptoms at 2 months postpartum.

Stress-Related Factors Psychosocial stressors have been linked to the onset (Daley, Hammen, & Rao, 2000; Kendler, Karkowski, & Prescott, 1999), severity (Hammen, Davila, Brown, Ellicott, & Gitlin, 1992), and course of depression (Burke, Davis, Otte, & Mohr, 2005). Occupational stress as well as economic pressures associated with low social class and income have been linked to postpartum depression in fathers (Wang & Chen, 2006). Zelkowitz and Milet (1997) found that work-related stress is associated with fathers perceiving their marriage, role as parents, and infants' behaviors as more negative. In addition, fathers who report excessive parenting stress (Bergström, 2013) and distress (deMontigny et al., 2013) during pregnancy and postpartum are more likely to experience significant depressive symptoms.

Complications of pregnancy and delivery have also been associated with paternal prenatal and postpartum depression. DeMontigny and colleagues (2013) reported that proportionally more depressed fathers had experienced previous perinatal loss than their nondepressed counterparts. Infants born at very low birth weight (Helle et al.,

2015) and admission to neonatal intensive care unit (NICU; Gönülal, Yalaz, Altun-Köroğlu, & Kültürsay, 2014) are also predictors of paternal depression.

Resilience/Protective Factors In addition to risk factors, it is important to examine protective factors for paternal prenatal and postpartum depression. Limited research has explored specific protective factors for women at risk of perinatal depression, and even fewer studies have investigated this in father populations. For both mothers and fathers, suggested protective factors span individual and social factors. Individual factors such as better education, employment, and higher social class and income have been reported to be generally protective against depression, and this effect may also be at work in pregnancy and in the postpartum (Davé et al., 2010; Sethna, Murray, & Ramchandani, 2012). Higher socioeconomic status can provide parents with access to better healthcare, healthy foods, opportunities for exercise, and other resources that facilitate healthy behavior (Everson, Maty, Lynch, & Kaplan, 2002; Lorant et al., 2003). In addition, maintaining a work-life balance may also play a protective role against paternal perinatal depression (Koh et al., 2014). Koh and colleagues (2014) reported that higher levels of work-family conflict were associated with poor self-esteem as well as paternal postpartum depression, suggesting that balancing attention between work and family may be important in protecting against paternal depression during the prenatal and postpartum periods.

While partner depression and poor relationship satisfaction seem to be vulnerability factors, interpersonal factors such as higher perceived social support from relatives, friends, colleagues, and partners play a protective role against depression in both the prenatal and postpartum periods (Wee et al., 2011; Yim et al., 2015). This interpersonal support may serve a protective function during the transition to parenthood by preserving or enhancing self-esteem and buffering the impact of daily demands and stress for parents (Yim et al., 2015). Preliminary research has also highlighted the protective role played by certain cultural factors (e.g., traditions, beliefs/values, and rituals) in maternal prenatal depression (Bina, 2008; Yim et al., 2015). For example, cultures that emphasize family support to the mother over the first month postpartum have been associated with lower postpartum depression rates and delayed onset of symptoms (Halbreich, 2005; Yim et al., 2015). Research looking at father populations has reported that progressive cultural values that diverge from gendered parenting roles promote father qualities such as warmth and involvement in parenting tasks that are often associated with traditional "feminine" gender roles (Saracho & Spodek, 2007) and that these progressive beliefs may buffer against paternal depression (Roubinov et al., 2014). While research has begun to identify the protective role of culture in paternal perinatal depression, further exploration of these cultural factors is needed.

Outcomes Associated with Paternal Prenatal and Postpartum Depression

Partner and Marital Functioning Depression in fathers has been linked to problems related to relationship satisfaction for both the father and his partner (Gawlik et al., 2014; Ramchandani et al., 2011). A longitudinal study of 102 German fathers found that relationship satisfaction during the second and third trimester of their partner's pregnancy predicted depression, anxiety, and partner satisfaction at 6 months postpartum (Gawlik et al., 2014). Other studies have found the reciprocal of this, that earlier depression is predictive of later decreases in relationship satisfaction. Moreover, higher levels of paternal depression have been associated with decreased confidence in the relationship's longevity (Ramchandani et al., 2011). Another study found that both maternal postpartum depression and paternal postpartum depression are indirectly associated with decreased social support and relationship satisfaction, which then leads to further decreases in relationship satisfaction in both partners and subsequent increases in paternal depression (Don & Mickelson, 2012).

Child Development A range of problem outcomes in children and adolescents have been identified as being related to earlier paternal depression, particularly when it occurs in infancy and early childhood. These problem outcomes have ranged from poor school performance to an increased risk of developing other psychiatric disorders (Gentile & Fusco, 2017). In terms of more immediate impacts on children, paternal depression has been associated with excessive crying in infancy and toddlerhood (Van den Berg et al., 2009), hyperactivity and overall conduct problems during the preschool ages (Ramchandani et al., 2005), poorer global child psychological impairment, and more frequent psychiatric diagnosis in school age (Gutierrez-Galve, Stein, Hanington, Heron, & Ramchandani, 2015).

These negative outcomes may in part be mediated by impaired father-infant interactions. A study observing face-to-face interactions between fathers and infants reported that depressed fathers' speech included more negative and critical statements and focused more on their own experiences as opposed to infants' experiences (Sethna et al., 2012). A related study found that when engaging in face-to-face interactions with their infants, depressed fathers had less active engagement and playfulness when compared to their nondepressed counterparts (Sethna, Murray, Edmondson, Iles, & Ramchandani, 2018). While these studies highlight differences among depressed versus nondepressed fathers in their interactions with their infant, the manner in which these interactions impact infant development has not been directly studied.

The effects of paternal prenatal and postpartum depression have also been examined in school-aged children (i.e., ages 5–15 years). Paternal depression has been correlated with problems in social functioning (Ringoot et al., 2015), negative affect and depression (Fletcher, Feeman, Garfield, & Vimpani, 2011; Kryski et al., 2018) as well as other psychiatric disorders (Ramchandani et al., 2008), and behavioral problems (Fletcher et al., 2011) among school-aged children. A longitudinal study, which included an assessment of child development at 3.5 years and a follow-up of children age 7, indicated that impaired child development among children with fathers suffering from postpartum depression was detectible even several years after birth (Gutierrez-Galve et al., 2015). These findings suggest that paternal prenatal and postpartum depression may have long-term effects on child outcomes. In addition, Ramchandani and colleagues (2008) reported that school-aged children of depressed fathers during the postpartum period have a doubled risk for developing psychiatric disorders, specifically oppositional defiant disorder and conduct disorder, compared to children of nondepressed fathers. The literature suggests that these negative outcomes may be mediated by paternal positivity (Rice, Lewis, Harold, & Thapar, 2013), dual exposure to paternal and maternal depression (Gutierrez-Galve et al., 2015), marital conflict (Gutierrez-Galve et al., 2015; Hanington, Heron, Stein, & Ramchandani, 2012), and child cortisol reactivity to depressed fathers (Mackrell et al., 2014).

Negative child outcomes such as depression and anxiety (Mikkonen, Moustgaard, Remes, & Martikainen, 2016; Pearson et al., 2013; Reeb et al., 2015) and poor academic performance (Shen et al., 2016) among adolescent populations have also been linked to paternal depression. A longitudinal study reported that paternal postpartum depression had effects that were similar to maternal postpartum depression on 18-year-old adolescents. The study also reported that paternal depression that occurred in the child's early adolescence continued to predict that child's own symptoms of depression and anxiety as late as age 21 (Pearson et al., 2013). In addition, Shen and colleagues (2016) reported that maternal and paternal perinatal depression were both independently associated with poor academic performance among adolescents age 16 years.

Parenting and Family While these findings highlight the negative effects of paternal prenatal and postpartum depression on child outcomes, there are some inconsistencies within the literature with respect to the mechanisms by which paternal depression may lead to child outcomes. Gentile and Fusco (2017) highlighted this limitation in their systematic review of untreated paternal prenatal and postpartum depression and child outcomes. While some studies suggested that fathers who experienced a weakened marital relationship were less likely to form successful bonds with their infant (Gutierrez-Galve et al., 2015; Kerstis et al., 2016), other studies reported that marital conflict only partially mediated the relationship between postpartum depression and behavioral and emotional problems in children, suggesting that there may be other pathways explaining this relationship (Carro, Grant, Gotlib, & Compas, 1993; Gentile & Fusco, 2017; Hanington et al., 2012). In studies of maternal depression's impact on mother-infant interactions, parenting behavior has been implicated as an important dynamic subsystem within the family, which conveys her depression's effects to child outcomes. In particular, deficits in maternal responsiveness and positive affect have been linked to relatively poorer emotion regulation in young children (Feng et al., 2008), with problematic emotion regulation being implicated as one developmental process that can lead to later child psychopathology (Keenan, 2000). A growing parallel to these findings appears in the father literature, with good evidence that paternal depression is associated with decreased paternal warmth and sensitivity, increased hostility and disengagement, (O'Brien et al., 2017; Wilson & Durbin, 2010), and decreased paternal responsiveness (Sethna et al., 2018). Some investigators have identified system-level impacts of paternal depression, pointing to increases in co-parenting conflict and decreases in co-parenting coordination and support in families where the father is depressed during the postpartum (Solmeyer & Feinberg, 2011; Tissot, Favez, Ghisletta, Frascarolo, & Despland, 2017). While these parallels with the maternal literature suggest that these pathways from paternal depression to child development may be important, they have yet to be thoroughly investigated.

An Integrative Model of Perinatal Paternal Depression

Taken together, the literature describes the position of paternal prenatal and postpartum depression as a phenomenon that is multiply predicted and which results in a variety of short-and long-term outcomes. While some of this literature connects to the broader evidence base on individual-level risks for depression, such as family history (e.g., Kendler, Gardner, & Prescott, 2002, 2006), this literature highlights the strong role of the individual's context, particularly with respect to familial and romantic relationships and stressful events. When looking specifically at what we understand of risk and causation of paternal prenatal and postpartum depression, the case for focusing on relationships, family, and transitions becomes far stronger. In particular, we propose viewing relationship disturbance as a function of either parent's depression and a mechanism through which depression in one parent evokes depression in the other as a needed step in building an understanding of early parental depression as a family systems phenomenon. Because of this, we propose a model that places paternal prenatal and postpartum depression in a relational context, in which parental relationship and co-parenting during pregnancy and the transition to parenthood plays a central role.

We combine four conceptual approaches to compose our proposed framework for contextualizing prenatal and postpartum depression in both fathers and mothers: The first approach comes from the work by Kendler and colleagues that has led to two expansive biopsychosocial models of the development of depression utilizing a large sample of monozygotic and dizygotic twins, specified separately by sex (Kendler et al., 2002, 2006). Among other causes (including genetic risk, substance misuse, personality, and early history), Kendler and colleagues' models for both genders place a strong emphasis on stressful life events and marital difficulties but also account for somewhat smaller effects in the genetic and distal factors domains.

Second, we utilize the contextual approach to understanding marital adjustment proposed by Simpson and colleagues, which relies heavily on adult attachment theory. Developed with maternal depression in mind, Simpson and colleagues' work suggests that an individual's success in transitioning to parenthood is mediated by a strong relationship with their spouse and associated spousal support (Simpson, Rholes, Campbell, Tran, & Wilson, 2003). This perspective is based on the premise from attachment theory, which posits that successful and resilient relationships buffer an individual's vulnerability to stressors, enabling them to navigate those stressors in a manner that produces more favorable and adaptive outcomes. Belsky and Rovine formerly found that perceived marital love and intimacy declined linearly across the 3 years after the transition to parenthood (with a sharper quadratic decline for new mothers), while marital ambivalence and conflict increased (Belsky & Rovine, 1990). However, there was considerable variability among trends, with some couples remaining level while others experienced increased marital quality over this time period. Some of this variation may be explained by the dynamics of depression in early parenthood (Dudley, Roy, Kelk, & Bernard, 2001; Hall & Long, 2007; Paulson et al., 2006). Extending these findings into the co-parenting domain, marital attachment in both parents has been negatively associated with co-parenting conflict in the postpartum. Interestingly, some evidence suggests that co-parenting engagement during infancy is negatively predicted by earlier depression, but only for fathers (Elliston, McHale, Talbot, Parmley, & Kuersten-Hogan, 2008).

The third approach, Belsky's determinants of parenting (1984), is a model of parenting determinants that specifies three domains of influence: personal psychological resources of the parent, contextual stress and support (e.g., marital relationship), and child characteristics (e.g., infant temperament). According to Belsky, the three domains combine to influence parenting behavior. This model has been applied in many studies addressing both parents and provides a broader systems context through which parenting, co-parenting, and child outcomes can be conceptually connected.

Finally, the literature on the development of emotion regulation (ER) describes a pathway through which children, via both expanded cognitive and motor capacities and through learned strategies, become increasingly capable of monitoring their own behavior, interpreting the behavior of others, and responding to social demands (Calkins & Hill, 2007). Although this capacity develops rather predictably, there is considerable individual variability in how an infant learns ER and the strategies that they develop to regulate themselves, much of this is attributable to caregiving. Maternal depression has been associated with problematic ER strategies and a mediated pathway to internalizing problems (Silk, Shaw, Forbes, Lane, & Kovacs, 2006), and some authors have tied ER as an important early mechanism through which depression-associated parenting disturbances lead to the child emotional and behavioral problems (Cummings et al., 2005).

Together, these models emphasize partner relations during pregnancy and the postpartum as a dynamic that is both sensitive to and predictive of depression. This, combined with the growing evidence on relational ties in early parental depression, leads to our working model (Fig. 15.1). In this model, emphasis is placed on the parental relationship and co-parenting quality. We suggest that, in the postnatal period, the parental relationship is negatively impacted by depression in either parent. Moreover, problems in the parental relationship may increase the risk for depression in both partners, through either increased stress or eroded support. Parental relationship problems have direct negative effects on co-parenting, which, when disrupted, may further expose both parents to depressive risk. Relationship and co-parenting negatively impact individual parenting experiences. Together, these disrupted systems lead to inconsistent or miscoordinated parent-infant interactions. Rather than providing the sense of security that infants gain when parents are united (Barrows, 2004), this disrupted context poses a threat to the healthy development of child emotion regulation, predisposing the child to emotional and behavioral problems as he or she ages. Additionally, prebirth parental relationship quality is also important as a moderator of the stresses surrounding new parenthood, protecting against declines in relationship quality, poor co-parenting quality, and depression. This model also accepts that each partner may be susceptible, at the individual level, to other individual risks for depression (Kendler et al., 2002, 2006), such as the personal history of depression and stressful life events.

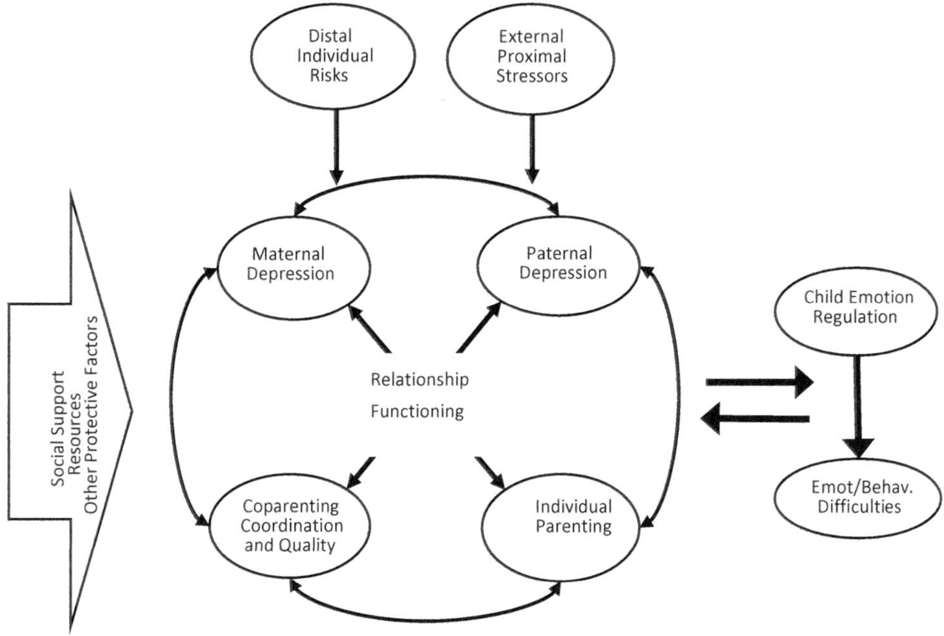

Fig. 15.1 A process model of the impacts of paternal and maternal depression on early parent and child functioning

Screening and Treatment

Because paternal depression has been documented as occurring at above base rates in general population of adult men, much like maternal depression (e.g., Paulson & Bazemore, 2010), clinicians who work with or meet men during this time period should make efforts to screen for depression in a general population. Several brief screening tools are available for this purpose, including the widely used Edinburgh Postnatal Depression Scale (EPDS), which has been validated for use during pregnancy and the postpartum (Cox, Holden, & Sagovsky, 1987) and has been used in samples of expecting and new fathers (Matthey, Barnett, Kavanagh, & Howie, 2001). Alternatively, the two-item PHQ-2 is promising for even more rapid screening of depression and can easily be incorporated into the general patient intake and screening practices in primary care and other medical settings (Löwe, Kroenke, & Gräfe, 2005).

As prenatal and postpartum depression in fathers and mothers is effectively a special case of major depressive disorder, healthcare professionals have access to many evidence-based interventions for most individuals with depression. These include the cognitive behavioral therapies with their rich evidence base (e.g., Butler, Chapman, Forman, & Beck, 2006), brief problem-solving approaches, and pharmacotherapy. Although the literature on treatment of depression in expecting and postpartum parents is small, promising evidence points to relative advantages of interpersonal therapy for individuals (O'Hara, Stuart, Gorman, & Wenzel, 2000) and couple-based intervention that aims to increase partner support of the depressed parent (Misri, Kostaras, Fox, & Kostaras, 2000). Both of these two postpartum-specific interventions contain elements of enhancing relationship functioning of the depressed parent, with the couple-based approach doing so explicitly, whereas interpersonal therapy focuses on the individual's navigation of social relationships as part of the experience of depression and stress during transitions. In brief, this evidence points at treatment that is attuned to the family system as having a unique advantage to other modalities.

Summary and Key Points

Including fathers in prenatal and postpartum depression research is a relatively new and still developing trend that has yet to penetrate deeply in clinical practice. As of this writing, all of the three major medical associations devoted to primary prenatal and postpartum care, The American College of Obstetricians and Gynecologists, The American Academy of Pediatrics, and The American Academy of Family Physicians, provide screening guidelines for pregnant and postpartum mothers. Although the American Academy of Pediatrics' guidelines mention the possibility of screening expecting and postpartum fathers for depression, none of these organizations offer a specific recommendation to do so. The building body of evidence argues strongly that fathers are at increased risk for depression during pregnancy and in the postpartum and that when depression occurs, it increases the risk for a range of negative outcomes in the child and family. With the availability of a range of evidence-based treatments for depression, there is a clear case for healthcare professionals to screen for, counsel, and treat/refer to depression in this population. Corresponding with this suggestion, researchers should consider more systematic studies of the long-term outcomes of depression screening, counseling, and referral, particularly in terms of which factors make the screening to intervention process more or less effective.

Paralleling the evidence base in mothers, research on prenatal and postpartum depression in fathers suggests that this phenomenon is best understood within a family systems perspective that contextualizes its risks, protective factors, and ultimate impacts in terms of the partner and developing child(ren). Evidence is building to suggest that paternal depression disrupts the partner relationship and father-child interactions, with some preliminary findings that it may also negatively impact the overall quality of co-parenting. While an important foundation for understanding the complex pattern of impacts and interactions of depression and the family system, this evidence base is still in its early stages. It will benefit from research examining how depression interacts with specific aspects of relationship functioning (e.g., conflict, intimacy, support), co-parenting (e.g., coordination, conflict, maternal gatekeeping), parenting, and how these mechanisms combine to impact child emotion regulation, attachment, and eventual emotional and behavioral functioning.

Studying how depression plays out in a family system necessarily requires the inclusion of both parents, a need that is underscored by its apparently contagious nature during this time period. Researchers should consider designs that include parents and elements of the extended family system wherever possible. This approach should be extended to intervention efficacy and effectiveness designs, insofar as the impact of any prenatal and postpartum intervention is rightly evaluated in terms of its impact on the whole family.

- Expecting and new fathers experience depression at higher rates than what is seen in the general population of adult men.
- Postpartum depression in fathers is associated with a range of negative child and family outcomes.
- It is important to understand prenatal and postpartum depression in parents from a family systems perspective, as depression disrupts and is influenced by stresses in this system.
- Researchers should seek out ways to include mothers and fathers in the study of prenatal and postpartum depression in order to better reflect its nature as being embedded in the family system.
- Screening, counseling, referral, and intervention should be a priority for clinicians who encounter fathers during their partners' pregnancy and through early fatherhood.

References

American Psychiatric Association. (2013). *Diagnostic and statistical manual of mental disorders (DSM-5)*. Arlington, VA: American Psychiatric Pub.

Anderson, A. M. (1996). Factors influencing the father-infant relationship. *Journal of Family Nursing, 2*(3), 306–324.

Barrows, P. (2004). Fathers and families: Locating the ghost in the nursery. *Infant Mental Health Journal, 25*(5), 408–432.

Baumeister, R. F. (Ed.). (2013). *Self-esteem: The puzzle of low self-regard*. Springer Science & Business Media, New York.

Belsky, J. (1984). The determinants of parenting: A process model. *Child Development, 55*, 83–96.

Belsky, J., & Rovine, M. (1990). Patterns of marital change across the transition to parenthood: Pregnancy to three years postpartum. *Journal of Marriage and the Family, 52*, 5–19.

Bennett, H. A., Einarson, A., Taddio, A., Koren, G., & Einarson, T. R. (2004). Prevalence of depression during pregnancy: Systematic review. *Obstetrics & Gynecology, 103*(4), 698–e709.

Berg, S. J., & Wynne-Edwards, K. E. (2001, June). Changes in testosterone, cortisol, and estradiol levels in men becoming fathers. In *Mayo Clinic proceedings* (Vol. 76, No. 6, pp. 582–592). Elsevier.

Bergström, M. (2013). Depressive symptoms in new first-time fathers: Associations with age, sociodemographic characteristics, and antenatal psychological well-being. *Birth, 40*(1), 32–38.

Bielawska-Batorowicz, E., & Kossakowska-Petrycka, K. (2006). Depressive mood in men after the birth of their offspring in relation to a partner's depression, social support, fathers' personality and prenatal expectations. *Journal of Reproductive and Infant Psychology, 24*(1), 21–29.

Bina, R. (2008). The impact of cultural factors upon postpartum depression: A literature review. *Health Care Women International, 29*(6), 568–592.

Bronte-Tinkew, J., Moore, K. A., Matthews, G., & Carrano, J. (2007). Symptoms of major depression in a sample of fathers of infants: Sociodemographic correlates and links to father involvement. *Journal of Family Issues, 28*(1), 61–99.

Burke, H. M., Davis, M. C., Otte, C., & Mohr, D. C. (2005). Depression and cortisol responses to psychological stress: a meta-analysis. *Psychoneuroendocrinology, 30*(9), 846–856.

Butler, A. C., Chapman, J. E., Forman, E. M., & Beck, A. T. (2006). The empirical status of cognitive-behavioral therapy: A review of meta-analyses. *Clinical Psychology Review, 26*(1), 17–31.

Calkins, S. D., & Hill, A. (2007). Caregiver influences on emerging emotion regulation. In *Handbook of emotion regulation* (Vol. 229248).

Cameron, E. E., Sedov, I. D., & Tomfohr-Madsen, L. M. (2016). Prevalence of paternal depression in pregnancy and the postpartum: An updated meta-analysis. *Journal of Affective Disorders, 206*, 189–203.

Carro, M. G., Grant, K. E., Gotlib, I. H., & Compas, B. E. (1993). Postpartum depression and child development: An investigation of mothers and fathers as sources of risk and resilience. *Development and Psychopathology, 5*(4), 567–579.

Cox, J. L., Holden, J. M., & Sagovsky, R. (1987). Detection of postnatal depression: Development of the 10-item Edinburgh Postnatal Depression Scale. *The British Journal of Psychiatry, 150*(6), 782–786.

Cummings, E. M., Keller, P. S., & Davies, P. T. (2005). Towards a family process model of maternal and paternal depressive symptoms: Exploring multiple relations with child and family functioning. *Journal of Child Psychology and Psychiatry, 46*(5), 479–489.

Daley, S. E., Hammen, C., & Rao, U. (2000). Predictors of first onset and recurrence of major depression in young women during the 5 years following high school graduation. *Journal of abnormal psychology, 109*(3), 525.

Davé, S., Nazareth, I., Sherr, L., & Senior, R. (2005). The association of paternal mood and infant temperament: A pilot study. *British Journal of Developmental Psychology, 23*(4), 609–621.

Davé, S., Petersen, I., Sherr, L., & Nazareth, I. (2010). Incidence of maternal and paternal depression in primary care: A cohort study using a primary care database. *Archives of Pediatrics & Adolescent Medicine, 164*(11), 1038–1044.

deMontigny, F., Girard, M. E., Lacharité, C., Dubeau, D., & Devault, A. (2013). Psychosocial factors associated with paternal postnatal depression. *Journal of Affective Disorders, 150*(1), 44–49.

deMontigny, F., & Lacharité, C. (2004). Fathers' perceptions of the immediate postpartal period. *Journal of Obstetric, Gynecologic, & Neonatal Nursing, 33*(3), 328–339.

Don, B. P., & Mickelson, K. D. (2012). Paternal postpartum depression: The role of maternal postpartum depression, spousal support and relationship satisfaction. *Couple & Family Psychology: Research and Practice, 1*(4), 323–334.

Dudley, M., Roy, K., Kelk, N., & Bernard, D. (2001). Psychological correlates of depression in fathers and mothers in the first postnatal year. *Journal of Reproductive and Infant Psychology, 19*(3), 187–202.

Edhborg, M., Matthiesen, A. S., Lundh, W., & Widstrom, A. M. (2005). Some early indicators for depressive symptoms and bonding 2 months postpartum: A study of new mothers and fathers. *Archives of Women's Mental Health, 8*(4), 221–231.

Elliston, D., McHale, J., Talbot, J., Parmley, M., & Kuersten-Hogan, R. (2008). Withdrawal from coparenting interactions during early infancy. *Family Process, 47*(4), 481–499.

Everson, S. A., Maty, S. C., Lynch, J. W., & Kaplan, G. A. (2002). Epidemiologic evidence for the relation between socioeconomic status and depression, obesity, and diabetes. *Journal of Psychosomatic Research, 53*(4), 891–895.

Falah-Hassani, K., Shiri, R., & Dennis, C. L. (2017). The prevalence of antenatal and postnatal co-morbid anxiety and depression: A meta-analysis. *Psychological Medicine, 47*(12), 2041–2053.

Feng, X., Shaw, D. S., Kovacs, M., Lane, T., O'Rourke, F. E., & Alarcon, J. H. (2008). Emotion regulation in preschoolers: The roles of behavioral inhibition, maternal affective behavior, and maternal depression. *Journal of Child Psychology and Psychiatry, 49*(2), 132–141.

Fleming, A. S., & Anderson, V. (1987). Affect and nurturance: Mechanisms mediating maternal behavior in two female mammals. *Progress in Neuro-Psychopharmacology and Biological Psychiatry, 11*(2-3), 121–127.

Fleming, A. S., Corter, C., Stallings, J., & Steiner, M. (2002). Testosterone and prolactin are associated with emotional responses to infant cries in new fathers. *Hormones and Behavior, 42*(4), 399–413.

Fleming, A. S., O'Day, D. H., & Kraemer, G. W. (1999). Neurobiology of mother–infant interactions: Experience and central nervous system plasticity across development and generations. *Neuroscience & Biobehavioral Reviews, 23*(5), 673–685.

Fletcher, R. J., Feeman, E., Garfield, C., & Vimpani, G. (2011). The effects of early paternal depression on children's development. *Medical Journal of Australia, 195*(11-12), 685–689.

Gao, L. L., Chan, S. W. C., & Mao, Q. (2009). Depression, perceived stress, and social support among first-time Chinese mothers and fathers in the postpartum period. *Research in Nursing & Health, 32*(1), 50–58.

Gawlik, S., Müller, M., Hoffmann, L., Dienes, A., Wallwiener, M., Sohn, C., et al. (2014). Prevalence of paternal perinatal depressiveness and its link to partnership satisfaction and birth concerns. *Archive of Women's Mental Health, 17*(1), 49–56.

Gentile, S., & Fusco, M. L. (2017). Untreated perinatal paternal depression: Effects on offspring. *Psychiatry Research, 252*, 325–332.

Gönülal, D., Yalaz, M., Altun-Köroğlu, Ö., & Kültürsay, N. (2014). Both parents of neonatal intensive care unit patients are at risk of depression. *Turkish Journal of Pediatrics, 56*(2), 171–176.

Gutierrez-Galve, L., Stein, A., Hanington, L., Heron, J., & Ramchandani, P. (2015). Paternal depression in the postnatal period and child development: Mediators and moderators. *Pediatrics, 135*(2), e339–e347.

Halbreich, U. (2005). The association between pregnancy processes, preterm delivery, low birth weight, and postpartum depressions—the need for interdisciplinary integration. *American journal of obstetrics and gynecology, 193*(4), 1312–1322.

Hall, W. A., & Long, B. C. (2007). Relations among prenatal role quality, life satisfaction, and dual-earner parents' postnatal depression. *Journal of Prenatal & Perinatal Psychology & Health, 21*(3), 231–248.

Hammen, C., Davila, J., Brown, G., Ellicott, A., & Gitlin, M. (1992). Psychiatric history and stress: predictors of severity of unipolar depression. *Journal of Abnormal Psychology, 101*(1), 45.

Hanington, L., Heron, J., Stein, A., & Ramchandani, P. (2012). Parental depression and child outcomes–is marital conflict the missing link? *Child: Care, Health and Development, 38*(4), 520–529.

Helle, N., Barkmann, C., Bartz-Seel, J., Diehl, T., Ehrhardt, S., Hendel, A., et al. (2015). Very low birthweight as a risk factor for postpartum depression four to six weeks postbirth in mothers and fathers: Cross-sectional results from a controlled multicentre cohort study. *Journal of Affective Disorders, 180*, 154–161.

Hübner-Liebermann, B., Hausner, H., & Wittmann, M. (2012). Recognizing and treating peripartum depression. *Deutsches Ärzteblatt International, 109*(24), 419–424.

Kamalifard, M., Hasanpoor, S., Kheiroddin, J. B., Panahi, S., & Payan, S. B. (2014). Relationship between fathers' depression and perceived social support and stress in postpartum period. *Journal of Caring Sciences, 3*(1), 57–66.

Keenan, K. (2000). Emotion dysregulation as a risk factor for child psychopathology. *Clinical Psychology: Science and Practice, 7*(4), 418–434.

Kendler, K. S., Karkowski, L. M., & Prescott, C. A. (1999). Causal relationship between stressful life events and the onset of major depression. *American Journal of Psychiatry, 156*(6), 837–841.

Kendler, K. S., Gardner, C. O., & Prescott, C. A. (2002). Toward a comprehensive developmental model for major depression in women. *American Journal of Psychiatry, 159*(7), 1133–1145.

Kendler, K. S., Gardner, C. O., & Prescott, C. A. (2006). Toward a comprehensive developmental model for major depression in men. *American Journal of Psychiatry, 163*(1), 115–124.

Kernis, M. H. (1993). *The roles of stability and level of self-esteem in psychological functioning. In self-esteem* (pp. 167–182). Boston: Springer.

Kerstis, B., Aarts, C., Tillman, C., Persson, H., Engström, G., Edlund, B., et al. (2016). Association between parental depressive symptoms and impaired bonding with the infant. *Archives of Women's Mental Health, 19*(1), 87–94.

Kim, P., & Swain, J. E. (2007). Sad dads: paternal postpartum depression. *Psychiatry (Edgmont), 4*(2), 35–47.

Koh, Y. W., Chui, C. Y., Tang, C. S. K., & Lee, A. M. (2014). The prevalence and risk factors of paternal depression from the antenatal to the postpartum period and the relationships between antenatal and postpartum depression among fathers in Hong Kong. *Depression Research and Treatment, 2014*, 127632.

Kozorovitskiy, Y., Hughes, M., Lee, K., & Gould, E. (2006). Fatherhood affects dendritic spines and vasopressin V1a receptors in the primate prefrontal cortex. *Nature Neuroscience, 9*(9), 1094–1095.

Kryski, K. R., Olino, T. M., Dyson, M. W., Durbin, C. E., Klein, D. N., & Hayden, E. P. (2018). Associations between observed temperament in preschoolers and parent psychopathology. *Personality and Mental Health, 12*(2), 131–144.

Lamb, M. E., Pleck, J. H., & Levine, J. A. (1985). The role of the father in child development. In Advances in clinical child psychology (pp. 229–266). Springer, Boston, MA.

Lorant, V., Deliège, D., Eaton, W., Robert, A., Philippot, P., & Ansseau, M. (2003). Socioeconomic inequalities in depression: A meta-analysis. *American Journal of Epidemiology, 157*(2), 98–112.

Löwe, B., Kroenke, K., & Gräfe, K. (2005). Detecting and monitoring depression with a two-item questionnaire (PHQ-2). *Journal of Psychosomatic Research, 58*(2), 163–171.

Mackrell, S. V., Sheikh, H. I., Kotelnikova, Y., Kryski, K. R., Jordan, P. L., Singh, S. M., et al. (2014). Child temperament and parental depression predict cortisol reactivity to stress in middle childhood. *Journal of Abnormal Psychology, 123*(1), 106–116.

Massoudi, P., Hwang, C. P., & Wickberg, B. (2016). Fathers' depressive symptoms in the postnatal period: Prevalence and correlates in a population-based Swedish study. *Scandinavian Journal of Public Health, 44*(7), 688–694.

Matthey, S., Barnett, B., Kavanagh, D. J., & Howie, P. (2001). Validation of the Edinburgh Postnatal Depression Scale for men, and comparison of item endorsement with their partners. *Journal of Affective Disorders, 64*(2-3), 175–184.

Mikkonen, J., Moustgaard, H., Remes, H., & Martikainen, P. (2016). Intergenerational transmission of depressive symptoms–the role of gender, socioeconomic circumstances, and the accumulation of parental symptoms. *Journal of Affective Disorders, 204*, 74–82.

Misri, S., Kostaras, X., Fox, D., & Kostaras, D. (2000). The impact of partner support in the treatment of postpartum depression. *The Canadian Journal of Psychiatry, 45*(6), 554–558.

Morse, C. A., Buist, A., & Durkin, S. (2000). First-time parenthood: Influences on pre-and postnatal adjustment in fathers and mothers. *Journal of Psychosomatic Obstetrics and Gynecology, 21*(2), 109–120.

O'Brien, A. P., McNeil, K. A., Fletcher, R., Conrad, A., Wilson, A. J., Jones, D., et al. (2017). New fathers' perinatal depression and anxiety—Treatment options: An integrative review. *American Journal of Men's Health, 11*(4), 863–876.

O'Hara, M. W., Stuart, S., Gorman, L. L., & Wenzel, A. (2000). Efficacy of interpersonal psychotherapy for postpartum depression. *Archives of General Psychiatry, 57*(11), 1039–1045.

O'Hara, M. W., Wisner, K. L., Asher, N., & Asher, H. (2014). Perinatal mental illness: Definition, description and aetiology. *Best Practice & Research Clinical Obstetrics & Gynaecology, 28*(1), 3–12.

Paulson, J. F., & Bazemore, S. D. (2010). Prenatal and postpartum depression in fathers and its association with maternal depression: A meta-analysis. *JAMA, 303*(19), 1961–1969.

Paulson, J. F., Dauber, S. E., & Leiferman, J. A. (2006). Individual and combined effects of maternal and paternal depression on parenting behavior. *Pediatrics, 118*(2), 659–668.

Paulson, J. F., Dauber, S. E., & Leiferman, J. A. (2011). Parental depression, relationship quality, and nonresident father involvement with their infants. *Journal of Family Issues, 32*(4), 528–549.

Pearson, R. M., Evans, J., Kounali, D., Lewis, G., Heron, J., Ramchandani, P. G., et al. (2013). Maternal depression during pregnancy and the postnatal period: Risks and possible mechanisms for offspring depression at age 18 years. *JAMA Psychiatry, 70*(12), 1312–1319.

Ramchandani, P., Stein, A., Evans, J., O'Connor, T. G., & ALSPAC Study Team. (2005). Paternal depression in the postnatal period and child development: A prospective population study. *The Lancet, 365*(9478), 2201–2205.

Ramchandani, P. G., O'Conner, T. G., Evans, J., Heron, J., Murray, L., & Stein, A. (2008). The effects of pre- and postnatal depression in fathers: A natural experiment comparing the effects of exposure to depression on offspring. *Journal of Child Psychology and Psychiatry, 49*(10), 1069–1078.

Ramchandani, P. G., Psychogiou, L., Vlachos, H., Iles, J., Sethna, V., Netsi, E., et al. (2011). Paternal depression: An examination of its links with father, child and family functioning in the postnatal period. *Depression and Anxiety, 28*(6), 471–477.

Ramchandani, P. G., Stein, A., O'connor, T. G., Heron, J. O. N., Murray, L., & Evans, J. (2008). Depression in men in the postnatal period and later child psychopathology: A population cohort study. *Journal of the American Academy of Child & Adolescent Psychiatry, 47*(4), 390–398.

Reeb, B. T., Wu, E. Y., Martin, M. J., Gelardi, K. L., Chan, S. Y. S., & Conger, K. J. (2015). Long-term effects of fathers' depressed mood on youth internalizing symptoms in early adulthood. *Journal of Research on Adolescence, 25*(1), 151–162.

Rice, F., Lewis, G., Harold, G. T., & Thapar, A. (2013). Examining the role of passive gene–environment correlation in childhood depression using a novel genetically sensitive design. *Development and Psychopathology, 25*(1), 37–50.

Ringoot, A. P., Tiemeier, H., Jaddoe, V. W., So, P., Hofman, A., Verhulst, F. C., et al. (2015). Parental depression and child Well-being: Young children's self-reports helped addressing biases in parent reports. *Journal of Clinical Epidemiology, 68*(8), 928–938.

Roberts, S. L., Roberts, S. L., Bushnell, J. A., Roberts, S. L., Bushnell, J. A., Collings, S. C., et al. (2006). Psychological health of men with partners who have post-partum depression. *Australian & New Zealand Journal of Psychiatry, 40*(8), 704–711.

Roubinov, D. S., Luecken, L. J., Crnic, K. A., & Gonzales, N. A. (2014). Postnatal depression in Mexican American fathers: Demographic, cultural, and familial predictors. *Journal of Affective Disorders, 152*, 360–368.

Saracho, O., & Spodek, B. (Eds.). (2007). Contemporary perspectives on socialization and social development in early childhood education. IAP.

Schulster, M., Bernie, A. M., & Ramasamy, R. (2016). The role of estradiol in male reproductive function. *Asian Journal of Andrology, 18*(3), 435.

Seidman, S. N., & Walsh, B. T. (1999). Testosterone and depression in aging men. *The American Journal of Geriatric Psychiatry, 7*(1), 18–33.

Sethna, V., Murray, L., Edmondson, O., Iles, J., & Ramchandani, P. G. (2018). Depression and playfulness in fathers and young infants: A matched design comparison study. *Journal of Affective Disorders, 229*, 364–370.

Sethna, V., Murray, L., & Ramchandani, P. G. (2012). Depressed fathers' speech to their 3-month-old infants: A study of cognitive and mentalizing features in paternal speech. *Psychological Medicine, 42*(11), 2361–2371.

Shen, H., Magnusson, C., Rai, D., Lundberg, M., Le-Scherban, F., Dalman, C., et al. (2016). Associations of parental depression with child school performance at age 16 years in Sweden. *JAMA Psychiatry, 73*(3), 239–246.

Silk, J. S., Shaw, D. S., Forbes, E. E., Lane, T. L., & Kovacs, M. (2006). Maternal depression and child internalizing: The moderating role of child emotion regulation. *Journal of Clinical Child and Adolescent Psychology, 35*(1), 116–126.

Simpson, J. A., Rholes, W. S., Campbell, L., Tran, S., & Wilson, C. L. (2003). Adult attachment, the transition to parenthood, and depressive symptoms. *Journal of Personality and Social Psychology, 84*(6), 1172.

Solmeyer, A., & Feinberg, M. E. (2011). Mother and father adjustment during early parenthood: The roles of infant temperament and coparenting relationship quality. *Infant Behavior and Development, 34*(4), 504–514.

Storey, A. E., Walsh, C. J., Quinton, R. L., & Wynne-Edwards, K. E. (2000). Hormonal correlates of paternal responsiveness in new and expectant fathers. *Evolution and Human Behavior, 21*(2), 79–95.

Tissot, H., Favez, N., Ghisletta, P., Frascarolo, F., & Despland, J. N. (2017). A longitudinal study of parental depressive symptoms and coparenting in the first 18 months. *Family Process, 56*(2), 445–458.

Tuszyńska-Bogucka, W., & Nawra, K. (2014). Paternal postnatal depression–a review. *Archives of Psychiatry and Psychotherapy, 2*, 61–69.

Uher, R., Payne, J. L., Pavlova, B., & Perlis, R. H. (2014). Major depressive disorder in DSM-5: Implications for clinical practice and research of changes from DSM-IV. *Depression and Anxiety, 31*(6), 459–471.

Van den Berg, M. P., van der Ende, J., Crijnen, A. A., Jaddoe, V. W., Moll, H. A., Mackenbach, J. P., et al. (2009). Paternal depressive symptoms during pregnancy are related to excessive infant crying. *Pediatrics, 124*(1), e96–e103.

Wang, S. Y., & Chen, C. H. (2006). Psychosocial health of Taiwanese postnatal husbands and wives. *Journal of Psychosomatic Research, 60*(3), 303–307.

Wang, Z., Ferris, C. F., & De Vries, G. J. (1994). Role of septal vasopressin innervation in paternal behavior in prairie voles (Microtus ochrogaster). *Proceedings of the National Academy of Sciences, 91*(1), 400–404.

Wee, K. Y., Skouteris, H., Pier, C., Richardson, B., & Milgrom, J. (2011). Correlates of ante- and postnatal depression in fathers: A systematic review. *Journal of Affective Disorders, 130*(3), 358–377.

Wilson, S., & Durbin, C. E. (2010). Effects of paternal depression on fathers' parenting behaviors: A meta-analytic review. *Clinical Psychology Review, 30*(2), 167–180.

Yim, I. S., Tanner Stapleton, L. R., Guardino, C. M., Hahn-Holbrook, J., & Dunkel Schetter, C. (2015). Biological and psychosocial predictors of postpartum depression: Systematic review and call for integration. *Annual Review of Clinical Psychology, 11*, 99–137.

Young, L. J. (1999). Oxytocin and vasopressin receptors and species-typical social behaviors. *Hormones and Behavior, 36*, 212–221.

Zarrouf, F. A., Artz, S., Griffith, J., Sirbu, C., & Kommor, M. (2009). Testosterone and depression: Systematic review and meta-analysis. *Journal of Psychiatric Practice®, 15*(4), 289–305.

Zelkowitz, P., & Milet, T. H. (1997). Stress and support as related to postpartum paternal mental health and perceptions of the infant. *Infant Mental Health Journal: Official Publication of The World Association for Infant Mental Health, 18*(4), 424–435.

Is It Easier the Second Time Around? Fathers' Roles Across the Transition from One Child to Two

16

Brenda L. Volling, Emily J. Steinberg, and Patty X. Kuo

The transition following the birth of a second child can be a stressful time for parents and their firstborn children (Volling, 2012). Some firstborn children experience externalizing problems such as aggression or hostility toward the mother or newborn (Field & Reite, 1984; Kolak & Volling, 2013; Volling, Gonzalez, Yu, & Oh, 2017), whereas others exhibit increases in internalizing behavior problems such as anxiety, behavioral inhibition, and withdrawal (Kuo, Volling, Gonzalez, Oh, & Yu, 2017; Oh, Song, Gonzalez, Volling, & Yu, 2017; Thomason, Oh, Volling, Gonzalez, & Yu, 2017). Other children have disturbed sleep (Field & Reite, 1984; Safyer, Stevenson, Gonzalez, Volling, Oh, & Yu, 2017) or revert back to behaviors from earlier developmental periods, with increases in toileting accidents or wanting a pacifier or bottle once weaned (Kayiatos, Adams, & Gilman, 1984; Stewart, Mobley, Van Tuyl, & Salvador, 1987). Changes in eating, toileting, sleeping, and frequency of physical complaints (e.g., stomachaches, headaches) have also been reported (Beyers-Carlson, Stevenson, Gonzalez, Oh, Volling, & Yu, 2017; Safyer et al., 2017). Yet, most children show little to no disruptive behaviors after the birth of their infant siblings (Volling, Gonzalez, Oh, Song et al., 2017), providing far more support for variability in children's reactions to the birth of a second child than a universal pattern of developmental crisis or psychological disturbance. It has been suggested in both professional and scholarly writings that fathers play an essential role in helping children adjust to the birth of their infant sibling by stepping in to care and provide emotional support for firstborn children when mothers are busily engaged with the care of a newborn (Kreppner, 1988; Stewart, 1990). As such, fathers' engagement in child care during this time might help explain these individual differences in children's adjustment across the transition to siblinghood. The primary goal of this chapter was to review extant research supporting this claim by focusing on the many family relationships in which fathers are embedded (father-child, co-parenting, marital) across the transition from one child to two, as well as paternal characteristics (parental competence, mental health) that are also affected or change across the transition, and

Author Note
The research reported herein was supported by grants from the *Eunice Kennedy Shriver* National Institute of Child Health and Human Development (R01HD042607, K02HD047423) to Brenda L. Volling.

B. L. Volling (✉)
Department of Psychology, University of Michigan, Ann Arbor, MI, USA
e-mail: volling@umich.edu

E. J. Steinberg
Department of Psychology, Fordham University, Bronx, NY, USA

P. X. Kuo
Department of Child, Youth and Family Studies, University of Nebraska-Lincoln, Lincoln, NE, USA

H. E. Fitzgerald et al. (eds.), *Handbook of Fathers and Child Development*,
https://doi.org/10.1007/978-3-030-51027-5_16

what ramifications these changes have for fathers, mothers, and children.

The fertility rate across the globe has declined significantly over the past several decades; yet, fertility rates average 2.5 children per woman globally (United Nations, 2015), with wide regional differences, ranging from 1.6 children per woman in Europe to 4.7 children per woman in Africa. Given that most families worldwide have two or more children, it is surprising how little attention developmental and family scientists have devoted to understanding the transition period surrounding the birth of second or subsequent children in the family. This lack of attention to one of the most significant developmental milestones in the lives of children and their parents is most likely a direct result of traditional developmental models emphasizing a "mother and one child only" research design. As such, the review that follows is by necessity limited in a number of ways. First, there are a surprisingly small number of studies that have addressed changes in family life after the birth of a second child, in general (see reviews by Fouts & Bader, 2016 and Volling, 2012), and even fewer including any information on fathers. Second, with a few exceptions (e.g., Kojima, Irisawa, & Wakita, 2005; Pereira, da Silva, Piccinini, & Lopez, 2015), most of the research on the pregnancy and birth of a second child has been conducted in the United States and Europe. But, here too, most, if not all, have included mothers' perceptions of pregnancy and firstborn adjustment, and not the perspectives of fathers. As such, most studies including fathers have focused on white, middle-class families in Europe and the United States, and this is also reflected in the review that follows. There is a clear need for more research on the transition period from one to two children, in general, and from a global family perspective. Because there are so few studies addressing the transition from one child to two and even fewer that have included fathers, this chapter also includes recent findings looking at mothers' and fathers' reports of changes in firstborn children's behavioral adjustment across the first year using data from the Family Transitions Study (FTS), a longitudinal investigation of changes in family and child functioning before and after the birth of a second child conducted in the United States. The FTS intentionally included fathers in the research design and is one of the only studies that allows an investigation into whether fathers' involvement in caregiving with the firstborn child before the infant's birth protects children from the development of problem behaviors (e.g., sleep problems, oppositional behavior, separation anxiety) after the birth of an infant sibling.

Father Involvement and Children's Adjustment Across the Transition

Fathers are hypothesized to be an important source of emotional and instrumental support for firstborn children during the transition to siblinghood, the period when only children become older siblings. This is a time when mothers are often busy with the care of a newborn and have less time and attention to dedicate to their firstborn children (Kreppner, 1988; Stewart et al., 1987). Confrontations between mothers and firstborns increase after the infant sibling's birth (Dunn & Kendrick, 1980; Kojima et al., 2005), as do increases in mothers' harsh and punitive physical discipline directed at their first child (Baydar, Hyle, & Brooks-Gunn, 1997). Indeed, Baydar et al. (1997) found it was the increases in harsh maternal discipline that mediated the effects of the birth of the sibling on children's problematic behaviors. In one study conducted in Japan, Kojima and colleagues (2005) reported that 46.8% mother-child dyads showed more negative interactions after the birth of a second child, but a comparable percentage (46.8%) showed no change in the mother-child relationship, and even a small number of mother-child dyads (6.4%) experienced an actual increase in positive interactions after the birth. These results are important for several reasons. First, Kojima et al.'s (2005) results are from one of the only studies to date conducted outside the United States and Europe. Second, the results reveal heterogeneity in the mother-child relationship after the birth of a second child showing that for many mothers and children, the transition period is not fraught with rivalry and negative firstborn behaviors. Finally, this variability in mother-child relationships across the transition may very well be explained by the supports to mothers in their new role of caring for two young children, which could certainly include fathers' involvement in the family.

Fathers may buffer their children from these changes in the mother-child relationship by increasing their involvement in child care activities and, in turn, supporting children, as well as decreasing the burden on mothers to care for two children (Kreppner, 1988; Kuo, Volling, & Gonzalez, 2018; Legg, Sherick, & Wadland, 1974). Indeed, Gottlieb and Mendelson (1990) found that girls receiving little emotional support from their fathers before the sibling's birth were the most distressed afterward, suggesting that fathers' involvement and support before the infant's birth was protective and could mitigate children's adjustment issues over the transition to siblinghood. These findings are similar to others finding that father's support during the perinatal period does in some cases compensate for the effects of maternal depression on mother-infant interaction and children's behavior problems in the United States (Mezulis, Hyde, & Clark, 2004), Israel (Vakrat, Apter-Levy, & Feldman, 2018), and Brazil (de Mendonça, Bussab, Rodrigues, Siqueira, & Cosette, 2013), even though others have not always found this to be the case (e.g., Goodman, 2008). In any event, future research may want to consider how fathers' support to firstborns and mothers may ease the stresses of this transition period.

Recently, Volling and her colleagues (Volling, Gonzalez, Oh, Song et al., 2017) conducted one of the few longitudinal investigations of children's adjustment after the birth of an infant sibling that included fathers by recruiting 241 two-parent families (mothers and fathers) to test specifically (1) whether there were changes in children's adjustment over the transition to siblinghood and (2) whether child (i.e., age, gender, temperament) and family characteristics, including father involvement, co-parenting between fathers and mothers, and couple relationship quality, predicted these individual differences in children's problem behaviors (e.g., aggression, withdrawal, sleep problems). These authors found that there were a number of areas in which fathers appeared to have an influential role in predicting children's problem behavior and family relationship functioning. Specifically, fathers' sense of competence in managing children's difficult behavior and disciplining children was incredibly important in predicting individual differences in trajectories of children's aggression over the year following the sibling's birth; the more competent and confident fathers felt in dealing with difficult child behavior, the less likely children were to engage in aggressive behavior before and after birth (Volling, Gonzalez, Yu, & Oh, 2017). Similarly, how well fathers and mothers worked together as co-parents before the infant was born predicted children's aggression and withdrawal after birth. When parents engaged in more undermining co-parenting, children were much higher in aggression and withdrawal even before the infant sibling was born and throughout the year following birth (Volling, Gonzalez, Oh, & Yu, 2017: Oh et al., 2017). Further, when spouses reported more marital conflict before the birth of the infant sibling, children had higher scores on separation anxiety and depressed mood than when spouses reported less marital negativity (Thomason et al., 2017). In addition, when couples reported less positive marital relations prenatally, their children were more withdrawn than children whose parents reported more marital positivity (Oh et al., 2017). Finally, children with difficult temperaments (i.e., negative emotionality) were more likely to experience somatic complaints (e.g., headaches, stomachaches) than children low on negative emotionality, but only if they also had insecure attachments to their fathers before birth (Beyers-Carlson et al., 2017). Notably, children's gender or the gender of the infant sibling played no role in predicting children's adjustment, even though popular writings often underscore both gender and birth order as important determinants of sibling rivalry. The age space between siblings, again often considered a primary determinant of children's adjustment after the sibling's birth, was only significant in predicting parent's reports of children's depression and anxiety, with older children more likely to be depressed and anxious than younger children. As Dunn (1983) noted long ago, family functioning is a stronger predictor of sibling relationship quality than structural family characteristics such as gender constellation and birth order, and we would argue the same here for children's adjustment after the birth of a sibling. Although few studies currently exist that address the transition period surrounding the birth of a second child, evidence is beginning to emerge suggesting that fathers' support as parent, co-parent, and spouse, as well as their confidence in parenting, predicts fewer behavior problems for their firstborn children, both before and after the birth of the infant sibling.

Fathers and Children's Jealousy of the Infant Sibling

Parents and professionals are often concerned about the firstborn's jealousy and rivalry toward the new baby. In one of the first studies to examine changes in older sibling's behaviors after the birth of an infant sibling, Dunn and Kendrick (1982) interviewed British mothers about their children's jealousy of the new baby. Mothers stated that children appeared to be more jealous and upset when fathers interacted with the newborn infant than when mothers did, although there is little observational research available to confirm these statements.

Only one study has directly observed children's behavior in response to father-infant interaction with a newborn sibling to address whether children are more jealous when fathers interact with the infant compared to mothers. Volling et al. (2014) investigated 241 two-parent, heterosexual parents observed during 15 minutes of mother-infant and father-infant interaction 1 month after the infant sibling' birth and undertook a person-centered approach (i.e., latent profile analysis) to uncover behavioral profiles of children's jealousy in response to parent-infant interaction. Using an attachment theoretical framework, they argued that when children watched their parents interact with their newborn sibling, strong attachment behaviors (e.g., fretting, clinging, approach) would be elicited, and these behaviors would be organized in a manner that reflected children's internal working models of attachment security with mothers and fathers. Children's behaviors such as monitoring, approach, interference, aggression, and protest in response to mother-infant and father-infant interactions were coded and then used in latent profile analysis to determine if distinct behavioral profiles emerged and whether these profiles were similar or different in response to mother-infant versus father-infant interaction.

Four distinct profiles of children's behavior in response to mother-infant interaction were found, with the majority of children (61%) exhibiting a *regulated-exploration* pattern in which children monitored the interaction of mothers with their infant siblings closely while they engaged in exploratory play nearby, intermittently joining positively in triadic mother-child-sibling interactions, but rarely disrupting the interactions or protesting and demanding attention. A second group of children (31%) was labeled *approach-avoidant* because they, too, monitored the interactions between mothers and infants closely, but they did not engage in functional exploration of toys, nor did they approach to join the mother-infant interaction or attempt to disrupt or protest the interaction. It was as if they were "frozen" in place with an intense interest in what was transpiring between the mother and infant, but unable to disengage that interest and focus on other aspects of the physical and social environment, whether positively or negatively. A third smaller group (5.8%) of children was referred to as *anxious-clingy* because they spent most of their time in close proximity to the mother and infant, sometimes joining positively in interaction, but also interfering and protesting in response to the parents' involvement with their infant sibling. Many of these children were younger than the other children in the sample. Finally, a small group (2.7%) was considered *disrupted-dysregulated,* because they also monitored interactions closely but also protested and interfered in those interactions, sometimes approaching to join positively in interaction but also displaying an overall pattern of disruptive and dysregulated behavior. One of the important implications of this research was to demonstrate that very few children actually displayed disruptive jealous behavior in response to mother-infant interaction. These disrupted-dysregulated children did display high levels of aggression and attention problems 3 months later when the infant sibling was 4 months of age. However, it was the children labeled approach-avoidant who clearly had far more internalizing and externalizing behavior problems 4 months after the birth than the other groups, underscoring the need to attend to the emotional issues of these more withdrawn children, whose quiet and nonconfrontational demeanor may be masking levels of anxiety and fear that are going unnoticed and unaddressed during a stressful period when the family may be undergoing significant change.

Volling and her colleagues (2014) also found very similar groups of children when considering the father-infant sessions with four clear profiles resembling the *regulated-exploration*, *approach-avoidant*, *anxious-clingy*, and *disrupted-dysregulated*, with similar percentages of children in each profile class. A fifth profile labeled *attention-seeking* was also found in which children monitored father-infant interaction closely but also appeared to be content to interact with their fathers from a distance and employed more attention-seeeking strategies. Again, *approach-avoidant* children with fathers were higher on emotional reactivity, anxiety-depression, sleep problems, and aggression than *regulated-exploration* children at 4 months after the birth. *Anxious-clingy* children were more withdrawn and aggressive and had more sleep problems, and *attention-seeking* children were more anxious-depressed than *regulated-exploration* children at 4 months. Even though similar behavioral profiles emerged for children across the mother and father sessions, children often did not behave similarly when mothers were interacting with the infant and when fathers were doing so (e.g., approach-avoidant children with mothers may be in the regulated-exploration group with fathers). This initial study is informative in showing that there are both differences and similarities in children's reactions to mother-infant and father-infant interaction shortly after the infant sibling's birth, but clearly, far more research is needed.

Change in Father-Child Interaction

One of the most consistently documented family changes after the birth of a second child is the change in mother-firstborn interaction, with an increase in confrontations and harsh discipline and decreases in attachment security (see Volling, 2012, for a summary). Are similar changes apparent for the father-firstborn relationship? It is difficult to know for certain, given there are currently so few studies available that have included fathers. Stewart and colleagues (Stewart, 1990; Stewart et al., 1987) were some of the first to actually observe family interactions between US parents and their firstborn children both before the infant sibling's birth and at 1, 4, 8, and 12 months after during home visits to determine if there were changes in father-child interactions similar to changes reported between mothers and firstborn children. Parents of 40 families were instructed to engage in a building or construction task (e.g., blocks), and nine different interactive behaviors (e.g., talk, exploration, show, refusals, rewards, commands) were coded. Stewart (1990) found there were dramatic declines in mothers' behaviors from the prenatal to 1-month postnatal session that remained relatively stable throughout the remainder of the year; yet, this was not the case for fathers. There were no noticeable changes in fathers' behaviors directed toward firstborns during home visits from pre-birth to 1 month post-birth, but there was a gradual decline over the year. Children also directed more behaviors (exploration, refusals, talking, showing) to their fathers over time with a corresponding decrease in these behaviors toward their mothers from pre- to 1-month post-birth. These initial findings suggested that changes in mother-child interaction after the transition, even though quite dramatic, did not represent what was occurring in father-child interactions over this same time. Not only did fathers maintain involvement with firstborns in the early months after the sibling's birth, but also children were directing more social behavior toward their fathers, possibly because fathers were more available to respond to their children once mothers were more engaged in the care of the newborn. Understanding how children fare over the transition and how parenting by mothers and fathers plays a role in children's adjustment will require a family systems perspective wherein children, fathers, and mothers are viewed as interdependent, influencing one another both directly and indirectly.

Father Involvement in Child Care

Because parents making the transition from one child to two are now confronted with balancing the care of two young children, understanding fathers' role in child care requires an examination of parental involvement in the care of both children and infants. In these newly created two-child families, mothers and fathers may need to engage in a "divide and conquer" strategy (Murphy, 2018), whereas one parent is responsible for the care of one child and the other specializes in the care of the other. Kreppner, Paulsen, and Schuetze (1982) reported there were three different ways by which couples could distribute child care responsibilities after the birth of a second child: (a) fathers focus on housework and leave child care to mothers, (b) fathers *specialize* in the care of the firstborn, allowing mothers to bond with the infant, and (c) mothers and fathers *juggle* the care of both children. Kuo et al. (2018) examined couple reports of the division of child care for both the firstborn and infant at 1, 4, 8, and 12 months postpartum and were interested in knowing whether there was more support for the *specialization* or *juggling* hypothesis. Further, they asked whether there were differences in fathers' child care involvement in dual-earner and single-earner families because fathers' child care roles may differ considerably in households with two working parents versus households with a traditional breadwinner father and stay-at-home mother.

The findings revealed that fathers, in general, did specialize in the care of their firstborns immediately after birth at 1 month and were less involved in the care of the infant who was cared for almost exclusively by mothers in the first month. But fathers' involvement showed change over the year so that child care with the older child declined and care of the infant gradually increased over the year. By 12 months, fathers were involved similarly in the care of older siblings and infants. Interesting patterns of change in child care were also evident based on family-earner status. One month following the birth, there were no differences in dual-earner and single-earner fathers' involvement in child care with both children, but by 4 months, differences became apparent, and there was further divergence over the year after the birth, with dual-earner fathers steadily increasing their involvement in child care, and single-earner fathers decreasing child care involvement from 1 to 4 months and remaining at this level of involvement across the year. Finally, Kuo and colleagues (2018) considered how egalitarian gender role beliefs and work-family conflict reported by fathers predicted men's involvement in child care. Overall, difficulty balancing work and family obligations predicted less father involvement in infant care directly after birth for both single-earner and dual-earner fathers. Egalitarian gender roles predicted greater father involvement with firstborns 1 month after the birth, but only in dual-earner families. Greater involvement in infant care 1 month after childbirth predicted an increase in fathers' involvement in the older siblings' care during the year, providing some support for the juggling hypothesis for both dual- and single-earner fathers.

Results emanating from this research indicated that flexible parental leave policies that support fathers' involvement in child care after childbirth may assist families in the transition to reduce conflict and stress between work and family roles because work-family conflict was a stronger predictor of care than men's gender role ideologies. In China, where the birth of a second child is of major interest owing to the lifting of the one-child policy in 2015, a recently published study by Liu and Zhou (2019) reported that the husband's emotional support during the pregnancy, as well as an increase in shared housework after the birth, was related to an increase in mothers' life satisfaction after the birth. It is interesting to note that fathers' involvement in the division of child care is also a significant predictor of pregnancy intentions, with women more likely to have a second child sooner when fathers/partners are more involved in child care with the first child, and this is the case in a number of countries, including the United States (Szabó, Dubas, Volling, & van Aken, 2017), Norway (Dommermuth, Hohmann-Marriott, & Lappegård, 2017), Italy (Pinnelli & Fiori, 2008), the United Kingdom (Schaffnit & Sear, 2017), and Korea (Park, 2012). Similarly, Szabo and colleagues (2017) found shorter birth intervals between first and second children when mothers reported more support from extended family and relatives. Because grandparents are relied upon in many countries (e.g., Condon, Corkindale, Luszcz, & Gamble, 2013; Hoang & Kirby, 2019; Hunts & Avery, 1998; Zamberletti, Cavrini, & Tomassini, 2018) for child care, future research needs to consider how fathers' and other's involvement in child care lends insights into the decisions and timing of the birth of the second child, as well as the adjustment of mothers and children, and suggests research needs to attend to the intricate relations between members of the family system and external social support systems during the transition.

Co-Parenting and the Transition After the Second Child

As fathers and mothers learn to navigate the needs of two children after the birth of a second child, parents may also experience changes in co-parenting quality (e.g., support, cooperation, conflict, undermining) during this transition. A few studies suggest that cooperative and supportive co-parenting relationships mitigate firstborns' behavior problems after the birth (Kolak & Volling, 2013) and foster positive sibling interactions (Song & Volling, 2015), whereas undermining and high-conflict co-parenting contributes to firstborn's behavioral difficulties (Kolak & Volling, 2013; Song & Volling, 2015). As such, understanding the nature of co-parenting during this period and the factors that shape this relationship may be critical to elucidating how two-parent families manage the transition. Both Szabó, Dubas, and van Aken (2012) and Kuo, Volling, and Gonzalez (2017) investigated co-parenting quality with the firstborn before and after the birth of a second child. Whereas Kuo, Volling, and Gonzalez (2017) examined immediate change across the transition (from the last trimester to 4 months postpartum) in a sample of US families, Szabó et al. (2012) studied changes from the last trimester to 1 year postpartum in a sample of Dutch families. Analysis of the immediate transition period showed that mothers and fathers reported increased co-parenting conflict and decreased cooperation (Kuo, Volling, Gonzalez, Oh, & Yu, 2017), whereas the comparison of 12 months postpartum co-parenting quality with prepartum quality evinced stability across the year (Szabó et al., 2012). Perhaps, the immediate transition period requires adjustment and adaptation before returning to prepartum levels, similar to marital quality trajectories after the birth of a second child (Volling, Oh, Gonzalez, Kuo, & Yu, 2015). Interestingly, both studies found that the difficult temperaments of both the infant and the firstborn were risk factors for greater co-parenting problems and more so for mothers, compared to fathers (Kuo, Volling, & Gonzalez, 2017; Szabó et al., 2012). Specifically, infant siblings with more difficult temperaments contributed to mothers' lowered perceived stability in co-parenting quality for the firstborn across the year (Szabó et al., 2012) and mothers' increased co-parenting conflict 4 months postpartum (Kuo, Volling, & Gonzalez, 2017). In contrast, firstborn children's difficult temperament was related to lower levels of co-parenting cooperation during the immediate transition period (Kuo, Volling, & Gonzalez, 2017), but not at the end of the first year (Szabó et al., 2012). Mothers may experience more caregiving stress when children have highly negative temperaments due to having a greater share of childcare responsibilities compared to fathers (Kuo et al., 2018). Taken together, these studies highlight the heterogeneity in the couple's co-parenting relationship during the transition to second-time parenthood and a need for further investigation into these family dynamics.

Marital Relationships and the Transition After the Second Child

Given the prevalence of studies examining marital change across the transition to parenthood, it is noteworthy how few studies have examined marital change across second-time parenthood, even though a meta-analysis by Twenge, Campbell, and Foster (2003) found that marital quality continued to decline after the birth of subsequent children. There are studies that have looked at partner relationship quality after the birth of an infant based on parity (first or subsequent children). However, studies considering marital relationship quality and parity have not found consistent findings, with some reporting greater decreases in marital satisfaction and relationship quality for multiparous couples (Belsky, Spanier, & Rovine, 1983; Krieg, 2007; Lindblom et al., 2014) and others reporting similar declines in marital quality for both primiparous and multiparous couples (O'Brien & Peyton, 2002).

A recent study by Canário and Figueiredo (2016) examined marital relationship changes among first-time and second-time Portuguese parents in both positive and negative aspects across the first trimester of pregnancy to 30 months postpartum and found that from the first trimester of pregnancy to 3 months postpartum, there were greater declines in partner relationships for second-time parents and women. When considering the postpartum period from 3 to 30 months after birth, however, there was a greater deterioration of relationship quality for first-time parents. It is not clear what is responsible for these different patterns of change at different points in pregnancy and the postpartum for men and women and for first- and second-time parents. Canário and Figueiredo (2016) concluded that the partner relationship deteriorated over this time from early pregnancy to 30 months with an increase in negative and a decrease in positive relationship quality for both men and women, as well as for first- and second-time parents, leaving a less than positive impression on the effects of children on the couple relationship. Attempts to examine between-group differences for first- and second-time parents, with respect to the partner relationship after the birth of an infant, overlooks the individual differences that exist in couple relationship quality for parents making the transition from one child to two children. Further, there is little evidence in research studies on the transition to parenthood, whether for first-time or second-time parents, that any decline in positive or increase in negative dimensions of partner relationship quality is a cause for clinical concern or a call for action. These changes may be normative in response to the addition of a new member to the family and may simply reflect a period of adjustment for children, parents, and couples.

Only one study has looked at within-group heterogeneity in marital relationship change by focusing on the trajectories of positive and negative marital relations in a sample of US husbands and wives after the birth of their second child, acknowledging that not all marriages of second-time parents are the same and that research needs to capture this heterogeneity for couples having a second child. To address this possibility, Volling et al. (2015) conducted a person-centered analysis using growth mixture modeling to search for different patterns of marital change at the dyadic level by examining change in both negative and positive martial relations simultaneously for husbands and wives in the same analyses. Volling et al. (2015) identified five distinct patterns of marital relationship change from before birth to a year after the birth of a second child. Most of the 229 couples were distributed across two different patterns of relationship change. The largest group exhibited a gradual decrease in positive relations for wives over the year with husbands showing a honeymoon effect (i.e., a decline in negative marital relations from prenatal to 1 month after that then rebounded back by 4 months; 44% of couples). In these marriages, both husbands and wives reported significantly higher positive than negative marital relationships. A second group

(34.5%) had wives showing a gradual increase in negative marital relations over the year and husbands showing a pattern of adjustment and adaptation (i.e., a decline in positive relations from pre-birth to 1 month post-birth that rebounded by 4 months). Still, these couples had higher scores on positive than negative relationship quality, and there was no indication that these couples were on the brink of marital dysfunction. The remaining four groups, comprising approximately 21% of the sample, demonstrated different patterns of marital relationship change, suggesting that couples in these marriages struggled with maintaining the quality of their relationships, with husbands and wives having discrepant views (e.g., husbands more negative than wives), greater declines for wives than husbands, and wives experiencing a honeymoon period of increasing positivity and decreasing negativity that did not last past the first month (see Volling et al., 2015, for a detailed presentation and discussion of these results). When examining differences across the different marital trajectory groups, Volling et al. (2015) found that the manner in which couples discussed disagreements around child care was a key aspect of differentiating the better functioning marriages (husbands and wives had similar positive views of their marriages) from the more troubled marriages (husbands and wives had very different views of their marriages, often reporting increases in marital negativity over time). Couples in troubled marriages were more likely to use destructive marital communication (e.g., scolding, blaming, yelling, cursing) in solving child care disagreements than couples in well-functioning marriages, who were more likely to engage in constructive marital communication to solve disagreements. There was also evidence suggesting that parents reported more depressive symptomatology in "troubled marriages" than in more positively functioning marriages. Future research would benefit by studying the heterogeneity in partner relationships within families undergoing the transition, taking into consideration socioeconomic status, sexual orientation of the parents, marital status, blended families, and father residence, as just a few examples.

Paternal Well-Being and Parental Competence

Because there are so few studies on the transition after the second child and even fewer that have included fathers, there are also few studies that have examined paternal characteristics such as parental efficacy and mental health (e.g., depression, anxiety) and how these characteristics affect their children and family relations across the transition. Ferketich and Mercer (1995) examined experienced (2 or more children) and inexperienced (first-time) fathers with respect to parental competence, self-esteem, sense of mastery, depression, and anxiety at birth and at 1, 4, and 8 months after the birth of their infants. There were no differences for experienced and inexperienced fathers for self-esteem, and experienced fathers reported more mastery but only at 1 month after the birth and not later. Experienced fathers did report less anxiety and depression at both 4 and 8 months compared with inexperienced fathers. Further, lower depression and more partner relationship support were significant predictors of paternal competence for experienced fathers in the first 8 months after the infant's birth. Condon and Esuvaranathan (1990) have also found in an Australian study that fathers of multiparous women reported more postpartum depression than fathers of primiparous women.

A more recent study looking at parity effects for mothers and fathers in 260 Portuguese couples during the pregnancy (first, second, and third trimester), at childbirth, and at 3 months postpartum found significant parity effects at some, but not all, timepoints (Figueiredo & Conde, 2011). For instance, second-time parents reported more anxiety and depressive symptoms in the second and third trimester and 3 months postpartum but not at childbirth. Yet, different patterns of change in anxiety and depression appeared to be the case for first- and second-time parents over the course of the study, with both first- and second-time parents experiencing higher levels of both anxiety and depression during the pregnancy than after the birth, and women reporting higher anxiety and depressive symptoms, in general, than men, regardless of parity.

Research on parity effects, particularly those in women, do not paint a consistent picture, as some studies find that primiparous women report more anxiety and depression than multiparous women (e.g., Gameiro, Moura-Ramos, & Canavarro, 2009; Giakoumaki, Vasilaki, Lili, Skouroliakou, & Liosis, 2009), more depression in second-time mothers than first-time mothers (e.g., DiPietro, Costigan, & Sipsma, 2008; Figueiredo & Conde, 2011), or no differences (e.g., Breitkopf et al., 2006). Such inconsistencies in the literature may have more to do with the focus on between-group differences based on parity than individual or within-group differences (focusing only on second-time parents). Further, analyzing men and women separately does not take into account the couple- or family-level dynamics that may be important for understanding not only how children adjust to the transition but also how parents do.

Only one study to date has considered a within-family perspective and analyzed mothers' and fathers' depressive symptoms simultaneously from before to a year after the birth of their second child. Volling, Yu, Gonzalez, Tengelitsch, and Stevenson (2018) conducted a latent class growth analysis on 231 families in a longitudinal study (prenatal, 1, 4, 8 and 12 months) and found four different family patterns of depression: (1) both mothers and fathers low in depressive symptoms (40.7%), (2) mothers low and fathers high (24.7%); (3) fathers low and mothers high (21.5%), and (4) both mothers and fathers high (9.5%). Utilizing a cumulative risk model, Volling and colleagues (2018) found that children had far more externalizing and internalizing behavior problems after the birth of their sibling when both mothers and fathers were high in depressive symptoms, compared with children who had only one or no parent high on depressive symptoms. Further, parents also struggled when both parents had high depressive symptoms; both mothers and fathers reported more negative marital relations and parenting stress and less positive marital relations and parenting efficacy compared with parents in families with either one or no parent being high on depressive symptoms. Once again, there is heterogeneity within families undergoing the transition to a second child with women having higher depressive symptoms than men in some families and men having higher depressive symptoms than women in others. More research is needed that attempts to examine heterogeneity among families making the transition from one child to two because such studies will allow us to identify risk and protective factors that predict individual differences in children's problem behavior and family stress that can be used to inform parent education and intervention efforts.

The Family Transitions Study (FTS)

Because there are few studies available to directly test the supportive role of fathers for firstborn children across the transition to siblinghood, the remainder of this chapter presents recent analyses examining children's adjustment after the birth of an infant sibling and whether fathers' involvement in the care of firstborn children before the birth is a protective factor that mitigates increases in children's problem behavior once the infant sibling is born. Data are from the Family Transitions Study, a longitudinal investigation of 241 families visited at five timepoints starting in the third trimester of the mothers' pregnancy with their second child and 1, 4, 8, and 12 months after the birth of the infant sibling to address individual variation in children's adjustment across the year and what child and family factors predict problematic outcomes for children.

The sample included 241 two-parent, heterosexual couples in the United States with fathers of the infant residing in the home (see Volling, Gonzalez, Oh, Song, et al., 2017 for complete details of recruitment criteria, protocols, and sample characteristics). The mean age of mothers at the prenatal timepoint was 31.60 years (SD = 4.22) and 33.20 years (SD = 4.78) for fathers. The majority of mothers (83.9%) and fathers (79.2%) earned a bachelor's degree or higher. Most couples (98%) reported being married (M = 5.77 years, SD = 2.74). Most families were European American (85.9% of mothers,

86.3% of fathers), and most (37.8%) had incomes ranging from $60,000 to $99, 999. Firstborns included 131 female and 110 male children and were 31.17 months (SD = 10.13) at the time of the infant's birth. Attrition over the study was 15% resulting in 203 families at 12 months. For the current analysis, firstborn children were grouped into one of three age groups based on their age at the time of the infant sibling's birth: 1- to 2-year-olds ($M = 20.15$ months, SD = 2.38), 2- to 3-year-olds ($M = 29.26$ months, SD = 3.40), and 3- to 4-year-olds ($M = 40.88$ months, SD = 3.31). Only 10 children were older than 4 years, so they were excluded from further analysis.

Table 16.1 FTS scales of children's adjustment after the birth of a sibling

1. Sleep problems ($\alpha = 0.63$ to 0.78)
1. Wakes frequently at night
2. Needs help to fall asleep
3. Makes a fuss or cries when going to bed at night
4. Has bad dreams or wakes at night crying
2. Separation anxiety ($\alpha = 0.60$ to 0.71)
5. Follows mother/father around the house
6. Wants to spend time with mother/father
7. Tries hard to get mother's/father's attention
8. Fears mother/father leaving him/her
3. Oppositional behavior ($\alpha = 0.59$ to 0.69)
9. Confrontations with mother/father involving hitting, slapping, biting, or other inappropriate physical acts
10. Breaks toys or other objects
11. Challenges mother/father when she/he requests child to do something
12. Withdraws from social interaction with mother/father
13. Is naughty or does things child knows he/she should not do
4. Emotional distress ($\alpha = 0.62$ to 0.75)
14. Cries/is weepy or tearful
15. Has temper tantrums
16. Whines a lot
5. Toileting accidents ($\alpha = 0.50$ to 0.77)
17. Wets the bed at night
18. Has daytime toileting accidents

Firstborn Adjustment

Both parents completed 36 items of children's behavior using a 5-point scale, ranging from (1) *almost never* to (5) *almost always* to assess firstborn children's adjustment. Items were created based on a review of the literature with attention to reports of problematic behaviors after the birth of a sibling (e.g., "makes a fuss about eating," "has temper tantrums," and "has bad dreams or wakes at night crying"). A series of exploratory factor analyses (EFA) were conducted, deleting any items that did not load greater than 0.40 on factors with eigenvalues greater than 1.00. This resulted in 18 items that loaded onto five factors, which were used to create five scales of children's adjustment, with fair to good internal consistency across the five timepoints: *sleep problems*, *separation anxiety*, *oppositional behavior*, *emotional distress*, and *toileting accidents* (see Table 16.1), which were also fairly stable over time for both mothers and fathers, $r = 0.15$–0.76, all p's < 0.05.

In an effort to validate the subscales, we ran correlations between the subscales of children's adjustment at each timepoint and the broadband dimensions of externalizing and internalizing behavior problems completed by parents on the widely-used Child Behavior Checklist 1.5–5 years (Achenbach & Rescorla, 2000). Internalizing and externalizing scores were significantly correlated with mothers' and fathers' reports of separation anxiety, sleep problems, opposition, and emotional distress at each time point. Fathers' reported toileting accidents were significantly correlated with externalizing at 1, 4, and 12 months and internalizing at 1 and 4 months. Mothers' reported toileting problems were correlated significantly with externalizing at prenatal, 1, 4, and 12 months and internalizing at prenatal and 1 month only. Thus, there was convergent evidence to suggest that subscales of the current measure were valid indicators of children's behavioral adjustment as reported by mothers and fathers.

Father Involvement

During a joint couple interview conducted during the prenatal home visit, mothers and fathers were asked to jointly agree on who did 11 different child care tasks from the *Child Care Checklist* (Ehrenberg, Gearing-Smll, Hunter, & Small, 2001) on a scale of (1) *always wife* to (5) *always husband*, with (3) *both equally* (e.g., "making snack for child," "taking child to the doctor," and "staying home when child is sick"; α = 0.73, M = 2.35, SD = 0.50).

Results: Age and Gender Differences in Children's Adjustment Over Time

Because mothers and fathers may have different perceptions of their children's problematic behaviors (Burney & Leerkes, 2010; Ventura & Stevenson, 1986) and because of the lack of information on fathers' perspectives across the transition from one to two children, both mothers' and fathers' reports were analyzed separately. The first descriptive analysis used mixed-model ANOVAs: 5 (time: pre-birth, 1, 4, 8, 12 months) × 2 (parent: father, mother) × 2 (gender: boy, girl) × 3 (age group: 1–2 years, 2–3 years, 3–4 years) with time and parent as repeated factors, age and gender as between-group factors, and each of the five behavior problem scales as dependent variables. Table 16.2 summarizes the results for these analyses.

There were significant main effects of the age group for emotional distress and toileting accidents with 2-year-olds having more problems than 1- and 3-year-olds (see Table 16.2). All 1-year-olds were still in diapers at the time, so parents often reported toileting accidents were not a problem or did not occur with these young children, but they started to consider soiling and bed-wetting problematic starting when children were 2 years of age. Because parents often start toilet training between 18 and 24 months (Van Aggelpoel, Vermandel, Fraeyman, Massart, & Van Hal, 2019; van Nunen, Kaerts, Wyndaele, Vermandel, & Van Hal, 2015), this increase in reported toileting accidents for 2-year-olds may very well reflect the normative timeline for toilet training and not necessarily any direct result of the birth of a sibling. In fact, toilet training is experienced as difficult and time-consuming by many parents (Van Aggelpoel et al., 2019), in general, so attempting to do so while also caring for a newborn infant may be perceived as problematic and stressful. The fact that parents reported that 2-year-olds experienced more emotional distress than 1-year-olds may reflect the significant changes occurring over 2–3 years in which children are developing a sense of self, an understanding of others, and critical skills for behavioral and emotional regulation (Thompson, 2006).

There was only one gender difference, with boys showing more oppositional behavior than girls. This finding is consistent with research reporting that aggression and conduct problems are often more common among boys than girls of this age (Baillargeon et al., 2007; Shaw, Keenan, & Vondra, 1994; Zahn-Waxler, Shirtcliff, & Marceau, 2008) and that boys increased in deliberate naughty behavior after the birth of a sibling (Kendrick & Dunn, 1980). Again, these findings may very well reflect normative differences in aggression in early childhood and have nothing to do with the birth of a sibling. For instance, Baillargeon et al. (2007) found toddler boys were higher on aggression than toddler girls and that there was stability in toddler aggression from 17 to 29 months of age. We also did not find abundant gender differences when examining changes in children's behaviors over the year. Indeed, there were no significant time x gender interactions for any of the behaviors, indicating that none of the behaviors changed differently for boys and girls. We also performed a follow-up analysis to determine whether the gender of the infant mattered as some have suggested that there are more or less problems when the older child is the same or opposite gender of the infant. Again, only one significant main effect was found for children's emotional distress, F (2,160) = 4.74, p = 0.03, η_p^2 = 0.03, with children in same-gender dyads, M = 2.42, SD = 0.06, more distressed than children in opposite-gender dyads, M = 2.25, SD = 05, although it should be underscored that

Table 16.2 Parents' reports of firstborn children's behavior problems by age, gender, parent, and time

Variables	Age			*F*	Gender		*F*	Parent		*F*	Time					*F*
	1 year *M(SE)*	2 years *M(SE)*	3 years *M(SE)*		Girls *M(SE)*	Boys *M(SE)*		Father *M(SE)*	Mother *M(SE)*		Prenatal *M(SE)*	1 month *M(SE)*	4 months *M(SE)*	8 months *M(SE)*	12 months *M(SE)*	
Sleep problems	2.01 (.09)	2.26 (.08)	2.19 (.11)	NS	2.14 (.07)	2.16 (.08)	NS	2.16 (.06)	2.15 (.06)	NS	2.21_a (.06)	2.10_b (.06)	2.18_a (.06)	2.20_a (.06)	2.08_b (.06)	3.24*
Separation anxiety	2.92 (.06)	2.94 (.05)	2.84 (.07)	NS	2.92 (.04)	2.87 (.05)	NS	2.88 (.04)	2.92 (.04)	NS	2.97_a (.05)	2.82_b (.05)	2.89 (.04)	2.90 (.05)	2.91 (.05)	4.67**
Opposition	1.84 (.05)	1.95 (.04)	1.94 (.06)	NS	1.84 (.04)	1.98 (.04)	6.79*	1.91 (.03)	1.91 (.27)	NS	1.92_a (.04)	1.93_a (.04)	1.85_b (.03)	1.95_a (.04)	1.90 (.03)	3.93**
Emotional distress	2.23_a (.07)	2.45_b (.06)	2.26 (.08)	3.71*	2.34 (.05)	2.29 (.06)	NS	2.30 (.04)	2.32 (.04)	NS	2.28_{ac} (.06)	2.28_{ac} (.06)	2.21_a (.05)	2.43_b (.05)	2.36_{bc} (.05)	5.52***
Toileting accidents	1.52_a (.08)	1.78_b (.06)	1.50_a (.09)	5.02**	1.61 (.06)	1.58 (.07)	NS	1.61 (.04)	1.59 (.05)	NS	1.60 (.07)	1.60 (.06)	1.65_a (.06)	1.50_b (.06)	1.64_a (.06)	NS

Note. Means designated with different subscripts are significantly different from each other based on post-hoc comparisons ($p < .05$)
NS nonsignificant
$^*p < .05$, $^{**}p < .01$, $^{***}p < .001$

gender differences in children's adjustment are not consistently reported across studies examining the transition to siblinghood (see Volling, 2012).

There were significant main effects of time for children's sleep problems, separation anxiety, oppositional behavior, and emotional distress, indicating these behaviors often differed across timepoints (see Table 16.2). Many prior studies of the transition to siblinghood have only considered short-term change (1 month before to 1 month after the birth) or post-birth adjustment with no pre-birth assessment (Volling, 2012). Based on the current findings from before to 1 year following the infant's birth, in only two instances, sleep problems and separation anxiety, were there significant changes across the prenatal and 1 month timepoints. Children actually showed significant declines in their sleep problems and separation anxiety in the first month, with subsequent increases by 4 months. Some children may actually experience a period of adjustment and adaptation and perhaps improvement in their behavior, even if only for a short period of time, which is consistent with some of the early work by Dunn and Kendrick (1982) reporting that some children actually evinced more mature behaviors after birth (e.g., relinquishing a pacifier), a finding that stands in strong contrast to popular conceptions of the birth of a sibling as a time of developmental crisis and intense rivalry.

There were no significant differences in mothers' and fathers' reports of any of the adjustment issues, suggesting that both parents, on average, rated their children's behavior similarly. There were, however, two significant parent x time interactions for separation anxiety, $F(4,158) = 6.81$, $\eta_p^2 = 0.15$, $p < 0.001$, and oppositional behavior, $F(4,158) = 3.49$, $\eta_p^2 = 0.08$, $p < 0.01$, and these are depicted in Fig. 16.1. *Post hoc* comparisons (all p's < 0.05) revealed separation anxiety, as reported by fathers pre-birth, was significantly higher at 1, 4, and 8 months and significantly lower at 4 months compared to 1 month. For mothers, separation anxiety was significantly higher at 4 months compared to 1, 8, and 12 months and significantly higher pre-birth compared to 1 month. For oppositional behavior, fathers reported significantly fewer opposition problems at 4 months compared to 1 and 8 months, whereas mothers reported significantly more opposition pre-birth compared to 4 and 12 months (all p's < 0.05).

There was also a significant two-way interaction between parent and child age for oppositional behavior, $F(2,161) = 4.28$, $\eta_p^2 = 0.05$, $p < 0.05$. *Post hoc* comparisons ($p < 0.05$) revealed that mothers of 2- and 3-year-olds reported significantly more opposition problems than mothers of 1-year-olds, whereas fathers of 2-year-olds reported significantly more opposition problems than fathers of 1-year-olds. Such differences may reflect the different views that fathers and mothers have about their children's problem behaviors, either because they are not spending equal amounts of time interacting with their children (e.g., mothers were more involved overall in the care of their children than fathers) or parents simply have different expectations for children's behaviors (e.g., fathers may be less concerned about opposition than mothers).

Father Involvement as a Protective Factor

To address whether fathers' involvement in child care before the birth might buffer children's maladjustment such that children with more involved fathers would demonstrate better adjustment trajectories over time (see Kreppner, 1988), we computed a median split on the division of child care measure at the prenatal timepoint resulting in two groups: high and low father involvement (below and above 2.35). Recall that a score of 3 corresponds to both husband and wife doing the task equally, so high and low father involvement here is relative to other fathers in the sample, and not in relation to mothers' involvement in child care. We then conducted 5(time) × 2(parent) × 2 (high/low father involvement) mixed-model ANOVAs with time and parent as repeated factors and father involvement as a between-group factor for each of the five behavior problems. Because time and parent effects were reported

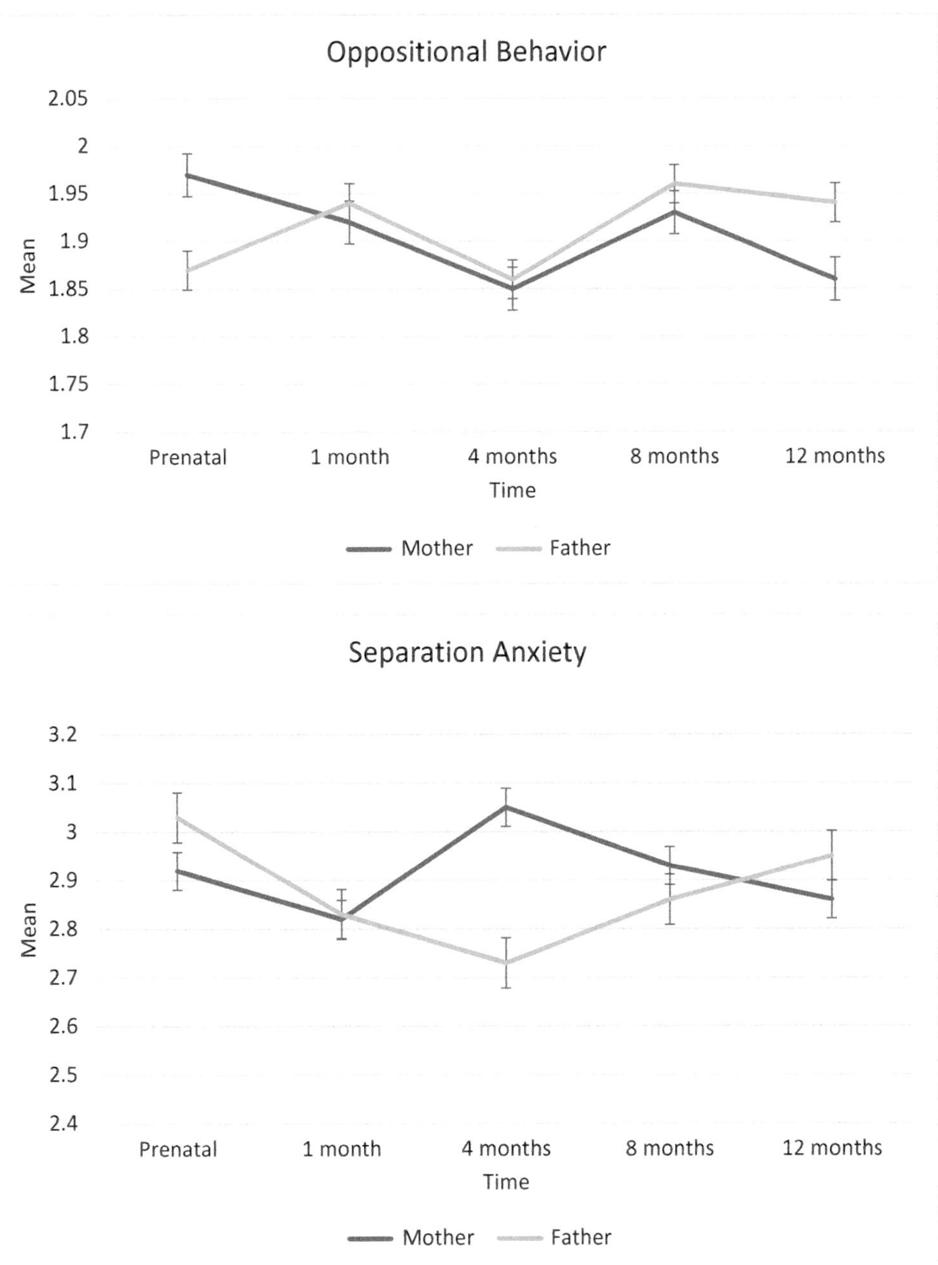

Fig. 16.1 Parent x time interactions for mothers' and fathers' reports of children's oppositional behavior and separation anxiety

earlier, we only report the main effects of father involvement or interactions with father involvement here. A significant interaction between parent (father, mother) and father involvement was found for separation anxiety, $F(1,165) = 4.19$, $\eta_p^2 = 0.03$, $p < 0.05$, revealing that mothers reported significantly more separation anxiety, $M = 2.97$, SE = 0.05, than fathers, $M = 2.90$, SE = 0.05, in families with low father involvement, but not in high father involvement families. There was also a significant time x father involvement interaction for separation anxiety,

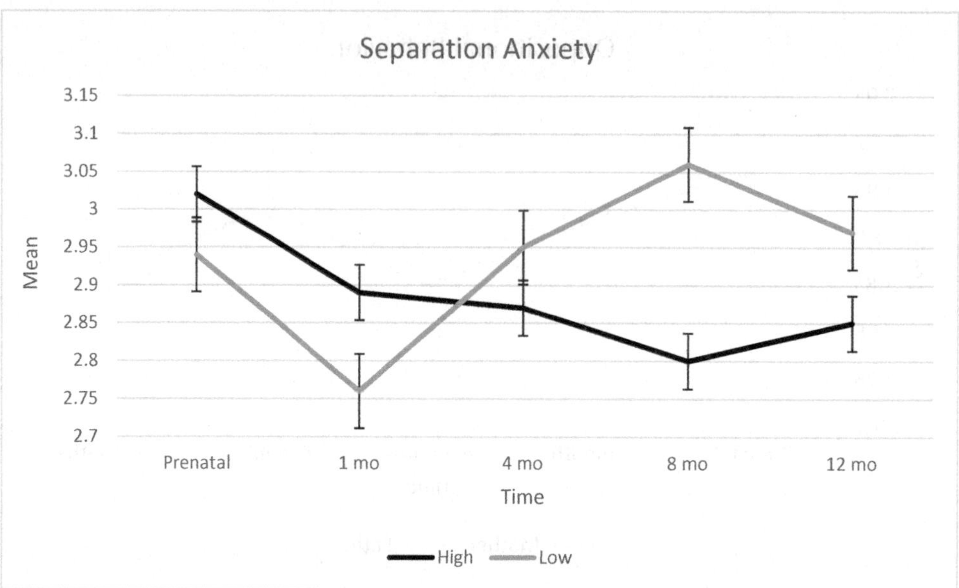

Fig. 16.2 Time x father involvement (high/low) interaction for children's separation anxiety

$F(4,162) = 3.05$, $\eta_p^2 = 0.07$, $p < 0.05$, which is depicted in Fig. 16.2, and shows that separation anxiety changed differently over time for children with low and high father involvement. For children in families with low father involvement before the birth, children's separation anxiety started high, dropped significantly at 1 month shortly after the birth, but then increased consistently through 12 months; children had significantly lower separation anxiety at 1 month than any other timepoint, all p's < 0.01. For children in families with high father involvement before the birth, separation anxiety decreased steadily throughout the year (see Fig. 16.2), with children having significantly higher separation anxiety at the pre-birth timepoint than any other timepoint, all p's < 0.05.

One of the main aims of FTS was to consider the protective role of fathers for children undergoing the transition to siblinghood. Only in the case of separation anxiety did we find evidence that fathers' involvement in child care was influential. Children's separation anxiety decreased over the year in families in which fathers were highly involved in child care before the infant sibling was born. Even though separation anxiety also declined from prenatal to 1 month after birth for children with fathers low in child care involvement, these children experienced a sudden increase in separation anxiety from 1 to 8 months, before experiencing a modest decline again, 1 year after the birth. Fathers' increased attention and support may indeed buffer children's separation anxiety, at a time when changes in the mother-child relationship are many and attachment security declines (Stewart, 1990; Teti, Sakin, Kucera, Corns, & Eiden, 1996). It is noteworthy that the effects of father involvement emerged for separation anxiety, which is a more relationship-based aspect of social functioning (e.g., following parents around the house, seeking attention, wanting to spend time with parents) than children's sleep problems, emotional distress, oppositional behaviors, or toileting accidents, which may be far more dependent on children's developmental level or their individual psychological characteristics such as temperament. Parents as well as health-care providers may want to consider how fathers can play a more active role in their children's care and the benefits of such involvement during the transition from one child to two.

Summary and Key Points

For the vast majority of families in the United States and across the globe, parents often decide to have more than one child, indicating that siblings are an important part of family life for most children. The transition from one child to two is a significant life event for both the firstborns who have gone from being an only child to becoming an older sibling and their parents, who must now reorganize family life to care for two young children, as well as extended family members who may be called upon to provide child care. Despite the prominence of families undergoing this important developmental transition, there are few longitudinal studies that have attempted to address how children and their parents adjust after the birth of an infant sibling, in general, yet alone entertain how this transition might differ for families from different racial and ethnic backgrounds, different cultures, different economic circumstances, and diverse family structures. One of the key points to be made here is the need for more research to understand these complexities in family formation for individuals from diverse backgrounds when having a second child, which may be intentional and carefully planned or unintentional and unwanted, with one or two parents, within extended family support networks or an isolated nuclear family, with resident or nonresident fathers, or in the United States or elsewhere around the world. The manner in which families manage the birth of second and subsequent children is a topic about which we know very little, a point also emphasized recently by Fouts and Bader (2016) in their review of the role of culture for understanding the transition to becoming an older sibling. These authors noted that currently, there are no focused cross-cultural studies addressing this issue which "limits our understanding of the extent to which culture (i.e., socially transmitted knowledge, beliefs, and practices) may influence the transition to becoming an older sibling (p. 221)." The few examples they found in the ethnographic record with respect to becoming an older sibling suggests that children in different parts of the world experience both jealousy and joy at the arrival of their baby sibling, highlighting the large individual differences in how children react and respond to the birth of a sibling. Pereira and colleagues (2015) interviewed a sample of 24 Brazilian mothers expecting their second child and focused on the rivalry and jealousy of the firstborn toward the mother and the new baby already during pregnancy. As research on the transition to siblinghood begins to capture the diverse cultural and family circumstances that make meaning of this transition for children and their families, we need to be mindful to focus on both the positive (affection, joy, interest, pride) and negative (jealousy, opposition, distress) behaviors of young children in response to a new sibling in the family and not overemphasize the transition as a period of developmental crisis (see Volling, Gonzalez, Oh, Song et al., 2017, for a rebuttal of this position).

Even though the research base on the transition from one child to two is sparse and even sparser when you consider the role of the father, there are several key points worth noting. First, in contrast to popular opinion and earlier writings about firstborn children's adjustment when a new baby arrives on the scene, the transition to siblinghood is not a time of developmental crisis for firstborn children. Most children and their parents may experience a brief period of disruption shortly after the birth as both parents and children reorganize and renegotiate family routines and family life, but eventually, families adapt and new routines replace the old ones. Both men and women move on in their new roles as the parents of two children instead of one. We must be aware, however, that some parents and their children do struggle with the transition, and life with two children may be more challenging and difficult to manage than life with only one child. There is a need to develop interventions, parent education classes, or just written materials that accurately reflect what we know to date about this transition and how health-care professionals and parents can best prepare children for the impending birth of a second child. Given the fact that the transition is still portrayed in many child-rearing books and on parenting websites as a time of crisis for young children, developing such materials is an important next step in helping parents and their children across this major life event.

Second, there does appear to be evidence that fathers' involvement in the care of firstborn children helps offset stress for children and mothers after the birth of a sibling. In the results reported here from the FTS, fathers' emotional support and involvement in the care of their first child even before the birth of the second helped alleviate children's distress and separation anxiety in the months and years after the birth. Further, the extent to which fathers felt confident in their abilities to discipline children and manage disruptive child behavior before and after the birth appeared to be particularly important in whether or not older siblings engaged in aggressive behavior. Providing information and parenting skills to assist fathers in managing children's difficult and challenging behavior may ease the transition for both children and their parents.

Finally, fathers' roles as both a co-parent and a spouse also played a part in how both parents and children flourish over the transition. Our research demonstrated that whether fathers were supportive co-parents or spouses, they played some role in how smooth the transition was for their children, themselves, and the mothers of their children. When fathers and mothers engaged in cooperative co-parenting before the infant was born, older siblings experienced less internalizing and externalizing behavior problems and showed more positive interest in the care of their infant sibling compared to children whose parents were unsupportive and undermining in their co-parenting roles. When parents disagreed about child care arrangements and engaged in destructive rather than constructive conflict resolution, this ineffective means of problem-solving did not bode well for marriages or parental mental health. Overall, the interdependent nature of family and ecological systems highlights the complexity of fathers' and mothers' roles as parents, co-parents, and spouses, which, in the end, contribute to the well-being of children, mothers, and fathers across the transition from one child to two.

References

Achenbach, T. M., & Rescorla, L. A. (2000). *Manual for the ASEBA preschool forms & profiles*. Burlington, VT: University of Vermont, Research Center for Children, Youth and Families.

Baillargeon, R. H., Zoccolillo, M., Keenan, K., Côté, S., Pérusse, D., Wu, H.-X., et al. (2007). Gender differences in physical aggression: A prospective population-based survey of children before and after 2 years of age. *Developmental Psychology, 43*, 13–26. https://doi-org.proxy.lib.umich.edu/10.1037/0012-1649.43.1.13

Baydar, N., Hyle, P., & Brooks-Gunn, J. (1997). A longitudinal study of the effects of the birth of a sibling during preschool and early grade school years. *Journal of Marriage and the Family, 59*, 957–965.

Belsky, J., Spanier, G. B., & Rovine, M. (1983). Stability and change in marriage across the transition to parenthood. *Journal of Marriage and the Family, 45*(3), 567–577. https://doi-org.proxy.lib.umich.edu/10.2307/351661

Beyers-Carlson, E., Stevenson, M. M., Gonzalez, R., Oh, W., Volling, B. L., & Yu, T. (2017). Developmental trajectories of children's adjustment across the transition to siblinghood: Pre-birth predictors and sibling outcomes at one year: IX. Developmental trajectories of children's somatic complaints after the birth of a sibling. *Monographs of the Society for Research in Child Development, 82*(3), 118–129, Serial No. 326.

Breitkopf, C. R., Primeau, L. A., Levine, R. E., Olson, G. L., Wu, Z. H., & Berenson, A. B. (2006). Anxiety symptoms during pregnancy and postpartum. *Journal of Psychosomatic Obstetrics and Gynecology, 27*(3), 157–162. https://doi-org.proxy.lib.umich.edu/10.1080/01674820500523521

Burney, R. V., & Leerkes, E. M. (2010). Links between mothers' and fathers' perceptions of infant temperament and coparenting. *Infant Behavior and Development, 33*(2), 125–135. https://doi.org/10.1016/j.infbeh.2009.12.002

Canário, C., & Figueiredo, B. (2016). Partner relationship from early pregnancy to 30 months postpartum: Gender and parity effects. *Couple and Family Psychology: Research and Practice, 5*(4), 226–239. https://doi-org.proxy.lib.umich.edu/10.1037/cfp0000066

Condon, J. T., & Esuvaranathan, V. (1990). The influence of parity on the experience of pregnancy: A comparison of first- and second-time expectant couples. *British Journal of Medical Psychology, 63*(4), 369–377. https://doi-org.proxy.lib.umich.edu/10.1111/j.2044-8341.1990.tb01632.x

Condon, J., Corkindale, C., Luszcz, M., & Gamble, E. (2013). The Australian first-time grandparents study: Time spent with the grandchild and its predictors. *Australasian Journal on Ageing, 32*, 21–27. https://doi-org.proxy.lib.umich.edu/10.1111/j.1741-6612.2011.00588.x

de Mendonça, J. S., Bussab, V. S. R., Rodrigues, A., Siqueira, J., & Cosette, L. (2013). Postpartum depression, father's involvement, and marital and co-parental relationships from mothers' and fathers' perspectives in a low-income Brazilian sample. *Family Science*.. https://doi.org/10.1080/19424620.2012.783423

DiPietro, J. A., Costigan, K. A., & Sipsma, H. L. (2008). Continuity in self-report measures of maternal anxiety, stress, and depressive symptoms from pregnancy through two years postpartum. *Journal of Psychosomatic Obstetrics and Gynecology, 29*(2), 115–124. https://doi-org.proxy.lib.umich.edu/10.1080/01674820701701546

Dommermuth, L., Hohmann-Marriott, B., & Lappegård, T. (2017). Gender equality in the family and childbearing. *Journal of Family Issues, 38*(13), 1803–1824. https://doi-org.proxy.lib.umich.edu/10.1177/0192513X15590686

Dunn, J. (1983) Sibling relationships in early childhood. Child Development, 54, 787–811. https://doi-org.proxy.lib.umich.edu/10.2307/1129886

Dunn, J., & Kendrick, C. (1980). The arrival of sibling: Changes in patterns of interaction between mother and first-born child. *Journal of Child Psychology and Psychiatry, 21*(2), 119–132.

Dunn, J., & Kendrick, C. (1982). *Siblings: Love, envy and understanding*. Cambridge, MA: Harvard University Press.

Ehrenberg, M. F., Gearing-Smll, M., Hunter, M. A., & Small, B. J. (2001). Childcare task division and shared parenting attitudes in dual-earner families with young children. *Family Relations: An Interdisciplinary Journal of Applied Family Studies, 50*(2), 143–153. https://doi-org.proxy.lib.umich.edu/10.1111/j.1741-3729.2001.00143.x

Ferketich, S. L., & Mercer, R. T. (1995). Predictors of role competence for experienced and inexperienced fathers. *Nursing Research, 44*(2), 89–95. https://doi-org.proxy.lib.umich.edu/10.1097/00006199-199503000-00005

Field, T., & Reite, M. (1984). Children's responses to separation from mother during the birth of another child. *Child Development, 55*(4), 1308–1316.

Figueiredo, B., & Conde, A. (2011). Anxiety and depression symptoms in women and men from early pregnancy to 3-months postpartum: Parity differences and effects. *Journal of Affective Disorders, 132*(1–2), 146–157. https://doi-org.proxy.lib.umich.edu/10.1016/j.jad.2011.02.007

Fouts, H. N., & Bader, L. R. (2016). Transitions in siblinghood: Integrating developmental, cultural, and evolutionary perspectives. In D. Narvaez, J. M. Braungart-Rieker, L. E. Miller-Graff, L. T. Gettler, & P. D. Hastings (Eds.), Contexts for young child flourishing: Evolution, family, and society. (pp. 215–230). Oxford University Press. https://doi-org.proxy.lib.umich.edu/10.1093/acprof:oso/9780190237790.003.0011

Gameiro, S., Moura-Ramos, M., & Canavarro, M. C. (2009). Maternal adjustment to the birth of a child: Primiparity versus multiparity. *Journal of Reproductive and Infant Psychology, 27*(3), 269–286. https://doi-org.proxy.lib.umich.edu/10.1080/02646830802350898

Giakoumaki, O., Vasilaki, K., Lili, L., Skouroliakou, M., & Liosis, G. (2009). The role of maternal anxiety in the early postpartum period: Screening for anxiety and depressive symptomatology in Greece. *Journal of Psychosomatic Obstetrics and Gynecology, 30*(1), 21–28. https://doi-org.proxy.lib.umich.edu/10.1080/01674820802604839

Goodman, J. H. (2008). Influences of maternal postpartum depression on fathers and on father-infant interaction. *Infant Mental Health Journal, 29*(6), 624–643. https://doi-org.proxy.lib.umich.edu/10.1002/imhj.20199

Gottlieb, L. N., & Mendelson, M. J. (1990). Parental support and firstborn girls' adaptation to the birth of a sibling. *Journal of Applied Developmental Psychology, 11*(1), 29–48.

Hoang, N.-P. T., & Kirby, J. N. (2019). A meta-ethnography synthesis of joint care practices between parents and grandparents from asian cultural backgrounds: Benefits and challenges. *Journal of Child and Family Studies*. https://doi-org.proxy.lib.umich.edu/10.1007/s10826-019-01553-y

Hunts, H. J. H., & Avery, R. J. (1998). Relatives as child care givers: After hours support for nontraditional workers. *Journal of Family and Economic Issues, 19*, 315–341. https://doi-org.proxy.lib.umich.edu/10.1023/A:1022925815835

Kayiatos, R., Adams, J., & Gilman, B. (1984). The arrival of a rival: Maternal perceptions of toddlers' regressive behaviors after the birth of a sibling. *Journal of Nurse Midwifery, 29*(3), 205–213.

Kendrick, C., & Dunn, J. (1980). Caring for a second baby: Effects on interaction between mother and firstborn. *Developmental Psychology, 16*(4), 303.

Kojima, Y., Irisawa, M., & Wakita, M. (2005). The impact of a second infant on interactions of mothers and firstborn children. *Journal of Reproductive and Infant Psychology, 23*, 103–114.

Kolak, A. M., & Volling, B. L. (2013). Coparenting moderates the association between firstborn children's temperament and problem behavior across the transition to siblinghood. *Journal of Family Psychology, 27*(3), 355.

Kreppner, K. (1988). Changes in parent-child relationships with the birth of the second child. *Marriage & Family Review, 12*(3–4), 157–181.

Kreppner, K., Paulsen, S., & Schuetze, Y. (1982). Infant and family development: From triads to tetrads. *Human Development, 25*(6), 373–391. https://doi-org.proxy.lib.umich.edu/10.1159/000272821

Krieg, D. B. (2007). Does motherhood get easier the second-time around? Examining parenting stress and marital quality among mothers having their first or second child. *Parenting: Science and Practice, 7*(2), 149–175. https://doi-org.proxy.lib.umich.edu/10.1080/15295190701306912

Kuo, P. X., Volling, B. L., & Gonzalez, R. (2017). His, hers, or theirs? Coparenting after the birth of a second child. *Journal of Family Psychology, 31*(6), 710–720.

Kuo, P. X., Volling, B. L., & Gonzalez, R. (2018). Gender role beliefs, work-family conflict, and father involvement after the birth of a second child. *Psychology of Men & Masculinity, 19*(2), 243–256.

Kuo, P. X., Volling, B. L., Gonzalez, R., Oh, W., & Yu, T. (2017). Developmental trajectories of children's adjustment across the transition to siblinghood: Pre-birth predictors and sibling outcomes at one year: VII. Developmental trajectories of children's emotional reactivity after the birth of a sibling. *Monographs of the Society for Research in Child Development, 82*(3), 93–105, Serial No. 326.

Legg, C., Sherick, I., & Wadland, W. (1974). Reaction of preschool children to the birth of a sibling. *Child Psychiatry and Human Development, 5*(1), 3–39.

Lindblom, J., Flykt, M., Tolvanen, A., Vänskä, M., Tiitinen, A., Tulppala, M., et al. (2014). Dynamic family system trajectories from pregnancy to child's first year. *Journal of Marriage and Family, 76*(4), 796–807. https://doi-org.proxy.lib.umich.edu/10.1111/jomf.12128

Liu, J., & Zhou, Z. (2019). Mothers' subjective well-being after having a second child in current China: A case study of Xi'an City. *International Journal of Environmental Research and Public Health, 16*, 3823. https://doi.org/10.3390/ijerph16203823

Mezulis, A. H., Hyde, J. S., & Clark, R. (2004). Father involvement moderates the effect of maternal depression during a child's infancy on child behavior problems in Kindergarten. *Journal of Family Psychology, 18*, 575–588. https://doi-org.proxy.lib.umich.edu/10.1037/0893-3200.18.4.575

Murphy, S. E. (2018). *We can work it out: Mothers' and fathers' coparenting of two children*. Unpublished doctoral dissertation. University of Texas at Austin, TX, USA.

O'Brien, M., & Peyton, V. (2002). Parenting attitudes and marital intimacy: A longitudinal analysis. *Journal of Family Psychology, 16*(2), 118–127. https://doi-org.proxy.lib.umich.edu/10.1037/0893-3200.16.2.118

Oh, W., Song, J. H., Gonzalez, R., Volling, B. L., & Yu, T. (2017). Developmental trajectories of children's adjustment across the transition to siblinghood: Pre-birth predictors and sibling outcomes at one year: VIII. Developmental trajectories of children's withdrawal after the birth of a sibling. *Monographs of the Society for Research in Child Development, 82*(3), 106–117. Serial No. 326.

Park, S.-M. (2012). Social networks and second-childbirth intentions of Korean married women. *Journal of Reproductive and Infant Psychology, 30*, 398–412.

Pereira, C. R. R., da Silva, D. G., Piccinini, C. A., & Lopez, R. (2015). Rivalidade fraterna durante a gesação materna do segundo filho: Manifestações e estratégias de manejo (Sibling rivalry during second-child pregnancy: Manifestations and management strategies). *Estudios de Psicología, 32*, 653–662. https://doi-org.proxy.lib.umich.edu/10.1590/0103-166X2015000400008

Pinnelli, A., & Fiori, F. (2008). The influence of partner involvement in fatherhood and domestic tasks on mothers' fertility expectations in Italy. *Fathering, 6*(2), 169–191. https://doi-org.proxy.lib.umich.edu/10.3149/fth.0602.169

Safyer, P., Stevenson, M. M., Gonzalez, R., Volling, B. L., Oh, W., & Yu, T. (2017). Developmental trajectories of children's adjustment across the transition to siblinghood: Pre-birth predictors and sibling outcomes at one year: X. Developmental trajectories of children's sleep problems after the birth of a sibling. *Monographs of the Society for Research in Child Development, 82*(3), 130–141. Serial No. 326.

Schaffnit, S. B., & Sear, R. (2017). Support for new mothers in the United Kingdom: Not all support is equal in the decision to having a second child. *Population Studies, 75*, 345–361. https://doi.org/10.1080/00324728.2017.1349924

Shaw, D. S., Keenan, K., & Vondra, J. I. (1994). Developmental precursors of externalizing behavior: Ages 1 to 3. *Developmental Psychology, 30*(3), 355.

Song, J.-H., & Volling, B. L. (2015). Coparenting and children's temperament predict firstborns' cooperation in the care of an infant sibling. *Journal of Family Psychology, 29*(1), 130–135. https://doi-org.proxy.lib.umich.edu/10.1037/fam0000052

Stewart, R. B. (1990). *The second child: Family transition and adjustment*. Thousand Oaks, CA: Sage Publications.

Stewart, R. B., Mobley, L. A., Van Tuyl, S. S., & Salvador, M. A. (1987). The firstborn's adjustment to the birth of a sibling: A longitudinal assessment. *Child Development, 58*(2), 341–355.

Szabó, N., Dubas, J. S., & van Aken, M. A. G. (2012). And baby makes four: The stability of coparenting and the effects of child temperament after the arrival of a second child. *Journal of Family Psychology, 26*(4), 554–564.

Szabó, N., Dubas, J. S., Volling, B. L., & van Aken, M. A. G. (2017). The effect of paternal and alloparental support on the interbirth interval among contemporary North American families. *Evolutionary Behavioral Sciences, 11*(3), 272–280. https://doi-org.proxy.lib.umich.edu/10.1037/ebs0000093

Teti, D. M., Sakin, J. W., Kucera, E., Corns, K. M., & Eiden, R. D. (1996). And baby makes four: Predictors of attachment security among preschool-age firstborns during the transition to siblinghood. *Child Development, 67*(2), 579–596.

Thomason, E., Oh, W., Volling, B. L., Gonzalez, R., & Yu, T. (2017). Developmental trajectories of children's adjustment across the transition to siblinghood: Pre-birth predictors and sibling outcomes at one year: VI. Developmental Trajectories of children's anxiety and depression after the birth of a sibling. *Monographs of the Society for Research in Child Development, 82*(3), 82–92. Serial No. 326.

Thompson, R. A. (2006). The development of the person: Social understanding, relationships, conscience, self. In N. Eisenberg, W. Damon, & R. M. Lerner (Eds.), Handbook of child psychology: Social, emotional, and personality development., Vol. 3, 6th ed. (pp. 24–98). Hoboken, NJ: John Wiley & Sons, Inc.

Twenge, J. M., Campbell, W. K., & Foster, C. A. (2003). Parenthood and marital satisfaction: A meta-analytic review. *Journal of Marriage and Family, 65*(3), 574–583. https://doi-org.proxy.lib.umich.edu/10.1111/j.1741-3737.2003.00574.x

United Nations, Department of Economic and Social Affairs, Population Division. (2015). *World Fertility Patterns 2015 – Data Booklet* (ST/ESA/ SER.A/370).

Vakrat, A., Apter-Levy, Y., & Feldman, R. (2018). Sensitive fathering buffers the effects of chronic maternal depression on child psychopathology. *Child Psychiatry and Human Development, 49*(5), 779–785. https://doi-org.proxy.lib.umich.edu/10.1007/s10578-018-0795-7

Van Aggelpoel, T., Vermandel, A., Fraeyman, J., Massart, M., & Van Hal, G. (2019). Information as a crucial factor for toilet training by parents. *Child Care Health and Development, 45*, 457–462. https://doi.org/10.1111/cch.12653462

van Nunen, K., Kaerts, N., Wyndaele, J. J., Vermandel, A., & Van Hal, G. (2015). Parents' views on toilet training (TT): A quantitative study to identify the beliefs and attitudes of parents concerning TT. *Journal of Child Health Care, 19*, 265–274. https://doi.org/10.1177/1367493513508232

Ventura, J. N., & Stevenson, M. B. (1986). Relations of mothers' and fathers' reports of infant temperament, parents' psychological functioning, and family characteristics. *Merrill-Palmer Quarterly, 32*, 275–289.

Volling, B. L. (2012). Family transitions following the birth of a sibling: An empirical review of changes in the firstborn's adjustment. *Psychological Bulletin, 138*(3), 497–528. https://doi.org/10.1037/a0026921

Volling, B. L., Gonzalez, R., Oh, W., Song, J., Yu, T., Rosenberg, L., et al. (2017). Developmental trajectories of children's adjustment across the transition to siblinghood: Pre-birth predictors and sibling outcomes at one year. *Monographs of the Society for Research in Child Development, 82*(3). Serial No. 326.

Volling, B. L., Gonzalez, R., Yu, T., & Oh, W. (2017). Developmental trajectories of children's adjustment across the transition to siblinghood: Pre-birth predictors and sibling outcomes at one year: IV. Developmental trajectories of children's aggressive behaviors after the birth of a sibling. *Monographs of the Society for Research in Child Development, 82*(3), 53–71. Serial No. 326. https://doi-org.proxy.lib.umich.edu/10.1111/mono.12310

Volling, B. L., Oh, W., Gonzalez, R., Kuo, P. X., & Yu, T. (2015). Patterns of marital relationship change across the transition from one child to two. *Couple and Family Psychology: Research and Practice, 4*(3), 177–197. https://doi-org.proxy.lib.umich.edu/10.1037/cfp0000046

Volling, B. L., Yu, T., Gonzalez, R., Kennedy, D. E., Rosenberg, L., & Oh, W. (2014). Children's responses to mother–infant and father–infant interaction with a baby sibling: Jealousy or joy? *Journal of Family Psychology, 28*(5), 634–644. https://doi-org.proxy.lib.umich.edu/10.1037/a0037811

Volling, B. L., Yu, T., Gonzalez, R., Tengelitsch, E., & Stevenson, M. M. (2018). Maternal and paternal trajectories of depressive symptoms predict family risk and children's emotional and behavioral problems after the birth of a sibling. *Development and Psychopathology*. https://doi-org.proxy.lib.umich.edu/10.1017/S0954579418000743

Zahn-Waxler, C., Shirtcliff, E. A., & Marceau, K. (2008). Disorders of childhood and adolescence: Gender and psychopathology. *Annual Review of Clinical Psychology, 4*, 275–303. https://doi-org.proxy.lib.umich.edu/10.1146/annurev.clinpsy.3.022806.091358

Zamberletti, J., Cavrini, G., & Tomassini, C. (2018). Grandparents providing childcare in Italy. *European Journal of Ageing, 15*, 265–275. https://doi-org.proxy.lib.umich.edu/10.1007/s10433-018-0479-y

Part III

Father-Child Transaction in Early Development

17 Overview to Part III: Father-Child Transactions in Early Development

Natasha J. Cabrera

The main question linking the chapters in this part is: How do fathers matter to children? This is a bold question that is firmly rooted in theoretical perspectives as well as empirical evidence that fathers are parents and as such are integral part of the family system (Cabrera et al., 2014). The family system is composed of individuals (mothers, fathers, children) as well as subsystems (co-parenting, parenting) that are interdependent and influence each other in particular ways. In these systems, relationships are the mechanisms through which parents and children influence each other in transactional and dynamic interactions (Bronfenbrenner & Morris, 2006). Thus, the parent-child relationship is not driven by the parent or by the child but rather by the reciprocal interaction of both, parents and children. In turn, each individual brings to the relationship a set of predispositions, genetically and environmentally determined. These transactional relationships between individuals in a family system change over time as both parents and children get older, giving us a long-term view of human development.

The father-child relationship is best understood as being nested in a network of other relationships, both proximal and distal that develop in different contexts (Bronfenbrenner & Morris, 2006). Important adult caregivers at home and in child care and school settings, also referred to as microsystems, are the most proximal to the child, especially in the early years, and thus the most consequential for children's development. The interaction of these microsystems, the mesosystem, also impacts children's development in expected ways. As children get older, other relationships beyond the home and the school, such as romantic partners and colleagues, become more proximal and important. All these relationships are also impacted by other macrolevel influences at the broader cultural and social levels. The study of fathers, then, at its core is the study of relationships between children and fathers, between fathers and their partners, and between fathers and other adults.

The research on how fathers matter for children has produced significant empirical evidence that fathers' contributions to children's development are over and above mothers' contributions and that father effects can be both direct as well as indirect and moderated by important contextual variables. The chapters in this part offer excellent summaries of the progress we have made as a field in documenting father effects in important domains of development.

In Chap. 19, Paquette, Gagnon, and Macario de Medeiros review the empirical evidence testing activation relationship theory, including the activation relationship, challenging parenting

N. J. Cabrera (✉)
Department of Human Development and Quantitative Methodology, University of Maryland, College Park, MD, USA
e-mail: ncabrera@umd.edu

H. E. Fitzgerald et al. (eds.), *Handbook of Fathers and Child Development*,
https://doi.org/10.1007/978-3-030-51027-5_17

behaviors, and rough-and-tumble play. Paquette and colleagues also examine the complementarity of attachment relationships (CAR) project to determine the prevalence of the types of activation relationships in father-child and mother-child dyads and verify gender differences in parent-child activation relationship with toddlers.

In Chap. 20, Bergmann and Klein focus on fathers' emotional availability (EA), that is, the overall affective quality of the father-child interaction or the observed global emotional climate of the interaction as well the emotional responsiveness of father and child. They summarize the current state of research on fathers' EA with their children up to pre-K age. They then discuss empirical evidence on the differences between fathers' EA and mothers' EA, the determinants of fathers' EA, the associations between fathers' EA and child development, and ways to improve fathers' EA.

In Chap. 21, Hennigar, Cabrera, and Chen focus on the impact that fathers have on the development of children's social competence, broadly defined as the possession of an array of skills such as self-control and interpersonal communication that help children learn to recognize, form, and sustain positive relationships (Denham, 2006; Ladd, Herald, & Kochel, 2006; La Paro & Pianta, 2000; Raver, 2002). They provide a short review of the ways children's social development has been defined and operationalized in the literature and discuss key theoretical frameworks for understanding social development. They then review the current literature on the association between fathers' parenting and their children's social development from birth through 8 years and conclude with a summary discussing the limitations of this work and offer future directions for research.

In Chap. 22, Vallotton, Foster, Harewood, Cook, and Adekoya examine how play, especially during infancy and early childhood, contributes in important ways to children's development. They present theoretical perspectives on the central role of play in fathering and how mothers and fathers function together within their family systems in ways that are different, alike, and complementary. They then explore the differences and similarities between father-child and mother-child play and the associations between father-child play and young children's developmental outcomes. In Chap. 23, Pancsofar focuses on the theoretical models guiding research on fathers' language input during early childhood and then presents an overview of the empirical evidence that compares mothers' and fathers' language input; shows the contributions of fathers' language input to early language development; and, examines the factors associated with fathers' language input to young children. Pancsofar then highlights emerging scholarship on the role of fathers' linguistic input in the language development of young children with disabilities.

Closely related to how fathers' linguistic input is associated with children's language skills, Duursma, Jialing Ho, Townsend, Grenyer, and Herbert examine the importance of father shared book reading on children's language and literacy development in Chap. 24. They focus particularly on how fathers and children engage in conversations during shared book reading. They review current knowledge about the importance of the home literacy environment and shared book reading on children's language and literacy development and then present evidence that links father engagement in shared book reading to children's language and literacy skills. They conclude by presenting preliminary data showing the diversity and responsiveness in with which fathers in two-parent families and their 3-year-olds talk about the story and respond to each other during a book reading interaction.

In Chap. 25, Meuwissen focuses on how fathers matter for the development of their children's executive function (EF), a set of higher-level thinking skills that enable children to control their behavior and emotions and direct them toward long-term goals. To this end, she reviews theoretical frameworks that link parenting generally and, fathers specifically, to child EF development. She also presents empirical evidence for links between mother and father parenting and EF, highlighting these processes for families facing risks and challenges.

References

Bronfenbrenner, U., & Morris, P. A. (2006). The bioecological model of human development. In P. Mussen (Ed.), *Handbook of child psychology*. Hoboken, NJ: Wiley.

Cabrera, N., Fitzgerald, H. E., Bradley, R. H., & Roggman, L. (2014). The ecology of father-child relationships: An expanded model. *Journal of Family Theory and Review, 6*, 336–354.

Denham, S. A. (2006) Social-Emotional Competence as Support for School Readiness: What Is It and How Do We Assess It?, Early Education and Development, 17:1, 57-89, DOI: 10.1207/s15566935eed1701_4

Ladd, G., Herald, S. L., & Kochel, K. P. (2006). School readiness: Are there social prerequisites? Early education and development, 17(1), 115–150. https://doi.org/10.1207/s15566935eed1701_6

La Paro, K. M., & Pianta, R. C. (2000). Predicting Children's Competence in the Early School Years: A Meta-Analytic *Review. Review of Educational Research, 70*(4), 443–484. https://doi.org/10.3102/00346543070004443

Raver, C. C. (2002). Emotions Matter: Making the Case for the Role of Young Children's Emotional Development for Early School Readiness. *Social Policy Report, 16*, 1–20. https://doi.org/10.1002/j.2379-3988.2002.tb00041.x

18 Father-Child Attachment Relationships

Geoffrey L. Brown and Hasan Alp Aytuglu

Attachment theory has long been the predominant framework for conceptualizing parent-child relationships in infancy and early childhood. Beginning with John Bowlby's classic work (Bowlby, 1969), attachment theory has articulated the fundamental nature and purpose of the parent-child relationship for the infant's survival, security, and subsequent socio-emotional growth. A voluminous body of conceptual and empirical research has been devoted to elucidating the nature and origins of individual differences in mother-child attachment relationships and the consequences of these individual differences for development throughout the lifespan (Thompson, 2000).

Despite its undeniable impact on our understanding of relationships between parents and young children, both attachment theory and empirical research arising from an attachment theoretical perspective have generally underrepresented fathers. As a result, the extent to which fathers serve as attachment figures for their children, as well as the consequences of these attachments for children, is relatively unknown. Although father-child attachment relationships remain vastly overlooked relative to mothers, an emerging body of research has begun to document the developmental sequelae of father-child attachment relationships. In the following sections, we (1) summarize relevant historical context for the study of father-child attachment relationships, (2) document patterns of attachment in father-child dyads, (3) review empirical support for the correlates of father-child attachment security in early childhood, (4) review empirical support for the developmental consequences of father-child attachment security in early childhood, and (5) turn to a discussion of current and future directions in research on father-child attachment relationships.

G. L. Brown (✉) · H. A. Aytuglu
Department of Human Development and Family Science, University of Georgia, Athens, GA, USA
e-mail: glbrown@uga.edu

Historical Context on Father-Child Attachment Relationships

In Bowlby's classic attachment volumes, he articulates the developmental course of early attachment relationships from an ethological perspective (Bowlby, 1969/1982). Briefly, infants are predisposed to engage in attachment behaviors, including proximity seeking, preferential desire for contact with the caregiver, and use of the caregiver as a "secure base" from which to explore the environment. These affiliative behaviors are thought to be particularly important during times of threat or distress, when the infant's "attachment system" is acti-

H. E. Fitzgerald et al. (eds.), *Handbook of Fathers and Child Development*,
https://doi.org/10.1007/978-3-030-51027-5_18

vated. In this way, attachment relationships serve an evolutionary purpose for very young children of many species by protecting young children and maximizing their likelihood of survival.

The pioneering work by Mary Ainsworth in both Uganda and the United States helped to further refine the conceptualization and measurement of attachment relationships in infancy (e.g., Ainsworth, 1967), including the development of the Strange Situation Procedure (SSP; Ainsworth, Blehar, Waters, & Wall, 1978) as a method for assessing infant-parent attachment security. Infants and young children develop a sense of felt security in the attachment relationship when they use their caregiver as a safe haven to explore their environments and regulate emotions during times of distress. In the context of the SSP, for example, securely attached infants are often distressed by the departure of a caregiver but greet the caregiver warmly at the time of reunion and settle quickly after gaining proximity and/or contact. As such, attachment security represents the infant's trust and confidence in the caregiver to meet his or her needs. In contrast, children who are insecurely attached fail to use the caregiver to regulate emotions. In the SSP, this occurs via several different insecure patterns, which are most clearly evident immediately following reunions: avoidance of the caregiver (insecure-avoidance), a mixture of proximity-seeking and ambivalent or angry behavior toward the caregiver (insecure-resistance), or failure to mount a coherent strategy toward the caregiver's return (disorganization).

Broadly speaking, attachment relationships are hypothesized to form through early patterns of interaction between the caregiver and child (Ainsworth, Bell, & Stayton, 1974). When a caregiver is sensitive and responsive to the needs of the infant (e.g., responding promptly to cries), then the infant comes to see the parent as a trustworthy source of support and direct attachment behaviors toward them. This theoretical proposition is supported by numerous empirical studies documenting associations between early parental sensitivity and infant-parent attachment security (e.g., De Wolff & van Ijzendoorn, 1997). In turn, secure attachment relationships in infancy are posited to shape individual and interpersonal functioning throughout childhood and beyond (Sroufe, 2000). Theoretical writings on attachment hypothesize that early attachment relationships serve as an "internal working model" (IWM) that is carried forward into other important relationships and social interactions (e.g., Bretherton & Munholland, 2008), such that infants who are securely attached to caregivers in infancy should form a secure representation of attachment relationships that leads to more adaptive social-emotional functioning across the life course than those with insecure early relationships. This proposition is supported by meta-analytic evidence that attachment security predicts socio-emotional development in many domains (Groh, Fearon, van IJzendoorn, Bakermans-Kranenburg, & Roisman, 2017).

Early work in developmental science focused almost entirely on the contributions of mother-child relationships, and parenting research today has continued to study mothers far more than fathers (e.g., Cabrera, Volling, & Barr, 2018). Consistent with this approach, Bowlby's early writings emphasized the concept of monotropy – the notion that infants attach to a single, primary caregiver who is responsible for meeting the child's needs in early infancy. Given that this role has been traditionally reserved for mothers in human and non-human species, relatively little of his early work discussed fathers explicitly. However, Bowlby did suggest a hierarchy of attachment figures in children's lives (with the primary caregiver at the top) and argued that children were at least capable of forming attachments to non-maternal figures who provide regular care. When Bowlby's attachment volume was reedited in 1982, he not only maintained that mothers were necessarily the child's first attachment relationship but also acknowledged that *slightly later* in infancy fathers serve as important attachment figures. This claim was supported by early attachment research revealing that many infants are likely to be distressed upon separation from either parent (Field et al., 1984; Kotelchuck,

1976) and that they direct attachment-related behaviors toward both mothers and fathers upon reunion (Lamb, 1976a, 1976b, 1977a, 1977b).

Thus, theorizing on the father-child attachment relationship suggests that most children whose fathers are involved in their lives should form attachment relationships to them during infancy. Understanding how and when these attachment relationships emerge and the extent to which father-child attachment security vs. insecurity might be lawfully related to children's outcomes can shed necessary light on the contributions of early father-child relationship quality for developmental consequences in early childhood and beyond.

To better elucidate father-child attachment relationships necessitates bringing to bear a family systems theoretical perspective on the study of these relationships (Cowan, 1997; Cowan & Cowan, 2019). A family systems perspective on father-child attachment requires considering the extent to which characteristics at all levels of the family system (e.g., couple relationship quality, triadic family processes, child temperament) might affect the father-child attachment relationship. Moreover, a family system lens argues for examining unique contributions of father-child attachment security to child outcomes over and above mothers' contributions. Finally, research on father-child attachment relationships should examine the ways in which father-child and mother-child attachment security interact to affect child outcomes, including compensatory (e.g., father-child attachment security may protect against deleterious consequences of an insecure mother-child relationship) and accumulative (e.g., secure attachments to both parents may be more adaptive than a secure attachment to only one) models (e.g., Dagan & Sagi-Schwartz, 2018). Although father-child attachment research remains limited relative to studies including mothers, empirical evidence addressing each of these issues has begun to emerge over the last several decades. This evidence is reviewed in the sections that follow.

Patterns of Father-Child Attachment

Father-child attachment relationships – like mother-child relationships – can theoretically emerge at any point in the life course or shift as a function of changes in caregiving or other environmental experiences throughout childhood (e.g., Palm, 2014). Nonetheless, the vast majority of research on attachment to mother or father has focused on the relationship between parents and their infants or young children. The literature reviewed in this chapter largely reflects this research focus (consistent with Bowlby's claims) on early childhood as a sensitive period for the development of father-child attachments.

Though results vary substantially based on variations in measurement and sample characteristics, distributions of attachment classifications in the SSP using both four-category (secure, insecure-avoidant, insecure-resistant, and disorganized) and secure vs. insecure distinctions are roughly similar for mother-child and father-child dyads in most studies (Ahnert, Pinquart, & Lamb, 2006). Although infants seem to form secure attachment relationships to fathers with roughly the same frequency that they do for mothers, it could be (as Bowlby hypothesized) that infants still prefer mothers over fathers as attachment figures. However, data bolstering the proposal of a possible attachment hierarchy among multiple attachment relationships is very much mixed. Some early studies in the field of father-child attachment showed clear preferences for children to display attachment behaviors toward mothers over fathers in dyadic interaction (Cohen & Campos, 1974; Lamb, Frodi, Hwang, & Frodi, 1983) and to turn to mothers preferentially when distressed during triadic interaction (Lamb, 1977a, 1977b). However, other early findings failed to find this attachment preference and argued that it may only occur during a specific developmental period (12–18 months) (Lamb, 1976a, 1976b; Sagi et al., 1985). The lack of clarity with respect to infants' strong preferential treatment of mothers over fathers reinforces the idea that fathers could be prominent attachment figures for young children. Thus, since this early work on attachment preferences, there has been a shift in the field away from studies attempting to identify the most prominent or important attachment figure and toward understanding the determinants and consequences of children's attachments to multiple caregivers (e.g., Dagan & Sagi-Schwartz, 2018).

Conceptually, attachments to multiple caregivers are thought to develop largely independent of one another, so that some children could develop a secure relationship with one parent and an insecure relationship with the other (e.g., Sroufe, 1985). However, there does appear to be significant, albeit modest, concordance between mother-child and father-child attachment (Fox, Kimmerly, & Schafer, 1991), such that children who are securely attached to their mothers are somewhat more likely to also be securely attached to their fathers. Meta-analytic evidence has found an overall correlation of .17 between infant attachment to mother and father (van Ijzendoorn & de Wolff, 1997). Numerous explanations may account for the similarity in infants' attachments to their mother and father. This includes mate selection tendencies, or the tendency of parents to select mates with personalities and parenting beliefs and behaviors that are similar to their own. Concordance between children's attachment security with mother and father may then get higher beyond infancy, given that parents who stay in a committed relationship may show increasingly convergent parenting attitudes and parenting styles.

Predictors of Father-Child Attachment Security

Consistent with the tenets of attachment theory and empirical research with mothers, the most commonly examined correlate of father-child attachment security is paternal sensitivity. Sensitivity refers to the extent to which caregiving is prompt and responsive to the child's cues, affectively warm, and provides appropriate levels of stimulation (Ainsworth et al., 1974). Despite its prominence in attachment theory and research with mothers, the evidence linking sensitivity to father-child attachment security is decidedly mixed, with numerous studies finding small and nonsignificant associations (Hazen, McFarland, Jacobvitz, & Boyd-Soisson, 2010; Volling, McElwain, Notaro, & Herrera, 2002). Overall, meta-analyses indicate that paternal sensitivity is significantly related to attachment security (van Ijzendoorn & de Wolff, 1997). However, this effect size of .12 is approximately half the size of the meta-analytic association between maternal sensitivity and mother-child attachment security (Lucassen et al., 2011). Notably, the association between sensitivity and father-child attachment is larger as children age into preschool and middle childhood periods, suggesting that this effect may only be smaller in infancy when the infant-father attachment bond is still developing. The discrepancy between mothers' vs. fathers' effect sizes may also in part emerge because of fathers' unique interactional styles with young children, which may not be captured by conceptualizations and measurements of parental sensitivity that are commonly used in research with mothers (e.g., Grossmann et al., 2002). Moreover, the extant literature has looked at correlates beyond sensitive parenting by considering a number of parenting, personal and psychological, sociocultural, and child characteristics that may account for variation in the quality of father-child attachment relationships.

Characteristics of Fathers' Parenting

Several studies have examined other elements of fathers' parenting (beyond sensitivity) as potential correlates of father-child attachment. Perhaps, the most widely studied of these has been the construct of father involvement, most often conceptualized as the quantity or frequency of time spent with children (Schoppe-Sullivan & Fagan, 2020). Although father involvement is a critical construct in the literature on fatherhood and appears to have significant benefits for children (see Sarkadi, Kristiansson, Oberklaid, & Bremberg, 2008; Cabrera et al., 2018; Schoppe-

Sullivan & Fagan, 2020 for reviews), it has historically not been considered as a determinant of attachment security. Nonetheless, it seems likely that fathers must spend a threshold of time with children to serve as attachment figures (Lamb, 2012), and several investigations find associations between the quantity of fathers' involvement and attachment security. For instance, higher levels of self-reported father involvement at 3 months have been linked to a greater likelihood of secure infant-father attachment classification in the Strange Situation Procedure at 12 months (Cox, Owen, Henderson, & Margand, 1992). Moreover, self-reported involvement was concurrently related to higher Attachment Q-Sort (AQS; Waters & Deane, 1985) scores among father-child dyads with 14-month-old children (Caldera, 2004) and more secure representations of father-child attachment relationships among school-aged children (Coyl-Shepherd & Newland, 2013).

Two recent studies have shown that the magnitude of association between involvement and attachment may depend on the specific types of activities in which fathers engage with their children. Fuertes, Faria, Beeghly, and Lopes-dos-Santos (2016) demonstrated that fathers' self-reported quantity of involvement in play activities (but not caregiving activities such as bathing or feeding) predicted attachment quality at 12 months, although involvement in both play and caregiving predicted attachment quality at 18 months. Brown, Mangelsdorf, Shigeto, and Wong (2018) found that associations between father involvement as reported on a retrospective time-diary interview and father-child attachment differed as a function of the type of activity and when those activities occurred. Specifically, fathers' greater involvement in play activities on non-workdays and caregiving on workdays were related to attachment security as rated on the AQS with 3-year-old children, over and above the contribution of observed paternal sensitivity.

Other investigations have found that the interaction between quality (i.e., observational assessments of fathers' parenting) and quantity (i.e., self-reports of fathering) is a better predictor of father-child attachment quality than either variable alone (Brown, Mangelsdorf, & Neff, 2012; Brown, McBride, Shin, & Bost, 2007). In both cases, when the quality of parenting was high, then there was no significant association between involvement and attachment security, such that most sensitive fathers developed secure relationships with their children regardless of the quantity of time they spent together. In contrast, greater involvement has been linked to lower levels of attachment security when fathers engaged in negative or intrusive parenting behavior (Brown et al., 2007).

Among other studies that examine fathers' parenting behavior as a correlate of attachment security, some attention has been devoted to fathering that is characterized by the quality of physically stimulating play. In the groundbreaking work by Grossmann et al. (2002), fathers' sensitivity in challenging play contexts was related to a greater likelihood of attachment security. More recently, Bureau et al. (2017) also found that fathers' observed play sensitivity was related to attachment security in preschoolers even after accounting for numerous contextual variables such as parenting stress and child gender. Another recent investigation found that fathers' stimulation (i.e., physical and/or object stimulation) at 9 months was subsequently associated with greater odds of a secure father-infant attachment classification in the Strange Situation (Olsavsky, Berrigan, Schoppe-Sullivan, Brown, & Kamp Dush, 2019). Despite considerable theorizing on the prominence of physically stimulating play for father-child relationships (Paquette, 2004), however, studies linking these fathering behaviors to attachment quality remain scarce, with others failing to find an association between rough-and-tumble play and attachment (Paquette & Dumont, 2013).

Parental Characteristics and Psychological Resources

Consistent with recent conceptual models of the determinants of fathering (e.g., Cabrera, Fitzgerald, Bradley, & Roggman, 2014), several studies have examined the extent to which fathers' personal characteristics and developmental histories affect father-child attachment security. For instance, the personality characteristics of extroversion and agreeableness measured when children were 10 months old were related to a greater likelihood of secure father-child attachment 3 months later, presumably because these characteristics foster more positive, proximal interactions between fathers and infants (Belsky, 1996). Although parental beliefs have rarely been considered as correlates of attachment, beliefs and attitudes toward the parental role may interact with other factors to concurrently predict father-child attachment security. In one study, fathers who viewed the paternal caregiving role as important were more likely to develop secure relationships when infant fussiness or marital quality was high (Wong, Mangelsdorf, Brown, Neff, & Schoppe-Sullivan, 2009). Another recent study found that fathers' pleasure in parenting, as coded from fathers' interviews about their parenting experiences, moderated the association between sensitivity and attachment and that the degree of congruence between reported parenting pleasure and observed sensitivity was significantly related to infant-father attachment classifications (Brown & Cox, 2019).

One intrapersonal antecedent of father-child attachment considered in prior research is fathers' recollections of their early caregiving histories in the family of origin. Volling and Belsky (1992) found that men's more positively recollected child-rearing histories were related to a greater likelihood of secure attachment with their children. Furthermore, fathers' own attachment styles on the Adult Attachment Interview (Main & Goldwyn, 1995) also appear to be a robust predictor of father-child attachment security in the next generation. Specifically, men with secure-autonomous states of mind with respect to their early caregiving experiences are more likely to develop secure attachment relationships with their own children in two-parent families (McFarland-Piazza, Hazen, Jacobvitz, & Boyd-Soisson, 2012; Psouni, 2019; Steele, Steele, & Fonagy, 1996). Although little is known about the mechanisms that may mediate or moderate these associations, the extant literature supports the notion that fathers who can discuss their past experiences in coherent, balanced, and flexible ways are likely to foster a sense of felt security in their own children.

Socio-Contextual Characteristics

Consistent with the proposition that fathering and father-child relationships are likely to be affected by family and contextual factors (Doherty, Kouneski, & Erickson, 1998), past studies have documented associations between the quality of the father-child attachment relationship and contextual variables both within and outside the family system. The most attention has been devoted to associations between the quality of the marital or interparental relationship and father-child attachment. Numerous studies indicate that fathers in marital relationships characterized by higher levels of reported satisfaction, more positive interactions, and less conflict in infancy are more likely to form secure attachment relationships with their children later in infancy and early childhood (Cox et al., 1992; Frosch, Mangelsdorf, & McHale, 2000; Owen & Cox, 1997). Further, more recent evidence suggests that the quality of the co-parenting partnership may also be a unique predictor of father-child attachment. In particular, several studies have found that both parental reports and observations of more supportive and less competitive co-parenting behavior were related to a greater likelihood of concurrent security in the father-child relationship in infancy (Brown, Schoppe-Sullivan, Mangelsdorf, & Neff, 2010; Caldera & Lindsey, 2006) and elementary school (Coyl-Shepherd & Newland, 2013).

In considering contextual factors beyond the family system, characteristics of the work-family interface have been implicated in the developing father-child attachment relationship. Belsky (1996), for example, documented that more positive emotional spillover between work and family was related to a greater likelihood of father-child attachment security, perhaps because men with satisfying work lives are also more inclined to be positively engaged with their children. Other investigations have posited that different processes may be responsible for the development of father-child attachment in single-earner (i.e., families in which only one parent is employed outside the home) vs. dual-earner families (i.e., families in which both parents are employed outside the home) (e.g., Volling & Belsky, 1992). Lickenbrock and Braungart-Rieker (2015) found that the frequency of self-reported father involvement measured at 3–7 months child age was related to attachment security at 14 months only when family resources (e.g., parental education, family income) were high and that this was especially likely among dual-earner but not single-earner households. Interestingly, several studies found that boys from dual-earner families were more likely to develop insecure relationships in the SSP at 13 months with their fathers but not with their mothers (Belsky & Rovine, 1988; Braungart-Rieker, Courtney, & Garwood, 1999). Despite the consistency of these findings, however, there is little evidence over the last 20 years to indicate that maternal employment status or the quantity of non-maternal care that children are exposed to affect the quality of father-child attachment.

Child Characteristics

The primary focus of research linking child characteristics to father-child attachment has been on individual differences in emotionality. Given that Strange Situation classifications are in part characterized by clear variation in infant's emotional reactivity (i.e., little crying or distress in insecure-avoidant dyads, intense crying and distress in insecure-resistant dyads), attachment theory and research has long been concerned with the connection between individual differences in temperament and attachment. In general, reviews of this literature have determined that temperamental characteristics may play a role in attachment subclassifications, but are unlikely to affect security vs. insecurity of attachment to either parent (Mangelsdorf & Frosch, 1999; Vaughn & Bost, 2008). Father-child attachment research specifically has also found few associations between temperament and attachment. Braungart-Rieker, Garwood, Powers, and Wang (2001) found that infant affect predicted attachment classifications for mother-child but not father-child dyads. Volling and Belsky (1992) found that maternal reports of infant difficulty at 3 months were related to infant-father attachment security, but this association was nonsignificant when measuring infant difficulty at 9 months. One exception comes from work by Planalp and Braungart-Rieker (2013) who found that infants classified as ambivalent with fathers were rated by mothers as higher in perceptual sensitivity and cuddliness than other infants. Wong et al. (2009) also found that the relation between attitudes toward the paternal role and father-child attachment security was only significant when infant fussiness was high. Collectively, these findings suggest that father-child attachment quality is at best modestly related to infants' innate temperamental tendencies.

Similarly, despite qualitative differences between father-son and father-daughter interactions, there is little indication of gender differences in rates of security for boys vs. girls. Nonetheless, child gender may interact with other parenting or socio-contextual variables, as exemplified by aforementioned evidence documenting that dual-earner family status was a risk factor for father-child insecurity for boys but not girls (Belsky & Rovine, 1988; Braungart-Rieker et al., 1999). Schoppe-Sullivan, Mangelsdorf, Brown, and Sokolowski (2007) found that although mothers and fathers in two-parent families were similarly sensitive to daughters and sons, daughters' attachment security with fathers and mothers was similar, whereas sons' was not, suggesting the utility of future research examining unique patterns of attachment as a function of both parent and child gender. Recent models of fatherhood emphasize the need to blend research on individual characteristics (of both fathers and children) with ecological contexts (Cabrera et al.,

2014). Future directions may include the examination of other child characteristics, including child health status and developmental delays, that may expand the realm of father-child attachment research to children with special needs and those in hospitalized settings. Such an approach may continue to shed light on the complex interplay between early child development, social context, and father-child relationships.

Developmental Consequences of Father-Child Attachment

Given that many children use fathers as attachment figures, it is critically imporant to understand the contributions of father-child attachment to children's developmental outcomes. Research in this domain faces a number of methodological challenges, and many studies linking father-child attachment to child outcomes fail to examine the independent effects of mother-child and father-child attachment. Family systems approaches to attachment, however, have begun to elucidate both the independent and interactive contributions of father-child attachment relationships to multiple domains of development. These empirical studies are reviewed in the sections that follow.

Socio-Emotional Functioning

Consistent with attachment's theoretical underpinnings, a limited body of evidence suggests that father-child attachment plays a role in children's early social relationships. For example, in a sample of 267 Canadian high school students, father-child attachment security (as well as mother-child attachment) was related concurrently to children's reports of positive friendship qualities and the lack of conflict with best friends (Lieberman, Doyle, & Markiewicz, 1999). Similarly, in a prospective longitudinal study of over 200 families, mother-child and father-child attachment assessed at ages 2–4 were both significant, independent predictors of social competence at age 5 (Neppl, Wedmore, Senia, Jeon, & Diggs, 2019). These studies report very similar effect sizes for mother-child and father-child attachment, suggesting that the relative predictive power of attachment for social outcomes may be similar across parent gender. These results dovetail with claims in the broader fatherhood literature that fathers play a particularly critical role – one that may be on par with mothers – in preparing children for social relationships in the outside world beyond the microsystem of the immediate family (Parke, 1996).

Other studies report links between father-child attachment and aspects of early-emerging emotion and self-concept development. Diener, Mangelsdorf, McHale, and Frosch (2002), for instance, found that infant-father attachment (but not infant-mother attachment) was related to patterns of child emotion regulation, such that infants in insecure-avoidant relationships were more likely to distract themselves and children in insecure-resistant relationships were more likely to engage in self-soothing during a stressful laboratory task. Children's representations of the security of both the mother-child and father-child attachment relationships were also associated with lower emotional understanding concurrently at age 5 (Psychogiou et al., 2018). These findings suggest a potential role of father-child attachment in the emotional underpinnings of personality and self-development. Moreover, father-child attachment security at 2 years has been found to be a unique predictor (over and above mother-child attachment security) of children's self-esteem at age 5 (Pinto, Veríssimo, Gatinho, Santos, & Vaughn, 2015). In sum, this body of research suggests that the quality of the early father-child attachment relationship may have a small to modest impact on multiple domains of normative socio-emotional development. But results overall paint a mixed picture regarding the relative strength of mother-child and father-child attachment and the independent effects of each on socio-emotional outcomes. Further, the extent to which attachments to fathers in infancy and early childhood continue to influence social and emotional well-being into the school years is not yet well known.

Psychopathology and Behavior Problems

Research has identified early father-child attachment quality as an antecedent of some forms of psychopathology. In general, these findings suggest that attachment quality is particularly likely to have an effect on dysregulated and problematic child behavior in early and middle childhood. Bureau, Deneault, and Yurkowski (2019), for example, found that father-child attachment security in preschoolers predicted greater self-esteem in middle-childhood, even after controlling for the quality of the mother-child attachment relationship, and lower levels of nonclinical externalizing behavior problems when children were also securely attached to mothers. Similarly, Kochanska and Kim (2013) reported that infants insecurely attached to both parents in infancy exhibited more internalizing and externalizing behavior problems in elementary school. Moreover, attachment insecurity in toddlerhood among father-child dyads has been linked to elevated levels of parent-reported antisocial behavior at age 12 (Goffin, Boldt, & Kochanska, 2018) and in one study was a better concurrent predictor of child conduct problems among preschoolers than mother-child attachment (Bureau et al., 2017).

In addition to affecting child outcomes directly, father-child relationship quality and child characteristics may also interact to explain variance in child behavior. One example of such an interaction comes from Brock and Kochanska (2018) who found that elevated levels of infant anger predicted both father- and teacher-reported oppositional behavior in the early school years in insecure (but not secure) father-child dyads. These findings suggest that father-child attachment may not necessarily predict child behavior problems directly, but instead that the association could be moderated by child characteristics or perhaps other aspects of family systems. Moving away from exclusively main effects models to consider these moderating effects in future research could help to elucidate the cumulative impact of father-child attachment security and other family system characteristics on both normative and atypical development of young children.

Cognitive and Language Development

Consistent with the theoretical propositions of attachment and meta-analytic empirical data from mother-child dyads (Groh et al., 2017), the preponderance of studies examining the consequences of father-child attachment have focused on social and emotional domains. It stands to reason that early relationships with both fathers and mothers would affect emotional and personality development, functioning in close relationships, and dysregulated patterns of child behavior. Though it is not addressed explicitly in attachment theory, early attachment relationships may provide a context for cognitive and linguistic growth as well. In the context of loving and secure early relationships, both parents and children may be more comfortable engaging in verbal communication with one another. Further, parents of securely attached children may be likely to support children's exploration of their environments and the cognitive growth that accompanies this exploration. Finally, the back-and-forth turn-taking interactions that often characterize parental sensitivity may play a role in promoting linguistic competence.

Nonetheless, the extent to which father-child attachment affects cognitive and language development has rarely been examined empirically. Belsky, Garduque, and Hrncir (1984) documented associations between attachments to both parents and children's executive capacity in play. One recent study also found that father-child attachment predicted receptive language skills in early childhood, even controlling for mother-child attachment and parental education (Teufl, Deichmann, Supper, & Ahnert, 2019). These two areas seem particularly ripe for further explanation, given evidence that father-child interaction quality makes unique contributions to the prediction of children's executive functioning (Hertz, Bernier, Cimon-Paquet, & Regueiro, 2019) and language development (Lankinen, Lähteenmäki, Kaljonen, & Korpilahti, 2019). Given the seemingly important role of fathers in facilitating language development, future investigations should consider whether the reach of father-child attachment may extend to impact cognitive and language domains and examine the mechanisms by which attachment quality affects these domains.

Future Directions

The state of research and theory building on the father-child attachment relationship is perhaps best captured by recognizing two historical trends in this domain. The first is the clear increase in attachment research (and family research in general) that has included fathers in recent decades, which represents an undeniably important form of progress. The second is the lingering paucity of studies that include fathers relative to those that assess attachment relationships in mother-child dyads (Cabrera et al., 2018). Overall, the studies discussed in this chapter rely on homogenous and relatively small sample sizes ranging from less than 50 to no more than 125. Clearly, the field would benefit from larger samples with increased power to detect significant findings. Similarly, effect sizes (even when significant) are in the low to modest range (approximately .1 to .3) in all cases, suggesting that more comprehensive models of the determinants and consequences of father-child attachment should be pursued. Much important work has been done, but much remains to elucidate the correlates, consequences, and societal implications of father-child attachment. In the sections that follow, we outline some suggestions and promising new directions for conceptual and empirical work on early father-child attachment relationships.

Expanding Determinants of Father-Child Attachment

Particularly given the lack of studies consistently linking sensitivity to attachment to fathers, the field would benefit from examining a more diverse range of predictors to better explain variance in father-child attachment security. To some extent, this approach could capitalize on already existing advances being made in our understanding of fathering from other perspectives. Despite both distant (Cowan, 1997) and recent (Fagan, 2019) calls for father-child attachment to more fully integrate family context (e.g., co-parenting, maternal gatekeeping), still relatively few investigations apply a family systems approach to the study of attachment (Cowan & Cowan, 2019). Developmental science as a whole has made great strides in characterizing the complexity of family life, family relationships, and interactions within the family over the last several generations. The father-child relationship is inevitably embedded within these complexities, and research examining the development of this relationship should continue to incorporate comprehensive assessments of family functioning and important ecological contexts that reside outside the family (Cabrera et al., 2014; Palkovitz & Hull, 2018).

Moreover, although an extensive body of literature has been devoted to explicating the construct of father involvement (e.g., quantity or frequency of parenting behaviors), few studies have integrated assessments of both father involvement and father-child attachment simultaneously. The development of parallel literatures in these domains is in part a result of distinct methodological traditions. Namely, father involvement is typically assessed using survey or time-diary measures assessing the quantity or frequency of fathers' engagement in various parenting activities. In contrast, attachment research is largely grounded in a tradition based on observational assessments of parent-child interactions and relationship quality. Nonetheless, bridging the gap between these research traditions can yield promising results (Brown et al., 2007; Brown et al., 2012) that have much to tell us about the mechanisms underlying father-child attachment formation. As such, future work that incorporates father involvement and father-child attachment quality can help to push forward our understanding of the multifaceted dynamics of father-child relationships.

Father-Specific Conceptualizations of Parenting

The evidence reviewed in this chapter supports the continued study of fathers from an attachment theoretical perspective. Nonetheless, father-child attachment research has by and large relied on methodological tools and theoretical concepts that were originally designed for use with mothers exclusively. The application of these methods and concepts to the study of fathers has proven fruitful but may fail to capture exhaustively the characteristics of father-child interactions and relationship quality. The utility of attachment theory as a paradigm for conceptualizing fathering may depend on the field's ability to successfully integrate the fundamental tenets of attachment with new methodological tools, coding systems, and conceptualizations designed to capture aspects of early parent-child relationships that are unique to fathers.

One prime example of a generative, father-centric conceptualization is the development of "activation theory," as outlined by Daniel Paquette (Paquette, 2004). The recognition that father-child relationships may be organized around the central purpose of activating children both physically and emotionally is an important observation that has in part contributed to advances in experimental paradigms (i.e., "the risky situation") (Paquette & Bigras, 2010) and observational coding systems of father-child interactions (i.e., rough and tumble play quality) (Fletcher, StGeorge, & Freeman, 2013). These measures have, in general, focused solely on fathers' activating and stimulating behaviors and have not yet been applied in varying cultural contexts. Nonetheless, these advances have allowed the field to better – or at least more fully – characterize some of the qualitative differences between father-child and mother-child relationships in early childhood and the potential consequences of father-centric parenting practices for children.

It seems clear that fathers often engage with children in stimulating and activating ways and that those interactions are a common and likely important context for the developing father-child relationship. But how (or whether) these parenting behaviors contribute to attachment quality specifically remains to be seen. Although preliminary data linking patterns of activation and attachment are rather mixed (e.g., Gaumon, Paquette, Cyr, Émond-Nakamura, & St-André, 2016; Paquette & Dumont, 2013), this area of inquiry serves as a promising exemplar of ways in which attachment research can be broadened to more fully encapsulate fathers' contributions. Some progress is apparent in calls for new attachment measures to be validated with both fathers and mothers (Solomon & George, 2016), a practice that is increasingly common (e.g., Boldt, Kochanska, Grekin, & Brock, 2016; Deneault, Bureau, Yurkowski, & Moss, 2019). However, the next generation of father-child attachment research would benefit from further attempts to develop novel, father-centric conceptualizations of early parent-child interactions and relationships.

Expanding Outcomes of Father-Child Attachment

Future efforts to document the unique effects of father-child attachment for children's development would also benefit from a broadened scope of developmental outcomes. One primary challenge is disentangling the independent contributions of the father-child attachment relationship to child well-being from mother-child relationship quality and other family system characteristics. More investigations assessing mother-child and father-child relationships within the same family, as well as broader aspects of family functioning (e.g., interparental relationship quality, co-parenting), would help to establish the contributions of the father-child relationship above and beyond other important family systems elements.

Another fruitful approach may be to more systematically consider constellations of mother-child and father-child attachment quality as determinants of development. Despite the undeniable importance of the IWM as a conceptual mechanism for transmitting the effects of early life experiences, the ways in which the IWM operates in the context of multiple attachment figures are not yet well known. Does the IWM emerge in response to experiences with a single, primary caregiver? Are multiple attachment relationships integrated into a single IWM representation? Is a secure relationship with a father enough to compensate for insecurity in the mother-child relationship or vice versa? Do children form multiple IWMs that may serve different purposes in different contexts? These and other questions are ripe for exploration as research continues to adopt a family systems approach to the study of attachment.

Dagan and Sagi-Schwartz (2018) discuss this issue at length and note the critical importance of examining integrative effects of attachment to mother and father on children's outcomes while acknowledging that studies accomplishing this goal are few, based on small samples, and not well-designed longitudinally. One notable exception comes from Kochanska and Kim (2013), who found that those children with insecure relationships with both parents (i.e., "double-insecurity") had more externalizing problems than those who were securely attached to at least one parent. Security with one parent provided protective effects, and security with both provided no additional benefits. This approach of considering the combined effects of attachments to mother, father, and potentially other attachment figures could further elucidate the ways in which multiple attachments conspire to impact a range of child outcomes.

Another promising direction for father-child attachment research includes an increased emphasis on biological and health outcomes for children (and perhaps fathers). Numerous recent calls in the scientific literature have advocated for a greater understanding of the neurobiology of fathering (Abraham & Feldman, 2018) as well as the relations between attachment and physical health (Ehrlich & Cassidy, 2019). Although this body of literature lags behind parenting research with mothers, recent studies have increasingly examined the biological underpinnings of fatherhood, including the neural basis of fathers' parenting (Rilling & Mascaro, 2017), neuroendocrine functioning among fathers (Gordon, Zagoory-Sharon, Leckman, & Feldman, 2010), and epigenetic processes that may underlie the intergenerational transmission of fathers' parenting (Soubry, 2018). This line of work demonstrates that early fathering is in some ways biologically embedded, but studies documenting the unique biological effects of father-child attachment for fathers and/or children are still quite rare. One excellent model of such work, however, comes from Kuo, Saini, Tengelitsch, and Volling (2019), who found that infants who were securely attached to only fathers (but not mothers) had higher cortisol levels and a blunted cortisol response relative to infants that were securely attached to their mother. That this study failed to find a protective effect of father-child attachment security is in and of itself intriguing. Future investigations that integrate measures of attachment with physiological, neurological, and biological assessments will continue to shed much-needed light on the ways in which early father-child attachment relationships may get under the skin to affect both psychosocial and physical well-being in father-child dyads.

Social Policy and Father-Child Attachment Research

A final, overarching goal for father-child attachment research is to broaden the social policy impact of this work by addressing issues that are relevant for policies and practice serving fathers and young children. A logical starting point could consist of expanding the scope of the populations included in this body of literature (Volling, 2019) to include greater representation of low SES, ethnic minority, and nonresident fathers in research on attachment. Indeed, research on father-child attachment suffers from a striking lack of diversity. Notably, the entirety of the dozens of empirical studies on father-child attachment reviewed in this chapter focused on (a) populations from the United States, Canada, or Western Europe, (b) samples that were predominantly Caucasian or European American, (c) families in which two married, biological parents resided with the child, and (d) households that were middle to high in socioeconomic status. As such, one must take great caution in generalizing conclusions from these findings to other populations. The case of ethnic minority families in the United States provides one useful test case. There is no theoretical reason, for example, to predict that the correlates of attachment security differ among African American vs. European American father-child dyads. However, African American fathers are (a) less likely to reside in the same home as their child relative to European American fathers and (b) more involved in children's lives than European American fathers when they are nonresidential (Jones & Mosher, 2013). As such, nonresidential African American fathers may well serve as attachment figures for their young children, but the determinants and consequences of father-child attachment security for African American and/or nonresidential fathers are not yet known.

One particularly promising avenue for expanding diversity in this area of research is the study of father-child attachment among gay father families. Establishing the processes that underlie attachment in same-sex families – and the consequences of these attachment relationships for children – is both a pressing scientific question and one with implications for changing social stigmas and perhaps legal rights for same-sex and adoptive parents. An initial step in this regard comes from the work by McConnachie et al. (2019), who found that children in adoptive gay father families were actually more likely to develop secure relationships than children in lesbian mother and heterosexual households. Future investigations of attachment in same-sex households should continue to inform both our scientific understanding of father-child attachment formation and the development of policies to support best practices in family formation.

Finally, relatively little attachment research has focused on applications of attachment theory to interventions and preventive interventions with fathers and young children. Given the prominence of attachment theory over the last 50 years and the relative dearth of empirical studies that have included fathers during that time, it is wholly appropriate that the field has been concerned with addressing questions of basic science and theory testing. However, mounting evidence of the importance of father-child relationships suggests that the next steps in the study of father-child attachment could include evaluation of interventions specifically targeting the father-child attachment relationship.

Although this work is rare, the very few intervention studies that have targeted fathers' sensitivity, for example, suggest that paternal sensitivity may be even more amenable to intervention effects than is maternal sensitivity (Bakermans-Kranenburg, Van Ijzendoorn, & Juffer, 2003). In a recent study Walter, Landers, Quehenberger, Carlson, and Brisch (2019) utilized a randomized control trial to assess the efficacy of a primary prevention program designed to promote infant-parent attachment. They found a significant difference between program and control participants in the rates of infant-father but not infant-mother attachment security, suggesting that the program was particularly effective in promoting father-child attachment. Similarly strong effects have been shown for a preventive intervention focused on father involvement that led (particularly when mothers also participated) to reduced parenting stress and child behavior problems and increased couple relationship quality (Pruett, Pruett, Cowan, & Cowan, 2017), suggesting the utility of targeted prevention work with fathers. The subsequent development of programming specifically to support father-child attachment relationships – and rigorous evaluations of those programs – is a critical new direction for those interested in fostering high-quality attachments between fathers and their young children.

Summary and Key Points

Despite being the predominant theoretical framework for conceptualizing early parent-child relationships, fathers in attachment theory and research have been overlooked historically. Nonetheless, an emerging body of research on father-child attachment has begun to elucidate patterns of early father-child attachment, as well as the personal and contextual correlates and developmental consequences of attachment security in predominantly White, middle-class, and residential father-child dyads. Most children form attachments to these fathers, with rates of security generally similar to what has been observed in mother-child dyads, and typically modest to moderate concordance between mother-child and father-child attachment within families.

Father-child attachment security is only weakly correlated with paternal sensitivity. As such, research on the predictors of attachment security has identified other parenting behaviors (e.g., involvement, stimulation) that appear to play a role in fostering father-child attachment security. Overall, family socio-contextual variables (e.g., marital quality, co-parenting) are collectively among the strongest and most consistent predictors of attachment security. Employment characteristics (e.g., single vs. dual-earner families) may play a role both as a direct and moderating influence on father-child attachment. Child characteristics (e.g., temperament and gender) are not generally related to father-child attachment security, with a few notable exceptions.

Disentangling the unique effects of father-child attachment on children's developmental outcomes remains a challenging task. Extant data suggests, however, that early father-child attachment security may have beneficial consequences for children's social and emotional outcomes in early and middle childhood. Children in secure father-child dyads exhibit elevated emotion regulation capacities and social competence and reduced psychopathology and externalizing behavior problems. Links to other outcomes, including cognitive and language development, are still tenuous.

With fathers more commonly considered in attachment theory and research in recent years, the unique correlates and consequences of the father-child relationship have begun to come into focus. These findings provide a roadmap for important future directions in the study of this critical early relationship. In order to more fully understand the generalizability of these results, research with more diverse samples (in terms of race/ethnicity, SES, and family structure) and greater attention to sociocultural contexts is essential. Further, study designs that more fully incorporate a family systems perspective with the goal of distinguishing unique, interactive, and cumulative effects of father-child and mother-child attachment relationships are sorely needed to establish the mechanisms whereby father-child attachment in the context of the family leads to positive developmental trajectories. Greater diversity in the selection of predictors and outcomes – with an emphasis on unique, father-centric processes – in attachment research can continue to shed light on the full range of fathers' contributions. As the body of basic science on father-child attachment relationships continues to grow, there are opportunities for both scientists and practitioners to inform applied efforts such as family policy, parent education, prevention and intervention programming, and clinical work targeting father-child relationships.

References

Abraham, E., & Feldman, R. (2018). The neurobiology of human allomaternal care; implications for fathering, coparenting, and children's social development. *Physiology & Behavior, 193*, 25–34.

Ahnert, L., Pinquart, M., & Lamb, M. E. (2006). Security of children's relationships with nonparental care providers: A meta-analysis. *Child Development, 77*, 664–679.

Ainsworth, M. D. S. (1967). *Infancy in Uganda: Infant care and the growth of love*. Baltimore: The Johns Hopkins Press.

Ainsworth, M. D. S., Bell, S. M., & Stayton, D. F. (1974). Infant-mother attachment and social development: Socialization as a product of reciprocal responsiveness to signals. In *The integration of a child into a social world*. Cambridge: Cambridge University Press.

Ainsworth, M. D. S., Blehar, M. C., Waters, E., & Wall, S. N. (1978). *Patterns of attachment: A psychological study of the strange situation*. Oxford: Erlbaum.

Bakermans-Kranenburg, M. J., Van Ijzendoorn, M. H., & Juffer, F. (2003). Less is more: Meta-analyses of sensitivity and attachment interventions in early childhood. *Psychological Bulletin, 129*, 195–215.

Belsky, J. (1996). Parent, infant, and social-contextual antecedents of father-son attachment security. *Developmental Psychology, 32*, 905–913.

Belsky, J., Garduque, L., & Hrncir, E. (1984). Assessing performance, competence, and executive capacity in infant play: Relations to home environment and security of attachment. *Developmental Psychology, 20*, 406–417.

Belsky, J., & Rovine, M. J. (1988). Nonmaternal care in the first year of life and the security of infant-parent attachment. *Child Development, 59*, 157–167.

Boldt, L. J., Kochanska, G., Grekin, R., & Brock, R. L. (2016). Attachment in middle childhood: Predictors, correlates, and implications for adaptation. *Attachment & Human Development, 18*, 115–140.

Bowlby, J. (1969). *Attachment and loss: Attachment*. New York: Basic Books.

Braungart-Rieker, J., Courtney, S., & Garwood, M. M. (1999). Mother–and father–infant attachment: Families in context. *Journal of Family Psychology, 13*, 535–553.

Braungart-Rieker, J. M., Garwood, M. M., Powers, B. P., & Wang, X. (2001). Parental sensitivity, infant affect, and affect regulation: Predictors of later attachment. *Child Development, 72*, 252–270.

Bretherton, I., & Munholland, K. A. (2008). Internal working models in attachment relationships: A construct revisited. In J. Cassidy & P. R. Shaver (Eds.), *Handbook of attachment: Theory, research, and clinical applications* (pp. 102–127). New York: The Guilford Press.

Brock, R. L., & Kochanska, G. (2018). Anger in infancy and its implications: History of attachment in mother–child and father–child relationships as a moderator of risk. *Development and Psychopathology, 31*, 1353–1366.

Brown, G. L., & Cox, M. J. (2019). Pleasure in parenting and father-child attachment security. *Attachment and Human Development, 22*, 51.

Brown, G. L., Mangelsdorf, S. C., & Neff, C. (2012). Father involvement, paternal sensitivity, and father–child attachment security in the first 3 years. *Journal of Family Psychology, 26*, 421–430.

Brown, G. L., Mangelsdorf, S. C., Shigeto, A., & Wong, M. S. (2018). Associations between father involvement and father–child attachment security: Variations based on timing and type of involvement. *Journal of Family Psychology, 32*, 1015–1024.

Brown, G. L., McBride, B. A., Shin, N., & Bost, K. K. (2007). Parenting predictors of father-child attachment security: Interactive effects of father involvement and fathering quality. *Fathering, 5*, 197–219.

Brown, G. L., Schoppe-Sullivan, S. J., Mangelsdorf, S. C., & Neff, C. (2010). Observed and reported supportive coparenting as predictors of infant-mother and infant-father attachment security. *Early Child Development and Care, 180*, 121–137.

Bureau, J.-F., Deneault, A.-A., & Yurkowski, K. (2019). Preschool father-child attachment and its relation to self-reported child socioemotional adaptation in middle childhood. *Attachment and Human Development., 22*, 90.

Bureau, J.-F., Martin, J., Yurkowski, K., Schmiedel, S., Quan, J., Moss, E., et al. (2017). Correlates of child–father and child–mother attachment in the preschool years. *Attachment and Human Development, 19*, 130–150.

Cabrera, N. J., Fitzgerald, H. E., Bradley, R. H., & Roggman, L. (2014). The ecology of father-child relationships: An expanded model. *Journal of Family Theory & Review, 6*, 336–354.

Cabrera, N. J., Volling, B. L., & Barr, R. (2018). Fathers are parents, too! Widening the lens on parenting for children's development. *Child Development Perspectives, 12*, 152–157.

Caldera, Y. M. (2004). Paternal involvement and infant-father attachment: A Q-set study. *Fathering, 2*, 191–210.

Caldera, Y. M., & Lindsey, E. W. (2006). Coparenting, mother-infant interaction, and infant-parent attachment relationships in two-parent families. *Journal of Family Psychology, 20*, 275–283.

Cohen, L. J., & Campos, J. J. (1974). Father, mother, and stranger as elicitors of attachment behaviors in infancy. *Developmental Psychology, 10*, 146–154.

Cowan, P. A. (1997). Beyond meta-analysis: A plea for a family systems view of attachment. *Child Development, 68*, 601–603.

Cowan, P. A., & Cowan, C. P. (2019). Introduction: Bringing dads back into the family. *Attachment and Human Development., 21*, 419.

Cox, M. J., Owen, M. T., Henderson, V. K., & Margand, N. A. (1992). Prediction of infant-father and infant-mother attachment. *Developmental Psychology, 28*, 474–483.

Coyl-Shepherd, D. D., & Newland, L. A. (2013). Mothers' and fathers' couple and family contextual influences, parent involvement, and school-age child attachment. *Early Child Development and Care, 183*, 553–569.

Dagan, O., & Sagi-Schwartz, A. (2018). Early attachment network with mother and father: An unsettled issue. *Child Development Perspectives, 12*, 115–121.

De Wolff, M. S., & Van Ijzendoorn, M. H. (1997). Sensitivity and attachment: A meta-analysis on parental antecedents of infant attachment. *Child Development, 68*, 571–591.

Deneault, A. A., Bureau, J. F., Yurkowski, K., & Moss, E. (2019). Validation of the Preschool Attachment Rating Scales with child-mother and child-father dyads. *Attachment & Human Development, 15*, 1–23.

Diener, M. L., Mangelsdorf, S. C., McHale, J. L., & Frosch, C. A. (2002). Infants' behavioral strategies for emotion regulation with fathers and mothers: Associations with emotional expressions and attachment quality. *Infancy, 3*, 153–174.

Doherty, W. J., Kouneski, E. F., & Erickson, M. F. (1998). Responsible fathering: An overview and conceptual framework. *Journal of Marriage and the Family, 60*, 277–292.

Ehrlich, K., & Cassidy, J. (2019). Attachment and physical health: Introduction to the special issue. *Attachment and Human Development, 21*, 1.

Fagan, J. (2019). Broadening the scope of father-child attachment research to include the family context. *Attachment and Human Development., 22*, 139.

Field, T., Gewirtz, J. L., Cohen, D., Garcia, R., Greenberg, R., & Collins, K. (1984). Leave-takings and reunions of infants, toddlers, preschoolers, and their parents. *Child Development, 55*, 628–635.

Fletcher, R., StGeorge, J., & Freeman, E. (2013). Rough and tumble play quality: Theoretical foundations for a new measure of father–child interaction. *Early Child Development and Care, 183*, 746–759.

Fox, N. A., Kimmerly, N. L., & Schafer, W. D. (1991). Attachment to mother/attachment to father: A meta-analysis. *Child Development, 62*, 210–225.

Frosch, C. A., Mangelsdorf, S. C., & McHale, J. L. (2000). Marital behavior and the security of preschooler–parent attachment relationships. *Journal of Family Psychology, 14*, 144–161.

Fuertes, M., Faria, A., Beeghly, M., & Lopes-dos-Santos, P. (2016). The effects of parental sensitivity and involvement in caregiving on mother–infant and father–infant attachment in a Portuguese sample. *Journal of Family Psychology, 30*, 147–156.

Gaumon, S., Paquette, D., Cyr, C., Émond-Nakamura, M., & St-André, M. (2016). Anxiety and attachment to the mother in preschoolers receiving psychiatric care: The father–child activation relationship as a protective factor. *Infant Mental Health Journal, 37*, 372–387.

Goffin, K. C., Boldt, L. J., & Kochanska, G. (2018). A secure base from which to cooperate: Security, child and parent Willing Stance, and adaptive and maladaptive outcomes in two longitudinal studies. *Journal of Abnormal Child Psychology, 46*, 1061–1075.

Gordon, I., Zagoory-Sharon, O., Leckman, J. F., & Feldman, R. (2010). Prolactin, oxytocin, and the development of paternal behavior across the first six months of fatherhood. *Hormones and Behavior, 58*, 513–518.

Groh, A. M., Fearon, R. P., van IJzendoorn, M. H., Bakermans-Kranenburg, M. J., & Roisman, G. I. (2017). Attachment in the early life course: Meta-analytic evidence for its role in socioemotional development. *Child Development Perspectives, 11*, 70–76.

Grossmann, K., Grossmann, K. E., Fremmer-Bombik, E., Kindler, H., Scheuerer-Englisch, H., & Zimmermann, P. (2002). The uniqueness of the child-father attachment relationship: Fathers' sensitive and challenging play as a pivotal variable in a 16-year longitudinal study. *Social Development, 11*, 307–331.

Hazen, N. L., McFarland, L., Jacobvitz, D., & Boyd-Soisson, E. (2010). Fathers' frightening behaviours and sensitivity with infants: Relations with fathers' attachment representations, father–infant attachment, and children's later outcomes. *Early Child Development and Care, 180*, 51–69.

Hertz, S., Bernier, A., Cimon-Paquet, C., & Regueiro, S. (2019). Parent–child relationships and child executive functioning at school entry: The importance of fathers. *Early Child Development and Care, 189*, 718–732.

Jones, J., & Mosher, W. D. (2013). Fathers' involvement with their children: United States, 2006–2010. *National Health Statistics Reports, 71*, 1–21.

Kochanska, G., & Kim, S. (2013). Early attachment organization with both parents and future behavior problems: From infancy to middle childhood. *Child Development, 84*, 283–296.

Kotelchuck, M. (1976). The infant's relationship to the father: Experimental evidence. In M. E. Lamb (Ed.), *The role of the father in child development* (pp. 329–344). New York: Wiley.

Kuo, P. X., Saini, E. K., Tengelitsch, E., & Volling, B. L. (2019). Is one secure attachment enough? Infant cortisol reactivity and the security of infant-mother and infant-father attachments at the end of the first year. *Attachment and Human Development, 21*, 426.

Lamb, M. E. (1976a). Interactions between 2-year-olds and their mothers and fathers. *Psychological Reports, 38*, 447–450.

Lamb, M. E. (1976b). Parent-infant interaction in 8-month-olds. *Child Psychiatry and Human Development, 7*, 56–63.

Lamb, M. E. (1977a). The development of parental preferences in the first two years of life. *Sex Roles, 3*, 495–497.

Lamb, M. E. (1977b). Father-infant and mother-infant interaction in 1st year of life. *Child Development, 48*, 167–181.

Lamb, M. E. (2012). Infant–father attachments and their impact on child development. In N. J. Cabrera & C. S. Tamis-LeMonda (Eds.), *Handbook of father involvement* (pp. 109–133). New York: Routledge.

Lamb, M. E., Frodi, M., Hwang, C. P., & Frodi, A. M. (1983). Effects of paternal involvement on infant preferences for mothers and fathers. *Child Development, 54*, 450–458.

Lankinen, V., Lähteenmäki, M., Kaljonen, A., & Korpilahti, P. (2019). Father–child activities and paternal attitudes in early child language development: The STEPS study. *Early Child Development and Care, 189*, 1–15.

Lickenbrock, D. M., & Braungart-Rieker, J. M. (2015). Examining antecedents of infant attachment security with mothers and fathers: An ecological systems perspective. *Infant Behavior and Development, 39*, 173–187.

Lieberman, M., Doyle, A. B., & Markiewicz, D. (1999). Developmental patterns in security of attachment to mother and father in late childhood and early adolescence: Associations with peer relations. *Child Development, 70*, 202–213.

Lucassen, N., Tharner, A., Van IJzendoorn, M. H., Bakermans-Kranenburg, M. J., Volling, B. L., Verhulst, F. C., et al. (2011). The association between paternal sensitivity and infant–father attachment security: A meta-analysis of three decades of research. *Journal of Family Psychology, 25*, 986–992.

Main, M., & Goldwyn, R. (1995). Interview-based adult attachment classifications: Related to infant-mother and infant-father attachment. *Developmental Psychology, 19*, 227–239.

Mangelsdorf, S. C., & Frosch, C. A. (1999). Temperament and attachment: One construct or two? *Advances in Child Development and Behavior, 27*, 181–220. Elsevier.

McConnachie, A. L., Ayed, N., Jadva, V., Lamb, M., Tasker, F., & Golombok, S. (2019). Father-child attachment in adoptive gay father families. *Attachment and Human Development., 22*, 110.

McFarland-Piazza, L., Hazen, N., Jacobvitz, D., & Boyd-Soisson, E. (2012). The development of father–child attachment: Associations between adult attachment representations, recollections of childhood experiences and caregiving. *Early Child Development and Care, 182*, 701–721.

Neppl, T. K., Wedmore, H., Senia, J. M., Jeon, S., & Diggs, O. N. (2019). Couple interaction and child social competence: The role of parenting and attachment. *Social Development, 28*, 347–363.

Olsavsky, A. L., Berrigan, M. N., Schoppe-Sullivan, S. J., Brown, G. L., & Kamp Dush, C. M. (2019). Paternal stimulation and father-infant attachment. *Attachment and Human Development, 22*, 15.

Owen, M. T., & Cox, M. J. (1997). Marital conflict and the development of infant–parent attachment relationships. *Journal of Family Psychology, 11*, 152–164.

Palkovitz, R., & Hull, J. (2018). Toward a resource theory of fathering. *Journal of Family Theory & Review, 10*, 181–198.

Palm, G. (2014). Attachment theory and fathers: Moving from "being there" to "being with". *Journal of Family Theory & Review, 6*, 282–297.

Paquette, D. (2004). Theorizing the father-child relationship: Mechanisms and developmental outcomes. *Human Development, 47*, 193–219.

Paquette, D., & Bigras, M. (2010). The risky situation: A procedure for assessing the father-child activation relationship. *Early Child Development and Care, 180*, 33–50.

Paquette, D., & Dumont, C. (2013). Is father–child rough-and-tumble play associated with attachment or activation relationships? *Early Child Development and Care, 183*, 760–773.

Parke, R. D. (1996). *Fatherhood*. Cambridge, MA: Harvard University Press.

Pinto, A., Veríssimo, M., Gatinho, A., Santos, A. J., & Vaughn, B. E. (2015). Direct and indirect relations between parent–child attachments, peer acceptance, and self-esteem for preschool children. *Attachment and Human Development, 17*, 586–598.

Planalp, E. M., & Braungart-Rieker, J. M. (2013). Temperamental precursors of infant attachment with mothers and fathers. *Infant Behavior and Development, 36*, 796–808.

Pruett, M. K., Pruett, K., Cowan, C. P., & Cowan, P. A. (2017). Enhancing father involvement in low-income families: A couples group approach to preventive intervention. *Child Development, 88*, 398–407.

Psouni, E. (2019). The influence of attachment representations and co-parents' scripted knowledge of attachment on fathers' and mothers' caregiving representations. *Attachment and Human Development., 21*, 485.

Psychogiou, L., Nath, S., Kallitsoglou, A., Dimatis, K., Parry, E., Russell, A. E., et al. (2018). Children's emotion understanding in relation to attachment to mother and father. *British Journal of Developmental Psychology, 36*, 557–572.

Rilling, J. K., & Mascaro, J. S. (2017). The neurobiology of fatherhood. *Current Opinion in Psychology, 15*, 26–32.

Sagi, A., Lamb, M. E., Lewkowicz, K. S., Shoham, R., Dvir, R., & Estes, D. (1985). Security of infant-mother, infant-father, and infant-metapelet attachments among Kibbutz-Reared Israeli Children. *Monographs of the Society for Research in Child Development, 50*, 257–275.

Sarkadi, A., Kristiansson, R., Oberklaid, F., & Bremberg, S. (2008). Fathers' involvement and children's developmental outcomes: A systematic review of longitudinal studies. *Acta Paediatrica, 97*, 153–158.

Schoppe-Sullivan, S. J., & Fagan, J. (2020). The evolution of fathering research in the 21st century: Persistent challenges, new directions. *Journal of Marriage and Family, 82*, 175–197.

Schoppe-Sullivan, S. J., Mangelsdorf, S. C., Brown, G. L., & Sokolowski, M. S. (2007). Goodness-of-fit in family context: Infant temperament, marital quality, and early coparenting behavior. *Infant Behavior and Development, 30*, 82–96.

Solomon, J., & George, C. (2016). *Handbook of attachment*. New York: Guilford.

Soubry, A. (2018). Epigenetics as a driver of developmental origins of health and disease: Did we forget the fathers? *BioEssays, 40*, 1700113.

Sroufe, L. A. (1985). Attachment classification from the perspective of infant-caregiver relationships and infant temperament. *Child Development, 56*, 1–14.

Sroufe, L. A. (2000). Early relationships and the development of children. *Infant Mental Health Journal, 21*, 67–74.

Steele, H., Steele, M., & Fonagy, P. (1996). Associations among attachment classifications of mothers, fathers, and their infants. *Child Development, 67*, 541–555.

Teufl, L., Deichmann, F., Supper, B., & Ahnert, L. (2019). How fathers' attachment security and education contribute to early child language skills above and beyond mothers: Parent-child conversation under scrutiny. *Attachment and Human Development, 22*, 71.

Thompson, R. A. (2000). The legacy of early attachments. *Child Development, 71*, 145–152.

van Ijzendoorn, M. H., & de Wolff, M. S. (1997). In search of the absent father—meta-analyses of infant-father attachment: A rejoinder to our discussants. *Child Development, 68*, 604–609.

Vaughn, B. E., & Bost, K. K. (2008). Attachment and temperament: Redundant, independent, or interacting influences on interpersonal adaptation and personality development? In J. Cassidy & P. R. Shaver (Eds.), *Handbook of attachment: Theory, research, and clinical applications* (pp. 192–216). New York: The Guilford Press.

Volling, B. L. (2019). Widening the lens on family processes and the development of parent-child attachment relationships. *Attachment and Human Development, 22*, 1.

Volling, B. L., & Belsky, J. (1992). Infant, father, and marital antecedents of infant father attachment security in dual-earner and single-earner families. *International Journal of Behavioral Development, 15*, 83–100.

Volling, B. L., McElwain, N. L., Notaro, P. C., & Herrera, C. (2002). Parents' emotional availability and infant emotional competence: Predictors of parent-infant attachment and emerging self-regulation. *Journal of Family Psychology, 16*, 447–465.

Walter, I., Landers, S., Quehenberger, J., Carlson, E., & Brisch, K. (2019). The efficacy of the attachment-based SAFE® prevention program: A randomized control trial including mothers and fathers. *Attachment and Human Development, 21*, 510.

Waters, E., & Deane, K. E. (1985). Defining and assessing individual differences in attachment relationships: Q-methodology and the organization of behavior in infancy and early childhood. *Monographs of the Society for Research in Child Development, 50*, 41–65.

Wong, M. S., Mangelsdorf, S. C., Brown, G. L., Neff, C., & Schoppe-Sullivan, S. J. (2009). Parental beliefs, infant temperament, and marital quality: Associations with infant-mother and infant-father attachment. *Journal of Family Psychology, 23*, 828–838.

19 Fathers and the Activation Relationship

Daniel Paquette, Carole Gagnon, and Julio Macario de Medeiros

This chapter begins with a look at theoretical perspectives before presenting research findings from the past 15 years, since the activation relationship theory was published in 2004. The studies will be examined in four respective sections: (a) the activation relationship and activative fathering, (b) paternal behaviors of openness to the world, (c) challenging parenting behavior, and (d) rough-and-tumble play. Next, we draw on the complementarity of attachment relationships (CAR) project to determine the prevalence of the three types of activation relationships in father-child and mother-child dyads and to verify the sex differences in parent-child activation relationship with toddlers. Finally, we conclude with potential future lines of research.

Theoretical Perspectives

This first portion of this chapter is intended as a complement to the activation relationship theory published by Paquette (2004a). We begin by revisiting the adaptive value of attachment for survival and reproduction. Next, we distinguish between the maternal and paternal functions in our species and suggest that these functions emerged in our hunter-gatherer ancestors. We also explain why mothers also activate their children, even if fathers are generally the primary activation figure. Finally, we discuss the importance of father-child and mother-child relationships in the differential socialization of the sexes, according to evolutionary perspectives, and make predictions regarding the activation relationship and the attachment relationship.

The Gregarious Nature of Our Species and the Mother-Child Attachment Relationship

Parenting is a reproductive strategy adopted through natural selection mainly in birds and mammals. With a few exceptions, fish, amphibians, and reptiles produce many eggs, which are abandoned after being laid by the mother. This "quantitative" reproductive strategy increases the odds that a certain number of offspring will survive their environmental hazards so they can, in turn, reproduce in the future. Birds and mammals, in contrast, have espoused a "qualitative" strategy by producing few offspring but caring for and protecting them to ensure they survive to adult age. Imprinting in altricial birds and attachment in mammals are analogous mechanisms that emerged in the course of evolution to help develop a mother-child bond that maintains the

D. Paquette (✉) · C. Gagnon
J. Macario de Medeiros
École de psychoéducation, Université de Montréal, Montréal, QC, Canada
e-mail: daniel.paquette@umontreal.ca

H. E. Fitzgerald et al. (eds.), *Handbook of Fathers and Child Development*, https://doi.org/10.1007/978-3-030-51027-5_19

proximity required to feed and protect offspring efficiently.

The survival strategy of sociality, or living in groups, emerged in a number of species, delivering numerous advantages such as protection from predators and the possibility of leveraging the learning of others (cultural transmission). In the social species of mammals (such as wolves, lions, elephants, and primates), attachment bonds are also forged with other individuals in the group, throughout development from infancy to adulthood, to foster social cohesion (Paquette, 2015). Humans live in more extended groups than do other primates, and human beings considerably set themselves apart from other primates by their ability to cooperate with others (Tomasello, 2014). In our nomadic ancestors, large groups enabled, among others things, the emergence of collective large-game hunting, our ecological niche.

Previous studies in humans have mainly succeeded in demonstrating that the attachment relationship is a mechanism that fosters the development of social competencies (sociability, reciprocity, popularity, positive social orientation, synchrony, communication, etc.), emotion regulation, and willingness to explore the environment: children who have a secure relationship with their mother tend to have stronger social competencies and to explore their environment more than their insecure peers (Moss, Bureau, Cyr, Mongeau, & St-Laurent, 2004; Weinfield, Sroufe, Egeland, & Carlson, 2008 for a review).

Fathers and Maternal Functions

The effects of mothers' parenting behaviors on the development of children have been studied exhaustively given that, across the globe, mothers are more involved in upbringing than fathers (Geary, 2010; Gray & Anderson, 2010). This greater involvement is fundamentally due to the fact that, in mammals, females are responsible for their children's caretaking after pregnancy (Geary, 2010). The attachment theory (Bowlby, 1969) has helped shed light on the importance for children of having an emotional bond with a significant person who will be able to meet their basic needs. In many cultures, fathers give their children scarce or no direct care (Hewlett, 2000), but they do generally assume important roles for the family as providers and protectors (Paquette, 2004a). Moreover, around the end of childhood, fathers generally take on various responsibilities related to boys' adaptation to the physical and social environment, depending on the culture (Paquette, 2004a). In industrialized Western societies, women's entry into the workforce in conjunction with smaller families has led fathers to become more involved with children. They first engaged in physical play with boys, which mothers in North America sometimes viewed as superfluous or useless to children's development, and even a behavior to banish if the physical play involved fighting (Panksepp, 1993). Next, fathers gradually engaged in general caretaking of younger and younger children (Bianchi, 2000), and probably as much with girls as boys in the case of babies, although fathers scored significantly higher on the parental involvement index for sons than for daughters at 11–16 months (Harris, Furstenberg, & Marmer, 1998). Studies on the effects of fathers' parenting behaviors are thus much more recent and initially tended to focus on paternal behaviors from a perspective of maternal functions. The Strange Situation Procedure (SSP) developed by Mary Ainsworth and colleagues (1978) made it possible to assess the quality of 12–18-month-old children's attachment with their primary caregiver. This procedure, which was validated with mothers, was also used with fathers (who are generally children's secondary attachment figures). The low stability, low transmissibility, and low predictability of father-child attachment led a growing number of researchers to question the relevance of using this procedure with fathers who had little involvement in daily caregiving (Suess, Grossmann, & Sroufe, 1992; van IJzendoorn, 1995; Youngblade, Park, & Belsky, 1993). Grossmann et al. (2002) showed paternal sensitivity during play with 2-year-old children to be a better predictor of attachment 14 years later than father-child attachment as measured by the strange situation. The activation relationship theory, as explained below, was developed by Paquette (2004a, 2004b) precisely to better understand paternal functions.

The Paternal Function of Openness to the World

Le Camus (2000) has examined a marginal literature showing that fathers prompt children to take initiatives in unfamiliar situations, to explore, to take chances, to overcome obstacles, to be braver in the presence of strangers, and to stand up for themselves. His conclusion is that the various parental roles played by the father, including authority figure, are part of a broader function of opening the child up to the world. Along these lines, Paquette (2004a, 2004b) defined the activation relationship as the emotional bond that fosters children's openness to the world, with special focus on parental behavior during the child's exploration and especially parental stimulation and control.

According to the evolutionary perspective, the division of maternal and paternal functions in parents occurred in the days of our hunter-gatherer ancestors. The very wide majority of primate species live in multi-male/multi-female groups (promiscuous species) or are polygynous. Only the mothers take care of the children; the adult males mainly assume a group protection role, even if they occasionally can be found playing with youths (not necessarily their own offspring, since they are unable to recognize them), but they provide no paternal care. Children are therefore mainly socialized via contact with the mother and then with peers, especially during rough-and-tumble play (RTP). RTP consists of a variety of vigorous behaviors, such as wrestling, grappling, jumping, tumbling, and running that would appear aggressive if not for the play contexts in which they occur (Pellegrini & Smith, 1998). It is more common in males than in females across primate species (Chalmers, 1983) and across human cultures starting from 3 years of age (Carson, Burks, & Parke, 1993). Rough-and-tumble play among peers begins in humans at preschool age, peaks between 8 and 10 years, and trails off at the beginning of adolescence (Pellegrini & Smith, 1998). Hence, as in the case of our primate cousins, human girls and boys interact with same-sex peers more frequently than with opposite-sex peers, starting from 3 years of age (Rose & Rudolph, 2006).

The human system of reproduction features a mix of union types. Although polygynous marriages can be found in most human societies, monogamy remains predominant across the globe given that, in most polygynous societies, only a small portion of men have more than one wife (Chapais, 2008). Humans lived in hunter-gatherer societies for over 99% of the evolutionary history of the genus *Homo* (Chapais, 2011). This division of labor increased the reproductive success of the human species by enhancing children's likelihood of survival while reducing mortality and the lapse of time between births (1–3 years for humans versus 5–6 years for chimpanzees). In sum, this means it is possible that in our primate ancestors, mothers assumed both attachment and activation functions with their offspring, and the emergence of the hunter-gatherer lifestyle among our hominid ancestors—and hence the sexual division of labor—led to differentiated maternal and paternal functions. This in turn could legitimize the hypothesis of the emergence of psychological mechanisms mainly promoting the learning of maternal function-related skills in mother-daughter dyads and paternal function-related skills in father-son dyads, consistent with the tendency of peers to interact with the same sex.

Fathers' ways of activating their children vary depending on the culture and the physical and social environments that must be adapted to. Father-child RTP is not universal but rather a fairly recent development in our individualistic and competitive Western industrialized societies (Allès-Jardel, Schneider, Goldstein, & Normand, 2009; Paquette, 2004a). We posit that many decades ago, when families had large numbers of children, it was the older brothers who played with younger boys, preparing them to interact with their peers outside the home, and women's entry into the workforce and the advent of smaller families led fathers to replace brothers in play with boys. In light of the great plasticity of human behavior, and the current ideological and social context, it may be hypothesized that parental differences between mothers and fathers are on the wane, at least in terms of frequency of parental behaviors. However, relations between parental behavior and child development may be expected to continue to differ depending on the sex of the parent and the child. We know that a given parental behavior may have different effects on the child depending on whether the behavior is enacted by the father or the mother (Roggman, Bradley, & Raikes, 2013). Moreover, the quality of the behavior can vary depending on the parent's sex. Fathers likely have a more dynamic and transient way of changing children's diapers than mothers (disruptive harmony in fathers vs. homeostatic harmony in mothers: see Herzog, 1992), and fathers are more stimulative and directive with their children in the context of RTP than mothers (see Paquette, Carbonneau, Dubeau, Bigras, & Tremblay, 2003).

Maternal and paternal functions in couples are here seen as complementary, whether the couple is composed of same- or different-sex parents. Although children develop both types of relationships with each parent, generally speaking, women will tend to act as the primary attachment figure (performing maternal functions), while men will tend to serve as the primary activation figure (performing paternal functions). In a minority of cases, the woman will be the primary activation figure in a heterosexual couple, just as a man may be the primary attachment figure. It may be hypothesized that complementary functions also exist in homosexual couples for the same reason, that is, to be able to optimally meet the child's many needs.

Attachment and Activation Relationships

According to Bowlby (1969), the attachment theory consists of two complementary behavior systems: (1) the proximity behavior system, which ensures the child's protection; and (2) the exploration system, which fosters the child's acquisition of knowledge and adaptation to unfamiliar environments. The parent acts as a "safe haven" by providing comfort to the children when tired, hungry, sick or afraid, or when feeling insecure in the presence of novelty, and this comfort provides them with the necessary confidence to further explore their environment (indirect role). The parent also acts as a "secure base" by being available and encouraging the autonomy during their exploration (direct role). The activation relationship theory is complementary to attachment theory and places greater focus on the exploration pole: parents promote their children's exploration by actively stimulating them during the process, and their encouragements foster the confidence for the child's risk-taking.

As proposed by Grossmann, Grossmann, Kindler, and Zimmermann (2008), we distinguish between attachment in the broad sense and attachment in the strict sense. Broadly speaking, the attachment relationship refers to the adult-child emotional bond resulting from daily interaction and ensuring the child's protection. In the strict sense of the term, children's feelings of confidence result from parental sensitivity to their comfort-seeking in times of distress (as assessed by the Strange Situation Procedure), with parents protecting their children by maintaining a close distance with them (Bowlby, 1973). Furthermore, the activation relationship concerns the safety of exploration (see Grossmann et al., 2008) as evaluated by the Risky Situation Procedure (Paquette & Bigras, 2010). According to the activation relationship theory (Paquette, 2004a), children's feelings of confidence result from parents' encouragement of risk-taking during children's exploration of their environment, with parents also protecting their children through discipline (limit-setting, control). In sum, the activation relationship is also an attachment bond but develops with a parent particularly engaged in the parental dimensions of stimulation and control.

The activation relationship could also be described as the parent-child attachment bond that is developed to foster regulation of risk-taking in children as a function of the child's temperament (Paquette & Bigras, 2010). The activation relationship theory considers risk-taking to be a basic need that enables children to develop their motor and competitive skills, explore their physical and social environments, and adapt as needed. Given that men have a universal tendency to take more psychological and physical risks on average than women in all spheres of daily life (Baker & Maner, 2008; Byrnes, Miller, & Schaffer, 1999; Farthing, 2007; Pawlowski, Atwal, & Dunbar, 2008), fathers may be better suited than mothers to helping their children, especially boys, learn to control their risk-taking, provided that they have learned to regulate their own risk-taking. Men's greater risk-taking is the result of sexual selection, that is, preservation of the anatomical and behavioral characteristics that provide an individual with a reproductive advantage over others of the same sex (Darwin, 1871). Through risk-taking, men are able to show women their skill as protectors and resource providers, as well as demonstrate to other men that they are adversaries to be reckoned with (Wilke, Hutchison, Todd, & Kruger, 2006). Studies have shown that women prefer men who take risks, but not when the risks are so high as to cost the man his life—unless in an act of heroism—since they would then be alone in raising their offspring (Farthing, 2007).

The use of the risky situation procedure has shown the existence of three types of activation (Paquette & Bigras, 2010). Underactivated children tend to engage in little exploration, be passive, and withdraw from novelty or stay close to the parent. Activated children are confident and prudent in their exploration and obey when the parent sets a limit. Finally, overactivated children are reckless and noncompliant when the parent sets limits. According to life history theory (Aimé, Paquette, Déry, & Verlaan, 2018; Paquette, 2015), a child's overactivation proves adaptive in a setting fraught with competition over immediate access to unpredictable resources; the child is then inclined to take greater risks to capture as many resources as possible in the short term. In theory, overactivated children will tend to use aggression and other antisocial behaviors, regardless of the context, and to strive for high social dominance status in order to maximize immediate access to resources. This profile may be expected to develop mainly in boys living, for example, in situations of poverty and when the parents have a high number of children, to the detriment of their parental involvement with each child. This reproductive strategy is referred to as "quantitative," since it involves having as many children as possible as early as possible (early reproduction). In contrast, the two other profiles bring into play a "qualitative" reproductive strategy that consists in preparing the individual for later reproduction. The activated profile is adaptive in a context of sufficient and stable resources. The child is able to take calculated risks to acquire resources. Theoretically, activated children develop a varied repertory of behaviors to cope with diverse competitive situations: they may be expected to use assertiveness, and, if necessary, aggression in confrontational contexts with threatening children, but prefer to use cooperation whenever possible. According to Charlesworth's (1988) evolutionary model, cooperation is the best competitive strategy for obtaining more resources in the long term. Child underactivation would be adaptive in a dangerous social or physical environment. This danger can be real or merely perceived by the parents. The underactivated profile could result from parent overprotection, for example, due to the interaction between the lower number of children per family in Western societies today and the overrepresentation of various dangers in the media. This profile may be expected to develop mainly in girls, in order to avoid injury or even death, given that their reproductive success strongly depends on their ability to bear children. Underactivated children will tend to avoid conflicts, submit to others, and leave resources to those who demand them. Although these individuals will delay their reproduction, they can still increase their reproductive success indirectly through kin selection (Hamilton, 1964), that is, by helping or caring for relatives, especially their siblings. In short, while the activation relationship can be theoretically associated with competition and power relationships (e.g., dominance and leadership), the attachment relationship can be associated with empathy and intimacy in friendships, romantic relationships and parent-child relationships (Paquette, 2015).

Double Moderation by Parent's Sex and Child's Sex

Evolutionary perspectives call for simultaneously taking into account the sex of parent and child within child development research (Möller, Majdandzic, de Vente, & Bögels, 2013). Very few studies have taken into account the interaction effect between parent's sex and child's sex on the development of psychological gender differences (Bornstein, 2013; Pomerantz, Fei-Yin Ng, & Wang, 2004). Yet given that fathers and mothers can have different effects on children, and boys and girls influence parents differently, it is essential, according to Bornstein (2013), to compare the four types of dyads (mother-son, father-son, mother-daughter, and father-daughter). Pomerantz et al. (2004) suggest that the match between children's and parents' sex may play an important role in the gender socialization process, since it is easier to identify with a parent of the same sex. The socialization process could therefore be more effective in father-son and mother-daughter dyads. This greater effectiveness could be rooted in gender segregation, a robust and cross-culturally universal preference for affiliating with children of the same sex, emerging as early as age two (Edwards & Whiting, 1993). In fact, in families with children of both sexes, fathers spend more time with boys, and mothers spend more time with girls (Crouter, Helms-Erickson, Updegraff, & McHale, 1999).

The parent-child attachment relationship being known to have important implications for children's emotional development and social competence, Eisenberg, Spinrad, and Cumberland (1998) have suggested that the secure relationship could make children relatively receptive to parental socialization attempts. Given the gregarious nature of our species, we go a step further by maintaining that the parent-child attachment relationship (in the broad sense, resulting from parent-child interaction history, taking into account the personal characteristics of parents and children) is an essential pillar of effective socialization. If this is the case, one might predict that the quality of parent-child relationship will be more predictive of children's gender differences than parenting behaviors. Hence, the parent-child relationship—attachment and activation—would consist of proximal mechanisms by which biologically predisposed sex differences in children may diminish or increase according to the socio-cultural values of the current environment. Children's gender differences in behavior and emotional expression would then be associated with and preceded by sex differences in the parent-child relationships, more so than by father or mother parenting. According to our model, the moment of the emergence of significant sex differences in parent-child relationships would depend on the kind of relationship. Given that the attachment relationship (in the strict sense of maternal functions) serves the base function of ensuring children's survival through the provision of care and parental protection during the period of maximal dependence on parents, there is no reason to expect to find a sex difference in the prevalence of attachment types in infancy and early childhood. Indeed, no such difference appears in the literature (van IJzendoorn et al., 2000). However, with regard to the maternal function of caretaking, it would be logical for there to be a sex difference in attachment just before puberty. Del Giudice (2009) recently proposed that sex differences in attachment emerge in middle childhood (7–10 years of age), become stronger in young adulthood, and finally decline markedly toward middle age. Hence, in the attachment relationship, the mother could be expected to influence the child's development more than the father, and both parents may have a greater influence on girls than on boys; thus, the descending order would be mother-daughter, father-daughter, mother-son, and father-son. In the activation relationship (paternal functions), one could expect the father to activate children more than the mother, yielding a descending order of father-son, mother-son, father-daughter, and mother-daughter. These sex differences in the parent-child activation relationship should already be significant with toddlers, since competition over resources (food, toys, warmth from adults, social rank, friends, etc.; Charlesworth, 1988) begins early, judging by the peak in 2-year-olds' physical aggression (Tremblay et al., 1999), with boys becoming significantly more physically aggressive than girls and girls displaying more indirect aggression than boys, starting from age three (Archer & Côté, 2005; Vaillancourt, 2005).

The Research to Date

This section presents studies inspired by the activation relationship theory that have developed instruments (the risky situation procedure, openness to the world, challenging parenting behavior, etc.) to be able to explore the effects of paternal behaviors on children's development. We will also address physical play, and especially rough-and-tumble play, since it is theoretically associated with activation (see Paquette, 2004a). The reader should be advised that this section will sometimes be in the form of a flowing list of findings as opposed to a series of logically connected paragraphs. We have intentionally omitted sociodemographic data from most of the studies given their significant volume and their low relevance to our analysis. Finally, the section puts special emphasis on the presence or absence of sex differences in parents and children.

(a) The Activation Relationship and Activative Fathering

Drawing inspiration from the Strange Situation Procedure (SSP; Ainsworth et al., 1978), Paquette and Bigras (2010) validated the Risky Situation (RS) with fathers and mothers, a 20-minute standard observation procedure assessing 12–18–month-olds' activation relationship. In the RS, the child is invited to take progressive risks, first social and then physical. The parent is asked not to interact with the child and especially not to encourage the child to explore. However, the parent may comfort the child at any time and is asked to ensure the child' safety and protection. After instructions have been given to the parent, the child is seated on the floor in front of available toys, while the parent reads a magazine on a chair behind the child (Episode 1). Then, a male stranger enters the room, sits on the floor, and starts playing with the toys without interacting with the child or the parent (Episode 2). After 3 minutes, or earlier if the child initiates interaction with him, the male stranger starts playing with the child and becomes increasingly stimulating and intrusive (Episode 3). Toys are put away and a big colorful set of stairs that was hidden behind drapes is revealed (Episode 4); the parent is instructed to get up from the chair to make sure the child is safe during exploration only if the latter starts to climb the stairs. The parent is then told to ask the child to go up and down the stairs (Episode 5). Finally, the parent is asked to forbid the child to climb the stairs (Episode 6). The coding grid permits children to be classified as activated, underactivated, or overactivated and also provides three scores from 0 to 5; a high activation score is indicating the degree to which the child is optimally activated (with 5 being the most positive activation relationship). As previously introduced, in the RS, underactivated children tend to engage in little exploration, be passive, and withdraw from novelty or remain close to the parent. Activated children are confident and prudent in their exploration and obey when the parent sets a limit. Overactivated children are reckless and noncompliant when the parent sets limits. In theory, underactivation is related to parental overprotection, and overactivation is related to a lack of parental discipline. The coding system with its five criteria was designed for ease of use by clinicians as well as researchers, requiring an average of 30 minutes per case. The Preschool Risky Situation (PRS), an RS adaptation that essentially involves presenting toys suitable for children 2–5 years old (replacing the set of stairs with a stepladder), was subsequently created for children of this age (Gaumon & Paquette, 2013).

Administering the SSP and the RS to a small sample of father-child dyads with toddlers has revealed both measures as being orthogonal, since only 24% of children had both a secure relationship and an activated relationship with the same parent (Paquette & Dumont, 2013a). Observational studies on the activation relationship have systematically shown that parents activate boys more than girls at age 12–18 months (Dumont & Paquette, 2013; Paquette & Bigras, 2010) and at preschool age (Gaumon & Paquette, 2013). The use of the RS has also uncovered associations between father-child activation and internalizing problems in toddlers (Dumont & Paquette, 2013) and preschoolers (Gaumon & Paquette, 2013): underactivated children with fathers have significantly more internalizing problems.

There were significant associations between some dimensions of temperament and the activation relationship, but the paternal stimulation of risk-taking explains activation once child sex and temperament, the father-child attachment relationship, and emotional support are taken into account (Paquette & Dumont, 2013a). Moreover, discipline (punishment) and stimulation (comprising items from the physical play, emotional support, and opening to the world scales) are moderator variables of the activation—social competence association (Dumont & Paquette, 2013). When paternal involvement in punishment was low, the more children were positively activated, the more socially competent they were. The same result was obtained when paternal involvement in stimulation was low.

Moffette (2013) found no significant association between father's parental stress and father-child activation and attachment relationships. Hamel (2014) verified the stability of the father-child activation relationship with 39 dyads who underwent the RS and the PRS. The findings highlighted that only 46% of the children remained in the same category. However, the percentage of activated children climbed from 44 to 77, suggesting an improvement in the activation relationship over time. Bueno, Vieira, Crepaldi, and Faraco (2017) recently confirmed the validity of PRS in evaluating the father-child activation relationship in Brazil and concluded that fathers have a greater tendency to activate boys and to protect girls.

Gaumon, Paquette, Cyr, Emond-Nakamura, and St-André (2016) administered the preschool SSP to mother-child dyads and the PRS to father-child dyads in the same family in a clinical sample (82% of boys). They found (1) no significant correlation between activation scores and anxiety scores, (2) no significant association between the attachment relationship with the mother and the activation relationship with the father, and (3) the status of the father-child activation relationship as a protective factor in the relation between disorganized attachment to mother and child anxiety: disorganized attachment with the mother is predictive of fewer anxiety symptoms in children when the quality of the activation relationship with the father is good (high activation score). In the same sample, unpublished results showed that overactivated preschoolers displayed significantly more externalizing problems than did children with either an activated or an underactivated relationship with their father. The use of a larger sample of the general population will help verify in the future if activation is associated with competition, externalizing problems, and physical and relational aggression in children.

Rather than evaluate activation in terms of dyads, a recent approach has been to focus on the activative behaviors of the parents. In the United States, Stevenson and Crnic (2013) have used four variables arising from observation of preschool-age children (low detachedness, high intrusiveness, high opportunity for interaction, and high cognitive stimulation) to obtain a latent factor called "activative fathering." Results showed, among other things, that high activative fathering was associated with later lower levels of behavior dysregulation during a problem-solving task as well as higher levels of child sociability. Contrary to expectations, paternal control did not moderate these relations. According to the authors, it would have been preferable to evaluate control during specific tasks related to risk-taking rather than with respect to activities such as play with friends and bedtime routines.

Also, in the United States, Volling, Stevenson, Safyer, Gonzalez, and Lee (2019) observed 12-month-old infants during three challenging teaching tasks with fathers and mothers. The use of a person-centered approach highlighted four similar parenting profiles in fathers and mothers, but fathers outnumbered mothers in the activation profile. These fathers engaged in moderate intrusiveness and cognitive stimulation, with moderately high levels of sensitivity and positive regard. Moreover, 30% of infants had an activation profile with both fathers and mothers.

Future research would benefit from exploring new avenues for evaluating activation. For example, in the course of their participation in the Jacobs Foundation residence Program in September 2015, Brenda Volling, Matthew Stevenson, Natasha Cabrera, and Daniel Paquette developed an observation grid to be able to evaluate the activation relationship based on parent-child play. The grid is intended to be more user- and environmentally friendly than the RS, which requires the use of precise materials in a laboratory. The instrument is composed of three Likert 5-level questions (very low to very high or consistent): active challenging behavior, excitation/arousal/destabilization, and proper limit-setting/control. It is currently being validated with various types of play (free vs. structured, physical vs. pretend, etc.). The second version with four scales has recently been tested by Daniel Paquette and Carole Gagnon, first with 8-minute father-child RTP and second with the 2-minute laughing task, completed after the RS. The first scale, the active challenging behavior scale, focuses on parental behaviors of stimulating exploration and risk-taking. The second deals with parental behaviors that surprise or momentarily destabilize the child, thus raising their level of excitement. The control dimension was divided into two scales to distinguish between (a) parental behaviors of discipline and limit-setting that ensure the child's safety in high-risk situations and (b) parental behaviors seeking to structure the game and guide the activity. The scale used here for each of the dimensions has four levels: 0 = no parental behavior; 1 = low level; 2 = optimal level; 3 = excessive level. Compared to the previous version and to the observational CPB of Majdandzic, de Vente, and Bögels (2016), the two main advantages of this new grid, currently being validated, are the following: (1) better evaluating the parent's level of behavior according to the child's reactions and (2) taking into account the fact that "too much" is just as detrimental to the child as "not enough." For example, it is well known that children develop behavior problems in cases of "too much discipline" (overcontrol) as in cases of "too little" (permissiveness).

(b) Paternal Behaviors of Openness to the World

Paquette, Eugène, Dubeau, and Gagnon (2009) created the Openness to the World Questionnaire (OWQ) to evaluate paternal behaviors linked to the activation relationship with preschool-age children. The factor analysis revealed three dimensions explaining 42% of total variance: stimulation of perseverance, punishment, and stimulation of risk-taking. The average scores on the three scales were not significantly different between boys and girls.

Michel Martin Eugène, Daniel Paquette, and Amélie Dubé created the Adolescent Openness to the World Questionnaire (AOWQ), a self-report questionnaire for teenagers, regarding the "openness to the world" their father demonstrated during their childhood. The factor analysis brought to light five factors explaining 49% of total variance (Eugène, Paquette, & Claes, 2010). Stimulation of exploration includes items related to environmental exploration, the invention of new games, and the use of new words. Stimulation of competition has to do with encouragement to compete and achieve victory in sports and other activities. Stimulation of risk-taking consists in encouraging the child to engage in risky activities and giving them significant autonomy in exploring their environment. Stimulation of perseverance consists in encouraging the child to successfully carry out difficult undertakings and to persevere in the face of adversity. Finally, punishment refers to punishing the child when he/she disobey an order or act inappropriately. The boys were found to be more stimulated to take risks and compete than the girls.

Bachand (2013) adapted the QOMA to create the Parent Openness to the World Questionnaire (POWQ) for children of primary school age. It is made up of four factors: stimulation of competition, stimulation of risk-taking, stimulation of perseverance, and discipline and teaching of responsibilities. Results showed that stimulation of perseverance and discipline and responsibilities are significantly positively associated with the total score for quality of father-child attachment relationship (assessed with the child's attitude toward the father; Giuli & Hudson, 1977) and with the score for father's sense of parental competence.

Paraventi et al. (2017) adapted the OWQ for adults without children, regarding their perception of parents in general. They asked university students in Southern Brazil to successively fill out a father-son version and a father-daughter version of the questionnaire, using a counterbalanced approach. Brazilian university students perceive fathers as more strongly stimulating risk-taking, stimulating perseverance as well as punishment in boys as opposed to girls.

Vandystadt (2017) has created a global index of openness to the world by combining three scales from the Montreal Father's Involvement Questionnaire (Paquette, Bolté, Turcotte, Dubeau, & Bouchard, 2000): introduction to novelty, physical play, and discipline. Findings showed that this index of openness to the world is not associated with the level of activation by fathers in children aged 12–18 months and that the parental alliance does not moderate this association.

In sum, questionnaires completed by fathers on encouraging openness to the world in their preschool-age children showed no differences according to child's sex, be it in Canada (Paquette et al., 2009) or in Brazil (Bueno et al., 2018). However, retrospective questionnaires completed by adolescents or young adults have shown sex differences in children both in Canada (Eugène, 2008; Eugène et al., 2010) and in Brazil (Paraventi et al., 2017; Schulz, 2015).

A few specific dimensions of parental behavior seem to more readily highlight differences according to child's sex and parent's sex. Adolescents revealed that Canadian fathers stimulate their sons to take more risks and to compete than their daughters and stimulate risk-taking more than mothers (Eugène et al., 2010). However, mothers stimulated exploration and perseverance more than fathers and stimulated competition more strongly in boys than in girls (Eugène et al., 2010). Adolescents revealed that Brazilian fathers stimulate more risk-taking and competition in boys but more exploration in girls (Schulz, 2015). Brazilian university students perceive fathers as more strongly stimulating risk-taking, stimulating perseverance as well as punishment in boys as opposed to girls (Paraventi et al., 2017). To date, few studies have explored the link between parents' openness to the world and youths' development. A study in Canada showed that only paternal stimulation (and not maternal stimulation) is associated with adolescent homelessness after controlling for emotional deprivation and sexual abuse: the homeless received less stimulation of openness to the world from their fathers than the nonhomeless (Eugène, 2008). In Brazil, stimulation of perseverance and stimulation of risk-taking as reported by fathers are not associated with prosocial behaviors but are associated with fewer behavior problems in preschoolers, with family functioning also playing a moderating role between stimulation of perseverance and behavior problems (Bueno et al., 2018). When family functioning is positive (high balanced cohesion or high balanced flexibility), the more stimulation of perseverance is associated to less emotional symptoms in the child. It is worth noting that da Silva (2017) used the "Big Five" personality traits with this sample to shed light on the four personality profiles of fathers with respect to dimensions of openness to the world. Two profiles proved to be associated with greater stimulation of risk-taking: the first was more associated with punishment, whereas the second was more associated with more stimulation of perseverance. In Belgium, no significant parent sex differences were found on the challenge/encouragement scale (Fliek, Daemen, Roelofs, & Muris, 2015).

Finally, for future research, it is important to stress that the punishment scale is inadequate and should be replaced with a real measurement of positive control focused on parental limit-setting and guidance to ensure children's safety during exploration of their environment. Punishment has been positively associated with behavior problems in children (Bueno et al., 2018), has not been found to significantly contribute to the phenomenon of adolescent homelessness (Eugène, 2008), and has not been associated with children's injury-risk behavior, whereas encouragement of perseverance and less risk-taking stimulation have predicted lower injury-risk behavior in preschoolers (StGeorge, Fletcher, Freeman, Paquette, & Dumont, 2015).

(c) Challenging Parenting Behavior

Paquette (2004a, 2004b) suggested that fathers are primarily engaged in an activation relationship with their children, that is, challenging them to confront and master unfamiliar and unpredictable elements in the outside world.

Majdandzic et al. (2016) have created and validated self-report questionnaires and observational procedures to evaluate challenging parenting behavior (CPB) in fathers and mothers when their children are, respectively, aged 4 months, 1 year, and 2.5 years. The CPB questionnaires assess the degree to which the parent encourages the child socio-emotionally and physically to exhibit risky behavior, or behavior that causes the child to go beyond his/her comfort zone. It includes seven subscales: teasing, RTP, encouragement of risk-taking, social daring, competition, encouragement of assertiveness, and challenging modeling. It should be mentioned that the RTP scale contains only one item on rough-and-tumble-play, with the others being physical play.

Questionnaires completed by Dutch parents showed that fathers have a significantly higher score than mothers on global CPB only for children 2.5 years and above and only on physical (not verbal) CPB (Lazarus et al., 2016; Majdandzic et al., 2016). However, according to Majdandzic, Möller, de Vente, Bögels, and van den Boom (2014), fathers were significantly more challenging toward their 2-year-old child than mothers and did not differ toward the 4-year-old. At 1 year of age, fathers set themselves apart only for more physical play than mothers, and mothers, by more challenging modeling than fathers (Majdandzic et al., 2016). Observations of challenging behavior did not reveal a clear pattern of differences between fathers and mothers, likely owing to the types of tasks that were chosen. For example, Majdandzic et al. (2016) used varied tasks, while Majdandzic et al. (2014) used risk-free tasks focused on verbal components (puzzle and game tasks). These studies found no differences between girls and boys on global CPB score, with the exception of one study that found more stimulation of competition in father-son dyads than in father-daughter dyads with 3- to 4-year-old children (Majdandzic et al., 2018). The fathers engaged in more physical play and stimulation of competition than the mothers with 2.5-year-old children (Majdandzic et al., 2016).

Studies on challenging behavior showed that the factorial structure of the CPB questionnaire is equivalent for fathers and mothers, in two different countries, in Dutch and Australian families (Majdandzic et al., 2016; for the 4–6 years version: Majdandzic, Lazarus, et al., 2018). The CPB scores obtained by questionnaire and by observation were also positively correlated together. The scores of the fathers and the mothers were also positively correlated together. Only paternal (not maternal) CPB was associated with less behavioral inhibition (Majdandzic et al., 2014) and less fear in children when controlling for parental anxiety (Möller, Majdandzic, & Bögels, 2015). Finally, the CPB scores of both parents were associated with less anxiety in children (Lazarus et al., 2016), but only the father's score was significantly associated with anxiety when both scores were entered into the same model (Majdandzic, de Vente Colonnesi, & Bögels, 2018).

(d) Rough-and-Tumble Play (RTP)

In the seminal article on the theory of the activation relationship, Paquette (2004a) posited that the activation relationship develops primarily through physical play. The catalyst behind this theory is the fact that fathers are generally less involved than mothers in all dimensions of parenting with the exception of physical play. Research over the last few years in Brazil, Belgium, Netherlands, and Canada have, indeed, confirmed that fathers engage in vigorous physical contact play more frequently than mothers do (Fliek et al., 2015; Gomes, 2015; Majdandzic et al., 2016). Paquette (2004a), primarily interested in the socialization of aggression in children 2–5 years old, focused more specifically on RTP (the most frequent type of physical play) as a possible mechanism for regulating aggression. The article also postulated that the father's control in father-child RTP promotes children's obedience and that role reversals enable the development of competition skills in children.

Fathers generally report more often engaging in RTP with their young children than mothers and more so with boys than with girls (Flanders, Leo, Paquette, Pihl, & Séguin, 2009; Paquette et al., 2003). However, still according to questionnaires, mothers do not engage in more RTP with boys than with girls (Flanders, 2008). Our observational pilot study entitled *Père-En-Jeux* (see Paquette et al., 2003) uncovered greater differences in the frequency and duration of father-son RTP than father-daughter RTP, but the most recent observational study by Dubé (2011) found no significant differences.

The use of self-report questionnaires by parents has shown that father-child and mother-child RTP frequencies are positively correlated with each other (Flanders et al., 2007). The same is true of physical play (Fliek et al., 2015). None of the studies on father-child RTP frequency has turned up direct significant associations with behavior problems or prosocial behaviors, except for one positive correlation with physical aggression in boys (Paquette et al., 2003). Dubé (2011) also obtained no direct significant correlations between duration or frequency of father-child RTP as self-reported by fathers in a questionnaire and the social adjustment of children in daycare (social competence, anxiety/withdrawal, aggression/irritability) evaluated by the educator. However, Gomes (2015) showed that a higher frequency of father-child physical play in Brazil predicted fewer externalizing behaviors in children. In this comparative study, the Canadian fathers engaged in more physical play than the Brazilian fathers, but the latter disciplined their children more than the former. Moreover, according to StGeorge et al. (2015), father-child RTP duration (but not frequency), assessed by questionnaire, was negatively associated with injury-risk behaviors in children.

Flanders (2008) has reported some questionnaire-based studies on mother-child RTP conducted by the GRIP (research unit on children's psychosocial maladjustment). Two studies have shown that mother-child RTP frequency is not associated with behavior problems (physical aggression, hyperactivity, and opposition) (Flanders, 2008; Flanders et al., 2007); two studies have found that it is positively associated with prosocial behaviors (see Flanders, 2008); and one study has found that it is positively associated with hyperactivity and inattention in children (see Flanders, 2008). In addition, frequency of mother-child RTP may be associated with physical aggression when taking into account child age and aggression trajectories: mother-child RTP is negatively associated with physical aggression for children under 60 months of age in the high trajectory and appears to be positively associated with physical aggression for older children, also in the high trajectory (Flanders, 2008). In other words, if these results are confirmed by other research, it might mean that mother-child RTP is effective in regulating emotions in preschool-age children who have longitudinally maintained a high aggression score but has a negative effect for school-aged children in the high trajectory. It is worth pointing out that researchers have not attempted to verify these results for the children's trajectories with fathers.

Fletcher, StGeorge, and Freeman (2013) have developed an observational measure of RTP quality (RTP-Q), which they used in Australia in two contexts enabling the occurrence of RTP, namely, get-up and sock wrestle games, and showed that high-quality father-child RTP is negatively associated with behavior problems (especially conduct problems and peer problems) in children after controlling for father involvement in caregiving tasks. The RTP-Q score was not associated with prosocial behavior. The fact that the behavior problems were not associated with another type of traditional play, such as toy play (StGeorge, Fletcher, & Palazzi, 2017), confirms that RTP is a better context than other types of games for teaching children to regulate their emotions and hence diminish behavior problems.

Significant associations appear when play quality indices act as moderating variables. Observational studies have shown that the dominance relationship during play is an important indicator of quality for predicting aggressive behavior, at least in China and in Canada (Anderson, Qiu, & Wheeler, 2017; Flanders et al., 2009, 2010). Thus, when the father exerts more dominance over his child, frequency of RTP is negatively associated with physical aggression and emotion regulation problems. Two other moderating variables have been brought to light, but only in boys (Dubé, 2011). The hierarchy of the father with respect to the boy must be coupled with mutuality: when interactions tend to be two-way, long duration of RTP is associated with greater social competence and less aggression in the boy. In other words, to enable reciprocity between the play partners, the hierarchy must not be too pronounced. The other moderating variable is the boy's fear during the play. Activation consists in provoking emotions in the child and then helping him regulate them. To do so, the father must be sensitive to the optimal margin of excitement depending on the specific characteristics of his child (e.g., temperament). It has been shown that when the boy is slightly but not overly frightened, duration of father-child is associated with greater social competence. This supports the idea of an optimal level of excitement and that, as noted previously, "too much" is just as detrimental to the child as "not enough." Finally, father-child RTP frequency at 3 years of age has been positively associated with the activation score only in boys (Paquette & Dumont, 2013b).

Sex Differences in Parent-Child Activation Relationship with Toddlers

The primary objective of this section is to verify, using a larger sample than prior studies, the presence of sex differences in the parent-child activation relationship at 12–18 months, and more specifically the prediction that fathers activate children more than mothers but that both parents activate boys more than girls. The secondary purpose of this section is to verify whether the activation relationship is associated with sociodemographic characteristics. To this end, we use data from the complementarity of attachment relationships (CAR) project and more particularly the RS coding for 12–18-month-olds, which has recently been made available.

The main goal of the CAR project in Montreal (Canada) is to verify whether the mother-child attachment and father-child activation relationships are complementary in predicting socio-affective development and risk-taking in the children of two-parent families in the general population. Children may be expected to be better adjusted to their environment when the parental functions between the two parents are complementary. Both the attachment relationship and the activation relationship of children are evaluated respectively using the SSP and the RS with each of the two parents, first between 12 and 18 months of age and then between 3.5 and 4 years old. The children's social adjustment is evaluated at age 4 by the daycare educator. This project will also allow for verifying the stability and predictive validity of RS. The activation relationship is anticipated to better predict externalizing problems (especially aggression) and internalizing problems (particularly anxiety) than the attachment relationship (ABC system). It is also expected that the activation relationship will predict children's competition at daycare, whereas attachment will predict their empathy and ability to forge positive and lasting relationships with others. The father is expected to activate the children more than the mother, and both parents are expected to activate boys more than girls. Hence, the primary activation figure is expected to have a greater influence on the children's development than the secondary; the same goes for attachment. Finally, associations are expected to be found between children's temperament and the activation relationship, but stimulation of risk-taking is anticipated to more strongly explain activation after controlling for children's characteristics (sex and temperament).

Interrater agreement was obtained for the entire sample by two raters (one man and one woman) and stands at 81% (Kappa = .66) for classification. The intraclass correlations are, respectively, 0.92 for the underactivation scale, 0.83 for the activation scale, and 0.91 for the overactivation scale. Disagreements were discussed with a third judge until a consensus was reached. RS procedural flaws were observed in 9.7% of mother-child dyads and 11.9% of father-child dyads, but they are not significantly associated with the three activation scores. Counterbalancing the RS (at a 1-month interval) with the father and the RS with the mother is significantly correlated with the father-child activation score ($r = -.197$, $p = .008$), such that the father-child activation score is lower when the RS with the father comes first.

Table 19.1 outlines the demographic characteristics of the sample, 49.7% of which is composed of boys (89/179). A total of 75% of the fathers and 53% of the mothers have an annual personal income of $40,000CAN or more. In the sample, 23% of the fathers and 24% of the mothers were born outside Canada.

Table 19.1 Sociodemographic characteristics of the sample ($n = 179$)

	Mean (SD)	Min-max
Mother's age	32.7 (4.5)	17–46
Father's age	34.6 (4.7)	23–45
Mother's education	16.2 (2.8)	9–27
Father's education	15.6 (2.8)	6–23
Mother's number of hours worked per week	26.4 (15.3)	0–55
Father's number of hours worked per week	37.8 (13.6)	0–80
Child's age at the RS with the mother (months)	15.3 (1.8)	12–19
Child's age at the RS with the father (months)	15.4 (1.8)	12–20
No. of children in family	1.5 (.8)	1–5

Table 19.2 shows that the prevalence of the activated relationship is relatively similar in the father-child dyads and mother-child dyads, that is, respectively 63.7% and 59.2%. The same is true of the underactivated relationship, that is, respectively 21.8% and 20.7%. However, the prevalence of the overactivated relationship is greater in the mother-child dyads (20.1%) than in the father-child dyads (14.5%).

Table 19.2 also shows that 41.9% of the children have an activated relationship with both parents. The crossed distribution between fathers and mothers differs significantly compared to random distribution ($chi^2 = 29.30$, $df = 4$, $p < .001$). In particular, there are more children under/under, fewer act/under and under/act, and more act/act and over/over than would be random.

The results of the paired T-test show that the underactivation and activation scores are significantly higher in the father-child dyads than in the mother-child dyads, while the overactivation score is significantly higher in the mother-child dyads (Table 19.3).

Table 19.4 presents the three mother-child and father-child scores according to child's sex. Neither fathers nor mothers activate boys more than girls. However, mothers and fathers (and more so the latter) underactivate girls more than boys. In addition, mothers and fathers (and more so the former) overactivate boys more than girls. The results of Tables 19.3 and 19.4 did not change when using residuals after controlling for the counterbalancing of the two RS procedures.

According to Table 19.5, more boys than girls are overactivated, for both mother-child and father-child dyads. However, more girls than boys are underactivated in the father-child dyads.

We conducted analyses to determine whether the activation relationship was associated with sociodemographic variables. The father's income is associated with the father-child activation relationship, whereas the mother's income is associated neither with mother-child activation nor with father-child activation (although both incomes are significantly correlated: $r = .18$, $p = .017$). More specifically, the father's income is slightly correlated with underactivation score

Table 19.2 Prevalence (%) of father-child and mother-child types of activation relationship in 179 families

Mother-child	Father-child			Total
	underactivated	activated	overactivated	
Underactivated	10.6	8.9	1.1	20.7
Activated	9.5	41.9	7.8	59.2
Overactivated	1.7	12.8	5.6	20.1
Total	21.8	63.7	14.5	100

Table 19.3 Paired T-tests on activation scores between mother-child and father-child dyads

Scores	Mother-child	Father-child	t (df = 178)	p
Underactivation	2.11 (1.34)	2.37 (1.18)	−2.69	.008
Activation	3.15 (.99)	3.35 (.98)	−2.11	.037
Overactivation	2.16 (1.29)	1.86 (1.17)	3.07	.002

Table 19.4 Comparison of means (SD) of mother-child (M-C) and father-child (F-C) scores between boys and girls

Scores	Boys (n = 89)	Girls (n = 90)	t (df = 177)	p
M-C underactivation	1.90 (1.34)	2.30 (1.30)	−2.03	.044
M-C activation	3.10 (1.06)	3.21 (.91)	−.73	.464
M-C overactivation	2.43 (1.21)	1.89 (1.31)	2.88	.004
F-C underactivation	2.17 (1.15)	2.56 (1.17)	−2.26	.025
F-C activation	3.37 (.94)	3.33 (1.04)	.24	.815
F-C overactivation	2.08 (1.21)	1.65 (1.10)	2.51	.013

Table 19.5 Percentage (%) of boys in mother-child and father-child according to activation types

	Underactivated	Activated	Overactivated
Mother-child dyads	45.9	47.2	61.6
Father-child dyads	33.3	51.8	65.4

(r = .15, p = .050) and overactivation score (r = −.17, p = .024). The three father-child activation scores are not associated with the father's education, age, number of hours worked per week, number of children in the family, or immigration factor (born outside of Canada). The same is true of the three mother-child activation scores, except for a significant correlation between activation score and number of children in the family (r = .15, p = .047). Moreover, the mother-child activation score is significantly correlated with the father's number of hours worked per week (r = −.22, p = .003): the mother mainly activates the children when the father works less.

Discussion

As Möller et al. (2013) have noted, fathers and mothers prepare their children for their future gender roles. Our results support the conclusion that sex differences in the parent-child activation relationship emerge very early on, that is, well before children's behaviors differ significantly according to sex. The paternal function, whether assumed by either or both parents, could open the child up to the world by enabling them to explore their physical environment and to cope with social competition.

The analyses conducted with this larger sample of toddlers show for the first time that fathers activate children more than mothers when the child's sex is not taken into account, and starting at an early age (12–18 months old). However, in contrast with what has been found with smaller samples to date, fathers and mothers do not activate boys more than girls, at least according to activation score. This is confirmed by the equal number of girls and boys in the activation category.

Above all, our results bring to light that fathers underactivate children more than mothers, and both underactivate girls more than boys; this yields a descending order of father-daughter, mother-daughter, father-son, and mother-son. Additionally, mothers overactivate children more than fathers, and both overactivate boys more than girls, for a descending order of mother-son, father-son, mother-daughter, and father-daughter. This translated into more boys in the overactivation category and more girls in the father-child underactivation category. In other words, fathers have a tendency to overprotect girls more than boys, whereas mothers exhibit greater difficulty setting limits for boys. Rather than contradicting the theory, these results clarify which scales of the activation relationship are important for shedding light on sex differences.

Research has uncovered that both maternal and paternal overprotection are associated with more child anxiety and with less challenging parenting behavior (Majdandzic, de Vente Colonnesi, & Bögels, 2018). Fathers appear to engage in less overprotection than mothers (Möller et al., 2015), but more challenging parenting behavior than mothers (Lazarus et al., 2016). Our results on underactivation nevertheless support the idea that fathers' overprotection has a greater impact on children's development than mothers' overprotection. Along these lines, Majdandzic, de Vente Colonnesi, and Bögels (2018) have shown that only paternal CPB predicts anxiety when maternal and paternal CPB are entered into the same model.

Fathers' greater overprotection of daughters could magnify girls' biological predisposition to be more cautious, that is, more risk-aversive, on average than boys (Eckel & Grossman, 2008), and potentially to develop anxiety problems. Mothers' greater difficulty with disciplining and setting limits on boys during exploration than fathers could magnify boys' biological predispositions to take more risks on average and potentially to have more accidents and to develop aggression problems. A meta-analysis by Else-Quest, Hyde, Goldsmith, and van Hulle (2006) has shown significant differences between sexes with respect to young children's temperament: an average effect size in favor of boys for the "surgency" factor (level of activity, impulsiveness, enjoyment associated with high-intensity stimuli, etc.) and a large effect size in favor of girls for the "effortful control" factor (sustained attention, inhibitory control, enjoyment associated with low-intensity stimuli, etc.). Girls express fear earlier than boys and show more hesitation and greater distress in approaching novel objects (Campbell, 2009). According to Campbell (2009), the sex difference in fear accounts for a considerable portion of differences observed in aggressive behavior.

Finally, the prediction that overactivation would be associated with a quantitative reproductive strategy is partly confirmed. Father-child overactivation is indeed correlated with a lower paternal income. In addition, as predicted, we obtained more overactivated boys than overactivated girls. However, more siblings were expected to be found in this profile than in the two other profiles, which did not turn out to be the case. It would be worth verifying, in the future, if overactivated boys use more physical aggression than children in the two other profiles. The fact that mother-child activation score is associated with more children at home and a spouse who works less often may potentially be explained by the fact that the presence of peers and the greater presence of the spouse at home promote optimal mother-child activation—either directly, via the modelling of the spouse and older children, or indirectly, via a fairer distribution of parental tasks between the two spouses, which would enable mothers to be more active in paternal functions. It would also be worthwhile to verify if fathers engage more in daily tasks when they work less outside the home. Another aspect to be investigated would be whether the quality of the mother-child activation relationship is lower in single-parent families. Finally, we confirmed the presence of more girls than boys in the underactivated profile, but only for the father-child activation relationship. This result once more confirms that more paternal overprotection likely has a greater impact on children's development than maternal overprotection.

Summary and Key Points

To sum up, fathers appear to play a greater role than mothers when it comes to activating children, whether via RTP, openness to the world, or challenging behavior. The activation relationship as evaluated by the RS helps bring to light the presence, already in toddlers, of double moderation by parent's sex and child's sex, while parental behaviors related to activation (RTP, openness to the world, and challenging behavior) are showing differences between girls and boys only starting from preschool age (3 years old) when there are differences. The results of studies on openness to the world as well as challenging parenting behavior indicate that the most important dimensions of paternal functions in highlighting sex differences are stimulation of competition and stimulation of risk-taking.

It would be important in the future to diversify the outcome variables. For example, the openness to the world questionnaires and quality of RTP observations could be used in connection with internalizing problems in children and anxiety in particular. The challenging behavior instruments could help verify associations with competition, risk-taking, and externalizing problems in children, especially aggression. Finally, it is important to avoid confusing physical play and RTP given that different types of physical play can in theory serve different functions in children's development.

It is important to note that prosocial behaviors do not seem to be associated with father-child activation. The only association found has been between father-son RTP and social competence in Canadian boys but only when the boy's fear is low during the RTP (Dubé, 2011). No association was found in Brazil between fathers' openness to the world and prosocial behaviors in children (Bueno et al., 2018). Research has shown prosocial behaviors as being associated with mother-child RTP in Canada (Flanders, 2008), and not with father-child RTP in Australia (Fletcher et al., 2013). An association has been found between the activation relationship and the social competence of Canadian children, but only when the fathers displayed little involvement in stimulation or in punishment (Dumont & Paquette, 2013). In the United States, Stevenson and Crnic (2013) have found an association between their concept of activative fathering and sociability, but the use of puzzle tasks rather than risk-taking tasks may have influenced the results. In other words, the play context and the dimensions observed are of paramount importance in shedding light on father-mother differences and their differential impact on children's development. Bureau et al. (2014) have shown that mothers are in greater synchrony with their child during the laughing task without toys than are fathers. If these researchers have found no other differences between the mothers and fathers of preschool-age children, it might be because the scales used to establish the factors were based on concepts of collaboration, sensitivity (in the traditional sense of the term), and respect for the child's rhythm in a context of caring (snack time) and quiet play. It may be supposed that the use of scales based on a definition of sensitivity adapted to the exciting physical play concept, and on concepts of competition, intrusiveness, risk-taking, and surprising the child, could reveal differences in favor of the fathers. In their discussion, these last authors mention having had the impression that fathers mainly tended to engage in physical play and intrusiveness, and their children tended to "express a wider variety of emotional states such as surprise and momentary discomfort while also becoming hysterically happy and hyperaroused."

In our view, prosocial behaviors should normally be mainly associated with maternal functions. Logically, we should also expect to find more sex differences for emotions respectively associated with the maternal functions and the paternal functions. As the principal agents of socialization up through the end of preschool age, parents help children learn to modulate their emotional expressions according to the everyday contexts they encounter and the values embraced by society. Gender socialization arises from societal constructions of gender and from distinct biological predispositions of girls and boys (Pomerantz et al., 2004). Parents often show differential attention to boys and girls that reinforce biological predispositions toward different gender roles (in the same direction). In the United States, women are expected to express more emotions that support relationships than men, and men are expected to be more assertive and even overtly aggressive if needed (Chaplin, Cole, & Zahn-Waxler, 2005).

The field dedicated to emotion socialization could, in the future, be examined in light of maternal and paternal functions as presented in activation relationship theory. Indeed, mothers and fathers are both invested in their children' emotional lives, but their roles differ depending on child's sex and the type of emotion the child is displaying (Kennedy Root & Rubin, 2010). Mothers seem to play a much greater role in communication and the expression of emotions, both of which are key elements of the attachment relationship. Compared to fathers, mothers elaborate more on emotional experiences during conversations with children, are more intensely expressive of both positive and some negative emotions, are more apt to experience a wider variety of emotions, and are more accurate decoders of emotions (Denham, Bassett, & Wyatt, 2010; Leaper, Anderson, & Sanders, 1998; Premo & Kiel, 2014; van der Pol et al., 2015; Zaman & Fivush, 2013). Moreover, mothers engage in more conversational, supportive, and interpretative communication with daughters than with sons from infancy through at least elementary school (Lovas, 2011). Mothers and fathers use a greater number and variety of emotion words with daughters than with sons during the preschool years (Fivush, Brotman, Buckner, & Goodman, 2000). During childhood and adolescence, mothers focus with daughters on internal feeling states and with sons on the causes and consequences of their actions and on practical problem-solving skills (Fivush, 1989, 1991; Kuebli, Butler, & Fivush, 1995).

Fathers use more instrumental language, such as directives and informing statements (Leaper et al., 1998). In case of perceived difficulties in the child, fathers have been found to engage in more discussion of emotional antecedents (causes of sadness) than mothers, whereas mothers have devoted more of the discussion to emotional states (Cassano & Zeman, 2010). There is burgeoning evidence that under conditions of risk, fathers may play a particularly important role in emotion socialization (Garside, 2004). We posit that anger may be more closely associated with the activation relationship whereas sadness may be more closely associated with the attachment relationship. Parents tolerate anger expressions more in boys than in girls, while sadness and fear are discouraged more in boys than in girls (see van der Pol et al., 2015). Mothers respond attentively to their toddler boys' expression of anger but tend to ignore or attempt to inhibit their girls' anger (Radke-Yarrow & Kochanska, 1990). Mothers even encourage anger in boys, since they demonstrate more positive emotional responses to their preschool-age sons' anger displays than their daughters' anger (Cole, Teti, & Zahn-Waxler, 2003). Mothers and fathers have discussed sadness more frequently with daughters than with sons, even though girls did not initiate conversations about sadness more than boys (Adams, Kuebli, Boyle, & Fivush, 1995; Fivush et al., 2000). Finally, fathers are particularly punitive in response to their son's displays of negative emotions, especially vulnerable emotions such as sadness and fear (Eisenberg et al., 1999). In future research, it would be especially important to undertake observational studies since, according to Leaper et al.'s (1998) meta-analysis, parents are more likely to treat girls and boys differently when behavioral observations are used rather than self-report methods. This could be explained by social desirability. It could also be explained by the primary role of indirect socialization (interactions and behaviors that do not especially reflect a socializer's beliefs, values, and goals), which has its roots in our primate ancestors, well before the development of human consciousness and hence direct socialization. Educators know that children tend more strongly to do what we do ourselves, as opposed to what we tell them to do.

Acknowledgments We thank the parents and children for their participation, the students for collecting and coding the data, and the three coordinators who successively planned the entire project, namely, Jessica Vaillancourt, Jessica Vandystadt, and Nathalie Dumas. This study was supported by a grant from Social Sciences and Humanities Research Council of Canada, number 435-2014-0448. The researchers associated with this project are Marc Bigras and Chantal Cyr of Université du Québec à Montréal; Karine Dubois-Comtois of Université du Québec à Trois-Rivières; Jean-Pascal Lemelin of Université de Sherbrooke; Sophie Couture of the Institut universitaire Jeunes en difficulté, the Centre intégré universitaire de santé et de services sociaux du Centre-Sud-de-l'île-de-Montréal; and Fabien Bacro of Université de Nantes (France).

References

Adams, S., Kuebli, K., Boyle, P. A., & Fivush, R. (1995). Gender differences in parent-child conversations about past emotions: A longitudinal investigation. *Sex Roles, 33*, 309–323.

Aimé, C., Paquette, D., Déry, M., & Verlaan, P. (2018). Predictors of childhood trajectories of overt and indirect aggression: An interdisciplinary approach. *Aggressive Behavior, 44*(4), 382–393.

Ainsworth, M. D. S., Blehar, M., Waters, E., & Wall, S. (1978). *Patterns of attachment*. Hillsdale, NJ: Erlbaum.

Allès-Jardel, M., Schneider, B. H., Goldstein, E., & Normand, S. (2009). Les origines culturelles de l'agressivité pendant l'enfance. In D. B. H. Schneider, S. Normand, M. Allès-Jardel, M. A. Provost, & G. M. Tarabulsy (Eds.), *Conduites agressives chez l'enfant : Perspectives développementales et psychosociales* (pp. 101–222). Québec, Canada: Les Presses de l'Université du Québec.

Anderson, S., Qiu, W., & Wheeler, S. J. (2017). The quality of father-child rough-and-tumble play and toddlers' aggressive behavior in China. *Infant Mental Health Journal, 38*(6), 726–742.

Archer, J., & Côté, S. (2005). Sex differences in aggressive behaviour: A developmental and evolutionary perspective. In R. E. Tremblay, W. W. Hartup, & J. Archer (Eds.), *Developmental origins of aggression* (pp. 425–443). New York/London: The Guilford Press.

Bachand, Y. (2013). *Sentiment de compétence parentale, qualité de la relation d'attachement et la fonction paternelle d'ouverture sur le monde chez des pères d'enfant d'âge scolaire*. Unpublished master's thesis. University of Montreal, Canada. https://papyrus.bib.umontreal.ca/xmlui/handle/1866/9975

Baker, M. D., & Maner, J. K. (2008). Risk-taking as a situationally sensitive male mating strategy. *Evolution and Human Behavior, 29*, 391–395.

Bianchi, S. E. (2000). Maternal employment and time with children : Dramatic change or surprising continuity? *Demography, 37*(4), 401–414.

Bornstein, M. H. (2013). Parenting X gender X culture X time. In W. Wilcox & K. Kline (Eds.), *Gender and parenthood: Biological and social scientific perspectives* (pp. 91–119). New York/Chichester, UK: Columbia University Press.

Bowlby, J. (1969). *Attachment and loss: Vol. 1 - Attachment*. London: Hogarth.

Bowlby, J. (1973). *Attachment and Loss: Vol. 2. Separation*. New-York: Basics Books.

Bueno, R. K., Kaszubowski, E., Bossardi, C. N., de Souza, C. D., Paquette, D., Crepaldi, M. A., et al. (2018). Relations between openness to the world, family functioning and child behaviour. *Early Child Development and Care*. https://doi.org/10.1080/03004430.2018.1527327

Bueno, R. K., Vieira, M. L., Crepaldi, M. A., & Faraco, A. M. X. (2017). Father–child activation relationship in the Brazilian context. *Early Child Development and Care*. https://doi.org/10.1080/03004430.2017.1345894

Bureau, J.-F., Yurkowski, K., Schmiedel, S., Martin, J., Moss, E., & Pallanca, D. (2014). Making children laugh: Parent-child dyadic synchrony and preschool attachment. *Infant Mental Health Journal, 35*(5), 482–494.

Byrnes, J., Miller, D., & Schaffer, W. (1999). Gender differences in risk-taking: A meta-analysis. *Psychological Bulletin, 125*, 367–383.

Campbell, A. (2009). Gender and crime: An evolutionary perspective. In A. Walsh & K. M. Beaver (Eds.), *Biosocial criminology: New directions in theory and research* (pp. 117–136). New York: Taylor & Francis.

Carson, J. L., Burks, V., & Parke, R. D. (1993). Parent-child physical play: Determinants and consequences. In K. MacDonald (Ed.), *Parent-child play: Descriptions and implications* (pp. 195–220). Albany, NY: State University of New York Press.

Cassano, M. C., & Zeman, J. L. (2010). Parental socialization of sadness regulation in middle childhood : The role of expectations and gender. *Developmental Psychology, 46*(5), 1214–1226.

Chalmers, N. (1983). The development of social relationships. In T. R. Halliday & P. J. B. Slater (Eds.), *Animal Behaviour, Vol. 3. Genes, development and learning* (pp. 114–148). Oxford: Blackwell Science Ltd..

Chapais, B. (2008). *Primeval kinship: How pair-bonding gave birth to human society*. Cambridge/London: Harvard University Press.

Chapais, B. (2011). The evolutionary history of pair-bonding and parental collaboration. In C. Salmon & T. K. Shackelford (Eds.), *Oxford handbook of evolutionary family psychology* (pp. 33–50). Oxford: Oxford University Press.

Chaplin, T. M., Cole, P. M., & Zahn-Waxler, C. (2005). Parental socialization of emotion expression: Gender differences and relations to child adjustment. *Emotion, 5*(1), 80–88.

Charlesworth, W. R. (1988). Resources and resource acquisition during ontogeny. In K. B. MacDonald (Ed.), *Sociobiological perspective on human development* (pp. 24–77). New York: Springer-Verlas.

Cole, P., Teti, L., & Zahn-Waxler, C. (2003). Mutual emotion regulation and the stability of conduct problems between preschool and early school age. *Development and Psychopathology, 15*, 1–18.

Crouter, A. C., Helms-Erickson, H., Updegraff, K., & McHale, S. M. (1999). Conditions underlying parents' knowledge about children's daily lives in middle childhood: Between-and within-family comparisons. *Child Development, 70*, 246–259.

da Silva, M. L. I. (2017). *A relação entre a personalidade paterna e a abertura ao mundo em pais de criança de 4 a 6 anos*. Unpublished master's thesis. Universidade federal de Santa Catarina, Florianopolis, Brazil.

Darwin, C. (1871). *The descent of man and selection in relation to sex*. London: John Murray.

Del Giudice, M. (2009). Sex, attachment, and the development of reproductive strategies. *Behavioral and Brain Sciences, 32*, 1–67.

Denham, S. A., Bassett, H. H., & Wyatt, T. M. (2010). Gender differences in the socialization of preschoolers' emotional competence. In A. K. Root & S. Denham (Eds.), *The role of gender in the socialization of emotion: Key concepts and critical issues.*. New directions for child and adolescent development (Vol. 128, pp. 29–49). San Francisco: Jossey-Bass.

Dubé, A. (2011). *Qualité des jeux de bataille père-enfant et adaptation sociale de l'enfant d'âge préscolaire*. Unpublished doctoral thesis. University of Montreal, Canada. https://papyrus.bib.umontreal.ca/xmlui/handle/1866/6269

Dumont, C., & Paquette, D. (2013). What about the child's tie to the father? A new insight into fathering, father–child attachment, children's socio-emotional development and the activation relationship theory. *Early Child Development and Care, 183*(3–4), 430–446.

Eckel, C. C., & Grossman, P. J. (2008). Men, women and risk aversion: Experimental evidence. In C. Plott & V. Smith (Eds.), *Handbook of experimental economics results* (pp. 1061–1073). Amsterdam: Elsevier North-Holland.

Edwards, C. P., & Whiting, B. B. (1993). Mother, older sibling, and me: The overlapping roles of caretakers and companions in the social world of 2-3 year olds in Ngeca, Kenya. In K. MacDonald (Ed.), *Parent-child: Descriptions and implications* (pp. 305–329). Albany, NY: State University of New York.

Eisenberg, N., Fabes, R. A., Shepard, S. A., Guthrie, I. K., Murphy, B. C., & Reiser, M. (1999). Parental reactions to children's negative emotions: Longitudinal relations to quality of children's social functioning. *Child Development, 70*, 513–534.

Eisenberg, N., Spinrad, T. L., & Cumberland, A. (1998). The socialization of emotion: Reply to commentaries. *Psychological Inquiry, 9*(4), 317–333.

Else-Quest, N. M., Hyde, J. S., Goldsmith, H. H., & van Hulle, C. A. (2006). Gender differences in temperament: A meta-analysis. *Psychological Bulletin, 132*(1), 33–72.

Eugène, M. M. (2008). *La fonction d'ouverture au monde par le père et l'itinérance à l'adolescence.* Unpublished doctoral thesis. University of Montreal, Canada. https://papyrus.bib.umontreal.ca/xmlui/handle/1866/6392

Eugène, M. M., Paquette, D., & Claes, M. (2010). Construction et validation d'une mesure de l'engagement paternel : le Questionnaire d'Ouverture au Monde pour Adolescents (QOMA). *Revue Québécoise de Psychologie, 31*(2), 201–214.

Farthing, G. W. (2007). Neither daredevils nor wimps: Attitudes toward physical risk takers as mates. *Evolutionary Psychology, 5*(4), 754–777.

Fivush, R. (1989). Exploring sex differences in the emotional content of mother child conversations about the past. *Sex Roles, 20*, 675–691.

Fivush, R. (1991). Gender and emotion in mother-child conversations about the past. *Journal of Narratives & Life History, 1*, 325–341.

Fivush, R., Brotman, M., Buckner, J., & Goodman, S. (2000). Gender differences in parent-child emotion narratives. *Sex Roles, 42*, 233–253.

Flanders, J. (2008). *Rough-and-tumble play and externalizing behaviour*. Unpublished doctoral thesis. McGill University, Montreal, Canada.

Flanders, J., Leo, V., Paquette, D., Pihl, R. O., & Séguin, J. R. (2009). Rough-and-tumble play and the regulation of aggression: An observational study of father-child play dyads. *Aggressive Behavior, 35*, 285–295.

Flanders, J. L., Séguin, J. R., Parent, S., Pihl, R. O., Zelazo, P. D., & Tremblay, R. E. (2007). *Psychometric properties of the Rough-and-Tumble Play Questionnaire*. Presented at the Society for Research on Child Development Biennial Meeting, April 2007, Boston, MA, USA.

Flanders, J. L., Simard, M., Paquette, D., Parent, S., Vitaro, F., Pihl, R. O., et al. (2010). Rough-and-tumble play and the development of physical aggression and emotion regulation: A five-year follow-up study. *Journal of Family Violence, 25*, 357–367.

Fletcher, R., StGeorge, J., & Freeman, E. (2013). Rough and tumble play quality: Theoretical foundations for a new measure of father-child interaction. *Early Child Development and Care, 183*(6), 746–759.

Fliek, L., Daemen, E., Roelofs, J., & Muris, P. (2015). Rough-and-tumble play and other parental factors as correlates of anxiety symptoms in preschool children. *Journal of Child and Family Studies, 24*, 2795–2804.

Garside, R. B. (2004). *Parental socialization of discrete positive and negative emotions: Implications for emotional functioning*. Doctoral dissertation, The Catholic University of America, 2003. Dissertation Abstracts International, 65, 4828.

Gaumon, S., & Paquette, D. (2013). The father–child activation relationship and internalizing disorders at preschool age. *Early Child Development and Care, 183*(3–4), 447–463.

Gaumon, S., Paquette, D., Cyr, C., Emond-Nakamura, M., & St-André, M. (2016). Anxiety and attachment to the mother in children receiving psychiatric care: The father-child activation relationship as a protective factor. *Infant Mental Health Journal, 37*(4), 372–387.

Geary, D. C. (2010). *Male, female. The evolution of human sex differences*. Washington, D.C: APA.

Giuli, C. A., & Hudson, W. W. (1977). Assessing parent-child relationship disorders in clinical practice: The child point of view. *Journal of Social Service Research, 1*, 77–92.

Gomes, L. (2015). *Envolvimento parental, desenvolvimento social e temperamento de pré-escolares: um estudo comparativo com famílias residentes em Santa Catarina e em Montreal*. Unpublished doctoral thesis. Universidade federal de Santa Catarina, Florianopolis, Brazil.

Gray, P. B., & Anderson, K. G. (2010). *Fatherhood: Evolution and human paternal behavior*. Cambridge/London: Harvard University Press.

Grossmann, K., Grossmann, K. E., Fremmer-Bombik, E., Kindler, H., Scheuerer-Englisch, H., & Zimmerman, P. (2002). The uniqueness of the child-father attachment relationship: Fathers' sensitive and challenging play as a pivotal variable in a 16-year longitudinal study. *Social Development, 11*(3), 307–331.

Grossmann, K., Grossmann, K. E., Kindler, H., & Zimmermann, P. (2008). A wider view of attachment and exploration: The influence of mothers and fathers on the development of psychological security from infancy to young adulthood. In *Handbook of attachment: Theory, research, and clinical applications* (2nd ed., pp. 857–879). New York: Guilford Press.

Hamel, S. (2014). *Stabilité de la relation d'activation père-enfant entre 12–18 mois et 3–5 ans et les facteurs associés à l'instabilité*. Unpublished master's thesis. University of Montreal, Canada. https://papyrus.bib.umontreal.ca/xmlui/handle/1866/11520

Hamilton, W. D. (1964). The genetical evolution of social behaviour. *Journal of Theoretical Biology, 7*, 1–52.

Harris, K. M., Furstenberg, F. F., & Marmer, J. K. (1998). Paternal involvement with adolescents in intact families: The influence of fathers over the life course. *Demography, 35*, 201–216.

Herzog, J. M. (1992). L'enseignement de la langue maternelle: Aspects du dialogue développemental fille-père. *Journal de la Psychanalyse de l'Enfant, 11*, 47–60.

Hewlett, B. S. (2000). Culture, history, and sex: Anthropological contributions to conceptualizing father involvement. In E. Peters & R. D. Day (Eds.), *Fatherhood : Research, interventions and policies* (Vol. 29(2/3), pp. 59–73).

Kennedy Root, A., & Rubin, K. H. (2010). Gender and parents' reactions to children's emotion during the preschool years. In A. K. Root & S. Denham (Eds.), *The role of gender in the socialization of emotion: Key concepts and critical issues. New Directions for Child and Adolescent Development* (Vol. 128, pp. 51–64). San Francisco: Jossey-Bass.

Kuebli, J., Butler, S., & Fivush, R. (1995). Mother-child talk about past emotions: Relations of maternal language and child gender over time. *Cognition & Emotion, 9*, 265–283.

Lazarus, R. S., Dodd, H. F., Majdandzic, M., de Vente, W., Morris, T., Byrow, Y., et al. (2016). The relationship between challenging parenting behaviour and childhood anxiety disorders. *Journal of Affective Disorders, 190*, 784–791.

Le Camus, J. (2000). *Le vrai rôle du père*. Paris: Éditions Odile Jacob.

Leaper, C., Anderson, K. J., & Sanders, P. (1998). Moderators of gender effects on parents' talk to their children: A meta-analysis. *Developmental Psychology, 34*, 3–27.

Lovas, G. S. (2011). Gender and patterns of language development in mother-toddler and father-toddler dyads. *First Language, 31*(1), 83–108.

Majdandzic, M., de Vente Colonnesi, C., & Bögels, S. M. (2018). Fathers' challenging parenting behavior predicts less subsequent anxiety symptoms in early childhood. *Behaviour Research and Therapy, 109*, 18–28.

Majdandzic, M., de Vente, W., & Bögels, S. M. (2016). Challenging parenting behavior from infancy to toddlerhood : Etiology, measurement, and differences between fathers and mothers. *Infancy, 21*(4), 423–452.

Majdandzic, M., Lazarus, R. S., Oort, F. J., van der Sluis, C., Dodd, H. F., Morris, T. M., et al. (2018). The structure of challenging parenting behavior and associations with anxiety in Dutch and Australian children. *Journal of Clinical Child & Adolescent Psychology, 47*(2), 282–295.

Majdandzic, M., Möller, E., de Vente, W., Bögels, S. M., & van den Boom, D. C. (2014). Fathers' challenging parenting behavior prevents social anxiety development in their 4-year-old children : A longitudinal observational study. *Journal of Abnormal Child Psychology, 42*, 301–310.

Moffette, V. (2013). *Le lien entre le stress parental du père et le développement de la relation d'activation chez les enfants âgés entre 12 et 18 mois*. Unpublished master's thesis. University of Montreal, Canada. https://papyrus.bib.umontreal.ca/xmlui/handle/1866/10595

Möller, E. L., Majdandzic, M., & Bögels, S. M. (2015). Parental anxiety, parenting behavior, and infant anxiety: Differential associations for fathers and mothers. *Journal of Child and Family Studies, 24*, 2626–2637.

Möller, E. L., Majdandzic, M., de Vente, W., & Bögels, S. M. (2013). The evolutionary basis of sex differences in parenting and its relationships with child anxiety in western societies. *Journal of Experimental Psychopathology, 4*(2), 88–117.

Moss, E., Bureau, J. F., Cyr, C., Mongeau, C., & St-Laurent, D. (2004). Correlates of attachment at age 3: Construct validity of the preschool attachment classification system. *Developmental Psychology, 40*(3), 323–334.

Panksepp, J. (1993). Rough-and-tumble play: A fundamental brain process. In Dans K. MacDonald (Dir.) (Ed.), *Parent-child play: Descriptions and implications* (pp. 147–184). Albany, NY: State University of New York Press.

Paquette, D. (2004a). Theorizing the father-child relationship: Mechanisms and developmental outcomes. *Human Development, 47*(4), 193–219.

Paquette, D. (2004b). La relation père-enfant et l'ouverture au monde. *Enfance, 56*(2), 205–225.

Paquette, D. (2015). An evolutionary perspective on antisocial behavior: Evolution as a foundation for criminological theories, Chapter 20. In J. Morizot & L. Kazemian (Eds.), *The development of criminal and antisocial behavior: Theory, research and practical applications* (pp. 315–330). NewYork: Springer.

Paquette, D., & Bigras, M. (2010). The risky situation: A procedure for assessing the father-child activation relationship. *Early Child Development and Care, 180*(1–2), 33–50.

Paquette, D., Bolté, C., Turcotte, G., Dubeau, D., & Bouchard, C. (2000). A new typology of fathering : Defining and associated variables. *Infant and Child Development, 9*, 213–230.

Paquette, D., Carbonneau, R., Dubeau, D., Bigras, M., & Tremblay, R. E. (2003). Prevalence of father-child rough-and-tumble play and physical aggression in preschool children. *European Journal of Psychology of Education, 18*(2), 171–189.

Paquette, D., & Dumont, C. (2013a). The father-child activation relationship, sex differences and attachment disorganization in toddlerhood. *Child Development Research*. https://doi.org/10.1155/2013/102860

Paquette, D., & Dumont, C. (2013b). Is father-child rough-and-tumble play associated with attachment or activation relationships? *Early Child Development and Care, 183*(6), 760–773.

Paquette, D., Eugène, M. M., Dubeau, D., & Gagnon, M.-N. (2009). Les pères ont-ils des influences spécifiques sur le développement des enfants? In D. Dubeau, A. Devault, & G. Forget (Eds.), *Prospère, la paternité du 21e siècle* (pp. 99–122). Québec, Canada: Presses de l'Université Laval.

Paraventi, L., Bittencourt, I. G., Schulz, M. L. C., de Souza, C. D., Bueno, R. K., & Vieira, M. L. (2017). A percepçao de pessoas sem filhos sobre a funçao paterna de abertura ao mundo. *Psico, 48*(1), 1–11.

Pawlowski, B., Atwal, R., & Dunbar, R. I. M. (2008). Sex differences in everyday risk-taking behavior in humans. *Evolutionary Psychology, 6*(1), 29–42.

Pellegrini, A. D., & Smith, P. K. (1998). Physical activity play: The nature and function of a neglected aspect of play. *Child Development, 69*(3), 577–598.

Pomerantz, E. M., Fei-Yin Ng, F., & Wang, Q. (2004). Gender socialization: A parent X child model, Chapter 6. In A. H. Eagly, A. E. Beall, & R. J. Sternberg (Eds.), *The psychology of gender* (pp. 120–144). New York/London: The Guilford Press.

Premo, J. E., & Kiel, E. J. (2014). The effect of toddler emotion regulation on maternal emotion socialization: Moderation by Toddler gender. *Emotion, 14*(4), 782–793.

Radke-Yarrow, M., & Kochanska, G. (1990). Anger in young children. In N. L. Stein, B. Leventhal, & T. Trabasso (Eds.), *Psychological and biological approaches to emotion* (pp. 297–310). Hillsdale, NJ: Erlbaum.

Roggman, L. A., Bradley, R. H., & Raikes, H. H. (2013). Fathers in family context, Chapter 11. In N. J. Cabrera & C. S. Tamis-LeMonda (Eds.), *Handbook of father involvement: Multidisciplinary perspectives* (pp. 186–201). New York/London: Routledge.

Rose, A. J., & Rudolph, K. D. (2006). A review of sex differences in peer relationship processes: Potential trade-offs for the emotional and behavioral development of girls and boys. *Psychological Bulletin, 132*(1), 98–131.

Schulz, M. L. C. (2015). *A funçao paterna de abertura ao mundo na percepçao de adolescentes*. Unpublished master's thesis. Universidade federal de Santa Catarina, Florianopolis, Brazil.

Stevenson, M. M., & Crnic, K. A. (2013). Activative fathering predicts later children's behaviour dysregulation and sociability. *Early Child Development and Care, 183*(6), 774–790.

StGeorge, J., Fletcher, R., Freeman, E., Paquette, D., & Dumont, C. (2015). Father-child interactions and children's risk of injuries. *Early Child Development and Care*. http://www.tandfonline.com/http://dx.doi.org/10.1080/03004430.2014.1000888

StGeorge, J., Fletcher, R., & Palazzi, K. (2017). Comparing fathers' physical and toy play and links to child behaviour: An exploratory study. *Infant and Child Development, 26*, e1958.

Suess, G. J., Grossmann, K. E., & Sroufe, L. A. (1992). Effects of infant attachment to mother and father on quality of adaptation in preschool: From dyadic to individual organization of self. *International Journal of Behavioral Development, 15*, 43–65.

Tomasello, M. (2014). *A natural history of human thinking*. Cambridge/London: Harvard University Press.

Tremblay, R. E., Japel, C., Pérusse, D., Boivin, M., Zoccolillo, M., Montplaisir, J., et al. (1999). The search of the age of 'onset' of physical aggression: Rousseau and Bandura revisited. *Criminal Behavior and Mental Health, 9*, 8–23.

Vaillancourt, T. (2005). Indirect aggression among humans. In R. E. Tremblay, W. W. Hartup, & J. Archer (Eds.), *Developmental origins of aggression* (pp. 158–177). New York: The Guilford Press.

van der Pol, L. D., Groeneveld, M. G., van Berkel, S. R., Endendijk, J. J., Hallers-Haalboom, E. T., Bakermans-Kranenburg, M. J., et al. (2015). Fathers' and mothers' emotion talk with their girls and boys from toddlerhood to preschool age. *Emotion, 15*(6), 854–864.

van IJzendoorn, M. H. (1995). Adult attachment representations, parental responsiveness, and infant attachment: A meta-analysis on the predictive validity of the Adult Attachment Interview. *Psychological Bulletin, 117*, 387–403.

van IJzendoorn, M. H., Moran, G., Belsky, J., Pederson, D., Bakermans-Kranenburg, M. J., & Kneppers, K. (2000). The similarity of siblings' attachments to their mother. *Child Development, 71*, 1086–1098.

Vandystadt, J. (2017). *L'engagement paternel et la relation d'activation père-enfant chez l'enfant âgé entre 12 et 18 mois : l'effet modérateur de l'alliance parentale*. Unpublished master's thesis. University of Montreal, Canada. https://papyrus.bib.umontreal.ca/xmlui/handle/1866/19123

Volling, B. L., Stevenson, M. M., Safyer, P., Gonzalez, R., & Lee, J. Y. (2019). In search of the father-infant activation relationship: A person-centered approach. In B. Volling & N. J. Cabrera (Eds.), *Advancing research and measurement on fathering and childrens' development* (Vol. 84(1), pp. 50–63). Monographs of the Society for Research in Child Development. Serial no 332.

Weinfield, N. S., Sroufe, L. A., Egeland, B., & Carlson, E. (2008). Individual differences in infant–caregiver attachment: Conceptual and empirical aspects of security. In J. Cassidy & P. R. Shaver (Eds.), *Handbook of attachment: Theory, research, and clinical applications* (pp. 78–101). New York: Guilford.

Wilke, A., Hutchison, J. M. C., Todd, P. M., & Kruger, D. J. (2006). Is risk taking used as a cue in mate choice? *Evolutionary Psychology, 4*, 367–393.

Youngblade, L. M., Park, K. A., & Belsky, J. (1993). Measurement of young children's close friendship: A comparison of two independent assessment systems and their associations with attachment security. *International Journal of Behavioral Development, 16*, 563–587.

Zaman, W., & Fivush, R. (2013). Gender differences in elaborative parent-child emotion and play activities. *Sex Roles, 68*, 591–604.

Fathers' Emotional Availability with Their Children: Determinants and Consequences

20

Sarah Bergmann and Annette M. Klein

Enormous changes during the past 60 years in the societies of many Western industrialized countries have contributed to reshaping the traditional division of labour in the family, particularly with respect to the role of the father and his role in parenting and childcare. This is reflected by the rising numbers of fathers making use of parental leave, becoming primary caregivers and in general increasing the amount of time they spend in childcare activities (e.g. Lamb, Pleck, Charnov, & Levine, 1987). These societal changes promoted great interest in efforts to understand fathers' quantity, quality and patterns of interaction with their children and to comprehend how fathers directly and indirectly affect their children's development. To this end, in order to describe the quality of the parent-child relationship, research on fatherhood relied on concepts, which originally had been developed for assessing the child's relationship with the mother as the traditional primary caregiver, such as sensitivity, responsiveness and attachment security (e.g. Kochanska & Aksan, 2004; Lucassen et al., 2011). One of these concepts is emotional availability (EA), which refers to the overall affective quality of a dyadic interaction and describes the extent to which caregivers and children share a healthy dyadic relationship (Biringen, 2000). As a theoretical construct, EA partly originates from attachment theory (Ainsworth, Blehar, Waters, & Wall, 1978; Bowlby, 1973). However, in contrast to attachment theory, EA sets a greater emphasis on the observed global emotional climate of an interaction and the emotional responsiveness of caregiver and child (Biringen, Derscheid, Vliegen, Closson, & Easterbrooks, 2014). Other attachment-related concepts describing caregiver-child interactions target individual behaviour of the caregiver (mainly the mother) rather than viewing adult and child in a relational context (Biringen & Robinson, 1991). In contrast, EA is based on a bidirectional or dyadic approach; adult and child are considered as individuals but viewed within their specific dyadic relationship as affecting one another (Biringen et al., 2014). In addition, EA takes the contributions to the interaction provided by both partners of a dyad into consideration. Hence, the behaviour of the child is taken into account when judgements on caregiver's EA are made. For example, if the child avoids his or her mother, the mother will not be considered as highly emotionally available (Biringen et al., 2014). However, particularly in cases in which children suffer from disabilities or

S. Bergmann (✉)
Department of Child and Adolescent Psychiatry, Psychotherapy and Psychosomatics, University of Leipzig, Leipzig, Germany

International Psychoanalytic University Berlin, Berlin, Germany
e-mail: sarah.bergmann@medizin.uni-leipzig.de

A. M. Klein
International Psychoanalytic University Berlin, Berlin, Germany

H. E. Fitzgerald et al. (eds.), *Handbook of Fathers and Child Development*,
https://doi.org/10.1007/978-3-030-51027-5_20

in the context of adoptive or foster families, scores on adult and child dimensions can differ, i.e. parents show greater emotional availability than children (Biringen et al., 2014). Moreover, EA takes the role of covert emotions into account and encompasses various aspects of the caregivers' behaviour rather than focusing on sensitivity only. Therefore, EA presents a broader picture of interactive exchange. As EA has shown to be associated with children's attachment security or attachment classifications in relationship towards their mothers (e.g. Easterbrooks, Biesecker, & Lyons-Ruth, 2000; Feniger-Schaal & Joels, 2018; Ziv, Aviezer, Gini, Sagi, & Koren-Karie, 2000) as well as with caregivers in substitute care (Altenhofen, Clyman, Little, Baker, & Biringen, 2013), it seems to be a relevant contributing factor to the nature of attachment relationships.

Being also partly rooted in family systems theory (e.g. Guttman, 1991), the EA construct reaches beyond the mother-child relationship and encompasses a variety of relationships, including the father-child relationship (Biringen, 2008; Saunders, Kraus, Barone, & Biringen, 2015). Though research measuring fathers' EA still remains scarce compared to the wealth of studies focusing on maternal EA in various contexts, the body of research addressing father-child EA has been significantly growing especially during the last 10 years. Therefore, in this chapter we want to summarize the current state of research on fathers' EA with their children up to prekindergarten age regarding the following four questions: (1) Is fathers' EA different from mothers' EA? (2) Which factors are determinants of fathers' EA? (3) Does fathers' EA affect child development? (4) How can fathers' EA be improved? Moreover, we want to provide suggestions for future research. However, before doing so we briefly give an introduction on how EA is operationalized and assessed in the following section.

Operationalization of EA

In order to provide an operationalization of EA assessed in dyadic mother-child interactions, Biringen and Robinson (1991) suggested composite scores derived from observing mothers and children to capture different components of EA. These were referred to as "emotional availability scales" (EAS; Biringen, Robinson, & Emde, 1998). Since then the EAS have been revised several times, so that the 4th edition is currently available (Biringen, 2008). The EAS can be flexibly used across various contexts (e.g. laboratory or home observations, unstructured or structured tasks, stressful contexts) with children of different age (e.g. infants, toddlers, children, young adolescents) and various caregivers (e.g. mother, father, childcare professionals) (Biringen et al., 2014). Usually, the coding of the EAS is based on filmed adult-child interactions with a recommended minimum length of 20 minutes (Biringen, 2008). However, due to time constraints, it is not uncommon for researchers to use shorter periods of observation: for example, Ziv et al. (2000) used 6 minutes of observation, and the results of their study indicate validity by showing small significant associations between the mother-child EA with attachment security and attachment classifications. In accordance with the definition of EA as mirroring the overall emotional climate between adult and child, the EAS reflect a macroanalytic holistic approach towards assessing the quality of the caregiver-child interactions (Bornstein, Hahn, Suwalsky, & Haynes, 2011) in a multidimensional way. Four dimensions refer to the adult's contributions to the interaction, and two dimensions refer to the child's contributions to the interaction. According to the 4th edition of the EAS (Biringen, 2008), sensitivity encompasses the adult's ability to create a general positive emotional climate within the interaction, which is characterized by authenticity and genuineness, and the adult's ability to correctly recognize the child's emotional cues and signals and to respond appropriately and promptly. Structuring refers to the adult's ability to adequately frame the child's activities and to provide appropriate mentoring, scaffolding and guidance, which support the child's autonomous attempts and are successfully picked up by the child. Nonintrusiveness captures the absence of overly suggestive, overly directive or overly protective tendencies shown by the adult as well as of behavioural or verbal interferences and overstimulation. Nonhostility refers to the absence of open (behaviour or statements that are clearly hostile) or covert (e.g. subtle signs of impatience, frustration) hostility shown by the adult in the interaction. Child responsiveness reflects the child's desire and ability to respond to the caregiver in emotionally available ways and to show joy and enjoyment during the interaction with the adult rather than negative emotions and behaviours. Child involvement describes the capacity as well as the interest of the child to involve the caregiver into the child's activity, e.g. by using eye contact, verbal means and physical positioning, while keeping a healthy balance between involving behaviours and age-appropriate autonomy.

The internationally widely used EAS reflect the most validated, reliable and objective operationalization of the EA construct. Hence, when alluding to EA in this chapter, we only refer specifically to studies using the EAS.

Is Fathers' EA Different from Mothers' EA? Current Evidence Comparing Fathers and Mothers

In Western industrialized societies, fathers have been attributed a different style of interaction with their children as compared to mothers. Their behaviour towards their children appears particularly physical, challenging, animating and stimulating including less predictability during the interaction as well as rough-and-tumble play (Crawley & Sherrod, 1984; Paquette, Carbonneau, Dubeau, Bigras, & Tremblay, 2003; St George & Freeman, 2017; Yogman, 1981). Hence, the question arose if fathers in Western societies would also differ from mothers regarding aspects of the relationship quality towards their children. As pointed out before, when studying fathers' relationship with their children, research often relies on measures, which have originally been developed for assessing the child's relationship with the mother as the traditional primary caregiver despite the fact that fathers may also share different activities with their children (e.g. Cabrera, Volling, & Barr, 2018). This may be one reason why studies regarding this question yielded inconsistent results, on the one hand suggesting that fathers are no different from mothers in terms of sensitivity and responsiveness towards their children (e.g. Cabrera, Shannon, & Tamis-LeMonda, 2007; Malmberg et al., 2016) and on the other hand reporting fathers to be less sensitive and responsive towards their children (e.g. Kochanska & Aksan, 2004) as assessed by observational instruments other than the EAS. To find out whether these differences between fathers and mothers would also emerge when the emotional connection between parent and child is considered in a more global way, researchers started to investigate EA in fathers as well as in mothers (e.g. Lovas, 2005) and compared them regarding their mean levels of EA. To the best of our knowledge, 14 publications compared fathers' to mothers' EA so far (sometimes conducting secondary analyses of data sets). The samples, which were investigated, included typically developing children but also children with Down syndrome, feeding disorders and sleeping disorders, children of refugees and clinically referred children (see Table 20.1). Seven of these 14 studies indicate that fathers appear to achieve lower EA scores than mothers in typically developing children (Bergmann et al., 2013; Hallers-Haalboom et al., 2017; Hallers-Haalboom et al., 2014; Lovas, 2005) and in samples partly including children with feeding disorders or developmental disabilities (Atzaba-Poria et al., 2010; John et al., 2013; Menashe-Grinberg & Atzaba-Poria, 2017). Lower sensitivity in fathers compared to mothers was observed consistently in these studies except for one (John et al., 2013); differences regarding other dimensions of EA were observed less constantly. For example, Lovas (2005) prospectively investigated effects of parent and child gender on EA in the USA when children were 19 (n = 113) and 24 months (n = 90) old. Fathers in this study were reported not only to be less sensitive but also to be less structuring than mothers at both points of assessment and more intrusive at 19 months. In line with these results, Bergmann et al. (2013) also found fathers in Germany to be less sensitive,

Table 20.1 Overview on studies comparing parent-child EA in fathers and mothers (studies presented according to child age)

Study	Sample	Context	Results
Martins, Mateus, Osorio, Martins and Soares (2014)	*N* = 52 (31 boys, 59.6%) Child age: 9–11 months (*M* = 10.38, SD = .36) Sample from Portugal Middle to middle-upper class	Home observations, 30 min (20 min usual routines, 10 min free play) EAS: 3rd edition	Sensitivity: no difference Nonintrusiveness: fathers > mothers (no other EA dimensions assessed/reported)
Martins, Soares, Martins and Osório (2016)	*N* = 50 (31 boys, 62%) Child age: 10 months old (*M* = 10.38, SD = .36) Sample from Portugal Middle to middle-upper class	Home observations, 30 min (20 min usual routines, 10 min free play) EAS: 3rd edition	Father total EA (sum of all subscales) > mother total EA (sum of all subscales)
Wiefel et al. (2005)	*N* = 68 (42 boys, 61.8%) Child age: 6 weeks–3 years 10 months (*M* = 1.11 years) Sample of clinically referred children (mainly attachment disorders, feeding disorders, regulatory disorders according to DC 0–3; no organic disorders) in Germany, predominantly middle class	Laboratory observation, 5 min for infants aged 2–9 months and 10 min for older infants in free play; feeding situation instead of free play for some children with feeding disorders EAS: 3rd edition	No difference between fathers and mothers regarding total EA (sum of all 6 subscales)
Lovas (2005)	*N* = 113 (63 boys, 55.8%) Child age: t1, 18–20 months (*M* = 19.2, SD = 0.41), t2: 23.9–25.9 months (*M* = 24.5, SD = 0.42) Sample from the USA (89% Caucasian, 6% Hispanic, 4% Asian American and 1% African American; 14% of the families were multi-ethnic), predominantly middle class	Laboratory observation, 12 min (7 min free play, 5 min of clean-up) EAS: 3rd edition	Sensitivity: fathers < mothers at t1, t2 Structuring: fathers < mothers at t1, t2 Nonintrusiveness: fathers < mothers at t1 Nonhostility: no difference Child responsiveness: fathers < mothers at t2 Child involvement: fathers < mothers at t2
Atzaba-Poria et al. (2010)	*n* = 28 children diagnosed with feeding disorder and *n* = 28 children without developmental or feeding disorders (control group) Child age: 1–3 years (*M* = 1.97, SD = .86) Sample from Israel Mainly (group with feeding disorders/control group) high school education (61%/64% of mothers, 61%/63% of fathers) and post-secondary school education (39%/50% of mothers, 39%/36% of fathers)	Home observation, 12 min play (5 min structured and 5 min unstructured play, 2 min clean-up session), 12 min one-to-one feeding EAS: 3rd edition	Sensitivity: fathers < mothers in the group with feeding disorders No significant difference in other EA dimensions in the group with feeding disorders No significant differences in the control group
Menashe and Atzaba-Poria (2016)	*N* = 65 (22 boys, 34%) Child age: 1–3 years (*M* = 1.97, SD = 0.86) Sample from Israel, about half of the children suffered from feeding problems Mainly high school education (62% of parents)	Home observation, 12 min play (5 min structured and 5 min unstructured play, 2 min clean-up session) EAS: 3rd edition	Sensitivity: no difference Nonintrusiveness: no difference No other dimensions reported

(continued)

Table 20.1 (continued)

Study	Sample	Context	Results
Menashe-Grinberg and Atzaba-Poria (2017)	$N = 111$ (47 boys, 42.0%) Child age: 1–3 years ($M = 1.91$, SD = 0.76) Sample from Israel, about half of the children suffered from feeding or sleeping problems Mainly high school education (45% of mothers and 40% of fathers) and post-secondary school education (37% of mothers and 36% of fathers)	Home observation, 12–15 min (structured and unstructured play, clean-up session) EAS: 3rd edition	Sensitivity: fathers < mothers Structuring: no difference, only trend for fathers < mothers Nonintrusiveness: no difference (No other EA dimensions reported)
van Ee, Sleijpen, Kleber and Jongmans (2013)	$N = 80$ children (37 boys, 46%), 29 fathers, 51 mothers, both parents participated for 18 children Child age: 18–43 months ($M = 27.14$, SD = 9.10) Sample of asylum seekers in the Netherlands from various geographic regions (Middle East, 43.8%; Africa, 32.5%; East Europe, 12.5%; Asia, 8.8%; South America, 2.6%) with experience of trauma, low socio-economic status, diverse education	Laboratory observation, 15 min free play EAS: 4th edition	No difference between fathers and mothers regarding sensitivity, structuring, nonintrusiveness and nonhostility, child dimensions not assessed/reported
de Falco, Venuti, Esposito and Bornstein (2009)	$N = 22$ children with Down syndrome and their parents Child age: 18–48 months (*M* chronological age = 35.32 months) Sample from Italy Low to middle socio-economic status in the Italian population	Laboratory observation, 10 min free play EAS: 3rd edition	No difference between fathers and mothers regarding all EA dimensions
Bergmann, Wendt, von Klitzing and Klein (2013)	$N = 48$ (25 boys, 52.1%) Child age: 7–46 months ($M = 25.19$, SD = 12.26) Sample from Germany Mainly well-educated: general qualification for university entrance, 83.8% of mothers and 79.2% of fathers; entrance qualification for studying at a university of applied sciences, 3 mothers (6.3%) and one father (2.1%); Certificate of Secondary Education, 10.4% of mothers and 18.8% of fathers	Laboratory observation, 16 min free play EAS: 4th edition	Sensitivity: fathers < mothers Structuring: fathers < mothers Nonintrusiveness: fathers < mothers Nonhostility: no difference Child responsiveness: no difference Child involvement: no difference
Hallers-Haalboom et al. (2014)	$N = 389$ families with 2 children: 107 boy-boy (28%), 91 girl-girl (23%), 98 boy-girl (25%) and 93 girl-boy (24%) Firstborn child age: 2.5–3.6 years at T1 ($M = 3.0$, SD = 0.3) Second-born child age: 12.0 months old (SD = 0.2) Sample from the Netherlands Mainly high educational level: 79% of mothers and 76% of fathers with completion of academic or higher vocational schooling	Home observation, 8 min free play EAS: 4th edition	Sensitivity: fathers < mothers Nonintrusiveness: fathers < mothers for younger child but no difference for older child (No other EA dimensions assessed/reported)

(continued)

Table 1 (continued)

Study	Sample	Context	Results
Hallers-Haalboom et al. (2017)	$N = 390$ families with 2 children: 99 boy-boy (27%), 86 girl-girl (24%), 90 boy-girl (25%) and 89 girl-boy (24%) Firstborn child age: 2.5–3.6 years at T1 ($M = 3.0$, SD = 0.3) Second-born child age: 12.0 months old (SD = 0.2) at T2 T2 and T3 followed when second-born child was 24.0 (SD = 0.3) and 36.0 months (SD = 0.7) old, respectively Sample from the Netherlands Mainly high educational level: 79% of mothers and 77% of fathers with completion of academic or higher vocational schooling	Home observation, 8 min free play EAS: 4th edition	Sensitivity: fathers < mothers (No other EA dimensions reported)
John, Halliburton and Humphrey (2013)	$N = 18$ (11 boys, 61.1%) Child age: 2–4.5 years ($M = 2$; 7 years; months) Sample from the USA Five children with diagnosis of a developmental disability varying in type and severity Household income: 10,000–200,000$ (median = 70,000$)	Home observation, semi-structured (18–20 min mother-child interaction followed by 12–15 min father-child interactions) at dinner or play table with a standardized set of toys EAS: 4th edition	Structuring: fathers < mothers No difference regarding all other EA dimensions
Piermattei, Pace, Tambelli, D'Onofrio and Di Folco (2017)	$N = 20$ (13 boys, 65%) Child age: 4.5–8.5 years ($M = 81.8$ months, SD = 13.4) Sample of late-adopted children and adoptive parents in Italy; age of adoption: $M = 63.5$ months, SD = 16.7; Min. = 37.0, Max. = 93.0; time spent by children in the family, 12–36 months; absence of special needs for all children Mainly well-educated: 50% of mothers with bachelor's degree, 60% fathers with high school diploma	Home observation, free play EAS: 4th edition	No difference between fathers and mothers regarding sensitivity, structuring, nonintrusiveness, nonhostility, child responsiveness and child involvement

less structuring and more intrusive in comparison to mothers when assessing EA in 48 families with children aged 7–46 months and controlling for the effects of child gender and age. Investigating 111 children of a similar age range (1–3 years) in interaction with their parents in Israel, Menashe-Grinberg and Atzaba-Poria (2017) reported only significantly lower levels of sensitivity for fathers, whereas there was just a trend for lower structuring in fathers and no difference regarding nonintrusiveness (other dimensions of EA were not reported). Notably, half of the children in this sample suffered from sleeping and feeding problems. When specifically comparing fathers and mothers of 28 children with feeding disorders aged 1–3 years, fathers achieved lower scores on the sensitivity scale but did not differ from mothers on any other of the EA dimensions (Atzaba-Poria et al., 2010). Using a within-family approach to study families with two children in the Netherlands, Hallers-Haalboom et al. (2014) explored differences between mothers and fathers in separate interactions with their youngest children aged 12 months as well as with their oldest children aged 2.5–3.6 years. Apart from lower sensitivity for fathers compared to mothers in interaction with both children, they also reported higher intrusiveness for fathers compared to mothers in interaction with the younger child; however, no difference regarding nonintrusiveness occurred in interaction with the older child. Last but not least, no differences between fathers and mothers regarding sensitivity occurred in a small sample of 18 preschoolers and their parents in the USA; however, fathers showed lower levels of structuring as compared to mothers (John et al., 2013). Notably, almost one third of the 18 children in this sample (i.e. five children) had a diagnosis of a developmental disorder.

Taken together, studies reporting differences between fathers and mothers regarding the adult dimensions of EA indicate that – in addition to lower sensitivity scores – fathers also tend to show lower structuring and lower nonintrusiveness compared to mothers, though not all studies found significant differences in the latter two dimensions (Atzaba-Poria et al., 2010; Menashe-Grinberg & Atzaba-Poria, 2017). Remarkably, studies including the assessment of nonhostility reported no significant differences between mothers and fathers regarding their covert or overt hostile behaviour (Atzaba-Poria et al., 2010; Bergmann et al., 2013; de Falco et al., 2009; Lovas, 2005).

In contrast to these results, other studies did not find any differences between mothers and fathers regarding EA. For example, in a sample of 68 clinically referred German children aged 6 weeks to 46 months with mainly attachment disorders, eating disorders and regulatory disorders, no significant differences between mother-child and father-child interactions regarding total EA (sum of all EA subscales) were reported (Wiefel et al., 2005). Likewise, when assessing 22 children with Down syndrome from 18 to 48 months in interaction with their parents in Italy, de Falco et al. (2009) did not observe any significant difference between mothers and fathers on the six EA dimensions. In the same vein, in a sample of 28 children aged 1–3 years without developmental disorders (who served as a control group to a group with feeding disorders) from Israel, Atzaba-Poria et al. (2010) did not find any differences between mothers and fathers regarding adult dimensions of EA. Similarly, fathers and mothers were equally sensitive and nonintrusive (no other dimensions reported) in a sample of 65 children between 1 and 3 years investigated by Menashe and Atzaba-Poria (2016) in Israel. Again, half of the children in this sample suffered from sleeping and feeding problems like in their study from 2017, which did report differences regarding sensitivity in a greater sample of N = 111. No differences between non-biological mothers and fathers in any of the six EA dimensions were reported for a small sample of 20 families with late-adopted children between 4.5 and 8.5 years in Italy (Piermattei et al., 2017). Moreover, in a sample of 80 asylum-seeking families in the Netherlands who showed high rates of parental post-traumatic stress symptoms, no differences between fathers and mothers regarding adult EA dimensions were reported in interaction with their children aged 18–42 months (child dimensions were not assessed; van Ee et al., 2013). However, this study is limited by the inclusion of only 29 fathers. Moreover, though 18 children participated with both mother and father, the study did not provide comparisons between these 18 fathers and 18 mothers interacting with the same child.

Apart from either observing higher EA in mothers compared to fathers or observing no significant differences at all, there is only one study reporting greater EA in fathers compared to mothers: in a sample from Portugal, Martins et al. (2014) found fathers to show lower intrusiveness than mothers in interaction with their 10-month-old infants, whereas mothers and fathers did not differ regarding their level of sensitivity (see also Martins et al., 2016).

Although EA is a dyadic construct, which underlines the importance of considering the child's contributions to the interaction when evaluating the adult's behaviour (and vice versa), the question of whether children are more or less responsive to and involving of their mothers than their fathers did not receive much attention in the EA literature so far. Those few studies dealing with this topic mainly indicate no significant differences between fathers and mothers regarding the child dimensions of EA (Atzaba-Poria et al., 2010; Bergmann et al., 2013; de Falco et al., 2009; John et al., 2013). Only in the sample investigated longitudinally by Lovas (2005), children at the age of 24 months were more responsive to and involving of mothers than of fathers.

To summarize, several studies point towards differences between fathers and mothers with respect to both the adult dimensions and child dimensions of EA. However, as not all studies reported these differences, the base of evidence appears relatively inconsistent. This inconsistency in results might be due to several factors, e.g. the lack of power to detect differences resulting from small sample sizes (see below). Another factor in particular might be the variety of samples included in the studies, which differ in culture and children's age range and developmental characteristics (e.g. typically developing children vs. clinically referred children). Interestingly, almost all of the studies (except for Atzaba-Poria et al., 2010, when investigating the control group) reporting no differences in fathers' compared to mothers' EA included children with a need of intense parenting and caregiving due to severe psychological or developmental problems. As de Falco et al. (2009) pointed out, fathers might develop a mechanism of compensation when being faced with challenges, which put their children's development at risk. This mechanism of compensation might involve a greater focus on affective exchanges in the father-child interaction. Moreover, these fathers may pay more attention to their children's signals and needs, which yields a level of EA comparable to that of mothers. Similar conclusions have been drawn by van Ee et al. (2013) for the fathers in their refugee sample who are also confronted with a situation that bears a potential risk for their children's development. As these fathers were not allowed to work or study due to their status as asylum seekers, it could even be speculated that the time fathers spent with their children in shared activities or even in caregiving tasks might have increased. As greater paternal involvement is a factor that is associated with higher EA (see below), fathers in the refugee sample may therefore show no difference in EA compared to mothers. However, this assumption seems refuted by the fact that in the sample of van Ee and colleagues, fathers were four times less involved in caregiving and activity tasks than mothers. Another potential reason for non-significant differences in EA between fathers and mothers in these at-risk samples might also be that mothers who are confronted with a child who shows severe impairment in his or her functional abilities diminish in their EA especially when affected by depressive symptoms (Barfoot, Meredith, Ziviani, & Whittingham, 2017). To further investigate the phenomenon that fathers' EA does not differ from mothers' EA when their children bear a considerably severe risk for their development and functioning, future research is necessary. In this context, it would be a good starting point to compare father-child EA in at-risk samples with control groups.

Regarding the question of whether fathers' EA differs from mothers' EA, it is important to keep the following things in mind: First, including fathers in studies tends to be associated with great difficulties and particular effort by researchers (e.g. Mitchell et al., 2007). Given the dearth of research on father-child EA, all of the studies mentioned above make significant contributions to the advancement in this field of research. However, some of the samples examined might have not been large enough to provide sufficient power to detect small differences between fathers and mothers regarding EA. Thus, continuous effort, sufficient resources and effective recruitment strategies are needed to extend the number of fathers participating in research. Second, all of the studies mentioned above contrasted mean levels of fathers' and mothers' EA, i.e. even for those studies which found significant differences on average between fathers and mothers regarding the EA dimensions, a proportion of fathers were presumably as emotionally available as mothers. In this context, research on father-child EA might benefit from different data analysis approaches, which take various patterns of the EA dimensions into account. For example, when focusing on other constructs than EA, Karberg, Cabrera, Malin and Kuhns (2019) showed that for fathers periods of intrusive behaviours towards their children were characterized by more positive affect on the side of the father and on the side of the child compared to periods of intrusive behaviours displayed by mothers. For the child, this might indicate a different meaning of the situation. Moreover, when comparing fathers and mothers regarding various aspects of parenting in a challenging context, another study reported significant differences regarding sensitivity, positive regard, stimulation of cognitive development (lower scores for fathers) and detachment (higher scores for fathers) but none regarding intrusiveness (Volling, Stevenson, Safyer, Gonzalez, & Lee, 2019). However, when analysing latent profiles based on these aspects of parenting, this study found similar profiles in mothers and fathers rather than unique ones. For example, an activation parenting profile (moderate to high sensitivity, positive regard and stimulation, moderate intrusiveness, low detachment) was observed in both parents, with a greater proportion of fathers (58%) showing this profile compared to mothers (49%) (Volling et al., 2019). Hence, complex methodological approaches may be a fruitful way to detect similarities and differences between mothers and fathers regarding EA with their children. This may also be underlined by the fact that for most studies presented in this section, the differences in maternal and paternal EA mean scores were small, which raises the question whether these differences would in fact affect children's development, and if they do so, to which degree. Finally, yet importantly, it remains unclear why differences between father-child and mother-child EA can be observed at least in some studies and which factors contribute to these differences. In general – despite rich research on predictors of mother-child EA – there is a lack of studies investigating determinants of father-child EA. In the following section, we provide an overview on the existing empirical evidence regarding this question. As a framework, we follow Belsky's (1984) process model of parenting.

What Are the Determinants of Father-Child EA?

In the following section, Belsky's model of parenting (Belsky, 1984) is used as a framework to review the current literature on determinants of fathers' EA. This model conceptualizes parenting as being multiply determined by the three major subsystems of determinants: (1) characteristics of the parent, such as psychopathology or personality; (2) characteristics of the child, such as temperament; and (3) characteristics of the family's social context, such as social support and quality of the marital relationship. The influential factors, which are discussed below following the three levels of Belsky's model, are not meant to be exhaustive in theoretically predicting father-child EA but specifically reflect the current state of empirical evidence on potential determinants.

Fathers' Characteristics and Involvement

Though Belsky's assumption that parents' own psychological and personality characteristics as well as their developmental history significantly affect parenting has found continuous empirical support (e.g. Belsky & Jaffee, 2006), not much is known on how these aspects relate to father-child EA. Whereas mother-child EA has shown to be linked to several aspects, e.g. mothers' psychopathology, age, experiences of trauma or maltreatment, attachment representations or attachment styles (see Biringen et al., 2014 for a review), investigating these and other aspects as predictors of father-child EA has been strongly neglected by the EA literature. So far the little evidence indicates that fathers' post-traumatic stress relates to father-child EA: in a study including refugees and asylum seekers, parental sensitivity, structuring and nonhostility and by trend nonintrusiveness were negatively associated with the extent of parental post-traumatic stress independent of parental gender (van Ee et al., 2013). However, due to the small sample size (only 29 fathers participated) and broad parental cultural diversity, generalization of these findings is impeded. To the best of our knowledge, only Rossen et al. (2018) utilized a longitudinal design to investigate potential risk and protective factors regarding EA for n = 191 (biological and social) fathers and n = 191 mothers. Potential predictors, such as substance use (alcohol, tobacco), self-reported bonding, depression, stress and anxiety, were assessed at 8 weeks after birth of the child, and parent-child EA was assessed when the child was 12 months old. Results of this study indicate that higher levels of paternal tobacco use predicted lower father-child EA when children were 12 months old. The authors suggest either that tobacco use could be an indicator for factors associated with low socio-economic status and therefore relates to father-child EA (social context, see below) or that it could be an indicator of difficulties in emotion regulation, which contribute to the development of tobacco addiction. Difficulties in emotion regulation in turn may impede the father from connecting emotionally with the child and from contributing to the child's affect regulation, which is reflected by low EA. Contrary to the expectations, depression only predicted later parent-child EA in dyadic analyses combined for mothers and fathers (by applying generalized estimating equations analysis, which allows to control for clustering based on the dependence of observations by mothers and fathers of the same child and offers more power). The same was true for parental age, which was positively associated with parent-child EA. This result dovetails other studies showing that adolescent parenthood is a risk factor for the quality of parent-child interactions (e.g. Riva Crugnola & Ierardi, 2018), which might be due to less implicit and explicit knowledge about childcare and child development, to lower emotional maturity or to their greater socio-economic disadvantages (see below; Rossen et al., 2018).

Apart from psychological symptoms, greater paternal involvement (i.e. the time fathers spend with their children absolutely or relatively to mothers) could contribute to a higher extent of EA in fathers: Atzaba-Poria et al. (2010) found mothers of children with feeding disorders only to be more sensitive than fathers, when father involvement in caregiving tasks (e.g. dressing, feeding) and their responsibility in childrearing – relative to mothers involvement – was low. If father involvement was high, no difference between the mothers and fathers regarding sensitivity could be observed. One explanation for this finding might be that due to a larger amount of time spent with their children, fathers gain a greater level of familiarity, routine and practice with them and therefore may find it easier to recognize emotional cues and needs exhibited by their children and to respond to those appropriately. Support for this assumption may be gained from former research showing that the extent of convergence between mothers' and fathers' perceptions of child problem behaviour increased if fathers spent more time with their children (Fitzgerald, Maguin, Zucker, & Reider, 1994). Another explanation might be that fathers who are more involved with their children– such as men who choose to take parental leave – are characterized by certain health-related or sociodemographic aspects, which might predispose them for showing higher EA with their children (e.g. Mansdotter, Fredlund, Hallqvist, & Magnusson, 2010). However, the generalizability of this finding is put into question as in another sample of 26 children with sleep problems and 25 children without sleep problems, the correlation between parental involvement and paternal sensitivity was even negative (Millikovsky-Ayalon, Atzaba-Poria, & Meiri, 2015). Hence, future research is needed not only to explore mechanisms underlying the possible association between paternal involvement and father-child EA but also to investigate potential paternal determinants of father-child EA in general.

Characteristics of the Child: Gender, Age, Temperament and Regulatory Problems

When discussing contributions of the child to parenting in the context of his model, Belsky (1984) did not give a broad overview but rather focused on child temperament as one specific characteristic, which he asserts shapes the way parents treat their children. Research since then has taken additional characteristics of the child into account and provided information on more complex associations between these characteristics and parenting, such as bidirectional, moderated or mediated pathways, and on how children – depending on their individual characteristics – differ in their susceptibility to environmental influences including positive and negative parenting (e.g. Belsky & Pluess, 2009). Thus, in the following we will review characteristics of the child, which have been investigated in relation to father-child EA, namely, gender, age, temperament and regulatory problems.

Child Gender

Child gender is one of the most widely investigated determinants of parenting behaviour. It is assumed that parents treat sons and daughters differently and therefore contribute to gender-differentiated behaviour exhibited by their children later in life (e.g. Leaper, 2002; Lovas, 2005). The literature which explored differences in EA depending on child gender mainly focused on mother-child dyads so far and showed mixed results: On the one hand, no differences in EA between boys and girls were found – neither on the adult dimensions nor on the child dimensions of EA (Biringen et al., 1999; Bornstein et al., 2006; Bornstein, Gini, Suwalsky, Putnick, & Haynes, 2006; Cornish, McMahon, & Ungerer, 2008; Hallers-Haalboom et al., 2014; Wiefel et al., 2005). On the other hand, studies indicate higher sensitivity and structuring for mothers of girls than for mothers of boys (Bornstein et al., 2008; Celia, Stack, & Serbin, 2018) and higher responsiveness and involvement for girls in comparison to boys (Bornstein et al., 2008; Celia et al., 2018; Stack et al., 2012; Ziv et al., 2000). In contrast to these results indicating higher EA for interactions with girls, Biringen et al. (2000) reported mothers to show less hostility with their sons rather than with their daughters, and Kim and Teti (2014) reported higher maternal EA (i.e. sum score of sensitivity, structuring, nonintrusiveness and nonhostility) in interactions with male infants than female infants.

Only five studies investigated fathers' EA with their sons and daughters. Similarly to the findings on mother-child EA, a recent study from Australia showed that fathers of sons tended to be less sensitive, more intrusive and more hostile compared to fathers of daughters when children were 12 months old (age was corrected for preterm infants) (McMahon et al., 2019). These differences might diminish over time as indicated by a longitudinal study investigating the development of parental sensitivity in firstborn and second-born children. In this study, fathers were more sensitive in interaction with second-born daughters than with second-born sons aged 12 months. However, from age 12 to 36 months, fathers' sensitivity in interaction with sons showed a greater increase than their sensitivity towards daughters. Also, no significant effect of child gender was observed for the firstborn children who were on average 2 years older than their second-born siblings, i.e. aged 2.5–3.6 years at the first wave of assessment (Hallers-Haalboom et al., 2017). Moreover, Lovas (2005) reported a significant effect of child gender on parent-child EA: In a global analysis, parents were less optimally structuring at 19 months of age and less sensitive at 24 months of age towards sons than towards daughters, and daughters were more responsive and involving than sons at both points of measurement. Specific dyadic comparisons of father-son with father-daughter interactions, however, did not reveal any significant differences. This is in line with two other studies that did not find any differences between sons and daughters regarding father-child (as well as mother-child) EA in children aged 7–46 months (Bergmann et al., 2013) and regarding paternal sensitivity in children aged 12 months and their older siblings aged 2.5–3.6 years (Hallers-Haalboom et al., 2014).

Due to these inconsistencies in the results reported above, it would be premature to draw any conclusions regarding the effect of child gender on father-child EA. Future studies are needed, which explore differences in EA between father-son and father-daughter dyads (as well as mother-son and mother-daughter dyads) within the same families and explore the stability of potential differences over time.

Child Age

Developmental achievements regarding children's social and emotional competences or motoric mobility might also come along with a reorganization of the relationship to the caregiver. Therefore, the question whether there are differences in caregiver and child dimensions of EA depending on child age and whether EA changes across time as children grow older has concerned research in the EA field since its early days (e.g. Biringen, Emde, Campos, & Appelbaum, 1995).

Regarding the association between child age and adult dimensions, results of longitudinal research including mother-child dyads are somewhat inconsistent, reporting increasing maternal EA with increasing child age on the one hand (e.g Biringen et al., 1999) and no change over time (Celia et al., 2018; Stack et al., 2012) or even decreases (Bornstein et al., 2010) on the other hand. Another cross-sectional study also reported a negative correlation between child age and mother-child EA (sum of all scales; Martins et al., 2016). The few studies on fathers' EA in association with child age more consistently report fathers to exhibit greater EA with older children: In a cross-sectional study with children aged 7–46 months, fathers showed higher levels of sensitivity and structuring if children were older, whereas for mothers these dimensions seemed to be similarly pronounced regardless of child age (Bergmann et al., 2013). These results dovetail a study on families with two children where fathers were more sensitive towards their older child as compared to their younger child. The same was true for nonintrusiveness; however, fathers were only more intrusive towards their younger child if it was a boy (Hallers-Haalboom et al., 2014). As these results could also reflect an effect of birth order rather than of child age, the authors conducted further analyses in a follow-up longitudinal study and compared sensitivity in parent-child interactions when the first- and second-born child were 3 years of age. The results revealed no significant differences, indicating an effect of child age rather than of birth order (Hallers-Haalboom et al., 2017). Moreover, in this longitudinal study, mothers' as well as fathers' sensitivity was reported to change in relation to child age, showing an increase from 12 to 24 months and staying stable between 24 and 36 months (Hallers-Haalboom et al., 2017). Taken together, the positive association between fathers' EA and child age could be a reflection of an enhanced routine of fathers in interaction with the respective child (see above), which also might be due to the fact that fathers get more involved as children grow older (e.g. Yeung, Sandberg, Davis-Kean, & Hofferth, 2001). Furthermore, the mentioned results could also be a reflection of children's growing language and motor abilities, social-emotional competences and clearer communication, which may make it easier for fathers to be a more emotionally available partner of interaction. However, in contrast to these results, Wiefel et al. (2005) did not find any significant association between child age and father-child EA (sum score of all EA dimensions) in a child psychiatric population consisting of children aged 6 weeks up to 3 years 10 months. Hallers-Haalboom et al. (2017) even reported fathers' (and mothers') sensitivity in interaction with 3-year-old firstborn children to decrease over the following two years. Thus, longitudinal research including several waves is needed to explore trajectories of father-child EA in typically developing children as well as in high-risk dyads using appropriate methodological approaches (e.g. growth modelling), which have already been applied to research on mother-child EA (Celia et al., 2018; Kim, Chow, Bray, & Teti, 2017).

Developmental changes in children as reflected by children's age do play a role not only for changes in adult dimensions of EA but also for child dimensions of EA. In general, cross-sectional research on parent-child EA as well as short-term longitudinal studies across infancy and toddlerhood consistently report that children show higher degrees of responsiveness to and involvement of their mothers with increasing age (e.g. Bergmann et al., 2013; Lovas, 2005; Stack et al., 2012; see Martins et al., 2016 for a contrary finding). More specifically, assessing long-term stability of mother-child EA using the 2nd edition of EAS across four waves, Celia et al. (2018) showed that between infancy (6 months and 12 months, respectively) and preschool age (55 months), children's levels of responsiveness to and involvement of their mothers increased by 0.01 and 0.03 points on the scales per month, respectively. This growth in children's EA can be explained by the fact that – especially during the first years of life – children's skills and competences in many areas of their development, such as emotion regulation, motor skills, language and social competences, advance significantly, which makes it easier for them to be adequately responsive to and involving of their caregivers. Therefore, it is not surprising that the same patterns were observed for father-child interactions in cross-sectional (Bergmann et al., 2013; de Falco et al., 2009) and short-term longitudinal studies (Lovas, 2005) as well. However, there is a lack of studies investigating patterns of long-term change regarding child responsiveness to and involvement of their fathers. This could be even more of interest as the increase in children's responsiveness and involvement does depend not only on the achievement of milestones in children's development but also on other factors, such as caregivers' EA. In this regard, Stack et al. (2012) showed that especially greater maternal sensitivity and structuring contributed to higher child responsiveness and involvement. The specific contribution of fathers' EA to children's dimensions of EA remains unclear, and as to the best of our knowledge, no study has investigated these associations so far.

Child Temperament

When underlining the importance to take the influence on parenting exerted by the child into account, Thomas, Chess and Birch (1968) postulated that the "goodness of fit" or "poorness of fit" between characteristics of the child, such as temperament, and contextual or environmental factors predict optimal or distorted development in children, respectively. If children show behaviours or characteristics, which do not conform to the expectations or demands of parents, they are at risk to experience negative social interactions and an unfavourable development in consequence. In the same vein, Belsky (1984) referred to the child's temperament, which makes it either easier or more difficult for parents to care for and rear their child. Within a psychobiological framework, three factors of temperament are often considered in infancy: surgency/extraversion, an orienting/regulatory capacity and negative affectivity (Gartstein & Rothbart, 2003). Surgency is described as the infant's tendency to react with positive affect, vocal reactivity and engagement with (rather than withdrawal from) stimuli. The factor orienting/regulatory capacity involves the duration of orienting, low-intensity pleasure, cuddliness and soothability and seems to be a precursor of effortful control later in life (Putnam, Rothbart, & Gartstein, 2008). Negative affectivity refers to the child's reaction to stressors, which is characterized by high levels of anger, frustration, discomfort and fear/anxiety. In general, if children show a more difficult temperament, such as high negative affectivity, parents are more likely to show less positive, less supportive and harsher behaviour, whereas higher levels of positive affect and self-regulation in children are associated with more responsive caregiving (Belsky & Jaffee, 2006). Based on these results, it can only be expected that parent-child EA should also be associated with child temperament. However, empirical evidence is scarce and mainly focused on mother-child EA, yielding mixed findings (Aviezer, Sagi, Joels, & Ziv, 1999; Jian & Teti, 2016; Kaplan, Evans, & Monk, 2008; Kiang, Moreno, & Robinson, 2004; Licata et al., 2014; Martins et al., 2016; Moreno, Klute, & Robinson, 2008). Similar inconsistencies occur for the few studies investigating father-child EA in relation to child temperament. Whereas in one study no association between father-child EA, such as sensitivity, with child temperament was found (Martins et al., 2016), another study reports children's fussy-difficult temperament to be negatively correlated with fathers' sensitivity during feeding (no other EA dimensions assessed; Millikovsky-Ayalon et al., 2015). In another study, which additionally investigated the links between fathers' structuring and nonintrusiveness with child negativity (includes oppositional behaviour, such as disobedience and lack of cooperation, and negative affect such as sadness, fear, anger), higher child negativity was associated with lower sensitivity, structuring and nonintrusiveness (Menashe-Grinberg & Atzaba-Poria, 2017). However, due to the cross-sectional nature of the mentioned studies, we cannot draw any conclusions on the causal relationships between fathers' (as well as mothers') EA and child temperament. In line with Belsky (1984), it could be assumed that children with a more difficult temperament are more likely to elicit lower EA in father-child interactions. However, lower EA may also increase difficult aspects of temperament in children. Moreover, empirical data point to a bidirectional association between negative parenting and difficult temperament, potentially yielding a cascading effect over time (e.g. Micalizzi, Wang, & Saudino, 2017). This could also apply to the association between EA and child temperament but has to be further investigated. Taken together, there is an enormous gap of research regarding the relation between child temperament and parent-child EA (Biringen et al., 2014).

Child Regulatory Problems

Regulatory problems in children, such as feeding or sleeping problems, can represent a risk factor for more negative parent-child relationships or interactions (e.g. Feldman, Keren, Gross-Rozval, & Tyano, 2004; Morrell & Steele, 2003). Indeed, mother-child EA in children with feeding disorders has shown to be lower compared to mother-child EA in typically developing children (i.e. lower sensitivity, structuring, nonintrusiveness, child responsiveness and child involvement during feeding and lower sensitivity, child responsiveness and child involvement during play; Atzaba-Poria et al., 2010). In another study mother-child EA in children with feeding disorders was even lower than mother-child EA in children with other clinical diagnoses, e.g. sleeping and crying or externalizing disorders (Wiefel et al., 2005). Moreover, lower quality of infant sleep has been associated with lower maternal EA assessed during bedtime (Philbrook & Teti, 2016; Teti, Kim, Mayer, & Countermine, 2010). Similar results can also be found in the scarce evidence including fathers, both in the context of feeding problems as well as sleeping problems of children. In a study comparing father-child EA in 1–3-year-old children with a diagnosed feeding disorder (i.e. nonorganic failure to thrive) and father-child EA in typically developing children, Atzaba-Poria et al. (2010) reported lower sensitivity and lower nonintrusiveness during feeding as well as lower structuring and nonintrusiveness during play for fathers of children with a feeding disorder. Moreover, children with feeding disorders were less responsive and involving when interacting with their fathers during both contexts. Thus, these results may mark spillover effects from difficulties around feeding to other situations (play) or relationships (as mothers' EA was also lower). Further explanations could be that deficits in father-child EA may contribute to the development of feeding disorders in children or that both aspects influence each other reciprocally.

Not only children with feeding disorders are more likely to experience lower EA in interaction with their fathers but also children with sleep disturbances. Compared to fathers of children without sleep disturbances, fathers (but not mothers) of children with sleep disturbances showed lower sensitivity during feeding interactions (no other EA dimensions assessed; Millikovsky-Ayalon et al., 2015). This finding could implicate that as parents are challenged by children's problems with sleeping during the night, it is more difficult for fathers to show sensitive behaviour during the day, potentially because their own quality of sleep and well-being is adversely affected (e.g. McDaniel & Teti, 2012). Of course, it is also possible that deficits in fathers' sensitivity contribute to the prospective development of sleeping problems in children (e.g. Bordeleau, Bernier, & Carrier, 2012) or that reciprocal associations between parent-child EA and children's sleep patterns occur (Philbrook & Teti, 2016).

However, considering that current evidence regarding the association between children's regulatory problems and father-child EA is – to the best of our knowledge – limited to two studies only, further research is needed to replicate these results and to investigate how father-child EA and the persistence of regulatory problems in children affect each other over time.

Social Context

Just as the mother-child relationship is embedded within a broader family system, so too is the father-child relationship (Cabrera, Karberg,

Malin, & Aldoney, 2017), which therefore cannot be viewed isolated but only in the broader context of other relationships, especially the spousal relationship. For example, the quality of the marital relationships, i.e. the level of discord which fathers perceive in the relationship to the mother, is negatively associated with the quality of the father-child interaction (e.g. Bernier, Jarry-Boileau, & Lacharité, 2014; Schacht, Cummings, & Davies, 2009). This is potentially due to the adverse effect which marital conflicts exert on fathers' psychological well-being (e.g. Cheung, Theule, Hiebert-Murphy, & Piotrowski, 2019) or by creating spillover effects of detriments from the marital relationship to the father-child relationship (Erel & Burman, 1995). Thus, by adopting an ecological perspective, Belsky (1984) reviewed the influence of sources of stress and support in the social environment in which the parent-child relationship is embedded on parenting. Specifically, he focused on the marital relationship, support provided by the social network and the experienced level of occupational stress. In accordance with his model, we will give an overview on the scarce empirical evidence, viewing father-child EA in the context of family relationships (mother-child EA, co-parenting quality) as well as in association with socio-economic aspects.

Mother-Child EA, Co-Parenting Quality

A large amount of studies provide empirical evidence that within the family microsystem the father-child relationship is interrelated with other relationships (e.g. Cabrera, Fitzgerald, Bradley, & Roggman, 2014; Cabrera, Shannon, & La Taillade, 2009; Cox & Paley, 2003; Cox, Paley, & Harter, 2001; Holland & McElwain, 2013). However, not much is known about how family subsystems influence each other regarding parent-child EA. Research on mothers showed that father presence (i.e. whether the father resided in the home or not) and marital status (i.e. whether the mother was married or not) seem to be positively associated with mother-child EA (Bornstein, Putnick, & Suwalsky, 2012). Moreover, high quality of co-parenting (experiencing increased closeness, support, endorsement) as reported by mothers predicts greater EA in mother-infant interaction as compared to when mothers report conflicts or competition in the relationship to the father (Kim & Teti, 2014). However, it is unclear whether this applies to fathers in the same way, yet what is striking is that in many studies taking both mothers' EA and fathers' EA in interaction with their children into account, moderate to strong positive correlations between maternal and corresponding paternal EA dimensions were reported (e.g. Atzaba-Poria et al., 2010; de Falco et al., 2009; Hallers-Haalboom et al., 2014; Martins et al., 2016; Millikovsky-Ayalon et al., 2015). Even when investigated longitudinally, fathers' sensitivity positively related to mothers' sensitivity over time (Hallers-Haalboom et al., 2017). There are several explanations for these findings. First, parent-child EA does not reflect a fixed characteristic of either parent or child but rather an aspect of their relationship (Biringen et al., 2014). Thus, convergences between father-child and mother-child EA could be an indicator of the overall family climate, such as the level of conflict, cohesion or emotional atmosphere (e.g. Yoo, Popp, & Robinson, 2014) and spillover effects from one dyadic relationship to another. Second, positive associations between father-child and mother-child EA could be due to "assortative mating", i.e. persons choose those individuals as partners who resemble them regarding their level of EA or potential determinants of EA, e.g. certain emotional competences (Bergmann, von Klitzing, et al., 2016). Third, the positive association could also be based on the fact that both parents interacted with the same children who due to their own characteristics (see above) trigger similar emotional exchanges with both their parents.

Taken together, despite current findings on associations between father-child and mother-child EA, we still lack knowledge on how EA in father-child relationships relates to the quality of other familial relationships and on processes underlying these associations.

Aspects of Socio-economic Status

The socio-economic conditions experienced by families impact the way in which mothers and fathers parent their children in complex manners, e.g. by affecting parental well-being and health or by reflecting disparate access to material resources (e.g. Roubinov & Boyce, 2017). Socio-economic status (SES) consists of multiple facets but is often operationalized using indicators such as income, level of educational attainment and occupation. Though low SES appears to be a relevant contextual risk factor for lower maternal EA, e.g. lower sensitivity, structuring and nonhostility in some studies (e.g. de Falco et al., 2014; McCarthy et al., 2003; Ziv et al., 2000), the association of aspects of SES with father-child EA seems less clear. Whereas in a study of families with two children, higher education in fathers was associated with higher paternal sensitivity in interaction with the youngest child (Hallers-Haalboom et al., 2014), no association between family SES and father-child EA was found in other samples (de Falco et al., 2009; Martins et al., 2016). Furthermore, fathers' EA with infants of 12 months was not related to family social risk which besides including aspects of SES also included further risks such as maternal age at birth and language spoken at home (McMahon et al., 2019). In contrast to these cross-sectional findings, in the longitudinal study by Rossen et al. (2018), greater socio-economic disadvantage assessed 8 weeks after childbirth significantly negatively predicted father-child EA when children were 12 months old. Hence, future research is needed to explore whether or not SES influences father-child EA and to further investigate mechanisms of this potential association.

Does Fathers' EA Affect Child Outcomes?

Fathers significantly impact their children's development – often independently from mothers' influence on child outcomes (Volling & Cabrera, 2019). Positive aspects of fathers' behaviour when interacting with their children (e.g. supportiveness, mutual responsiveness etc.) predict greater socio-emotional competence, emotion regulation and language development in children, whereas negative aspects (e.g. intrusiveness, negativity, etc.) are associated with negative child outcomes such as externalizing or internalizing symptoms (e.g. Volling & Cabrera, 2019).

Despite this base of evidence, studies investigating if and how father-child EA affects child development remain scarce. From studies on mother-child dyads, we know that high mother-child EA significantly predicts a variety of positive child outcomes, such as greater social competence (e.g. Bergmann, Schlesier-Michel, et al., 2016; Biringen et al., 2005) and emotion regulation (Little & Carter, 2005) as well as increased cognitive and language development (e.g. Austin et al., 2017). In addition, high mother-child EA seems to be a protective factor against the development of child psychopathology (e.g. Biringen et al., 2005; Bödeker et al., 2018). These findings have only recently been extended to fathers in a prospective study in Australia, which investigated the effect of fathers' EA (i.e. sensitivity, structuring, nonintrusiveness, nonhostility) with 81 preterm and 39 full-term infants at 12 months of corrected age on child development at 24 months of corrected age. This study demonstrated that – after controlling for child sex, family social risk and preterm vs. full term birth – high paternal sensitivity as well as high structuring at 12 months predicted greater child language development at 24 months. Moreover, a high level of structuring predicted greater child cognitive development, whereas greater paternal intrusiveness (i.e., lower nonintrusiveness) at 12 months predicted a greater extent of child externalizing symptoms at 24 months. No effect of fathers' EA on children's motor development was found (McMahon et al., 2019). A potential mechanism that could underlie the association between father-child EA and child development could involve children's emotion regulation, which evolves within the early relationship with the caregiver: If children experience adequate regulation of their arousal and emotional state by a responsive and attuned caregiver, they are more likely to develop healthy emotion regulation competences, which in turn could protect them from maladaptive development (e.g. Sroufe, 2000). Thus, fathers' EA might also contribute to children's development of emotion regulation. This assumption is supported by a study, which investigated if EA (sum of all scales) in mother-child and father-child dyad would be associated with emotion regulation exhibited by 10-month-old infants across parents. When father-child EA was high, children were more likely to show adaptive emotion regulation with both parents than adaptive emotion regulation with just one parent. Likewise, when father-child EA was low, children were more likely to show maladaptive emotion regulation with both parents than adaptive emotion regulation with one parent. Mother-child EA, however, was not associated with emotion regulation concordance (Martins et al., 2016). In line with this result, findings of other studies suggest that deficits in father-child EA could promote the development of regulatory problems in children (Atzaba-Poria et al., 2010; Millikovsky-Ayalon et al., 2015; see also above: child characteristics as determinants of EA).

To summarize, there are first indications that young children benefit from high father-child EA. However, as there is still a lack of studies which replicate these results, more research investigating the contribution of fathers' EA on various aspects of child development is needed. Beyond that, due to a potential benefit of children from high father-child EA, the question arises how EA in father-child dyads can be improved.

How Can Fathers' EA Be Improved?

In general, there are several interventions, which seem to increase EA in various populations, though not all of them have been investigated yet in randomized controlled trials (RCTs). The majority of interventions use relationship- or attachment-based approaches, which can be part of home-visit programmes and usually focus on mothers and their children ranging from infancy up to prekindergarten age (e.g. Flierman et al., 2016; Nicolson, Judd, Thomson-Salo, & Mitchell, 2013; Olds et al., 2002; Ziv, Kaplan, & Venza, 2016). As indicated by evidence-based research, interventions based on video feedback are particularly effective (Bakermans-Kranenburg, van Ijzendoorn, & Juffer, 2003). One specific example is the Video-feedback Intervention to promote Positive Parenting (VIPP; Juffer, Bakermans-Kranenburg, & van Ijzendoorn, 2008), which integrates aspects of attachment theory and social learning theory. Within a strength-based approach, it aims to promote responsive and sensitive parental behaviour by providing supportive feedback to parents on positive aspects of their behaviour (e.g. sensitivity, empathy) in (video-recorded) interactions with their children. Though previous studies indicate that video feedback is feasible with father-child dyads and well-accepted by fathers (Iles, Rosan, Wilkinson, & Ramchandani, 2017; Lawrence, Davies, & Ramchandani, 2013), its effect on EA has not yet been explicitly investigated in father-child dyads so far. Still, small numbers of fathers are included in studies investigating effectiveness of video-feedback interventions on parent-child EA: An RCT by Poslawsky et al. (2015) included fathers (n = 8, i.e. 10% of parents) as primary caregivers when examining the effect of VIPP opposed to care as usual (control condition) on parent-child EA in children with autism. After the intervention, parents who had received VIPP showed an increase in EA: Parental nonintrusiveness was significantly higher than before the intervention. In the control group, however, nonintrusiveness decreased. Likewise, a tele-intervention approach using videoconferencing (i.e. Skype) to deliver a programme (EA2 intervention) was applied to mothers (n = 12) as well as fathers (n = 3) with adoptive children. Of these families, n = 8 received the intervention immediately, whereas the control group of $n = 7$ families received the intervention after a waiting period of 6 weeks. The intervention included various elements with group discussions on videotaped interactions of other parent-child interactions and video feedback among them (Baker, Biringen, Meyer-Parsons, & Schneider, 2015). Though due to the very small sample size, caution is warranted when interpreting the results, this pilot study suggests an increase of EA (all adult dimensions and child responsiveness) in parents who immediately received the intervention compared to a randomized wait-list group, which showed slight decreases in structuring, nonintrusiveness and nonhostility (Baker et al., 2015). As the number of fathers was small in both cases – in the study by Poslawsky et al. (2015) as well as in the study by Baker et al. (2015) – these studies did not provide separate analyses for mothers and fathers regarding the effects of the intervention on parent-child EA. Hence, we cannot draw any conclusion whether the interventions reported above are equally effective regarding an improvement of father-child-EA as they are regarding mother-child EA. However, an answer to this question would be helpful as there seems to be a tendency to apply the same templates of interventions that have been developed to improve mothers' EA likewise to fathers. In order to develop interventions specifically tailored to improve EA in fathers, a greater evidence base regarding determinants of father-child EA and its effect on child development is needed.

Summary and Key Points

Parallel to fathers' growing active role in parenting and childcare in Western countries, they have also increasingly become a focus of research. It was and is of great interest how fathers interact with their children, which aspects are favourable or impeding for positive interactions and relationships between fathers and their children, which domains of child development are affected by the way fathers and children shape their relationships and whether there are opportunities to positively influence father-child interactions and thus also child development. Contributing to the continuously growing literature in the field of fatherhood research, the aim of this chapter was to give an overview of the current state of research on the affective quality of father-child interactions, i.e. as assessed by father-child EA. Although the number of studies dealing with EA in father-child interactions is comparably low, considering the plethora of studies assessing mother-child EA, which currently encompasses a number of 300 studies and more, the information accumulated in publications on father-child EA and summarized in this chapter could serve as a starting point for future research based on the following key points.

First, studies contrasting mean levels of father-child and mother-child EA are common within the EA literature but inconsistent regarding their results. The reasons for this inconsistency may be found in methodological aspects (e.g. characteristics of the sample, sample size, statistical approach) but so far remain unclear. Hence, future research is needed to shed some more light on the question under which circumstances fathers are different from mothers regarding EA and whether or not potential differences would result in any consequences for child development.

Second, though studies investigating EA in fathers have grown in number throughout recent years, not much is known on potential determinants of father-child EA, due to both the lack of studies and inconsistent results across studies. The majority of available evidence regarding this issue is based on results derived from cross-sectional, correlational and non-experimental studies, which do not allow any conclusions regarding the causality of effects. Using longitudinal study designs and gaining understanding and knowledge on which factors influence father-child EA and what makes it more difficult for some fathers than others to exhibit high EA is of utmost relevance not only for identifying potential risk factors for child development but also for the development of means of prevention and intervention, which effectively improve EA in fathers and their children.

Third, there is a dearth of studies investigating the effect of father-child EA on different domains of child development. Again, cross-sectional and correlational studies are not sufficient to gain an idea about the direction of effects; thus, longitudinal studies are necessary. Moreover, an advantage of the EA framework over other observational instruments is that parent-child interactions are assessed using a multidimensional approach. Knowing which EA dimension of father-child interactions predicts which domain in child development could contribute to the development of specific prevention or intervention programmes for fathers. Additionally, investigating both parents' interactions with their children could help to elucidate the relative impact of mothers' and fathers' EA on prospective child development including potential buffering or exacerbating effects.

Fourth, our evaluation in this chapter revealed that the empirical base for knowing how to specifically improve EA in fathers is not sufficient. This is due to the phenomenon that interventions which on theoretical and empirical grounds are designed to improve mother-child EA are also used for a small number of fathers, which is not sufficiently large enough to allow specific subgroup analyses (i.e. effectiveness of the intervention regarding mothers' vs. fathers' EA). Hence, it would be premature to conclude that these interventions were successful in improving father-child EA. Thus, apart from including a greater number of fathers in randomized controlled studies to test the effectiveness of interventions, which are currently available to improve EA, more knowledge and understanding of factors, which affect father-child EA, are imperative in order to design successful interventions. As there is a good chance that father-child EA may represent a relevant avenue to improve child development, addressing the gaps of research summarized in this chapter should be given a greater priority.

References

Ainsworth, M. D. S., Blehar, M., Waters, E., & Wall, S. (1978). *Patterns of attachment: a psychological study of the Strange Situation*. Hillsdale, NJ: Erlbaum.

Altenhofen, S., Clyman, R., Little, C., Baker, M., & Biringen, Z. (2013). Attachment security in three-year-olds who entered substitute care in infancy. *Infant Mental Health Journal, 34*(5), 435–445.

Atzaba-Poria, N., Meiri, G., Millikovsky, M., Barkai, A., Dunaevsky-Idan, M., & Yerushalmi, B. (2010). Father-child and mother-child interaction in families with a child feeding disorder: the role of paternal involvement. *Infant Mental Health Journal, 31*(6), 682–698.

Austin, M. P., Christl, B., McMahon, C., Kildea, S., Reilly, N., Yin, C., et al. (2017). Moderating effects of maternal emotional availability on language and cognitive development in toddlers of mothers exposed to a natural disaster in pregnancy: The QF2011 Queensland Flood Study. *Infant Behavior & Development, 49*, 296–309.

Aviezer, O., Sagi, A., Joels, T., & Ziv, Y. (1999). Emotional availability and attachment representations in kibbutz infants and their mothers. *Developmental Psychology, 35*(3), 811–821.

Baker, M., Biringen, Z., Meyer-Parsons, B., & Schneider, A. (2015). Emotional attachment and emotional availability tele-intervention for adoptive families. *Infant Mental Health Journal, 36*(2), 179–192.

Bakermans-Kranenburg, M. J., van Ijzendoorn, M. H., & Juffer, F. (2003). Less is more: meta-analyses of sensitivity and attachment interventions in early childhood. *Psychological Bulletin, 129*(2), 195–215.

Barfoot, J., Meredith, P., Ziviani, J., & Whittingham, K. (2017). Parent-child interactions and children with cerebral palsy: An exploratory study investigating emotional availability, functional ability, and parent distress. *Child: Care, Health and Development, 43*(6), 812–822.

Belsky, J. (1984). The determinants of parenting: A process model. *Child Development, 55*(1), 83–96.

Belsky, J., & Jaffee, S. R. (2006). The multiple determinants of parenting. In D. Cicchetti & D. J. Cohen (Eds.), *Developmental psychopathology: Risk, disorder, and adaptation* (pp. 38–85). Hoboken, NJ: Wiley.

Belsky, J., & Pluess, M. (2009). Beyond diathesis stress: Differential susceptibility to environmental influences. *Psychological Bulletin, 135*(6), 885–908.

Bergmann, S., Schlesier-Michel, A., Wendt, V., Grube, M., Keitel-Korndörfer, A., Gausche, R., et al. (2016). Maternal weight predicts children's psychosocial development via parenting stress and emotional availability. *Frontiers in Psychology, 7*, 1156.

Bergmann, S., von Klitzing, K., Keitel-Korndörfer, A., Wendt, V., Grube, M., Herpertz, S., et al. (2016). Emotional availability, understanding emotions, and recognition of facial emotions in obese mothers with young children. *Journal of Psychosomatic Research, 80*, 44–52.

Bergmann, S., Wendt, V., von Klitzing, K., & Klein, A. M. (2013). Emotional availability of father–child dyads versus mother–child dyads in children aged 0-3 years. *Family Science, 3*(3–4), 145–154.

Bernier, A., Jarry-Boileau, V., & Lacharité, C. (2014). Marital satisfaction and quality of father-child interactions: The moderating role of child gender. *The Journal of Genetic Psychology, 175*(2), 105–117.

Biringen, Z. (2000). Emotional availability: Conceptualization and research findings. *American Journal of Orthopsychiatry, 70*(1), 104–114.

Biringen, Z. (2008). *The emotional availability (EA) scales* (4th ed.). Boulder, CO. emotionalavailability.com

Biringen, Z., Brown, D., Donaldson, L., Green, S., Krcmarik, S., & Lovas, G. (2000). Adult Attachment Interview: Linkages with dimensions of emotional availability for mothers and their pre-kindergarteners. *Attachment & Human Development, 2*(2), 188–202.

Biringen, Z., Damon, J., Grigg, W., Mone, J., Pipp-Siegel, S., Skillern, S., et al. (2005). Emotional availability: Differential predictions to infant attachment and kindergarten adjustment based on observation time and context. *Infant Mental Health Journal, 26*(4), 295–308.

Biringen, Z., Derscheid, D., Vliegen, N., Closson, L., & Easterbrooks, M. A. (2014). Emotional availability (EA): Theoretical background, empirical research using the EA Scales, and clinical applications. *Developmental Review, 34*(2), 114–167.

Biringen, Z., Emde, R. N., Brown, D., Lowe, L., Myers, S., & Nelson, D. (1999). Emotional availability and emotion communication in naturalistic mother-infant interactions: Evidence for gender relations. *Journal of Social Behavior and Personality, 14*(4), 463–478.

Biringen, Z., Emde, R. N., Campos, J. J., & Appelbaum, M. I. (1995). Affective reorganization in the infant, the mother, and the dyad: The role of upright locomotion and its timing. *Child Development, 66*(2), 499–514.

Biringen, Z., & Robinson, J. (1991). Emotional availability in mother-child interactions: A reconceptualization for research. *American Journal of Orthopsychiatry, 61*(2), 258–271.

Biringen, Z., Robinson, J., & Emde, R. (1998). *Emotional availability scales,* (3rd ed.) Unpublished manual for the EAS-training. www.emotionalavailability.com.

Bödeker, K., Fuchs, A., Fuhrer, D., Kluczniok, D., Dittrich, K., Reichl, C., et al. (2018). Impact of maternal early life maltreatment and maternal history of depression on child psychopathology: Mediating role of maternal sensitivity? *Child Psychiatry & Human Development, 50,* 278.

Bordeleau, S., Bernier, A., & Carrier, J. (2012). Longitudinal associations between the quality of parent-child interactions and children's sleep at preschool age. *Journal of Family Psychology, 26*(2), 254–262.

Bornstein, M. H., Gini, M., Putnick, D. L., Haynes, O. M., Painter, K. M., & Suwalsky, J. T. D. (2006). Short-term reliability and continuity of emotional availability in mother-child dyads across contexts of observation. *Infancy, 10*(1), 1–16.

Bornstein, M. H., Gini, M., Suwalsky, J. T. D., Putnick, D. L., & Haynes, O. M. (2006). Emotional availability in mother-child dyads: short-term stability and continuity from variable-centered and person-centered perspectives. *Merrill-Palmer Quarterly-Journal of Developmental Psychology, 52*(3), 547–571.

Bornstein, M. H., Hahn, C. S., Suwalsky, J. T. D., & Haynes, O. M. (2011). Maternal and infant behavior and context associations with mutual emotion availability. *Infant Mental Health Journal, 32*(1), 70–94.

Bornstein, M. H., Putnick, D. L., Heslington, M., Gini, M., Suwalsky, J. T., Venuti, P., et al. (2008). Mother-child emotional availability in ecological perspective: three countries, two regions, two genders. *Developmental Psychology, 44*(3), 666–680.

Bornstein, M. H., Putnick, D. L., & Suwalsky, J. T. D. (2012). A longitudinal process analysis of mother-child emotional relationships in a rural Appalachian European American community. *American Journal of Community Psychology, 50*(1–2), 89–100.

Bornstein, M. H., Suwalsky, J. T., Putnick, D. L., Gini, M., Venuti, P., de Falco, S., et al. (2010). Developmental continuity and stability of Emotional Availability in the family: two ages and two genders in child-mother dyads from two regions in three countries. *International Journal of Behavioral Development, 34*(5), 385–397.

Bowlby, J. (1973). *Attachment and loss. Volume I: Attachment* (2nd ed.). New York: Basic Books.

Cabrera, N. J., Fitzgerald, H. E., Bradley, R. H., & Roggman, L. (2014). The ecology of father-child relationships: an expanded model. *Journal of Family Theory & Review, 6*(4), 336–354.

Cabrera, N. J., Karberg, E., Malin, J. L., & Aldoney, D. (2017). The magic of play: Low-income mothers' and fathers playfulness and children's emotion regulation and vocabulary skills. *Infant Mental Health Journal, 38*(6), 757–771.

Cabrera, N. J., Shannon, J. D., & La Taillade, J. J. (2009). Predictors of co-parenting in Mexican American families and direct effects on parenting and child social emotional development. *Infant Mental Health Journal, 30*(5), 523–548.

Cabrera, N. J., Shannon, J. D., & Tamis-LeMonda, C. (2007). Fathers' influence on their children's cognitive and emotional development: from toddlers to pre-K. *Applied Developmental Science, 11*(4), 208–213.

Cabrera, N. J., Volling, B. L., & Barr, R. (2018). Fathers are parents, too! Widening the lens on parenting for children's development. *Child Development Perspectives, 12*(3), 152–157.

Celia, M. G., Stack, D. M., & Serbin, L. A. (2018). Developmental patterns of change in mother and child emotional availability from infancy to the end of the preschool years: a four-wave longitudinal study. *BioMed Research International, 52*, 76–88.

Cheung, K., Theule, J., Hiebert-Murphy, D., & Piotrowski, C. (2019). Paternal depressive symptoms and marital quality: A meta-analysis of cross-sectional studies. *Journal of Family Theory & Review, 11*(3), 449–467.

Cornish, A. M., McMahon, C., & Ungerer, J. A. (2008). Postnatal depression and the quality of mother-infant interactions during the second year of life. *Australian Journal of Psychology, 60*(3), 142–151.

Cox, M. J., & Paley, B. (2003). Understanding families as systems. *Current Directions in Psychological Science, 12*(5), 193–196.

Cox, M. J., Paley, B., & Harter, K. (2001). Interparental conflict and parent-child relationships. In J. H. Grych & F. D. Fincham (Eds.), *Interparental conflict and child development: Theory, research, and applications* (pp. 249–272). New York: Cambridge University Press.

Crawley, S. B., & Sherrod, K. B. (1984). Parent-infant play during the first year of life. *Infant Behavior and Development, 7*(1), 65–75.

de Falco, S., Emer, A., Martini, L., Rigo, P., Pruner, S., & Venuti, P. (2014). Predictors of mother-child interaction quality and child attachment security in at-risk families. *Frontiers in Psychology, 5*, 898.

de Falco, S., Venuti, P., Esposito, G., & Bornstein, M. H. (2009). Mother-child and father-child emotional availability in families of children with Down Syndrome. *Parenting-Science and Practice, 9*(3–4), 198–215.

Easterbrooks, M. A., Biesecker, G., & Lyons-Ruth, K. (2000). Infancy predictors of emotional availability in middle childhood: the roles of attachment security and maternal depressive symptomatology. *Attachment & Human Development, 2*(2), 170–187.

Erel, O., & Burman, B. (1995). Interrelatedness of marital relations and parent-child relations: A meta-analytic review. *Psychological Bulletin, 118*(1), 108–132.

Feldman, R., Keren, M., Gross-Rozval, O., & Tyano, S. (2004). Mother-child touch patterns in infant feeding disorders: Relation to maternal, child, and environmental factors. *Journal of the American Academy of Child and Adolescent Psychiatry, 43*(9), 1089–1097.

Feniger-Schaal, R., & Joels, T. (2018). Attachment quality of children with ID and its link to maternal sensitivity and structuring. *Research in Developmental Disabilities, 76*, 56–64.

Fitzgerald, H. E., Maguin, E. T., Zucker, R. A., & Reider, E. E. (1994). Time spent with child and parental agreement about preschool children's behavior. *Perceptual and Motor Skills, 79*(1), 336–338.

Flierman, M., Koldewijn, K., Meijssen, D., van Wassenaer-Leemhuis, A., Aarnoudse-Moens, C., van Schie, P., et al. (2016). Feasibility of a preventive parenting intervention for very preterm children at 18 months corrected age: A randomized pilot trial. *The Journal of Pediatrics, 176*, 79–85.e71.

Gartstein, M. A., & Rothbart, M. K. (2003). Studying infant temperament via the revised infant behavior questionnaire. *Infant Behavior and Development, 26*(1), 64–86.

Guttman, H. A. (1991). Systems theory, cybernetics, and epistemology. In A. S. Gurman & D. P. Kniskern (Eds.), *Handbook of family therapy* (Vol. 2, pp. 41–62). New York: Brunner/Mazel.

Hallers-Haalboom, E. T., Groeneveld, M. G., van Berkel, S. R., Endendijk, J. J., van der Pol, L. D., Linting, M., et al. (2017). Mothers' and fathers' sensitivity with their two children: A longitudinal study from infancy to early childhood. *Developmental Psychology, 53*(5), 860–872.

Hallers-Haalboom, E. T., Mesman, J., Groeneveld, M. G., Endendijk, J. J., van Berkel, S. R., van der Pol, L. D., et al. (2014). Mothers, fathers, sons and daughters: parental sensitivity in families with two children. *Journal of Family Psychology, 28*(2), 138–147.

Holland, A. S., & McElwain, N. L. (2013). Maternal and paternal perceptions of coparenting as a link between marital quality and the parent-toddler relationship. *Journal of Family Psychology, 27*(1), 117–126.

Iles, J. E., Rosan, C., Wilkinson, E., & Ramchandani, P. G. (2017). Adapting and developing a video-feedback intervention for co-parents of infants at risk of externalising behaviour problems (VIPP-Co): A feasibility study. *Clinical Child Psychology and Psychiatry, 22*(3), 483–499.

Jian, N., & Teti, D. M. (2016). Emotional availability at bedtime, infant temperament, and infant sleep development from one to six months. *Sleep Medicine, 23*, 49–58.

John, A., Halliburton, A., & Humphrey, J. (2013). Child–mother and child–father play interaction patterns with preschoolers. *Early Child Development and Care, 183*(3–4), 483–497.

Juffer, F., Bakermans-Kranenburg, M. J., & van Ijzendoorn, M. H. (Eds.). (2008). *Promoting positive parenting: an attachment-based intervention.* New York: Taylor & Francis.

Kaplan, L. A., Evans, L., & Monk, C. (2008). Effects of mothers' prenatal psychiatric status and postnatal caregiving on infant biobehavioral regulation: Can prenatal programming be modified? *Early Human Development, 84*(4), 249–256.

Karberg, E., Cabrera, N. J., Malin, J., & Kuhns, C. (2019). Longitudinal contributions of maternal and paternal intrusive behaviors to children's sociability and sustained attention at prekindergarten. *Monographs of the Society for Research in Child Development, 84*(1), 79–93.

Kiang, L., Moreno, A. J., & Robinson, J. L. (2004). Maternal preconceptions about parenting predict child temperament, maternal sensitivity, and children's empathy. *Developmental Psychology, 40*(6), 1081–1092.

Kim, B. R., Chow, S. M., Bray, B., & Teti, D. M. (2017). Trajectories of mothers' emotional availability: Relations with infant temperament in predicting attachment security. *Attachment & Human Development, 19*(1), 38–57.

Kim, B. R., & Teti, D. M. (2014). Maternal emotional availability during infant bedtime: an ecological framework. *Journal of Family Psychology, 28*(1), 1–11.

Kochanska, G., & Aksan, N. (2004). Development of mutual responsiveness between parents and their young children. *Child Development, 75*(6), 1657–1676.

Lamb, M. E., Pleck, J. H., Charnov, E. L., & Levine, J. A. (1987). A biosocial perspective on paternal behavior and involvement. In J. B. Lancaster, J. Altman, A. S. Rossi, & L. R. Sherroa (Eds.), *Parenting across the life span* (pp. 111–142). New York: Aldine de Gruyter.

Lawrence, P. J., Davies, B., & Ramchandani, P. G. (2013). Using video feedback to improve early father-infant interaction: a pilot study. *Clinical Child Psychology and Psychiatry, 18*(1), 61–71.

Leaper, C. (2002). Parenting girls and boys. In M. H. Bornstein (Ed.), *Handbook of parenting. Volume 1: Children and parenting* (2nd ed., pp. 189–226). Mahwah, NJ: Lawrence Erlbaum.

Licata, M., Paulus, M., Thoermer, C., Kristen, S., Woodward, A. L., & Sodian, B. (2014). Mother-infant interaction quality and infants' ability to encode actions as goal-directed. *Social Development, 23*(2), 340–356.

Little, C., & Carter, A. S. (2005). Negative emotional reactivity and regulation in 12-month-olds following emotional challenge: Contributions of maternal-infant emotional availability in a low-income sample. *Infant Mental Health Journal, 26*(4), 354–368.

Lovas, G. S. (2005). Gender and patterns of emotional availability in mother-toddler and father-toddler dyads. *Infant Mental Health Journal, 26*(4), 327–353.

Lucassen, N., Tharner, A., Van Ijzendoorn, M. H., Bakermans-Kranenburg, M. J., Volling, B. L., Verhulst, F. C., et al. (2011). The association between paternal sensitivity and infant-father attachment security: A meta-analysis of three decades of research. *Journal of Family Psychology, 25*(6), 986–992.

Malmberg, L. E., Lewis, S., West, A., Murray, E., Sylva, K., & Stein, A. (2016). The influence of mothers' and fathers' sensitivity in the first year of life on children's cognitive outcomes at 18 and 36 months. *Child: Care, Health and Development, 42*(1), 1–7.

Mansdotter, A., Fredlund, P., Hallqvist, J., & Magnusson, C. (2010). Who takes paternity leave? A cohort study on prior social and health characteristics among fathers in Stockholm. *Journal of Public Health Policy, 31*(3), 324–341.

Martins, C., Mateus, V., Osorio, A., Martins, E. C., & Soares, I. (2014). Joint attention with the mother and the father at 10 months of age. *European Journal of Developmental Psychology, 11*(3), 319–330.

Martins, E. C., Soares, I., Martins, C., & Osório, A. (2016). Infants' style of emotion regulation with their mothers and fathers: Concordance between parents and the contribution of father-infant interaction quality. *Social Development, 25*(4), 812–827.

McCarthy, P., Walls, T., Cicchetti, D., Mayes, L., Rizzo, J., Lopez-Benitez, J., et al. (2003). Prediction of resource use during acute pediatric illnesses. *Archives of Pediatrics & Adolescent Medicine, 157*(10), 990–996.

McDaniel, B. T., & Teti, D. M. (2012). Coparenting quality during the first three months after birth: the role of infant sleep quality. *Journal of Family Psychology, 26*(6), 886–895.

McMahon, G. E., Spencer-Smith, M. M., Pace, C. C., Spittle, A. J., Stedall, P., Richardson, K., et al. (2019). Influence of fathers' early parenting on the development of children born very preterm and full term. *Journal of Pediatrics, 205*, 195–201.

Menashe, A., & Atzaba-Poria, N. (2016). Parent–child interaction: Does parental language matter? *British Journal of Developmental Psychology, 34*(4), 518–537.

Menashe-Grinberg, A., & Atzaba-Poria, N. (2017). Mother–child and father–child play interaction: The importance of parental playfulness as a moderator of the links between parental behavior and child negativity. *Infant Mental Health Journal, 38*(6), 772–784.

Micalizzi, L., Wang, M., & Saudino, K. J. (2017). Difficult temperament and negative parenting in early childhood: A genetically informed cross-lagged analysis. *Developmental Science, 20*(2).

Millikovsky-Ayalon, M., Atzaba-Poria, N., & Meiri, G. (2015). The role of the father in child sleep disturbance: Child, parent, and parent–child relationship. *Infant Mental Health Journal, 36*(1), 114–127.

Mitchell, S. J., See, H. M., Tarkow, A. K. H., Cabrera, N., McFadden, K. E., & Shannon, J. D. (2007). Conducting studies with fathers: Challenges and opportunities. *Applied Developmental Science, 11*(4), 239–244.

Moreno, A. J., Klute, M. M., & Robinson, J. L. (2008). Relational and individual resources as predictors of empathy in early childhood. *Social Development, 17*(3), 613–637.

Morrell, J., & Steele, H. (2003). The role of attachment security, temperament, maternal perception, and caregiving behavior in persistent infant sleeping problems. *Infant Mental Health Journal, 24*(5), 447–468.

Nicolson, S., Judd, F., Thomson-Salo, F., & Mitchell, S. (2013). Supporting the adolescent mother-infant relationship: Preliminary trial of a brief perinatal attachment intervention. *Archives of Women's Mental Health, 16*(6), 511–520.

Olds, D. L., Robinson, J., O'Brien, R., Luckey, D. W., Pettitt, L. M., Henderson Jr., C. R., et al. (2002). Home visiting by paraprofessionals and by nurses: a randomized, controlled trial. *Pediatrics, 110*(3), 486–496.

Paquette, D., Carbonneau, R., Dubeau, D., Bigras, M., & Tremblay, R. E. (2003). Prevalence of father-child rough-and-tumble play and physical aggression in preschool children. *European Journal of Psychology of Education, 18*(2), 171–189.

Philbrook, L. E., & Teti, D. M. (2016). Bidirectional associations between bedtime parenting and infant sleep: parenting quality, parenting practices, and their interaction. *Journal of Family Psychology, 30*(4), 431–441.

Piermattei, C., Pace, C. S., Tambelli, R., D'Onofrio, E., & Di Folco, S. (2017). Late adoptions: attachment security and emotional availability in mother–child and father–child dyads. *Journal of Child and Family Studies, 26*(8), 2114–2125.

Poslawsky, I. E., Naber, F. B. A., Bakermans-Kranenburg, M. J., van Daalen, E., van Engeland, H., & van Ijzendoorn, M. H. (2015). Video-feedback Intervention to promote Positive Parenting adapted to Autism (VIPP-AUTI): a randomized controlled trial. *Autism, 19*(5), 588–603.

Putnam, S. P., Rothbart, M. K., & Gartstein, M. A. (2008). Homotypic and heterotypic continuity of fine-grained temperament during infancy, toddlerhood, and early childhood. *Infant and Child Development: An International Journal of Research and Practice, 17*(4), 387–405.

Riva Crugnola, C., & Ierardi, E. (2018). Reflective functioning, maternal attachment, mind-mindedness, and emotional availability in adolescent and adult mothers at infant 3 months. *Attachment & Human Development, 20*(1), 84–106.

Rossen, L., Mattick, R. P., Wilson, J., Burns, L., Macdonald, J. A., Olsson, C., et al. (2018). Mother-infant and partner-infant emotional availability at 12 months of age: Findings from an Australian longitudinal study. *Infancy, 23*(6), 893–916.

Roubinov, D. S., & Boyce, W. T. (2017). Parenting and SES: Relative values or enduring principles? *Current Opinion in Psychology, 15*, 162–167.

Saunders, H., Kraus, A., Barone, L., & Biringen, Z. (2015). Emotional availability: theory, research, and intervention. *Frontiers in Psychology, 6*, 1069.

Schacht, P. M., Cummings, E. M., & Davies, P. T. (2009). Fathering in family context and child adjustment: A longitudinal analysis. *Journal of Family Psychology, 23*(6), 790.

Sroufe, L. A. (2000). Early relationships and the development of children. *Infant Mental Health Journal, 21*(1–2), 67–74.

St George, J., & Freeman, E. (2017). Measurement of father-child rough-and-tumble play and its relations to child behavior. *Infant Mental Health Journal, 38*(6), 709–725.

Stack, D. M., Serbin, L. A., Girouard, N., Enns, L. N., Bentley, V. M., Ledingham, J. E., et al. (2012). The quality of the mother-child relationship in high-risk dyads: application of the Emotional Availability Scales in an intergenerational, longitudinal study. *Development and Psychopathology, 24*(1), 93–105.

Teti, D. M., Kim, B. R., Mayer, G., & Countermine, M. (2010). Maternal emotional availability at bedtime predicts infant sleep quality. *Journal of Family Psychology, 24*(3), 307–315.

Thomas, A., Chess, S., & Birch, H. G. (1968). *Temperament and behavior disorders in children*. New York: New York University Press.

van Ee, E., Sleijpen, M., Kleber, R. J., & Jongmans, M. J. (2013). Father-involvement in a refugee sample: relations between posttraumatic stress and caregiving. *Family Process, 52*(4), 723–735.

Volling, B. L., & Cabrera, N. J. (2019). Advancing research and measurement on fathering and child development: Introducing the issues and a conceptual framework. *Monographs of the Society for Research in Child Development, 84*(1), 7–17.

Volling, B. L., Stevenson, M. M., Safyer, P., Gonzalez, R., & Lee, J. Y. (2019). In search of the father–infant activation relationship: a person-centered approach. *Monographs of the Society for Research in Child Development, 84*(1), 50–63.

Wiefel, A., Wollenweber, S., Oepen, G., Lenz, K., Lehmkuhl, U., & Biringen, Z. (2005). Emotional availability in infant psychiatry. *Infant Mental Health Journal, 26*(4), 392–403.

Yeung, W. J., Sandberg, J. F., Davis-Kean, P. E., & Hofferth, S. L. (2001). Children's time with fathers in intact families. *Journal of Marriage and Family, 63*(1), 136–154.

Yogman, M. W. (1981). Games fathers and mothers play with their infants. *Infant Mental Health Journal, 2*(4), 241–248.

Yoo, Y. S., Popp, J., & Robinson, J. (2014). Maternal distress influences young children's family representations through maternal view of child behavior and parent-child interactions. *Child Psychiatry & Human Development, 45*(1), 52–64.

Ziv, Y., Aviezer, O., Gini, M., Sagi, A., & Koren-Karie, N. (2000). Emotional availability in the mother-infant dyad as related to the quality of infant-mother attachment relationship. *Attachment & Human Development, 2*(2), 149–169.

Ziv, Y., Kaplan, B. A., & Venza, J. (2016). Practicing attachment in the real world: improving maternal insightfulness and dyadic emotional availability at an outpatient community mental health clinic. *Attachment & Human Development, 18*(3), 292–315.

The Role of Fathers and Their Young Children's Social Development

21

Avery Hennigar, Natasha J. Cabrera, and Yu Chen

Social competence, broadly defined, is the possession of an array of social skills (e.g., self-control, interpersonal communication) that help children learn to recognize, form, and sustain positive relationships (Denham, 2006; La Paro & Pianta, 2000; Ladd, Herald, & Kochel, 2006; Raver, 2002). Social skills are important for children's success in life and are particularly critical in school settings where children are required to cooperate, follow instructions, persevere in school tasks, and get along with others (Longoria, Page, Hubbs-Tait, & Kennison, 2009). The development of social skills is the result of a confluence of epigenetic and early life experiences, and it begins in infancy, when attachment formation is critical for parent-child relationship (Ainsworth & Bowlby, 1991; Smith & Hart, 2004). In these environments, children interact with their fathers, mothers, siblings, peers, and the community at large in dynamic, stimulating, and complex ways (Hinde, 1979; Smith & Hart, 2004), through which they begin to learn to take turns and take the perspective of others (Hinde, 1979). This developmental dance between a child and his/her environment unfolds in a dynamic cultural context and results in the most significant socialization experiences in a child's life (Corsaro, 2017; Parke & Buriel, 2007; Rogoff, 2003). Yet, research on how social development unfolds has primarily focused on mothers. However, the role that fathers play in children's social development has been steadily emerging over the last few decades.

In this chapter, we first provide a short review of the ways children's social development has been defined and operationalized in the literature. We follow with a discussion of key theoretical frameworks for understanding social development and then review the current literature on the associations between fathers and their children's social development from birth through 8 years. We conclude with a summary discussing the limitations, future directions, and key points.

Defining Social Development

Social development is most often conceptualized as the ability to integrate thoughts, feelings and emotions, and behaviors to achieve interpersonal goals that are valued within a social context (Rubin & Rose-Krasnor, 1992). Children develop social skills from birth. At about 12 months of age when attachment formation becomes critical for the developing child and parents, children reach their first milestone in social development. During the preschool years, children begin to

A. Hennigar · Y. Chen
Department of Human Development and Computational Methodology, University of Maryland, College Park, MD, USA

N. J. Cabrera (✉)
Department of Human Development and Quantitative Methodology, University of Maryland, College Park, MD, USA
e-mail: ncabrera@umd.edu

H. E. Fitzgerald et al. (eds.), *Handbook of Fathers and Child Development*,
https://doi.org/10.1007/978-3-030-51027-5_21

develop friendships with other children of their same age. These early relationships at first lack well-developed perspective taking, but between the ages of 5 and 9, children begin to nurture enduring friendships, engage in social comparison, and are able to take the perspective of others, thus sharing and taking turns in peer and play interactions (Smith & Hart, 2004).

Children develop social skills in the early years during meaningful, reciprocal, and dynamic interactions with their parents. Such socialization helps children adapt to culturally appropriate values and behaviors that enable them to develop key competencies and act effectively as a member of a social group (Weisner, 2002). Socially competent children exhibit social skills (e.g., have positive interactions with others, express emotions effectively), are able to establish relationships, and have certain individual attributes, such as showing empathy and utilizing coping skills. Additionally, they exhibit self-regulatory skills, engage in planning and decision-making, exhibit positive self-identity and interpersonal skills (e.g., maintain positive relationships, resolve conflict), and demonstrate cultural competence (Han & Kemple, 2006; Ma, 2012; McCay & Keyes, 2002; Raver & Zigler, 1997).

Socially competent children behave in ways that represent culturally appropriate values and norms of the specific cultural context in which children grow up (Hussong, Zucker, Wong, Fitzgerald, & Puttler, 2005). Although there are universally accepted social behaviors, cultural groups prioritize different social skills that may be of particular importance to that group and may emphasize competencies that are reflected in different behaviors. The challenge for scholars to understand how culture is implicated in social development is defining the key dimensions of culture for a particular group. In the United States and elsewhere, children who are first or second generation live in bicultural contexts that expose them to the values and norms of their heritage country as well as the values and norms of the host country through different institutions (e.g., ethnic social clubs) and organizations. For the most part, social competencies in the social development literature are defined from a Western perspective, and thus, little is known about the social competencies that children develop while growing up in bicultural environments (Cabrera, 2012).

Theoretical Frameworks

Attachment theory (Bowlby, 1982) is the most commonly used framework to understand children's social development; in particular, scholars have examined how positive and adaptive patterns of parent-child interactions during early childhood promote later social adjustment. At the core, attachment theory posits that children seek security in relationships with their caregivers, who are most often their parents, and it suggests that individual differences in later life functioning and personality are shaped by these child's early experiences (Ainsworth, 1973). During parent-child interactions, children learn to trust their caregivers, making it possible to safely and comfortably explore their environments. Secure relationships with caregivers enable children to develop mental representations of themselves as worthy of love and respect, which shape the basis for forming loving and reciprocal relationships with peers and adults in the future. Thus, most children's earliest relationships with their mothers, fathers, siblings, extended family members, and others (i.e., friends, teachers) serve as the foundation for the development of social competency skills. While other adult caregivers who young children interact with (e.g., neighbors, preschool teachers, childcare providers) also assist in the development of children's social competencies, those that are most proximal to the child yield the greatest influence. The empirical evidence on caregivers has mostly focused on mothers rather than fathers; consequently, we know more about attachment between mothers and children than we do about fathers and children (see Brown & Aytuglu, this volume, for a review).

More recently, scholars have argued that children develop social competencies in a context of exploration. Building on attachment and evolutionary theories, Paquette's (2004) activation theory posits that fathers encourage children to take risks and engage in interactions that cause them to feel momentarily destabilized. In contrast, mothers primarily soothe and calm their children. Although there is not a lot of empirical support for this theory, fathers' "activating" approach in playing with their children, that is, exciting or shocking them during physical play, greatly benefits the early development of regulatory skills. Further, this activation is only effective for children who have an established emotional bond with their fathers. Therefore, having a secure attachment relationship is key for children and their fathers when engaging in rough-and-tumble play and other activating interactions.

According to Bronfenbrenner's ecological model, young children are socialized directly through their microsystem or their immediate and proximate environments—home and childcare—and through interactions with parents and other caregivers (Bronfenbrenner & Morris, 2006). This model also hypothesizes that children are influenced by the interrelation between microsystems, known as the mesosystem. The interactions between home and school are important for supporting children's optimal growth and development. In addition, the exosystem (e.g., parents' work environment) and macrosystems (e.g., culture, norms, government, policies) indirectly influence the child. The cascading influences of policies, cultural values, and customs reach the child through the interactions of the other subsystems. Although less studied, this model has been used in previous literature specifically to examine the father-child subsystem (e.g., Julion et al., 2016; Varghese & Wachen, 2016).

Cultural theories complement ecological systems theories by prioritizing the cultural context in which development unfolds. Cultural theorists focus on understanding the origins of social competencies in particular settings and then determining whether or not they transfer to other settings, such as school (Wainryb, 2004). Culture is composed of the ways in which people process and make sense of their experiences and includes prescriptions about individuals' roles within families, decision-making patterns, and cognitions and practices about childrearing and child development (Rogoff, 2003). These cultural theories are not parent gender specific but may act as a useful theoretical foundation for studying fathers' cultural variation as it relates to their children's social development. Further, some cultural theories may also help explain differences in parents' behavior or beliefs around socialization practices due to certain cultural norms around what it means to be a father or a man, more generally.

An often-neglected topic in the study of children's social development is the socialization processes of ethnic minority children. There is little information about how parental socialization practices, influenced by racism and discrimination, are used to shape children's development (Cabrera, Kuhns, Malin, & Aldoney, 2016). Ethnic minority children in the United States are socialized in particular ways that address the social status of their group, which is rooted in a history of racism and discrimination (Garcia Coll et al., 1996; Roosa, Morgan-Lopez, Cree, & Specter, 2002). How do children growing up in such conditions develop social competencies? What are those social competencies? Are there social competencies more important for one group than for another group? How do parents socialize their children to the values and behaviors of both cultures? How do they align? Which values have changed, and which values have been adapted? These questions remain largely unexamined. In these efforts, the integrative model for the study of developmental competencies in minority children (aka the Integrative Model; Garcia Coll et al., 1996) can help us understand how the unique characteristics of the socialization experiences of ethnic minority children develop and the ways in which they might influence developmental trajectories. According to the Integrative Model, when thinking about the multiple developmental competencies of minority children (i.e., cognitive, social, emotional, bilingualism, bicultural competencies, and coping mechanisms for racism), we must include a different set of proximal and distal factors and processes. These processes include (a) social position (race, social class, ethnicity, and gender); (b) race-based factors such as racism, prejudice, discrimination, and oppression; (c) residential, economic, social, and psychological segregation; (d) promoting and inhibiting environments such as neighborhoods and health-care facilities; (e) adaptive culture, including traditional and cultural legacies, economic and political factors, migration and acculturation, and current context demands; (f) child characteristics, including age, temperament, health status, biological factors, and physical characteristics; and (g) family structure and roles, values, beliefs, and goals, racial socialization, and economic status.

Another theoretical framework used to understand how children develop social skills in cultural contexts is the ecocultural niche framework, in the tradition of Vygotsky's sociocultural theory (Weisner, 1996). This framework is used to examine children's participation in culturally structured activities, and families' efforts to sustain daily routines over time help children internalize the values of the cultural group and behave accordingly. Vygotsky's theory highlights the role of settings and routines (e.g., cultural scripts, tasks and activities, motivations, and cultural goals and beliefs) of daily life as a mechanism of cultural transmission and as a measure of family adaptation and transmission of social values and expectations (Harkness, Hughes, Muller, & Super, 2004; Rogoff, 1982). All parents aim to establish sustainable and meaningful daily routines that are compatible with family member and community competencies (Weisner, Matheson, & Bernheimer, 1996). Children develop social competencies by participating in routine activities (e.g., chores, taking care of siblings), family rituals (e.g., going to church), and culturally regulated customs of childrearing. Caretakers bring their cultural beliefs and "ethnotheories" (e.g., beliefs and views on what promotes development; Harkness et al., 2004) into these quotidian activities, through which young children implicitly or explicitly learn about appropriate social behaviors, expected norms, linguistic conventions, and cognitive skills (Sameroff & Fiese, 2000). These daily routines are shared with and initiated by parents, siblings, and grandparents who use their views about childrearing to transmit particular cultural values (Rogoff, 2003).

As children grow up, the ecological niche expands to include peers, friends, and other adults operating in the larger society, creating a dynamic context for development. For children living in immigrant families, the ecological niche consists of a combination of the practices and customs of their parents' heritage culture as well as of the practices and norms of the receiving society. As time goes by, both sets of beliefs/practices will change, providing a dynamic and complex environment for children's development. Collectively, these interactions form an ecological network of social and reciprocal relationships that support the developing child (Sroufe, Coffino, & Carlson, 2010). When there is a lack of consistent sensitive care, children will feel insecure in their relationship with their caregivers and unable to see the attachment figure as a source of emotional security. Thus, these early parent-child interactions are the most significant socialization experiences in a child's life that have enduring effects (Sroufe, 2005; Vondra, Shaw, Swearingen, Cohen, & Owens, 2001).

One of the few theoretical foundations or conceptual frameworks to specifically address the role of both mothers and fathers suggests that fathers can make both equal and unique contributions to their children's development compared to mothers (Cabrera, Fitzgerald, Bradley, & Roggman, 2014). This framework considers both the transactional and reciprocal nature of father-child relationships. In contrast to other theories, such as ecological theory, it suggests that all factors of the model (i.e., fathers' characteristics and parenting, the father-child relationship, child outcomes) occur synergistically, rather than hierarchically.

Taken together, these theories show that children develop social skills by interacting with their environments in dynamic, transactional, stimulating, and complex ways within their families (Smith & Hart, 2004). The influence of these parent-child interactions on social development is dependent upon a group of contextual factors, including cultural values (e.g., racial and ethnic beliefs), family structure and resources (e.g., paternal residency, education, and income), as well as characteristics of the child (e.g., child gender and genetic and biological traits). Specifically, secure attachment with parents (and other family members) during the first years serves as a cornerstone for children's social competence. As they grow older and become more cognitively advanced, children extend their socialization experiences with parents to their relationships in other settings (i.e., how they act around their peers and teachers). In this chapter, we take a developmental perspective to demonstrate how everyday parent-children interactions, with a particular focus on those between fathers and children, shape different domains of social development.

Fathers' Influence on Children's Social Development

The earliest research on how fathers influence their children's social adjustment primarily focused on the effects of fathers' absence on children's social adaptation (Cabrera, Ryan, Mitchell, Shannon, & Tamis-LeMonda, 2008; Danzinger & Radin, 1990). This work showed that father absence was associated with a host of behavioral problems and maladjustment (McLanahan, Tach, & Schneider, 2013). Over the past recent decades, however, researchers have begun to pay attention to understanding how fathers who are *present* in their children's lives influence children's social development (e.g., Baker, Fenning, & Crnic, 2011; Cabrera et al., 2008; Roskam, Meunier, & Stievenart, 2016). Given space considerations, we do not include a systematic review of the literature but rather focus on a select set of notable studies published over the last decade to synthesize the most recent, emerging literature on this topic. We categorize this literature into studies that have tested *direct effects* and those that have tested *indirect effects* or the processes through which direct father involvement matters for children (Cabrera, 2012; Cabrera & Bradley, 2012; Flouri & Buchanan, 2004).

Direct Effects

Ecocultural theories suggest that the most proximal influence on children's development is their parents and other caregivers (Bronfenbrenner, 1979; Cabrera, Hofferth, & Hancock, 2014). Fathers and mothers *directly* influence their children's social development during daily interactions (Flouri, 2010). Through these daily reciprocal interactions, fathers socialize their children to develop regulatory skills, get along with other adults and peers, understand and express emotions, and learn the norms and values of belonging to a particular ethnic and racial group. In the following sections, we review the literature that examines the direct effects of fathers on a variety of children's social development outcomes, including social and emotional skills, behavior problems, emotion socialization, racial and ethnic socialization, and peer relationships.

Social and Emotional Skills

The quality of children's attachment with their parents sets the stage for the development of social skills. Children who are securely attached to their caregivers are likely to engage in positive, reciprocal, and loving interactions (Cabrera, 2019). When children interact with their parents and caregivers in nurturing ways, they are more likely to learn to positively interact with others, take turns in conversations and social interactions, and enjoy social exchanges (Berscheid & Reis, 1998). Through interactions and daily activities, parents also model behaviors, reward socially accepted behaviors, and punish problem behaviors (McKee et al., 2007). A consistent finding in this literature is that through direct responsive daily engagements with their children, fathers directly influence the development of regulatory and social skills (e.g., Cabrera, Karberg, Malin, & Aldoney, 2017; Cabrera, Shannon, West, & Brooks-Gunn, 2006; Martin, Ryan, & Brooks-Gunn, 2010).

The degree to which parents engage in sensitive and reciprocal, co-regulated, parent-child interactions has been found to be positively related to the development of social competence (Feldman, Bamberger, & Kanat-Maymon, 2013; Feldman & Masalha, 2010). An observational study of Israeli and Palestinian parents that assessed paternal reciprocity—that is, the ability to engage in mutual, back-and-forth social exchanges—found that reciprocity during infancy was positively related to preschoolers' prosocial behaviors and social competence. They also found that paternal reciprocity was negatively related to aggression, while maternal reciprocity was significantly related only to social competence and aggression (Feldman et al., 2013).

The context of play, especially with young children, is an important setting for the development of children's social skills (e.g., Kroll, Carson, Redshaw, & Quigley, 2016; Lee & Schoppe, 2017). Fathers who exhibit high levels of positive physical play with their children and use less directive or coercive tactics during play are more likely to have children who are rated as less aggressive and more competent than fathers who do not (McDowell & Parke, 2009). In particular, paternal engagement in creative play (e.g., drawing, listening to or playing music, dancing, telling stories, etc.) with young children seems to be a long-term predictor of fewer behavior problems, controlling for a group of socioeconomic status characteristics, and child temperament, age, and health (Kroll et al., 2016).

Studies that have focused on the quantity, opposed to the quality, of parenting behaviors have also found similar patterns of associations. Baker (2013) conducted an analysis of the Early Childhood Longitudinal Study-Birth Cohort (ECLS-B), a nationally representative probability sample of children born in 2001. She found that controlling for a host of demographic characteristics (e.g., parents' education, work hours, race and ethnicity, marital status, family income), on average, fathers who reported reading, telling stories, and singing to their toddlers more frequently had preschoolers who had better social emotional skills. These social emotional skills were measured as the degree to which children were observed to engage with their mother, sustain attention during play, and express negativity toward the mother via direct observations (Baker, 2013).

Using positive and developmentally appropriate discipline strategies (e.g., reasoning) can help children comply with family and social norms and guidelines about appropriate behaviors (Pinderhughes, Dodge, Bates, Pettit, & Zelli, 2000). Parents who use positive disciplinary approaches, such as indirect commands, giving choices, and reasoning, can help children regulate their behaviors (Eaton, 1997). However, to our knowledge, there are virtually no studies of fathers' discipline and children's social development. A small-scale study of low-income families and their toddlers found that fathers overwhelmingly used commands (e.g., "Do that") to promote compliance in their 24-month-old children. Controlling for maternal supportiveness, fathers' regulatory behaviors (e.g., physically removing the child from the situation) at 24 months predicted children's sustained attention at pre-K, whereas fathers' regulatory language (e.g., commands, prohibitions) at 24 months predicted children's emotion regulation at pre-K (Malin, Cabrera, Karberg, Aldoney, & Rowe, 2014).

Neurobiological evidence seems to support findings based on behavioral measures of parenting that positive parent-child interactions are key for social development. Apter-Levi, Zagoory-Sharon, and Feldman (2014) examined the hormonal effects of oxytocin and vasopressin on mother- and father-child social synchrony (i.e., co-regulation, coordination, and mutual responsiveness). Overall, mothers and fathers who had high levels of oxytocin were found to be more affectionate and more likely to initiate social engagement with children than parents with lower levels. While mothers provided more affectionate contact, fathers provided more stimulatory contact and were more likely to increase object salience (i.e., parent responds to a child's gaze or joint attention to an object) when their infants showed bids for social engagement.

The presence of the father in the family, in addition to what they do, might change the dynamics of family life in a way that supports or jeopardizes children's development (Bocknek, Brophy-Herb, Fitzgerald, Schiffman, & Vogel, 2014). Using the National Longitudinal Survey of Youth—1979, Cabrera, Hofferth, and Hancock (2014) found that children who lived with their fathers at age 4 were rated by their teachers as exhibiting fewer externalizing problem behaviors when they were 4–6 and 8–10 years old. For children who lived with a stepfather at ages 4 and 8, the benefits of having a stepfather were found only for children who were less regulated. Less regulated children living with a stepfather at ages 4 and 8 exhibited fewer externalizing behavior problems when they were between 4 to 6 and 8 to 10 years old than more regulated children.

Collectively, though limited in scope, the empirical evidence from survey, observational, and neurobiological studies suggests that positive interactions between fathers and their children are uniquely important for children's social and emotional skills.

Behavior Problems

Understanding the development of externalizing problems is one of the areas of research that has had enduring attention from the research community. Consequently, there is solid theoretically grounded empirical evidence that negative parenting (e.g., intrusive, disengaged, rejecting, controlling, using harsh discipline) is detrimental for social adjustment (Roskam et al., 2016). In a sample of 419 families and their children (56% boys), Roskam and colleagues (2016) found that children were more likely to exhibit internalizing behaviors (e.g., sadness, depression, withdrawal, anxiety, and loneliness) and externalizing behaviors (e.g., aggression and delinquency) when parents interacted with them in a harsh and controlling manner. These negative behaviors on the part of the child, in turn, lead to heightened level of negative parenting from their parents in subsequent interactions. This bidirectional effect between children's behavior problems and negative parenting has significant implications for children's social adjustment over time.

Negative fathering behaviors carry unique risk for the development of problem behaviors in school-age children. A study of fathers who were observed to be intrusive (i.e., impose their agendas on the child despite signals that the child prefers a different activity) with their 4-year-old children had children who exhibited decreased social skills (i.e., cooperation, self-control, and assertiveness) 2 years later, controlling for mothers' intrusiveness and maternal reports of children's behavior problems at 54 months (Stevenson & Crnic, 2013). At the other extreme, fathers who are disengaged also impact their children negatively. A study of fathers and their children found that infants who had the most disengaged fathers (i.e., father was silent or not engaged during the interaction) were five times more likely to demonstrate early externalizing behavior problems (i.e., parent report on the child behavior checklist) by 1 year of age than those with fathers who were not disengaged (Ramchandani et al., 2012). Grounded in attachment theory that poor attachment relationships are more likely to be related to psychosocial maladaptation, Putnick and colleagues (2015) conducted a longitudinal study of children across nine different countries. They found that children who reported feeling rejected by their fathers when they were 8 years old were more likely to exhibit internalizing and externalizing behaviors 1 and 2 years later, even after controlling for paternal age, education, and social desirability bias.

The associations between fathers and children's development are not just parent driven; rather, they are dynamic and show that children also play a role in their own development. Controlling parenting behaviors and the use of harsh discipline have been found to be bidirectionally related to children's problem behaviors (McKee et al., 2007; Patterson, DeBaryshe, & Ramsey, 1989). A large-scale study of French-speaking fathers and mothers from Belgium found that children's externalizing behavior at age 4 predicted fathers' controlling behavior at age 5. Fathers' controlling behaviors were measured via their responses to items such as "When my child becomes too agitated or bothersome, I punish him/her" (Roskam et al., 2016). In turn, fathers' controlling behavior at age 5 significantly predicted children's externalizing behavior at age 6. The same pathways were observed between mothers and children, but there was limited support for an interaction between fathers' and mothers' behaviors. Similarly, Zarra-Nezhad et al. (2014) analyzed data from a larger study of Finnish children with their parents and found that children who were rated by their kindergarten teachers as having high levels of social withdrawal were more susceptible to the negative effects of low maternal affection on externalizing behavior during grades 1 through 3. Interestingly, for these socially withdrawn children, mothers' and fathers' psychological control (e.g., "I believe my child should be aware of how much I have done for him/her") was associated with more prosocial behaviors and few externalizing behaviors; however, mothers' psychological control, at the same time, predicted more internalizing behaviors. It is possible that parenting control provides the necessary structure for avoidant and fearful children to engage in social interactions.

The association between negative fathering and children's externalizing behavior problems seems to hold across cultural groups. In small-scale, concurrent study of Chinese families and their children, Yu, Volling, and Niu (2015) found that fathers' controlling emotion socialization practices (e.g., punitive and minimization behaviors) were significantly and positively associated with children's internalizing and externalizing problem behaviors, but only when mothers' control also was low. There is also some evidence that father involvement might be more beneficial for the development of social competence among ethnic minority children. Analysis from the ECLS-B revealed that the association between paternal control and discipline was related to fewer problem behaviors and higher engagement scores only among African American boys (Baker, 2017).

Emotion Socialization

The ability to label and express emotions, understand them in oneself and others, and behave accordingly is central to the development of empathy and of reciprocal and nurturing relationships (Murray & Palaiologou, 2018). What we know about how children are socialized to express emotions in a socially pro-active way comes mostly from studies of mothers (e.g., De Rosnay & Harris, 2002), but a handful of studies that have included fathers show similar associations. Children who are insecurely attached to their mothers and fathers are more likely to exhibit lower emotion understanding (e.g., ability to match a facial expression to the emotion of a character depicted in a specific scenario), even after controlling for parents' depressive symptoms and child age (Psychogiou et al., 2018). Having deficient emotion understanding would then impair children's ability to make and keep friends (Denham et al., 2003).

The few studies that have examined how fathers socialize their children to understand emotions, to express them, and to react appropriately to other people's display of emotions report similar results. One such study found that fathers who used emotion coaching with their children's expressions of emotions had children who were rated by parents and teachers as being more socially competent and demonstrating responsibility, cooperation, self-control, and assertiveness at age 8 (Baker et al., 2011). Parents who reported responding in supportive ways to their children's emotion of sadness (e.g., telling the child it is okay to cry) reported that their children exhibited higher social competence (Baker et al., 2011). In contrast, mothers and fathers who reported feeling uncomfortable or embarrassed by their children's emotional behavior and reprimanded or punished children also reported more child negativity, emotional intensity, and dysregulation (Shewark & Blandon, 2015).

Ethnic and Racial Socialization

Through ethnic and racial socialization practices, parents play a significant role in giving children the tools they need to be part of a diverse society in a way that reflects values of justice, fairness, and equality for all (Derlan, Umana-Taylor, Updergraff, & Jahromi, 2017; Hughes, 2003). Ethnic and racial socialization typically refers to the way parents transmit cultural information, attitudes, and ideas about race and ethnicity to their children (Brown, Tanner-Smith, Lesane-Brown, & Ezell, 2007; Hughes et al., 2006; Knight, Bernal, Garza, Cota, & Ocampo, 1993; Umaña-Taylor, Alfaro, Bámaca, & Guimond, 2009). Children with strong ethnic and racial identities help children understand how others, who are not like them, might perceive them and, consequently, how they might engage and interact with them.

In the United States, the cultural context and history of racism and discrimination against African American and other ethnic minorities has resulted in a body of work that has focused primarily on how ethnic minority parents prepare their children for bias and discrimination (Boykin & Toms, 1985; Hughes, 2003). In particular, the bulk of this work has been done with African American mothers of school-age children (e.g., Caughy, O'Campo, Randolph, & Nickerson, 2002; Hughes & Chen, 1997; Marshall, 1995). This literature shows that mothers avail themselves of a set of strategies that include cultural socialization, preparation for bias, promotion of mistrust, and egalitarianism but are silent about race (Hughes et al., 2006).

In contrast, the body of work on how White families socialize their children to understand the rights and privileges of being White is virtually nonexistent (Karberg, Cabrera, Malin, & Kuhns, 2019). The limited work on non-minority parents shows that they typically endorse a color-blind approach in socializing their children to live in a diverse society. A color-blind approach is one where attention is not drawn to racial differences but rather to racial similarities. This can be problematic because it also negates racial inequality (Pahlke, Bigler, & Suizzo, 2012). Using a color-blind approach may also diminish opportunities to facilitate the development of cross-race friendships, which decrease levels of bias, discrimination, and prejudice and increase intergroup contact (Crystal, Killen, & Ruck, 2008; Killen, Hitti, Cooley, & Elenbaas, 2015; Thijs & Verkuyten, 2008; Tropp & Prenovost, 2008; Turner & Cameron, 2016). There is little evidence that majority parents' socialization practices include strategies to increase intergroup contact across racial and ethnic groups (Loyd & Gaither, 2018).

Comparatively, we know less about how fathers of any ethnic group transmit cultural values to their children. We found only one study indicating that African American fathers employ four themes during their discussion about values with their sons: cultural messages (e.g., cultural pride and managing racism), education (e.g., social intelligence and educational attainment), respect, and responsibility (Doyle, Magan, Cryer-Coupet, Goldston, & Estroff, 2016). This is an area that needs further research.

Peer Relationships

The ability to make and keep friends is a strong predictor of children's social adjustment (Hymel, Rubin, Rowden, & LeMare, 1990). From the early years, parents, including fathers, play a key role in helping children form friendships that are meaningful and long-lasting (Davidson, Updegraff, & McHale, 2011; Updegraff, Kim, Killoren, & Thayer, 2010). A study of low-income fathers and their fifth graders found that children who perceived their fathers to be close to them were more likely to report positive peer relationships and were rated as exhibiting fewer behavioral problems than their counterparts (Cabrera, Cook, McFadden, & Bradley, 2011). A large-scale study of Finnish first-grade children and their parents found that mothers' and fathers' psychological control (e.g., "my child needs to know the sacrifices I make for him/her") and self-reported depressive symptoms uniquely predicted children's risk of friendship dissolution. In contrast, parental affection (e.g., "I often show my child that I love him/her") did not alter the stability of friendship from grade 1 to grade 6 (Dickson, Huey, Laursen, Kiuru, & Nurmi, 2018). Overall, these findings are consistent with those based on White European samples that positive father-child relationship is associated with less negative friendships, whereas more negative father-child relationships forecast less satisfactory friendships over time (Youngblade & Belsky, 1992).

Indirect Effects

Studies that have examined indirect effects have taken a family systems perspective, positing that families are composed of interrelated subsystems (e.g., father-child; father-mother) that have reciprocal influences on each other. A mechanism through which one subsystem (e.g., father-child) influences individuals (e.g., children) is through (indirect) other subsystems (mother-father, mother-child). This literature points to multiple pathways.

First, fathers might influence their children's social development through the *mother-father relationship*. Fathers who participated in the Fragile Families and Child Wellbeing Study (FFCWS) and reported being highly involved with their children had children who scored higher on tests assessing cognitive and social skills because they reported having a more positive relationship with their partners (Cabrera et al., 2008). Dette-Hagenmeyer and Reichle (2014) found that fathers' inconsistent parenting at age 7 mediated the relation between paternal depressive symptoms and children's hyperactivity and social-emotional competence 6 months later. Fathers' inconsistent parenting also mediated the relation between paternal depressive symptoms and oppositional-defiant child behavior. The co-parenting relationship is another mechanism that explains why parental involvement explains variation in children's social skills. Using the FFCWS, co-parenting support between mothers and fathers was found to mediate the association between union stability (i.e., number of residential romantic partner changes from the child's birth until they were 5 years old) and children's externalizing problem behaviors at age 5 (Karberg & Cabrera, 2017). In this paper, union instability acts as a proxy for consistent father presence in their children's lives. Thus, when fathers are not consistently present in their children's lives, it has a negative impact on children's behavior problems, through the decreased quality of the co-parenting relationship between mothers and fathers.

A second pathway of influence is through the *parent-child relationship*. An analysis of data from the ECLS-B revealed that high levels of maternal and paternal risks (i.e., teen parenting, no high school degree, low English proficiency, unemployment, poor health, etc.) at infancy were indirectly linked to toddlers' social behaviors (i.e., engagement of the mother, quality of play, and negativity toward their mother) at 24 months through decreased *maternal supportiveness* and *father engagement* (Cabrera, Fagan, Wight, & Schadler, 2011). Studies of fathers who had an alcohol diagnosis were found to be less warm and sensitive with their children, which, in turn, predicted lower self-regulation a year later (Eiden, Colde, Edwards, & Leonard, 2010) and overall deficits in social competence from early childhood to adolescence (Hussong et al., 2005). In a sample of Korean fathers, Chae and Lee (2011) found that fathers' own childhood attachment representations had a significant impact on their boys' social competence through their parenting behaviors (e.g., self-report on parent involvement, limit setting, responsiveness, reasoning guidance, and intimacy).

Father effects might also be compensatory, or protective. That is, high levels of father involvement can compensate for low levels of maternal behaviors, for example, maternal supportiveness (i.e., observed sensitivity, positive regard, and emotional supportiveness). Analysis of data from the NICHD Study of Early Child Care and Youth Development revealed that fathers' supportiveness during a parent-child play interaction was significantly associated with children's social skills only when mothers' supportiveness was scored at average or below, suggesting a compensatory effect (Martin et al., 2010). Father effects can also be promotive or strengthening. A strengthening effect occurs when a particular outcome is more likely to occur when the individual receives high levels of support from several sources. An observational study of families who participated in the Early Head Start Research and Evaluation Project revealed that resident fathers' high-quality play had a moderating (strengthening) effect on the association between mothers' quality of play and children's emotion regulation (i.e., scores on the Leiter International Performance Scale Social-Emotional Rating Scale). The association between maternal quality play and children's emotion regulation was significant only when fathers engaged in high-quality play with their children (Cabrera et al., 2017).

Another mechanism of how parenting influences children's social development is through *children* themselves. A small-scale study of fathers and their developmentally delayed children found that the association between father intrusiveness at age 4 and children's social skills (i.e., cooperation, self-control, and assertiveness) at 6 years was mediated through children's behavioral dysregulation at 5 years (Stevenson & Crnic, 2013). Another study found that the association between negative parenting and children's skills varied by child gender. Fathers and mothers who were permissive at age 5 had children who exhibited more physical aggression at age 8 only when they were boys (Braza et al., 2015). Children's physiological traits may also strengthen or mitigate the association between fathering and their behavior problems. Erath, El-Sheikh, and Mark Cummings (2009) measured 8-year-olds' skin conductance level reactivity (SCLR), a measure of the degree to which an individual responds to stress. They found that the association between harsh parenting (averaged between mother and father) and externalizing behaviors was stronger among children with lower SCLR, suggesting that children's own biological responses shape the parent-child relationship.

Summary and Key Points

The study of how fathers influence children's social development has come a long way: from studies that focused merely on the effects of father *absence* on children's development to studies that focused on how *present* fathers make a difference in their children's social development. Although still limited in scope, the emerging research points to a consistent conclusion. Fathers' involvement in their children's lives is instrumental in shaping children into socially competent individuals who can adapt to social norms, make and keep friends, and contribute in positive ways to the social fabric of our society. The evidence supports the conclusion that fathers have both direct and indirect effects on an array of social developmental outcomes. Although the literature examining indirect effects is relatively limited, it points to several pathways of influence. Fathers influence their children through the impact they have on the relationship with their partners, the relationship with their children, and through children's own skills and behaviors. The next generation of studies on how fathers matter for children's development needs to focus on better understanding the complex processes through which fathers make a difference on children's development. This information would be essential to aid in developing more targeted interventions and to better inform policy decisions.

The literature on how fathers influence children's social competencies suffers from various limitations. First, there are more studies on how father negative behaviors are related to children's behavior problems than studies on how positive father involvement leads to social adaptation. Second, there is little information on how ethnic minority fathers engage in ethnic and racial socialization strategies with their young children and, similarly, how White fathers, and White parents more generally, approach ethnic and racial socialization with their children. Third, there is a lack of diversity in the target populations in the studies reviewed. The majority of the samples were Caucasian, middle-class families. Due to differences in culture, class, opportunity, and context, it cannot be assumed that the processes that lead to certain developmental outcomes in majority children have the same effects in minority children (Garcia Coll et al., 1996). Consequently, there is a substantial gap in measurement of culturally specific variables and social development outcomes. Fourth, the studies reviewed for this chapter largely excluded the cultural context in which children develop, which underestimates the role that culturally specific mechanisms have on the ways in which fathers socialize their children. Future work that includes this cultural context would provide a fuller understanding in the ways in which fathers, ethnic minority and White, help their children develop the social skills they need to live in a racially, economically, and culturally diverse society.

Fifth, there is a noted inconsistency in the studies reviewed in how maternal and paternal variables were used analytically. Some researchers ran separate models for mothers and fathers; however, this was often done without testing the comparability between the two models, making it difficult to compare these processes between mothers and fathers. Other researchers included maternal and paternal variables in the same model or controlled for maternal characteristics while examining the effect of fathers. These analytical approaches may lead to distinct conclusions about how fathers and mothers uniquely (main effects) or interactively (indirect effects) influence children's social development. Lastly, many studies did not include key covariates in their models such as parents' psychological well-being and parenting stress, which are consistently associated with negative parenting and children's behavioral and emotional difficulties (Cohen & Wills, 1985; Conger & Elder, 1994; Dette-Hagenmeyer & Reichle, 2014).

In conclusion, the research on understanding the specific and unique role that fathers have in their children's social adaptation points in a clear future direction. We need more studies of fathers and their children across the developmental spectrum and across cultural and family contexts. We need to pay better attention to how culture shapes the context of social development for children and conduct rigorous studies that are framed within theoretical frameworks that can both describe and explain development and that clearly model the unique influences that each parent has on their children's development. New research that addresses these gaps in the literature will be critical to designing interventions and programs that can help mothers and fathers provide their children with opportunities for optimal social development.

References

Ainsworth, M. D. S. (1973). The development of infant-mother attachment. In B. Cardwell & H. Ricciuti (Eds.), *Review of child development research* (pp. 1–94). Chicago: University of Chicago Press.

Ainsworth, M. D. S., & Bowlby, J. (1991). An ethological approach to personality development. *American Psychologist, 46*, 333–341. https://doi.org/10.1037/0003-066X.46.4.333

Apter-Levi, Y., Zagoory-Sharon, O., & Feldman, R. (2014). Oxytocin and vasopressin support distinct configurations of social synchrony. *Brain Research, 1580*, 124–132. https://doi.org/10.1016/j.brainres.2013.10.052

Baker, C. E. (2013). Fathers' and mothers' home literacy involvement and children's cognitive and social emotional development: Implications for family literacy programs. *Applied Developmental Science, 17*, 184–197. https://doi.org/10.1080/10888691.2013.836034

Baker, C. E. (2017). Father-son relationships in ethnically diverse families: Links to boys' cognitive and social emotional development in preschool. *Journal of Child and Family Studies, 26*, 2335–2345. https://doi.org/10.1007/s10826-017-0743-3

Baker, J. K., Fenning, R. M., & Crnic, K. A. (2011). Emotion socialization by mothers and fathers: Coherence among behaviors and associations with parent attitudes and children's social competence. *Social Development, 20*, 412–430. https://doi.org/10.1111/j.1467-9507.2010.00585.x

Berscheid, E., & Reis, H. T. (1998). Attraction and close relationships. In D. T. Gilbert, S. T. Fiske, & G. Lindzey (Eds.), *Handbook of social psychology* (Vol. 1, 2nd ed.). New York: McGraw-Hill.

Bocknek, E. L., Brophy-Herb, H. E., Fitzgerald, H. E., Schiffman, R. F., & Vogel, C. (2014). Stability of biological father presence as a proxy for family stability: Cross-racial associations with the longitudinal development of emotion regulation in toddlerhood. *Infant Mental Health Journal, 35*, 309–321. https://doi.org/10.1002/imhj.21454

Bowlby, J. (1982). Attachment and loss: Retrospect and prospect. *American Journal of Orthopsychiatry, 52*, 664–678. https://doi.org/10.1111/j.1939-0025.1982.tb01456.x

Boykin, A. W., & Toms, F. D. (1985). Black child socialization: A conceptual framework. In H. P. McAdoo & J. L. McAdoo (Eds.), *Black children: Social, educational, and parental environments* (pp. 33–52). Newbury Park, CA: Sage.

Braza, P., Carreras, R., Muñoz, J., Braza, F., Azurmendi, A., Pascual-Sagastizábal, E., et al. (2015). Negative maternal and paternal parenting styles as predictors of children's behavioral problems: Moderating effects of the child's sex. *Journal of Child and Family Studies, 24*, 847–856. https://doi.org/10.1007/s10826-013-9893-0

Bronfenbrenner, U. (1979). *The ecology of human development*. Cambridge, MA: Harvard University Press.

Bronfenbrenner, U., & Morris, P. A. (2006). The bioecological model of human development. In R. M. Lerner & W. Damon (Eds.), *Handbook of child psychology: Theoretical models of human development* (pp. 793–828). Hoboken, NJ: Wiley.

Brown, T. N., Tanner-Smith, E. E., Lesane-Brown, C. L., & Ezell, M. E. (2007). Child, parent, and situational correlates of familial ethnic/race socialization. *Journal of Marriage and Family, 69*, 14–25. https://doi.org/10.1111/j.1741-3737.2006.00339.x-i1

Cabrera, N., Fagan, J., Wight, V., & Schadler, C. (2011). Influence of mother, father, and child risk on parenting and children's cognitive and social behaviors. *Child Development, 82*, 1985–2005. https://doi.org/10.1111/j.1467-8624.2011.01667.x

Cabrera, N., Kuhns, C., Malin, J., & Aldoney, D. (2016). Helping children navigate a diverse world: Parents' contributions. *Advances in Child Development and Behavior, 51*, 81–102. https://doi.org/10.1016/bs.acdb.2016.05.002

Cabrera, N. J. (2012). An ecological view of the socialization process of Latino children. In S. L. Odom, E. P. Pungello, & N. Gardner-Neblett (Eds.), *Infants, toddlers, and families in poverty: Research implications for early child care* (pp. 257–280). New York: Guilford Press.

Cabrera, N. J. (2019). Father involvement, father-child relationship, and attachment in the early years. *Attachment & Human Development, 1-5*, 1–5. https://doi.org/10.1080/14616734.2019.1589070

Cabrera, N. J., & Bradley, R. H. (2012). Latino fathers and their children. *Child Development Perspectives, 6*, 232–238. https://doi.org/10.1111/j.1750-8606.2012.00249.x

Cabrera, N. J., Cook, G. A., McFadden, K. E., & Bradley, R. (2011). Father residence and father-child relationship quality: Peer relationships and externalizing behavioral problems. *Family Science, 2*, 109–119. https://doi.org/10.1080/19424620.2011.639143

Cabrera, N. J., Fitzgerald, H. E., Bradley, R. H., & Roggman, L. (2014). The ecology of father-child relationships: An expanded model. *Journal of Family Theory Review, 6*, 336–354. https://doi.org/10.1111/jftr.12054

Cabrera, N. J., Hofferth, S. L., & Hancock, G. (2014). Family structure, maternal employment, and changes in children's externalizing problem behavior: Differences by age and self-regulation. *European Journal of Developmental Psychology, 11*, 136–158. https://doi.org/10.1080/17405629.2013.873716

Cabrera, N. J., Karberg, E., Malin, J. L., & Aldoney, D. (2017). The magic of play: Low-income mothers' and fathers' playfulness and children's emotion regulation and vocabulary skills. *Infant Mental Health Journal, 38*, 757–771. https://doi.org/10.1002/imhj.21682

Cabrera, N. J., Ryan, R. M., Mitchell, S. J., Shannon, J. D., & Tamis-LeMonda, C. S. (2008). Low-income, nonresident father involvement with their toddlers: Variation by fathers' race and ethnicity. *Journal of Family Psychology, 22*, 643–647. https://doi.org/10.1037/0893-3200.22.3.643

Cabrera, N. J., Shannon, J. D., West, J., & Brooks-Gunn, J. (2006). Parental interactions with Latino infants: Variation by country of origin and English proficiency. *Child Development, 77*, 1190–1207. https://doi.org/10.1111/j.1467-8624.2006.00928.x

Caughy, M. O., O'Campo, P. J., Randolph, S. M., & Nickerson, K. (2002). The influence of racial socialization practices on the cognitive and behavioral competence of African American preschoolers. *Child Development, 73*, 1611–1625. https://doi.org/10.1111/1467-8624.00493

Chae, J., & Lee, K. Y. (2011). Impacts of Korean fathers' attachment and parenting behavior on their children's social competence. *Social Behavior and Personality: An International Journal, 39*, 627–643. https://doi.org/10.2224/sbp.2011.39.5.627

Cohen, S., & Wills, T. A. (1985). Stress, social support, and the buffering hypothesis. *Psychological Bulletin, 98*, 310–357. https://doi.org/10.1037/0033-2909.98.2.310

Conger, R. D., & Elder, G. H. (1994). *Families in troubled times: Adapting to change in rural America*. New York: Aldine de Gruyter.

Corsaro, W. A. (2017). *The sociology of childhood*. Thousand Oaks, CA: Sage Publications.

Crystal, D. S., Killen, M., & Ruck, M. (2008). It is who you know that counts: Intergroup contact and judgments about race-based exclusion. *The British Journal of Developmental Psychology, 26*, 51–70. https://doi.org/10.1348/026151007X198910

Danzinger, S. K., & Radin, N. (1990). Absent does not equal uninvolved: Predictors of fathering in teen mother families. *Journal of Marriage and Family, 52*, 636–642. https://doi.org/10.2307/352930

Davidson, A., Updegraff, K., & McHale, S. (2011). Parent/peer relationship patterns among mexican-origin adolescents. *International Journal of Behavioral Development, 35*, 260–270. https://doi.org/10.1177/0165025410384926

De Rosnay, M. D., & Harris, P. L. (2002). Individual differences in children's understanding of emotion:

The roles of attachment and language. *Attachment and Human Development, 4*, 39–54. https://doi.org/10.1080/14616730210123139

Denham, S. A. (2006). Social-emotional competence as support for school readiness: What is it and how do we assess it? *Early Education and Development, 17*, 57–89. https://doi.org/10.1207/s15566935eed1701_4

Denham, S. A., Blair, K. A., DeMulder, E., Levitas, J., Sawyer, K., Auerbach-Major, S., et al. (2003). Preschool emotional competence: Pathway to social competence? *Child Development, 74*, 238–256. https://doi.org/10.1111/1467-8624.00533

Derlan, C. L., Umana-Taylor, A. J., Updergraff, K. A., & Jahromi, L. B. (2017). Longitudinal relations among Mexican-origin mothers' cultural characteristics, cultural socialization, and 5-year-old children's ethnic-racial identification. *Developmental Psychology, 53*, 2078–2091. https://doi.org/10.1037/dev0000386

Dette-Hagenmeyer, D. E., & Reichle, B. (2014). Parents' depressive symptoms and children's adjustment over time are mediated by parenting, but differentially for fathers and mothers. *European Journal of Developmental Psychology, 11*, 196–210. https://doi.org/10.1080/17405629.2013.848789

Dickson, D. J., Huey, M., Laursen, B., Kiuru, N., & Nurmi, J. E. (2018). Parent contributions to friendship stability during the primary school years. *Journal of Family Psychology, 32*, 217–228. https://doi.org/10.1037/fam0000388

Doyle, O., Magan, I., Cryer-Coupet, Q. R., Goldston, D. B., & Estroff, S. E. (2016). "Don't wait for it to rain to buy an umbrella:" The transmission of values from African American fathers to sons. *Psychology of Men & Masculinity, 17*, 309–319. https://doi.org/10.1037/men0000028

Eaton, M. (1997). Positive discipline: Fostering the self-esteem of young children. *Young Children, 52*, 43–46.

Eiden, R. D., Colde, C., Edwards, E. P., & Leonard, K. E. (2010). A longitudinal study of social competence among children of alcoholic and non-alcoholic parents: Role of parental psychopathology, parental warmth, and self-regulation. *Psychological Addictive Behavior, 23*, 36–46. https://doi.org/10.1037/a0014839

Erath, S. A., El-Sheikh, M., & Mark Cummings, E. (2009). Harsh parenting and child externalizing behavior: Skin conductance level reactivity as a moderator. *Child Development, 80*, 578–592. https://doi.org/10.1111/j.1467-8624.2009.01280.x

Feldman, R., Bamberger, E., & Kanat-Maymon, Y. (2013). Parent-specific reciprocity from infancy to adolescence shapes children's social competence and dialogical skills. *Attachment & Human Development, 15*, 407–423. https://doi.org/10.1080/14616734.2013.782650

Feldman, R., & Masalha, S. (2010). Parent-child and triadic antecedents of children's social competence: Cultural specificity, shared process. *Developmental Psychology, 46*, 455–467. https://doi.org/10.1037/a0017415

Flouri, E. (2010). Fathers' behaviors and children's psychopathology. *Clinical Psychology Review, 30*, 363–369. https://doi.org/10.1016/j.cpr.2010.01.004

Flouri, E., & Buchanan, A. (2004). Early father's and mother's involvement and child's later educational outcomes. *British Journal of Educational Psychology, 74*, 141–153. https://doi.org/10.1348/000709904773839806

Garcia Coll, C., Crnic, K., Lamberty, G., Wasik, B. H., Jenkins, R., Garcia, H., et al. (1996). An integrative model for the study of developmental competencies in minority children. *Child Development, 67*, 1891–1914. https://doi.org/10.1111/j.1467-8624.1996.tb01834.x

Han, H. S., & Kemple, K. M. (2006). Components of social competence and strategies of support: Considering what to teach and how. *Early Childhood Education Journal, 34*, 241–246. https://doi.org/10.1007/s10643-006-0139-2

Harkness, S., Hughes, M., Muller, B., & Super, C. M. (2004). Entering the developmental niche: Mixed methods in an intervention program for inner city children. In T. Weisner (Ed.), *Discovering successful pathways in children's development: New methods in the study of childhood and family life* (pp. 329–358). Chicago: University of Chicago Press.

Hinde, R. A. (1979). *Towards understanding relationships*. London, UK: Academic Press.

Hughes, D. (2003). Correlates of African American and Latino parents' messages to children about ethnicity and race: A comparative study of racial socialization. *American Journal of Community Psychology, 31*, 15–33. https://doi.org/10.1023/A:1023066418688

Hughes, D., & Chen, L. (1997). When and what parents tell children about race: An examination of race-related socialization among African American families. *Applied Developmental Science, 1*, 200–214. https://doi.org/10.1207/s1532480xads0104_4

Hughes, D., Rodriguez, J., Smith, E. P., Johnson, D. J., Stevenson, H. C., & Spicer, P. (2006). Parents' ethnic-racial socialization practices: A review of research and directions for future study. *Developmental Psychology, 42*, 747–770. https://doi.org/10.1037/0012-1649.42.5.747

Hussong, A. M., Zucker, R. A., Wong, M. M., Fitzgerald, H. E., & Puttler, L. I. (2005). Social competence in children of alcoholic parents over time. *Developmental Psychology, 41*, 747–759. https://doi.org/10.1037/0012-1649.41.5.747

Hymel, S., Rubin, K. H., Rowden, L., & LeMare, L. (1990). Children's peer relationships: Longitudinal prediction of internalizing and externalizing problems from middle to late childhood. *Child Development, 61*, 2004–2021. https://doi.org/10.1111/j.1467-8624.1990.tb03582.x

Julion, W. A., Sumo, J., Bounds, D. T., Breitenstein, S. M., Schoeny, M., Gross, D., et al. (2016). Study protocol for a randomized clinical trial of a fatherhood intervention for African American non-resident fathers: Can we improve father and child outcomes? *Contemporary Clinical Trials, 49*, 29–39. https://doi.org/10.1016/j.cct.2016.05.005

Karberg, E., & Cabrera, N. J. (2017). Family change and co-parenting in resident couples and children's behavior problems. *Journal of Family Studies, 8*, 1–17. https://doi.org/10.1080/13229400.2017.1367714

Karberg, E., Cabrera, N. J., Malin, J., & Kuhns, C. (2019). Longitudinal contributions of maternal and paternal intrusive behaviors to Children's sociability and sustained attention at Prekindergarten. *Monographs of the Society for Research in Child Development, 84*, 79–93.

Killen, M., Hitti, A., Cooley, C., & Elenbaas, L. (2015). Morality, development, and culture. In M. Gelfand, C. Y. Chiu, & Y. Y. Hong (Eds.), *Advances in culture and psychology* (pp. 161–220). New York: Oxford University Press.

Knight, G. P., Bernal, M. E., Garza, C. A., Cota, M. K., & Ocampo, K. A. (1993). Family socialization and the ethnic identity of Mexican-American children. *Journal of Cross-Cultural Psychology, 24*, 99–114. https://doi.org/10.1177/0022022193241007

Kroll, M. E., Carson, C., Redshaw, M., & Quigley, M. A. (2016). Early father involvement and subsequent child behaviour at ages 3, 5 and 7 years: Prospective analysis of the UK Millennium Cohort Study. *PLoS One, 11*, 1–17. https://doi.org/10.1371/journal.pone.0162339

La Paro, K. M., & Pianta, R. C. (2000). Predicting Children's competence in the early school years: A meta-analytic review. *Review of Educational Research, 70*, 443–484. https://doi.org/10.3102/00346543070004443

Ladd, G. W., Herald, S. L., & Kochel, K. P. (2006). School readiness: Are there social prerequisites? *Early Education and Development, 17*, 115–150. https://doi.org/10.1207/s15566935eed1701_6

Lee, J., & Schoppe, S. S. J. (2017). Resident fathers' positive engagement, family poverty, and change in child behavior problems. *Family Relations, 66*, 484–496. https://doi.org/10.1111/fare.12283

Longoria, A. Q., Page, M. C., Hubbs-Tait, L., & Kennison, S. M. (2009). Relationship between kindergarten children's language ability and social competence. *Early Child Development and Care, 179*, 919–929. https://doi.org/10.1080/03004430701590241

Loyd, A. B., & Gaither, S. E. (2018). Racial/ethnic socialization for White youth: What we know and future directions. *Journal of Applied Developmental Psychology, 59*, 54–64. https://doi.org/10.1016/j.appdev.2018.05.004

Ma, H. K. (2012). Social competence as a positive youth development construct: A conceptual review. *The Scientific World Journal, 2012*. https://doi.org/10.1100/2012/287472

Malin, J. L., Cabrera, N. J., Karberg, E., Aldoney, D., & Rowe, M. L. (2014). Low-income, minority fathers' control strategies and their children's regulatory skills. *Journal of Infant Mental Health, 35*, 462–472. https://doi.org/10.1002/imhj.21467

Marshall, S. (1995). Ethnic socialization of African American children: Implications for parenting, identity development, and academic achievement. *Journal of Youth and Adolescence: A Multidisciplinary Research Publication, 24*, 377–396. https://doi.org/10.1007/BF01537187

Martin, A., Ryan, R. M., & Brooks-Gunn, J. (2010). When fathers' supportiveness matters most: Maternal and paternal parenting and children's school readiness. *Journal of Family Psychology, 243*, 145–155. https://doi.org/10.1037/a0018073

McCay, L. O., & Keyes, D. W. (2002). Developing social competence in the inclusive primary classroom. *Childhood Education, 78*, 70–78. https://doi.org/10.1080/00094056.2002.10522707

McDowell, D. J., & Parke, R. D. (2009). Parental correlates of children's peer relations: An empirical test of a tripartite model. *Developmental Psychology, 45*, 224–235. https://doi.org/10.1037/a0014305

McKee, L., Roland, E., Coffelt, N., Olson, A. L., Forehand, R., Massari, C., et al. (2007). Harsh discipline and child problem behaviors: The roles of positive parenting and gender. *Journal of Family Violence, 22*, 187–196. https://doi.org/10.1007/s10896-007-9070-6

McLanahan, S., Tach, L., & Schneider, D. (2013). The causal effects of father absence. *Annual Review of Sociology, 39*, 399–427. https://doi.org/10.1146/annurev-soc-071312-145704

Murray, J., & Palaiologou, J. (2018). Young children's emotional experiences. *Early Child Development and Care, 188*, 875–878. https://doi.org/10.1080/03004430.2018.1449839

Pahlke, E., Bigler, R., & Suizzo, M. (2012). Relations between colorblind socialization and children's racial bias: Evidence from European American mothers and their preschool children. *Child Development, 83*, 1164–1179. https://doi.org/10.1111/j.1467-8624.2012.01770.x

Paquette, D. (2004). Theorizing the father-child relationship: Mechanisms and developmental outcomes. *Human Development, 47*, 193–219. https://doi.org/10.1159/000078723

Parke, R. D., & Buriel, R. (2007). Socialization in the family: Ethnic and ecological perspectives. In W. Damon, R. M. Lerner, & N. Eisenberg (Eds.), *Handbook of child psychology (volume 3)*. Hoboken, NJ: Wiley. https://doi.org/10.1002/9780470147658.chpsy0308

Patterson, G., DeBaryshe, B. D., & Ramsey, E. (1989). A developmental perspective on antisocial behavior. *American Psychologist, 44*, 329–335. https://doi.org/10.1037/0003-066X.44.2.329

Pinderhughes, E. E., Dodge, K. A., Bates, J. E., Pettit, G. S., & Zelli, A. (2000). Discipline responses: Influences of parents' socioeconomic status, ethnicity, beliefs about parenting, stress, and cognitive-emotional processes. *Journal of Family Psychology, 14*, 380–400. https://doi.org/10.1037/0893-3200.14.3.380

Psychogiou, L., Nath, S., Kallitsoglou, A., Dimatis, K., Parry, E., Russell, A. E., et al. (2018). Children's emotion understanding in relation to attachment to mother and father. *British Journal of Developmental*

Psychology, 36, 557–572. https://doi.org/10.1111/bjdp.12239

Putnick, D. L., Bornstein, M. H., Lansford, J. E., Malone, P. S., Pastorelli, C., Skinner, A. T., et al. (2015). Perceived mother and father acceptance-rejection predict four unique aspects of child adjustment across nine countries. *Journal of Child Psychology & Psychiatry, 56*, 923–932. https://doi.org/10.1111/jcpp.12366

Ramchandani, P. G., Domoney, J., Sethna, V., Psychogiou, L., Vlachos, H., & Murray, L. (2012). Do early father-infant interactions predict the onset of externalizing behaviors in young children? Findings from a longitudinal cohort study. *Journal of Psychology and Psychiatry, 54*, 56–64. https://doi.org/10.1111/j.1469-7610.2012.02583.x

Raver, C. C. (2002). Emotions matter: Making the case for the role of young children's emotional development for early school readiness. *Social Policy Report, 16*, 1–20. https://doi.org/10.1002/j.2379-3988.2002.tb00041.x

Raver, C. C., & Zigler, E. F. (1997). Social competence: An untapped dimension in evaluating head start's success. *Early Childhood Research Quarterly, 12*, 363–385. https://doi.org/10.1016/S0885-2006(97)90017-X

Rogoff, B. (1982). Integrating context and cognitive development. In M. E. Lamb & A. L. Brown (Eds.), *Advances in developmental psychology* (Vol. 2). Hillsdale, NJ: Erlbaum.

Rogoff, B. (2003). *The cultural nature of human development.* New York: Oxford University Press.

Roosa, M. W., Morgan-Lopez, A. A., Cree, W. K., & Specter, M. M. (2002). Ethnic culture, poverty, and context: Sources of influence on Latino families and children. In J. M. Contreras, K. A. Kerns, & A. M. Neal-Barnett (Eds.), *Latino children and families in the United States* (pp. 27–44). Westport, CT: Praeger Publishers.

Roskam, I., Meunier, J., & Stievenart, M. (2016). Do mothers and fathers moderate the influence of each other's self-efficacy beliefs and parenting behaviors on children's externalizing behavior? *Journal of Child and Family Studies, 25*, 2034–2045. https://doi.org/10.1007/s10826-016-0365-1

Rubin, K. H., & Rose-Krasnor, L. R. (1992). Interpersonal problem solving and social competence in children. In V. B. van Hasslet & M. Hersen (Eds.), *Handbook of social development: A lifespan perspective*. New York: Plenum Press.

Sameroff, A. J., & Fiese, B. H. (2000). Transactional regulation: The developmental ecology of early intervention. In J. P. Schonkoff & S. J. Meisels (Eds.), *Handbook of early childhood intervention* (pp. 135–159). New York: Cambridge University Press.

Shewark, E. A., & Blandon, A. Y. (2015). Emotion socialization and children's emotion regulation. *Social Development, 24*, 266–284. https://doi.org/10.1111/sode.12095

Smith, P. K., & Hart, C. H. (Eds.). (2004). *Blackwell handbook of social development.* Oxford: Blackwell.

Sroufe, L. A. (2005). Attachment and development: A prospective, longitudinal study from birth to adulthood. *Attachment & Human Development, 7*, 349–367. https://doi.org/10.1080/14616730500365928

Sroufe, L. A., Coffino, B., & Carlson, E. A. (2010). Conceptualizing the role of early experiences: Lessons from the Minnesota longitudinal study. *Developmental Review, 30*, 36–51. https://doi.org/10.1016/j.dr.2009.12.002

Stevenson, M., & Crnic, K. (2013). Intrusive fathering, children's self-regulation and social skills: A mediation analysis. *Journal of Intellectual Disability Research, 57*, 500–512. https://doi.org/10.1111/j.1365-2788.2012.01549.x

Thijs, J., & Verkuyten, M. (2008). Peer victimization and academic achievement in a multiethnic sample: The role of perceived academic self-efficacy. *Journal of Educational Psychology, 100*, 754–764. https://doi.org/10.1037/a0013155

Tropp, L. R., & Prenovost, M. A. (2008). The role of intergroup contact in predicting children's interethnic attitudes: Evidence from meta-analytic and field studies. In S. R. Levy & M. Killen (Eds.), *Intergroup attitudes and relations in childhood through adulthood* (pp. 236–248). New York: Oxford University Press.

Turner, R. N., & Cameron, L. (2016). Confidence in contact: A new perspective on promoting cross-group friendship among children and adolescents. *Social Issues and Policy Review, 10*, 212–246. https://doi.org/10.1111/sipr.12023

Umaña-Taylor, A. J., Alfaro, E. C., Bámaca, M. Y., & Guimond, A. B. (2009). The central role of familial ethnic socialization in Latino adolescents' cultural orientation. *Journal of Marriage and Family, 71*, 46–60. https://doi.org/10.1111/j.1741-3737.2008.00579.x

Updegraff, K. A., Kim, J., Killoren, S. E., & Thayer, S. M. (2010). Mexican American parents' involvement in adolescents' peer relationships: Exploring the role of culture and adolescents' peer experiences. *Journal of Research on Adolescence, 20*, 65–87. https://doi.org/10.1111/j.1532-7795.2009.00625.x

Varghese, C., & Wachen, J. (2016). The determinants of father involvement and connections to children's literacy and language outcomes: Review of the literature. *Marriage & Family Review, 52*, 331–359. https://doi.org/10.1080/01494929.2015.1099587

Vondra, J. I., Shaw, D. S., Swearingen, L., Cohen, M., & Owens, E. B. (2001). Attachment stability and emotional and behavioral regulation from infancy to preschool age. *Development and Psychopathology, 13*, 13–33. https://doi.org/10.1017/S095457940100102X

Wainryb, C. (2004). The study of diversity in human development: Culture, urgencies, and perils. *Human Development, 47*, 131–137. https://doi.org/10.1159/000077986

Weisner, T. S. (1996). Why ethnography should be the most important method in the study of human development. In R. Jessor, A. Colby, & R. Shweder (Eds.), *Ethnography and human development: Context and meaning in social inquiry* (pp. 305–324). Chicago: University of Chicago Press.

Weisner, T. S. (2002). Ecocultural understanding of children's developmental pathways. *Human Development, 45*, 275–281. https://doi.org/10.1159/000064989

Weisner, T. S., Matheson, C., & Bernheimer, L. (1996). American cultural models of early influence and parent recognition of developmental delays: Is earlier always better than later? In S. Harkness, C. M. Super, & R. New (Eds.), *Parents' cultural belief systems* (pp. 496–531). New York: Guilford Press.

Youngblade, L. M., & Belsky, J. (1992). Parent-child antecedents of 5-year-olds' close friendships: A longitudinal analysis. *Developmental Psychology, 28*, 700–713. https://doi.org/10.1037/0012-1649.28.4.700

Yu, T., Volling, B. L., & Niu, W. (2015). Emotion socialization and children's behavior problems in China and the United States. *Journal of Comparative Family Studies, 46*, 419–434. Retrieved from http://www.jstor.org/stable/43613126

Zarra-Nezhad, M., Kiuru, N., Aunola, K., Zarra-Nezhad, M., Ahonen, T., Poikkeus, A., et al. (2014). Social withdrawal in children moderates the association between parenting styles and the children's own socioemotional development. *Journal of Child Psychology & Psychiatry, 55*, 1260–1269. https://doi.org/10.1111/jcpp.12251

Fathers and Young Children at Play: A Scoping Review of Studies of Fathers' Play with Sons and Daughters from Birth to Preschool

22

Claire D. Vallotton, Tricia Foster, Tamesha Harewood, Jody Cook, and Anike R. Adekoya

There are few activities that are more representative of early childhood than play. Play itself takes different forms from infancy throughout childhood, but regardless of the age of the player, it can be defined as an activity that is self-directed, inherently enjoyable, spontaneous, and free from the constraints of goals or rules imposed by others (Whitebread, 2012). And while play is often undertaken for its own sake, it nonetheless contributes in important ways to children's development; by creating a motivating opportunity to focus on means rather than the end, children can try out new behaviors, modify their actions, and adapt accordingly, leading to skill development and problem-solving capabilities (Pellegrini, 2009). Especially during infancy and early childhood, parents have opportunities to engage in play together with their children, capitalizing on the inherent opportunities that play offers for making positive connections and engendering cultural learning (Tomasello, 2008). The degree to which parents support children's play, and engage in play themselves, varies across cultures; in Western cultures, parents tend to regard play as beneficial to children and as an important activity for parents to participate in (Whitebread, 2012).

While both mothers and fathers in many cultures play with their children, play may be a particularly salient feature of fathers and fathering. American fathers spend proportionally more of their time playing with their young children, as compared to mothers (Bianchi, Robinson, & Milke, 2006; Nelson-Coffey, Killingsworth, Layous, Cole, & Lyubomirsky, 2019). But perhaps even more important than the amount of time spent playing is the possibility that play itself is closely tied to what it means to be a father. Paquette (2004) proposes a theoretical model that emphasizes play as central to fathering, just as nurturing is central to mothering. This theory offers a unique paternal extension to attachment frameworks, proposing that fathers provide a complement to mothers' nurturance by engaging in stimulating, active play with their young children, supporting children to explore their worlds and expand their skills in a structured, safe way. Play is a primary way that fathers interact with their children in ways that tend to excite and temporarily destabilize them, which is

C. D. Vallotton (✉) · T. Harewood · J. Cook
A. R. Adekoya
Human Development and Family Studies, Michigan State University, East Lansing, MI, USA
e-mail: vallotto@msu.edu

T. Foster
Occupational Therapy Program, School of Health Sciences, Eastern Michigan University, Ypsilanti, MI, USA

H. E. Fitzgerald et al. (eds.), *Handbook of Fathers and Child Development*,
https://doi.org/10.1007/978-3-030-51027-5_22

beneficial to children as long as it is done in the context of a caring father-child relationship, described as the "father-child activation relationship." This is contrasted with the mother-child attachment relationship, which centers on nurturing and calming children in times of stress (Paquette, 2004).

Differences between mothers and fathers are evident not only in the quantity of parent-child play (Craig, 2006; Lindsey, Mize, & Pettit, 1997a, 1997b) but also in the qualities of the play. Many studies suggest that fathers engage in more rough and tumble, stimulating play with their children (Carson, Burks, & Parke, 1993), and do so in more challenging ways (Labrell, 1996). Fathers and mothers play may support distinct skills in children (Flanders, Leo, Paquette, Pihl, & Seguin, 2009). But there are similarities as well – both moms and dads from European-American families have similarly favorable views of, and engagement in, pretend play with their toddlers (Haight, Parke, & Black, 1997).

The similarities and differences between mothers and fathers, evident in the realm of parent-child play, may reflect how the larger context of family processes and relationships unfold. Cabrera, Fitzgerald, Bradley, and Roggman (2014) proposed a model of family relationships, relevant to both mothers and fathers, highlighting the various ways that mothers and fathers are alike, different, and also complementary in the ways they interact within their family systems. Parents are alike in that they are both sensitive and responsive to their children – behaviors that benefit children, regardless of from whom they come. At the same time, mothers and fathers are different – in the ways they spend time with children (e.g., Bianchi et al., 2006), and the qualities of the interactions themselves (Carson et al., 1993). Furthermore, parents have the capacity to complement one another. Even if particular behaviors may be more typical for mothers or fathers, they can each assume roles not typically enacted if the situation demands, or they may provide compensatory effects when necessary, as is the case when fathers "buffer" their children from the effects of maternal depression (Mezulis, Hyde, & Clark, 2004).

Despite the growing involvement of fathers in children's lives over recent decades (Bianchi et al., 2006) and the understanding that fathers contribute in important ways to children's development and well-being, there remain gaps in the literature on fathers, in general, and the role of father-child play, in particular (Cabrera & Roggman, 2017). Informed by theories of play's contributions to children's development (Pellegrini, 2009), the central role of play in fathering (Paquette, 2004), and with the understanding that mothers and fathers operate together within their family systems in ways that are different, alike, and complementary (Cabrera et al., 2014), this chapter explores the differences and similarities between father-child and mother-child play and the associations between father-child play and young children's developmental outcomes.[1] To this end, we examined the existing literature to address the following questions:

1. How is father-child and mother-child play similar and different during early childhood?
2. How do the qualities of father-child play in early childhood distinctly affect child development?

We utilized a scoping review methodology to answer the proposed research questions. Scoping reviews follow a systematic approach of searching and evaluating the available literature on a given topic. As described by Arksey and O'Malley

[1]A note on definitions and sociocultural context. The 50 articles reviewed in depth span several decades, from 1977 (i.e., Weinraub & Frankel, 1977) to 2017 (i.e., Ahnert et al., 2017), reflecting predominant theories of the authors' time and space. As such, sex and gender concepts (e.g., male female vs man woman vs son daughter vs boy girl) may have been used interchangeably, and sex and gender binaries may have been assumed without the context of current understandings of sex and gender diversity and interactivity. For clarity in reporting, this section also uses sex and gender binaries and assumes that these were appropriately reported in each article. However, here, "sex" refers to one's biological sex (i.e., male, female); "gender" refers to the sociocultural representations of "man" and "woman," "boy" and "girl," including prescriptive symbols of masculinity and femininity across the lifespan (e.g., toy trucks as masculine, and primarily for boys; dolls as feminine, and primarily for girls).

(2005), a scoping review study is undertaken for one of four purposes: (1) to describe the range or nature of research activity on a given topic, (2) to determine whether it is worth doing a more extensive systematic literature review, (3) to summarize the findings of current research, or (4) to identify gaps in the current research. This scoping review is focused primarily on the first and third of these purposes: describing the range of research on observed qualities of father-child play during early childhood and summarizing what we know from the findings in the current literature. In addition, we also aim to identify methodological and sampling limitations in the existing work on father-child play, which limit generalizability of the conclusions we can draw from the current literature.

Methodology

We used an inductive approach to accomplish our aims by following the stages of conducting a scoping review laid out by Arksey and O'Malley (2005); these include the following: "Stage 1: identifying the research question; Stage 2: identifying relevant studies; Stage 3: study selection; Stage 4: charting the data; Stage 5: collating, summarizing and reporting the results" (p. 22).

Identifying the Research Questions

Defining our initial questions as listed above was done iteratively in discussion among the five authors, each of whom come from different perspectives regarding this topic. Some authors focus on community populations of families with demographically based vulnerabilities, while others focus on clinical populations of either parents or children from the lenses of public health, mental health, or early intervention. All authors share an interest in fathers and fathering, early childhood, and longitudinal effects of parenting on child development, with a focus on the unique effects of fathers' relationships with their children on children's development. Our research questions were refined as we debated substantive issues related to the nature of fatherhood and of play. We sought to define our questions and purposes narrowly enough to be able to draw conclusions about the existing literature regarding our questions: How is father-child and mother-child play similar and different during early childhood? And, how do the qualities of father-child play in early childhood distinctly affect child development? For each of these questions, we address three aims:

1. To describe the range of research that currently exists
2. To summarize the findings of this body of research
3. To identify gaps in the research related to methodological and sampling limitations

Identifying the Relevant Studies

Our specific research questions shaped how we searched for and selected relevant articles in the subsequent stages of searching literature, screening abstracts, and, finally, screening full text for inclusion in the review. Overall, our primary foci were studies that included fathers and father figures, regardless of their biological relationship to the child or their residential status, and parent-child play as a meaningful construct, rather than just as a context in which to measure other aspects of parenting or child development. Relevant studies also included comparisons of father-child to mother-child play with young children. Methodologically, we targeted studies that were quantitative in nature and captured direct observations of parent-child play. The criteria for study inclusion are described in full in Table 22.1 of the Appendix.

To identify the set of relevant studies, we searched three databases: PsycInfo including PsycArticles within ProQuest, Family and Society Studies Worldwide, and Core Collection in Web of Science. We included studies published in English only for the feasibility of understanding and reporting on results. We included only peer-reviewed studies to ensure a minimum level

Table 22.1 Inclusion/exclusion criteria: definitions and rationale

Criterion	Definition	Rationale
Father figure included	Study must include fathers, defined as any father figure involved in the child's life	The extant literature has drawn no clear conclusions about the differential effects of involved fathers on children's development; thus, a more inclusive approach is warranted. Further, biological status of fathers is rarely confirmed in studies, and using coresidence as a criterion may systematically exclude more fathers in minority groups and those with lower income and education. We determined that if a father figure was identified as such in a study, the level of involvement in the child's life is sufficient to have a substantial influence
Mother included	Study must include mothers, defined as any mother figure involved in the child's life, and must measure the same play behaviors, as were measured for fathers, and include them in analyses	In order to answer our question about the distinct effects of fathers most directly, it became clear that each study would need to contrast or control for the effects of mother-child interaction on child development
Child age	Studies must include young children under 5 years but can include older children. For studies with a range of child ages that include children >5 years, the mean age of children at the wave where parent-child play is observed must be <61 months	Birth to age five is the period of early childhood, when the most rapid development occurs, and before formal schooling begins in many countries from which the studies are expected to come. Parent-child interactions during this time are central to child development
Observed interactions	Studies must include observed (live or recorded) parent-child interactions; recording could be audio, visual, transcriptions, or any combination	We are interested in what may be subtle and unconscious aspects of parents' behaviors with their children, which are best captured via direct observation. Play is an elusive concept, and notoriously hard to define, and parents may have difficulty reporting about play behaviors with any consistency. Thus, we focused only on observed interactions of parent-child play
Play as the construct of interest	Parent-child play had to be a salient construct in the design and measurement of the study. Studies could meet this criterion in one of the following ways: 1. Examine types of play parents generate 2. Contrast parent behavior across multiple contexts including play 3. Observe naturally occurring play vs. researcher-contrived play task 4. Define play as a meaningful construct or context, and measure parents' play-relevant behaviors. To exclude studies that used play as the "default" context for measuring other parenting behaviors, we required the word "play" or "playful" to be in the title of the study	Play is an important context for child development, and a context in which many aspects of the parent-child relationship and parenting behaviors are revealed. An initial scan of the literature led us to conclude that our discipline relies heavily on the context of play to measure a vast array of the qualities of parenting. But, because of the centrality of play to our question, we required play itself to be the focus of the study, rather than only a context in which to examine general parenting behaviors
Quantitative	Studies must measure and report on parent behaviors quantitatively	Observations of behavior lend themselves to quantitative descriptions (rating or coding) and may enable us to compare some aspects across studies. Further, quantitative methodology allows for direct comparisons between fathers and mothers, which is necessary to answer our primary research question exploring differences between fathers and mothers

of quality. We did not exclude studies based on year of publication.

In each of the three databases, we used the search terms:

- "father*[2]" AND "mother*" in the abstract or title
- AND "child*" OR "infan*" OR "toddler*" in the abstract or title
- AND "play*" in the title

Initial searches yielded 389 articles (PsycInfo and PsycArticles, 172; Core Collection in Web of Science, 132; Family and Society Studies Worldwide, 85).

Study Selection

After removing duplicates from the 389 studies identified in our search, 238 articles remained. We used the criteria in Table 22.1 to further refine our selections of the final articles to be reviewed. After an initial training and revision process for coding the abstracts, each of the abstracts were reviewed by two members of the author team for inclusion/exclusion based on the review criteria detailed in Table 22.1; inter-author agreement was 85%. All disagreements (32 in all) were discussed by the full team and determined by consensus. At the abstract review stage, 155 studies were excluded (83 remained), and then at the full text level, an additional 33 studies were removed, leaving the final list of 50; there was 88% agreement between authors on which studies should be included in the final review, and all disagreements were resolved through discussion and consensus. Disagreements centered largely on whether the concept of play was sufficiently meaningful in the study, a challenge anticipated in our initial criteria and an ongoing challenge in the research in our discipline. Figure 22.1 shows the number of articles identified, and those excluded, at each step in our procedures.

Charting and Summarizing the Data

In the fourth stage, we coded the 50 selected studies for the variables of interest, including research questions proposed, sample characteristics, methodology (including procedures for the play observations and the aspects of play that were measured), and child outcomes. Definitions of codes were derived among the authors initially and refined in an iterative process as the full set of articles were coded using each set of codes. Authors each took responsibility for a set of variables on which they reviewed all articles, and coding was checked by other authors. The results of this coding enable us to accomplish our first aim: to describe the range of the current literature examining the nature of father-child play (as compared to mother-child play) in early childhood and, within that, the range of studies that address the effects of father-child play on children's behavior and development.

Once all data were coded, subsets of articles were identified based on their research questions, the aspects of play they measured, or their inclusion of child outcomes. Teams of authors read the full text of these subsets of articles to address our second aim: to summarize the empirical evidence that addresses our research questions on the nature and effects of father-child play.

In our coding process, we created a table charting the demographic characteristics of the samples from each article. We use this chart to report the sample characteristics and identify the limitations therein, of each subset of articles, which addresses our third aim.

[2]Using an asterisk (*) in the search terms instructs the search to include all derivations of the word as long as the initial stem of the word is included. For example, "father*" included "fathering," "fatherhood," "father-child," "father-mother," etc. Likewise, the term "infan*" includes "infant," "infancy," "infant-parent," etc., and the term "play*" includes "playful," "playing," etc.

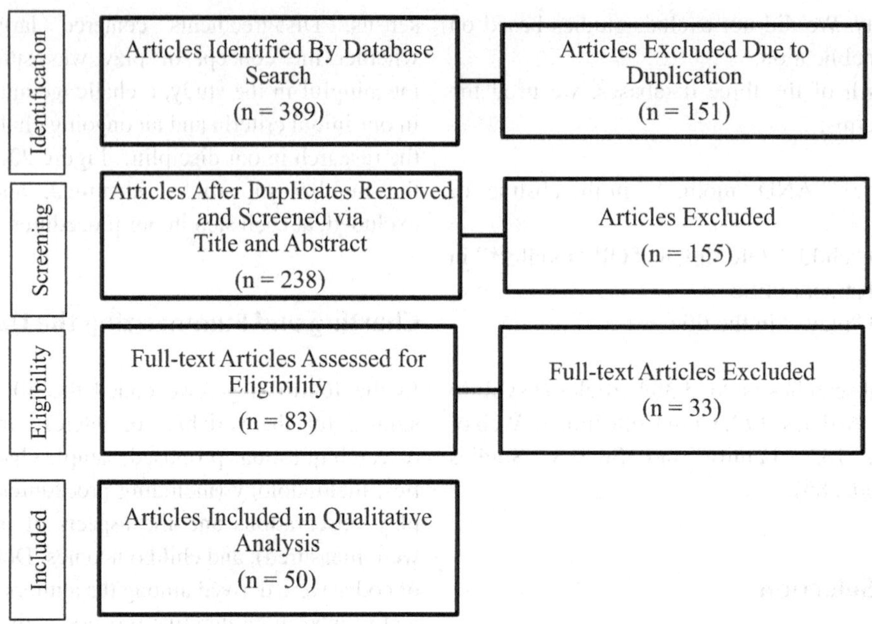

Fig. 22.1 Flow chart of procedures for identifying included articles

Findings

Question 1: Differences in Father-Child and Mother-Child Play

Aim 1: Describe the Range of Studies Observing Father- and Mother-Child Play in Early Childhood First, we describe the range of research studies that met our criteria for answering our first research question: What can our current literature say about the nature of father-child play, how it is similar or different from mother-child play? For each, we describe the features of the current set of literature available to address these questions; in so doing, this helps us to address our third aim of identifying gaps and limitations of the current empirical literature on father-child play. Importantly, two of the features that we describe inform the way that we report results to address aim 2: the research questions addressed by the articles and the aspects of parent-child play that were observed organize the way we summarize the findings to address our second aim.

The full set of 50 articles reviewed in this study are listed and described in Appendix Table 22.2, including the authors and year of the publication, the nationality of the sample, whether the study design included families or dyads, the research questions, the procedures for observing play, and the aspects of play measured by observation. Here, we describe the main findings regarding the nature of the range of studies identified in this review.

Year of Publication Though we put no date restrictions in our search, the earliest articles identified by our search were published in 1977 and 1979. The most prolific decade for these studies was the 1980s in which 17 of the articles were produced, followed by the 1990s which produced 14 of the articles, with studies waning to 10 in the 2000s. This earlier interest in the 1980s may reflect the gender revolution of the earlier decade in which issues of gender roles and socialization became a greater interest to child development researchers.

Table 22.2 Article characteristics for final set of articles

Article author/year	Population country	Study design	Research questions	Observation location	Level of structure and toy description	Parent play behaviors observed
Ahnert et al. (2017)	Austria and Germany	Family and dyad	PD; CSD; OCE	Home	Structured; specific set of toys used	INT:S
Arco (1983)	USA	Dyad	PD	Lab	Semi-structured/structured; no toys used	Temporal bouts of play
Bradley and Gobbart (1989)	Australia	Family	PD; CSD	Home	Semi-structured; specific set of toys provided	TOYS
Bright and Stockdale (1984)	USA	Family	PD; CSD	Lab	Semi-structured; specific set of toys provided	COM:VOC; INT:E,D; BEHAV; ENJOY; TOYS
Cabrera et al. (2017)	USA	Family	PD; OCE; CO	Home	Structured; toys provided by researcher	ENJOY
Caldera et al. (1989)	USA	Family	PD; CSD	Lab	Structured; specific set of toys provided	COM:PRAG; INT:E; BEHAV; TOYS
Caldera and Sciaraffa (1998)	USA	Family	PD; CSD	Lab	Structured; specific set of toys provided	BEHAV; TOYS
Chiarello et al. (2006)	USA	Family	PD; OCE	Home	Semi-structured; family's toys used	INT:R,D; BEHAV; ENJOY
Crawley and Sherrod (1984)	USA	Dyads	PD	Home	Semi-structured; family's toys used	TYPES
de Falco et al. (2010)	USA	Family	PD; CO	Lab	Semi-structured; specific set of toys provided	TYPES
Dickson et al. (1997)	USA	Family	PD	Home	Natural; family's toys used	TYPES; ENJOY
El-Ghoroury and Romanczyk (1999)	USA	Family	PD; OCE; CO	Home	Natural; family's toys used	COM:PRAG; INT:E,S,D; BEHAV
Field (1979)	USA	Family	PD; OCE	Lab	Semi-structured; no toys were used	TYPES
Flippin and Watson (2011)	USA	Family	PD; CO	Lab	Semi-structured; toys provided by researcher	INT:R,S
Grossmann et al. (2002)	Germany	Family	PD; CO	Home	Semi-structured; toys provided by researcher	INT:R,S
Haight et al. (1997)	USA	Family	PD	Home	Semi-structured; family's toys were used	TYPES; INT:E
Idle et al. (1993)	Canada	Family	PD; CSD	Lab	Structured; specific set of toys provided	TOYS
Kazura (2000)	USA	Family	PD; OCE	Lab	Semi-structured/structured; toys provided by researcher	TYPES; INT:R,S,D
Keren et al. (2005)	Israel	Family	PD; CSD; CO	Home	Semi-structured; toys provided by researcher	COM:VOC; INT:D; BEHAV; ENJOY

(continued)

Table 22.2 (continued)

Article author/year	Population country	Study design	Research questions	Observation location	Level of structure and toy description	Parent play behaviors observed
Kerns and Barth (1995)	USA	Family	PD; CSD; CO	Lab	Structured; no toys were used	COM:PRAG; INT:E,R,D
Kwon et al. (2013)	USA	Family	PD; IC	Lab	Semi-structured/structured; toys provided by researcher/specific set of toys provided	COM:VOC; INT:R,S,D
Laflamme et al. (2002)	Canada	Family	PD; CSD	Lab	Semi-structured; toys provided by researcher	TYPES; COM:VOC; BEHAV
Lamb et al. (1982)	Sweden	Family	PD; CSD	Home	Natural; no toys used/family's toys	TYPES; COM:VOC; INT:E,R; BEHAV; ENJOY
Leaper and Gleason (1996)	USA	Family	PD; CSD; OCE; CO	Lab	Structured; specific set of toys provided	COM:PRAG; INT:D
Leaper (2000)	USA	Family	PD; CSD; OCE;	Home	Structured; specific set of toys provided	COM:PRAG; INT:D
Liddell et al. (1987)	South Africa	Dyads and triads	PD; CSD	Outside/ playground	Spontaneous; no toys were used	COM:VOC
Lindsey and Mize (2000)	USA	Family	PD; IC	Lab	Semi-structured; specific set of toys provided	TYPES; COM:PRAG; INT:E,R,D; TOYS
Lindsey et al. (1997a)	USA	Family	PD; CSD	Lab	Semi-structured; toys provided by researcher	TYPES; COM:PRAG; INT:E,R,D
Lindsey et al. (2010)	USA	Family	PD; IC	Lab	Structured; toys provided by researcher	COM:PRAG; INT:R,D
Lindsey and Mize (2001)	USA	Family	PD; IC	Lab	Semi-structured; specific set of toys provided	TYPES; COM:PRAG; INT:E,D
Lindsey et al. (1997b)	USA	Family	PD; CO	Lab	Semi-structured; toys provided by researcher	COM:PRAG; INT:R
MacDonald and Parke (1984)	USA	Family	PD; CSD; CO	Home	Natural/structured; family's toys were used	TYPES; COM:VOC; INT:E,D
McBride-Chang and Jacklin (1993)	USA	Family	PD; CSD; OCE; CO	Unreported	Unreported	TOYS
McGovern (1990)	USA	Family	PD	Lab	Semi-structured; toys provided by researcher	TYPES; INT:E,R; TOYS
Menashe-Grinberg and Atzaba-Poria (2017)	Israel	Family	PD; CO	Home	Semi-structured/structured; toys provided by researcher/specific set of toys provided	INT:R,S; ENJOY
O'Brien and Nagle (1987)	USA	Unreported	PD; CSD	Lab	Structured; specific set of toys provided	COM:PRAG; INT:D
Power (1985)	USA	Family	PD; CSD; OCE	Lab	Semi-structured; specific set of toys provided	TYPES; INT:S,D

Article author/year	Population country	Study design	Research questions	Observation location	Level of structure and toy description	Parent play behaviors observed
Roggman and Peery (1988)	USA	Family	PD	Lab	Semi-structured; no toys were used	BEHAV
Roggman and Peery (1989)	USA	Family	PD; CSD; OCE	Lab	Semi-structured; no toys were used	BEHAV
Roopnarine (1986)	USA	Family	PD; CSD; OCE	Lab	Semi-structured; specific set of toys provided	TOYS
Roopnarine et al. (1992)	India	Family	PD; CSD	Home	Spontaneous; family's toys were used	TYPES; BEHAV
Roopnarine and Mounts (1985)	USA	Family	PD; CSD; CO	Lab	Semi-structured; specific set of toys provided	TYPES
Roopnarine et al. (1990)	India	Family	PD; CSD	Home	Spontaneous; family's toys were used	TYPES; COM:VOC; BEHAV; ENJOY
Ryckebusch and Marcos (2004)	France	Family	PD; IC	Unreported	Semi-structured; specific set of toys provided	COM:PRAG; INT:D
Stevenson et al. (1988)	USA	Family	PD; CSD; OCE	Lab	Semi-structured; toys provided by researcher	TYPES
Tenenbaum and Leaper (1997)	USA	Family	PD; CSD	Home	Semi-structured; specific set of toys provided	COM:PRAG
Teti et al. (1988)	USA	Dyad	PD; CSD	Home	Natural; family's toys were used	TYPES; INT:S
Weinraub and Frankel (1977)	USA	Dyad	PD	Lab	Semi-structured; toys provided by researcher	COM:VOC; INT:E; BEHAV
Wood, Desmarais, and Gugula (2002)	Canada	Mixed	PD; CSD	Lab	Semi-structured; toys provided by researcher	TOYS
Yogman (1981)	USA	Family	PD	Lab	Structured; no toys were used	TYPES

Families Versus Dyads Most studies defined their study design for the comparison of fathers and mothers as either the comparison of two parents interacting with their child/ren from the same family (43; 86%) or dyads (6 studies; 12%), in which mother-child and father-child dyads in the sample that were not from the same family. The focus here on families, rather than parent-child dyads, means that the majority of studies in this sample exclude parents and children from single-parent homes.

Nationality of Sample We did limit our search to articles published in English, which likely limited the diversity of the populations represented in the studies selected for this review. Thirty seven of the 50 studies (74%) were conducted in the USA, with three additional studies North American studies conducted in Canada. Four studies were conducted in European countries; two in India, two in Israel, one in South Africa, and one in Australia.

Sample Characteristics Fifteen of the 50 articles (30%) consisted of Caucasian only samples, including four studies with samples from Canada and Australia. Nine other studies (18%) included international samples from Austria, Germany, France, Italy, India, Israel, Sweden, and South Africa. Eighteen studies (36%) had mixed samples, but a majority of participants were Caucasian, and eight studies (16%) did not disclose the race of the sample. Twenty articles (40%) indicated the mean age of fathers ranged from 24 to 39 years; one study (2%) indicated fathers' mean age as 19, and 29 (58%) did not indicate the ages of fathers. Twenty-eight (56%) studies did not explicitly state the biological status of parents, but language within these studies led us to assume the fathers included in the studies were the biological fathers of the children. Six studies (12%) specifically mentioned biological fathers; one study (2%) had mixed statuses of biological, other, and nonbiological; and 16 studies (32%) did not indicate a status. Only six studies (12%) indicated fathers were the secondary caregivers for their children, three studies (6%) indicated mixed caregiving roles, and the remaining 41 (82%) did not indicate a role. There were three studies (6%) which examined samples with disabilities only, four (8%) with mixed-ability samples, 16 (32%) with typically developing samples, and 26 (52%) which did not disclose this information. Of the 50 articles, 10 (20%) included infants (0–12 months) only, 16 (32%) included toddlers only (12–36 months), and 13 (26%) included preschoolers only (36+ months). Three articles (6%) included both infants and toddlers, five (10%) included toddlers and preschoolers, and three (6%) included infants, toddlers, and preschoolers. A majority of the studies had even samples of males and females, two studies had very uneven samples of more than 55% males, and two studies (4%) did not disclose the sex of the sample. Two studies (4%) included low-income samples only, 15 studies (30%) included middle income only, 1 study (2%) included high income only, 7 (14%) had low-to-middle-income samples, 14 (28%) had mid- to high-income samples, and 11 (22%) did not indicate the sample's SES. The 50 articles included in this review were largely conducted in the USA and consisted primarily of intact families that were predominantly Caucasian and falling within a middle to high SES. There was an often implicit assumption that fathers and mothers hold traditional parenting roles within their families, with fathers as the secondary caregiver to their young children. Samples of children generally included even numbers of males and females, focusing on different age ranges including infants, toddlers, and/or preschoolers, and generally reported children as typically developing.

Research Questions All studies posed research questions on play differences (PD; 100%), or how similarly/differently fathers and mothers play with their children, which is consistent with our selection criteria for this study. In addition, we coded any other research questions posed by each study, with many articles including more than one additional research question (see the fourth column of Table 22.2 for the questions posed by each study). The other research questions can be grouped into one of the following categories: interaction contexts (IC; 10%), comparing parenting behaviors across different interaction context including play; child outcomes (CO; 26%), effects of parent play on child behavior or development (this set of articles will be used to address our second research question); child effects, effects of child characteristics, such as age, sex, or ability, on parent-child play; within child effects, we identified a substantial set of articles focusing on child sex differences (CSD; 54% of all articles): whether parents play differently with sons and daughters; because of the predominance of studies looking at child sex differences, in the table, we identify child effects questions as either CSD or other child effects (OCE; 26% of all articles). Thus, after basic comparisons of play between fathers and mothers (a criterion for inclusion in this scoping review), the most common research questions posed by the authors were effects of child sex or other characteristics on parent-child play, followed by the effects of parent-child play on child outcomes, and, distantly, how qualities of parent-child interaction in play differ from interactions in other contexts. These research questions provide a primary way to organize our study results as we address the second aim of this scoping review.

Procedures for Observing Play Studies differed in their data collection procedures including where data collection took place, how the play observation was set up, and whether and which toys were used. Twenty-nine (58%) of the studies (which is the majority) conducted observations in lab settings (e.g., a play room with one-way mirrors at a university), 18 (36%) conducted observations in the homes of the families or dyads, one (2%) observed outside or on a playground, and two (4%) did not report where the data collection occurred. There were a variety of ways that studies structured the play, and the toys used during observed play; researchers often included more than one level of structure, and/or more than one set of toys, in the design of their study. The levels of structure, from least to most structured, include the following: spontaneous play (6%), natural play (10%) in family's space, and with family's toys but researcher determines timing; semi-structured (60%) where the researcher provides materials, space, and time, but few instructions (e.g., "play as you normally would"); and structured (32%) in which the researcher provides materials, space, timing, and instructions for how to proceed, for example, 3-bag task, 2-box, etc. The toys used were described as follows: No toys were used (12%); family's toys were used (20%); toys were provided by researcher and included a variety (30%); and a specific set of toys were provided by researcher to test specific responses or behaviors (38%). With the majority of studies observing structured or semi-structured play in the lab, and even those in the home using toys provided by the researchers, the second finding from across these studies is the lack of studies designed to understand the nature and effects of spontaneous play between parents and children in their own homes.

Aspects of Play Observed We coded the methodology section of each article for the aspects of play that were measured from the parent-child play observation (see the final column of Table 22.2 for the aspects of play coded in each article). In most studies, these coded aspects of play were addressing the primary study questions posed in each article regarding the differences and similarities between father-child and mother-child play. However, there was variation in how focused these behaviors were on play itself. Aspects of parents' play that were focused on play itself included the types of play (TYPES) that parents create or engage in, such as rough and tumble, pretense, face-to-face games, and construction; and enjoyment of play (ENJOY), including positive affect and playfulness. Another play-focused aspect of play was parents' behaviors with toys (TOYS), including their reactions to toys, their choices of toys, and their comments on children's behaviors with toys; toy-focused coding was primarily used in the studies addressing gender socialization. Other studies measured play-related parenting behaviors which were less focused on play but still argued to be meaningful aspects of the play itself. These included parent-child interaction qualities of involvement/engagement (INT:E), responsiveness (INT:R), scaffolding/stimulation (INT:S), and directiveness (INT:D); communication during and about play, including aspects of pragmatics (COM:PRAG) and vocalization/speech frequency (COM:VOC); and parents' physical behaviors (BEHAV) during play, microanalytically coded, such as touch, gaze, and proximity.

These aspects of parents' play that were measured provide a secondary way to organize the findings across studies to summarize what we know about father-child play, which answers the primary research questions of the studies reviewed and addresses the second aim of this scoping review. Figure 22.2 depicts the frequency of these major categories of the aspects of play observed, as well as the subcategories, which will be described further when the results of these studies are summarized to address the second aim of this scoping review.

Aim 2: Summary of Results From Studies of Father-Child and Mother-Child Play in Early Childhood We organize our summary of study results based on our findings from coding aspects of play measured from observations, which answers the main research question addressed by all of our studies: How does father-child play differ from mother-child play? After that, we organize the remaining findings according to the common research questions posed in the articles: how play differs from other contexts and how child characteristics (sex and other) affect play. Within each section, we contextualize the findings given the characteristics of the study sam-

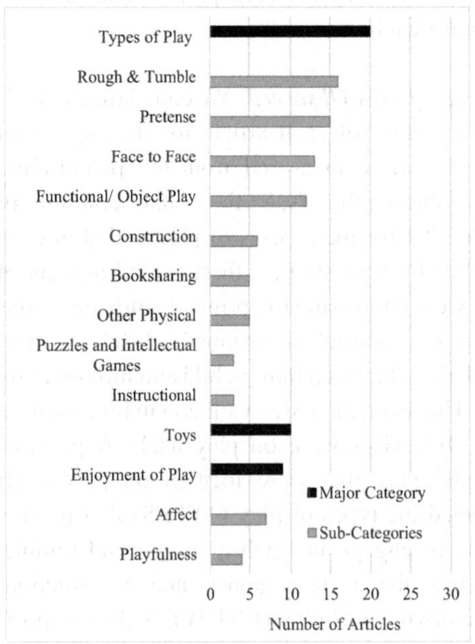

Panel A. *Studies measuring play-specific behavior.*

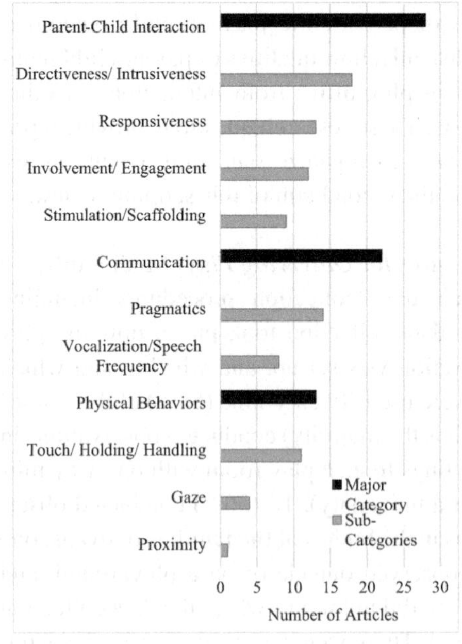

Panel B. Studies measuring play-related parenting behaviors.

Fig. 22.2 Number of articles that measured each aspect of parents' play. (**a**) Studies measuring play-specific behavior. (**b**) Studies measuring play-related parenting behaviors

ples and describe limitations to the conclusions that can be drawn, which addresses our third aim for this scoping review.

Of the 50 articles reviewed, which each included play as a meaningful construct in the study, either as a context/predictor or an outcome, about half (26) measured one or more concepts of play itself, including the types of play that fathers and mothers generated or engaged in (e.g., rough and tumble, pretend), their enjoyment of play or playfulness, and fathers' and mothers' behavior toward toys. Because 90% of the articles that measured parents' behavior toward toys were focused on child sex differences and gender socialization, we address these in the section on child sex differences in parents' play behaviors. After summarizing parent gender differences in these play-focused behaviors, we review the subsets of articles that measured parents' play-related behaviors, including parent-child interaction qualities in play, parents' communication during and about, and parents' physical behaviors during play. We review each of these sets of articles to address the question of similarities and differences in fathers' and mothers' play with young children.

Types of Play Parents Generated or Engaged In Twenty studies examined one or more types of play. One pattern that arises in these studies is how they framed whose play behavior – the parent or the child – they were measuring. Studies of parents with their infants and toddlers examined the play types that parents generated, while those studies of parents with children 3–5 years measured parents' engagement in children's play, or jointly constructed play. Thus, we organize the results regarding differences in fathers' and mothers' play types by age of child.

Play Types with Young Infants Of the six studies that included young infants (4–8 months), there were more similarities than differences in the amount and types of play parents do with their infants. Fathers and mothers play games with infants at similar rates, and parents generated similar types of games with their babies, such as peekaboo, tell-me-a-story, and so big (Field, 1979). Fathers and mothers are similar in conventional visual and verbal games (Yogman, 1981) and physical and object play (Crawley & Sherrod, 1984; McGovern, 1990). However, fathers engaged in more rough physical play (Crawley & Sherrod, 1984) and created more proximal, arousing physical play (Yogman, 1981) and more social play that included repetitive, turn-taking games, such as imitating facial expressions or sounds (McGovern, 1990), while mothers created more distal, visual, and attention-maintaining games (Yogman, 1981). Further, Field (1979) found that fathers played more games than mothers specifically with their boys (mothers were the same across sexes) and only when the boys were born at term (compared to preterm). Interestingly, Lamb, Frodi, Hwang, Frodi, and Steinberg (1982) found that the effects of parent sex on engaging in games with 8-month-olds were moderated by parents' involvement in caregiving, such that for the total amount of play, stimulus play, coordinate play, and conventional play, less involved fathers engaged in more play than involved fathers, whereas the reverse was true among mothers (more involved mothers engaged in more of these types of play than did less involved mothers). Across these studies, fathers and mothers generate the same amounts and types of games with young infants, but fathers tend to also engage in more highly arousing behaviors, including both physical and social interchanges.

Play with Older Infants and Toddlers There were more similarities than differences in the types of play fathers and mothers generated or engaged across the 11 studies that examined parents' play with older infants (e.g., 9–15 months) and toddlers (e.g., 18–36 months, or developmental equivalents for de Falco, Esposito, Venuti, & Bornstein, 2010). Functional, or object-mediated, play was examined in nine studies and was the most common type of play for both parents in several studies (Crawley & Sherrod, 1984;

Roopnarine, Ahmeduzzaman, Hossain, & Riegraf, 1992). The study with the oldest children in this group (24–36 months) identified pretense as the most common type of play for both fathers and mothers (Haight, Parke, & Black, 1997), which reflects both parents' responsiveness to children's growing symbolic skills and interests and counters the common idea that fathers' primarily engage in physical play with their children.

In two studies, fathers spent a lower percent of time than mothers in object-mediated play with their older infants and toddlers (Roopnarine, Talukder, Jain, Joshi, & Srivastav, 1990; Teti et al., 1988). To add nuance to these findings, fathers engaged in more functional and exploratory play (de Falco et al., 2010; Stevenson et al., 1988), while mothers engaged in more instructive play with objects (Stevenson et al., 1988); one might interpret these findings to mean that fathers' play is more *playful* and less focused on the learning opportunities inherent in play. Fathers also generated more conventional play as children got older (e.g., 13 months as compared to 7 or 10 months), while mothers' conventional play decreased with child age (Laflamme, Pomerleau, & Malcuit, 2002), indicating that both fathers and mothers adjust their play to children's changing abilities, but in different ways.

In five of six studies looking at physical play at this age, such as rough and tumble, tickling, and bouncing, fathers generated more physical play (Crawley & Sherrod, 1984; Dickson, Walker, & Fogel, 1997; Roopnarine et al., 1990, 1992; Teti et al., 1988). In three of seven studies, mothers generated more pretend play or symbolic behaviors (Crawley & Sherrod, 1984; de Falco et al., 2010; Power, 1985), and did more book sharing in two of four studies (Crawley & Sherrod, 1984; Dickson et al., 1997). On the other hand, in one study, fathers engaged in more symbolic play behaviors in a structured pretense setting, whereas they were similar to mothers in unstructured pretense and free play (Stevenson et al., 1988). Of the seven studies examining social, face-to-face games, there were no apparent differences between moms and dads in five of them, but two studies found that mothers generated more peekaboo (Roopnarine et al., 1990, 1992) and in one study did more language play (Teti, Bond, & Gibbs, 1988). Overall, there are more parent gender differences in the play with older infants and toddlers than with younger infants, as play itself begins to differentiate in response to changes in children's development; fathers begin to engage in more physical and socially arousing play, while mothers engage in more symbolic and language-mediated play.

Play Types with Preschool-Aged Children Six studies examined the types of play that parents engaged in with their preschool-aged children, 3–5 years old. All six studies examined physical play; of these, four studies found that fathers engaged in more vigorous physical play with their children than did mothers. Further, two of these also identified child sex differences such that dads engaged in more joint physical play with sons than with daughters (Lindsey & Mize, 2000, 2001).

Five of six studies looked at parents' engagement in pretense with their preschoolers; three of these studies found that mothers engaged in more pretense with their children than did fathers. However, Lindsey and colleagues also identified child sex differences in these results such that girls were more likely to generate pretense than were boys (Lindsey et al., 1997a, 1997b), both parents were more likely to be involved in pretense with their girls than boys (Lindsey & Mize, 2000), and moms were engaged in more joint play with daughters than with sons during pretense than other types of play (Lindsey & Mize, 2001).

There were fewer parent-gender differences in the other types of play examined at this age. Four studies included object-mediated or functional play (a specific type of object-mediated play); one found that mothers engaged in more object-mediated play MacDonald and Parke (1984), while another found that fathers engaged in more functional play (Stevenson et al., 1988). The three studies that examined construction found no differences. Only one of the three studies that looked at parents' instructive play found that mothers did more of this type (Stevenson et al., 1988).

Summary and Discussion of Play Types Looking across the 20 studies examining fathers' and mothers' types of play with their children, there is a developmental progression in the parent gender differences that emerge. There are very few parent gender differences in early infancy in the ways parents play with their babies, when play is focused on dyadic exchange (rather than objects), but fathers play in more somewhat more arousing ways. In later infancy and toddlerhood, toys become a focus of much of parent-child play for both fathers and mothers, but fathers and mothers differentiate here in the other types of play that are most common: physical play for fathers and symbolic play for mothers. In the third year of life and on, pretense becomes a much more common play type for children as children's symbolic and communication skills begin to drive the types of play. This is especially true for preschool-aged girls, and this is when child sex begins to drive parent gender differences in the types of play parents engage in: both parents engage in more symbolic play with their daughters, but especially mothers, and fathers engage in more physical play with their sons. It is possible that this is, in part, driven by differences in boys' and girls' language skills (e.g., Huttenlocher, Haight, Bryk, Seltzer, & Lycns, 1991), which are associated with different interests in play (Karrass, Braungart-Rieker, Mullins, & Lefever, 2002; Lyytinen, Laakso, Poikkeus, & Rita, 1999) and draw different play behaviors from parents and caregivers (Barnett, Gustafsson, Deng, Mills-Koonce, & Cox, 2012; Gleason, 1987; Vallotton, 2009). Because pretense is also rich with social roles, which draw on gender norms, this could also be the time at which parents' explicit and implicit gender socialization efforts emerge more fully; this will be addressed further in the section describing the set of studies that examined the effects of child gender on fathers' and mothers' play, including a set of articles focused on gender socialization processes.

The results on fathers' and mothers' play types can be contextualized in understanding that the demographic characteristics of these 20 articles, which were somewhat more diverse than the overall set of 50 articles in this scoping review. Seven articles consisted of Caucasian-only participants; five included samples with a mix of racial or ethnic backgrounds; four studies were conducted outside of the USA; and four were of unknown race and nationality. The articles represented some variation in SES, with the majority of samples falling in the middle- to high-SES range. Though this is one of the more diverse subsets of articles in our review, the analyses conducted in the articles do not enable us to compare how these results may differ across families with different demographic characteristics.

Enjoyment of Play Six studies examined parents' enjoyment of play, including four articles that measured their affect (e.g., affect/animation or expressions of excitement during play) and four that coded aspects related to parents' playfulness. Parental playfulness as a construct was surprisingly rare across the studies and not consistent in the way it was described or measured. Chiarello, Huntington, and Bundy (2006) measured parents' inventiveness in play using the Maternal Behavior Rating Scale (Mahoney, 1992); Keren, Feldman, Namdari-Weinbaum, Spitzer, and Tyano (2005) examined creativity as part of their rating of parental play quality; and both Cabrera, Karberg, Malin, and Aldoney (2017) and Menashe-Grinberg and Atzaba-Poria (2017) used the Parental Playfulness System (Atzaba-Poria et al., 2014). Four articles explored aspects related to affect including animation or excitement (Caldera, Huston, & O'Brien, 1989; Chiarello et al., 2006), enthusiasm (Bright & Stockdale, 1984), and positive affect (Keren et al., 2005). Most of the studies were conducted in the USA, although one was based in Israel and one was unknown in terms of location. Three of the samples were middle to high SES, and two of these three had a predominantly White sample. One exception was the study of Cabrera et al. (2017), focusing on low-income ethnic minority families enrolled in Early Head Start.

Collectively, none of the articles examining the overall concept of parental enjoyment of play demonstrated any significant differences between fathers and mothers. Two articles that considered parental playfulness, as defined by their creativity, curiosity, and humor during play, found that mothers and fathers exhibited similar levels of playfulness when playing with their toddlers (Cabrera et al., 2017; Menashe-Grinberg & Atzaba-Poria, 2017). Similarly, Chiarello et al. (2006) found that mothers and fathers showed comparable levels of animation, a construct measured as acceptance, enjoyment, warmth, expressiveness, and inventiveness, while playing with their infants and toddlers with motor delays. The same was true for parents of older children; mothers and fathers had similar levels of creative play and positive affect, when engaged in symbolic play with their preschoolers (Keren et al., 2005), and were alike in their enthusiasm levels during a structured play task (Bright & Stockdale, 1984). However, Caldera et al. (1989) found that mothers and fathers were excited about different things during play – each was more likely to show excitement when encountering toys considered to be "same-sex" stereotyped toys, for example, fathers and sons were more excited when opening a box that contained trucks than one containing dolls.

While fathers and mothers demonstrate similar levels of playfulness and affect, two of the studies suggest that their influence on children's outcomes differs by parent sex. Cabrera et al. (2017) showed that fathers' and mothers' level of playfulness is similar; however, fathers' playfulness predicted children's later language skills, while mothers' playfulness was related to children's later emotional regulation skills. And the findings of Menashe-Grinberg and Atzaba-Poria (2017) offer a view of fathers' playfulness as being uniquely important to children – child outcomes were positive only when fathers were both supportive in their parenting and playful in their interactions, what the authors described as a "double buffer" effect. This effect was not evident for mothers, whose supportive behaviors predicted positive child outcomes, even if they had low levels of playfulness.

Summary and Discussion of Enjoyment of Play Taken together, these studies do not support the notion that fathers are inherently more playful or that they are any more capable than mothers of being imaginative, creative, and fun in their play with their children, despite the tendency for family members to consider dad as the preferred playmate (Lamb, 1977; Paquette, 2004). Instead, perceived differences may relate more to the ways that parents spend their time; dads spend proportionally more of their time spent in playful activities with their children, and, when they do, it is more physically stimulating and vigorous, as compared to mothers. The meaningful differences between moms and dads may lie more in the mechanism of playfulness as it relates to important outcomes – father playfulness may relate to different child outcomes than mother playfulness (Cabrera et al., 2017). And, playfulness may be especially important to the role of fathering, as there is at least limited evidence that it is a necessary ingredient in father-child interactions in supporting child outcomes (Menashe-Grinberg & Atzaba-Poria, 2017). Whether this is related to the distinct role of fathers as parents who "specialize" in play, or is a by-product of the ways that fathers and mothers spend their time within the families, has yet to be determined. The majority of the families in the subset were American, and middle to high SES, reflecting a particular cultural belief in the value and enjoyment of parental play with children (Whitebread, 2012).

Parent-Child Interaction Qualities During Play Twenty-eight articles examined the aspects of parent-child interaction qualities in play; these were conceptualized by the authors as qualities of the play interactions between parents and children, though the same constructs could potentially be measured in other contexts as well. These studies were conducted mostly in the USA (71%); others were conducted in Germany, Israel, Sweden, and France. Forty-three percent (43%) of these studies included racially mixed samples, 21% Caucasians only, and 3% each Israeli, German/Austrian, Swedish, and French; 14% of studies did not report on sample demographics. A large percentage of these studies (64%) consisted of middle- to high-income samples. Thirty-nine percent of the studies included preschoolers only, 32% included toddlers only, 11% included infants only, and 18% included mixed samples of infants, toddlers, and preschoolers.

Each of these studies examined one or more of the following play interaction qualities: degree of engagement or involvement in play (14), responsiveness to children's play (13), scaffolding or stimulation of play (10), and directiveness or intrusiveness in play (19). However, many of these aspects of play were those already considered in the types of play (e.g., parents' engagement in pretense and physical play) and the communication during and about play (e.g., using directives in communication, responding to child communication). Thus, in this section, we focus on results of similarities and differences in fathers' and mothers' interaction qualities during play that are not otherwise described and then link these to other findings.

Engagement and Involvement Fourteen articles focused on parents' engagement or involvement in children's play, including measures of quality, such as the intensity of parents' play, to simple measures of the amount of time they percent of observed time they spent playing with their child. Three of these were already described in types of play (Lindsey et al., 1997a, 1997b; Lindsey & Mize, 2001; MacDonald & Parke, 1984), and one did not report direct comparisons of fathers and mothers (Kerns & Barth, 1995). Of the ten remaining articles, seven found no differences in mothers' and fathers' involvement in children's play (Ahnert et al., 2017; Caldera et al., 1989; El-Ghoroury & Romanczyk, 1999; Haight et al., 1997; Lamb et al., 1982; Lindsey & Mize, 2000; Weinraub & Frankel, 1977). The other three articles found slight differences indicating that fathers were slightly less involved or engaged in children's play than mothers. McGovern (1990) found that fathers demonstrated lower reciprocity with 4-month-old infants. Bright and Stockdale (1984) found that mothers observed their preschool-aged children more than fathers did and also spent more time doing their own thing, but there was no difference in fathers and mothers actively following their children's leads in play. And Leaper (2000) found that mothers were higher in affiliation with their preschool-aged children during play than were fathers; however, this difference was specific to one particular activity (toy track activity) and did not generalize to the other (play food activity). Further, although Weinraub and Frankel (1977) found no overall mean differences between parents in involvement, they found that mothers and fathers sat with, talked with, and played with same-sex infants more than opposite-sex infants.

Stimulation and Scaffolding Of the 10 articles that examined some aspect of parents' stimulation or scaffolding of children's play, one did not report direct comparisons of fathers and mothers (Keren et al., 2005), and one was already described in the play types above (Teti et al., 1988). Of the remaining eight articles that tested parent gender differences in stimulation or scaffolding, seven reported no differences between fathers and mothers. However, Menashe-Grinberg and Atzaba-Poria (2017) found tentative evidence that mothers' structuring of their toddlers' play was higher than fathers' structuring ($p = 0.07$). Although Power (1985) found no main effect of parent gender on parents' effectiveness in supporting infant play, there was an interaction of parent gender and infant age such that at 13 months (but not 7 or 10), mothers' attempts to influence infant behavior were more successful than were fathers'. Power (1985) found no main effects of parent gender in the ways they attempted to influence infant's behaviors, but they did find an interaction between parent gender, infant age, and infant sex, such that as infants aged (from 7, to 10, to 13 months), mothers spent more and more time directing the exploration of their girls, but less and less time directing the exploration of their boys. Further, as reported in the play types results, Teti et al., (1988) found that 18-month-olds (but not 12-month-olds) experienced more opportunities for language mastery and object play with mothers than with dads. Thus, it appears that there are few differences in the attempts or success of mothers' and fathers' efforts to scaffold and stimulate their infants' play and no evidence of differences during preschool. But during the transition from infancy to toddlerhood, mothers make more attempts to scaffold their children's play and are more successful, but these attempts may vary by toddlers' sex.

Responsiveness Of the 13 papers that examined parental responsiveness in some way, one did not report a direct father-mother comparison (Kerns & Barth, 1995), and six found no differences between mothers and fathers (Grossman et al., 2002; Kazura, 2000; Kwon, Bingham, Lewsader, Jeon, & Elicker, 2013; Lindsey & Mize, 2000; Lindsey et al., 1997a, 1997b). Five of the remaining six articles found that mothers were more responsive than fathers across a range of different types of measures, including verbal responsiveness, identifying and responding to infants' cues, and responding to versus ignoring children (Chiarello et al., 2006; Flippin & Watson, 2011; Lindsey, Cremeens, & Caldera, 2010; McGovern, 1990; Menashe-Grinberg & Atzaba-Poria, 2017). Further, Lamb and colleagues (1982) found no difference in fathers' and mothers picking up infants in response to infants' initiations, but they did find mothers were more likely to hold to soothe. Interestingly, Lindsey and colleagues (2010) found that fathers of girls were more likely to ignore their daughter's play initiations, compared to fathers with boys or mothers with either boys or girls; further, both parents were more likely to either comply with or reject their boys' initiations than girls', whereas they were more likely to ignore girls' initiations than boys'. Thus, overall, there is consistent evidence that fathers are less responsive to their children's cues and communications, and this evidence is more robust in infancy and toddlerhood than when children are preschool age.

Directiveness and Intrusiveness Nine of the 19 articles that examined directiveness were measuring aspects of parents' communication, such as assertive communication and the use of directives and commands, which will be described below; of these, four did not identify parent gender differences, but five found that fathers were more assertive and directive in their communication. Of the remaining ten articles, three did not directly compare mothers and fathers on these qualities (Keren et al., 2005; Kerns & Barth, 1995; Lindsey & Mize, 2000). Of the seven unique articles reporting comparisons of mothers' and fathers' intrusiveness, four reported no differences in fathers' and mothers' interaction behavior (Chiarello et al., 2006; El-Ghoroury & Romanczyk, 1999; Kwon et al., 2013; Menashe-Grinberg & Atzaba-Poria, 2017). However, Power (1985) found that fathers were more likely than mothers to offer their infants an object, when the infant was already playing with a different one, and to change the infant's behavior with the object they were playing with. Kazura (2000) found that fathers were more directive than mothers with their toddlers. And Bright and Stockdale (1984) found that fathers controlled and directed their preschool-aged children's play more than mothers did, particularly with their boys; children controlled and directed their fathers more than their mothers and engaged in more lead-taking behavior with fathers than mothers. Thus, there is ample evidence that fathers are more assertive and directive in communication, but there is more evidence of similarities than differences between fathers and mothers in intrusiveness. However, there is some evidence across ages in early childhood that fathers are more intrusive than mothers.

Summary and Discussion of Parent-Child Interaction Qualities The majority of findings across the 28 articles examining qualities of parent-child interaction identified no differences between mothers and fathers in most dimensions. However, where there were differences identified, these were consistent across studies; for example, while only 5 of 13 studies identified parent gender differences in responsiveness, all differences favored mothers. Thus, these sets of findings indicate that fathers are slightly less engaged in children's play than are mothers, mothers are more responsive than fathers, fathers are more directive of children's play than are mothers, and mothers provided somewhat more successful scaffolding of infants' play, but no differences were apparent in preschool. Importantly, some studies identified child characteristics, including age and sex, as well as contexts that exerted bigger influences on parents' interaction qualities than did parent gender. Further, children's age and sex, along with their play and communication behaviors, also influenced parents' interaction qualities; these influences were usually the same across mothers and fathers, but sometimes the effects differed.

Although this sample included several studies from other countries, it was dominated by studies conducted in the USA with mostly middle- to high-income samples. However, many of these US studies included samples of a mix of racial and ethnic backgrounds. Once again, where there was a mix of racial or ethnic backgrounds, or family income, the analyses rarely enabled differences to be detected.

Communication During and About Play Although 28 articles coded some aspect of parents' communication with children during and about play, 22 focused on the communication qualities, whereas others used communication behaviors or speech to measure other constructs (such as vocal games as a play type generated by parents or the verbal responsiveness as a way to assess responsiveness more generally). The majority of the studies were conducted throughout the USA (73%), and the remaining 27% were conducted internationally in France, India, Israel, Canada, Sweden, and South Africa. Families examined were largely intact and consisted mainly of preschool age children (50%). Fifty-nine percent of the studies included middle- to high- income, Caucasian samples; 27% of the samples did not report race or ethnicity; and 14% included Indian, Mexican, and Swedish samples.

Of the 22 studies focusing on communication, eight measured the rate or frequency of vocalizations or speech; these were mostly studies of parents' play with preverbal infants, often in the context of face-to-face vocal or verbal games. Fourteen studies, mostly with toddlers and preschoolers, coded the pragmatics of parents' speech, that is, the functions of speech or what is communicated during and about play. For example, some looked at how parents and children used communication to initiate or change the play and how they responded to each other's messages regarding play.

Vocalization/Speech Frequency Six of the eight articles described parents' vocalizations with preverbal or newly verbal children (e.g., under 2 years old), typically in the context of face-to-face exchanges that parents have with infants that are early bouts of parent-infant play. Among these articles, three found that mothers vocalized more frequently (Kwon et al., 2013; Laflamme et al., 2002; Lamb et al., 1982; Liddell, Henzi, & Drew, 1987), one study found no difference in the rate of vocalizations between fathers and mothers (Roopnarine et al., 1990), and one found that fathers and mothers spoke with the same frequency during play, but that fathers spoke more to infants during departure in the strange situation task (Weinraub & Frankel, 1977). Further, Weinraub & Frankel, (1977) also found that both fathers and mothers spoke more to infants of their same-sex than to opposite-sex infants. Interestingly, two studies observed children across ages and found that fathers increased their vocalizations as infants got older (e.g., from 9 to 15 months; Laflamme et al., 2002) and that there were no differences in their rates of speech when children were older than 2 years (Liddell et al., 1987). Kwon and colleagues (2013) found that while mothers vocalized more and used more diverse vocabularies overall, fathers used richer language (type/token ratio) than did mothers. Between 3 and 5 years old, Bright & Stockdale, (1984) found that mothers spent more time being quiet than did fathers, particularly with boys, but there were no differences in the number of comments made; and MacDonald and Parke (1984) found no differences between the verbal behaviors of mothers and fathers, but both parents talked more to girls than to boys. Thus, there is consistent evidence that mothers vocalize more during play than do fathers, particularly with younger infants. The evidence is less consistent of these parent gender differences after children begin speaking.

Purpose, Content, and Forms of Speech Fourteen articles examined aspects of communication beyond simple frequency to assess the purpose, content, or form of communication; this included several studies that coded all communication as either initiating play or responding to others' initiations and others that examined numerous different types of speech (e.g., declaratives including comments, praise, suggestions, interpretations; questions including closed and open-ended; attentionals; expressives), or parts of speech (e.g., nouns, pronouns, verbs). Overall, there were few parent gender differences identified; four articles found no parent gender differences at all (Caldera et al., 1989; Leaper & Gleason, 1996; Lindsey & Mize, 2000; Ryckebusch & Marcos, 2004), and two additional articles did not directly test parent gender differences in speech acts (Kerns & Barth, 1995; Lindsey et al., 1997a, 1997b). Fathers engaged in more shared conversation (Bright & Stockdale, (1984), while mothers made more statements (El-Ghoroury & Romanczyk, 1999). Mothers used more affiliative language than fathers, while fathers used more assertive language than mothers (Leaper, 2000). This use of assertive communication by fathers is also evidenced by a series of studies by Lindsey and colleagues. Fathers provided more play initiations overall (Lindsey et al., 1997a, 1997b; Lindsey et al., 2010) and specifically more play directives to children than did mothers; additionally, fathers used more imperatives (an initiation that offers no choice, e.g., "Put that down.") and polite commands (e.g., "Why don't you stack that here?"), whereas mothers gave more play leads (initiations that offer the other a choice, e.g., "Want to play cars?") than did fathers (Lindsey et al., 2010; Lindsey & Mize, 2001). Thus, fathers are more assertive in guiding children's play, and mothers and fathers have different styles of supporting children's play, with fathers being more commanding and mothers more suggesting.

Despite that mothers use more suggestions and fewer commands than do fathers, few studies found differences in the rates of questions overall. No studies found parent gender differences in the overall frequency or rate of parents' use of questions. However, O'Brien and Nagle (1987) found that fathers asked more Wh-questions than did mothers but were no different in yes/no questions. On the other hand, Tenenbaum and Leaper (1997) investigated parents' use of didactic questions (questions that teach) and found that mothers asked more conceptual didactic questions (e.g., causal or comparative questions, such as "What would happen if…" or "Which one does…?"), but there was no difference in perceptual didactic questions, which often include labeling and focus on what is perceivable in the present (e.g., "What is this animal called?").

Investigating parts of speech, O'Brien and Nagle (1987) also found that fathers used more pronouns and referred to objects more than did mothers; but otherwise parents were the same in utterance/min, mean length of utterance (MLU), noun-pronoun ratio, natives, repetitions, exact variations, nouns, verbs, modifiers, person references, and variety of nouns, verbs, and modifiers, which were influenced more by play context than parent gender.

Responses to Communication in Play Communication is not just about the messages one sends but about reciprocal responses. A series of studies found parent gender differences in parent and child responses to each other's communications during and about play. Children produced more directives with fathers than with mothers and particularly for the subtype of action requests (Ryckebusch & Marcos, 2004). However, mothers were more likely to comply with children's play directives than were fathers (Lindsey et al., 1997a, 1997b; Lindsey et al.,

2010), and children complied with more of fathers' play directives than they did with mothers' directives. To add further complexity, there were child sex differences in these response patterns as well. Lindsey and colleagues (2001) found that fathers gave more imperatives to boys and more polite commands and play leads to girls; whereas mothers gave more leads, polite commands, and imperatives to boys than to girls. But both parents complied with more of girls' play leads than boys' leads. Thus, fathers use more polite and relationship-enhancing communications with girls than with boys, including both how they initiate and respond, and use more assertive and instrumental communication with boys. Mothers are more likely than fathers to comply overall to the leads of boys or girls but used more relationship-enhancing leads with their boys than with girls. Thus, there appears to be a cross-gender effect for gentle communication that reinforces relationships.

Summary and Discussion of Communication in Play Before children begin speaking, fathers talk less to babies than do mothers. After children begin speaking, they start to influence parents' communication, drawing more language from fathers and reducing the parent gender difference in frequency of speech. Once the difference in frequency has diminished, slight differences in style begin to emerge – fathers are more assertive in communication than are mothers, with fathers providing more directives or instrumental speech and mothers providing more suggestions and using more affiliative language. However, there are sex differences in children's communication patterns which then exert influences on fathers' and mothers' communication, sometimes in different directions, such as the cross-gender use of more relationship-enhancing forms of communication. Of the small subset of studies focusing on vocal frequency, half were conducted in the USA with mostly Caucasian samples, and half were from other countries (Sweden, South Africa, and India). Among the larger set of studies examining the growing parent- and child-sex differences in communication, the majority of studies came from the USA and reflect Caucasian middle- to high-income samples. Thus, this set of studies likely does not reflect the variation in communication patterns that may emerge in more economically and racially diverse families, and thus it may underestimate the differences that are characteristic of the intersection of racial and gender socialization that is apparent in parent-child interactions with somewhat older children (e.g., Brown, Linver, & Evans, 2010; Howard, Rose, & Barbarin, 2013; Thomas & King, 2007).

How the Context of Play Influence Parenting Behaviors. Five articles addressed questions around how the context of play influenced various parenting behaviors and parent-child interactions and if these influences varied by parent gender. For instance, do parents engage in different responsive behaviors in play contexts versus caregiving contexts? Or, do parents interact in different ways in pretend play versus free play contexts? And, do these contextual influences differ for mothers and fathers? In effect, the play context in these studies served as the predictor variable for some important parent behavior or parent-child interaction while also exploring differences between mothers and fathers. These articles do not include articles that examined how play contexts, often some gender-typed toy choice, affect parent behavior in relation to gender socialization with children, as these articles were specifically addressed in the gender socialization question below. Four out of five of these studies were conducted in the USA, and included mixed samples, wherein European Americans or non-Hispanic white participants represented at least 82% of the samples, with predominately middle SES families. All of the studies were conducted with toddlers and/or preschoolers; none of the studies included infants in its sample.

The results of these studies indicate that, not surprisingly, context influences the ways that parents interact with their children. All five studies found similar main effects of context on parent behaviors, regardless of parent gender or child age. With toddlers, both moms and dads provided more cognitive scaffolding, less negativity, and more complex language during free play than during a structured task (Kwon et al., 2013) and more action requests during object building and more information requests during free play (Ryckebusch & Marcos 2004). With preschoolers, physical play yielded greater parent-child mutuality – an important predictor of children's social emotional competence (Lindsey & Mize, 2000) – along with more imperatives from both fathers and mothers (Lindsey & Mize, 2001), while pretend play elicited more requests for permission and play leads across the board (Lindsey & Mize, 2001). Both moms and dads were more likely to follow the child's lead during free play than during a caregiving task (Lindsey & Mize, 2001).

Although context influenced parents in similar ways, one study by Lindsey et al. (2010) found an important interaction between parent sex and context in that most of the differences between fathers and mothers were apparent during free play, while caregiving yielded similar types of behaviors across parent sex. During free play with their toddler, fathers were more assertive and instrumental, while mothers were more facilitative and cooperative. But a caretaking task of sharing a snack with their child elicited similar behaviors across parent sex; both fathers and mothers were more likely to give directives and imperatives during the caregiving context. Both fathers and mothers demonstrated a greater variety of behaviors during free play when compared to physical play (Lindsey & Mize, 2000). Ryckebusch and Marcos (2004) found a parent gender by context interaction, but only for older children in their study, as the influence of context became more important as children approached 22 months.

Summary and Discussion of Contextual Influences Context influences parenting behaviors in general, and in similar ways regardless of parent gender, but also the degree to which parents are differentiated in their behaviors. This has important implications when we consider the way mothers and fathers spend their time with their children. We know mothers and fathers vary in this regard; fathers spend more of their time in play and other enriching activities with their children, while mothers spend more of their time in other routine, instrumental caretaking activities with children. These various contexts allow for distinct interaction patterns with children, differentially influencing parent-child interactions. In these studies, free play in particular yielded a wider variety of behaviors and allowed for parent gender differences to emerge; activities such as free play set the stage for more horizontal egalitarian exchanges between parents and children, as opposed to caregiving tasks which tend to be more parent-centered, driven by an agenda. And even the type of play makes a difference in behaviors: object and structured play, which is often goal-directed, tended to promote more directive language and interactions from parents, who were more likely to follow the child's lead during pretend or free play. The situational demands of the task itself influences parenting behaviors, and some tasks may intensify the gender differentiated behaviors of mothers and fathers with children more than others. None of these studies investigated parents of infants; given that some parenting behaviors become more differentiated as children get older (e.g., Lindsey et al., 1997a, 1997b), the differential effects of context may become increasingly more pronounced over time as well.

These findings are relevant when considering the methodology used to understand differences and similarities between mothers and fathers – the way we design research studies may put artificial constraints on the ways that mothers and fathers interact with children, with some contexts allowing for more varied and individualized behaviors, while others generate a more homogenous set of behaviors. Of the 50 studies analyzed in this review, only five considered interaction of context with parent gender on our variables of interest. Context is a relevant variable when understanding behaviors, in general, but also important to consider when we are trying to understand differences between groups, in particular, and assessing parenting across multiple contexts may be necessary to understand a fuller scope of parents' play- or playful-parenting behaviors. Further, given the sample limitations, this limited set of studies cannot speak to the ways mothers' and fathers' play-relevant behaviors differ across contexts for infants, nor how these may differ for diverse families or those with lower incomes. Importantly, for families with fewer financial resources and less time to spend with their children in play-focused activities (Ishizuka, 2019), incorporating playfulness into other activities may be more important and predictive of children's development than the qualities of stand-alone play. This could be a valuable direction for future study.

How Child Characteristics Affect Father- and Mother-Child Play Overall, 32 articles posed questions about the effects of child characteristics, such as age, sex, and ability, on mothers' and fathers' play with their children. In addition, other articles included child characteristics of some kind in their analyses of fathers' and mothers' play, even if they had not posed these as initial research questions. The most common child characteristic examined was child sex (27 articles), and this includes a set of articles focused on questions of parents' socialization of child gender-related behavior via play. Thus, we first summarize the results of the articles focused on child sex differences and then address the other child characteristics that influence mothers' and fathers' play.

Child Sex Differences in Fathers' and Mothers' Play Of the 27 articles measuring child effects, 13 (48%) specifically evaluated child gender. The majority of those 13 articles were concentrated in North America, with 9 (69%) in the USA and 2 in Canada; the remaining two studies were located in Australia and Israel. Four (31%) of the articles did not clearly describe the race or ethnicity of their participants, including one with an Israeli sample. Otherwise, most studies included primarily (31%) or entirely (31%) Caucasian samples; one American study focused exclusively on participants of Mexican descent. Seven (54%) studies were comprised of middle or middle-to-high SES samples. Infants appeared in only two studies, while preschoolers and toddlers were sampled in eight (62%) and nine (69%) studies, respectively. It is important to note that while only 13 (26%) of the 50 articles reviewed here explicitly stated research questions related to gender socialization, nearly two-thirds of the articles in this scoping review assessed whether fathers and mothers play differently with their sons and daughters. In this section, we take into consideration all of the articles which tested these child sex differences in mothers' and fathers' play. Although the articles typically cited more similarities than differences (e.g., Lindsey et al., 2010; Roopnarine & Mounts, 1985; Stevenson, Leavitt, Thompson, & Roach, 1988), the findings of more than half (20) illustrate that sex-of-the-child plays some significant role in the observed play behaviors of fathers and mothers.

Roggman and Peery's (1989) study of nonverbal indicators of playfulness between parents and 4-month-old infants revealed interesting variations in behavior toward sons. The less interest their infant sons showed in play (as a function of babies' gaze toward parents), the more parents exhibited physical playfulness by touching them: fathers showed a longer duration of touch, and mothers a higher frequency of touch. The researchers found no significant father-daughter and mother-daughter associations for parent tactile behaviors. However, when parent gaze was examined, there were significant results for mother-daughter interactions that were not significant for other parent-child dyads: mothers gazed more at daughters who gazed more at them. From this, Roggman and Peery (1989) assert that parent-son pairs exhibit a complementary style of play (i.e., decreased engagement from son, increased engagement via physical touch from father and mother) while mother-daughter pairs use a more reciprocal style of play (i.e., increased engagement from daughter, increased engagement from mother via gaze). Further, the study notes that such dissimilar play behaviors point more broadly to the unique gender-typed social environments presented even to infants through the process of gender socialization. The gender socialization that Roggman and Peery (1989) saw in early infancy has been established as an important factor in parent-child play throughout early childhood; in fact, 16 other articles offer gender socialization theories as an explanation of their results.

Much of the differential treatment of parents toward their sons and daughters appears to be contextual. For example, Roopnarine's (1986) analyses of parents' responses to children's toy play found fathers tended to present dolls more frequently to their infant daughters than to infant sons and were more attentive to their toddler daughters than to toddler sons when their children were interacting with dolls. However, when engaged in block play, sons were more likely to receive their fathers' attention than were daughters; no significant effects were found for mothers in either context.

In their examination of parent-child play patterns, Idle, Wood, and Desmarais (1993) gave parents a survey where – absent their children – parents identified which conventionally gender-typed (i.e., masculine, feminine, neutral) toys would be most desirable for their sons and daughters. The survey showed that mothers and fathers broadly agreed that for their sons, the conventionally masculine toys were most desirable, and feminine toys the least; and for their daughters, that neutral toys were most desirable, and masculine toys the least. Still, when it came to their sons, fathers' responses regarding sons were more clearly gender-typed than were mothers'. Surprisingly, when they were observed in actual play with their children, these parents' patterns of play were much less gender-typed than their surveys might have predicted. Instead, the child's own toy preferences appeared to be more influential than child sex, with fathers spending equal amounts of time engaged with masculine and neutral toys, and mothers spending most of their time with neutral toys, followed by masculine, and the least amount of time with feminine toys. The contrast in the parents' more gender-traditional self-reports and their less traditional play behaviors may reflect both a cultural shift in gender norms and the psychological tension between parents' awareness of socially accepted gender behaviors and the realities of responsive play with a young child.

That said, child toy choice did not seem to erase all evidence of gender-typed play behaviors. Parents in this study were still observed steering sons away from some cross-gender-typed play (i.e., play with traditionally feminine toys); however, parents also seemed to avoid same-gender-typed, feminine toy play with their daughters (Idle et al., 1993). Once again, these results suggest that – even with evidence of a shift in gender norms – gender socializing environments may be uniquely constructed for males versus females: in Idle and colleagues' (1993) study, that meant sons may have encountered some resistance regarding cross-gendered play (indirectly reinforcing play with non-feminine toys), while girls may have experienced more flexibility; or seen another way, playing like a girl (i.e., with feminine toys) was seen as less desirable for both sexes.

Summary of effects of child sex differences. Results from the articles in this review, spanning several decades, suggest that, overall, fathers and mothers typically display similar play behaviors with their sons and daughters. However, where differential child-sex-based treatment is strongly implicated, play context remains an important factor, with gender socialization theories appearing to be a popular explanation appearing to offer the most cogent rationale. Given that this sample is dominated by studies conducted in North America with primarily Caucasian, middle-income samples, this body of literature does not address questions of the intersection between racial and gender socialization, which each begins within the early childhood period.

Effects of Other Child Characteristics on Fathers' and Mothers' Play Twelve articles included effects of child characteristics, other than gender, on parent behaviors during play. This included seven articles focused on child age, two on child ability (conceptualized as a motor delay or preterm birth), two on attachment and temperament, and one on child positive affect. The vast majority (92%) of these studies were conducted in the USA; one (8%) was conducted in Austria and Germany. Nearly half (46%) of these studies include racially homogenous, or nearly homogenous, white Caucasian samples. Two (15%) studies include a more diverse sampling of the population, with one (8%) comprised primarily of African Americans and Latinx Americans and another (8%) where one-third of its sample is Latinx American. Five (38%) of the articles were unclear about the race or ethnicity of their participants. Where SES was defined (62% of articles), most samples were of middle (54%) or middle-to-high (8%) SES, with one of primarily low SES (8%). Five (38%) of the studies are comprised of some mixture of infants, toddlers, and/or preschoolers; three (23%) include only infants; three (23%) include only toddlers; and two (15%) include only preschoolers.

Results from nine of the 12 studies revealed that parents' play behaviors are affected by children's age, ability, attachment, and affect. Findings showed that fathers and mothers with younger children demonstrated more physical and functional play, while those with older children engaged in more pretense and higher-quality play (Ahnert et al., 2017; Lindsey & Mize, 2000; Power, 1985; Roopnarine, 1986; Stevenson et al., 1988). Also, parents played significantly less, held children longer, and had lower quality of play with children having a disability or considered high risk, that is, preterm (Ahnert et al., 2017; Chiarello et al., 2006; Field, 1979). Children's attachment to parents influenced their parents' facilitation and responsiveness during play (Kazura, 2000). And toddlers' positive affect during play sessions with their parents influenced their parents' playfulness (Cabrera et al., 2017).

Differences between mothers' and fathers' play behaviors related to these child effects were found in six of the above nine articles. Results showed fathers spent more time directing younger children's exploration during play while mothers spent more time directing older girls (Power, 1985) and engaged in higher-quality play with preschoolers, compared to toddlers, than fathers (Ahnert et al., 2017). Further, fathers played games more often than mothers but only with full-term male infants (Field, 1979) and held their children with motor delays on their laps for longer play intervals than did mothers (Chiarello et al., 2006). Fathers with insecure attachment relationships with their children were more facilitating than fathers with other attachment relationships, while mothers with secure attachment relationships were more facilitative and responsive than those with insecure attachment relationships (Kazura, 2000). Finally, children's affect during play with parents influenced mothers' playfulness but not fathers' (Cabrera et al., 2017).

Summary and Discussion of Child Effects For those studies that examine the effects of child abilities on parents' play behaviors, the presence of lower-quality or less frequent play may at first seem like a negative response from parents. However, it may in fact be beneficial for children with motor or other delays to experience a slower pace during play. Similarly, fathers holding their children with motor delays for longer intervals on their lap during play may be a protective behavior, especially if the two are engaging in more active play, which is characteristic of fathers playing with their infants and toddlers. Thus, there is evidence that both mothers' and fathers' play behaviors are adaptive to their children's abilities. Overall, results from these studies suggest that fathers' behaviors during play with their children are sensitive to children's ages, abilities, and attachment relationships, but not to their affect, which is supported by the finding discussed earlier than mothers who tend to be more responsive to their children than fathers. Taken together, these findings indicate that fathers are more attuned to stable and slow-moving child characteristics and less sensitive to in-the-moment states of their children.

Aim 3: Identify Gaps and Limitations in the Literature on Differences in Father- and Mother-Child Play As described in almost every subsection of the results for our first question, the populations sampled by the studies in this review are dominated by intact, middle-income, Caucasian families in the USA. While a substantial portion of studies come from other countries, providing some diversity in the sample, those studies in the USA tend to conflate socioeconomic with ethnic and racial diversity; that is, it is primarily the studies that had racial diversity that also had socioeconomic diversity among their samples. In addition to the limited diversity in the samples of these 50 articles, it was also rare that these studies included demographic characteristics in their analyses, other than as control variables. These limitations to generalizability likely differ by the research question and aspects of play observed; thus, as we summarize the findings of each subset of articles in the later section, we describe the samples predominant in each subset and the limitations thereof.

Further, most of the studies utilized structured or semi-structured play tasks in a lab setting, and even those that observed in the home often used toys provided by the researchers in order to provide some standardization in the procedures and facilitate making comparisons. However, this seems to reflect a preconceived notion of how parents and children play together, or what constitutes meaningful play, for example, that "play" is a specific set-aside time, separate from other aspects of child care and family life, and is child-centric in its use of toys. This child-centric concept of play as its own unique parenting task is consistent with the new American norm of "intensive parenting," which is really only accessible to families with the resources of time and money to invest themselves in child-centric play interactions (Ishizuka, 2019). It is possible, then, that these studies have entirely missed major aspects of what play means in families' everyday lives, for example, playful interactions during meals, playful ways of conducting housekeeping tasks together, etc., as well as many other types of spontaneous and natural play that may occur throughout the day. It is also likely that there are demographic differences in whether this child- and toy-centric view of play authentically reflects the ways that parents operate with their children (Ishizuka, 2019).

Finally, although there were quite a number of studies that examined the types of play generated by parents and others that examined their engagement in their children's play, there was surprisingly little research that measured parents' playfulness. If this line of research is to expand to attend to the myriad ways that play may be an aspect of families' everyday interactions with one another, rather than a separate time or task of parenting, measuring the playfulness of father-child and mother-child interactions will be a necessary tool in that endeavor.

Question 2: How Does Father-Child Play in Early Childhood Distinctly Affect Child Development?

Among the 50 articles identified for this study, a subset of articles addressed the second question of this scoping review by analyzing the effects of father- and mother-child play on children's concurrent behavior or subsequent developmental outcomes. In addition to the 13 articles whose research questions were coded for child outcomes, we include four articles that reported child outcomes within their results, even though they had not included child outcomes in their research questions. Other articles did report on effects of parental play on child outcomes but did not directly contrast or control for effects of mothers and fathers.

Aim 1: Describe the Range of Studies Testing the Unique Effects of Father-Child Play on Children's Development Of the 17 articles associating child outcomes with aspects of parents' play, six (35%) focused on types of play parents generated or engaged in, two (12%) parents' enjoyment in play, two (12%) parents' communication during and about play, and ten (59%) parent-child interaction qualities during play. Most (82%) of these studies were conducted in the USA, with two (12%) conducted in Israel and one (6%) in Germany. Although more than one-third of the studies do not identify the racial or ethnic makeup of their respective samples, one study conducted in Israel characterized its sample as predominantly Israeli-born; another American study noted that its sample was of Italian descent. In five (29%) studies, Caucasian participants made up at least 80% of the sample. Two studies (12%) involve a more diverse ethnic sample, including one identifying participants of white, Hispanic, and Asian heritage and the second involving mostly African Americans, followed by Latinx Americans, and others of minoritized heritage. Of the ten studies describing SES, samples were typically categorized as at least middle SES. Fifty-three percent of the 17 studies included only preschoolers, 29% were only toddlers, and another 18% were mixed groups of preschoolers, toddlers, and/or infants.

Aim 2: Summary of Results Comparing the Effects of Father-Child and Mother-Child Play on Child Development The results below are organized by aspects of parent-child play that were measured in the studies, examining the effects of these across the child outcomes these may influence.

Types of Play Parents Generated or Engaged In The type of play fathers engage in with their children appears to have some effect on their children's development. Of the six articles analyzed, it was physical and symbolic/pretense play that were of particular interest in relation to their children's emotional and social development.

Physical Play In general, fathers' involvement of physical and pretense play was positively correlated with their children's involvement in these types of play, respectively (Lindsey et al., 1997b). Fathers' physical play was positively associated with their children's positive affective expression (MacDonald & Parke, 1984) and negatively associated with their children's use of directives during play. Further, it appears that fathers' physical play is particularly important for their sons' social and emotional development. Fathers' mutuality with their sons during physical play was positively associated with sons' emotional knowledge (i.e., emotion recognition and understanding; Lindsey & Mize, 2000). When engaging in physical play, father-son dyads who showed a more balanced level of compliance in interactions (i.e., father or son follows the others' initiation) were associated with sons' being well-liked by peers, as rated by their teachers (Lindsey & Mize, 2000; MacDonald & Parke, 1984). Sons were also seen to be more competent, helpful, and involved by their teachers (Lindsey & Mize, 2000) as well as possessing leadership characteristics, better at communicating, and more willing to share (MacDonald & Parke, 1984). Such findings were not found between mothers' physical play and sons' social development (MacDonald & Parke, 1984). Additionally, fathers', but not mothers', physical play was associated with their daughters being better liked by peers, though also more likely to be more dominant and engage in more abrasive peer relationships (MacDonald & Parke, 1984). Daughters were also better at communicating; able to express positive emotions, as rated by their teachers; and more creative when their fathers engaged in more physical play with them (MacDonald & Parke, 1984). These findings suggest that fathers' physical play may influence their sons' and daughters' emotional expression and social-emotional development in unique ways, different from that of mothers, with particular import for boys.

Symbolic and Pretense Play Fathers' level of pretense or symbolic play is associated with their children's play behaviors as well as emotional and social development. Fathers' facilitation and creativity during pretend play predict children's level of complexity in pretend play (Keren et al., 2005), which is also true for mother-child pairs (Keren et al., 2005; Lindsey et al., 1997b). During pretend play, fathers elicited more speech, especially informative speech, from their children than did mothers; during construction play, however, fathers elicited more confirming speech from their children than mothers did during either pretend or construction play (Leaper & Gleason, 1996). With fathers of children with Down syndrome, de Falco and colleagues (2010) observed that although fathers engaged in less symbolic and more exploratory play with their children than mothers, children engaged in more symbolic play when playing with their fathers than with their mothers or alone. Although this relationship is examined within a specific sample, it illustrates that fathers' presence during children's play may have unique effects on children's pretense play behaviors.

Similar to the findings with physical play, father-child pretense play was associated with children's social competence, as rated by teachers, for both sons and daughters; with mothers, this association only held for mother-daughter pairs (Lindsey & Mize, 2000). Furthermore, Lindsey and Mize (2000) found that specifically for father-son pairs who engaged in more joint pretense play and those who had more balanced interactions during pretense play, sons had higher emotional knowledge; for mother-son pairs, only their balanced interactions were associated with their sons' emotional knowledge. This suggests that fathers' mutuality and connection with their sons in either pretense or symbolic play has unique effects on sons' emotional development, different from the effects of mothers' play with sons.

Enjoyment and Playfulness Fathers' enjoyment and playfulness in play affect their children's emotional development. While fathers and mothers demonstrate similar levels of playfulness and positive affect, two of the studies suggest that their influence on children's outcomes differs by parent sex. Cabrera et al. (2017) showed that fathers' and mothers' level of playfulness is similar; however, fathers' playfulness predicted children's later receptive language skills, while mothers' playfulness was related to children's later emotional regulation skills. And the findings of Menashe-Grinberg and Atzaba-Poria (2017) offer a view of fathers' playfulness as being uniquely important to children – child outcomes were positive only when fathers were both supportive in their parenting and playful in their interactions, what the authors described as a "double buffer" effect. This effect was not evident for mothers, whose supportive behaviors predicted positive child outcomes, even if they had low levels of playfulness. Although fathers' playfulness during play with their children does impact their children's emotional development in unique ways, it may not be the only characteristic of fathers' play needed to affect their children's behavior and development in the long term.

Communication During and About Play Fathers' communication during play affects children's language development. Fathers elicit more speech from children than mothers do during play (El-Ghoroury & Romanczyk, 1999; Leaper & Gleason, 1996), including eliciting more vocal or verbal initiations from their children with autism (El-Ghoroury & Romanczyk, 1999). In family-centered practices, parent-child play is often used as a context in which to implement early interventions for children with delays or disabilities; the effects of father-child play on children's development may be particularly important in this context.

Parent-Child Interaction Qualities During Play In addition to modest differences in fathers' and mothers' qualities of interaction during play, fathers' and mothers' play interaction qualities have somewhat different effects on their children's behavior and development. These include differential effects of engagement in play and responsiveness to children's play behaviors.

Engagement Fathers' engagement in play is associated with children's play behaviors and engagement in play. For example, children respond more positively to their fathers' than their mothers' play initiations (Kerns & Barth, 1995) but showed lower affiliation (i.e., the extent to which the two individuals played with one another; Leaper, 2000) and were less cooperative in play with their fathers than with mothers (Roopnarine & Mounts, 1985). This affiliation score was moderated by fathers' ethnicity, such that Latino father-child dyads had higher affiliation ratings than others (Leaper, 2000). To add, the more fathers engaged in play with daughters, the more distressed daughters were during separation; conversely, when mothers engaged more with daughters, their daughters showed less distress during separation (Weinraub & Frankel, 1977). On the other hand, the more fathers engaged in physical contact with their sons during play, the more distressed sons were during separation; the same was not true for mothers (Weinraub & Frankel, 1977). Thus, how fathers interact with their daughters and sons during play affects children's attachment-related behaviors.

Further, high levels of father-child mutuality during physical play supported sons', but not daughters', social competence as rated by their teachers (Lindsey & Mize, 2000). Furthermore, fathers' engagement in play with their sons also predicted sons' popularity, leadership skills, helpfulness, involvement, and communication while being negatively correlated with their sons' apprehension, inability to get along with others, and unwillingness to share (MacDonald & Parke, 1984). Similarly, father-daughter play engagement and play quality predicted teachers' ratings of daughters' friendly-cooperative behaviors; specifically, when fathers provided more suggestions and fewer negative responses, daughters had higher social skills (Kerns & Barth, 1995). However, qualities of mother-child play (i.e., number of play initiations, responses to play initiations, and play initiation that were directive, suggestion, or physical) are related to their children's popularity; specifically, mothers' who used fewer physical play initiations often had children who were more popular, and those who used more suggestions and positive responses during play had children with more friendly-cooperative behaviors (Kerns & Barth, 1995). Thus, while it was similar play engagement behaviors from fathers and mothers that predicted sons' and daughters' social skills, they predicted somewhat different skills in their male and female children.

Responsiveness and Sensitivity Fathers' responsive play behaviors elicited more symbolic play from their children, and their *verbal* responsiveness (as compared to responsive play behaviors) elicited more functional and symbolic play, whereas for mothers, it was only verbal responsiveness (not responsive play behaviors) that elicited these play behaviors from children (Flippin & Watson, 2011). With fathers of children with motor development delays, fathers' responsiveness elicited similar levels of motor behaviors and playfulness from their children as mothers did (Chiarello et al., 2006), and both parents' responsiveness during play were only moderately correlated with children's contributions to play (Chiarello et al., 2006). In a sample of middle-class Israeli parents, both fathers' and mothers' sensitivity, structuring, and nonintrusiveness were negatively correlated with children's negativity (i.e., negative affect, noncompliance, and non-on-task behaviors; Menashe-Grinberg & Atzaba-Poria, 2017). Furthermore, Grossmann and colleagues (2002) found that fathers' play sensitivity in toddlerhood was correlated with children's attachment security at 10 and 16 years of age, whereas mothers' play sensitivity was not correlated to children's later secure attachment (Grossmann et al., 2002). Thus, though fathers had somewhat lower levels of responsiveness compared to mothers, fathers' responsiveness affected their children in similar ways to mothers, with additional long-term effects on attachment, and unique effects of fathers' responsive play behaviors (as opposed to verbal responsiveness) on aspects of children's play that affect their development.

Overall, fathers' levels of engagement and responsiveness in play affect the level of engagement of their children in play, as well as a number of social and emotional outcomes, with some evidence of effects on children's communication skills. Despite some differences in parents' overall levels of these play interaction qualities, fathers and mothers have largely similar effects on children's behaviors and outcomes. However, fathers' engagement and responsiveness have unique effects on their children's engagement in play; their social and emotional skills, particularly for sons; and their attachment both concurrently and later in childhood.

Summary and Discussion of Fathers' Effects on Children's Behavior and Development The context of play is an important context in which fathers support their children's development. The types of play fathers engage in as well as their enjoyment and playfulness, communication, and interaction qualities (i.e., engagement, responsiveness, directiveness) all affect their children's play behaviors as well as emotional, social, and language development. There is some consistent evidence for unique effects of fathers' play behaviors on children's social and emotional development, though less so in other domains; it would be productive for the field to develop this area of research further.

Aim 3: Identify Gaps and Limitations in the Literature on Unique Effects of Father-Child Play on Children's Development We identified only 17 of the total 50 articles that observed both father- and mother-child play and analyzed their unique relationships to children's development. Most of these studies examined the effects of the qualities of play interactions, rather than types of play, playfulness, or communication during play; and like most of this literature, the most common methodology was observation of structured or semi-structured play constructed by the researchers. Thus, the effects we may really be measuring here are that of fathers' and mothers' abilities to adapt their play behaviors to the constructed setting.

The most common child outcomes assessed were concurrent play behaviors and children's later social and emotional development; given the unique effects of father-child play in these domains, it would be valuable to further examine unique effects of father-child play on children's communication, cognitive, and physical play behaviors and development.

Summary and Key Findings

Overall, fathers and mothers are more alike than different in their play with young children, but their differences reflect fathers' unique roles and are important to children's development. Fathers and mothers are similar in their engagement in and enjoyment of play with children and, by and large, in the types of play they generate and engage in. There are more similarities than differences in the qualities of play, with no differences in engagement and scaffolding, and only moderate differences showing mothers to be higher in responsiveness, and fathers are higher in intrusiveness and more directive. The key differences in fathers' play are in the types of play that fathers generate, engaging in more arousing physical play and less symbolic play than mothers, and in the ways they interact during play, which is more directive and assertive than mothers. This distinct style of father-child play creates unique opportunities for children to develop language and social and emotional skills, especially for their sons. Additional key findings are summarized below.

- Fathers are *not* inherently more playful than mothers, nor do they enjoy play more than mothers. Perceived differences in this regard may be attributed to the way that parents spend time with their children – fathers spend a greater proportion of their time with children in play activities, while mothers are still doing more of the routine caregiving labor of parenting – and may thus experience more stress or limited pleasure from these tasks. But, for both parents, play is an enjoyable opportunity to connect with their children in a creative way.
- Dads are more demanding playmates (they initiate more and are more assertive), while moms are more responsive. Moms' greater responsiveness and more suggestive style of facilitating play do not demand that children respond, either vocally or behaviorally. Thus, dads elicit more symbolic behavior and speech from children, creating unique opportunities to support children's language development.
- Father-child and mother-child play become more differentiated over time – likely because both parents are responsive to developmental

changes in their children, but in different ways.

- Even if there are no mean level differences between fathers and mothers for a particular play behavior, there still may be differential influences on child development, in part at least because children respond differently to the same behaviors from their fathers and mothers.
- Certain contexts, by their very nature, elicit more similar patterns of play behaviors between fathers and mothers, whereas other contexts, such as free play, allow for a wider repertoire of behaviors, revealing more differences between fathers and mothers.
- Mothers and fathers are also more similar than different in how they treat their sons and daughters, and both contribute to similar processes of gender socialization. However, articles overtly interested in effects of child gender on parent-child play typically highlighted the experiences of a small slice of the possible population, often focusing on Caucasian, middle-SES samples with toddlers and preschoolers located in North America. This suggests a gap in the intentional study of the influence of child gender effects in low- and high-SES samples including fathers of color, fathers outside North America, and infants in general.
- What we currently know about father-child play is limited by how we measure it. We know that the context of the play is a significant influence on play behaviors, yet very few articles examine spontaneous or naturally occurring play in everyday contexts. Thus, we may be privileging here the types of play interactions engaged in by families, who can afford the time to interact with their children in child-focused activities, and misestimating the ways that play and playfulness may arise in other types of family interactions, such as family chores, meals, transportation, etc.
- Most parent-child interactions, including play, are measured as a dyad between parent and child. Yet, there is evidence that once both parents are present in the mother-father-child triad, the complex set of relationships influences parents' and children's play behaviors, with the triad becoming an entity in its own right. Families interact throughout their day in many different configurations, yet we almost exclusively measure important parenting behaviors in dyads.
- Fathers' demographic characteristics influence father-child play, including ethnicity and socioeconomic status, in ways that may reflect cultural differences in fathers' roles, father-child relationships, and perhaps socialization goals. However, most studies in our review were focused on white or Euro or Euro-American samples, and those with more variation often only controlled for, rather than examining, effects of demographic characteristics. This calls into question the generalizability of the collection of findings in this review and calls for more research on father-child interactions in diverse samples.
- We need more studies that can elucidate out children's own contributions, beyond child sex, to parent-child play interactions, including child temperament, abilities, and developmental skills; this would also help to reveal how child sex predicts other important child behaviors and skills (e.g., communication during play, physical behaviors, and toy choices and play themes) that in turn elicit different behaviors from parents.

Author Acknowledgments The authors wish to thank Carin Graves, Social Sciences Librarian at Michigan State University, for her guidance in using a scoping review, providing us with tools to conduct our review, and guiding the development of our protocol. This chapter will make a greater contribution to the field because of her expert assistance.

Appendix

Table 22.1 describes the inclusion and exclusion criteria by which inclusion in this chapter was determined, as well as the rationale.

Table 22.2 describes characteristics of the studies in each of the articles reviewed in this chapter.

References

Ahnert, L., Teufl, L., Ruiz, N., Piskernik, B., Supper, B., Remiorz, S., et al. (2017). Father-child play during the preschool years and child internalizing behaviors: Between robustness and vulnerability. *Infant Mental Health Journal, 38*, 743–756. https://doi.org/10.1002/imhj.21679

Arco, C. M. (1983). Pacing of playful stimulation to young infants: Similarities and differences in maternal and paternal communication. *Infant Behavior & Development, 6*, 223–228. http://dx.doi.org.proxy1.cl.msu.edu/10.1016/S0163-6383(83)80029-0

Arksey, H., & O'Malley, L. (2005). Scoping studies: Towards a methodological framework. *International Journal of Social Research Methodology, 8*, 19–32. https://doi.org/10.1080/1364557032000119616

Atzaba-Poria, N., Cabrera, N.J., Menashe, A., & Karberg, E. (2014). The parent-child playfulness system. Unpublished manuscript, Ben-Gurion University of the Negev, Beer Sheva, Israel.

Barnett, M. A., Gustafsson, H., Deng, M., Mills-Koonce, W. R., & Cox, M. (2012). Bidirectional associations among sensitive parenting, language development, and social competence. *Infant and Child Development, 21*, 374–393. https://doi.org/10.1002/icd.1750

Bianchi, S. M., Robinson, J. P., & Milke, M. A. (2006). *The changing rhythms of American family life*. New York: Russell Sage Foundation.

Bradley, B. S., & Gobbart, S. K. (1989). Determinants of gender-typed play in toddlers. *The Journal of Genetic Psychology: Research and Theory on Human Development, 150*, 453–455. http://dx.doi.org.proxy1.cl.msu.edu/10.1080/00221325.1989.9914612

Bright, M. C., & Stockdale, D. F. (1984). Mothers', fathers', and preschool children's interactive behaviors in a play setting. *The Journal of Genetic Psychology: Research and Theory on Human Development, 144*, 219–232. http://dx.doi.org.proxy1.cl.msu.edu/10.1080/00221325.1984.9923428

Brown, T. L., Linver, M. R., & Evans, M. (2010). The role of gender in the racial and ethnic socialization of African American adolescents. *Youth & Society, 41*(3), 357–381. https://doi.org/10.1177/0044118X09333665

Cabrera, N., Fitzgerald, H., Bradley, R., & Roggman, L. (2014). The ecology of father-child relationships: An expanded model. *Journal of Family Theory & Review, 6*, 336–354. https://doi.org/10.1111/jftr.12054

Cabrera, N., & Roggman, L. (2017). Father play: Is it special? *Infant Mental Health Journal, 38*, 706–708. https://doi.org/10.1002/imhj.21680

Cabrera, N. J., Karberg, E., Malin, J. L., & Aldoney, D. (2017). The magic of play: Low-income mothers' and fathers' playfulness and children's emotion regulation and vocabulary skills. *Infant Mental Health Journal, 38*, 757–771. https://doi.org/10.1002/imhj.21682

Caldera, Y. M., Huston, A. C., & O'Brien, M. (1989). Social interactions and play patterns of parents and toddlers with feminine, masculine, and neutral toys. *Child Development, 60*, 70–76. http://dx.doi.org.proxy1.cl.msu.edu/10.2307/1131072

Caldera, Y. M., & Sciaraffa, M. A. (1998). Parent–toddler play with feminine toys: Are all dolls the same? *Sex Roles: A Journal of Research, 39*, 657–668. http://dx.doi.org.proxy1.cl.msu.edu/10.1023/A:1018851932580

Carson, J., Burks, V., & Parke, R. D. (1993). Parent–child physical play: Determinants and consequences. In K. MacDonald (Ed.), *Children's play in society* (pp. 197–220). Albany, NY: State University of New York Press.

Chiarello, L. A., Huntington, A., & Bundy, A. (2006). A comparison of motor behaviors, interaction, and playfulness during mother-child and father-child play with children with motor delay. *Physical & Occupational Therapy in Pediatrics, 26*(1–2), 129–151.

Craig, L. (2006). Does father care mean fathers share? A comparison of how mothers and fathers in intact families spend time with children. *Gender & Society, 20*, 259–281. https://doi.org/10.1177/0891243205285212

Crawley, S. B., & Sherrod, K. B. (1984). Parent–infant play during the first year of life. *Infant Behavior & Development, 7*(1), 65–75. http://dx.doi.org.proxy1.cl.msu.edu/10.1016/S0163-6383(84)80023-5

de Falco, S., Esposito, G., Venuti, P., & Bornstein, M. H. (2010). Mothers and fathers at play with their children with down syndrome: Influence on child exploratory and symbolic activity. *Journal of Applied Research in Intellectual Disabilities, 23*, 597–605.

Dickson, K. L., Walker, H., & Fogel, A. (1997). The relationship between smile type and play type during parent-infant play. *Developmental Psychology, 33*, 925–933. http://dx.doi.org.proxy1.cl.msu.edu/10.1037/0012-1649.33.6.925

El-Ghoroury, N. H., & Romanczyk, R. G. (1999). Play interactions of family members towards children with autism. *Journal of Autism and Developmental Disorders, 29*, 249–258. https://doi.org/10.1023/A:1023036223397

Field, T. (1979). Games parents play with normal and high-risk infants. *Child Psychiatry & Human Development, 10*, 41–48. https://doi.org/10.1007/BF01433636

Flanders, J. L., Leo, V., Paquette, D., Pihl, R. O., & Seguin, J. R. (2009). Rough-and-tumble play and the regulation of aggression: An observational study of father-child play dyads. *Aggressive Behavior, 35*, 285–295. https://doi.org/10.1002/ab.20309

Flippin, M., & Watson, L. R. (2011). Relationships between the responsiveness of fathers and mothers and the object play skills of children with autism spectrum disorders. *Journal of Early Intervention, 33*, 220–234. http://dx.doi.org.proxy1.cl.msu.edu/10.1177/1053815111427445

Gleason, J. B. (1987). Sex differences in parent-child interaction. In S. U. Philips, S. Steele, & C. Tanz (Eds.), *Studies in the social and cultural foundations of language. Language, gender, and sex in comparative perspective* (pp. 189–199). New York: Cambridge University Press.

Grossmann, K., Grossmann, K. E., Fremmer-Bombik, E., Kindler, H., Scheuerer-Englisch, H., & Zimmermann, P. (2002). The uniqueness of the child-father attachment relationship: Fathers' sensitive and challenging play as a pivotal variable in a 16-year longitudinal study. *Social Development, 11*(3), 307–331.

Haight, W. L., Parke, R. D., & Black, J. E. (1997). Mothers' and fathers' beliefs about and spontaneous participation in their toddlers' pretend play. *Merrill-Palmer Quarterly, 43*(2), 271–290.

Howard, L. C., Rose, J. C., & Barbarin, O. A. (2013). Raising African American boys: An exploration of gender and racial socialization practices. *American Journal of Orthopsychiatry, 83*(2–3), 218–230. https://doi.org/10.1111/ajop.12031

Huttenlocher, J., Haight, W., Bryk, A., Seltzer, M., & Lycns, T. (1991). Early vocabulary growth: Relation to language input and gender. *Developmental Psychology, 27*, 236–248.

Idle, T., Wood, E., & Desmarais, S. (1993). Gender role socialization in toy play situations: Mothers and fathers with their sons and daughters. *Sex Roles: A Journal of Research, 28*, 679–691. http://dx.doi.org.proxy1.cl.msu.edu/10.1007/BF00289987

Ishizuka, P. (2019). Social class, gender, and contemporary parenting standards in the United States: Evidence from a national survey experiment. *Social Forces, 98*(1), 31–58. https://doi.org/10.1093/sf/soy107

Karrass, J., Braungart-Rieker, J. M., Mullins, J., & Lefever, J. B. (2002). Processes in language acquisition: The roles of gender, attention, and maternal encouragement of attention over time. *Journal of Child Language, 29*, 519–543. https://doi.org/10.1017/S0305000902005196

Kazura, K. (2000). Fathers' qualitative and quantitative involvement: An investigation of attachment, play, and social interactions. *The Journal of Men's Studies, 9*, 41–57. http://dx.doi.org.proxy1.cl.msu.edu/10.3149/jms.0901.41

Keren, M., Feldman, R., Namdari-Weinbaum, I., Spitzer, S., & Tyano, S. (2005). Relations between parents' interactive style in dyadic and triadic play and toddlers' symbolic capacity. *American Journal of Orthopsychiatry, 75*, 599–607.

Kerns, K., & Barth, J. (1995). Attachment and play – convergence across components of parent-child relationships and their relations to peer competence. *Journal of Social and Personal Relationships, 12*, 243–260. https://doi.org/10.1177/0265407595122006

Kwon, K.-A., Bingham, G., Lewsader, J., Jeon, H.-J., & Elicker, J. (2013). Structured task versus free play: The influence of social context on parenting quality, toddlers' engagement with parents and play behaviors, and parent–toddler language use. *Child & Youth Care Forum, 42*, 207–224. http://dx.doi.org.proxy1.cl.msu.edu/10.1007/s10566-013-9198-x

Labrell, F. (1996). Paternal play with toddlers: Recreation and creation. *European Journal of Psychology of Education, 11*, 43–54. https://doi.org/10.1007/BF03172935

Laflamme, D., Pomerleau, A., & Malcuit, G. (2002). A comparison of fathers' and mothers' involvement in childcare and stimulation behaviors during free-play with their infants at 9 and 15 months. *Sex Roles: A Journal of Research, 47*, 507–518. http://dx.doi.org.proxy1.cl.msu.edu/10.1023/A:1022069720776

Lamb, M., Frodi, A., Hwang, C., Frodi, M., & Steinberg, J. (1982). Mother-infant and father-infant interaction involving play and holding. *Developmental Psychology, 18*, 215–221. https://doi.org/10.1037//0012-1649.18.2.215

Lamb, M. E. (1977). The development of mother-infant and father-infant attachments in second year of life. *Developmental Psychology, 13*, 637–648.

Leaper, C. (2000). Gender, affiliation, assertion, and the interactive context of parent–child play. *Developmental Psychology, 36*, 381–393. http://dx.doi.org.proxy1.cl.msu.edu/10.1037/0012-1649.36.3.381

Leaper, C., & Gleason, J. B. (1996). The relationship of play activity and gender to parent and child sex-typed communication. *International Journal of Behavioral Development, 19*(4), 689–703.

Liddell, C., Henzi, S., & Drew, M. (1987). Mothers, fathers, and children in an urban park playground – a comparison of dyads and triads. *Developmental Psychology, 23*, 262–266. https://doi.org/10.1037/0012-1649.23.2.262

Lindsey, E. W., Cremeens, P. R., & Caldera, Y. M. (2010). Gender differences in mother-toddler and father-toddler verbal initiations and responses during a caregiving and play context. *Sex Roles: A Journal of Research, 63*, 399–411. http://dx.doi.org.proxy1.cl.msu.edu/10.1007/s11199-010-9803-5

Lindsey, E. W., & Mize, J. (2000). Parent-child physical and pretense play: Links to children's social competence. *Merrill-Palmer Quarterly-Journal of Developmental Psychology, 46*, 565–591. https://doi.org/10.1037/t58344-000

Lindsey, E. W., & Mize, J. (2001). Contextual differences in parent-child play: Implications for children's gender role development. *Sex Roles: A Journal of Research, 44*, 155–176. http://dx.doi.org.proxy1.cl.msu.edu/10.1023/A:1010950919451

Lindsey, E. W., Mize, J., & Pettit, G. S. (1997a). Differential play patterns of mothers and fathers of sons and daughters: Implications for children's gender role development. *Sex Roles, 37*, 643–661. https://doi.org/10.1007/BF02936333

Lindsey, E. W., Mize, J., & Pettit, G. S. (1997b). Mutuality in parent-child play: Consequences for children's peer competence. *Journal of Social and Personal Relationships, 14*(4), 523–538. http://dx.doi.org.proxy1.cl.msu.edu/10.1177/0265407597144007

Lyytinen, P., Laakso, M.-L., Poikkeus, A.-M., & Rita, N. (1999). The development and predictive relations of play and language across the second year. *Scandinavian Journal of Psychology, 40*, 177–186. https://doi.org/10.1111/1467-9450.00115

MacDonald, K., & Parke, R. D. (1984). Bridging the gap: Parent-child play interaction and peer interactive competence. *Child Development, 55*, 1265–1277. https://doi.org/10.2307/1129996

Mahoney, G. (1992). *Maternal behavior rating scale (revised)*. Tallmadge, OH: Family Child Learning Center.

McBride-Chang, C., & Jacklin, C. N. (1993). Early play arousal, sex-typed play, and activity level as precursors to later rough-and-tumble play. *Early Education and Development, 4*, 99–108. http://dx.doi.org.proxy1.cl.msu.edu/10.1207/s15566935eed0402_2

McGovern, M. A. (1990). Sensitivity and reciprocity in the play of adolescent mothers and young fathers with their infants. *Family Relations, 39*, 427–431. https://doi.org/10.2307/585223

Menashe-Grinberg, A., & Atzaba-Poria, N. (2017). Mother–child and father–child play interaction: The importance of parental playfulness as a moderator of the links between parental behavior and child negativity. *Infant Mental Health Journal, 38*, 772–784. http://dx.doi.org.proxy1.cl.msu.edu/10.1002/imhj.21678

Mezulis, A. H., Hyde, J. S., & Clark, R. (2004). Father involvement moderates the effect of maternal depression during a child's infancy on child behavior problems in kindergarten. *Journal of Family Psychology, 18*(4), 575.

Nelson-Coffey, S. K., Killingsworth, M., Layous, K., Cole, S. W., & Lyubomirsky, S. (2019). Parenthood is associated with greater well-being for fathers than mothers. *Personality and Social Psychology Bulletin, 45*(9), 1378–1390. https://doi.org/10.1177/0146167219829174

O'Brien, M., & Nagle, K. J. (1987). Parents' speech to toddlers: The effect of play context. *Journal of Child Language, 14*, 269–279. http://dx.doi.org.proxy1.cl.msu.edu/10.1017/S0305000900012927

Paquette, D. (2004). Theorizing the father-child relationship: Mechanisms and developmental outcomes. *Human Development, 47*, 193–219. https://doi.org/10.1159/000078723

Pellegrini, A. D. (2009). *The role of play in human development*. New York: Oxford University Press.

Power, T. G. (1985). Mother- and father-infant play: A developmental analysis. *Child Development, 56*, 1514–1524. https://doi.org/10.2307/1130470

Roggman, L. A., & Peery, J. C. (1988). Caregiving, emotional involvement, and parent-infant play. *Early Child Development and Care, 34*, 191–199. https://doi.org/10.1080/0300443880340114

Roggman, L. A., & Peery, J. C. (1989). Parent-infant social play in brief encounters: Early gender differences. *Child Study Journal, 19*, 65–79.

Roopnarine, J. L. (1986). Mothers' and fathers' behaviors toward the toy play of their infant sons and daughters. *Sex Roles: A Journal of Research, 14*, 59–68. http://dx.doi.org.proxy1.cl.msu.edu/10.1007/BF00287848

Roopnarine, J. L., Ahmeduzzaman, M., Hossain, Z., & Riegraf, N. B. (1992). Parent–infant rough play: Its cultural specificity. *Early Education and Development, 3*, 298–311. http://dx.doi.org.proxy1.cl.msu.edu/10.1207/s15566935eed0304_3

Roopnarine, J. L., & Mounts, N. S. (1985). Mother-child and father-child play. *Early Child Development and Care, 20*, 157–169. https://doi.org/10.1080/0300443850200205

Roopnarine, J. L., Talukder, E., Jain, D., Joshi, P., & Srivastav, P. (1990). Characteristics of holding, patterns of play, and social behaviors between parents and infants in New Delhi, India. *Developmental Psychology, 26*, 667–673. http://dx.doi.org.proxy1.cl.msu.edu/10.1037/0012-1649.26.4.667

Ryckebusch, C., & Marcos, H. (2004). Speech acts, social context and parent-toddler play between the ages of 1;5 and 2;3. *Journal of Pragmatics, 36*, 883–897. https://doi.org/10.1016/j.pragma.2003.10.019

Stevenson, M. B., Leavitt, L. A., Thompson, R. H., & Roach, M. A. (1988). A social relations model analysis of parent and child play. *Developmental Psychology, 24*, 101–108. http://dx.doi.org.proxy1.cl.msu.edu/10.1037/0012-1649.24.1.101

Tenenbaum, H. R., & Leaper, C. (1997). Mothers' and fathers' questions to their child in Mexican-descent families: Moderators of cognitive demand during play. *Hispanic Journal of Behavioral Sciences, 19*, 318–332. https://doi.org/10.1177/07399863970193005

Teti, D. M., Bond, L. A., & Gibbs, E. D. (1988). Mothers, fathers, and siblings: A comparison of play styles and their influence upon infant cognitive level. *International Journal of Behavioral Development, 11*, 415–432. https://doi.org/10.1177/016502548801100402

Thomas, A. J., & King, C. T. (2007). Gendered racial socialization of African American mothers and daughters. *The Family Journal: Counseling and Therapy for Couples and Families, 15*(2), 137–142. https://doi.org/10.1177/1066480706297853

Tomasello, M. (2008). *Origins of human communication*. Cambridge, MA: MIT Press.

Vallotton, C. D. (2009). Do infants influence their quality of care? Infants' communicative gestures predict caregivers' responsiveness. *Infant Behavior & Development, 32*, 351–365. https://doi.org/10.1016/j.infbeh.2009.06.001

Weinraub, M., & Frankel, J. (1977). Sex differences in parent-infant interaction during free play, departure, and separation. *Child Development, 48*, 1240–1249. https://doi.org/10.2307/1128481

Whitebread, D. (2012). *The importance of play*. Report prepared for Toy Industries of Europe. Retrieved from http://www.importanceofplay.eu/IMG/pdf/dr_david_whitebread_-_the_importance_of_play.pdf

Wood, E., Desmarais, S., & Gugula, S. (2002). The impact of parenting experience on gender stereotyped toy play of children. *Sex Roles: A Journal of Research, 47*, 39–49. http://dx.doi.org.proxy1.cl.msu.edu/10.1023/A:1020679619728

Yogman, M. W. (1981). Games fathers and mothers play with their infants. *Infant Mental Health Journal, 2*, 241–248. https://doi.org/10.1002/1097-0355(198124)2:4<241::AID-IMHJ2280020406>3.0.CO;2-8

23 Fathers' Language Input and Early Child Language Development

Nadya Pancsofar

Conceptions of fatherhood have been shaped by broad social changes over the last several decades, such as increases of women in the workforce, a rise in single-father households, and greater father involvement in family life and child care (Cabrera, Tamis-LeMonda, Bradley, Hofferth, & Lamb, 2000; Jones & Mosher, 2013; Livingston, 2013). In response, research has shifted from a focus on more traditional roles of fathers as financial providers and fathers' presence or absence to a closer consideration of characteristics of father-child interactions and their impact on child development (Pancsofar & Vernon-Feagans, 2006). Within the burgeoning body of literature addressing the roles of fathers in early child development, the scholarship on fathers' contributions to early child language development has been particularly active. Early oral language development is an important component of emergent literacy, with links to school readiness and early reading (NICHD Early Child Care Research Network, 2005; Walker, Greenwood, Hart, & Carta, 1994). The first 2 years of children's lives are characterized by rapid changes in children's language development, and young children learn language in social contexts in which their caregivers play an important role (Kuhl, 2007; Tomasello, 1992). Emerging research focused on fathers' talk to young children has added to the more well-established links between maternal language input and child language development to provide a deeper understanding of the role of parent-child language interactions in the language development of young children (Hoff-Ginsberg, 1991; Huttenlocher, Haight, Bryk, Seltzer, & Lyons, 1991; Reynolds, Vernon-Feagans, Bratsch-Hines, Baker, & The Family Life Project Investigators, 2018; Tamis-LeMonda, Baumwell, & Cristofaro, 2012; Weizman & Snow, 2001).

This chapter addresses theoretical foundations guiding research on fathers' language input during early childhood and then presents an overview of the findings from key research in the following areas: comparisons of mothers' and fathers' language input, contributions of fathers' language input to early language development, and factors associated with fathers' language input to young children. This chapter then considers an emerging area of scholarship that is focused on the role of fathers' language input in the language development of young children with disabilities, an example one area for future research that builds upon the extant findings to address an aspect of diversity in child language development. This chapter concludes with a consideration of other areas for future research, implications for practice, and key summary points.

N. Pancsofar (✉)
Department of Special Education, Language, and Literacy, The College of New Jersey, Ewing, NJ, USA
e-mail: pancsofa@tcnj.edu

H. E. Fitzgerald et al. (eds.), *Handbook of Fathers and Child Development*,
https://doi.org/10.1007/978-3-030-51027-5_23

Theoretical Foundations

The acquisition of language skills occurs within social contexts (Bates, 1976; Bruner, 1981; Kuhl, 2007; Tomasello, 1992; Vygotsky, 1962). Children learn much of their earliest language in the context of social interactional routines, such as feeding, diaper changing, book activities, and social games (Tomasello, 1992). The people in a young child's environment support that child's language learning as conversational partners. Caregivers of very young children often focus their attention and feedback on how, when, and where to make appropriate utterances. Bruner (1981) argues that language acquisition involves a transaction between a novice with a high readiness to learn and an expert adult well-tuned to the needs of the novice that brings the child's efforts to communicate into an appropriate contextualization.

Caregivers also support early language learning through scaffolding and joint attention, in which children imitate and incorporate adult model utterances or phrases into their own lexicon in interactions in which caregivers expand upon child utterances and caregivers and children attend to the same thing (Ninio & Bruner, 1976; Snow, Perlman, & Nathan, 1987; Tamis-LeMonda, Kuchirko, & Song, 2014; Warren, Yoder, & Leew, 2001). When caregivers follow a child's attentional lead, they sustain a child's interest in activities and social interaction (Warren et al., 2001). Interactivity and reciprocity, in which caregivers' talk is contingent on the vocalizations of young language learners, are key components of speech and language development (Kuhl, 2007). Parents' timely and contingent responses to children's communicative bids can act as reinforcement to maintain or evoke further communication from the child (Dunst, Lowe, & Bartholomew, 1989).

Stimulating caregiver language that is attuned to the child's developmental level has been thought to be integral to early language development (Bruner, 1981; Snow, 1977). Parental language input provides young children with the tools of language structure and use. Parents modify their speech and language to their young children in ways that support their early language learning. These modifications include simplified, less complex, and more redundant language and speech with a higher pitch and exaggerated intonation pattern (Fernald, 1989; Kavanaugh & Jirkovsky, 1982; Kitamura & Burnham, 2003; McRoberts & Best, 1997; Rondal, 1980; Snow, 1977). Previous research on the influence of parental language input on children's language development has focused primarily on mothers. Research on maternal language input has consistently indicated that mothers' talk to their children is associated with their children's gains in linguistic abilities (Huttenlocher et al., 1991; Reynolds et al., 2018; Tamis-LeMonda et al., 2012). In particular, the diversity of maternal vocabulary has long been found to be a strong predictor of children's later language development and literacy (Bornstein, Haynes, & Painter, 1998; Hoff-Ginsberg, 1991; Pan, Rowe, Singer, & Snow, 2005; Weizman & Snow, 2001). However, focusing exclusively on maternal language input provides an incomplete understanding of the social interactional contexts in which children learn language, and over the past several decades, research has broadened the scope of analysis to include fathers. The extant literature on fathers' language input has considered several broad areas, including comparisons between mothers' and fathers' talk to young children, the contributions of early fathers' language input to child language development, and factors that shape fathers' language input.

Comparing Mothers' and Fathers' Language Input to Young Children

Research comparing the language use of fathers and mothers in interactions with their young children has generally found both similarities and differences (Kwon, Bingham, Lewsader, Jeon, & Elicker, 2013; Leaper, Anderson, & Sanders, 1998; Pancsofar & Vernon-Feagans, 2006; Roopnarine, Fouts, Lamb, & Lewis-Elligan, 2005; Rowe, Coker, & Pan, 2004; Tamis-LeMonda et al., 2012). The very early work in this area was synthesized in a meta-analysis conducted by Leaper et al. (1998), who found that fathers used less total language, less supportive language, less negative language, and more directive and informing language than did mothers. Leaper et al. found that effect sizes in the areas of supportive and negative parent language were significantly larger for parents of infants and toddlers than for parents of older children. However, it is possible that trends in fathers' language use, particularly in comparison to mothers' language use, may have changed over the past several decades since the Leaper et al. meta-analysis was conducted, as the number of dual-earner families continues to increase and fathers have taken on more direct child care responsibilities (Cabrera, Volling, & Barr, 2018; Jones & Mosher, 2013; Livingston, 2013).

Several more recent studies have considered differences in mothers' and fathers' language input to young children, and these studies have often included somewhat more diverse samples of families than earlier work included in the Leaper et al. meta-analysis. In a study of middle-class dual-earner families in which fathers held shared responsibility for the daily care of their children, Pancsofar and Vernon-Feagans (2006) compared mothers' and fathers' language input to their 24-month-old children in triadic free play interactions. They found that when considering measures of total verbal output, fathers talked less overall, had shorter turn lengths, and used fewer different word roots and fewer total wh-questions. However, when considering measures of parent talk, such as type-token ratio (a measure of lexical density, which is the ratio of the number of different word roots to the total words), mean length of utterance, and the proportion of questions asked, that controlled for total output, there were no significant differences found between mothers and fathers. These results from Pancsofar and Vernon-Feagans suggest that mothers and fathers differed on the quantity but not the quality of their language output. However, findings comparing mothers' and fathers' language input within middle-class families have not been wholly consistent. For example, in a more recent study of middle-class mothers and fathers in structured and free play dyadic interactions with their 2-year-old children, Kwon et al. (2013) found that mothers generally did more talking; however, they found that fathers demonstrated higher type-token ratios, indicating a more dense vocabulary use.

Other studies comparing mothers' and fathers' language use with young children in low-income families have generally found more similarities than differences. Roopnarine et al. (2005) considered a sample of African American families from lower, middle, and upper SES backgrounds and found that while mothers were more available to their infants and spent more time overall vocalizing to their young infants, fathers spent a greater proportion of their time with their young infants vocalizing than did mothers. There have been some indications from this research that fathers may make more requests for clarifications than do mothers (Rowe et al., 2004; Tamis-LeMonda et al., 2012). Rowe et al. (2004) compared fathers' and mothers' language input in a sample of rural low-income White families with 2-year-old children. While Rowe et al. found that mothers and fathers were similar in their amount of talk, diversity of vocabulary, and MLU, they did find that fathers used significantly more wh-questions and more requests for clarifications than did mothers. More recently, Tamis-LeMonda et al. (2012) studied the language use of mothers and fathers in dyadic play interactions with 24-month-old children from racial diverse, low-income families. Tamis-LeMonda et al. found that the language use by mothers and fathers was strongly correlated and largely similar, including across measures of total utterances, communicative diversity, word types, and MLU. However, they found that fathers used more action directives than mothers and were marginally more likely than mothers to ask their children to repeat utterances. The results of these studies of comparing parents' language input in low-income families suggest that while mothers' and fathers' language use is quite similar, fathers may be slightly more challenging linguistic partners for children and may request more clarifications or repetitions from their young children (Rowe et al., 2004; Tamis-LeMonda et al., 2012).

While most studies comparing mothers' and fathers' language input have been conducted within the United States, a study of Italian toddlers found some significant differences in parental language input across mothers and fathers, with mothers producing higher MLU and a higher number of tokens (Majorano, Rainieri, & Corsano, 2013). Majorano et al. (2013) also found fathers produced a lower number of didactic and asynchronous utterances and produced names in the Italian lexicon with a lower frequency than mothers. More research is needed that includes fathers with young children outside of the United States to better understand the roles of fathers in the language learning process across the structural characteristics and sociocultural aspects of different languages (Majorano et al., 2013).

Among studies that have compared the language use of mothers and fathers specifically in book reading interactions with their young children, some interesting differences have been found. In a study of low-income families, Duursma (2016) found that in book reading with their young children, fathers used more non-immediate talk (talk that goes beyond information in the text to, for example, make predictions or connections with the child's own world) than did mothers. Duursma suggests that this finding may indicate that fathers use more diverse strategies than mothers to engage their children in book reading and that their focus may be less on the book itself but more on engaging the child in the interaction. Malin, Cabrera, and Rowe (2014) also found that fathers used more metalingual talk (talk that is not related to the book/text) than did mothers in book reading interactions with their 2-year-old children. These findings suggest that within the context of book reading, fathers may structure these language interactions differently and use different linguistic strategies with their young children than do mothers.

Findings across studies comparing the language input of mothers and fathers have not always been consistent, and it is not clear from this research what meaning is carried by these differences nor how these differences may shape the unique contributions of mothers and fathers to their children's early language development. Some of the challenges to interpreting this body of research may be related to differences in the contexts of parent-child language interactions across these studies. For example, there may be differences in parental talk with children when engaging in different types of tasks. Salo, Rowe, Leech, and Cabrera (2016) found that fathers used a more diverse vocabulary and asked more questions during book reading tasks with their 2-year-old children than in toy play interactions. Kwon et al. (2013) also found differences in parent talk across different parent-child tasks. Specifically, both mothers and fathers used more complex language during free play tasks with their toddlers than they did during more structured tasks.

Pancsofar, Vernon-Feagans, Odom, and Roe (2008) have also hypothesized that triadic mother-father-child language interactions could create contexts in which the behavior and language use of one parent are constrained and influenced by the actions of the other. Family systems theory posits that families are comprised of smaller subsystems that may function in different ways (Minuchin, 1985), and the language use of mothers and fathers in dyadic interactions with their children may be qualitatively different than their language use in triadic language interactions. Bingham, Kwon, and Jeon (2013) examined the difference in fathers' language use across dyadic and triadic interactional contexts in predominantly middle-class families with toddlers. They found that differences between mothers' and fathers' language use in triadic contexts were greater than differences in language use in dyadic contexts. Notably, this trend was particularly salient for fathers, who demonstrated a greater decline in speech output in triadic contexts (as compared to dyadic contexts) than did mothers. Bingham et al. posit that fathers may speak less than mothers and use fewer vocabulary words in triadic settings because they may feel less responsible for interacting with their child when mothers are present or may feel less supported in their parenting role in that context.

Contributions of Early Father Language Input to Child Language Development

Research on the associations between fathers' language input and child language development has consistently identified significant contributions of fathers' talk to their children during early childhood and their children's subsequent language development. These associations have been found above and beyond the contributions made by mothers' language input to child language development, as well as family demographic characteristics. In one of the first larger-scale longitudinal studies to consider the contributions of fathers' language input to child language development during early childhood, Pancsofar and Vernon-Feagans (2006) found that fathers' language input made a significant and unique contribution to their children's later expressive language development in White two-parent middle-class dual-earner families. Specifically, fathers who used more different word roots in their observed interactions with their children at 24 months of age had children with better expressive language skills at 36 months of age than did children whose fathers used a less diverse vocabulary. These fathers' contributions to children's language development were found after controlling for parental level of education, quality of child care, and mothers' language input. Later, Pancsofar, Vernon-Feagans, and the Family Life Project Investigators (2010) found similar results when considering the contributions of fathers' language input in a larger, more ethnically diverse sample of two-parent families from low-income rural communities. Pancsofar et al. found fathers who used a more diverse vocabulary (number of different word roots) during picture-book interactions when children were 6 months of age had children who later demonstrated more advanced communication development at 15 months and expressive language development at 36 months of age. These associations were found after controlling for family demographics, child characteristics, and mothers' education and language input.

Associations between fathers' language input during early childhood and child language development have been supported by the findings of other recent research studies across diverse families. Tamis-LeMonda et al. (2012) found that in a sample of low-income, racially diverse families, fathers' communicative diversity, calculated as the number of different kinds of utterances used during dyadic play interactions when children were 24 months of age, was a unique predictor of children's overall language at that age, even after controlling for demographic factors and mothers' language input. Similarly, in work with international families, Majorano et al. (2013) found during free play interactions, fathers' noun frequency in the Italian lexicon was significantly associated with language production and comprehension in Italian toddlers.

In a study of low-income fathers and their children, Malin et al. (2014) found that controlling for parental education, mothers' and fathers' use of metalingual language (e.g., using wh-questions) significantly predicted children's receptive vocabulary skills at prekindergarten. Rowe, Leech, and Cabrera (2017) also found associations between fathers' use of wh- questions and children's early language skills among low-income African American families. Fathers' use of wh- questions in free play interactions with their 24-month-old children was concurrently positively associated with child vocabulary and verbal reasoning skills (Rowe et al., 2017).

The positive associations between fathers' language input and child language outcomes during early childhood have been found to sustain through the transition to formal schooling. Reynolds et al. (2018) found that fathers' MLU and use of wh- questions when children were 6–36 months of age were significantly associated with child vocabulary and math scores in kindergarten. In another study involving the same sample of families, Baker, Vernon-Feagans, and the Family Life Project Investigators (2015) found that fathers' MLU when children were 60 months of age independently contributed to children's vocabulary scores during the spring of their kindergarten year, above and beyond the contributions of mothers' language. Fathers with longer MLU had children with more advanced picture vocabulary scores during kindergarten.

This growing body of literature has consistently linked fathers' early language input in several contexts, including play and shared book reading, to their children's subsequent language development across racially and socioeconomically diverse families, and these father contributions have been found above and beyond the impact of mothers' language input and family and child demographic factors (Baker et al., 2015; Malin et al., 2014; Pancsofar et al., 2008; Pancsofar & Vernon-Feagans, 2006; Reynolds et al., 2018; Rowe et al., 2017; Tamis-LeMonda et al., 2012). In particular, fathers' early vocabulary, MLU, and use of wh-questions have been linked to later child language outcomes, including through the transition to formal schooling. These meaningful and enduring contributions of fathers' talk to young children have highlighted the need to better understand what factors may shape the language used by fathers in early interactions with their young children.

Factors Associated with Fathers' Language Input to Young Children

Research into the factors associated with fathers' language input to young children remains limited; however, this emerging work has begun to highlight some general areas of focus, including father demographic factors, fathers' work and employment experiences, fathers' relationships with mothers, and fathers' stress and depression. Transactional relationships between fathers' language input and child language development have also warranted closer attention to more deeply understand the factors that shape fathers' language use with young children.

Demographic Factors

Previous work on the demographic predictors of fathers' language input to young children has primarily considered fathers' education, ethnicity, and residential status. Among these demographic factors, fathers' education has been found to be the most consistent predictor of fathers' language use in interactions with their young children (Cabrera, Hofferth, & Chae, 2011; Malin et al., 2012; Pancsofar, Vernon-Feagans, Odom, & The Family Life Project Investigators, 2013; Zhang, Jin, Shen, Zhang, & Hoff, 2008). Cabrera et al. (2011) found that across race/ethnicity, fathers' education was significantly associated with fathers' verbal stimulation with their infants in low-income families. Fathers who had completed at least some college education engaged in more verbal stimulation with their infants than did fathers who finished high school, but did not attend college. In a study of the language use of African American fathers in low-income families with their 6-month-old infants, Pancsofar et al. (2013) found that fathers who had more years of education used a more diverse vocabulary with their infants. Malin et al. (2012) found that in a sample of low-income families with 2-year-old children, a higher level of education in fathers was associated with more child vocabulary diversity and more total child utterances, and this relationship was partially mediated by fathers' language input, with fathers with higher levels of education using more complex and diverse language when interacting with their children.

Fathers' education has also been found to be positively associated with other aspects of fathering that are related to fathers' language input, such as supportive father-child interactions (Cabrera, Shannon, & Tamis-LeMonda, 2007) and frequency of reading to young children (Duursma, Pan, & Raikes, 2008). While the mechanisms explaining the relationship between fathers' education and fathers' language input are not clear, fathers with more education may have more advanced language and literacy skills overall, and they may be more aware of the developmental needs of their children or more confident in their abilities to meet those developmental needs (Cabrera et al., 2007; Varghese & Wachen, 2016).

Research on fathers' language use with young children has found very few differences across racial or ethnic groups (Cabrera et al., 2011; Sims

& Coley, 2016). Researchers have found that fathers from ethnic minority groups are as involved and engaged in language activities with their young children as are White fathers (Varghese & Wachen, 2016). However, it is important to note that, as Varghese and Wachen (2016) point out, studies that include race and ethnicity as a predictor of fathers' language use with young children have focused primarily on African American, Latino, and White fathers, and far less is known about the experiences of fathers of other races or ethnicities.

The existing literature on the residential status of fathers has also found very few associations with the quality of father-child language interactions (Varghese & Wachen, 2016). Rowe et al. (2004) found few differences overall in how resident and nonresident fathers communicated with their toddlers, but they did find that nonresident fathers used more indirect forms of prohibitives with their children than did resident fathers. More research is needed in this area to further understand the nuances of how resident status could be related to father-child language interactions and the language input used by nonresident fathers of young children.

Work and Employment

According to ecological systems theory, child development and learning occur within and are affected by a variety of contexts, which are organized as nested systems that include, from most proximal to most distal, the microsystem, mesosystem, exosystem, and macrosystem (Bronfenbrenner, 1986; Bronfenbrenner & Morris, 1998). One key exosystem context (settings in which the child does not have an active role) for child development is fathers' work settings and experiences (Cabrera, Fitzgerald, Bradley, & Roggman, 2014). Many studies have found connections between fathers' work experiences and fathering (e.g., Aldous, Mulligan, and Bjarnason, 1998; Stewart and Barling, 1996; Yeung, Sandberg, Davis-Kean, and Hofferth, 2001). Grossman, Pollack, and Golding (1988) found that while fathers who expressed greater job satisfaction spent less time with their 5-year-old children than did less satisfied fathers, fathers with greater job satisfaction were more supportive and sensitive toward their children. Several studies have found that among two-parent families with children under the age of 5, greater work hours for fathers have been associated with less father participation in child care (Aldous et al., 1998; NICHD Early Child Care Research Network, 2000) and reading activities with their young children (Marsiglio, 1991). Further, studies looking at paternity leave across Europe, Australia, and the United States have found that fathers who take leave from work around childbirth are more likely to engage in child care-related activities with their young children than fathers who did not take leave (Huerta et al., 2014) and that paternity leave may positively impact later children's school performance (Cools, Fiva, & Kirkeboen, 2015). While a robust body of research has linked characteristics of fathers' work experiences to fathering during early childhood, very few studies have considered the associations between fathers' work and their language interactions with their young children.

In one of the only studies to consider links between fathers' work and fathers' language input with young children, Pancsofar et al. (2013) found that the work experiences of African American fathers living in low-income rural communities were significantly associated with their vocabulary use in picture-book interactions with their 6-month-old infants, even after controlling for fathers' education. Fathers who worked nonstandard shifts (work hours that fell outside of the traditional "9-to-5" workday) and who reported higher levels of job flexibility used more diverse vocabulary with their infants. These findings are in contrast to research on maternal shift work, which has been found to be negatively associated with parenting and to have a negative impact on early child cognitive and language development (Bratsch-Hines, Baker, & Vernon-Feagans, 2016; Han, 2005). However, because fathers traditionally have been considered the primary breadwinners of the family, work experiences may have a differential impact on fathering than on mothering (Doherty, Kouneski, &

Erickson, 1998). Pancsofar et al. (2013) hypothesized that for fathers of infants, particularly in low-income rural communities, nonstandard work hours and greater job flexibility may facilitate greater caregiving responsibilities and more opportunities for father-child language interactions. In a more recent study, positive associations were found between fathers' shift work when their children were 24 months old and their children's preschool reading skills among African American and Hispanic families (Baker, 2016). Further research is needed to better understand the associations between fathers' work experiences and father-child language interactions across families from diverse socioeconomic backgrounds.

Marital Quality

Another possible contributor to fathers' language input is the quality of the mother-father relationship (Cabrera et al., 2014). According to family systems theory, the family is comprised of smaller subsystems, such that members of the parent-child subsystem are simultaneously members of other dyads that support or stress them (Minuchin, 1985). In this way, the quality of the adult-adult parenting subsystem can support or stress the functioning of the parent-child subsystem. Minuchin (1985) argues that either patterns of interactions associated with marital relationships can provide complementary and cooperative resources for parenting or they can be a source of parenting difficulties.

Fathers in more harmonious, satisfied, and low-conflict relationships with their children's mothers have been found to have more positive attitudes toward their infants, participate in more caregiving activities, report greater satisfaction in fathering, and demonstrate more engagement, sensitivity, warmth, and support in father-child interactions (Baker, 2014; Belsky, Youngblade, Rovine, & Volling, 1991; Cabrera et al., 2007; Goldberg & Easterbrooks, 1984; Kitzmann, 2000; Volling & Belsky, 1991). A more limited body of research has specifically considered links between marital quality and parental language input. Pratt, Kerig, Cowan, and Cowan (1992) measured marital satisfaction and mothers' and fathers' language input during dyadic play sessions with children at 3.5 years of age. Pratt et al. found that mothers' and fathers' conversational styles were similar but that more satisfied parents spoke in longer utterances. Brody, Pellegrini, and Sigel (1986) also considered the relationship between parents' language input and marital quality. Brody et al. looked at marital stress and dyadic teaching interactions with mothers and fathers with children 5.5–7.5 years of age. The authors found that fathers in distressed families gave less positive feedback and were more intrusive in father-child interactions than were fathers in nondistressed families.

In a study of two-parent dual-earner middle-class families, Pancsofar et al. (2008) found that when marital relationships were high in love and broader family relationships were low in conflict when children were 12 months old, fathers later used a more diverse vocabulary in triadic play interactions when children were 2 years old. In a more recent study of a racial diverse sample of low-income families, Cabrera et al. (2011) found that fathers' reports of conflict with their child's mother were negatively associated with their verbal stimulation with their infants. This body of research suggests that the quality of the mother-father marital relationship is related to language used by fathers in interactions with their young children, such that more supportive, less conflictual marital relationships in families with young children may contribute to higher quality, more verbally stimulating language input from fathers (Cabrera et al., 2011; Pancsofar et al., 2008).

Fathers' Stress and Depression

While very few studies have examined links between fathers' stress and depression and fathers' language input, the extant literature links fathers' depression with related areas of parenting and parent-child interactions (Baker, 2014; Bronte-Tinkew, Moore, Matthews, & Carrano, 2007; Paulson, Keefe, & Leiferman, 2009), as well as directly to child language outcomes during early childhood (Paulson et al., 2009). Fathers' depression during the early childhood period has been associated with a lower frequency of father engagement with their young children (Bronte-Tinkew et al., 2007). Baker (2014) found that among African American fathers of 24-month-old children from low-income families, fathers who experienced fewer depressive symptoms participated in more frequent play, caregiving, and home literacy activities, which included book reading, storytelling, and singing songs. Paulson et al. (2009) examined relationships between parental depression and the frequency of parent-child reading during early childhood in low-income families. Paulson et al. found that for both mothers and fathers, depressive symptoms when infants were 9 months of age were negatively associated with frequency of concurrent parent-child book reading. For fathers only, depressive symptoms when infants were 9 months of age were negatively associated with later father-child book reading when children were 24 months of age and with children's expressive vocabulary development at 24 months of age.

In one of the few studies to examine links between fathers' depression and fathers' talk to young children, Sethna, Murray, and Rachandani (2012) found that depression in fathers of 3-month-old infants was associated with fathers' more frequent use of speech that focused on the fathers' experience and less on the infants' experience. Depressed fathers also used more negative and critical utterances with their infants, when compared with nondepressed fathers. Malin et al. (2012) found significant associations between fathers' depressive symptoms and child MLU, with fathers with more depressive symptoms having 2-year-old children with smaller MLUs. This relationship was partially mediated by fathers' language input, with fathers with more depressive symptoms using fewer utterances when interacting with their young children.

More research is needed to fully understand the role that fathers' depression and stress may have on their language use with their young children, particularly at the transition to parenthood, which has been identified as a time in which fathers are particularly at risk for depression (Garfield et al., 2014). Further investigation is also needed to consider the role that maternal depression may play in understanding father-child interactions. For example, Cabrera et al. (2007) found that African American fathers in low-income families whose partners reported higher levels of depressive symptoms were less engaged in verbally stimulating interactions with their infants; however, it was unclear what factors explained this association.

Child Language Skills

While most research on father-child language interactions has considered the contributions of fathers' talk to child language development, there is a bidirectional relationship in which child-level characteristics and skills may shape the language used by fathers in interactions with their young children (Cabrera et al., 2014). For example, in the area of child vocabulary, a transactional process has been identified in the literature in which children acquire words from parents, and parents' speech is influenced by children's vocabularies (Huttenlocher, Waterfall, Vasilyeva, Vevea, & Hedges, 2010). Therefore, it is important to explore the ways in which fathers' language input to young children may be shaped by the language skills that these children bring to father-child language interactions.

Rowe et al. (2004) found that fathers used fewer directives, a more diverse vocabulary, and longer utterances with 2-year-old children who talked more. Schwab, Rowe, Cabrera, and Lew-Williams (2018) found a similar trend in which fathers repeated words less often in interactions with children who had larger vocabularies at 24 months of age. Child language skills have been positively linked to other aspects of father-child interactions, such as frequency of father-child book reading (Duursma et al., 2008). Duursma et al. (2008) found that fathers were more likely to read to their children frequently if their children had better language skills.

The extant literature suggests that fathers shape their language use and language interactions with young children in response to the language skills demonstrated by their children (Duursma et al., 2008; Rowe et al., 2004; Schwab et al., 2018) and that fathers' language input, in turn, contributes to further growth in language skills for young children (Baker et al., 2015; Pancsofar et al., 2008; Pancsofar & Vernon-Feagans, 2006; Reynolds et al., 2018; Tamis-LeMonda et al., 2012). However, this relationship has been examined overwhelmingly for children who are typically developing. Only a very few studies have considered the relationship between fathers' talk and child language development for children with disabilities. However, such research is of critical importance as the early childhood period is a particularly important time for the language development of children with disabilities (Ratner, 2013).

Expanding the Lens: Fathers of Children with Disabilities

This growing literature on the role of fathers' language input in early child language development has considered comparisons between the language input of mothers and fathers, contributions of fathers' language input to child language development, and factors that may shape the quality and quantity of language used by fathers in interactions with their young children. However, this body of research has largely omitted fathers of children with disabilities, and this remains an important area for future research. Father involvement has been found to be a protective factor for children with disabilities, and fathers of children with disabilities have been found to be just as involved with their children's care, nurturing, and playtime as fathers of children without disabilities (Potter, 2017; Varghese & Wachen, 2016). However, literature suggests that the language input by parents of children with disabilities may differ qualitatively from parental language input to children without disabilities, and parental language input to children with disabilities may generally be more limited, more directive, and less complex (Ratner, 2013).

Little is known about the language interactions between fathers and young children with disabilities, the ways in which fathers' language input may contribute to linguistic gains in young children with disabilities, or the ways in which early intervention efforts may shape fathers' language use with their young children with disabilities. In a recent review of the literature on early intervention with children with autism, Flippin and Crais (2011) found that fathers were very underrepresented in this work. In particular, Flippin and Crais noted a lack of observational studies of interactions between fathers and children with disabilities. Regarding children with autism in particular, Flippin and Crais write, "Little knowledge exists as to how and why father-child interactions with a child with ASD may parallel or differ from the types of interactions fathers may have with their children who are typically developing" (p. 45).

One of the only studies to consider fathers' language use with young children with disabilities was conducted by Flippin and Watson (2015), who examined the verbal responsiveness of mothers and fathers in play interactions with their preschool-aged children with autism. They found that mothers demonstrated more verbal responsiveness than did fathers; however, fathers' verbal responsiveness was concurrently associated with more advanced child language skills even after controlling for children's nonverbal cognitive skills. It is not clear in this study the direction of the association between fathers' verbal responsiveness and child language, nor if these associations would be found over time for children with autism. More extensive, longitudinal studies are needed in this area.

While the connections between fathers' depression and stress and fathers' language input have not been well studied, there is some indication from the existing literature that fathers' depression and stress may negatively impact their language interactions with their young children (Baker, 2014; Malin et al., 2012; Paulson et al., 2009; Sethna et al., 2012). Fathers of children with disabilities have been found to have more elevated levels of stress than fathers of children without disabilities (MacDonald & Hastings, 2010), and there may be some instances in which the stress levels for fathers of children with disabilities may be particularly high. For example, fathers of children with autism have been found to experience higher levels of stress as compared to fathers of children with other disabilities (Flippin & Crais, 2011; Meadan, Halle, & Ebata, 2010), and levels of stress and anxiety have been related to the severity of children's disability for both mothers and fathers (Garcia-Lopez, Sarria, & Pozo, 2016). In particular, parents of children with disabilities who experience an array of changing behaviors have reported high levels of stress (Falk, Norris, & Quinn, 2014; Gray, 2006; Harper, Dyckes, Harper, Roper, & South, 2013; Hastings et al., 2005). For many parents of children with severe disabilities, the early childhood period may be particularly stressful as they move through the process of discovery and diagnosis of their child's disability (Meadan et al., 2010; Rivard, Terroux, Parent-Boursier, & Mercier, 2014). Research comparing depression and stress levels across mothers and fathers of children with disabilities has yielded mixed results, but it has indicated that fathers of children with autism may be particularly impacted by mothers' mental health, such that mothers' mental health has been found to predict fathers' positive parenting experiences (Flippin & Crais, 2011; Meadan et al., 2010).

Additionally, fathers of children with disabilities, who are primary financial providers for their families, may feel additional stress or strain in their parenting (Pancsofar, Petroff, Rao, & Mangel, 2019). In a recent qualitative study of 15 fathers of children with severe and complex disabilities that included deafblindness, autism, and fragile X syndrome, fathers articulated that their families experienced more extensive and longer-term financial demands related to their children's complex learning and developmental needs and that fathers' work was one way through which families could meet these unique financial needs (Pancsofar et al., 2019). These fathers articulated challenges in addressing multiple, sometimes conflicting responsibilities, including emotional demands of parenting a child with a complex disability, with more practical demands of their jobs. It is not clear how the unique interplay between fathers' work and parenting may relate to their language interactions with their young children with disabilities.

Very few studies have considered the involvement of fathers in early language interventions (Flippin & Crais, 2011). Among the existing research on fathers' involvement in interventions for children with disabilities or developmental delays, father participation has been associated with more positive child behavioral outcomes (Bagner, 2013). However, it is not known how early intervention experiences may shape the language used by fathers with their young children with disabilities.

The very limited findings from this body of research suggest much more work is needed to fully understand father-child language interactions for young children with disabilities. Some preliminary work in this area suggests that similar to what has been found with typically developing children, the language input of fathers of young children with autism may make meaningful contributions to their child's language development (Flippin & Watson, 2015) and that some of the factors found to be associated with father language input to young children, such as stress, may be experienced in unique ways by fathers of children with severe and complex disabilities (Pancsofar et al., 2019).

Future Research and Implications for Practice

Despite the growing recognition of the role of fathers in child language development and the consistent findings that fathers make important and long-lasting contributions to early language development, fathers are still underrepresented in research considering the role of parents in early language development (Cabrera et al., 2018; Zauche, Thul, Darcy Mahoney, & Stapel-Wax, 2016). Further research on fathers' contributions to early child language development is needed to better illuminate the explanatory mechanisms underlying these associations. Most research to date has either compared mothers' and fathers' language input or examined the contributions of fathers' language input, above and beyond the contributions of mothers (Baker et al., 2015; Duursma, 2016; Kwon et al., 2013; Leaper et al., 1998; Majorano et al., 2013; Malin et al., 2014; Pancsofar & Vernon-Feagans, 2006; Pancsofar et al., 2010; Reynolds et al., 2018; Roopnarine et al., 2005; Rowe et al., 2004; Tamis-LeMonda et al., 2012). Further research is needed that explores the interaction between fathers' and mothers' language input and crossover effects. Further work is also needed that explores how fathers' beliefs and knowledge on child-rearing and child development may shape their language interactions with their young children, as previous research has found important associations here for mothers' language input (Rowe, 2008).

Greater inclusivity is needed in future research on fathers' contributions to early language development, and this work must be expanded to better include fathers of children with disabilities. Future work should also address the diversity of fathering experiences during early childhood, including more culturally and linguistically diverse samples of fathers and more diverse family structures that include nonresident fathers for children both with and without disabilities (Cabrera et al., 2018). Further, the extant literature in this area has almost exclusively focused on heterosexual fathers from families headed by mother-father dyads. Future work into fathers' contributions to early child language development should be more inclusive of families parented by two fathers, as well as single-father families.

The limited research on factors that shape fathers' language input to young children highlights some important implications for practice. Programs that support the continuing higher education for fathers with young children may benefit fathers' language input to young children, as fathers' education has been positively associated with more stimulating talk to their young children (Cabrera et al., 2011; Pancsofar et al., 2013). Similarly, employer support for more flexible work arrangements for fathers of young children may support fathers' language input (Pancsofar et al., 2013). Professionals working with fathers of young children need to be aware of the possible constraints and opportunities that their job may apply on their interactions with their children. Professionals hoping to support high-quality father-child language interactions should also work to support fathers, develop their coping skills, and alleviate stress, particularly for fathers of young children with disabilities. Through these strategies, professional practice and home-school collaborations can expand to better include fathers and recognize the positive contributions that they make to early child language development (Pancsofar, Petroff, & Lewis, 2017).

Continued research on the factors that may be related to fathers' language input to young children is needed to better illuminate the bidirectional nature of father-child interactions and the ways in which child language skills may shape fathers' language use over time, particularly for young children with disabilities. Such research may be of particular importance in highlighting the ways in which fathers of children with disabilities shape their language interactions with children who experience challenges in underlying skills, such as joint attention. A better understanding of father-child language interactions in these contexts would highlight more effective approaches for professionals in supporting fathers' talk to their young children.

It is important that teachers and other professionals working with young children and their families recognize the important contributions of fathers to early language development and grow more inclusive of fathers in their professional practices. Literature on home-school collaborations in special education has found that professionals most frequently interact with mothers and that fathers have been left feeling like the "odd man out" in their child's educational plans and related services (Mueller & Buckley, 2014; Pancsofar et al., 2019). In their work with families, professionals should acknowledge and validate the contributions of fathers to their children's early language development (Pancsofar et al., 2017).

Summary and Key Points

Over the past several decades, there has been an increasingly robust consideration of the roles of fathers in child language development during the early childhood years. First, research in this area has considered comparisons between mothers' and fathers' language input to young children. This research has found many similarities between the language use of mothers and fathers in interactions with their children; however, some studies have indicated that fathers may produce less overall talk to their children and may, at times, use higher quality language and language with different communicative functions than mothers.

Second, the findings across this body of literature suggest that characteristics of fathers' language to their young children have positive associations with later child language skills, above and beyond the contributions of mothers' language input. These early positive contributions of father language input to child language development have been found to sustain through the transition to formal schooling. Third, research into the predictors of fathers' talk to their children has considered a variety of factors. This research suggests that fathers' education, work and employment, marital relationship, and stress and depression may shape the quality and quantity of fathers' talk to young children. Research also suggests that fathers may talk more to their children with more advanced language development.

Last, while the majority of studies in this area have considered the experiences of fathers of typically developing children, some emerging research suggests that fathers may play a similar role in shaping the language development of young children with disabilities. Further research is needed in this area to more fully understand the associations between father language input and child language development for children with disabilities.

References

Aldous, J., Mulligan, G. M., & Bjarnason, T. (1998). Fathering over time: What makes the difference? *Journal of Marriage and the Family, 60*, 809–820. https://doi.org/10.2307/353626

Bagner, D. M. (2013). Father's role in parent training for children with developmental delay. *Journal of Family Psychology, 27*, 650–657. https://doi.org/10.1037/a0033465

Baker, C. E. (2014). African American fathers' depression and stress as predictors of father involvement during early childhood. *Journal of Black Psychology, 40*, 311–333. https://doi.org/10.1177/0095798413486480

Baker, C. E. (2016). African American and Hispanic fathers' work characteristics and preschool children's cognitive development. *Journal of Family Issues, 37*, 1514–1534. https://doi.org/10.1177/0182513X15576198

Baker, C. E., Vernon-Feagans, L., & The Family Life Project Investigators. (2015). Fathers' language input during shared book activities: Links to children's kindergarten achievement. *Journal of Applied Developmental Psychology, 36*, 53–59. https://doi.org/10.1016/j.appdev.2014.11.0090193-3973

Bates, E. (1976). *Language and context: The acquisition of pragmatics*. New York: Academic Press.

Belsky, J., Youngblade, L., Rovine, M., & Volling, B. (1991). Patterns of marital change and parent-child interaction. *Journal of Marriage and the Family, 53*(2), 487–498. https://doi.org/10.2307/352914

Bingham, G. E., Kwon, K., & Jeon, H. (2013). Examining relations among mothers', fathers', and children's language use in a dyadic and triadic context. *Early Child Development and Care, 183*, 394–414. https://doi.org/10.1080/03004430.2012.711590

Bornstein, M. H., Haynes, M. O., & Painter, K. M. (1998). Sources of child vocabulary competence: A multivariate model. *Journal of Child Language, 25*, 367–393.

Bratsch-Hines, M., Baker, C., & Vernon-Feagans, L. (2016). Rural ethnic minority youth and families in the United States: Theory, research, and applications. In L. J. Crocket & G. Carlo (Eds.), *Minority families in the United States: Family processes, child care, and early schooling* (pp. 143–164). New York: Springer.

Brody, G. H., Pellegrini, A. D., & Sigel, I. E. (1986). Marital quality and mother-child and father-child interactions with school-aged children. *Developmental Psychology, 22*, 291–296. https://doi.org/10.1037/0012-1649.22.3.291

Bronfenbrenner, U. (1986). The ecology of the family as a context for human development: Research perspectives. *Developmental Psychology, 22*, 723–742.

Bronfenbrenner, U., & Morris, P. A. (1998). The ecology of developmental processes. In W. Damon (Ed.), *Handbook of child psychology* (pp. 993–1028). New York: Wiley.

Bronte-Tinkew, J., Moore, K. A., Matthews, G., & Carrano, J. (2007). Symptoms of major depression in a sample of fathers of infants. *Journal of Family Issues, 28*, 61–99. https://doi.org/10.1177/0192513X06293609

Bruner, J. (1981). The social context of language acquisition. *Language and Communication, 1*, 155–178. https://doi.org/10.1016/0271-5309(81)90010-0

Cabrera, N. J., Fitzgerald, H. E., Bradley, R. H., & Roggman, L. (2014). The ecology of father-child relationships: An expanded model. *Journal of Family Theory & Review, 6*, 336–354. https://doi.org/10.1111/jftr.12054

Cabrera, N. J., Hofferth, S. L., & Chae, S. (2011). Patterns and predictors of father-infant engagement across race/ethnic groups. *Early Childhood Research Quarterly, 26*, 365–375. https://doi.org/10.1016/j.ecresq.2011.01.001

Cabrera, N. J., Shannon, J. D., & Tamis-LeMonda, C. (2007). Fathers' influence on their children's cognitive and emotional development: From toddlers to pre-K. *Applied Developmental Science, 11*, 208–213. https://doi.org/10.1080/10888690701762100

Cabrera, N. J., Tamis-LeMonda, C. S., Bradley, R. H., Hofferth, S., & Lamb, M. E. (2000). Fatherhood in the twenty-first century. *Child Development, 71*, 127–136. https://doi.org/10.1111/1467-8624.00126

Cabrera, N. J., Volling, B. L., & Barr, R. (2018). Fathers are parents too! Widening the lens on parenting for children's development. *Child Development Perspectives, 12*, 152–157. https://doi.org/10.1111/cdep.12275

Cools, S., Fiva, J. H., & Kirkeboen, L. J. (2015). Causal effects of paternity leave on children and parents. *Journal of Economics, 117*, 801–828. https://doi.org/10.1111/sjoe.12113

Doherty, W. J., Kouneski, E. F., & Erickson, M. F. (1998). Responsible fathering: An overview and conceptual framework. *Journal of Marriage and the Family, 60*, 277–292.

Dunst, C. J., Lowe, L. W., & Bartholomew, P. C. (1989). Contingent social responsiveness and infant communicative competence. *National Student Speech Language Hearing Association Journal, 17*, 39–49. https://doi.org/10.2307/353848

Duursma, E. (2016). Who does the reading, who does the talking? Low-income fathers and mothers in the US interacting with their young children around a picture book. *First Language, 36*, 465–484. https://doi.org/10.1177/0142723716648849

Duursma, E., Pan, B. A., & Raikes, H. (2008). Predictors and outcomes of low-income fathers' reading with their toddlers. *Early Childhood Research Quarterly, 23*, 351–365. https://doi.org/10.1016/j.ecresq.2008.06.001

Falk, N. H., Norris, K., & Quinn, M. G. (2014). The factors predicting stress, anxiety and depression in the parents of children with Autism. *Journal of Autism and Developmental Disorders, 44*, 3185–3203. https://doi.org/10.1007/s10803-014-2189-4

Fernald, A. (1989). Intonation and communicative intent in mothers' speech to infants: Is the melody the message? *Child Development, 60*, 1497–1510.

Flippin, M., & Crais, E. R. (2011). The need for more effective father involvement in early Autism invention: A systematic review and recommendations. *Journal of Early Intervention, 33*, 24–50. https://doi.org/10.1177/1053815111400415

Flippin, M., & Watson, L. R. (2015). Fathers' and mothers' verbal responsiveness and the language skills of young children with Autism Spectrum Disorder. *American Journal of Speech-Language Pathology, 24*, 400–410. https://doi.org/10.1044/2015_AJSLP-13-0138

Garcia-Lopez, C., Sarria, E., & Pozo, P. (2016). Multilevel approach to gender differences in adaption in father-mother dyads parenting individuals with Autism Spectrum Disorder. *Research in Autism Spectrum Disorders, 28*, 7–16. https://doi.org/10.1016/j.rasd.2016.04.003

Garfield, C. F., Duncan, G., Rutsohn, J., McDade, T. W., Adam, E. K., Coley, R. L., et al. (2014). A longitudinal study of paternal mental health during transition to fatherhood as young adults. *Pediatrics, 133*, 836–842. https://doi.org/10.1542/peds.2013-3262

Goldberg, W. A., & Easterbrooks, M. A. (1984). Role of marital quality in toddler development. *Developmental Psychology, 20*, 504–514. https://doi.org/10.1037/0012-1649.20.3.504

Gray, D. E. (2006). Coping over time: The parents of children with Autism. *Journal of Intellectual Disability Research, 50*, 970–976. https://doi.org/10.1111/j.1365-2788.00933.x

Grossman, F. K., Pollack, W. S., & Golding, E. (1988). Fathers and children: Predicting the quality and quantity of fathering. *Developmental Psychology, 24*, 82–91. https://doi.org/10.1037/0012-1649.24.1.82

Han, W. (2005). Maternal nonstandard work schedules and child cognitive outcomes. *Child Development, 76*, 137–154. https://doi.org/10.1111/j.1467-8624.2005.00835.x

Harper, A., Dyckes, T. T., Harper, J., Roper, S. O., & South, M. (2013). Respite care, marital quality, and stress in parents of children with Autism Spectrum Disorders. *Journal of Autism and Developmental Disorders, 43*, 2604–2616. https://doi.org/10.1007/s10803-013-1812-0

Hastings, R. P., Kovshoff, H., Brown, T., Ward, N. J., Espinosa, F. D., & Remington, B. (2005). Coping strategies in mothers and fathers of preschool and school-age children with Autism. *Autism, 9*, 377–391. https://doi.org/10.1177/1363361305056078

Hoff-Ginsberg, E. (1991). Mother-child conversation in different social classes and communicative settings. *Child Development, 62*, 782–796. https://doi.org/10.2307/1131177

Huerta, M. C., Adema, W., Baxter, J., Han, W., Lausten, M., Lee, R., et al. (2014). Fathers' leave and fathers' involvement: Evidence from four OECD countries. *European Journal of Social Security, 16*, 308–346. https://doi.org/10.1177/138826271401600403

Huttenlocher, J., Haight, W., Bryk, A., Seltzer, M., & Lyons, T. (1991). Early vocabulary growth: Relation to language input and gender. *Developmental Psychology, 27*, 236–248. https://doi.org/10.1037/0012-1649.27.2.236

Huttenlocher, J., Waterfall, H., Vasilyeva, M., Vevea, J., & Hedges, L. V. (2010). Sources of variability in children' language growth. *Cognitive Psychology, 61*, 343–365. https://doi.org/10.1016/j.cogpsych.2010.08.002

Jones, J., & Mosher, W. D. (2013). Fathers' involvement with their children: United States, 2006–2010. *National Health Statistics Reports, 71*, 1–22. Retrieved from http://www.cdc.gov/nchs/data/nhsr/nhsr071.pdf

Kavanaugh, R. D., & Jirkovsky, A. M. (1982). Parental speech to young children: A longitudinal analysis. *Merrill-Palmer Quarterly, 28*, 297–311.

Kitamura, C., & Burnham, D. (2003). Pitch and communicative intent in mother's speech: Adjustments for age and sex in the first year. *Infancy, 4*, 85–110. https://doi.org/10.1207/S15327078IN0401_5

Kitzmann, K. M. (2000). Effects of marital conflict on subsequent triadic family interactions and parenting. *Developmental Psychology, 36*, 3–13. https://doi.org/10.1037/0012-1649.36.1.3

Kuhl, P. K. (2007). Is speech learning 'gated' by the social brain? *Developmental Science, 10*, 110–120. https://doi.org/10.1111/j.1467-7687.2007.00572.x

Kwon, K., Bingham, G., Lewsader, J., Jeon, H., & Elicker, J. (2013). Structure task versus free play: The influence of social context on parenting quality, toddlers' engagement with parents and play behaviors, and parent-toddler language use. *Child Youth and Care Forum, 42*, 207–224. https://doi.org/10.1007/s10566-013-9198-x

Leaper, C., Anderson, K. J., & Sanders, P. (1998). Moderators of gender effects on parents' talk to their children: A meta-analysis. *Developmental Psychology, 34*, 3–27. https://doi.org/10.1037/0012-1649.34.1.3

Livingston, G. (2013). The rise of single fathers: A ninefold increase since 1960. *Pew Research Center*. Retrieved from http://www.pewsocialtrends.org/2013/07/02/the-rise-of-single-fathers/

MacDonald, E. E., & Hastings, R. P. (2010). Fathers of children with developmental disabilities. In M. E. Lamb (Ed.), *The role of the father in child development* (pp. 486–516). Hoboken, NJ: Wiley.

Majorano, M., Rainieri, C., & Corsano, P. (2013). Parents' child-directed communication and child language development: A longitudinal study with Italian toddlers. *Journal of Child Language, 40*, 836–859. https://doi.org/10.1017/S0305000912000323

Malin, J. L., Cabrera, N. J., & Rowe, M. L. (2014). Low-income minority mothers' and fathers' reading and children's receptive vocabulary skills. *Early Childhood Research Quarterly, 29*, 425–432. https://doi.org/10.1016/j.ecresq.2014.04.010

Malin, J. L., Karberg, E., Cabrera, N. J., Rowe, M., Cristaforo, T., & Tamis-LeMonda, C. S. (2012). Father-toddler communication in low-income families: The role of paternal education and depressive symptoms. *Family Science, 3*, 155–163. https://doi.org/10.1080/19424620.2012.779423

Marsiglio, W. (1991). Paternal engagement activities with minor children. *Journal of Marriage and the Family, 53*, 973–986. https://doi.org/10.2307/353001

McRoberts, G. W., & Best, C. T. (1997). Accommodation in mean fo during mother-infant and father-infant vocal interactions: A longitudinal case study. *Journal of Child Language, 24*, 719–736.

Meadan, H., Halle, J. W., & Ebata, A. T. (2010). Families with children who have Autism Spectrum Disorders: Stress and support. *Exceptional Children, 77*, 7–36. https://doi.org/10.1177/001440291007700101

Minuchin, P. (1985). Families and individual development: Provocations from the field of family therapy. *Child Development, 56*, 289–302.

Mueller, T. G., & Buckley, P. C. (2014). Odd man out: How fathers navigate the special education system. *Remedial and Special Education, 35*, 40–49. https://doi.org/10.1177/0741932513513176

NICHD Early Child Care Research Network. (2000). Factors associated with fathers' caregiving activities and sensitivity with young children. *Journal of Family Psychology, 14*, 200–219. https://doi.org/10.1037/0893-3200.14.2.200

NICHD Early Child Care Research Network. (2005). Pathways to reading: The role of oral language in the transition to reading. *Developmental Psychology, 41*, 428–442. https://doi.org/10.1037/0012-1649.41.2.428

Ninio, A., & Bruner, J. (1976). The achievement and antecedents of labeling. *Journal of Child Language, 5*, 1–15. https://doi.org/10.1017/S0305000900001896

Pan, B. A., Rowe, M. L., Singer, J. D., & Snow, C. E. (2005). Maternal correlates of growth in toddler vocabulary production in low-income families. *Child Development, 76*, 763–782. https://doi.org/10.1111/j.1467-8624.2005.00876.x

Pancsofar, N., Petroff, J., & Lewis, A. (2017). Father friendly classrooms: Making a space for dads of children with disabilities. *Teaching Exceptional Children, 49*, 309–317. https://doi.org/10.1177/0040059916681826

Pancsofar, N., Petroff, J. G., Rao, S., & Mangel, A. (2019). "What I want to do as a father is be there:" constructions of school involvement for fathers of children with complex disabilities. *Research and Practice for Persons with Severe Disabilities, 44*, 153–168. https://doi.org/10.1177/1540796919843147

Pancsofar, N., & Vernon-Feagans, L. (2006). Mother and father language input to young children: Contributions to later language development. *Journal of Applied Developmental Psychology, 27*, 571–587. https://doi.org/10.1016/j.appdev.2006.08.003

Pancsofar, N., Vernon-Feagans, L., Odom, E., & Roe, J. R. (2008). Family relationships during infancy and later mother and father vocabulary use with young children. *Early Childhood Research Quarterly, 23*, 493–503. https://doi.org/10.1016/j.ecresq.2008.07.001

Pancsofar, N., Vernon-Feagans, L., Odom, E., & The Family Life Project Investigators. (2013). Work experiences and father vocabulary to infants in African American families in low-income rural communities. *Journal of Applied Developmental Psychology, 34*, 73–81. https://doi.org/10.1016/jappdev.2012.11.005

Pancsofar, N., Vernon-Feagans, L., & The Family Life Project Investigators. (2010). Fathers' early contributions to children's language development in families from low-income rural communities. *Early Childhood Research Quarterly, 25*, 450–463. https://doi.org/10.1016/j.ecresq.2010.02.001

Paulson, J. F., Keefe, H. A., & Leiferman, J. A. (2009). Early parental depression and child language development. *Journal of Child Psychology and Psychiatry, 50*, 254–262. https://doi.org/10.1111/j.1469-7610.2008.01973.x

Potter, C. A. (2017). Father involvement in the care, play and education of children with Autism. *Journal of Intellectual and Developmental Disability, 42*, 375–384. https://doi.org/10.3109/13668250.2016.1245851

Pratt, M. W., Kerig, P. K., Cowan, P. A., & Cowan, C. P. (1992). Family worlds: Couple satisfaction, parenting style, and mothers' and fathers' speech to young children. *Merrill-Palmer Quarterly, 38*, 245–262.

Ratner, N. B. (2013). Why talk with children matters: Clinical implications of infant- and child-directed speech research. *Seminars in Speech and Language, 34*, 203–2014. https://doi.org/10.1055/s-0033-1353449

Reynolds, E., Vernon-Feagans, L., Bratsch-Hines, M., Baker, C. E., & The Family Life Project Key Investigators. (2018). Mothers' and fathers' language input from 6 to 36 months in rural two-parent-families: Relations to children's kindergarten achievement. *Early Childhood Research Quarterly, 47*, 385–395. https://doi.org/10.1016/j.ecresq.2018.09.002

Rivard, M., Terroux, A., Parent-Boursier, C., & Mercier, C. (2014). Determinants of stress in parents of children with Autism Spectrum Disorders. *Journal of Autism and Developmental Disorders, 44*, 1609–1620. https://doi.org/10.1007/s10803-013-2028-z

Rondal, J. A. (1980). Fathers' and mothers' speech in early language development. *Journal of Child Language, 7*, 353–369. https://doi.org/10.1017/S0305000900002671

Roopnarine, J. L., Fouts, H. N., Lamb, M. E., & Lewis-Elligan, T. Y. (2005). Mothers' and fathers' behaviors toward their 3- to 4- month old infants in lower, middle, and upper socioeconomic African American families. *Developmental Psychology, 41*, 723–732. https://doi.org/10.1037/0012-1649.41.5.723

Rowe, M. L. (2008). Child-directed speech: Relation to socioeconomic status, knowledge of child development and child vocabulary skill. *Journal of Child Language, 35*, 185–205. https://doi.org/10.1017/S0305000907008343

Rowe, M. L., Coker, D., & Pan, B. A. (2004). A comparison of fathers' and mothers' talk to toddlers in low-income families. *Social Development, 13*, 278–291. https://doi.org/10.1111/j.1467-9507.2004.000267.x

Rowe, M. L., Leech, K. A., & Cabrera, N. (2017). Going beyond input quantity: *Wh*- questions matter for toddlers' language and cognitive development. *Cognitive Science, 41*, 162–179. https://doi.org/10.1111/cogs.12349

Salo, V. C., Rowe, M., Leech, K. A., & Cabrera, N. J. (2016). Low-income fathers' speech to toddlers during book reading versus toy play. *Journal of Child Language, 43*, 1385–1399. https://doi.org/10.1017/S0305000915000550

Schwab, J. F., Rowe, M. L., Cabrera, N., & Lew-Williams, C. (2018). Fathers' repetition of words is coupled with children's vocabularies. *Journal of Experimental Child Psychiatry, 166*, 437–450. https://doi.org/10.1016/j.jecp.2017.09.012022-0965

Sethna, V., Murray, L., & Rachandani, P. G. (2012). Depressed fathers' speech to their 3-month-old infants: A study of cognitive and mentalizing features in paternal speech. *Psychological Medicine, 42*, 2361–2371. https://doi.org/10.1017/S0033291712000487

Sims, J., & Coley, R. L. (2016). Independent contributions of mothers' and fathers' language and literacy practices: Associations with children's kindergarten skills across linguistically diverse households. *Early Education and Development, 27*, 495–512. https://doi.org/10.1080/10409289.2016.1091973

Snow, C. E. (1977). Mothers' speech research: From input to interaction. In C. E. Snow & C. A. Ferguson (Eds.), *Talk to children: Language input and acquisition* (pp. 31–49). Cambridge, MA: Cambridge University Press.

Snow, C. E., Perlman, R., & Nathan, D. (1987). Why routines are different: Toward a multiple-factors model of the relation between input and language acquisition. In K. E. Nelson & A. Van Kleek (Eds.), *Children's language* (Vol. 6, pp. 65–98). Hillsdale, NJ: Lawrence Erlbaum Associates.

Stewart, W., & Barling, J. (1996). Fathers' work experiences effect children's behaviors via job-related affect and parenting behaviors. *Journal of Organizational Behavior, 17*, 221–232. https://doi.org/10.1002/(SICI)1099-1379(199605)17:3%3C221::AID-JOB741%3E3.0.CO;2-G

Tamis-LeMonda, C., Baumwell, L., & Cristofaro, T. (2012). Parent-child conversations during play. *First Language, 32*, 413–438. https://doi.org/10.1177/0142723711419321

Tamis-LeMonda, C. S., Kuchirko, Y., & Song, L. (2014). Why is infant language learning facilitated by parental responsiveness? *Current Directions in Psychological Science, 23*, 21–126. https://doi.org/10.1177/0963721414522813

Tomasello, M. (1992). The social bases of language acquisition. *Social Development, 1*, 67–87. https://doi.org/10.1111/j.1467-9507.1992.tb00135.x

Varghese, C., & Wachen, J. (2016). The determinants of father involvement and connections to children's literacy and language outcomes: Review of the literature. *Marriage & Family Review, 52*, 331–359. https://doi.org/10.1080/01494929.2015.1099587

Volling, B. L., & Belsky, J. (1991). Multiple determinants of father involvement during infancy in dual-earner and single-earner families. *Journal of Marriage and the Family, 53*, 461–474. https://doi.org/10.2307/352912

Vygotsky, L. S. (1962). *Though and language*. Cambridge, MA: MIT Press.

Walker, D., Greenwood, C., Hart, B., & Carta, J. (1994). Prediction of school outcomes based on early language production and socioeconomic factors. *Child Development, 65*, 606–621. https://doi.org/10.2307/1131404

Warren, S. F., Yoder, P. J., & Leew, S. V. (2001). Promoting social-communicative development in infants and toddlers. In H. Goldstein, L. A. Kaczmarek, & K. M. English (Eds.), *Promoting social communication:*

Children with developmental disabilities from birth to adolescence (pp. 121–149). Baltimore, MD: Paul Brookes.

Weizman, Z. O., & Snow, C. E. (2001). Lexical input as related to children's vocabulary acquisition: Effects of sophisticated exposure and support for meaning. *Developmental Psychology, 37*, 265–279. https://doi.org/10.1037/0012-1649.37.2.265

Yeung, W. J., Sandberg, J. F., Davis-Kean, P. E., & Hofferth, S. L. (2001). Children's time with fathers in intact families. *Journal of Marriage and the Family, 63*, 136–154. https://doi.org/10.1111/j.1741-3737.2001.00136.x

Zauche, L. H., Thul, T. A., Darcy Mahoney, A. E., & Stapel-Wax, J. L. (2016). Influence of language nutrition on children's language and cognitive development: An integrated review. *Early Childhood Research Quarterly, 36*, 318–333. https://doi.org/10.1016/jecresq.2016.01.015

Zhang, Y., Jin, X., Shen, X., Zhang, J., & Hoff, E. (2008). Correlates of early language development in Chinese children. *International Journal of Behavioral Development, 32*, 145–151. https://doi.org/10.1177/0165025407087213

Fathers Talking and Reading with Their 3-Year-Olds During Shared Bookreading

24

Elisabeth Duursma, Cheryl Jialing Ho, Michelle L. Townsend, Brin F. Grenyer, and Jane S. Herbert

Children's language and literacy development benefits when adults engage with them in cognitively stimulating activities such as shared bookreading (e.g., Baker, Vernon-Feagans, and the Family Life Project Investigators, 2015; Mol and Bus, 2011). The vast majority of studies on shared bookreading have focused on mother-child interactions (REF). The small number of studies that have considered father engagement in reading have primarily compared reading frequency or vocabulary of fathers to that of mothers (Baker, 2013; Baker, Vernon-Feagans, & the Family Life Project Investigators, 2015). Given the growing recognition that there is a lack of research on father's unique contribution to child development (Cabrera, Volling, & Barr, 2018), and that the early learning opportunities provided in the home environment predict children's later academic achievement (Son & Morrison, 2010), it is important to better understand the ways in which fathers and children engage in conversations during shared bookreading.

In this chapter, we review what is currently known about the importance of the home literacy environment and shared bookreading on children's language and literacy development. We then turn our attention to emerging knowledge about fathers' engagement in shared bookreading with their children and the benefits that brings to children's language and literacy skills. Finally, we present preliminary data showing the diversity and responsiveness with which fathers in two-parent families and their 3-year-olds talk together during a bookreading interaction. We aim to provide new insight into how fathers and children talk about the story and respond to each other during this valuable learning activity.

The Home Literacy Environment

One of the key contributors to children's language and literacy development is the home literacy environment (HLE) (Hartas, 2012; Niklas & Schneider, 2013). The HLE refers to a range of diverse activities and experiences in the home such as shared bookreading, singing songs, telling stories, writing letters, and playing with alphabet blocks that promote children's literacy development (Van Tonder, Alison, & Nicholson, 2019). Researchers have distinguished the HLE as either *active* or *passive* (Bracken & Fischel,

E. Duursma (✉)
School of Education, University of Wollongong, Wollongong, NSW, Australia
e-mail: eduursma@uow.edu.au

C. J. Ho · J. S. Herbert
School of Psychology and Early Start, University of Wollongong, Wollongong, NSW, Australia

M. L. Townsend · B. F. Grenyer
Illawarra Health and Medical Research Institute and School of Psychology, University of Wollongong, Wollongong, NSW, Australia

H. E. Fitzgerald et al. (eds.), *Handbook of Fathers and Child Development*,
https://doi.org/10.1007/978-3-030-51027-5_24

2008; Myrtil, Justice, & Jiang, 2019). An active HLE refers to children's direct participation in and exposure to literacy activities such as shared bookreading, storytelling, and singing songs (Myrtil et al., 2019). Singing songs is known to help increase phonemic and phonological awareness (Hansen & Milligan, 2012). Additionally, singing can promote oral language skills as well as the understanding of concepts such as sequence and patterning (Connors, 2014) as well as children's lexical acquisition and semantic knowledge (Heydon, McKee, & O'Neill, 2018; Winters & Griffin, 2014). Telling stories can help children understand the world in which they live, and listening to stories and discussing them can support their literacy skills such as listening skills and learning about narratives (e.g., Büyüköztürk, Kiliç Çakmak, Akgün, Karadeniz, & Demirel, 2012; Justice & Kaderavek, 2002; Yazici & Bolay, 2017). The passive HLE refers to children's indirect learning through observing family members engaging in literacy activities such as parents reading for themselves, parental beliefs, and attitudes toward literacy (Myrtil et al., 2019). The active HLE is a stronger predictor of children's emergent literacy outcomes than the passive HLE (Burgess, Hech, & Lonigan, 2002; Foster, Froyen, Skibbe, Bowles, & Decker, 2016; Myrtil et al., 2019).

Shared bookreading is one of the most researched activities within the HLE literature as it is a common and highly valued practice in Western culture (e.g., Noble et al., 2019) and is associated with positive literacy development (Mol & Bus, 2011; Raikes et al., 2006; Van Tonder et al., 2019). Bookreading can support early language skills including vocabulary (Farrant & Zubrick, 2011), narrative and conversation skills (Thierry & Sparks, 2019), print awareness (Justice & Ezell, 2000), and phonological awareness (Lefebvre, Trudeau, & Sutton, 2011; Noble et al., 2019). Several meta-analyses have shown positive relationships between the amount of time children spend actively engaged in shared bookreading with an adult and emergent literacy skills, phonics, and reading comprehension (Barnes & Puccioni, 2017; Mol, Bus, & de Jong, 2009). Shared bookreading is also known to promote children's oral language and vocabulary skills (e.g., Mol et al., 2009; Wasik, Hindman, & Snell, 2016) and plays a crucial role in the development of the knowledge required for success in independent reading (Mol & Bus, 2011; Samuelsson et al., 2005).

Although several meta-analyses of the effects of shared bookreading (e.g., Mol & Bus, 2011; Noble et al., 2019) have shown small effect sizes, Noble et al. (2019) argue that shared bookreading often includes several potentially language-boosting behaviors which are linked to positive language outcomes. For example, adults tend to use more complex language when sharing a book with a child compared to a play situation (Cameron-Faulkner & Noble, 2013; Noble, Cameron-Faulkner, & Lieven, 2018), which is related to better language skills (Huttenlocher, Vasilyeva, Cymerman, & Levine, 2002). In addition, shared bookreading promotes high levels of joint attention, contingent talk, and responsiveness which are linked to positive language outcomes (Farrant & Zubrick, 2013; McGillion, Pine, Herbert, & Matthews, 2017; Noble et al., 2019).

Although a high frequency of shared bookreading is valuable, the quality or style of the interaction is perhaps even more important for children's language and literacy development (Reese, Cox, Harte, & McAnally, 2003). Different terms have been used to describe parent-child interactions around a book which promote early literacy by actively engaging the child with the story. Hindman, Connor, Jewkes, and Morrison (2008) call this *meaning-related talk* which focuses on labelling and description of illustrations, talking about new words and ideas, and connecting the text or illustrations to children's prior knowledge but also predictions and inferences. Whitehurst (1994) talks about *dialogic reading* or *interactive reading* that promotes children's language and literacy development (e.g., Whitehurst, 1994). When adults engage in dialogic reading, they create a "dialogue" with the child around the book by using techniques such as asking questions, giving feedback, and assisting in having the child become the narrator of the story (e.g., Duursma, 2016; Whitehurst, 1994).

When children are exposed to dialogic reading, they tend to have better expressive language skills and use more complex words and longer utterances compared to children whose parents simply read them the words in the book (Whitehurst, 1994; Zevenbergen & Whitehurst, 2003). Another term used for the interactive talk around bookreading is *non-immediate talk*. This is talk that goes beyond the text and the illustrations and is used to make connections with the child's own experiences to make predictions, offer explanations, or discuss the meaning of words. Non-immediate talk is known to be related to children's later vocabulary development and emergent literacy skills (De Temple & Snow, 2003). Non-immediate talk offers children the opportunity to understand and use more difficult words which are required to discuss the internal states of the characters, to evaluate the book, and to evaluate the story and the illustrations and make predictions (De Temple & Snow, 2003).

One of the most influential components of shared bookreading is that adults and children have the opportunity to engage in conversations which can contribute to the construction of meaning within the shared context (Barnes & Puccioni, 2017; Halliday, 2004). Wide and extensive shared bookreading provides the opportunity for the adult to support their child in explaining the meaning of words as children encounter many words that are used relatively infrequently in everyday conversations. Hayes and Ahrens (1988) showed that everyday conversations and popular TV shows seldom included rare words while picture books did, thereby offering a unique learning opportunity for children. Language input is the key predictor of the speed with which children acquire new words, so when children are exposed to more words per unit of time, and a greater variety of words, they will learn more words (De Temple & Snow, 2003; Henderson, Devine, Weighall, & Gaskell, 2015). Through repeated bookreading and discussion, young children become able to understand and use new words (Flack, Field, & Horst, 2018).

Children also more easily learn words that have high affective values. Words with high affective values are those referring to the names of people important to the child or enjoyable activities such as peekaboo (De Temple & Snow, 2003; Ninio & Snow, 1996). Words that are presented in isolation, or in very simple sentences, words that are stressed, and words that are in initial or final positions within utterances are also learned more easily (De Temple & Snow, 2003; Larragueta & Ceballos-Viro, 2018).

As children's vocabularies grow, it becomes easier for them to learn an increasing number of new words due to the *paradigm effect* (De Temple & Snow, 2003). This means that children start to understand pattern-like or paradigm relationships between words and are able to rapidly learn new words that fit within these models. For example, when children learn the words for different types of animals such as dog, cat, or rabbit, then less frequently used animal names such as octopus, flamingo, or wombat become easier to learn. This occurs because children already have a basic knowledge of animal names to which they can efficiently add new animal names (De Temple & Snow, 2003). Thus, shared bookreading quickly builds the child's vocabulary.

The contribution of shared bookreading to children's language and literacy development will depend on how parents engage with their child around a book (Aram, Bergman Deitcher, & Adar, 2017). Picture books with high-quality narratives support parent-child interactions around the book (Hoffman, Teale, & Yokota, 2015). These books are characterized by using unfamiliar words, as well as using familiar words in different ways, also called figurative language (Hoffman et al., 2015). When books contain complex language, adults might be more inclined to refer to this type of language during shared bookreading (Pentimonti, Zucker, & Justice, 2011).

Parent-child bookreading can be considered a three-way conversation with the parent, the child, and the book being the discourse partners (Breit-Smith, van Kleeck, Prendeville, & Pan, 2017; Fletcher & Reese, 2005). Parent and child work together to create the *fictional narrative* (Breit-Smith et al., 2017). Shared bookreading fits within Vygotsky's (1978) sociocultural theory where social interactions between children and more competent members of a culture provide the context in which children attain the knowledge and competencies to become a participant in their community (Sparks & Reese, 2012). Parent-child interactions form a key component of children's development, and variations in quantity and quality of these interactions can lead to different child outcomes (Sparks & Reese, 2012; Vygotsky, 1978). Bookreading fits within Vygotsky's Zone of Proximal Development which refers to the difference between what a child can do independently and what a child can do with the help of a more skilled other (Vygotsky, 1978). Parents help guide, or scaffold, children through the book using verbal utterances and gestures, adjusting for the child's developmental level. Scaffolding refers to the adult or more competent other helping the child expand the boundaries of what they can learn on their own (Barnyak & McNelly, 2016; Vygotksy, 1978). The book, even though inanimate, also serves as a discourse partner as the words used in the text contribute to the conversation between parent and child (Breit-Smith et al., 2017). Learning occurs within Vygotsky's Zone of Proximal Development via meaningful and scaffolded interactions with adults or other more competent others. However, adults do need to take the child's needs and knowledge into consideration and use different strategies (Barnyak & McNelly, 2016; Vygotsky, 1978). For example, the adult needs to have some idea of which words in a book the child understands and which words need an explanation. Bookreading provides an opportunity to expose children to decontextualized language (Snow, 1990) or language removed from the here and now (Rowe, 2012). When children are exposed to this more challenging type of talk, parents can help them practice for the language used in schools (Rowe, 2012).

Bruner (1981) argues that parents play an active role in children's language acquisition by fine-tuning their speech to the level of the child. They adapt their language to the level at which the child operates in terms of semantics, syntax, sentence length, and complexity and move ahead with the child at a rate that shows sensitivity to the child's progress (Bruner, 1981). Bookreading offers a unique opportunity to evaluate how parents, in this case fathers, "fine-tune" or adapt their speech to their child as they discuss the story line and meaning of new words or connect event in the book to the child's experiences.

Fathers and Bookreading

Fathers play a significant and unique role in children's development (Cabrera, Fitzgerald, Bradley, & Roggman, 2007; Cano, Perales, & Baxter, 2018; Sarkadi, Kristiansson, Oberklaid, & Bremberg, 2008). Family research originally focused primarily on the role of mothers, with fathers having been comparatively left out of research (Cabrera et al., 2018; Lamb, 2010). In the past two decades though, fathers have been recognized as playing a crucial role within the family context (Goeke-Morey & Cummings, 2007). It is important to include fathers' influence on child development as fathers could contribute more to some aspects of child development or in different ways than mothers (Goeke-Morey & Cummings, 2007). Father involvement contributes to family functioning and stability and also impacts child outcomes such as emotional regulation (Bocknek, Brophy-Herb, Fitzgerald, Schiffman, & Vogel, 2014), child literacy, and language development (Varghese & Wachen, 2016). Father involvement can be viewed within Bronfenbrenner's ecological systems theory which conceptualizes the developing child within its immediate as well as broader contexts of family, educational settings, community, and society (Bronfenbrenner, 1979, 1994). Bronfenbrenner (1979) described the ecological systems model "as a set of nested structures, each inside the next, like Russian dolls" (p. 3). The child is placed at the center and surrounded by the different systems: microsystem, mesosystem, exosystem, macrosystem, and chronosystem. Father-child interactions can be placed within Bronfenbrenner's theory of proximal processes (Bronfenbrenner & Morris, 2006). These processes are reciprocal and become increasingly more complex exchanges between individuals, and they are the drivers of development.

Foster et al. (2016) argue that the activities in which fathers engage with their children are important for children's development and essential to completely understand children's early experiences in the home. Research has shown that fathers and mothers engage in different ways with their children around a book (e.g., Baker, Vernon-Feagans, and the Family Life Project Investigators, 2015; Duursma, 2016). These differences can result in differences in child outcomes such as cognitive and language skills (Duursma, Pan, & Raikes, 2008) and are important to examine in order to better understand child development.

Most of the research on shared bookreading has focused on mothers' reading to their children as mothers are often considered the primary caregiver. To date, only small body of research has paid attention to fathers' reading to their children (Duursma, 2016; Baker, Vernon-Feagans, & the Family Life Project Investigators, 2015. It has also been suggested that men might be less likely to be involved in an activity that is seen as more "appropriate" or within the space of mother's involvement (Nutbrown, Clough, Stammers, Emblin, & Alston-Smith, 2019). Some researchers have suggested that fathers may not value reading with young children (Fletcher & Daly, 2002), and mothers might hold stronger beliefs regarding their own ability to help children in their literacy skills compared to fathers (Lynch, 2002). In a case study of two families conducted by Karther (2002), fathers reported leaving the bookreading to their wives as they considered her the primary caregiver or they did not feel confident enough in their reading abilities to read to children.

Research has demonstrated that when fathers read books with their children, they are less likely to do so on a frequent basis (Duursma et al., 2008) and tend to be less engaged during bookreading (Clark, 2009). However, fathers' reading to their children has been shown to be linked to children's outcomes, in particular language skills (e.g., Duursma et al., 2008; Foster et al., 2016). In a study of over 5000 children aged 24 months, Baker (2014) found that fathers who participated in more home literacy activities, which included shared bookreading, singing songs, and telling stories, had children with better reading, math, and social emotional outcomes at age 4. Foster et al. (2016) found in their study of 379 fathers of preschoolers that even though fathers engaged less frequently in home learning activities than mothers, their engagement in HLE activities (as measured by an HLE parenting questionnaire asking about helping children with literacy or maths activities) was a significant predictor of children's academic skills which included decoding, letter knowledge, and mathematics. In a study of 405 families, fathers and mothers from disadvantaged areas were asked about their engagement in literacy activities in the home with their 2-year-olds (Quach et al., 2018), including number of books in the home, frequency of reading each week, and type of parent-child reading interaction. Children's emergent literacy skills and language skills were assessed at age 4 using standardized assessments. Results showed that fathers' home reading practices at age 2 predicted children's expressive and receptive language at age 4, even after accounting for mothers' home reading practices and child vocabulary and communication skills at age 2 (Quach et al., 2018).

Most of these studies have focused on frequency of bookreading, while less is known about what fathers actually do during the shared bookreading interaction. Duursma (2016) reported that low-income fathers used more non-immediate talk and more engagement strategies during shared bookreading with their 2- and 3-year-olds than mothers did. Schwab, Rowe, Cabrera, and Lew-Williams (2018) reported that in their study of 24 low-income families, fathers of children with larger vocabularies used less repetition during shared bookreading, and repetition in fathers' input at child age 24 months was not predictive of children's receptive vocabulary at 24 months or verbal reasoning abilities at 36 months. The authors suggest that specific features of input are more or less helpful in promoting vocabulary at different stages in language development (Schwab et al., 2018). Low-income fathers talked more, used more diverse vocabulary, and asked more questions during bookreading than during toy play with their 2-year-olds, demonstrating that different contexts elicit particular qualities of paternal speech that could promote young children's language learning in different ways. In turn, children provided more labels (Salo, Rowe, Leech, & Cabrera, 2016). Fathers also used more metalingual talk than mothers during shared bookreading, and parental reading quality contributed to children's vocabulary. Children's interest in reading mediated the association between maternal and paternal metalingual talk and children's receptive vocabulary (Malin, Cabrera, & Rowe, 2014).

A study conducted by Baker, Vernon-Feagans, and the Family Life Project Investigators (2015) found that more educated fathers who also used more complex language during shared bookreading had children with better emergent literacy and numeracy-related skills in kindergarten compared to less educated fathers who used less complex language. However, a large gap remains in our knowledge of how fathers engage their children during bookreading. In our current research in this area, we have been looking at fathers' interactions with their children around picture books and examining the relationship between father and child talk, as well as the association with child language.

As mothers still tend to spend more time with their children engaged in learning activities such as shared bookreading, both mothers and fathers might not be aware of the significant contributions fathers can make in this area to children's development (Foster et al., 2016). Foster et al. (2016) argue that fathers could be an "untapped, and potentially highly influential resource," in particular in promoting academic competence.

To replicate and extend the findings of Duursma (2016), we recently conducted a study exploring the use of immediate and non-immediate talk in a different sample (Australian middle-class families). In this study, we focused on the ways fathers in two-parent families read and talk while sharing a book with their 3-year-olds. The research questions were as follows:

1. How do fathers use immediate and non-immediate talk while sharing a book with their 3-year-olds?
2. How do children respond to fathers' use of immediate and non-immediate talk?
3. What is the relationship between child and paternal language use (e.g., immediate and non-immediate talk) and child vocabulary?

In the final part of this chapter, we present the preliminary findings from this research.

Methods

Participants

Participating families were part of the Illawarra Born cross generational health study (for further details on this cohort, see Townsend et al., 2019). This longitudinal study recruited women during pregnancy and has conducted the following data collection waves: 22 and 30 weeks gestation during pregnancy, linkage with birth hospital records, and infant age 7–10 weeks, 6 months, 1 year, 2 years, and 3 years. Of the original cohort of 42 women, 36 were available to be contacted by phone and email, and 30 agreed to participate in a 3-year data collection wave. Fathers were then recruited through the participating mothers. All of the fathers resided with the mothers and were the biological father of the participating children. Of the 30 families, two families chose not to participate in the father-child activity recorded at home, two families did not return the recording devices, and one family did not have a father figure present in the home. An additional four father-child dyads participated but were excluded due to the presence of an additional sibling during the recorded activity. The final sample for the current study therefore consisted of 21 father-child dyads.

Fathers in the current study ranged in age from 31 to 50 years. Their highest level of educational qualification was 38% university degree, 42% TAFE/diploma degree (similar to American community college), 10% finished year 12, and 10% finished year 10. Children ranged in age from 37 to 46 months old ($M = 42.48$ months, $SD = 2.73$). There were 12 boys and 9 girls, who were all reported to be typically developing. All participating dyads were English speaking and were able to read the book together.

Child Assessments

Early Years Toolbox Expressive Vocabulary Test (EYT) Children's expressive language was assessed using the EYT. The EYT consists of 54 items and requires children to verbally produce the correct label for each shown stimulus (Howard & Melhuish, 2017). The EYT is administered using an app on an iPad where participants respond verbally and the data collector records the response on the app. When a participant labels a stimulus incorrectly, the data collector asks the participant "what else might this be called?" until the child either produces the correct answer or is unable to produce the correct response. After six incorrect responses, the app ceases automatically. The expressive vocabulary component of the EYT was found to demonstrate high test-retest reliability and convergent validity (Howard & Melhuish, 2017). This assessment has been used successfully with children aged 2.5–6 years, with good internal consistency and convergent validity in a large and demographically diverse Australian sample (Howard & Melhuish, 2017). Cronbach's alpha for the measure was $\alpha = 0.92$. The standardized *Mean* for children aged 3:0–3:5 was 16.68 ($SD = 7.20$), and for children ages 3:6–3:11, the *Mean* was 20.35 ($SD = 7.28$).

Picture Book For this study, we selected the developmentally appropriate picture book, *Mopoke* (2017) by Philip Bunting (Scholastic Australia). *Mopoke* is an Australian picture book about an owl (mopoke is the smallest owl species in Australia). The 48-page book won the Children's Book Council Australia's (CBCA) Picture Book of the Year Award-Honour Book in 2018. The book has few words, and each page shows a mopoke on a branch with a different outfit or appearance. For example, on one page, there is a small mopoke on the page, and the accompanying words read "a weepoke" where another page shows a mopoke in the snow and reads "a snowpoke." The book was chosen to elicit verbal responses from both father and child. In addition, the short storylines were also constructed such that readers can grasp the pattern of the book easily and encourage unique personal interpretation of the book when reading to the child.

Procedure

As part of the larger longitudinal study on health and well-being, mothers completed an online questionnaire pack on their psychological well-being and attended a 1-hour session at the University of Wollongong with their child (age 3). A range of tasks relating to mother-child interaction and children's social-emotional development were conducted during the lab session, with only the child's language measure included in the current analyses. At the end of the lab session, mothers were provided with a copy of *Mopoke,* father-child task instructions, and a digital voice recorder. Additional at-home activities (a father-child numeracy task and a dinnertime conversation task) were also explained at this point but are unrelated to the current study and not discussed further. A researcher arranged to collect the recording device, and the completed father informed consent form, the following day or at a convenient time.

Instructions provided for the fathers asked them to read the book with their child at home "as they normally would" and to record the entire bookreading session. No further instructions or suggested time limits were given. The duration taken for this shared bookreading activity ranged from 2.5 minutes to 14.36 minutes ($M = 5.07$, $SD = 2.59$).

Ethical approval was provided by the University of Wollongong Human Research Ethics Committee.

Transcription, Coding, and Analysis

All participants were identified by their participant number (ID). The recordings were then manually transcribed using the CHAT conventions of the Child Language Data Exchange System (CHILDES) (MacWhinney, 2000), and the written transcripts of both the father and the child's speech were then coded for data analysis. The unit of transcription was the utterance, which was determined by every pause, a change in conversational turn, or a change in intonational pattern (Demir, Applebaum, Levine, Petty, & Goldin-Meadow, 2011).

The transcripts were coded using the codes described in the next section. One author coded all of the transcripts, and a second author coded 25% of transcripts to determine reliability. Interrater reliability showed a Cohen's kappa between 0.6 and 0.9 and reliability of between 73% and 95%.

Coding Scheme

For the purpose of this study, we coded only talk focused on the bookreading. For example, talk not related to the book but focusing on where the child would sit was not coded. If a father read the book multiple times with his child, we coded only the first reading. We focused on immediate and non-immediate talk in the interactions. Based on De Temple and Snow's (2003) definitions, immediate talk is talk that directly related to the text or the book and includes labelling of pictures. Non-immediate talk is talk that goes beyond the book and can include references to the child's own experiences, making predictions and inferences.

Within the code of non-immediate talk, we differentiated between five different types of non-immediate talk. The first one referred to *making inferences and predictions* which referred to utterances or questions that involved making inferences or predictions about the characters or the story in the book. For example, "Where do you think mopoke went?" or "You think he is cold?" The second non-immediate talk code referred to *text-reader* links which involved making connections or links to the child's past experiences or the real world which includes experiences of people close to the child. For example, "You don't like combing your hair, don't you?" or "Looks like he's got a belly like daddy and mommy." *Requesting explanation or information* were utterances that involved requesting information or explanation from the child related to the storylines in the book such as "Why is he posh?" or "Why do you think he is called a highpoke?" *Explicitly explaining or rephrasing the meanings of difficult words or terms* included sentences such as "a yoyo is like a toy with a ball attached to a string" or "wee means small or tiny." The final code within non-immediate talk was *general knowledge* which included utterances that involved teaching or discussing knowledge that might be new to the child. Examples included the following: "Do you think snow is hot or cold?" or "What is a wombat doing in a tree?" Book-focused talk was related to the book itself and included engagement with the book, book handling, and story or book evaluations. Book extension activities included numeracy and external interactions such as high-fiving. Other codes included eliciting text and providing elicited text, written text, and communicative scaffolding which included repetition, directives, back channeling, praise, and clarification.

Table 24.1 describes all the different coding categories used for both father and child during bookreading and includes examples.

Results

Descriptive Statistics

Children's average vocabulary score was 24 (*SD* = 8.8; range = 3–38), which was higher than the standardized mean for children this age (*M* = 16.68–20:35; *SD* = 7.20–2.28 for ages 3:0–3:5 and 3:6–3:11). We also looked at father and child type (total number of different words), tokens (total number of words), and their ratio (type/token) produced during the bookreading

Table 24.1 Coding scheme

Category	Subcategory	Description	Example
Immediate talk: *Immediate talk focuses on the story, the pictures shown in the book, or on things that could be seen readily in the surrounding environment.* **IMM**	Labelling **IMM:LAB**	Utterances about the name of objects, pictures, or items shown in the book or utterances describing objects, pictures, or items shown in the book	That's a comb there. There's a suitcase and a monocle on him. See, there are two of them.
Non-immediate talk: *Non-immediate talk is talk that goes beyond the information in the text or the illustrations.* **NIM**	Making inferences/ predictions **NIM:INF**	Utterances that involve making inferences or predictions about the characters or the story in the book	Here, he is blowpoke, and then after that, he became a woahpoke! Where do you think mopoke went? It's gone! What do you think the wombat's doing up there?
	Text-reader links **NIM:TRL**	Utterances that involve making connections or links to the child's past experiences or to the real world, which includes experiences of people close to the child (e.g., mother, father, sibling, friend)	Daddy have a mo? Are you a little poke?
	Text-picture links/ explanations **NIM:EXP**	Utterances that involve interpreting storylines such as providing/ requesting/explaining the storylines and making links between the words and pictures in the book	Why do you think he is called a highpoke? He is called a mo'poke because he has a moustache. Can you see that?
	Explain the meanings of difficult words/ terms **NIM:MEA**	Utterances that attempt to explain terms/words that are a little more complex for children to understand	Fro is like when you have big fuzzy hair like this. It's called an Afro. A yoyo is like a toy with a ball attached to a string.
	General knowledge **NIM:GEN**	Utterances that involve general knowledge discussions with the child	What is a wombat doing on a tree? Wombats don't go on trees.

(continued)

Table 24.1 (continued)

Category	Subcategory	Description	Example
Book-focused talk: *Talks that are related to the book knowledge or the book itself* **BFT**	Concepts of print **BFT:CON**	Utterances that involve requesting or providing information on concepts of print such as holding the book, reading it from left to right, or those that explicitly mark the beginning or the end of the book	The end. That's it.
	Book engagement **BFT:ENG**	Utterances that involve engaging the child with the book or the reading activity itself	Do you want to turn the page? Shall we start? Do you want to read this book? Where shall we sit? Come, sit on my lap.
	Book handling **BFT:HAN**	Utterances that are related to the book itself, such as the title or name of the author, as well as the print-related utterances that are not part of the storylines	Mopoke by Philip Bunting. Read the last page of the book or the last page of the book cover.
	Book/story evaluation **BFT:EVA**	Utterances involving the overall evaluation of the story, character, or book	Did you like the book? It's a funny one, isn't it?
Book extension activity: *Activities that occur beyond the book itself* **BEA**	Numeracy **BEA:NUM**	Utterances that involve guiding the child's counting as well as the act of counting of objects, items, or pictures shown in the book	Can you count how many stars are there? 1, 2, 3, 4, 5, 6, 7, 8, 9, 10, 11! Can you count how many more pokes are there?
	External interaction **BEA:INT**	Utterances that involve external interactions that are being inspired by the book or storylines	Hi-fived!
Eliciting text/open-ended prompts	**ETP**	Utterances that elicit words or text from the child that are related to the book or utterances that encourage the child to guess the "pokes" based on the pictures so as to solicit the child's contribution	Look! This is a…?
Providing text that is elicited	**PTE**	Utterances that provide answers to the elicited text	This is a…. snowpoke.
Written text	**WRT**	Utterances that are related to reading the storyline itself	This is a mopoke.
Communicative scaffolding: *Verbal utterances that act as a support or to guide the children during bookreading* **COS**	Repetition/ expansion **COS:REP**	Utterances that involve repeating after the child or expanding the child's utterances in a proper sentence	Child: He's big! Dad: Yeah, he's big. Child: Big! Dad: Yeah, he's very big.
	Directives **COS:DIR**	Utterances that are related to giving instructions or commands to the child that are not related to the storyline	Let me turn the page. Let's finish the book first, shall we?

(continued)

Table 24.1 (continued)

Category	Subcategory	Description	Example
	Back channeling **COS:BCH**	Utterances that are related to those maintaining the conversation (e.g., minimal encouragement, verbal response)	Hmm. Uh-huh. Yeah.
	Clarification **COS:CLA**	Utterances that involve requesting for clarification or confirmation from the child	Child: Mommy. Dad: Hmm? You mean he's a baby and this is the mom?
Non-related talk	**NRT**	Utterances that do not fall into any of the above categories or are completely unrelated to bookreading	Can we play hide and seek? (before reading the book) Can we do the cooking activity first?
Unclear	**UNC**	Utterances that are unclear or hard to understand	(mumbling or inaudible)

session. Type-token ratio (TTR) is used in language development to study lexical variation, where a high-degree TTR indicates a higher level of lexical variation and a low TTR indicates a low level of lexical variation. The range falls between 0 and 1. The TTR for fathers was 0.60 and 0.39 for children (see Table 24.2 for more information).

Table 24.2 Mean, standard deviation, and range for child age, vocabulary score, and type and token for child and father

	Mean	SD	Range
Child age	42.48	2.73	37–46
Vocabulary score	24.05	8.79	3–38
Type child	51.19	23.40	13–96
Token child	95.81	58.47	17–229
TTR child	0.60	0.13	0–1
Type father	125	62.60	35–321
Token father	345.29	252.13	94–1252
TTR father	0.39	0.06	0–1

Correlations

Next, we ran correlations between child age, vocabulary score, type, and token. Table 24.3 shows a significant correlation between child age and vocabulary, indicating that older children tended to do better on the vocabulary assessment. There were no further significant correlations between vocabulary score and child or father types and tokens. However, there were significant correlations between father and child type ($r = 0.66$, $p < 0.01$) and father and child token ($r = 0.68$, $p < 0.01$). None of the child codes were significantly correlated with child vocabulary scores.

Table 24.4 shows the mean, standard deviation (SD), and range for all of the codes used by both father and child. As the book contained few words and relied heavily on the pictures, it was not surprising that all of the fathers read the entire text during the bookreading session.

Immediate and Non-immediate Talk

Labelling was the most common activity during the bookreading with an average of 17 labels for fathers and 8.5 for children. Labelling was coded as *immediate talk*. Fathers often asked their child to label a picture in the book (see example 1) or provided labels themselves (example 2).

Example 1

Father: What has he got there?
Father: Can you see that?

Example 2

Father: Yoyo.

Table 24.3 Correlations between child age, vocabulary score, and father and child type and token

	Child age	Vocabulary score	Child type	Child token	Child TTR	Father type	Father token
Child age		0.67**	0.06	0.19	−0.19	0.26	0.30
Vocabulary score			0.052	0.07	0.03	0.01	0.07
Child type				0.86**	−0.64**	0.66**	0.60**
Child token						0.72**	0.68**
Child TTR						−0.65**	−0.59**
Father type							0.96**
Father token							

**$p < 0.01$

Table 24.4 Mean, standard deviation, and range for all codes used by father and child

	Father		Child	
Code	Mean (SD)	Range	Mean (SD)	Range
IMM:LAB	17 (13)	1–64	8.5 (5.6)	2–24
NIM:INF	3 (2.6)	0–9	2.8 (4)	0–18
NIM:TRL	2.8 (6)	0–26	1.4 (2.2)	0–7
NIM:EXP	0.8 (1.9)	0–7	1.1 (1.9)	0–6
NIM:MEA	4.5 (5)	0–21	1.2 (2.6)	0–10
NIM:GEN	1.9 (3.9)	0–18	1.1 (2)	0–8
BFT:CON	1 (1)	0–4	0.33 (0.66)	0–2
BFT:ENG	2 (2)	0–7	0.24 (0.44)	0–1
BFT:HAN	3 (3.7)	0–15	1.1 (2.7)	0–11
BFT:EVA	1.8 (2)	0–8	0.90 (1.3)	0–4
BEA:NUM	2.9 (6.4)	0–30	3 (6.7)	0–31
BEA:EXI	0.7 (0.9)	0–3	0.2 (7)	0–31
ETP	1.2 (2)	0–8	0.14 (0.65)	0–3
PTE	0.33 (0.73)	0–2	0.85 (1.5)	0–6
WRT	19 (4.6)	0–22	0.9 (4.1)	0–19
COS:REP	1.5 (1.5)	0–5	5.8 (6.4)	0–21
COS:DIR	1.7 (3)	0–14	0.6 (0.9)	0–3
COS:BCH	4 (3.4)	0–13	4.1 (3.7)	0–12
COS:FIL	1.1 (2.7)	0–11	0.9 (1.1)	0–5
COS:PRA	2 (2.9)	0–11	0.2 (0.8)	0–4
COS:CLA	1.6 (1.5)	0–4	0.5 (0.8)	0–3
NRT	0.76 (0.94)	0–3	0.5 (0.8)	0–2
UNC	0.2 (0.40)	0–1	0.9 (1.2)	0–3

Child: It is a yoyo.

Children often engaged in labelling as well as can be seen from the next examples (examples 3 and 4):

Example 3

Child: That is a highpoke.
Child: And that is a lowpoke.

Example 4

Child: This is tiny.
Father: This is a weekpoke.

Correlations showed no significant relationship between father and child labelling ($r = 0.32$, $p = 0.15$), indicating that if fathers used a lot of labelling, children did not automatically do so as well.

Table 24.5 Correlations father and child code non-immediate talk

	Child				
Father	Inferences	Text-reader link	Explanation	Meanings	General knowledge
Inferences	0.76**	0.33	0.42	0.57**	0.46*
Text-reader link	−0.12	0.81**	0.50*	0.28	0.58
Explanation	−0.07	0.50*	−0.13	0.51*	0.37
Meanings	0.09	0.28	0.20	0.49*	0.12
General knowledge	−0.06	0.58**	0.15	0.05	0.94**

*$p < 0.05$
**$p < 0.01$

Non-immediate talk was commonly observed, in particular in regard to explaining difficult words or terms. For example, on one of the pages in the book, there is a picture of an owl (mopoke) with an Afro hairdo labelled "fropoke". Many fathers explained what a "fro" (Afro) was, sometimes explicitly (see example 6) and sometimes less explicit (example 7).

Example 6

Father: This is a fropoke (reads text).
Father: See, he has got a big hair fro hairdo.
Child: Yeah, he has got mopoke.
Child: Lots of funny hair.

Example 7

Father: It is a fropoke
Child: A fropoke?
Father: Afro hair with a little comb in there.

Correlations were conducted between father and child non-immediate talk and are displayed in Table 24.5. As shown, there were significant correlations between child and father use of *inferences* ($r = 0.76$, $p < 0.01$), *text-reader links* ($r = 0.81$, $p < 0.01$), *explaining meanings* ($r = 0.49$, $p < 0.05$), and *general knowledge* ($r = 0.94$, $p = <0.01$). These correlations indicate that when fathers used this type of non-immediate talk, children responded using similar non-immediate talk. There were also significant correlations between *text-reader links* and *explanations* ($r = 0.50$, $p < 0.05$) and *text-reader link* and *general knowledge* ($r = 0.58$, $p < 0.01$). This indicates that fathers who regularly make *text-reader links* often provide *explanations* as well and similarly with *text-reader links* and *general knowledge*. These fathers seem to ensure their child understands the storyline and the illustrations by explaining difficult words and relating things from the book to the child's own experiences. Father's use of *inferences* was significantly correlated with *meanings* ($r = 0.57$, $p < 0.01$) and *general knowledge* ($r = 0.46$, $p < 0.05$), indicating that fathers who used *inferences* tended to also use *meanings* and *general knowledge*, again attuning to children's developmental level.

Relating the text or pictures to the child's own experiences was not uncommon, with an average of three instances per interaction by fathers and about one by children (often in response to fathers' mentioning of child's own experience). When one father came across the picture of a wombat (a marsupial living in burrows in Australia), he related this animal to a child's recent trip to a local zoo (Symbio Zoo) (see example 8):

Example 8

Father: Do you know what a wombat is?
Father: The other time, did you see it in Symbio?
Child: No.
Father: You did not?
Child: No.
Father: No?
Father: Okay, not very good.

The yoyo in the story also evoked responses from fathers relating the story to the child's own experiences (see examples 9 and 10).

Example 9

Child: It is a yoyo.
Father: You are talking about a yoyo the other day, were you not?
Child: Yeah.
Father: Can you use a yoyo?
Child: No?
Father: No worries, you will get your own soon.

Example 10

Father: This is a yopoke.
Father: Have you ever seen a yoyo?
Child: No, yeah, yeah.
Father: You have?
Child: Jamie has one.
Father: Jamie has one?
Father: Is it on a string?
Child: Yeah.

One dyad had quite an elaborate discussion about the child's glow-in-the-dark pajamas after reading the page of the glowpoke where the owl glows in the dark (see example 11).

Example 11

Father: This is a glowpoke.
Father: So he is glowing in the dark like your pajamas.
Father: The skeleton ones.
Child: But they do not work.
Father: They do when you turn the lights off.
Child: But when we were at my nanny's, they do not work.
Father: I will show you later how they work.

On average, fathers made or requested three *inferences* during the bookreading session. This number was slightly lower for children as they did not often spontaneously make predictions or inferences but usually responded to an inference made by the father (see example 12).

Example 12

Father: Yeah, you think he is cold?
Child: Hm.
Father: He is like brr.
(makes shivering sound)

However, sometimes children made inferences or predictions as well as seen in example 13 where the child talked about the mopoke leaving a clue (in the form of a feather).

Example 13

Father: It is gone!
Child: Where is he?
Child: His feather!
Father: He fell down
Father: Maybe he flew away.
Child: A clue.
Child: There is a clue. I found his feather.

On average, fathers referred to general knowledge twice per session, with children, on average, responding once. Usually, fathers referred to some general knowledge in one sentence (see examples 14 and 15).

Example 14

Father: What is a wombat doing in a tree?
Child: The tree.
Father: A wombat does not go on a tree.

Example 15

Child: A turtle and a snail.
Father: YEAH, and they are slow animals, are they not?
Child: Yeah.

Book-Focused Talk

Book-focused talk was quite common, in particular *book handling* which referred to utterances related to the book itself such as the title of the book, the name of the author, or the print at the end of the book explaining what a mopoke is. On average, fathers used this type of talk three times per interactions, with children responding, on average, once per session. Most fathers read the title of the book. Reading the name of the author or the postscript (information on mopoke) was not common. Examples 16 and 17 show *book handling*.

Example 16

Father: Mopoke.
Child: Mopoke.
Father: by Philip Bunting

Example 17

Father: This book is called Mopoke.

Not many fathers talked about *concepts of print* as the average was only one per session.

Fathers, and sometimes children, primarily announced the end of the book (see examples 18 and 19).

Example 18

Father: The end.
Father: Is it the end?
Father: It is the end.
Father: That is it.

Example 19

Child: The end.
Father: Yes, the end.

On average, fathers *evaluated* the book or experience twice per session, often asking the child if they enjoyed the book (examples 20 and 21).

Example 20

Father: You like that child?
Child: Yes.
Father: Was that a funny book?
Child: Yes.

Example 21

Father: Did you enjoy that?
Child: Yeah.

Utterances referring to *engaging with the book*, such as "Do you want to turn the page?" or "One more page left mate!," occurred an average of three times per session for fathers and once for children (often in response to fathers).

Counting was quite a common practice during the bookreading session. This may be explained by the fact that fathers were asked to engage in a numeracy task in the same recorded session as the bookreading, although the specific book characteristics are also a likely contributor, as one page in the book featured many mopokes. On average, fathers engaged in counting three times per session. The same number was found for children (see examples 22 and 23).

Example 22

Father: This is more pokes.
Child: One, two, three.
Father: Try again.
Child: One, two, three, six, seven, eight.
Father: Count together. One, two, three, four, five, six, seven, eight.
Child: One, two, three, four, one, two, three, four, seven, six, nine, ten.

Example 23

Father: Do you want to try and count them?
Child: Okay.
Child: One, two, three, four, five, six, seven, eight, nine, ten, eleven.
Father: That is great.

Elicitations and Communicative Scaffolding
Elicitations of text, and subsequently providing text, was not very common with an average of one instance per session. This primarily involved fathers trying to elicit words or texts from their children (see example 24).

Example 24

Father: This is a yopoke.
Father: Because it has got a?
Child: Yoyo.

Communicative Scaffolding
Communicative scaffolding was quite common, in particular *back channeling* where the speaker tries to maintain the conversation by using utterances such as "yeah" or "mmhm."

Both fathers and children produced, on average, four instances of back channeling, usually used as some sort of acknowledgment of what the other speaker said (see example 25).

Example 25

Father: This is a lowpoke because he is low.
Child: Yeah.

In one instance, a father and a child entered a (somewhat heated) discussion about reading the text. The father read the text out loud, but the child did not seem to believe the father was actually reading the text and demanded the father "just read the text" (see example 26).

Example 26

Father: This is a poorpoke (reads the text).
Child: Can you just read it?
Father: I am reading it.
Child: That is not how you read it!
Father: Yeah, I am reading the words. See.
Child: Oh.

Praise was also quite common with fathers on average, using praise at least twice during the interaction (see examples 27 and 28).

Example 27

Father: That means it is big.
Child: One, two.
Father: That is right, a little one small one.

Example 28

Father: This is a?
Child: Snowpoke.
Father: Very good!

What was remarkable throughout the bookreading sessions is that several children created their own words based on the word "poke." Every page in the book shows a mopoke with a specific characteristic (e.g., a mopoke glowing in the dark is called a glowpoke; mopoke with monocle and suitcase is called poshpoke). One child guessed that the owl in one of the pictures was called a "sickpoke" as he did not look well or an "eatpoke" (see examples 29 and 30).

Example 29

Father: Woah, this one is a?
Child: Sick. What, uh, sickpoke?
Father: Sickpoke?
Child: Yeah.

The same child talked about an "eatpoke" a little later:

Example 30

Father: Oh, this one is a?
Child: Eatpoke?
Father: Slowpoke.

Another child came up with the word "greenpoke" (see example 31).

Example 31

Child: A greenpoke.
Father: No, it is a glowpoke.

Other "invented" poke words included a disappear poke, sad poke, and sickpoke.

In summary, the results show quite a diversity in how fathers engaged with their 3-year-olds around a book. Some fathers only read the text and spent little time conversing with their children, while other fathers engaged in elaborate conversations with their young children, explaining difficult words, discussing the pictures, and making connections with the child's own experiences.

Discussion

One of the most important sociocultural tools children in Western countries can attain is literacy, and it is one that can only be learned via social interaction (e.g., Duursma, 2016; Reese et al., 2003). Shared bookreading not only benefits children's early language development and emergent literacy skills (e.g., Mol & Bus, 2011) but reading a book together also has a high affective component, and these parent-child interactions can promote benefits in children's socio-emotional development (Aram & Aviram, 2009).

Many studies focusing on parental bookreading make comparisons between fathers and mothers. The findings in this area tend to be mixed with some studies reporting differences in how fathers and mothers engage with their children around a book (Lyytinen, Laakso, & Poikkeus, 1998; Vandermaas-Peeler, Sassine, Price, & Brilhart, 2011) and others finding no difference between fathers and mothers in style of reading (Van Kleeck, Gillam, Hamilton, & McGrath, 1997). As there is so little research in the area of fathers reading to their children, we wanted to put the spotlight on fathers, and instead of comparing them with mothers, we only focused on how fathers engaged their young children during a bookreading interaction. We propose that it is valuable for the bookreading literature to better understand the unique contribution of fathers in themselves rather than creating potential "deficit models" of how fathers differ in reading style from mothers.

Even within our relatively small sample ($n = 21$), there was diversity in how fathers and their children interacted around a picture book. In the interactions, we focused on immediate and non-immediate talk as this type of talk is known to be beneficial for children's language development (e.g., Beals, de Temple, and Dickinson, 1994; De Temple and Snow, 2003). However, we also looked at other types of language fathers used to engage their children, such as communicative scaffolding and book handling. Although we would have expected that the book used would stimulate conversations between fathers and children, it was remarkable to see how many of the children created their own words based on the information provided in the text. Each page of the picture book included a "made-up" word, and children were quick to pick up on this and create their own "made-up" words using the same patterns used in the book. It is known that children can learn new words after a single incidental exposure, but recent research has shown that repeated exposure to words within the same story helps children learning new words (e.g., Houston-Price, Howe, and Lintern, 2014; Williams and Horst, 2014). When readers provide children opportunities to engage in an interactive way with new vocabulary, asking questions that require the child to use the new word help promote learning (Blewitt, Rump, Shealy, & Cook, 2009; Sénéchal, 1997). Picture books are ideal for vocabulary acquisition as they provide pictures and text at the same time so children can process information visually and verbally (Larragueta & Ceballos-Viro, 2018). Children also recall a story better when text is supported by pictures (Greenfield & Beagles-Roos, 1988). Larragueta and Ceballos-Viro (2018) reported that children learned more words from picture books if the text consisted of simple sentences or even just a single word (as in *Mopoke*), compared to texts with more details. More details might place more cognitive demands on children and could make it more challenging for children to remember the words (e.g., Horst, 2013). The pictures also need to be quite legible in order for children to understand the story (Larragueta & Ceballos-Viro, 2018). When parents read picture books, their children are not only exposed to a wealth of words, but picture books also offer children novel words which are embedded in different phrases and sentences. Children can learn new words and concepts which they rarely encounter in daily conversations (Dickinson, Griffith, Golinkoff, & Hirsch-Pasek, 2012; Larragueta & Ceballos-Viro, 2018; Liu, 2014). The picture book used in this study had simple illustrations and text, facilitating word learning. Fathers in this study worked within Vygotsky's (1978) Zone of Proximal Development by helping their children navigate the text and illustrations by providing, for example, explanations, relating text and illustrations to child's own experiences, and actively engaging the child with the story. In turn, children showed an understanding of the story and illustrations by "inventing" their own words, similar to what the author of the book used does. This suggests that children can learn new words from books and can do so in a relatively short time as the spontaneous use of pokes demonstrated.

Dickinson et al. (2012) argue that children learn best when adults are responsive to them. A study conducted by Landry et al. (2012) showed that when mothers were more responsive during bookreading, the children became more engaged and used more complex language. In our study, we found associations between fathers' responses and child responses. The type of non-immediate talk used by fathers was associated with the type of non-immediate talk used by their children. For example, when fathers used inferences, children tended to respond to those inferences and similarly with other types of non-immediate talk. However, we also found that different types of non-immediate talk were related to one another; for example, when fathers used explanations, this was related to children's general knowledge use, and father's inferences were related to children's use/response to meanings. This suggests that one type of non-immediate talk used by fathers is not necessarily related to the same type of non-immediate talk used by children. One type of non-immediate talk used by fathers seems to generate similar but also different types of non-immediate talk produced by children. Salo et al. (2016) also reported that when fathers used more labels or elicited labels from their children during bookreading, children often repeated the label provided or responded to the elicitation with a label.

Haden, Reese, and Fivush (1996) characterized parental talk during shared bookreading in terms of the level of distance from the text itself and the level of demand on the child to go beyond the text, which we identified as non-immediate talk. When parents use strategies such as asking children to make predictions or inferences, Haden et al. (1996) label these as high-level distancing as they are more cognitively demanding for children (Vandermaas-Peeler et al., 2011). Low-distancing strategies include less demanding questions such as asking the child to label a picture. The high-level cognitive demands were related to children's story comprehension and receptive vocabulary (Haden et al., 1996). We did find that when fathers used more cognitively demanding strategies such as asking for explanations or predictions or relating events to the child's own experiences, children tended to respond to these questions as seen from correlations between father and child non-immediate talk.

In summary, this study showed fathers actively engaging their children in a bookreading interaction using a variety of strategies. Most fathers were very responsive to their children's developmental level and had a good understanding of what their child would and would not understand. Future studies could look at more longitudinal data to examine whether and how father-child interactions change over time and as the child's language development progresses.

Limitations

This study was rather small, and results should not be generalized to all fathers. Although all our recordings appeared to show fathers and children who were comfortable reading together, we did not ask fathers about the frequency with which they read to their child at home or their own reading patterns. Future studies could include more information on children's home learning environment, including paternal and maternal bookreading frequency.

In this study, fathers recorded themselves at home reading to their child with an audio recorder. We used this approach to minimize the potential intrusion of recording devices on the bookreading session. However, as there was no video available of the interaction, it was sometimes hard to determine precisely what fathers and children were doing (e.g., looking at a particular part of a picture). Future bookreading studies could include videotaping fathers and children, which would also provide opportunities to code the gestures produced during reading and talk and to capture social-emotional elements like how and where fathers and children chose to sit while reading together. Additional "familiarization" sessions may, however, be required to capture the naturalistic parent-child interaction style in the presence of a video camera.

Summary and Key Points

The last decades have seen an increase in father engagement literature with studies showing how father involvement benefits child development (Lamb, 2010). Within the bookreading literature, it is important to acknowledge that fathers interact differently with their children than mothers do (Duursma, 2016). Although comparisons between fathers and mothers can be helpful at times, they also run the risk of using mother-child interactions as the golden standard and comparing fathers alongside it. There are many differences but also similarities in how fathers engage their children around a book. As there is so little research on what fathers actually do during bookreading, it is essential to study fathers on their own and not necessarily compare them with mothers as this runs the risk of looking at fathers from a deficit perspective.

Our study showed that fathers were actively engaging their children during a shared reading session. Fathers used a variety of strategies to discuss the book and the story with their young children. Many fathers used non-immediate talk to link the book to their child's own experiences and to make inferences or provide general knowledge, thereby engaging their child at a cognitively challenging manner. Fathers were well attuned to children's language level as demonstrated by the questions fathers asked about the meaning of words or by the explanations provided about the story and difficult words.

It is important to enhance our understanding of how fathers are engaged with, and impact upon, their children's development. More longitudinal and in-depth studies on shared bookreading are needed, including as children's independent reading skills grow, to better understand the long-term impact of positive father involvement on children's language and literacy development.

References

Aram, D., & Aviram, S. (2009). Mothers' storybook reading and kindergartners; socioemotional and literacy development. *Reading Psychology, 30*, 175–194. https://doi.org/10.1080/02702710802275348

Aram, D., Bergman Deitcher, D., & Adar, G. (2017). Understanding parents' attitudes towards complexity in children's books. *Reading Horizons: A Journal of Literacy and Language Arts, 56*(4), 3. Retrieved from https://scholarworks.wmich.edu/reading_horizons/vol56/iss4/3

Baker, C. E. (2013). Fathers' and mothers' home literacy environment and children's cognitive and social emotional development: Implications for family literacy programs. *Applied Developmental Science, 17*(4), 184–197. https://doi.org/10.1080/10888691.2013.836034

Baker, C. E. (2014). African American fathers' contributions to children's early academic achievement: Evidence from two-parent families from the Early Childhood Longitudinal Study-Birth Cohort. *Early Education and Development, 25*, 19–35. https://doi.org/10.1080/10409289.2013.764225

Baker, C. E., Vernon-Feagans, L., & The Family Life Project Investigators. (2015). Fathers' language input during shared book activities: Links to children's kindergarten achievement. *Journal of Applied Developmental Psychology, 36*, 53–59. https://doi.org/10.1016/j.appdev.2014.11.009

Barnes, E., & Puccioni, J. (2017). Shared book reading and preschool children's academic achievement: Evidence from the Early Childhood Longitudinal Study-Birth Cohort. *Infant Child Development, 26*, e2035. https://doi.org/10.1002/icd.2035

Barnyak, N. C., & McNelly, T. A. (2016). The literacy skills and motivation to read of children enrolled in Title 1: A comparison of electronic and print nonfiction books. *Early Childhood Education Journal, 44*, 527–536. https://doi.org/10.1007/s10643-015-0745-0

Beals, D. E., De Temple, J. M., & Dickinson, D. (1994). Talking and listening that support early literacy development of children from low-income families. In D. Dickinson (Ed.), *Bridges to literacy: Approaches to supporting child and family literacy* (pp. 30–40). Cambridge, MA: Basil Blackwell.

Blewitt, P., Rump, K. M., Shealy, S. E., & Cook, S. A. (2009). Shared book reading: When and how questions affect young children's word learning. *Journal of Educational Psychology, 101*, 294–304. https://doi.org/10.1037/a0013844

Bocknek, E. L., Brophy-Herb, H. E., Fitzgerald, H. E., Schiffman, R. F., & Vogel, C. (2014). Stability of biological father presence as a proxy for family stability: Cross-racial associations with the longitudinal development of emotion regulation in toddlerhood. *Infant Mental Health Journal, 35*, 309–321. https://doi.org/10.1002/imhj.21454

Bracken, S. S., & Fischel, J. E. (2008). Family reading behavior and early literacy skills in preschool children from low-income backgrounds. *Early Education and Development, 19*(1), 45–67. https://doi.org/10.1080/10409280701838835

Breit-Smith, A., van Kleeck, A., Prendeville, J. A., & Pan, W. (2017). Preschool children's exposure to story grammar elements during parent-child book reading. *Journal of Research in Reading, 40*(4), 345–364. https://doi.org/10.1111/1467-9817.12071

Bronfenbrenner, U. (1979). *Ecology of human development: Experiments by nature and design*. Cambridge, MA: Harvard University Press.

Bronfenbrenner, U. (1994). Ecological models of human development. In T. Husen & T. N. Postelthwaite (Eds.), *International encyclopedia of education* (pp. 1642–1647). Oxford, UK: Pergamon Press.

Bronfenbrenner, U., & Morris, P. A. (2006). The bioecological model of human development. In R. M. Lerner & W. Damon (Eds.), *Handbook of child psychology: Theoretical models of human development* (pp. 793–828). Hoboken, NJ: Wiley.

Bruner, J. (1981). The social context of language acquisition. *Language & Communication, 1*(2/3), 155–178. https://doi.org/10.1016/0271-5309(81)90010-0

Bunting, P. (2017). *Mopoke*. Gosford, NSW: Scholastic Australia.

Burgess, S. R., Hech, S. A., & Lonigan, C. J. (2002). Relations of the home literacy environment (HLE) to the development of reading-related abilities: A one-year longitudinal study. *Reading Research Quarterly, 37*(4), 408–426. https://doi.org/10.1598/RRQ.37.4.4

Büyüköztürk, Ş., Kiliç Çakmak, E., Akgün, Ö., Karadeniz, E., & Demirel, F. (2012). *Scientific research methods*. Ankara: Pegem Publishing.

Cabrera, N., Fitzgerald, H. E., Bradley, R. H., & Roggman, L. (2007). Modeling the dynamics of paternal influences on children over the life course. *Applied Development Science, 11*(4), 185–189. https://doi.org/10.1080/10888690701762027

Cabrera, N. J., Volling, B. L., & Barr, R. (2018). Fathers are parents, too! Widening the lens on parenting for children's development. *Child Development Perspectives, 12*(3), 152–157. https://doi.org/10.1111/cdep.12275

Cameron-Faulkner, T., & Noble, C. (2013). A comparison of book text and child directed speech. *First Language, 33*, 268–279. https://doi.org/10.1177/0142723713487613.

Cano, Perales, & Baxter. (2018). A matter of time: Father involvement and child cognitive outcomes. *Journal of Marriage and the Family, 81*(1), 164–184. https://doi.org/10.1111/jomf.12532

Children's Book Council of Australia (CBCA). (2018). *Book of the year awards – Winners 2018*. Retrieved June 12, 2019, from https://cbca.org.au/winners-2018

Clark, C. (2009). *Why fathers matter to their children's literacy*. London: National Literacy Trust.

Connors, A. (2014). How music sets the tone for learning. *Teaching young children, 7*(5), 21–23.

De Temple, J., & Snow, C. E. (2003). Learning words from books. In A. van Kleeck, S. A. Stahl, & E. B. Bauer (Eds.), *On reading books to children: Parents and teachers* (pp. 16–36). Mahway, NJ: Lawrence Erlbaum.

Demir, Ö. E., Applebaum, L., Levine, S. C., Petty, K., & Goldin-Meadow, S. (2011). The story behind parent-child book-reading interactions: Specific relations to later language and reading outcomes. In *Proceedings of the... Annual Boston University Conference on Language Development. Boston University Conference on Language Development* (p. 157). NIH Public Access.

Dickinson, D. K., Griffith, J. A., Golinkoff, R. M., & Hirsch-Pasek, K. (2012). How reading books fosters language development around the world. *Child Development Research, 2012*, 1–15. https://doi.org/10.1155/2012/602807

Duursma, E. (2016). Who does the reading, who the talking? Low-income fathers and mothers in the US interacting around a picture book. *First Language, 36*(5), 456–484. https://doi.org/10.1177/0142723716648849

Duursma, E., Pan, B. A., & Raikes, H. (2008). Predictors and outcomes of low-income fathers' reading with their toddlers. *Early Childhood Research Quarterly, 23*(3), 351–365. https://doi.org/10.1016/j.ecresq.2008.06.001

Farrant, B. M., & Zubrick, S. R. (2011). Early vocabulary development: The importance of joint attention and parent-child book reading. *First Language, 32*, 343–364. https://doi.org/10.1177/0142723711422626

Farrant, B. M., & Zubrick, S. R. (2013). Parent-child book reading across early childhood and child vocabulary in the early school years: Findings from the Longitudinal Study of Australian Children. *First Language, 33*, 280–293. https://doi.org/10.1177/0142723713487617

Flack, Z. M., Field, A. P., & Horst, J. S. (2018). The effects of shared storybook reading on word learning: A meta-analysis. *Developmental Psychology, 54*(7), 1334–1346. https://doi.org/10.1037/dev0000512

Fletcher, K., & Reese, E. (2005). Picture book reading with young children: A conceptual framework. *Developmental Review, 35*, 64–103. https://doi.org/10.1016/j.dr.2004.08.009

Fletcher, R., & Daly, K. (2002). *Fathers' involvement in their children's literacy development*. Newcastle: Family Action Centre, University of Newcastle, Australia.

Foster, T. D., Froyen, L. A., Skibbe, L. E., Bowles, R. P., & Decker, K. B. (2016). Fathers' and mothers' home learning environments and children's early academic outcomes. *Reading & Writing, 29*, 1845–1863. https://doi.org/10.1007/s11145-016-9655-7

Goeke-Morey, M. C., & Cummings, E. M. (2007). Impact of father involvement: A closer look at indirect effects models involving marriage and child adjustment. *Applied Developmental Science, 11*, 221–225. https://doi.org/10.1080/10888690701762126

Greenfield, P., & Beagles-Roos, J. (1988). Radio vs. television: Their cognitive impact on children of different socioeconomic and ethnic groups. *Journal of Communication, 38*(2), 71–92. https://doi.org/10.1111/j.1460-2466.1988.tb02048.x

Haden, C. A., Reese, E., & Fivush, R. (1996). Mothers' Extratextual comments during Storybook Reading: Stylistic Differences over Time and Across Texts. *Discourse Processes, 21*(2), 135–169. https://doi.org/10.1080/01638539609544953

Halliday, M. A. K. (2004). The place of dialogue in children's construction of meaning. In R. B. Ruddell & N. J. Unrau (Eds.), *Theoretical models and processes of reading* (5th ed.). Newark, DE: International Reading Association.

Hansen, D., & Milligan, S. A. (2012). Aural skills at the juncture of research in early reading and music literacy. *Music Educators Journal, 99*(2), 75–80. https://doi.org/10.1177/0027432112462894

Hartas, D. (2012). Inequality and the home learning environment: Predictions about seven-year-olds' language and literacy. *British Educational Research Journal., 38*(5), 859–879. https://doi.org/10.1080/01411926.2011.588315

Hayes, D. P., & Ahrens, M. G. (1988). Vocabulary simplification for children: A special case of 'motherese?'. *Journal of Child Language, 15*(2), 395–410. https://doi.org/10.1017/S0305000900012411

Henderson, L., Devine, K., Weighall, A., & Gaskell, G. (2015). When the daffodat flew to the intergalactic zoo: Off-line consolidation is critical for word learning from stories. *Developmental Psychology, 51*(3), 406–417. https://doi.org/10.1037/a0038786

Heydon, R., McKee, L., & O'Neill, S. (2018). Singing our song: The affordance of singing in an intergenerational, multimodal literacy programme. *Literacy, 52*(3), 128–136.

Hindman, A. H., Connor, C. M., Jewkes, A. M., & Morrison, F. J. (2008). Untangling the effects of shared book reading: Multiple factors and their associations with preschool literacy outcomes. *Early Childhood Research Quarterly, 23*, 330–350. https://doi.org/10.1016/j.ecresq.2008.01.005

Hoffman, J., Teale, W. H., & Yokota, J. (2015). The book matters! Choosing narrative children's literature to support read aloud discussion of complex texts in the early grades. *Young Children, 70*(4), 8–15.

Horst, J. S. (2013). Context and repetition in word learning. *Frontiers in Psychology, 4*, 149. https://doi.org/10.3389/fpsyg.2013.00149

Houston-Price, C., Howe, J. A., & Lintern, N. J. (2014). Once upon a time there as a fabulous funambulist: What children learn about the "high-level" vocabulary they encounter while listening to stories. *Frontiers in Psychology, 5*, 75. https://doi-org.exproxy.uow.edu.au/10.3389/fpsyg.2014.00075

Howard, S. J., & Melhuish, E. (2017). An early years toolbox for assessing early executive function, language, self-regulation, and social development: Validity, reliability, and preliminary norms. *Journal of Psychoeducational Assessment, 35*(3), 255–275. https://doi.org/10.1177/0734282916633009

Huttenlocher, J., Vasilyeva, M., Cymerman, E., & Levine, S. (2002). Language input and child syntax. *Cognitive Psychology, 45*, 337–374. https://doi.org/10.1016/S0010-0285(02)00500-5

Justice, L. M., & Ezell, H. K. (2000). Enhancing children's print and word awareness through home-based parent intervention. *American Journal of Speech-Language Pathology, 9*, 257–269. https://doi.org/10.1044/1058-0360.0903.257

Justice, L. M., & Kaderavek, J. (2002). Using shared storybook reading to promote emergent literacy. *Teaching Exceptional Children, 34*(4), 8–13.

Karther, D. (2002). Fathers with low literacy and their young children. *The Reading Teacher, 56*, 184–193.

Lamb, M. E. (2010). *The role of the father in child development* (5th ed.). New York, NY: Wiley.

Landry, S. H., Smith, K. E., Swank, P. R., Zucker, T., Crawford, A. D., & Solaris, E. F. (2012). The effects of a responsive parenting intervention on parent-child interactions during shared book reading. *Developmental Psychology, 48*(4), 969–986. https://doi.org/10.1037/a0026400

Larragueta, M., & Ceballos-Viro, I. (2018). What kind of book? Selecting picture books for vocabulary acquisition. *The Reading Teacher, 72*(1), 81–87. https://doi.org/10.1002/trtr1681

Lefebvre, P., Trudeau, N., & Sutton, A. (2011). Enhancing vocabulary, print awareness and phonological awareness through shared storybook reading with low-income pre-schoolers. *Journal of Early Childhood Literacy, 11*, 453–479. https://doi.org/10.1177/1468798411416581

Liu, H. M. (2014). Lexical and acoustic features of maternal utterances addressing preverbal infants in picture book reading link to 5-year-old children's language development. *Early Education and Development, 25*, 1103–1117. https://doi.org/10.1080/10409289.2014.899887

Lynch, J. (2002). Parents' self-efficacy beliefs, parents' gender, children's reader self-perceptions, reading achievement and gender. *Journal of Research in Reading, 25*, 54–67. https://doi.org/10.1111/1467-9817.00158

Lyytinen, P., Laakso, M., & Poikkeus, A. (1998). Parental contribution to child's early language and interests in book. *European Journal of Psychology of Education, 13*, 297–308. https://doi.org/10.1007/BF03172946

MacWhinney, B. (2000). *The CHILDES project: Tools for analyzing talk*. Mahwah, NJ: Lawrence Erlbaum.

Malin, J. L., Cabrera, N. J., & Rowe, M. L. (2014). Low-income minority mothers' and fathers' reading and children's interest: Longitudinal contributions to children's receptive vocabulary skills. *Early Childhood Research Quarterly, 29*(4), 425–432. https://doi.org/10.1016/j.ecresq.2014.04.010

McGillion, M., Pine, J. M., Herbert, J. S., & Matthews, D. (2017). A randomized controlled trial to test the effect of promoting caregiver contingent talk on language development in infants from diverse socioeconomic status backgrounds. *Journal of Child Psychology and Psychiatry, 58*, 1122–1131. https://doi.org/10.1111/jcpp.12725

Mol, S. E., & Bus, A. (2011). To read or not to read: A meta-analysis of print exposure from infancy to early adulthood. *Psychological Bulletin, 137*(2), 267–296. https://doi.org/10.1037/a0021890

Mol, S. E., Bus, A. G., & de Jong, M. T. (2009). Interactive book reading in early education: A tool to stimulate print knowledge as well as oral language. *Review of Educational Research, 79*, 979–1007. https://doi.org/10.3102/0034654309332561

Myrtil, M. J., Justice, L. M., & Jiang, H. (2019). Home-literacy environment of low-income rural families: Associations with child- and caregiver-level characteristics. *Journal of Applied Developmental Psychology, 60*, 1–10. https://doi.org/10.1016/j.appdev.2018.10.002

Niklas, F., & Schneider, W. (2013). Home literacy environment and the beginning of reading and spelling. *Contemporary Educational Psychology, 38*(1), 40–50. https://doi.org/10.1016/j/cedpsych.2012.10.001

Ninio, A., & Snow, C. E. (1996). *Pragmatic development*. Boulder, CO: Westview.

Noble, C., Sala, G., Peter, M., Lingwood, J., Rowland, C., Gobet, F., et al. (2019). The impact of shared book reading on children's language skills: A meta-analysis. *Educational Research Review, 28*, 100290. https://doi.org/10.1016/j.edurev.2019.100290

Noble, C. H., Cameron-Faulkner, T., & Lieven, E. (2018). Keeping it simple: The grammatical properties of shared book reading. *Journal of Child Language, 45*(3), 753–766. https://doi.org/10.1017/S0305000917000447

Nutbrown, C., Clough, P., Stammers, L., Emblin, N., & Alston-Smith, S. (2019). Family literacy in prisons: Fathers' engagement with their young children. *Research Papers in Education, 34*(2), 169–191. https://doi.org/10.1080/02671522.2017.1402085

Pentimonti, J. M., Zucker, T. A., & Justice, L. M. (2011). What are preschool teachers reading in their classrooms? *Reading Psychology, 32*(2), 197–236. https://doi.org/10.1080/02702711003604484

Quach, J., Sarkadi, A., Napiza, N., Wake, M., Loughman, A., & Goldfeld, S. (2018). Do fathers' home reading practices at age 2 predict child language and literacy at age 4? *Academic Pediatrics, 18*, 179–187. https://doi.org/10.1016/j.acap.2017.10.001

Raikes, H., Alexander Pan, B., Luze, G., Tamis-LeMonda, C. S., Brooks-Gunn, J., Constantine, J., et al. (2006). Mother–child book reading in low-income families: Correlates and outcomes during the first three years of life. *Child Development, 77*(4), 924–953. https://doi.org/10.1111/j.1467-8624.2006.00911.x

Reese, E., Cox, A., Harte, D., & McAnally, H. (2003). Diversity in adults' style of reading books to children. In A. van Kleeck, S. A. Stahl, & E. B. Bauer (Eds.), *On reading books to children: Parents and teachers* (pp. 37–57). Mahwah, NJ: Lawrence Erlbaum.

Rowe, M. L. (2012). A longitudinal investigation of the role of quantity and quality of child-directed speech in vocabulary development. *Child Development, 83*(5), 1762–1774. https://doi.org/10.1111/j.1467-8624.2012.01805.x

Salo, V. C., Rowe, M. L., Leech, K. A., & Cabrera, N. J. (2016). Low-income fathers' speech to toddlers during book reading versus toy play. *Journal of Child Language, 43*, 1385–1399. https://doi.org/10.1017/S0305000915000550

Samuelsson, S., Byrne, B., Quain, P., Wadsworth, S., Corley, R., DeFries, J. C., et al. (2005). Environmental and genetic influences on prereading skills in Australia, Scandinavia, and the United States. *Journal of Educational Psychology, 97*, 705–722. https://doi.org/10.1037/0022-0663.97.4.705

Sarkadi, A., Kristiansson, R., Oberklaid, F., & Bremberg, S. (2008). Fathers' involvement and children's developmental outcomes: A systematic review of longitudinal studies. *Acta Paediatrica, 97*, 153–158. https://doi.org/10.1111/j.1651-2227.2007.00572.x

Schwab, J. F., Rowe, M. L., Cabrera, N., & Lew-Williams, C. (2018). Fathers' repetition of words is coupled with children's vocabularies. *Journal of Experimental Child Psychology, 166*, 437–450. https://doi.org/10/1016/j.jecp.2017.09.012

Sénéchal, M. (1997). The differential effect of storybook reading on preschoolers' acquisition of expressive and receptive vocabulary. *Child Language, 24*, 123–138. https://doi.org/10.1017/S0305000996003005

Snow, C. E. (1990). The development of definitial skill. *Journal of Child Language, 17*, 697710. https://doi.org/10.1017/S0305000900010953

Son, S.-H., & Morrison, F. J. (2010). The nature and impact of changes in home learning environment on development of language and academic skills in preschool children. *Developmental Psychology, 46*(5), 1103–1118.

Sparks, A., & Reese, E. (2012). From reminiscing to reading: Home contributions to children's developing language and literacy in low-income families. *First Language, 33*(1), 89–109. https://doi.org/10.1177/0142723711433583

Thierry, K. L., & Sparks, A. (2019). Latino families engage in elaborative conversations: Effects on children's recall and vocabulary. *Journal of Child and Family Studies, 28*, 2297–2311. https://doi.org/10.1007/210826-019-01446-0

Townsend, M. L., Kelly, M. A., Pickard, J. A., Larkin, T. A., Flood, V. M., Caputi, P., et al. (2019). Illawarra born cross-generational health study: Feasibility of a multi-generational birth cohort study. *Pilot and Feasibility Studies, 5*, 1–32. https://doi.org/10.1186/s40814-019-0418

Van Kleeck, A., Gillam, R. B., Hamilton, L., & McGrath, C. (1997). The relationship between middle-class parents' book-sharing discussion and their preschoolers' language development. *Journal of Speech, Language and Hearing Research, 40*, 1261–1271. https://doi.org/10.1044/jslhr.4006.1261

Van Tonder, B., Alison, A., & Nicholson, T. (2019). Not just storybook reading: Exploring the relationship between home literacy environment and literate cultural capital among 5-year-old children as they start school. *Australian Journal of Language and Literacy, 42*(2), 87–102. https://search.informit.com.au/documentSummary;dn=391279468267528;res=IELHSS>

Vandermaas-Peeler, M., Sassine, B., Price, C., & Brilhart, C. (2011). Mothers' and fathers' guidance behaviors during storybook reading. *Journal of Early Childhood Literacy, 12*, 415–442. https://doi.org/10.1177/1468798411417381

Varghese, C., & Wachen, J. (2016). The determinants of father involvement and connections to children's literacy and language outcomes: A review of literature. *Marriage & Family Review, 52*, 331–359. https://doi.org/10.1080/01494929.2015.1099587

Vygotsky, L. S. (1978). *Mind in society: The development of higher psychological processes*. Cambridge, MA: Harvard University Press.

Wasik, B. A., Hindman, A. H., & Snell, E. K. (2016). Book reading and vocabulary development: A systematic review. *Early Childhood Research Quarterly, 37*, 39–57. https://doi.org/10.1016/j.ecresl.2016.04.003

Whitehurst, G. J. (1994). A picture book reading intervention in day care and home for children from low-income families. *Developmental Psychology, 30*, 679–689. https://doi.org/10.1037/0012-1649.30.5.679

Williams, S. E., & Horst, J. S. (2014). Goodnight book: Sleep consolidation improves word learning via storybooks. *Frontiers in Psychology, 5*, 184. https://doi.org/10.3389/fpsyg.2014.00184

Winters, K. L., & Griffin, S. (2014). Singing is a celebration of language using music to enhance young children's vocabularies. *Language and Literacy, 16*(3), 78–91.

Yazici, E., & Bolay, H. (2017). Story based activities enhance literacy skills in preschool children. *Universal Journal of Educational Research, 5*(5), 815–823. https://doi.org/10.13189/ujer.2017.050528

Zevenbergen, A. A., & Whitehurst, G. J. (2003). Dialogic reading: A shared picture book reading intervention for preschoolers. In A. van Kleeck, S. A. Stahl, & E. B. Bauer (Eds.), *On reading books to children: Parents and teachers* (pp. 177–202). Mahwah, NJ: Lawrence Erlbaum.

Fathers and Children's Executive Function

25

Alyssa S. Meuwissen

Executive function (EF) is increasingly recognized as crucial for children's success. Therefore, establishing antecedents has become a high priority so that they can be leveraged to build EF skills (Blair, 2016; Diamond & Lee, 2011). Research linking the quality of parenting and child executive function (EF) has been rapidly accumulating over the last decade (Carlson, 2005). However, although there is robust correlational evidence that multiple dimensions of maternal parenting are linked to child EF, fathers and father figures rarely have been included in this research.

This is problematic because fathers are significant contributors to children's caregiving environments and thus need to be included in research to fully understand the family system in which a child develops. Sixty-nine percent of children in the USA live with two parents (U. S. Census Bureau, 2016), and 98% of nonresidential fathers have some contact with their children (Jones & Mosher, 2013). In 2016, there were approximately 28,000 same-sex male couples raising children in the USA. Sociological changes across the past 40 years, including substantial increases in the number of women in the workforce, have resulted in fathers becoming more involved with their young children (Cabrera, Volling, & Barr, 2018). These shifts have redefined the roles of both fathers and mothers as parents as they adapt to each other and to these new demands of the environment that require greater flexibility in role expectations (Cabrera, Fitzgerald, Bradley, & Roggman, 2014; Bianchi, Robinson, & Milkie, 2006).

Bioecological theory suggests that fathers are a part of the microsystem of family interrelationships that occur transactionally over time (Volling et al., 2019) and thus need to be included when studying child development. Additionally, mothers and fathers, as members of this microsystem, affect and adapt to each other, shaping the overall caregiving context (Bronfenbrenner & Morris, 2006). The current direct and indirect effects of both mothers and fathers need to be integrated into theory and research to fully understand parenting as a context of child development (Cabrera et al., 2018; Lucassen et al., 2015). This is also crucial to influence changes in policy away from gender-stereotyped expectations for parents (Panter-Brick et al., 2014). Recent research shows that fathers have direct and indirect effects on their children's development (reviewed in Barker, Iles, & Ramchandani, 2017; Cabrera et al., 2018) and that men's parenting styles and values are varied and nuanced (Panter-Brick et al., 2014). In sum, it is not a reasonable shorthand to make conclusions about "parenting" without studying both mothers and fathers, including in same-sex parenting couples, and

A. S. Meuwissen (✉)
Center for Early Education and Development, University of Minnesota, St. Paul, MN, USA
e-mail: asm@umn.edu

H. E. Fitzgerald et al. (eds.), *Handbook of Fathers and Child Development*, https://doi.org/10.1007/978-3-030-51027-5_25

giving both genders of parents their due as important influences on their children. Research that only includes mothers should be explicitly titled as such, and the exclusion of fathers should be acknowledged as a limitation.

This chapter focuses specifically on father impacts on executive function. Executive function (EF) refers to a set of higher level thinking skills that enable people to control their behavior and emotions and direct them toward long-term goals rather than what is automatic or easiest. The construct of EF is closely related to other terms such as self-regulation, effortful control, and emotion regulation. EF involves the ability to effectively integrate bottom-up (reactive) and top-down (reflective) processes (Blair, 2016; Zelazo, 2015). EF is commonly described in terms of three main components: working memory (holding and manipulating information in one's mind), cognitive flexibility (switching between rules and adapting thinking to different situations), and inhibitory control (stopping impulsive behaviors; for review, see Carlson, Zelazo, & Faja, 2013). Especially in younger children (ages 2–5), EFs have also been found to vary along a hot-cool dimension, with hot executive function activated in situations that are highly motivating and emotional, such as tasks in which one must delay or inhibit approaching a desirable reward, and cool executive function activated in situations that do not have a strong emotional component, such as rule switching or memory tasks (Carlson, White, & Davis-Unger, 2014; Kim, Nordling, Yoon, Boldt, & Kochanska, 2013; Willoughby, Kupersmidt, Voegler-Lee, & Bryant, 2011; Zelazo & Carlson, 2012). The development of executive function is tied to the development of the brain's prefrontal cortex, which lasts from birth into young adulthood, with a period of rapid development between ages 2 and 5. Executive function is influenced by a variety of factors, from biological to social (Blair & Diamond, 2008).

Executive function skills have a foundational role in academic readiness and behavioral and social competence. When children are unable to coordinate their emotional arousal and cognitive control systems, they cannot function effectively in school and peer contexts (Blair & Diamond, 2008). Supporting the development of EF in the early preschool years could have a cascading effect, promoting a variety of crucial skills such as math and literacy abilities, theory of mind, and emotion regulation (Masten et al., 2012; McClelland et al., 2007). Indeed, EF in early childhood is associated with outcomes across the life span, such as income, educational attainment, social skills, mental and physical health, and criminal offenses (Mischel et al., 2011; Moffitt et al., 2011).

Because EF has such significance in children's and adults' lives, it is important to understand causal influences on its development. To fully do so, we must include fathers as a contributor to children's development. When a family consists of two parents, using one parent as a proxy for the home environment limits the power to detect effects on children (Cowan, Cowan, Pruett, & Pruett, 2019), misses the opportunity for a nuanced understanding of the family system, and may overestimate the effects of mothers if they do not control for the influence of fathers.

This chapter reviews (1) theory around why parenting generally and fathers specifically matter for child EF development, (2) empirical evidence for links between mother and father parenting and EF, (3) research on these processes for families facing risks and challenges, and (4) implications for interventions. In this chapter, I will use the terms "father" and "fathering" to represent all male parenting figures, with the acknowledgment that one does not need to be a biological or legal father to have an impact on a child in one's care.

Theoretical Basis for a Link Between Parenting and Child EF

There are three major developmental theories that have proposed a link between parenting and child EF: Vygotsky's sociocultural theory, self-determination theory, and attachment theory. These theories are important in providing a foundation for understanding mechanisms by which parents, both mothers and fathers, may influence their children's cognitive development. While much of the research resulting from these theories has focused on mothers, many of the proposed mechanisms could generalize to fathers as well. These theories form a useful base from which to examine possible similarities and differences between mothers and fathers.

Vygotsky's Sociocultural Theory Vygotsky proposed that adult-child interactions are the foundational context for children to actively build their thinking and regulation abilities. By internalizing, transforming, and reorganizing the problem solving skills they use during these interactions, children are gradually able to use their own executive function to control their social, emotional, and cognitive processes without the help of the adult. Language is viewed as a crucial component of mental processes, in that children use speech to regulate their behavior. The adult's main role in the regulation of joint activity is to provide assistance at an appropriate level slightly ahead of the child's competence so that a child can progress toward independence (Vygotsky, 1978; Wood, Bruner, & Ross, 1976). Wood (1980) termed the role of the adult in this process "scaffolding," where the adult matches their help to the child's ability.

Self-Determination Theory Self-determination theory (SDT) has also focused on scaffolding-type behaviors, using the label autonomy support. This theory proposes that there are three universal human needs: autonomy, competence, and relatedness, which are necessary for motivation and well-being. Autonomy support is the component of parenting in self-determination theory research that has been most consistently associated with positive child outcomes (Grolnick & Farkas, 2002) and is predictive from infancy through adolescence (Joussemet, Landry, & Koestner, 2008). Similar to the construct of scaffolding, autonomy support involves meeting a child at their current developmental needs: allowing the child to do all they are capable of and then providing any additional support needed to meet a goal. Autonomy supportive behaviors include supporting children to be independent in problem-solving, providing reasons and explanations for requests, taking the child's perspective and acknowledging feelings, offering and encouraging choices, being low on controlling techniques, and allowing children to participate in decisions (Grolnick & Ryan, 1989; Joussemet et al., 2008).

Autonomy supportive parenting allows children to use their cognitive skills to their highest ability, provides experience with successful problem-solving, and gives opportunities to practice EF skills such as planning ahead, making decisions, and monitoring their own errors, which rely on reflective thinking and self-regulation (Zelazo, 2004). The opposite, controlling parenting, is thought to be detrimental to EF because it undermines internal motivation, denies children an active role, and prevents opportunities to cause and self-evaluate effects on the environment (Meuwissen & Carlson, 2015).

Attachment Theory Attachment theory provides another framework to consider why early relationships are a critical factor in the development of EF. One of Bowlby's main hypotheses was that high-quality parenting leads to secure attachment and thus a variety of positive developmental outcomes, whereas low-quality parenting results in an insecure attachment and negative outcomes (Bowlby, 1970). Ideally, children are first regulated by a sensitive, responsive parent who correctly identifies and interprets a child's signals and reacts contingently and appropriately (Eshel, Daelmans, Cabral de Mello, & Martines, 2006). This external regulation then becomes a prototype for later self-regulation (Sroufe, 1990).

For internalization to occur, attachment figures need to be both a secure base (a base from which the child can go out and explore the environment) and a safe haven (a place to return for comfort when exploring the environment becomes stressful or frightening; Bowlby, 1988). These two roles need to cycle back and forth: once the child is comforted, they are able to return to exploring the environment. Through this process, children gradually become less dependent on their parents as they learn self-regulation (Drake, Belsky, & Fearon, 2014). This is key for cognitive development because having a secure base in whom the child trusts allows the child to explore the environment, gain skills in problem-solving, and develop mastery motivation, rather than devoting resources to anxiously monitor their caregiver's availability (Bowlby, 1970; Moss, Gosselin, Parent, Rousseau, & Dumont, 1997). Although Bowlby (1969) recognized the development of secondary attachment figures, the majority of research in the attachment tradition has focused solely on mothers as primary attachment figures.

The three theories discussed above all propose that adult-child interactions are a primary context for children to learn regulation. Parents are initially responsible for regulation, and this must be gradually internalized by the child to achieve self-regulated behavior. The theories agree that the parent needs to carefully monitor and adjust to the child's state and that the parent leads the child toward self-regulation by giving the child appropriate responsibility and control over their actions (Grolnick & Farkas, 2002; Moss et al., 1997). A major weakness of this literature is a lack of inclusion of fathers in the research and little thinking about how mothers and fathers may work together or interact to support a child's developing self-regulation.

While these three theories continue to generate research, thinking on the relationship between caregiving and EF has more recently been bolstered by new research incorporating biological and neurological processes. EF is now thought to be transferred from parent to child through interdependent genetic and environmental processes, including parenting (Barker et al., 2017; Bridgett, Burt, Edwards, & Deater-Deckard, 2015). The protracted development of the brain regions involved in EF may indicate an extended period of sensitivity to social influences (Hackman & Farah, 2009), and these regions are indeed affected by the quality of parental care and the aspects of the home environment (Hackman, Gallop, Evans, & Farah, 2015). The plasticity of EF in the preschool years (about 3–5 years old) suggests that parenting may be especially critical during this period, and therefore, interventions during early childhood may have a greater effect than later in the child's life (Zelazo & Carlson, 2012).

Empirical Evidence for Mother and Father Effects on EF

In this section, I will first review what is known about mother impacts on child EF, to overview the current state of the field. Next, I will explore what is known about father effects.

Research Evidence for Maternal Autonomy Support/Scaffolding and Child EF

The Vygotskian and SDT theories have been supported in that autonomy support (vs. control), typically measured through observed mother-child interactions or self-report surveys, is the maternal parenting dimension that most consistently predicts child EF, both in lab tasks and rated behavior (Bernier, Carlson, & Whipple, 2010; Fay-Stammbach, Hawes, & Meredith, 2014; Karreman, van Tuijl, van Aken, & Dokovic, 2006). These findings hold even when controlling for other aspects of parenting such as warmth and cognitive stimulation (Bernier et al., 2010; Bindman, Pomerantz, & Roisman. 2015). Maternal autonomy support is related to children's performance on both cool (e.g., Bernier et al., 2010) and hot (e.g., Grolnick, Kurowski, McMenamy, Rivkin, & Bridges, 1998) EF tasks and predicts child EF above and beyond parent EF (Distefano, Gallinsky, McClelland, Zelazo, & Carlson, 2018). Multiple studies have found that autonomy support predicts child EF across the toddler and preschool years, with language at an intermediate time point mediating some of the relations (e.g., Hammond, Muller, Carpendale, Bibok, & Liebermann-Finestone, 2012; Matte-Gagne & Bernier, 2011). There is also evidence that autonomy supportive parenting predicts academic achievement into high school because of links with early EF, even when controlling for child temperament, mother education, and other dimensions of mother parenting (Bindman et al., 2015).

Research Evidence for Maternal Sensitivity/Responsivity/Attachment and Child EF

Early research found that securely attached toddlers and preschoolers showed more competence, persistence, problem-solving skills, and cooperation during mother-child problem-solving tasks compared to insecure counterparts (Matas, Arend, & Sroufe, 1978; Moss et al., 1997). While early research typically relied on small-scale studies with limited racial and socioeconomic diversity, recently, multiple large-scale longitudinal studies of more representative samples have found that attachment security and sensitive parenting in infancy (measured by observed parent-child interactions) predict EF performance through elementary school (Drake et al., 2014; Sulik et al., 2015). Findings have also linked sensitive/responsive parenting to EF in the preschool years in multiple samples facing heightened risk (Brophy-Herb, Stansbury, Bocknek, & Horodynski, 2012; Camerota et al., 2015). In a longitudinal study, adults with histories of secure attachment could better regulate frustration and aggression and showed coping patterns characterized by persistence and flexibility (Sroufe, 2005). These findings support attachment theory's hypothesis that children who have a stable, supportive caregiver early in life are more able to deploy their cognitive resources to exploration and problem-solving and can gradually internalize self-regulation. Additionally, animal literature has persuasively shown that sensitive, responsive care has lasting effects on offspring adjustment and behavioral and physiological regulation (reviewed in Bridgett et al., 2015).

Conclusions About Mother Parenting The links between child EF and both mother autonomy support and sensitivity have been corroborated by multiple high-quality, longitudinal studies, including large-sample studies. This research has been done in diverse populations with various risk factors. Meta-analyses show that there is solid evidence of a nontrivial relation between these maternal parenting dimensions and child EF (Fay-Stammbach et al., 2014; Karreman et al., 2006).

What We Know About the Father Parenting-Child EF Link

While the links between mother parenting and child EF have a solid evidence base, we still have much to learn about the effect fathers have on children's EF. Cabrera et al. (2014) have identified three ways in which issues related to father vs. mother parenting have been studied: focusing on similarities, focusing on differences, and focusing on how mothers and father complement each other. In the following sections, I have used these three themes, with the addition of focusing on quantity of father involvement, to organize the research that has been done around fathers and child EF. Because very few studies have examined father parenting in relation to EF specifically, I also draw on evidence from broader cognitive and social outcomes in this review.

Theme 1: Individual Variation in Quality of Father Parenting Affects Child Outcomes, in Similar Ways to Mothers This first theme reflects research suggesting that the impact of fathers may not be qualitatively different from that of mothers, but that fathers are similarly important (e.g., Grolnick & Farkas, 2002). It proposes that fathers meaningfully vary on parenting dimensions such as autonomy support and sensitivity, as mothers do, and these variations have implications for development. Shannon et al. (2002) argue that variations among fathers need to be emphasized rather than only looking at mean differences between mothers and fathers, which can lead to stereotyped views of fathers as only engaging in rough-and-tumble play.

Evidence for Similar Effects from Fathers and Mothers on General Development Both positive (e.g., sensitivity) and negative (e.g., restrictive, harsh parenting) father behaviors have been associated with a variety of cognitive and social outcomes (e.g., Cabrera et al., 2011, 2018; Grolnick & Farkas, 2002; Magill-Evans, Harrison, Rempel, & Slater, 2006), even in interactions with children as young as 3 months (Ramchandani et al., 2013). Fathers' and mothers' supportive parenting independently predict language and cognitive outcomes in early childhood (Shannon, Tamis-LeMonda, London, & Cabrera, 2002; Tamis-LeMonda, Shannon, Cabrera, & Lamb, 2004). Children develop independent attachments to their mother and father, and secure attachments to fathers have been linked to a variety of child outcomes (reviewed in Dagan & Sagi-Schwartz, 2018). In many cases, father parenting remains a significant predictor even when taking mother parenting into account (Coley et al., 2011; Cowan et al., 2019; Tamis-LeMonda et al., 2004). There is also evidence that the quality of father-child interactions has stronger effects on cognitive development than quantity of involvement (Easterbrooks & Goldberg, 1984; Meuwissen & Carlson, 2015; Shannon et al. 2002).

Evidence for Similar Effects from Fathers and Mothers on EF Development Most of the research that has been done tying father parenting to specific EF outcomes has focused on and found evidence for similarities between mother and father effects. Three studies have found that father sensitive/responsive parenting in toddlerhood during play interactions is linked to later preschool EF lab tasks (Bernier, Carlson, Deschenes, & Matte-Gagne, 2012; Kochanska, Askan, Prisco, & Adams, 2008; Towe-Goodman et al., 2014). On average, mothers and fathers show equivalent levels of autonomy support when doing a puzzle with their child (Connor et al., 1997; Meuwissen & Carlson, 2019), and one study found the effect of autonomy support on observed child self-regulation did not differ by parent gender (Meuwissen & Carlson, 2019). Meuwissen and Carlson (2015) found that father autonomy support with their 3-year-olds was linked to concurrent child EF lab tasks, independent of child general IQ and father EF, as well as predictive of a school readiness composite (including EF measures) 2 years later (Meuwissen & Carlson, 2018). Bernier et al. (2012) showed a combined measure of maternal- and paternal-child interactions contributed to the prediction of cool EF at 3 years old but did not examine effects of mother and father parenting separately. Self-reports of parenting behaviors (e.g., monitoring, discipline, and autonomy; bonding) from both mothers and fathers have been significantly linked to early childhood EF measured via lab tasks (de Cock et al., 2017; Roskam, Stievenart, Meunier, & Noel, 2014) and parent report (Lucassen et al., 2015). These findings support the idea that quality of fathering contributes to the development of child EF in the preschool years in similar ways to mothers.

Theme 2: Fathers Provide Unique Experiences, Especially in Play A second theme represents research on qualities of father-child interactions that are unique from mother-child interactions, which may promote cognitive and EF development (e.g., Grossmann, Grossmann, Kindler, & Zimmermann, 2008; Paquette, 2004). One of the most commonly studied differences between mothers and fathers is in the context of play. Paquette and colleagues have proposed a theory about the importance of father-child play in which they suggest that in contrast to the mother-child attachment relationship that focuses on comforting the child, the most important dimension of a father-child attachment relationship is the concept of activation (operationalized as stimulation and overcoming fears), especially present in rough-and-tumble play. Grossman et al. (2008) agree that in a review of studies, the key marker of secure attachment in father-child relationships is for the father to be a trusted, dependable companion when the child faces challenging situations in play.

Compared to mothers, fathers tend to have a stronger playmate role (Cabrera & Roggman, 2017), and their play tends to be more physical, vigorous, state disrupting, surprising, and unpredictable (Fletcher, St. George, & Freeman, 2013; John, Halliburton & Humphrey, 2013; Lamb, 2004). Interestingly, one study found that although these differences were present, fathers and mothers overall showed equal emotional availability (John et al., 2013). There also is evidence that mothers' and fathers' play has some similar characteristics, with mothers and fathers rated as having equal playfulness during free play (operationalized as creativity, imagination, humor, and curiosity; Cabrera et al., 2017). One key difference may be that father play gives children more experience with high levels of arousal, which may be important for cognitive stimulation and practice with skills such as regulating behavior, managing impulses and strong emotions, and coping with frustration (Fletcher et al., 2013; Grossmann et al., 2008). However, this literature has significant limitations in that mother rough-and-tumble play has not been observationally explored, so it is difficult to draw direct comparisons (Cabrera et al., 2017).

Evidence for Unique Effects of Fathers on General Development High-quality rough-and-tumble father-child play has been associated with fewer conduct, peer, and emotional problems in the early school years (Flanders, Leo, Paquette, Pihl, & Seguin, 2009; Fletcher et al., 2013; Grossmann et al., 2008). For father-child dyads, quality of physical play is a better predictor of child socioemotional outcomes than is attachment (Dumont & Paquette, 2013). Fathers who appropriately controlled and structured rough-and-tumble play in an observed interaction had children who were rated as less aggressive (by father report; Flanders et al., 2009).

Evidence for Unique Effects of Fathers on EF Development There has been very limited research on unique father contributions to child EF. In one study investigating physical play (Meuwissen & Carlson, 2018), fathers ($N = 89$, majority White, middle class) interacted with their 5-year-old children in two contexts. The first was an indoor gym with various playground equipment (e.g., monkey bars, slide, small basketball hoop), and the second was a seated puzzle task, which was coded for autonomy support (using a self-determination theory lens; Whipple, Bernier & Mageau, 2011). Children were assessed on a school readiness composite, which included lab tasks of EF, literacy, and numeracy. Findings showed that father overstimulation in gym play (an observational measure of fathers pushing children to do things the child found scary or overwhelming) was negatively correlated to the concurrent child school readiness composite, with a medium effect size. Previous measurement of father autonomy support at age 3 longitudinally predicted the age 5 school readiness composite, but concurrent autonomy support at age 5 did not. This suggests that the physical play context, where there are demands to regulate during exciting situations such as climbing or wrestling, may be more relevant for father-child dyads in the later preschool years than the calmer puzzle task. Recognizing fathers' role as an important regulator in exciting play interactions could lead to new intervention targets that have not previously been explored.

Theme 3: The Quantity of Father Involvement Is Important for Child Outcomes The third theme is that the amount of time fathers spend with children is associated with positive outcomes. Lamb (2004) suggested that children who have a lot of interaction with both parents, especially with parents who differ in their parenting styles, may be exposed to a wider range of stimulation. This could promote EF by requiring greater mental flexibility and frequent rule switching. This hypothesis suggests that children who have two highly involved parents should have the best cognitive and EF outcomes. Lower quantity of involvement is often cited as a possible reason when father behavior is more weakly linked to child outcomes than mother behavior, yet measures of maternal and paternal involvement are not often included in such studies (e.g., Kochanska et al., 2008, Magill-Evans et al., 1999). It will therefore be important to conduct studies that include the quality and quantity of parenting from both parents to separate out the effects of these two variables and assess the validity of these claims.

Evidence for Effects of Quantity of Father Involvement on General Development In a review of longitudinal evidence on the effect of father involvement, Sarkadi et al. (2008) concluded higher amounts of father-child interaction enhance cognitive, social, and behavioral outcomes. Children of more involved fathers show better problem-solving skills, less externalizing behavior (Grolnick & Farkas, 2002), and lower likelihood of cognitive delay (Bronte-Tinkew, Carrano, Horowitz, & Kinukawa, 2008). Preschoolers with two supportive parents score highest on cognitive outcomes like the Bayley Mental Development Index (Ryan, Martin, & Brooks-Gunn, 2006). Easterbrooks and Goldberg (1984) found that father involvement was related to optimal child development, independently of observed parenting characteristics, although including both types of measures accounted for the most variance. There is also some animal evidence for this hypothesis: when rhesus monkey infants were reared with both their mothers and fathers (not the typical arrangement for adult male monkeys), they were more intelligent, confident, and mentally flexible (Harlow, Harlow, & Suomi, 1971).

Evidence for Effects of Quantity of Father Involvement on EF Development I am not aware of any published studies that have linked quantity of father involvement to specific EF tasks. Meuwissen and Carlson (2015) found that in two-parent, mostly White middle class families, father involvement (measured via survey) was concurrently correlated with father autonomy support, and father autonomy support was associated with their 3-year-old children's EF, but there was no significant relation between father involvement and children's EF. This was contrary to previous literature showing positive effects of father involvement on cognitive development. Multiple interpretations of the correlation between father quality (e.g., autonomy support) and quantity of parenting are possible: that fathers who spend more time with their children are therefore able to develop higher-quality parenting skills, or that fathers with higher-quality parenting spend more time with their children, because they may find it more enjoyable or feel more effective. Additionally, related variables such as child temperament or mother behavior could be part of this relationship. More work needs to be done to understand the interrelations between father involvement, parenting quality, and child EF.

Theme 4: Fathers Have Effects on the Family System, Interdependent with Other Caregiver Effects This theme has arisen from family systems theory suggesting that the network of caregiving relationships a child has (which could include mothers, fathers, and other care providers) does not act independently but rather collectively to impact child outcomes (e.g., Dagan & Sagi-Schwartz, 2018). This view suggests that the most useful lines of research will integrate fathers and mothers into understanding overall family functioning. Palkovitz (2013) and colleagues note that the construct of co-parenting reflects a nuanced system where variables such as father involvement, mother-father relationships, parent gender roles, and child outcomes all interact across time. When Cowan et al. (2009) outlined aspects of family life related to father engagement, they included factors such as the quality of relationships between parents and the pattern of caregiver-child relationships transmitted across generations, indicating that relationships affect relationships and do not act on children independently. Fathers are important in father-child interactions, but also as partners and co-parents (Cowan et al., 2019). It should also be acknowledged that there is significant evidence of bidirectional relationships between parent and child behavior showing that a child shapes parents and vice versa (Kiel & Kalomiris, 2015; Meuwissen, & Carlson 2018).

Evidence for Interdependent Father/Mother Effects on General Development There is substantial evidence that the quality of the co-parenting relationship is important for child outcomes such as psychological adjustment and academic outcomes (Palkovitz, Fagan, & Hull, 2013; Teubert & Pinquart, 2010). In reviewing the literature and finding that father effects on emotion regulation tend to be weaker and are more often moderated by other family variables than mother effects, Kiel and Kalomiris (2015) have suggested that mother parenting has a direct impact on children whereas father parenting is absorbed into general family climate. Dagan and Sagi-Schwartz (2018) have identified unanswered questions in the field of attachment research about how attachments to multiple parenting figures may interact with one another, which are important to move the attachment field beyond a sole focus on mothers.

Overall, more research needs to be done to form a coherent picture of how mother and father effects work together to influence child outcomes.

Evidence for Interdependent Father/Mother Effects on EF Development Feinberg (2003) suggested that co-parents who have a hostile relationship may be less able to provide their children with external regulation, thus limiting children's ability to learn self-regulation. This idea has been supported by one study that found that toddlers from families characterized by higher co-parenting cooperation and warmth showed more positive and less negative affect when doing a frustrating lab task, compared to those in families with lower parental cooperation and warmth. The effects of the co-parenting relationship held above and beyond quality of maternal parenting (McHale, Kuersten, & Lauretti, 1996). While this suggests possible effects on emotion regulation, a correlate of EF, I am not aware of any published studies that have linked father effects on the family system to specific EF tasks. This is an important direction for future research.

Conclusions About Father Parenting This review showed that there is growing support around the first theme, that dimensions of father parenting (e.g., sensitivity, autonomy support) affect both children's EF development in ways that are similar to mothers. The other three themes, while supported by some studies on general social and cognitive outcomes, are theoretically plausible but lack a substantial evidence base specific to EF outcomes.

Families Facing Risks and Challenges

When discussing father effects on child EF, families facing risks and challenges are one population of specific interest. Fathers in low-income families are less likely to be married to their child's mother or living in the home with the child compared to families with more resources, and the lack of father involvement may be a particularly important risk factor in such contexts (Fitzgerald & Bocknek, 2013). There is also a well-established link between socioeconomic status (SES) and EF (Hackman et al., 2015; Holochwost et al., 2016; Merz et al., 2018), as well as specific risk factors such as low parent education (Matte-Gagne & Bernier, 2011), homelessness (Masten et al., 2012), and household chaos (Bridgett et al., 2015), with cumulative risk and chronic stress being especially detrimental to children's regulatory systems (Holochwost, et al., 2016; Merz et al., 2018). Statistically, SES (as a multidimensional construct) is more strongly related to EF than many other neurocognitive skills (Hackman & Farah, 2009; Merz et al., 2018). In a diverse, national sample, associations between SES and EF appear in early childhood and remain consistent through middle childhood (Hackman et al., 2015). Promoting EF skills in children from lower SES backgrounds is especially important as it is associated with academic outcomes. EF interventions hold promise for closing academic achievement gaps, as children with the lowest EF tend to benefit the most from universal interventions (Diamond & Lee, 2011).

Cumulative risk is associated with both lower-quality parenting and lower child EF (Holochwost et al., 2016). Risk factors of fathers, mothers, and children interact to influence both mother and father behavior (Cabrera et al., 2011). Research with mothers has established interrelations of

SES, parenting quality, and EF. Quality of mother parenting can explain significant variance in the link between SES and child EF (Hackman et al., 2015; Rhoades, Greenberg, Lanza, & Blair, 2011), and maternal scaffolding predicts child effortful control above and beyond cumulative risk factors (Lengua, Honorado, & Bush, 2007). The positive associations between mother autonomy support and child EF are consistent across levels of socioeconomic status (Distefano et al., 2018). However, genetic contributions, which could contribute to such links, were not included in these studies. Whereas parenting quality has been shown to transmit much of the influence of early risk on later EF (Rhoads et al., 2011), high-quality mother parenting can be a buffer between difficult environments and child EF (Rochette & Bernier, 2014). Indeed, a recent study showed that a preventive intervention focused on increasing supportive parenting (sample was 90% mothers) reduced the association between poverty and brain development in adolescents, indicating parenting interventions are a promising target to reduce social disparities (Brody et al., 2017).

Father Impacts on EF in Families Facing Risks and Challenges

Quantity and quality of father support are known to predict many outcomes in under-resourced families in both cognitive and social domains (e.g., Coley et al., 2011; Fitzgerald & Bocknek, 2013; Rowe & Cabrera, 2013). When looking at EF as an outcome, evidence shows that maternal parenting is a key mediator between SES and EF, but father parenting has often not been included in such studies. One barrier to this research is that father presence and involvement varies greatly in such samples, as fathers facing high levels of life stress tend to be less involved with their children (Rosenberg & Wilcox, 2006). In these families, it will be especially crucial to attend to both variables of quantity and quality of father parenting. Samples of father figures could be very mixed in terms of the type and duration of their relationship with the child. However, it is important that these considerations do not stop researchers from conducting these studies but instead are seen as key pieces of the research designs. Multiple studies using different conceptualizations of these research questions are necessary to begin to understand if and how fathers and father figures can be leveraged to support child EF in diverse contexts, which we know is critical for the well-being of these children.

In a study on Head Start low-income minority families, Malin et al. (2014) found that fathers' regulatory behavior and regulatory language with their 2-year-olds predicted sustained attention and emotion regulation, respectively, about 2 years later (before kindergarten entry). These effects held after controlling for maternal supportiveness, indicating unique effects of father-child interactions on child regulation outcomes. Interestingly, children's vocabulary skills also predicted fathers' regulatory behaviors, suggesting transactional effects. Using a sample from the same study, fathers' playfulness, but not mothers' (rated in a free-play activity on creativity, imagination, humor, and/or curiosity), predicted their 2-year-olds' prekindergarten vocabulary, while only mothers' playfulness predicted emotion regulation. Fathers' playfulness was more related to demographic factors than mothers', suggesting possible greater influence of context for fathers.

Meuwissen and Englund (2016) analyzed the contributions of both mother parenting and father-figure support (for any male who lived in the home, biologically related or not) on child EF using data from the Minnesota Longitudinal Study of Risk and Adaptation (Sroufe, Egeland, Carlson, & Collins, 2005). The study recruited mothers (58% White) with earning incomes at or below the poverty level, who were often young and single and had low levels of education. Results showed that quality of support from father figures (measured from extensive interviews with mothers at multiple time points) predicted child EF lab tasks in early childhood and teacher ratings of child EF skills in middle childhood, above and beyond demographics and observed quality of maternal parenting.

These studies indicate that quality of father figure/child interactions may play an important role in EF development in children facing challenges and will likely provide better information than simply the presence or absence of a father figure. More research is needed on how context and resources affect the quality of father parenting and how father parenting interacts with other variables in low-resourced families to influence child outcomes.

Interventions: Establishing a Causal Link

The research reviewed to this point has been almost exclusively correlational, measured either concurrently or longitudinally. Although this research substantiates a nontrivial link between mother parenting and child EF and suggests similar relations for fathers, correlational and longitudinal research has serious limitations. Because there is neither random assignment nor manipulation of variables, we cannot rule out the possibility that confounding variables have affected these results. Although many of the studies controlled for some important factors such as demographics and general child cognitive abilities, these correlational studies neglect crucial possible influences such as shared genetics or evocative effects from child to parent (e.g., children with higher EF may be easier to parent well). To make a causal claim about parenting affecting child EF development, researchers need to move beyond correlational studies to randomized control trials where quality of parenting is manipulated.

It has been established that early childhood EF is responsive to a variety of interventions with diverse methods and theoretical frameworks (see Diamond & Ling, 2016 for review). Training through real-life activities that continually increase in challenge seems to be most effective, which suggests that what parents do with their children on a day-to-day basis could be a crucial target for intervention (Diamond & Ling, 2016). School-based interventions may begin too late to catch a crucial window of plasticity, and adding earlier parenting components to EF interventions may boost their effectiveness (Holochwost et al., 2016), as patterns of both parenting and child behavior can stabilize early in development (Meuwissen & Carlson, 2018; Ramchandani et al., 2013; Sulik et al., 2015). Also, changes in parenting practices, attitudes, and expectations are known to be one important mechanism by which interventions can continue to have long-term effects for children after the intervention ends (Reynolds, Ou, & Topitzes, 2004). If our goal is to promote strong EF in children, parenting practices may be one of the strongest targets, yet little work has been done intervening with parents to promote EF development.

Parenting Interventions Measuring Child EF Outcomes

To my knowledge, there have been no full-scale parenting interventions designed to target child EF, but two parenting interventions (focused on mothers) have measured child EF as a secondary outcome. In both, the intervention targets were wide and varied, and it is therefore unclear which part of the intervention led to the increases in EF.

The Attachment Biobehavioral Catch-Up is an attachment-based ten-session parenting program, which provides developmental information, discussions of video-taped parent-child interactions, and an opportunity for parents to reflect on their own past caregiving experiences. In a randomized control trial, preschool-aged children whose parents (98% mothers; 61% African American) participated in the ABC intervention performed better on an EF task, the Dimensional Change Card Sort (DCCS), than children in the control intervention, even with covarying language ability (Lewis-Morrarty, Dozier, Bernard, Terracciano, & Moore, 2012). The DCCS was the only EF measure used. It will be important to replicate this finding with a more complete battery of EF tasks.

The second intervention study examined the effect of having a paraprofessional vs. a nurse provide regular home visits to the mother throughout pregnancy and the first 2 years of the child's life. The program promoted adaptive behaviors, improving relationships with family members, and use of services. Two years after the visits ended, when the children were 4 years of age, mothers who had been visited by nurses had children who performed better on EF lab tasks and language compared to controls, but there was no effect on maternal sensitivity or child emotion regulation (Olds et al., 2004).

There are major weaknesses in the literature around father interventions, including a dearth of robust evaluation for many interventions including fathers, and a lack of disaggregated results between mothers and fathers or between interventions delivered to one vs. both parents (Panter-Brick et al., 2014). However, there is evidence that father interventions have had positive impacts on father and child behavior (Cabrera et al. 2014; Magill-Evans et al., 2006).

In a proof of concept study for manipulating autonomy support behavior either upward or downward, mothers and fathers were both able to change their behavior during an interaction with their child in response to a set of instructions and an example video, suggesting that parents understood the concept presented and were able to implement them in the immediately following interaction. Also, children of parents who became less autonomy supportive/more controlling showed declines in self-regulation during that task. Although this study had a number of limitations, it shows promise that teaching parents (both mothers and fathers) to become more autonomy supportive could subsequently promote child EF development (Meuwissen & Carlson, 2019).

Working with Family Systems

To promote any child development outcomes, involving the whole family system seems likely to be more effective in creating change than working with either parent in isolation (Barker et al., 2017; Cabrera et al., 2014; and others). There is a small amount of evidence that including both mothers and fathers in interventions is most effective (reviewed in Bakermans-Kranenburg, van IJzendoorn, & Juffer, 2003; Panter-Brick et al., 2014). However, in the Magill-Evans et al. (2006) review on father interventions, they noted that in interventions that include both mothers and fathers, fathers tend to have lower participation rates, especially on homework assignments and discussions, and seem to prefer interventions focused on active involvement with their child. They concluded that active participation with or observation of the father's own child is crucial for interventions targeting fathers. Panter-Brick et al. (2014) make explicit a need to engage co-parents as the target of interventions rather than see fathers as an add-on to mother interventions. Calls are being made for creative approaches to engage fathers and confront the biases in our current approaches to research and policy (Barker et al., 2017; Panter-Brick et al., 2014).

Conclusions About Parenting Interventions

In sum, there is good evidence that interventions can change attitudes and behaviors, although most of this research has focused on mothers. There is still much work to be done exploring if changing parenting can change child EF outcomes and which dimensions of parenting have the greatest effect. There is a substantial body of research indicating that parent sensitivity/responsiveness can be affected by interventions and linked to positive child outcomes (Bakermans-Kranenburg et al., 2003; Eshel et al., 2006), but less research on parent autonomy support (mixed results: reviewed in Su & Reeve, 2011), or on EF as an outcome. There is also some evidence that father interventions can change father parenting behaviors and improve some child outcomes, but there is much to learn about what interventions may be most effective for fathers and what targets in father behavior are most useful to promote child EF.

Summary and Key Points

There is a growing evidence base that father parenting is related to early childhood EF development, yet there is still much to be investigated in this area. Aspects of mother parenting, such as sensitivity and autonomy support, have rich theoretical and strong empirical support. In this chapter, I reviewed four focus areas of research on fathers and child EF development. Multiple studies show that fathers impact child EF in similar ways as mothers, while research is still emerging on how father effects may differ from mothers, the importance of quantity of father involvement, and how father and mother effects interact to influence the family system. Each of these focus areas also highlights gaps and points to future directions in the research. First, it will be useful to replicate and extend what we know about mother parenting to father parenting, as many areas of research have exclusively relied on mothers. Second, it is also worthwhile to consider what contexts or processes may be more relevant for fathers specifically, such as rough-and-tumble play. Third, we need more studies that measure both father involvement and observe qualities of father parenting, to disentangle the effect of quantity and quality of father interactions. And fourth, it will be important to conduct studies that include both mothers and fathers of the same children and to examine systems-level effects of relationships on other relationships. There is a paucity of research investigating father impacts on child cognitive development for families facing risks and challenges. This will be an important gap to fill, as parenting appears to be a crucial buffer in such situations. And finally, interventions with fathers have been a neglected avenue of impact. Very few parenting interventions have measured child EF outcomes (and none that included fathers) or been specifically designed for the purpose of promoting child EF. However, parenting interventions show promise for improving child EF, and interventions that include the entire family are likely to be most effective.

Modern research needs to move away from the notion that a study of mothers fully captures a child's parenting environment. There are multiple lines of promising research reviewed in this chapter that have the potential to make substantial gains in our understanding of how fathers matter for the development of children's executive function. By addressing these issues, we can increasingly leverage fathers as part of building a strong foundation for children's success.

References

Bakermans-Kranenburg, M. J., van IJzendoorn, M. H., & Juffer, F. (2003). Less is more: Meta-analyses of sensitivity and attachment interventions in early childhood. *Psychological Bulletin, 129*(2), 195–215.

Barker, B., Iles, J. E., & Ramchandani, P. G. (2017). Fathers, fathering, and child psychopathology. *Current Opinion in Psychology, 15*, 87–92.

Bernier, A., Carlson, S. M., Deschenes, M., & Matte-Gagne, C. (2012). Social factors in the development of early executive functioning: A closer look at the caregiving environment. *Developmental Science, 15*(1), 12–24. https://doi.org/10.1111/j.1467-7687.2011.01093.x

Bernier, A., Carlson, S. M., & Whipple, N. (2010). From external regulation to self-regulation: Early parenting precursors of young children's executive functioning. *Child Development, 81*(1), 326–339.

Bianchi, S. M., Robinson, J. P., & Milkie, M. A. (2006). Parenting: How has it changed? In *Changing rhythms of American family life* (pp. 1–18). New York, NY: Russel Sage.

Bindman, S. W., Pomerantz, E. M., & Roisman, G. I. (2015). Do children's executive functions account for associations between early autonomy supportive parenting and achievement through high school? *Journal of Educational Psychology, 107*(3), 756–770.

Blair, C. (2016). Developmental science and executive function. *Current Directions in Psychological Science, 25*(1), 3–7.

Blair, C., & Diamond, A. (2008). Biological processes in prevention and intervention: The promotion of self-regulation as a means of preventing school failure. *Development and Psychopathology, 20*(3), 899–911. https://doi.org/10.1017/S0954579408000436

Bowlby, J. (1969). *Attachment and loss: Volume 1. Attachment*. New York: Basic Books.

Bowlby, J. (1970). Disruption of affectional bonds and its effects on behavior. *Journal of Contemporary Psychotherapy, 2*(2), 75–86.

Bowlby, J. (1988). *A secure base: Parent-child attachment and healthy human development* (Vol. xii). New York: Basic Books.

Bridgett, D. J., Burt, N. M., Edwards, E. S., & Deater-Deckard, K. (2015). Intergenerational transmission of self-regulation: A multidisciplinary review and integrative conceptual framework. *Psychological Bulletin, 141*(3), 602–654.

Brody, G. H., Gray, J. C., Yu, T., Barton, A. W., Beach, S. T., Galvain, A., et al. (2017). Protective prevention effects on the association of poverty with brain development. *JAMA Pediatrics, 171*, 46–52.

Bronfenbrenner, U., & Morris, P. A. (2006). The bioecological model of human development. In P. Mussen (Ed.), *Handbook of child psychology*. Hoboken, NJ: Wiley.

Bronte-Tinkew, J., Carrano, J., Horowitz, A., & Kinukawa, A. (2008). Involvement among resident fathers and links to infant cognitive outcomes. *Journal of Family Issues, 29*, 1211–1244. https://doi.org/10.1177/0192513X08318145

Brophy-Herb, H. E., Stansbury, K., Bocknek, E., & Horodynski, M. A. (2012). Modeling maternal emotion-related socialization behaviors in a low-income sample: Relations with toddler's self-regulation. *Early Childhood Research Quarterly, 27*, 352–364.

Cabrera, N., Fagan, J. V., Wight, V., & Schadler, C. (2011). The influence of mother, father, and child risk on parenting and children's cognitive and social behaviors. *Child Development, 82*, 1985–2005.

Cabrera, N. J., Fitzgerald, H. E., Bradley, R. H., & Roggman, L. (2014). The ecology of father-child relationships: An expanded model. *Journal of Family Theory Review, 6*, 336–354. https://doi.org/10.1111/jftr.12054

Cabrera, N. J., Karberg, E., Malin, J. L., & Aldoney, D. (2017). The magic of play: Low-income mothers' and fathers' playfulness and children's emotion regulation and vocabulary skills. *Infant Mental Health Journal, 38*(6), 757–771.

Cabrera, N. J., & Roggman, L. (2017). Father play: Is it special? *Infant Mental Health Journal, 38*(6), 706–708.

Cabrera, N. J., Volling, B. L., & Barr, R. (2018). Fathers are parents, too! Widening the lens on parenting for children's development. *Child Development Perspectives, 12*(3), 152–157.

Camerota, M., Willoughby, M. T., Cox, M., Greenberg, M. T., & the Family Life Project Investigators. (2015). Executive function in low birth weight preschoolers: The moderating effect of parenting. *Journal of Abnormal Child Psychology*. https://doi.org/10.1007/s10802-015-0032-9

Carlson, S. M. (2005). Developmentally sensitive measures of executive function in preschool children. *Developmental Neuropsychology, 28*(2), 595–616.

Carlson, S. M., White, R. E., & Davis-Unger, A. C. (2014). Evidence for a relation between executive function and pretense representation in preschool children. *Cognitive Development, 29*, 1–16.

Carlson, S. M., Zelazo, P. D., & Faja, S. (2013). Executive function. In P. D. Zelazo (Ed.), *Oxford handbook of developmental psychology* (Vol. 1, pp. 706–743). New York: Oxford University Press.

Coley, R. L., Lewin-Bizan, S., & Carrano, J. (2011). Does early paternal parenting promote low-income children's long-term cognitive skills? *Journal of Family Issues, 32*, 1522–1542. https://doi.org/10.1177/0192513X11402175

Connor, D. B., Knight, D. K., & Cross, D. R. (1997). Mothers' and fathers' scaffolding of their 2-year-olds during problem-solving and literacy interactions. *British Journal of Developmental Psychology, 15*, 323–338.

Cowan, P. A., Cowan, C. P., Pruett, M. K., & Pruett, K. (2019). Fathers' and mothers' attachment styles, couple conflict, parenting quality, and children's behavior problems: An intervention test of mediation. *Attachment and Human Development*. https://doi.org/10.1080/14616734.2019.1582600

Cowan, P. A., Cowan, C. P., Pruett, M. K., Pruett, K., & Wong, J. J. (2009). Promoting fathers' engagement with children: Preventive interventions for low-income families. *Journal of Marriage and Family, 71*(3), 663–679.

Dagan, O., & Sagi-Schwartz, A. (2018). Early attachment network with mother and father: An unsettled issue. *Child Development Perspectives, 12*(2), 115–121.

de Cock, E. S. A., Henrichs, J., Klimstra, T. A., Maas, J. B. M., Vreeswijk, C. M. J. M., Neeus, W. H. J., et al. (2017). Longitudinal associations between parental bonding, parenting stress, and executive functioning in toddlerhood. *Journal of Child and Family Studies, 26*(6), 1723–1733.

Diamond, A., & Lee, K. (2011). Interventions shown to aid executive function development in children 4 to 12 years old. *Science, 333*, 959–964.

Diamond, A., & Ling, D. S. (2016). Conclusions about interventions, programs, and approaches for improving executive functions that appear justified and those that, despite much hype, do not. *Developmental Cognitive Neuroscience, 18*, 34–48.

Distefano, R., Galinsky, E., McClelland, M. M., Zelazo, P. D., & Carlson, S. M. (2018). Autonomy-supportive parenting and associations with child and parent executive function. *Journal of Applied Developmental Psychology, 58*(2018), 77–85.

Drake, K., Belsky, J., & Fearon, R. M. P. (2014). From early attachment to engagement with learning in school: The role of self-regulation and persistence. *Developmental Psychology, 50*(5), 1350–1362. https://doi.org/10.1037/a0032779

Dumont, C., & Paquette, D. (2013). What about the child's tie to the father? A new insight into fathering, father-child attachment, children's socioemotional development and the activation relationship theory. *Early Child Development and Care, 183*(3–4), 430–446.

Easterbrooks, A. M., & Goldberg, W. A. (1984). Toddler development in the family: Impact of father involvement and parenting characteristics. *Child Development, 55*(3), 740–752.

Eshel, N., Daelmans, B., Cabral de Mello, M., & Martines, J. (2006). Responsive parenting: Interventions and outcomes. *Bulletin of the World Health Organization, 84*(12), 991–998.

Fay-Stammbach, T., Hawes, D. J., & Meredith, P. (2014). Parenting influences on executive function in early childhood: A review. *Child Development Perspectives, 8*(4), 258–264.

Feinberg, M. E. (2003). The internal structure and ecological context of coparenting: A framework for research and intervention. *Parenting: Science and Practice, 3*(2), 95–131.

Fitzgerald, H. E., & Bocknek, E. L. (2013). Fathers, children, and the risk-resilience continuum. In N. J. Cabrera & C. S. Tamis-LeMonda (Eds.), *Handbook of father involvment* (2nd ed., pp. 169–185). New York: Routledge.

Flanders, J. L., Leo, V., Paquette, D., Pihl, R. O., & Seguin, J. R. (2009). Rough-and-tumble play and the regulation of aggression: An observational study of father-child play dyads. *Aggressive Behavior, 35*, 285–295.

Fletcher, R., St. George, J., & Freeman, E. (2013). Rough and tumble play quality: Theoretical foundations for a new measure of father-child interaction. *Early Child Development and Care, 183*(6), 746–759. https://doi.org/10.1080/03004430.2012.723439

Grolnick, W. S., & Farkas, M. (2002). Parenting and the development of children's self-regulation. In M. H. Bornstein (Ed.), *Handbook of parenting, Vol V, Practical issues in parenting* (pp. 89–110). Mahwah, NJ: Lawrence Erlbaum Associates.

Grolnick, W. S., Kurowski, C. O., McMenamy, J. M., Rivkin, I., & Bridges, L. J. (1998). Mothers' strategies for regulating their toddlers' distress. *Infant Behavior & Development, 21*(3), 437–450.

Grolnick, W. S., & Ryan, R. M. (1989). Parent styles associated with children's self-regulation and competence in school. *Journal of Educational Psychology, 81*(2), 143–154.

Grossmann, K., Grossmann, K. E., Kindler, H., & Zimmermann, P. (2008). A wider view of attachment and exploration. In J. Cassidy & P. R. Shaver (Eds.), *Handbook of attachment: Theory, research, and clinical applications* (2nd ed., pp. 857–879). New York: The Guilford Press.

Hackman, D. A., & Farah, M. J. (2009). Socioeconomic status and the developing brain. *Trends in Cognitive Science, 13*(2), 65–73.

Hackman, D. A., Gallop, R., Evans, G. W., & Farah, M. J. (2015). Socioeconomic status and executive function: Developmental trajectories and mediation. *Developmental Science*, 1–17. https://doi.org/10.1111/desc.12246

Hammond, S. I., Muller, U., Carpendale, J. I. M., Bibok, M. B., & Liebermann-Finestone, D. P. (2012). The effects of parental scaffolding on preschoolers' executive function. *Developmental Psychology, 48*(1), 271–281.

Harlow, H. F., Harlow, M. K., & Suomi, S. J. (1971). From thought to therapy: Lessons from a primate laboratory: How investigation of the learning capability of rhesus monkeys has led to the study of their behavioral abnormalities and rehabilitation. *American Scientist, 59*(5), 538–549.

Holochwost, S. J., Gariepy, J.-L., Propper, C. B., Garnder-Neblett, N., Neblett, E., & Mills-Koonce, R. (2016). Sociodemographic risk, parenting, and executive functions in early childhood: The role of ethnicity. *Early Childhood Research Quarterly, 36*, 537–549.

John, A., Halliburton, A., & Humphrey, J. (2013). Child-mother and child-father play interaction patterns with preschoolers. *Early Child Development and Care, 183*(3–4), 483–497.

Jones, J., & Mosher, W. D. (2013). Fathers' involvement with their children: United States, 2006 2010. *National Health Stat Report, 20*(71), 1–21.

Joussemet, M., Landry, R., & Koestner, R. (2008). A self-determination theory perspective on parenting. *Canadian Psychology, 49*(3), 194–200.

Karreman, A., van Tuijl, C., van Aken, M. A. G., & Dokovic, M. (2006). Parenting and self-regulation in preschoolers: A meta-analysis. *Infant and Child Development, 15*, 561–579.

Kiel, E. J., & Kalomiris, A. E. (2015). Current themes in understanding children's emotion regulation as developing from within the parent-child relationship. *Current Opinion in Psychology, 3*, 11–16.

Kim, S., Nordling, J. K., Yoon, J. E., Boldt, L. J., & Kochanska, G. (2013). Effortful control in "hot" and "cool" tasks differentially predicts children's behavior problems and academic performance. *Journal of Abnormal Child Psychology, 41*(1), 43–56.

Kochanska, G., Askan, N., Prisco, T. R., & Adams, E. E. (2008). Mother-child and father-child mutually responsive orientation in the first 2 years and children's outcomes at preschool age: Mechanisms of influence. *Child Development, 79*(1), 30–44.

Lamb, M. E. (Ed.). (2004). *The role of the father in child development* (4th ed.). Hoboken, NJ: Wiley.

Lengua, L. J., Honorado, E., & Bush, N. R. (2007). Contextual risk and parenting as predictors of effortful control and social competence in preschool children. *Journal of Applied Developmental Psychology, 28*(1), 40–55. https://doi.org/10.1016/j.appdev.2006.10.001

Lewis-Morrarty, E., Dozier, M., Bernard, K., Terracciano, S. M., & Moore, S. V. (2012). Cognitive flexibility and theory of mind outcomes among foster children: Preschool follow-up results of a randomized clinical trial. *Journal of Adolescent Health, 51*, S17–S22.

Lucassen, N., Kok, R., Bakermans-Kranenburg, M. J., Van IJzendoorn, M. H., Jaddoe, W. V., Hofman, A., et al. (2015). Executive functions in early childhood: The role of maternal and paternal parenting practices. *British Journal of Developmental Psychology.* https://doi.org/10.1111/bjdp.12112

Magill-Evans, J., Harrison, M. J., & Burke, S. O. (1999). Parent-child interactions and development of toddlers born preterm. *Western Journal of Nursing Research, 21*(3), 292–312.

Magill-Evans, J., Harrison, M. J., Rempel, G., & Slater, L. (2006). Interventions with fathers of young children:

Systematic literature review. *Journal of Advanced Nursing, 55*(2), 248–264.

Malin, J. L., Cabrera, N. J., Karberg, E., Aldoney, D., & Rowe, M. (2014). Low-income, minority fathers' control strategies and their children's regulatory skills. *Infant Mental Health Journal, 35*(5), 462–472.

McHale, J. P., Kuersten, R., & Lauretti, A. (1996). New directions in the study of family-level dynamics during infancy and early childhood. *New Directions for Child and Adolescent Development, 1996*(74), 5–26.

Masten, A. S., Herbers, J. E., Desjardins, C. D., Cutuli, J. J., McCormick, C. M., Sapienza, J. K., et al. (2012). Executive function skills and school success in young children experiencing homelessness. *Educational Researcher, 41*(9), 375–384. https://doi.org/10.3102/0013189X12459883

Matas, L., Arend, R. A., & Sroufe, L. A. (1978). Continuity of adaptation in the second year: The relationship between quality of attachment and later competence. *Child Development, 49*(3), 547–556.

Matte-Gagné, C., & Bernier, A. (2011). Prospective relations between maternal autonomy support and child executive functioning: Investigating the mediating role of child language ability. *Journal of Experimental Child Psychology, 110*(4), 611–625.

McClelland, M. M., Cameron, C. E., Connor, C. M., Farris, C. L., Jewkes, A. M., & Morrison, F. J. (2007). Links between behavioral regulation and preschoolers' literacy, vocabulary, and math skills. *Developmental Psychology, 43*(4), 947–959.

Meuwissen, A. M., & Carlson, S. M. (2015). Fathers matter: The role of father parenting in preschoolers' executive function development. *Journal of Experimental Child Psychology, 140*, 1–15.

Meuwissen, A. S., & Carlson, S. M. (2018). The role of father parenting in children's school readiness: A longitudinal follow-up. *Journal of Family Psychology, 32*(5), 588.

Meuwissen, A. S., & Carlson, S. M. (2019). An experimental study of the effects of autonomy support on preschoolers' self-regulation. *Journal of Applied Developmental Psychology, 60*, 11–23.

Meuwissen, A. S., & Englund, M. M. (2016). Executive function in at-risk children: Importance of father-figure support and mother parenting. *Journal of Applied Developmental Psychology, 44*, 72–80.

Merz, E. C., Wiltshire, C. A., & Noble, K. G. (2018). Socioeconomic inequality and the developing brain: Spotlight on language and executive function. *Child Development Perspectives*. https://doi.org/10.1111/cdep.12305

Mischel, W., Ayduk, O., Berman, M. G., Casey, B. J., Gotlib, I. H., Jonides, J., et al. (2011). "Willpower" over the life span: Decomposing self-regulation. *Social Cognitive and Affective Neuroscience, 6*(2), 252–256.

Moffitt, T. E., Arseneault, L., Belsky, D., Dickson, N., Hancox, R. J., Harrington, H., et al. (2011). A gradient of childhood self-control predicts health, wealth, and public safety. *Proceedings of the National Academy of Sciences, 108*(7), 2693–2698.

Moss, E., Gosselin, C., Parent, S., Rousseau, D., & Dumont, M. (1997). Attachment and joint problem-solving experiences during the preschool period. *Social Development, 6*(1), 1–17.

Olds, D. L., Robinson, J., Pettitt, L., Luckey, D. W., Holmbergy, J., et al. (2004). Effects of home visits by paraprofessionals and by nurses: Age 4 follow-up results of a randomized trial. *Pediatrics, 114*, 1560–1568.

Palkovitz, R., Fagan, R., & Hull. (2013). Coparenting and children's well-being. In N. J. Cabrera & C. S. Tamis-LeMonda (Eds.), *Handbook of father involvement* (2nd ed., pp. 169–185). New York: Routledge.

Panter-Brick, C., Burgess, A., Eggerman, M., McAllister, F., Pruetty, K., & Leckman, J. F. (2014). Practitioner review: Engaging fathers—Recommendations for a game change in parenting interventions based on a systematic review of the global evidence. *Journal of Child Psychology and Psychiatry, 55*, 1187–1212.

Paquette, D. (2004). Theorizing the father-child relationship: Mechanisms and developmental outcomes. *Human Development, 47*(4), 193–219.

Ramchandani, P. G., Domoney, J., Sethna, V., Psychogious, L., Vlachos, H., & Murray, L. (2013). Do early father-infant interactions predict the onset of externalizing behaviours in young children? Findings from a longitudinal cohort study. *The Journal of Child Psychology and Psychiatry, 54*(1), 56–64.

Reynolds, A. J., Ou, S., & Topitzes, J. W. (2004). Paths of effects of early childhood intervention on educational attainment and delinquency: A confirmatory analysis of the Chicago Child-Parent Centers. *Child Development, 75*(5), 1299–1328.

Rhoades, B. L., Greenberg, M. T., Lanza, S. T., & Blair, C. (2011). Demographic and familial predictors of early executive function development: Contribution of a person-centered approach. *Journal of Experimental Child Psychology, 108*(2011), 638–662.

Rochette, E., & Bernier, A. (2014). Parenting, family socioeconomic status, and child executive functioning: A longitudinal study. *Merril-Palmer Quarterly, 60*(4), 431–460.

Rosenberg, J., & Wilcox, W. B. (2006). *The importance of fathers in the healthy development of children.* US Department Health and Human Services, Administration for Children and Families, Administration on Children, Youth and Families, Children's Bureau, Office of Child Abuse and Neglect.

Roskam, I., Stievenart, M., Meunier, J. C., & Noel, M. P. (2014). The development of children's inhibition: Does parenting matter? *Journal of Experimental Child Psychology, 122*, 166–182.

Rowe, M. L., & Cabrera, N. J. (2013). Father input and child vocabulary development: The importance of wh-questions and clarification requests. *Seminars in Speech and Language, 34*, 249–259.

Ryan, R. M., Martin, A., & Brooks-Gunn, J. (2006). Is one good parent good enough? Patterns of mother and father parenting and child cognitive outcomes at 24 and 36 months. *Parenting: Science and Practice,*

6(2), 211–228. https://doi.org/10.1080/15295192.2006.9681306

Sarkadi, A., Kristiansson, R., Oberklaid, F., & Bremberg, S. (2008). Fathers' involvement and children's developmental outcomes: A systematic review of longitudinal studies. *Acta Paediatrica, 97*(2), 153–158.

Shannon, J. D., Tamis-LeMonda, C. S., London, K., & Cabrera, N. (2002). Beyond rough and tumble: Low-income fathers' interactions and children's cognitive development at 24 months. *Parenting: Science and Practice, 2*(2), 77–104.

Sroufe, L. A. (1990). An organizational perspective on the self. In D. C. Cicchetti & M. Beeghly (Eds.), *The self in transition: Infancy to childhood* (pp. 281–307). Chicago: The University of Chicago Press.

Sroufe, L. A. (2005). Attachment and development: A prospective, longitudinal study from birth to adulthood. *Attachment & Human Development, 7*(4), 329–367. https://doi.org/10.1080/14616730500365928

Sroufe, L. A., Egeland, B., Carlson, E. A., & Collins, W. A. (2005). *The development of the person: The Minnesota study of risk and adaptation from birth to adulthood.* New York: Guilford Press.

Su, Y., & Reeve, J. (2011). A meta-analysis of the effectiveness of intervention programs designed to support autonomy. *Educational Psychology Review, 23*, 159–188.

Sulik, M. J., Blair, C., Mills-Koonce, R., Berry, D., Greenberg, M., & The Family Life Project Investigators. (2015). Early parenting and the development of externalizing behavior problems: Longitudinal mediation through children's executive function. *Child Development, 86*(5), 1588–1603.

Tamis-LeMonda, C. S., Shannon, J. D., Cabrera, N. J., & Lamb, M. E. (2004). Fathers and mothers at play with their 2- and 3-year-olds: Contributions to language and cognitive development. *Child Development, 75*(6), 1806–1820.

Teubert, D., & Pinquart, M. (2010). The association between coparenting and child adjustment: A meta-analysis. *Parenting: Science and Practice, 10*(4), 286–307.

Towe-Goodman, N. R., Willoughby, M., Blair, C., Gustafsson, H. C., Mills-Koonce, W. R., Cox, M. J., et al. (2014). Fathers' sensitive parenting and the development of early executive functioning. *Journal of Family Psychology, 28*(6), 867–876.

U. S. Census Bureau. (2016). *The majority of children live with two parents*, Census Bureau reports. United States Census Bureau. https://www.census.gov/newsroom/press-releases/2016/cb16-192.html

Volling, B. L., Cabrera, N. J., Feinberg, M. E., Jones, D. E., McDaniel, B. T., et al. (2019). Advancing research and measurement on fathering and children's development. *Monographs of the Society for Research in Child Development, 84*(1), 7–160.

Vygotsky, L. (1978). *Mind and society: The development of higher mental processes*. Cambridge, MA: Harvard University Press.

Whipple, N., Bernier, A., & Mageau, G. A. (2011). Broadening the study of infant security of attachment: Maternal autonomy-support in the context of infant exploration. *Social Development, 20*, 17–32.

Willoughby, M., Kupersmidt, J., Voegler-Lee, M., & Bryant, D. (2011). Contributions of hot and cool self-regulation to preschool disruptive behavior and academic achievement. *Developmental Neuropsychology, 36*(2), 162–180.

Wood, D. J. (1980). Teaching the young child: Some relationships between social interaction, language, and thought. In D. R. Olson (Ed.), *The social foundations of language and thought* (pp. 259–275). New York: WW Norton & Company.

Wood, D., Bruner, J., & Ross, S. (1976). The role of tutoring in problem solving. *British Journal of Psychology, 66*, 181–191.

Zelazo, P. D. (2004). The development of conscious control in childhood. *Trends in Cognitive Sciences, 8*(1), 12–17.

Zelazo, P. D. (2015). Executive function: Reflection, iterative reprocessing, complexity, and the developing brain. *Developmental Review.* https://doi.org/10.1016/j.dr.2015.07.001

Zelazo, P. D., & Carlson, S. M. (2012). Hot and cool executive function in childhood and adolescence: Development and plasticity. *Child Development Perspectives, 6*, 354–360. https://doi.org/10.1111/j.1750-8606.2012.00246.x

Part IV

Fathers' Involvement in Context

26 Overview to Part IV: Fathers' Involvement in Context

Júlia Scarano de Mendonça

The field of fathers and fathering needs more studies on the diversity of fathers and fathering practices in different parts of the world and in different social contexts in order to move forward towards a broader understanding of fathers and their relationships in diverse family systems. This is what this part intends to do. In the following pages, the reader will have the opportunity to learn about different ways fathers get involved with their children and families in different continents (Africa, South America, and North America), in minority ethnic groups within the USA (African and Latino Americans, American Indians, and Alaska Natives), and also in special groups of fathers such as stay-at-home fathers and fathers in the military service. Thus, this part provides the reader with a great range of the diversity of father involvement in different contexts and cultures.

Such an approach is important because it offers the opportunity to challenge findings from research done mostly in WEIRD populations (western, educated, industrial, rich, democratic), most often studied in the field. Unfortunately, research on families living outside North America and Europe and in minority groups is still rare in developmental psychology. Generalizations made from these samples should be treated with caution given that social interaction and human development are highly contingent on sociocultural influences (Henrich, Heine, & Norenzayan, 2010; Kärtner, Keller, Chaudhary, & Yovsi, 2012). In what follows, I will present the chapters in this part.

In Chap. 27, Rabie, Skeen, and Tomlinson offer a fascinating perspective of fathering and early childhood development in sub-Saharan Africa. They argue that the traditional Western framework of a biological father connected to the nuclear family is incongruent with many African cultures, where fatherhood, and parenting in general, is seen as a shared community responsibility with the involvement of extended families and community members in general. They point out, unfortunately, that fatherhood is still an under-researched area of inquiry in sub-Saharan Africa, with the exception of South Africa, and more research is needed.

Throughout the chapter, the authors provide interesting examples from the various countries in sub-Saharan Africa on the impacts of both absence and presence of father involvement on their children, reaffirming the important impact of fathers in the lives of their children even in societies that understand parenting as a shared community responsibility. The authors point out the exclusion of men from the educational, social, and health services in sub-Saharan Africa as strong barriers for engaging fathers in the lives of their young children in sub-Saharan Africa. They

J. S. de Mendonça (✉)
Graduate Program in Educational Psychology, Centro Universitário FIEO, Osasco, São Paulo, Brazil

H. E. Fitzgerald et al. (eds.), *Handbook of Fathers and Child Development*,
https://doi.org/10.1007/978-3-030-51027-5_26

end the chapter suggesting ways to promote father engagement in these countries.

In Chap. 28, De Mendonça and Bussab propose a provocative hypothesis based on previous analyses on a low-income Brazilian sample—that the main function of paternal depression, in the context of maternal PPD, is to promote fathers' proximity to the family. Using an evolutionary framework of depression and paternal care, the authors argue that variability in the environment can produce diverse adaptive responses, especially in fathers. Paternal depression can then be understood as an adaptation to a vulnerable family situation (maternal postpartum depression). Although this hypothesis still needs to be tested, the question that rises in this chapter is related to the universality of this possible mechanism. Is this a mechanism found only in families from cultures that put a strong value on family life, like Brazil, or is it a universal mechanism?

Chapters 29, 30, and 31 offer a very interesting account of how minority ethnic groups within the USA (African and Latino Americans, American Indians, and Alaska Natives) experience fatherhood. In Chap. 29, Gadsden and Iruka point out that research on African American fathers still has to account for the diversity of the group, emphasizing that most previous research focused almost exclusively on low-income African American fathers. The authors discuss how research has treated race and social class in an intertwined way which may have obscured results. In Chap. 30, Mogro-Wilson focuses on Latino American fathers from various countries of origin, including Mexico, Central and South America, and Puerto Rico. Together, Latinos comprise 18% of the US population (U.S. Bureau of Labor Statistics, 2017) with 25% of school-aged children in the USA coming from Latino families (U.S. Census Bureau, 2018). Applying the Bronfenbrenner's bio-ecological model, Mogro-Wilson provides an interesting picture of how cultural values of Latino fathers may influence their involvement with their children. Among the barriers to Latino father involvement is local and national policies with anti-immigrant rhetoric. Finally, in Chap. 31, Allison-Burbank and Collins provide a fascinating account of the sociocultural determinants of the so called "American Indian" (AI) and "Alaska Native" (AN) well-being, health status, and childrearing practices. The authors are from Diné, Acoma Pueblo, and Onk Akimel O'Odham tribal nations and fathers themselves who recognize the importance of sharing their journey in raising young Indigenous children. Allison-Burbank and Collins provide very interesting information about AI/AN culture in various aspects of life such as family traditions and structure, gender socialization, and the roles of AI/AN fathers in Indigenous societies. The chapter presents historical and social factors that are threats to responsive and conscious Indigenous fathering, emphasizing the trauma associated with violence, substance abuse, and poverty that AI/AN men frequently face, and also the intergenerational trauma due to past colonization.

In Chap. 32, Lee, Lee, and Chang provide a detailed account of the experience of stay-at-home fathers (SAHF) including socio-demographics, gender roles, masculine identity, work-life family conflict, social support, and mental health. In their literature review, the authors highlight the lack of representation of diverse fathers and families in the SAHF literature, with most studies focusing on the experience of middle- and upper-income, white, heterosexual men in the USA. Noteworthy is the lack of studies of SAHF from other parts of the world and also the impact of SAHF on child well-being and father-child relationships. According to the authors, the number of stay-at-home fathers has been rising in the past 15–20 years and more research is needed to better understand this specific population and family configuration.

Finally, in Chap. 33, Walsh and Rosenblum explore the experiences of fathers parenting young children across the military service "deployment cycle"—before, during, and after deployment. The authors address the specific challenges faced by military members that are fathers of young children and the limitations of existing resources for meeting their needs. Given that the total number of US military personnel is close to 3.5 million, and that nearly 40% of US service members are parents (most of them fathers) according to the U.S. Department of Defense (2018), Walsh and Rosenblum emphasize that there is a need for continued research and the expansion of services for this specific population.

References

Henrich, J., Heine, S. J., & Norenzayan, A. (2010). The weirdest people in the world? *Behavioral and Brain Sciences, 33*, 61–83.

Kärtner, J., Keller, H., Chaudhary, N., & Yovsi, R. (2012). The development of mirror self-recognition in different sociocultural contexts. *Monographs of the Society for Research in Child Development, 77*(4), 1–87.

U.S. Bureau of Labor Statistics. (2017). *Labor force characteristics by race and ethnicity*. Retrieved January 16, 2020 from https://www.bls.gov/

U.S. Census Bureau. (2018). *Current population survey, annual social and economic supplement, 2018*. Retrieved January 16, 2020 from https://www.census.gov/data/tables/2018/demo/hispanic-origin/2018-cps.html

U.S. Department of Defense. (2018). *Demographics report: Profile of the military community*. Retrieved January 16, 2020 from http://download.militaryonesource.mil/12038/MOS/Reports/2018-demographics-report.pdf

close to 4.3 million, and that nearly 40% of US service members are parents (most of them fathers). According to the U.S. Department of Defense (2018), Walsh and Rosenblum emphasize that there is a need for continued research and the expansion of services for this specific population.

References

Henry, S., Heim, S., & Nierenwold, A. (2010). The world's poorest ... Retrieved from ...

Paquette, D., Bolté, C., Turcotte, G., Dubeau, D., & Bouchard, C. (2012). The development of mirror self-recognition in different sociocultural contexts. Monographs of the Society for Research in Child Development, 77(4), 1–87.

U.S. Bureau of Labor Statistics. (2019). Employment characteristics by race and ethnicity. Retrieved January 16, 2020 from https://www.bls.gov/...

U.S. Census Bureau. (2018). Current population survey, annual social and economic supplement, 2018. Retrieved January 16, 2020 from https://www.census.gov/data/tables/2018/demo/families/cps-2018.html

U.S. Department of Defense. (2018). Demographics: Profile of the military community. Retrieved January 16, 2020 from https://download.militaryonesource.mil/12038/MOS/Reports/2018-demographics-report.pdf

Fatherhood and Early Childhood Development: Perspectives from Sub-Saharan Africa

27

Stephan Rabie, Sarah Skeen, and Mark Tomlinson

Globally, the nature and composition of modern families have evolved (Arnot, 2014). The promotion of gender rights in many countries has contributed to an increase in women's educational attainment, employment participation, and changes in family formation patterns, with both men and women establishing themselves in the labor market before starting a family (OECD, 2011; Oláh, Richter, & Kotowska, 2014). These new gender roles and family patterns have resulted in the transformation of fathers' roles in family responsibilities, with more emphasis placed on their involvement in caregiving activities (Oláh et al., 2014). Indeed, there has been a mounting call over the past decades for greater male involvement in their children's lives (Oláh et al., 2014; Richter, 2006). There is also a growing body of evidence showing the positive impact father involvement can have on child developmental outcomes (Barker, Levtov, & Heilman, 2018; McWayne, Downer, Campos, & Harris, 2013; Palm & Fagan, 2008; Sarkadi, Kristiansson, Oberklaid, & Bremberg, 2008). Research conducted in high-income countries (HIC) suggests that fathers' increased involvement and engagement during early childhood improve social, emotional, cognitive, and behavioral outcomes for young children (Sarkadi et al., 2008). For instance, having a father engaged in caregiving activities predicts improved cognitive achievement in preschool children and decreased behavioral problems in preschool boys (Barker et al., 2018; Jones & Mosher, 2013). Fathers involved from the start of their children's lives often establish a pattern of lifelong engagement, and this continued engagement may not only contribute to positive physical, socioemotional, cognitive, and behavioral development during childhood but also enhance developmental outcomes later in life (Panter-Brick et al., 2014). Beyond its impact on developmental outcomes, fathers' involvement in caregiving and household activities has also been shown to promote gender equality – children internalize notions of equality and mutual respect, and they are likely to pass these ideas onto their own children (Barker et al., 2018). Moreover, engaged fatherhood can aid in ensuring children's access to health and education and serve as a buffer against abuse, neglect, and violence (Barker et al., 2018).

Despite the substantial support for the importance of father involvement in improving early

S. Rabie
Institute for Life Course Health Research, Department of Global Health, Stellenbosch University, Stellenbosch, South Africa

S. Skeen (✉)
Institute for Child and Adolescent Health Research, Masiphulisane Research Centre, Stellenbosch University, Khayelitsha, South Africa
e-mail: skeen@sun.ac.za

M. Tomlinson
Department of Psychology, Stellenbosch University, Matieland, Stellenbosch, South Africa

H. E. Fitzgerald et al. (eds.), *Handbook of Fathers and Child Development*,
https://doi.org/10.1007/978-3-030-51027-5_27

childhood development (ECD) outcomes, these perspectives are dominated by evidence from Western, educated, industrialized, rich, and democratic (WEIRD) societies (Henrich, Heine, & Norenzayan, 2010; McAllister, Burgess, Kato, & Barker, 2012; Nsamenang, 2010). Why is this problematic? First, families across the globe vary in their cultural and psychological characteristics (Valiquette Tessier, Gosselien, Young, & Thomassin, 2019). More relevant for this chapter, recent research on fathering has emphasized cross-cultural variability in parenting (Lamb & Lewis, 2004; Madhavan & Roy, 2012) and highlights that definitions of fatherhood and father involvement vary from one culture to another (Townsend, 2013). Culture plays an important role in determining what is acceptable, manageable, and important for caregiving practices (Akilapa & Simkiss, 2012). Accordingly, fatherhood is expressed and understood within differing ideologies and cultural groups (Nsamenang, 2010). Within the context of sub-Saharan Africa's diverse cultural, linguistic, and ethnic composition, it is imperative to have contextually appropriate perspectives on fatherhood and father involvement.

It is within this context that we present a review of father involvement in the lives of young children in sub-Saharan Africa. Our review considers different conceptualizations of fatherhood in diverse cultural settings. We review the available evidence on the impact of father involvement on childhood developmental outcomes. This is followed by a discussion of the barriers and enabling factors for engaging fathers in ECD programs in sub-Saharan Africa. Finally, we consider lessons learned that are applicable across different contexts to improve father involvement in the lives of their young children.

Conceptualizations of Fatherhood in Sub-Saharan Africa

The traditional view of fathers in many sub-Saharan African cultures is that of the patriarchal head of the family (Jorosi-Tshiamo, Mogobe, & Mokotedi, 2013; Makusha & Richter, 2014; Mugadza, Mujeyi, Stout, Wali, & Renzaho, 2019). This adherence to the patriarchal system has perpetuated the idea that in many African societies, childcare is predominantly the responsibility of women (Ejuu, 2016; Mugadza et al., 2019). For instance, among the Kikuyu people in Kenya, fathers are generally not involved in the daily caregiving activities of their children (Mugadza et al., 2019). Rather, fathers are seen as protectors and providers – they are the custodians of ultimate power and responsibility in the family and community (Lasser, Fite, & Wadende, 2011). Similar gender stereotypes exist in many parts of Ethiopia, where mothers are viewed as the primary caregivers and confidantes to their children, and fathers are considered to be the disciplinarian and head of the household (Beatson, 2013). In Botswana and South Africa, patriarchal values have been found to contribute to fathers' inadequate involvement in childcare and caregiving activities (Jorosi-Tshiamo et al., 2013; Kang'ethe, 2009; Makusha & Richter, 2014). Most Botswanan men are raised by female caregivers (mothers, aunts, grandmothers, or sisters) and subsequently socialized to believe that women are the primary caregivers of children (Sabone, 2009). As a result, many fathers in Botswana and South Africa hold the view that their primary, and sometimes only contribution to the care of their children, is through providing financial support (Jorosi-Tshiamo et al., 2013; Madhavan, Richter, Norris, & Hosegood, 2014).

In contrast, it has recently been shown that fathers are becoming increasingly engaged and involved in caregiving activities in many sub-Saharan African communities (Ejuu, 2016; Jorosi-Tshiamo et al., 2013). As is the case elsewhere, African conceptualizations of fatherhood are in the process of evolving due to urbanization and exposure to other communities and belief systems (Mncanca, Okeke, & Fletcher, 2016; Ratele, Shefer, & Clowes, 2012). For instance, in South Africa, as more women enter both formal and informal employment, fathers are increasingly spending quality time with their children, attending school events and healthcare centers, and ensuring that their children arrive at school safely (Makusha & Richter, 2014).

Therefore, it is important to consider that the dominant literature conceptualizes fathering and fatherhood within the traditional Western framework of a biological father connected to the nuclear family (Mncanca et al., 2016). Mncanca et al. (2016, p. 203) assert that the "Eurocentric conceptualization of family constellation that reduces fatherhood in a nuclear family is insufficient to illuminate the complex assemblage of fatherhood" in most African settings. Moreover, this perspective is incongruent with many African cultures, where fatherhood, and parenting in general, is seen as a shared community responsibility (Mugadza et al., 2019). For example, childcare is viewed as a community task by the Nso of Cameroon (Keller, Borke, Lamm, Lohaus, & Dzeaye Yovsi, 2011); extended families among the Mijikenda of Kenya live together and share caregiving activities (Abubakar et al., 2013), and community members among the Efe in the Democratic Republic of Congo collectively care for all infants and children in the community (Bhana, Nzimakwe, & Nzimakwe, 2011). Furthermore, it is common practice in Botswana, Namibia, and South Africa for parents to send their children to reside with grandparents, extended family, or other community members (Mugadza et al., 2019). As such, collective fatherhood is a distinctive feature of many traditional African communities (Richter & Morrell, 2008). For example, in twenty-first-century sub-Saharan Africa, in cities and peri-urban settlements, the concept of fatherhood extends to an integrated network of cohesive social relationships between adult men and children – albeit their own biological children or not (Makusha & Richter, 2014; Richter, Chikovore, & Makusha, 2010). This highlights the concept of social fathers – maternal or paternal grandfathers, uncles, older brothers, or mothers' partners who engage in the caregiving of children and offer paternal affection and guidance (Makusha & Richter, 2014; Richter et al., 2010). For instance, Hunter (2006) and Mkhize (2006) highlight the significant role other male relatives can play in the lives of children, with these children often referring to other significant men in their lives as their fathers. According to Makusha and Richter (2014), this account of a family represents kinship, commitment, and security in African communities. Fatherhood, in the context of sub-Saharan Africa, is therefore considered not only biological but rather a social responsibility assumed by adult males within the proximal environment of children (Lesejane, 2006; Mkhize, 2006; Mncanca et al., 2016). Within this context, the current chapter extends the conceptualization of fatherhood beyond a biological connection situated within a nuclear family to include significant male figures that play important roles in caring for their children.

Father Involvement in the Early Lives of Children

Despite the mounting calls for research on men's roles in families across the globe (Oláh et al., 2014), and particularly in sub-Saharan Africa (Hosegood & Madhavan, 2012), there continues to be a dearth of research knowledge on African fathers, their involvement, and its influence on the physical, emotional, cognitive, social, and behavioral development of their children (Nsamenang, 2010). With the exception of South Africa, where increasing research attention has been paid to fatherhood in recent years (Anderson, 2015; Khewu & Adu, 2017; Lesejane, 2006; Madhavan & Roy, 2012; Makusha & Richter, 2014; Mncanca et al., 2016; Mncanca & Okeke, 2016; Ratele et al., 2012; Richter, 2006; Richter et al., 2010), fatherhood continues to be an under-researched area of inquiry in sub-Saharan Africa. Considering the evidence from HIC in support of the important role fathers play in the development of their children (Barker et al., 2018; McWayne et al., 2013; Sarkadi et al., 2008) and the diverse nature of fatherhood in the African context (Nsamenang, 2010), providing perspectives on fatherhood and childhood development in sub-Saharan Africa is imperative.

Much of the research attention that has been paid to fatherhood in sub-Saharan Africa focuses on the impact of father absence on child development. Fathers are often absent in one of two ways: they are absent from services that improve the well-being of their children (i.e., educational, social, and health services), or they are physically absent from the homes in which their children are raised (Richter & Morrell, 2008). According to Richter and Morrell (2008), men's absence from health and educational services is often due to their exclusion from these services – educators and health professionals often speak to women, citing feeling uncomfortable with men, and have subsequently failed to adapt their approach to include both male and female caregivers in these services (Richter & Morrell, 2008). In terms of physical absence, structural factors such as endemic poverty and unemployment, high premature mortality rates of men, and patterns of migrant labor have contributed significantly to fathers' absence from the lives of their children in sub-Saharan Africa (Anderson, 2015; Morrell & Richter, 2004). The latter holds especially true for Southern Africa, where, due to the entrenched migrant labor system, many fathers are absent from the homes their children live in (Richter & Morrell, 2008). For example, Namibia has the highest number of absent fathers in sub-Saharan Africa, where only an estimated 30% of preschool children reside with their fathers (Herbert & Princess, 2017). In South Africa, data from the 2018 General Household Survey indicate that nearly half of all children (43.1%) reside in households with absent fathers, a third of children (33.8%) reside in households with both parents, and only 3.3% of children reside with single-parent fathers (Statistics South Africa, 2018). In some of these communities, father involvement may be better characterized as *in flux* rather than *absent*, due to the transitionary and seasonal nature of the migrant labor system (Roy, 2008).

A number of studies assessing the impact of father absence on child development report significant patterns of family disruption (Lu & Treiman, 2011). In particular, fathers' absence has been shown to negatively influence the emotional care and nurture children receive (Spjeldnaes, Moland, Harris, & Sam, 2011), as well as negatively impact children's physical, behavioral, and cognitive development. In Botswana, for instance, Mahgoub, Nnyepi, and Bandeke (2006) found that children under the age of three years who live in single-mother households were significantly more underweight (15.8%) compared to children residing with both parents (13.6%). In fact, their findings indicate that living with both parents offered a protective effect on children's physical development (Mahgoub et al., 2006). Similarly, through examining the associations between household structure and child health in Botswana, Ntshebe (2013) found that children under the age of five raised in female-headed households had increased vulnerability to stunting and that the prevalence of diarrhea in toddlers and preschoolers was associated with the child's biological father's absence from the household. Comparable data on the impact of father absence and associated lack of engagement have been reported in Ghana (Rikimaru, Yartey, Taniguchi, Kennedy, & Nkrumah, 1998), where children of unemployed fathers were found to be severely malnourished compared to fathers with formal employment.

Father absence also appears to have a particularly detrimental effect on boys (Langa, 2010; Richter, 2006). For example, Ramphele (2002) found that in Cape Town, South Africa, boys who grew up without father figures were more susceptible to engaging in risk-taking behavior, such as substance use, violence, and gang activity. Morrell and Richter (2004) argue that the lack of positive male role models can contribute to a crisis in the development of masculinity for many boys, providing a possible explanation for their tendencies toward aggression and violence. Indeed, father presence appears to have a moderating effect on boys' aggression, as fathers may represent models for culturally appropriate behavior (Richter & Morrell, 2008).

In terms of cognitive development, Booth (1995), in her study on the impact of father absence on school preparedness, found a negative association between absent fathers who participated in migrant labor and Swazi children's vocabulary and fine motor skills development. When compared to children whose fathers were present at home, children of absent fathers did not possess the basic developmental skills required for schooling (Booth, 1995). This may be ascribed to the detrimental effect father absenteeism may have on the home environment, with some evidence suggesting that a negative home environment can contribute to impaired development, particularly in terms of language development, behavioral problems, and school readiness (Evans et al., 2010; Trentacosta et al., 2008; Vernon-Feagans et al., 2012). One study in Uganda found that among other socioeconomic variables, a positive home environment predicted positive cognitive development in children (Bangirana et al., 2009). Although the authors did not specify the family composition that contributed to positive home environments in this particular study, there is evidence signifying that children of single-parent households are at greater risk for a wide range of adverse developmental outcomes, as there are often fewer economic and emotional resources, which may thwart a single parent's ability to provide an environment that is conducive to learning and development (Carlson & Corcoran, 2001).

Despite the evidence for the impact of father absence on child development, other studies from sub-Saharan Africa suggest that father absence may not necessarily result in detrimental development outcomes during childhood. For instance, a study in the Nakuru Municipality in Kenya found no significant differences in children's levels of self-esteem between single-parent families, headed predominantly by single mothers, and dual-parent families (Kinga, Kimani, & Muriithi, 2014). They argue that the development of self-esteem is largely determined by the relationship between children and their parents, and a positive relationship with a single parent that is nurturing and engaging may be more beneficial than a potentially inaccessible, rejecting, or hostile dual-parent family (Kinga et al., 2014). In terms of migrant labor, studies in Ghana (Adams, Cuecuecha, & Page, 2008) and South Africa (Lu & Treiman, 2011) indicate that remittance from migrant fathers contributes to human capital investment and subsequently positively impacts children's educational aspirations and academic performance. That is, although fathers are physically absent in search of employment, they are psychologically present (Boss, 2007), connected to the household, and invested in its well-being (Madhavan, Schatz, Clark, & Collinson, 2012). One study in Mozambique found that children of successful migrant fathers (i.e., fathers who migrated from their homes and successfully secured employment) had the lowest under-five mortality rate when compared to children of unsuccessful migrant fathers and even nonmigrant fathers (Yabiku, Agadjanian, & Cau, 2012). This positive impact may be ascribed to the fact that in many African communities, when men are involved in the lives of their children, they are responsible for making important decisions and allocating resources that affect the care, well-being, and health of young children (Richter, 2006; Richter & Morrell, 2008). Within the communal nature of caregiving in sub-Saharan Africa, children may not necessarily be disadvantaged by the physical absence of their migrant fathers, but may rather be disadvantaged if they belong to a household that is without social status or financial support – something that used to be provided by men (Townsend, 2013). This phenomenon has changed in recent years. As more women in Africa enter the labor market, they are increasingly providing financially for the household (Madhavan et al., 2012) and subsequently transforming traditional gender roles and creating potential opportunities for men (albeit biological or social father figures) to be more involved and present in the lives of children. One qualitative study in South Africa that explored the experiences of young women raised in families with absent fathers (Makofane, 2015) found their grandfathers or maternal uncles fulfilled the fathering role in their lives, and as a result, "they did not miss the physical and emotional presence of their fathers" (Makofane, 2015, p. 30).

Although there has been substantial emphasis on father absence, there is also evidence demonstrating that increased father presence and the associated enhanced engagement have a direct influence on the developmental outcomes of children (Richter & Morrell, 2008). In particular, the amount of time fathers spend with their children and the different types of activities fathers engage in with their children have been shown to directly contribute to positive physical, psychological, emotional, and educational outcomes. In a large rural sample in KwaZulu-Natal in South Africa, father presence was associated with enhanced prenatal development (Cunningham, Elo, Herbst, & Hosegood, 2010). Infants with fathers present in the household were on average 59 g heavier at birth compared to infants whose fathers' resided elsewhere (Cunningham et al., 2010). Although these data are not causal, the findings suggest that co-residence with fathers may provide benefits beyond financial support, with the authors hypothesizing that the additional social support offered to mothers may contribute to these positive developmental outcomes (Cunningham et al., 2010). From a cultural viewpoint, the authors argue it is a customary belief that "the fetus is thought to belong to the father's lineage and the mother is only a channel through which the child enters the world" (Cunningham et al., 2010, p. 240). As a result, fathers may be more invested in ensuring the mother lives and the child is raised in a protected environment (Cunningham et al., 2010), which may potentially contribute to positive developmental outcomes.

Father presence has also been shown to significantly contribute to cognitive development, intellectual functioning, and educational performance (Lasser et al., 2011; Richter & Morrell, 2008). For example, in South Africa, Mboya and Nesengani (1999) found that South African family patterns were significantly related to academic achievement in children. In particular, children raised in households with both parents performed significantly better on scholastic achievement measures when compared to children who lived in father-absent homes (Mboya & Nesengani, 1999). Similarly, Southwood (2011) found that South African children who grew up with absent or uninvolved fathers had poorer language skills in the domains of syntax, pragmatics, and semantics when compared to children of present fathers. The author argues that the presence of a male primary caregiver has a positive influence, either direct or vicarious, on children's language development and skills (Southwood, 2011). Anderson, Kaplan, and Lancaster's (1999) paternal investment study on Xhosa men in South Africa may provide a possible explanation for fathers' positive impact on the cognitive development (Richter & Morrell, 2008). They found that residential fathers (biological, step-, or social fathers) were more likely to spend time with their children helping with homework compared to nonresidential fathers (Anderson et al., 1999). These findings align with the evidence indicating that fathers engage more in play activities with their toddlers and preschool children compared to mothers (Richter, 2006). More recently, Morrell, Dunkle, Ibragimov, and Jewkes (2016) found that in a sample of 2298 South African households, more than half of fathers participated in caregiving activities in the household, and over 80% engaged in play activities and assisted their children with their homework. These findings suggest that fathers may engage in different activities with their children compared to mothers, which may offer unique developmental benefits.

Barriers to Father Involvement and Potential Targets for Intervention in Sub-Saharan Africa

There is substantial research on the associations between contextual factors and barriers to father involvement in many African communities (Richter et al., 2010). As noted earlier in this chapter, cultural beliefs related to gender roles and the role of the father moderates the level of paternal involvement. Although in recent years there has been a gradual transformation in gender roles in some African communities, childcare and caregiving activities continue to largely be considered the responsibility of women (Ejuu, 2016; Mugadza et al., 2019). A number of studies have demonstrated that fathers have a desire to be involved in caring for their children (Mufutau & Okeke, 2017; Rolfe, 2006) and consider their involvement to be important, (Nkuoh, Cmmh, Meyer, Tih, & Nkfusai, 2010), yet pervasive patriarchal beliefs appear to stymie their involvement. For example, one study in Cameroon investigating father involvement in antenatal care found that some fathers viewed pregnancy as a "women's affair" (Nkuoh et al., 2010, p. 365). Moreover, the participants emphasized that accompanying their wife to antenatal care would be "shameful" and that it "was not their custom to participate in antenatal care" (Nkuoh et al., 2010, p. 365). Rather, providing financially for the family was considered to be more important (Nkuoh et al., 2010). Comparable findings related to cultural beliefs and father absence have been reported in South Africa. Richter et al. (2010) report that unmarried Black South African men are required to pay *ihlawulo* (a cultural obligation of paying damages) for fathering a child, or should they wish to marry, they are expected to pay *lobola* (bride-price). Since men are not allowed to reside with their child and their child's mother until they finalize *lobola* payment, the mother and her family facilitate the relationship between father and child (Makusha & Richter, 2016). These cultural practices, in combination with contexts of unemployment and endemic poverty, often regulate father involvement and prevent fathers' access to their children.

Relatedly, socioeconomic factors appear to pose significant barriers to fathers' involvement in the lives of their children (Mncanca et al., 2016). Considering the high rates of unemployment and poverty in sub-Saharan Africa (Fosu, 2015), many men are unable to provide what many consider to be the most important contribution to their children's lives – financial support (Kwambai et al., 2013). As such, men are discouraged from participating in the development of their children by the lack of employment or economic means to support the child (Mncanca et al., 2016). In addition, the feelings of failure and shame associated with fathers' inability to support their children further compound father absenteeism (Richter et al., 2010). The lack of employment opportunities in many sub-Saharan African countries and especially Southern Africa has created a migrant labor system, where traditionally fathers, and more recently an increasing number of mothers, leave the household to secure employment. As such, fathers are absent from the household for extended periods of time, which contributes to disrupted family life and, in some cases, compromised care (Mncanca et al., 2016). Although the migrant labor system represents a major barrier to father involvement, as noted previously in this chapter, there are mixed findings on father absence, migrant labor, and child development.

Another barrier to father involvement in child development is men's exclusion from health and educational services (Richter & Morrell, 2008). This exclusion should be considered from two perspectives. First, there is evidence to suggest that some fathers are often excluded from services that improve the health and well-being of their children through their own cultural beliefs and value systems. In particular, patriarchal views resulting in the belief that caregiving is the responsibility of women are detrimental to father involvement and place an increased burden on mothers to ensure that their children receive the healthcare and education they require. Although sub-Saharan Africa's diversity and varied belief systems should not be disregarded, the advancement of equal gender rights across cultures and communities could prove valuable to highlight the important role fathers play with respect to their children's access to health and education services.

Furthermore, Richter and Morrell (2008) argue that health practitioners and educators have failed to adapt their approach to include both male and female caregivers in their services. A South African study found that one of the key inhibitors to fathers' involvement in education in the early childhood period was fathers' weak relationships with their children's teachers (Mncanca & Okeke, 2016). In particular, many of the participants shared that there was no reasonable support for fathers in preschools, resulting in many of the fathers not being involved in their children's preschool education (Mncanca & Okeke, 2016). One participant claimed that he had no relationship with his child's teachers at all. In most sub-Saharan African countries, occupations such as teaching (preschool and schools more generally) are dominated by women. Ejuu (2016) contends that including more men in these occupations may provide a possible solution to increase father involvement, as fathers will have staff members to relate to and voice their concerns.

Further to this, involvement of fathers must be supported in a way that is respectful of women's autonomy and supportive of their decision-making ability for themselves and the health of their children (WHO 2015). There are examples in the literature of when the promotion of male participation has had unintended negative consequences for their female partners. For example, in Tanzania, researchers found that encouraging fathers to attend antenatal care appointments resulted in healthcare providers denying services to pregnant women attending clinics without their partners and that men attending antenatal care with their partners were fast-tracked to receive services (Peneza & Maluka, 2018). In another study from a low-resource setting, Papua New Guinea, some women noted a preference for attending some or all antenatal care appointments without their partner, in order to consult privately with healthcare providers and link with other pregnant women. This underscores the need to consider women's needs and preferences when designing interventions to promote father engagement (Davis et al., 2018).

What Should Be Done?

How, then, do we promote father involvement in the early years of their child's life in sub-Saharan Africa? With increasing global concern in promoting father involvement, a number of interventions have emerged on the continent (Morrell et al., 2016). For example, in Niger, Écoles des Maris (Schools for Husbands) aims to transform behavior and attitudes on a community level by training "model husbands" to promote the benefits of utilizing local health service (McAllister et al., 2012). Anecdotal evidence indicates that Écoles des Maris has improved men's attitudes toward healthcare utilization and increased rates of labor attendance (McAllister et al., 2012). Several interventions have also emerged in South Africa, with a number of interventions aimed at transforming gender relations and identities and emphasizing childcare work with fathers and men (Enderstein & Boonzaier, 2015; Morrell et al., 2016). The Fatherhood Project (Morrell & Richter, 2004) was one of the first South African interventions that targeted all men, not just fathers, to change notions related to fatherhood and encouraged them to become more involved in the lives of children. Since the Fatherhood Project, a number of interventions have emerged aimed at promoting responsible gender relations, with many implemented by Sonke Gender Justice, a local nongovernmental organization. Similar interventions, often targeted at HIV, have demonstrated efficacy in engaging men to participate in domestic and care work traditionally assumed by women (Dworkin, Colvin, Hatcher, & Peacock, 2012). In fact, McAllister et al. (2012) argue that father involvement can be promoted through engaging men in existing family support, maternal and child health, HIV prevention, and Prevention of Mother to Child Transmission (PMTCT) programs. The majority of funding for engaging men has been allocated to HIV prevention and PMTCT programs in sub-Saharan Africa. As such, with this existing infrastructure, fathers (biological or social) should be consulted to identify a point of departure to increase their involvement. Beardshaw (2006) argues that including fathers and men in health services can have a significant impact on their behavior. For instance, if health and reproductive services are exclusively targeted at women and subsequently excluding fathers and men, important societal expectations for male involvement are communicated that can determine their level of involvement.

Including fathers in health and reproductive services also creates potential opportunities for engaging fathers early. Establishing father involvement early in their children's lives, or even prenatally, is paramount, as it has enduring effects for father engagement across the life course and predicts lifelong involvement (Panter-Brick et al., 2014). Moreover, establishing paternity at birth has been found to increase fathers' involvement in a child's life (Richter et al., 2012). Brief interventions with fathers during the early stages of becoming a parent also promote father involvement in their children's lives and provide fathers with important skills to become better fathers (Doherty, Erickson, & LaRossa, 2006). However, these interventions should not necessarily target fathers alone. McAllister et al. (2012) argue that when interventions are specifically targeted at fathers, in comparison with wider engagement services or programs, fewer fathers may be reached, and outcomes may be less positive. There is some evidence that targeted interventions may not be more cost-effective or useful compared to universal family services (Bremberg, 2006), and the same may apply to engaging fathers (McAllister et al., 2012). Similarly, when fathers are excluded from universal services, as is the case in many health and educational services currently, vulnerable or problematic fathers who may require targeted interventions may remain difficult to reach (McAllister et al., 2012). This situation calls for interventions that are context-specific, considering the influence of social, economic, and cultural factors that may influence father involvement.

Summary and Key Points

With the exception of South Africa, scant research attention has been paid to father involvement in sub-Saharan Africa. Although there is some evidence in support of the important role fathers play in their children's lives, there is an urgent need for a robust fatherhood research agenda, informed by cultural, social, economic, and structural factors. Research initiatives that produce rigorous evidence are crucial for informing policies that can ultimately promote fathers' involvement in health and educational services and in the lives of their children. In this chapter, we presented a review of father involvement in the early years of their children's life in sub-Saharan Africa. We contest the traditional Western conceptualization of fatherhood and argue that in the diverse cultural contexts of sub-Saharan Africa, fatherhood, and parenting in general, is a shared community responsibility. As such, fatherhood extends beyond the biological and nuclear family and includes significant male figures that play important roles in caring for their children. Our chapter recognizes, in line with global literature, the important role fathers play in the well-being and development of their children. In particular, father involvement has a profound impact on children's physical, cognitive, socioemotional, and behavioral development. We identify the contextual factors that serve as barriers to fathers' involvement – most notably socioeconomic factors, cultural beliefs systems, and health and educational services that are catering predominantly for women. We argue that father engagement can be promoted through transforming gender stereotypes and creating equitable gender roles in child-rearing; by including more men in existing family support, maternal and child health, and HIV prevention and PMTCT programs; through involving fathers early in the lives of their children; and through implementing contextually sensitive interventions that account for cultural, social, economic, and structural dynamics. Most importantly, we emphasize the need for rigorous research evidence in sub-Saharan Africa that can be used to inform policy. Within this context, it is important to understand several key points:

- Fatherhood in sub-Saharan Africa extends beyond the biological and nuclear family and includes significant male figures that contribute to the well-being of children.
- Father involvement has a profound positive impact on the physical, cognitive, socioemotional, and behavioral development of children.
- Cultural beliefs, contexts of unemployment and endemic poverty, and the exclusion from health and educational services pose

significant barriers to father involvement in child development.

- Father engagement can potentially be promoted through the following:
  - Changing gender stereotypes and creating equitable gender roles in child-rearing
  - Including more men in existing health and educational services
  - Involving fathers early in the lives of their children
  - Implementing contextually sensitive interventions
- Father engagement should be promoted in a manner that does not compromise women's autonomy or decision-making ability for themselves or their children.
- Rigorous research evidence is required in sub-Saharan Africa to inform policy development and decision-making to improve father involvement in the lives of their children.

References

Abubakar, A., Van Baar, A., Fischer, R., Bomu, G., Gona, J. K., & Newton, C. R. (2013). Socio-cultural determinants of health-seeking behaviour on the Kenyan coast: A qualitative study. *PLoS One, 8*(11), e71998. https://doi.org/10.1371/journal.pone.0071998

Adams, R. H. J., Cuecuecha, A., & Page, J. (2008). *The impact of remittances on poverty and inequality in Ghana*. The World Bank.

Akilapa, R., & Simkiss, D. (2012). Cultural influences and safeguarding children. *Paediatrics and Child Health, 22*(11), 490–495. https://doi.org/10.1016/j.paed.2012.06.008

Anderson, K. G. (2015). Father absence, childhood stress, and reproductive maturation in South Africa. *Human Nature, 26*(4), 401–425. https://doi.org/10.1007/s12110-015-9243-6

Anderson, K. G., Kaplan, H., & Lancaster, J. (1999). Paternal care by genetic fathers and stepfathers I: Reports from Albuquerque men. *Evolution and Human Behavior, 20*(6), 405–431. https://doi.org/10.1016/S1090-5138(99)00022-7

Arnot, M. (2014). Families are changing: Are communities responding? *Journal of the Community Development Society, 6*(2), 36–44. https://doi.org/10.1080/15575330.1975.10878070

Bangirana, P., John, C. C., Idro, R., Opoka, R. O., Byarugaba, J., Jurek, A. M., et al. (2009). Socioeconomic predictors of cognition in Ugandan children: Implications for community interventions. *PLoS One, 4*(11), e7898. https://doi.org/10.1371/journal.pone.0007898

Barker, G., Levtov, R., & Heilman, B. (2018). Changing the global mindset on fathers. *ZERO TO THREE, 38*, 44.

Beardshaw, T. (2006). Taking forward work with men in families. In L. Richter & R. Morrell (Eds.), *Baba: Men and fatherhood in South Africa* (pp. 306–316). Cape Town, South Africa: HSRC Press.

Beatson, J. E. (2013). Supporting refugee Somali Bantu mothers with children with disabilities. *Pediatric Nursing*, (3), 39, 142–135.

Bhana, D., Nzimakwe, T., & Nzimakwe, P. (2011). Gender in the early years: Boys and girls in an African working class primary school. *International Journal of Educational Development, 31*(5), 443–448. https://doi.org/10.1016/j.ijedudev.2010.09.001

Booth, M. Z. (1995). Children of migrant fathers: The effects of father absence on Swazi children's preparedness for school. *Comparative Education Review, 39*(2), 195–210. https://doi.org/10.1086/447307

Boss, P. (2007). Ambiguous loss theory: Challenges for scholars and practitioners. *Family Relations, 56*, 105–111. https://doi.org/10.1111/j.1741-3729.2007.00444.x

Bremberg, S. (2006). *New tools for parents: Proposals for new forms of parent support*. Stockholm: Swedish National Institute of Public Health.

Carlson, M. J., & Corcoran, M. E. (2001). Family structure and children's behavioral and cognitive outcomes. *Journal of Marriage and Family, 63*(3), 779–792. https://doi.org/10.1111/j.1741-3737.2001.00779.x

Cunningham, S. A., Elo, I. T., Herbst, K., & Hosegood, V. (2010). Prenatal development in rural South Africa: Relationship between birth weight and access to fathers and grandparents. *Population Studies, 64*(3), 229–246. https://doi.org/10.1080/00324728.2010.510201

Davis, J., Vaughan, C., Nankinga, J., Davidson, L., Kigodi, H., Alalo, E., et al. (2018). Expectant fathers' participation in antenatal care services in Papua New Guinea: A qualitative inquiry. *BMC Pregnancy and Childbirth, 18*(1), 138.

Doherty, W. J., Erickson, M. F., & LaRossa, R. (2006). An intervention to increase father involvement and skills with infants during the transition to parenthood. *Journal of Family Psychology, 20*(3), 438. https://doi.org/10.1037/0893-3200.20.3.438

Dworkin, S. L., Colvin, C., Hatcher, A., & Peacock, D. (2012). Men's perceptions of women's rights and changing gender relations in South Africa: Lessons for working with men and boys in HIV and antiviolence programs. *Gender & Society, 26*(1), 97–120. https://doi.org/10.1177/0891243211426425

Ejuu, G. (2016). Celebrating African Men's role in child care and early childhood development programs. *Childhood Education, 92*(1), 29–35. https://doi.org/10.1080/00094056.2016.1134239

Enderstein, A. M., & Boonzaier, F. (2015). Narratives of young South African fathers: Redefining masculinity through fatherhood. *Journal of Gender Studies, 24*(5), 512–527. https://doi.org/10.1080/09589236.2013.856751

Evans, G. W., Ricciuti, H. N., Hope, S., Schoon, I., Bradley, R. H., Corwyn, R. F., et al. (2010). Crowding and cognitive development: The mediating role of maternal responsiveness among 36-month-old children. *Environment and Behavior, 42*(1), 135–148. https://doi.org/10.1177/0013916509333509

Fosu, A. K. (2015). Growth, inequality and poverty in Sub-Saharan Africa: Recent progress in a global context. *Oxford Development Studies, 43*(1), 44–59. https://doi.org/10.1080/13600818.2014.964195

Henrich, J., Heine, S. J., & Norenzayan, A. (2010). The weirdest people in the world? *Behavioral and Brain Sciences, 33*(2–3), 61–83. https://doi.org/10.1017/s0140525x0999152x

Herbert, Z., & Princess, G. (2017). Experiences of female university students who grew up in father absent homes. International Journal of Education and Psychology in the Community, 7(1/2), 16.

Hosegood, V., & Madhavan, S. (2012). Understanding fatherhood and father involvement in South Africa: Insights from surveys and population cohorts. *Fathering, 10*(3), 257. https://doi.org/10.3149/fth.1003.257

Hunter, M. (2006). Fathers without amandla: Zulu-speaking men and fatherhood. Baba: men and fatherhood in South Africa, 99–107.

Jones, J., & Mosher, W. D. (2013). *Fathers' involvement with their children: United States, 2006–2010 (National Health Statistics Reports, No. 71)*. Hyattsville, MD: National Center for Health Statistics.

Jorosi-Tshiamo, W. B., Mogobe, K. D., & Mokotedi, M. T. (2013). Male involvement in child care activities: A review of the literature in Botswana. *African Journal of Reproductive Health, 17*(4), 35–42.

Kang'ethe, S. M. (2009). Inadequate Male Involvement in Health Issues: The cause of gender-skewed HIV and AIDS situations in Botswana. In B. Osei-Huwedie, T. Maundeni, E. Mukamaambo, & P. Ntseane (Eds.), *Male involvement in sexual and reproductive health: Prevention of violence and HIV and AIDS in Botswana* (pp. 7–28). Cape Town, South Africa: Made Plain Communications.

Keller, H., Borke, J., Lamm, B., Lohaus, A., & Dzeaye Yovsi, R. (2011). Developing patterns of parenting in two cultural communities. *International Journal of Behavioral Development, 35*(3), 233–245. https://doi.org/10.1177/0165025410380652

Khewu, N., & Adu, E. O. (2017). Black fathers' involvement in the early education of their children and associated factors: South African context. *Journal of Social Sciences, 42*(1–2), 1–9. https://doi.org/10.1080/09718923.2015.11893388

Kinga, T. N., Kimani, J. M., & Muriithi, W. (2014). A comparative study of levels of self esteem among students of single and dual parent families. The case of students in selected secondary schools in Nakuru Municipality, Kenya. *Research on Humanities and Social Sciences, 4*(1), 55–58.

Kwambai, T. K., Dellicour, S., Desai, M., Ameh, C. A., Person, B., Achieng, F., et al. (2013). Perspectives of men on antenatal and delivery care service utilisation in rural western Kenya: A qualitative study. *BMC Pregnancy and Childbirth, 13*(1), 134. https://doi.org/10.1186/1471-2393-13-134

Lamb, M. E., & Lewis, C. (2004). The development and significance of father – Child relationships in two-parent families. In M. E. Lamb (Ed.), *The role of the father in child development* (4th ed., pp. 272–306). Hoboken, NJ: Wiley.

Langa, M. (2010). Adolescent boys' talk about absent fathers. *Journal of Psychology in Africa, 20*(4), 519–526. https://doi.org/10.1080/14330237.2010.10820410

Lasser, J., Fite, K., & Wadende, A. P. (2011). Fatherhood in Kenyan ethnic communities: Implication for child development. *School Psychology International, 32*(1), 49–57. https://doi.org/10.1177/0143034310396613

Lesejane, D. (2006). Fatherhood from an African cultural perspective. In L. Richter & R. Morrell (Eds.), *Baba: Men and fatherhood in South Africa* (pp. 173–182). Cape Town, South Africa: HSRC Press.

Lu, Y., & Treiman, D. J. (2011). Migration, remittances, and educational stratification among blacks in apartheid and post-apartheid South Africa. *Social Forces; a Scientific Medium of Social Study and Interpretation, 89*(4), 1119–1143. https://doi.org/10.1093/sf/89.4.1119

Madhavan, S., Richter, L., Norris, S., & Hosegood, V. (2014). Fathers' financial support of children in a low income community in South Africa. *Journal of Family and Economic Issues, 35*(4), 452–463. https://doi.org/10.1007/s10834-013-9385-9

Madhavan, S., & Roy, K. (2012). Securing fatherhood through kin work: A comparison of Black low-income fathers and families in South Africa and the United States. *Journal of Family Issues, 33*(6), 801–822. https://doi.org/10.1177/0192513X11426699

Madhavan, S., Schatz, E., Clark, S., & Collinson, M. (2012). Child mobility, maternal status, and household composition in rural South Africa. *Demography, 49*(2), 699–718. https://doi.org/10.1007/s13524-011-0087-3

Mahgoub, S. E. O., Nnyepi, M., & Bandeke, T. (2006). Factors affecting prevalence of malnutrition among children under three years of age in Botswana. *African Journal of Food Agriculture Nutrition and Development, 6*(1), 3–15.

Makofane, M. (2015). "Not all men are fathers": Experiences of African women from families with absent fathers. *Social Work, 51*(1), 22–44. https://doi.org/10.15270/51-1-426

Makusha, T., & Richter, L. (2014). The role of black fathers in the lives of children in South Africa: Child protection for Black South Africans is often a collective responsibility. *Child Abuse and Neglect, 38*(6), 982–992. https://doi.org/10.1016/j.chiabu.2014.05.003

Makusha, T., & Richter, L. (2016). Gatekeeping and its impact on father involvement among Black South Africans in rural KwaZulu-Natal. *Culture, Health and Sexuality, 18*(3), 308–320. https://doi.org/10.1080/13691058.2015.1083122

Mboya, M. M., & Nesengani, R. I. (1999). Migrant labor in South Africa: A comparative analysis of the academic achievement of father-present and father-absent adolescents. *Adolescence, 34*(136), 763–763.

McAllister, F., Burgess, A., Kato, J., & Barker, G. (2012). *Fatherhood: Parenting Programmes and policy – A critical review of best practice*. London: Fatherhood Institute.

McWayne, C., Downer, J. T., Campos, R., & Harris, R. D. (2013). Father involvement during early childhood and its association with children's early learning: A meta-analysis. *Early Education and Development, 24*(6), 898–922. https://doi.org/10.1080/10409289.2013.746932

Mkhize, N. (2006). African traditions and the social, economic and moral dimensions of fatherhood. In L. Richter & R. Morrell (Eds.), *Baba: Men and fatherhood in South Africa* (pp. 182–198). Cape Town, South Africa: HSRC Press.

Mncanca, M., & Okeke, C. I. O. (2016). Positive fatherhood: A key synergy for functional early childhood education in South Africa. *Journal of Sociology and Social Anthropology, 7*(4), 221–232. https://doi.org/10.1080/09766634.2016.11885720

Mncanca, M., Okeke, C. I. O., & Fletcher, R. (2016). Black fathers' participation in early childhood development in South Africa: What do we know? *Journal of Social Sciences, 46*(3), 202–213. https://doi.org/10.1080/09718923.2016.11893528

Morrell, R., Dunkle, K., Ibragimov, U., & Jewkes, R. (2016). Fathers who care and those that don't: Men and childcare in South Africa. *South African Review of Sociology, 47*(4), 80–105. https://doi.org/10.1080/21528586.2016.1204240

Morrell, R., & Richter, L. (2004). The fatherhood project: Confronting issues of masculinity and sexuality. *Agenda, 18*(62), 36–44.

Mufutau, M. A., & Okeke, C. I. O. (2017). Factors affecting rural men's participation in children's preschool in one rural education district in the eastern Cape Province. *Studies of Tribes and Tribals, 14*(1), 18–28. https://doi.org/10.1080/0972639x.2016.11886728

Mugadza, H. T., Mujeyi, B., Stout, B., Wali, N., & Renzaho, A. M. (2019). Childrearing practices among Sub-Saharan African migrants in Australia: A systematic review. *Journal of Child and Family Studies*, 1–15. https://doi.org/10.1007/s10826-019-01463-z

Nkuoh, G. N., Cmmh, D., Meyer, D. J., Tih, P. M., & Nkfusai, J. (2010). Barriers to men's participation in antenatal and prevention of mother-to-child HIV transmission care in Cameroon, Africa. *Journal of Midwifery & Women's Health, 55*(4), 363–369. https://doi.org/10.1016/j.jmwh.2010.02.009

Nsamenang, B. (2010). Fathers, families and children's well-becoming in Africa. In M. E. Lamb (Ed.), *The role of the father in child development* (pp. 388–412). Hoboken, NJ: John Wiley & Sons.

Ntshebe, O. (2013). Family complexity and child health in Botswana. *27th International Population Conference*, 26–31 August. Busan, Korea.

OECD. (2011). *Doing better for families*. OECD Publishing. https://doi.org/10.1787/9789264098732-en

Oláh, L. S., Richter, R., & Kotowska, I. E. (2014). The new roles of men and women and implications for families and societies. Families and societies. Working Paper Series

Palm, G., & Fagan, J. (2008). Father involvement in early childhood programs: Review of the literature. *Early Child Development and Care, 178*(7–8), 745–759. https://doi.org/10.1080/03004430802352137

Panter-Brick, C., Burgess, A., Eggerman, M., McAllister, F., Pruett, K., & Leckman, J. F. (2014). Practitioner review: Engaging fathers–recommendations for a game change in parenting interventions based on a systematic review of the global evidence. *Journal of Child Psychology and Psychiatry, 55*(11), 1187–1212. https://doi.org/10.1111/jcpp.12280

Peneza, A. K., & Maluka, S. O. (2018). 'Unless you come with your partner you will be sent back home': Strategies used to promote male involvement in antenatal care in Southern Tanzania. *Global Health Action, 11*(1), 1449724. https://doi.org/10.1080/16549716.2018.1449724

Ramphele, M. (2002). *Steering by the stars: Being young in South Africa*. Cape Town, South Africa: Tafelberg.

Ratele, K., Shefer, T., & Clowes, L. (2012). Talking South African fathers: A critical examination of men's constructions and experiences of fatherhood and fatherlessness. *South Africa Journal of Psychology, 42*(4), 553–563. https://doi.org/10.1177/008124631204200409

Richter, L. (2006). The importance of fathering for children. In L. Richter & R. Morrell (Eds.), *BABA: Men and fatherhood in South Africa*. Cape Town: HSRC Press.

Richter, L., Chikovore, J., & Makusha, T. (2010). The status of fatherhood and fathering in South Africa. *Childhood Education, 86*(6), 360–365. https://doi.org/10.1080/00094056.2010.10523170

Richter, L., Desmond, C., Hosegood, V., Madhavan, S., Makiwane, M., Makusha, T., et al. (2012). Fathers and other men in the lives of children and families. *Strategies to Overcome Poverty & Inequality: Towards Carnegie III*. Cape Town, South Africa.

Richter, L., & Morrell, R. (2008). Fathering: The role of men in raising children in Africa—Holding up the other half of the sky. In M. H. Garcia, A. Pence, & J. Evans (Eds.), *Africa's future, Africa's challenge: early childhood care and development in Sub-Saharan Africa* (pp. 151–166). The World Bank.

Rikimaru, T., Yartey, J. E., Taniguchi, K., Kennedy, D. O., & Nkrumah, F. K. (1998). Risk factors for the prevalence of malnutrition among urban children in Ghana.

Journal of Nutritional Science and Vitaminology, 44(3), 391–407.

Rolfe, H. (2006). Where are the men? Gender segregation in the childcare and early years sector. *National Institute Economic Review, 195*(1), 103–117. https://doi.org/10.1177/0027950106064038

Roy, K. (2008). A life course perspective on fatherhood and family policies in the United States and South Africa. *Fathering: A Journal of Theory, Research, and Practice about Men as Fathers, 6*(2), 92–112. https://doi.org/10.3149/fth.0602.92

Sabone, M. B. (2009). Transformations in Gender Roles and Relationships: Impact on childcare and socialisation. In B. Osei-Huwedie, T. Maundeni, E. Mukamaambo, & P. Ntseane (Eds.), *Male involvement in sexual and reproductive health: prevention of violence and HIV and AIDS in Botswana* (pp. 165–176). Cape Town, South Africa: Made Plain Communications.

Sarkadi, A., Kristiansson, R., Oberklaid, F., & Bremberg, S. (2008). Fathers' involvement and children's developmental outcomes: A systematic review of longitudinal studies. *International Journal of Paediatrics, 97*(2), 153–158. https://doi.org/10.1111/j.1651-2227.2007.00572.x

Southwood, F. (2011). The presence of a primary male caregiver affects children's language skills. *Stellenbosch Papers in Linguistics*. https://doi.org/10.5774/39-0-5

Spjeldnaes, I. O., Moland, K. M., Harris, J., & Sam, D. L. (2011). "Being man enough": Fatherhood experiences and expectations among teenage boys in South Africa. *Fathering, 9*(1), 3–21.

Statistics South Africa. (2018). General Household Survey Statistical Release. In *General household survey*. https://doi.org/10.1016/S0022-5223(12)00629-0

Townsend, N. (2013). Cultural contexts of father involvement. In N. J. Cabrera & C. S. Temis-LeMonda (Eds.), *Handbook for father involvement: Multidisciplinary perspectives* (pp. 249–277). New York: Routledge.

Trentacosta, C. J., Hyde, L. W., Shaw, D. S., Dishion, T. J., Gardner, F., & Wilson, M. (2008). The relations among cumulative risk, parenting, and behavior problems during early childhood. *Journal of Child Psychology and Psychiatry, 49*(11), 1211–1219. https://doi.org/10.1111/j.1469-7610.2008.01941.x

Valiquette-Tessier, S.-C., Gosselien, J., Young, M., & Thomassin, K. (2019). A literature review of cultural stereotypes associated with motherhood and fatherhood. *Marriage & Family Review, 55*(4), 299–329. https://doi.org/10.1080/01494929.2018.1469567

Vernon-Feagans, L., Garrett-Peters, P., Willoughby, M., Mills-Koonce, R., & Family Life Project Key Investigators. (2012). Chaos, poverty, and parenting: Predictors of early language development. *Early Childhood Research Quarterly, 27*(3), 339–351. https://doi.org/10.1016/j.ecresq.2011.11.001

WHO. Recommendations on Health Promotion Interventions for Maternal and Newborn Health. Geneva: World Health Organization, 2015.

Yabiku, S. T., Agadjanian, V., & Cau, B. (2012). Labor migration and child mortality in Mozambique. *Social Science & Medicine, 75*(12), 2530–2538. https://doi.org/10.1038/mp.2011.182

Father-Child Interactional Synchrony as a Function of Maternal and Paternal Depression in Low-Income Brazilian Families

28

Júlia Scarano de Mendonça
and Vera Sílvia Raad Bussab

Our goal in this chapter is to reflect on parental depression in new parents by looking at the functions that maternal and paternal depression may have in the family system, in line with the evolutionary approach of depression proposed by Hagen (1999). Analyses based on the functional adaptation of depression provide an alternative explanation for counterintuitive phenomena and may be viewed as an additional tool to understand the intriguing and sometimes paradoxical phenomena associated with depression. Moreover, it is our intention to provide a model of parental depression in new parents based on the interplay between mothers' and fathers' depression, consistent with family system theory (Minuchin, 1985).

In this chapter, we first present an overview of evolutionary theories of depression, especially Hagen's hypothesis, and family system theory. Subsequently, we present a brief account of the two previous studies whose results together are the focus of this reflection. We end the chapter with a discussion of the findings in the light of the theories presented.

The studies used in this reflection examined father-child interaction as a function of mother's postpartum depression (PPD) symptoms, mother's and father's later depression, and family relationships: specifically, the marital and co-parental relationship and paternal involvement. Results have shown greater father-child interactional synchrony when mothers reported PPD symptoms (De Mendonça, Bussab, Lucci, & Kärtner, 2015b) suggesting that fathers buffered mothers' impaired functioning due to depression, and when mothers and fathers reported depression symptoms at the child's third year (De Mendonça & Bussab, 2016). Fathers' buffering mechanism was interpreted as a way to compensate mothers' impaired functioning, a mechanism within the family that has also been reported when mothers present a history of drug abuse (McKelvey, Burrow, Mesman, Pemberton, Bradley, & Fitzgerald, 2012). However, the positive interaction found in the second study between depressed fathers and their children has rarely been reported in the literature and points out to the complex phenomena of paternal depression.

J. S. de Mendonça (✉)
Graduate Program in Educational Psychology, Centro Universitário FIEO, Osasco, São Paulo, Brazil

V. S. R. Bussab
Department of Experimental Psychology, Institute of Psychology, University of São Paulo, São Paulo, Brazil

H. E. Fitzgerald et al. (eds.), *Handbook of Fathers and Child Development*,
https://doi.org/10.1007/978-3-030-51027-5_28

Evolutionary Approaches to Depression

Evolutionary approaches to depression offer an alternative interpretation to the most current understanding of depression as a mood disturbance. From an evolutionary perspective, negative emotions, like the ones present in depression, can also be understood as defense mechanisms, functioning in the same way as body symptoms such as cough or fever, by signaling to the individual that a potential harmful mechanism is active within the organism or in the external environment (Nesse & Williams, 1997, 2012). In fact, several evolutionary approaches to depression offer functional analyses, highlighting its adaptive function[1] for an individual's protection mechanism against harsh environmental conditions (Hagen, 1999, 2002, 2011; Price, Sloman, Gradner, Gilbert, & Rohde, 1994).

Postpartum depression (PPD) has been traditionally defined as a mood disturbance, but it has also benefited from an analysis of the functions of emotions in the course of evolution (Luz & Bussab, 2009). Emotions are defined as subjective reactions to environmental events; they consist of physiological, perceptual, and behavioral changes in the individual's states (Sroufe, 1997). Emotions guide the individual's actions by mediating the external input and the individual's behavior, and they represent an important step in the evolutionary process (Ades, 2009). The modulation of the emotional experience includes mechanisms involving its perception and control and has, among its main functions, the promotion of changes in the individual's behavior, optimizing the individual's social adaptation.

Our discussion benefits mostly from Hagen's analysis of PPD. From this perspective, the low mood that characterizes depression mental states and the subsequent lack of one's energy would have a signaling function, indicating mother's need for extra support for the care of a newborn, and could be seen as a psychological functional adaptation to a situation evaluated as more costly than the mother can cope with. Once the mother evaluates the costs of caring for a new infant as very high (more than she can cope with), she may unconsciously develop a depression that will impair her capacity to care for the infant, increasing her chances of obtaining support from her local environment, especially from her partner, to promote the infant's survival and well-being. The theory predicts that (1) women who perceive a lack of social support are at greater risk of developing PPD, and (2) PPD will enhance partner's support and paternal investment.

Further studies provide empirical evidence to support Hagen's hypothesis. For example, Hagen (2002), in an American sample, reports marginally significant positive correlations between maternal PPD and an increase in paternal care behavior, suggesting an enhancement of paternal care investment when their partners present PPD, as predicted by the theory. Similarly, Edhborg, Lundh, Seimyr, and Widström (2003) demonstrated that fathers in Sweden families where the mothers scored high on the EPDS were more positively involved in the father-child interaction and presented a tendency toward more visual contact with the child 15–18 months postpartum in comparison to fathers whose partners did not score high on the EPDS. The authors found also that children of high EPDS scoring mothers were more likely to be securely attached to their fathers, in contrast to the children's attachment to their mothers. Additional evidence is provided by Spinelli (2009), whose research found a greater risk among low-income Brazilian women of developing PPD when they perceive that the financial support provided by their partners after childbirth was less than what they imaged during pregnancy, suggesting that the lack of partner's support (even if only instrumental) is a risk factor for PDD.

However, understanding maternal PPD as a condition with the potential to increase paternal investment presents a special challenge, considering the apparent paradox between the two forces that it represents. On the one hand, the

[1] "Adaptations, also known as biological functions, are organisms traits whose properties are best explained by the positive effects they had on the reproduction of the organism's ancestors over evolutionary time, that is, which evolved by natural selection" (Hagen, 2011, p. 717).

negative consequences it has for mother-child interaction are well documented (Field, 2010; Fonseca, Silva, & Otta, 2010; Stanley, Murray, & Stein, 2004). On the other hand, the potential it offers for obtaining extra support from the local environment, especially from the partner, is highlighted. This paradox can be understood in the light of an integrative analysis, considering ontogeny and phylogeny, and its proximal and ultimate levels of analysis. At the proximal level, the lack of mother's partner support is among the causes of PPD, while at the ultimate level, the increase in paternal investment is among its functions.

The evolutionary hypothesis of maternal PPD proposed by Hagen highlights its impact on fathers' behavior. However, to our knowledge, it does not include recent research findings showing that (1) the incidence of fathers' depression during the postnatal period is quite high and (2) that mothers' PPD has been found to be the main risk factor for fathers' depression. Moreover, it does not discuss the impact that fathers' depression may have on their potential support for depressed mothers and the increase in paternal investment. Are fathers capable of increasing their investment when they are also depressed? What is the relation between mothers' and fathers' depression in the postpartum period? In what follows, we look further into these questions.

The Family as a System

The *Family System Approach* (Minuchin, 1985) also guided the studies that are the focus of our analysis. It proposes that the family unit is a changing system, composed of various subsystems (mother-child dyad, father-child dyad, husband-wife, etc.) that are interrelated and influence each other (Favez, Frascarolo, & Tissot, 2017; Fivaz-Depeursinge & Corboz-Warnery, 1999; De Mendonça, Cossette, Lapointe, & Strayer, 2008). It predicts the influence of the larger social and cultural context on family interactive patterns, the reciprocal influences between the family subsystems, and a constant reorganization on the whole system's dynamics as adaptations to changes among its members.

Next, we briefly present the two studies that are the focus of the present discussion. We first present the objectives, hypothesis, and a brief summary of the results of each of the studies. Considering that both studies were conducted using the same sample, the method (participants, measures, and procedures) will be explained after.

Study 1 *Father-child interactional synchrony in Brazilian families with maternal depression* (De Mendonça et al., 2015b).

Past studies suggest that maternal depression can influence paternal behavior (Hagen, 1999, 2002; Hagen & Thornhill, 2017; Paulson, Dauber, & Leiferman, 2006). In addition, Gray and Anderson (2010) have shown that the quality of the marital relationship is one of the most powerful predictors of paternal behavior.

The main objective in this study was to examine the associations between maternal PPD and later depression, paternal behavior, and family relationships (marital and co-parental relationships and father involvement). The specific objectives were (1) to examine the effect of mother's depression from the postpartum period up to the child's 36th month of life on father-child interaction at the child's 36th month of life and (2) to examine the associations between mothers' and fathers' perceptions of their inter-parental relationship and father-child interaction at the child's 36th month of life. Two hypotheses were proposed: (1) Father-child interaction would be closer and more synchronized when mothers presented PPD and later depression compared to when mothers did not report depression symptoms, and (2) father-child interaction would be closer and more synchronized when the parental relationship was more satisfactory compared to when it was less so.

Our main interest in the present discussion is to reflect on the functions that maternal and paternal depression may have in the family system. Following this, the discussion in this chapter will be centered on the objective (1) of this study.

For this reason, results will only be provided for the first objective.

Results (1) The percentage of mothers with depression symptoms at 3 months was 36%; at 8 months, it was 29%; and it was even higher at 36 months, reaching 40% of the total sample. (2) Positive correlations were found between maternal depression assessments at 3, 8, and 36 months. (3) Maternal depression accounted for some of the father-child interaction total variance. Severity of maternal depression was associated with closer father-child interpersonal distance and more father-child visual synchronization, at the child's 36th month. Also, when mothers were depressed at the child's 8th and 36th months, fathers and children showed more visual synchronization at 36 months.

Study 2 *Father-child interactional synchrony as a function of paternal depression in a low-income Brazilian sample* (De Mendonça & Bussab, 2016).

Past research has shown that mothers and fathers can play different roles within the family system (De Mendonça, Cossette, Strayer, & Gravel, 2011; De Mendonça, Bussab, & Kärtner, 2019; Tamis-LeMonda, 2004). Thus, it is likely that the feelings elicited by depression in mothers and in fathers will also have a different impact on the family system.

A great amount of research has shown that maternal depression has negative effects on parenting behaviors. In contrast, our previous results using self-report measures showed that fathers with depression symptoms perceived themselves as more involved in the family at the child's third year (De Mendonça, Bussab, Rodrigues, Siqueira, & Cossette, 2012). Given that self-report measures can be influenced by the subjective experience of the individual, a direct observation of the nuclear family (mother-father-child) social interaction could provide new light on this issue.

The main objective in this study was to understand fathers' involvement with their 3-year-old children in the context of paternal depression by direct observation of father-child interaction.

Results Past research has derived three factors from the *Edinburgh Postnatal Depression Scale* (EPDS) total score, representing different dimensions of depression: (1) *depressive symptoms,* (2) *anhedonia,* and (3) *anxietal symptoms* (McVey & Tuohy, 2007). Further analysis using these factors showed a significant positive correlation between the factor *depressive symptoms* and father-child interpersonal distance (r = 0.324, p = 0.030), indicating that when fathers were depressed, they got closer to the child in a free play situation, in accordance with our previous results using self-report measures.

Method

The two studies used for this reflection were conducted in the context of a larger longitudinal research project at the University of São Paulo (Brazil) on the origins and consequences of PPD in low-income families (Otta, Bussab, & Morais, 2006). The larger project consisted of a four-year longitudinal study in which 400 low-income mothers were followed from the third trimester of pregnancy up to their child's third birthday. In total, seven meetings were held—at the third trimester of pregnancy, delivery, and child's 3rd, 8th, 12th, 24th, and 36th months—and several aspects of the mother-child interaction and of the child's development were evaluated over the years.

Participants

Forty-three couples participated in the two studies. Mothers were, on average, 26.3 years old (SD = 5.6; range = 16–43). Forty three percent of them (N = 20) had not finished secondary school, 43.5% (N = 20) had finished secondary school, and 4.3% (N = 2) had completed higher education. At their child's 36th month, 52.5% (N = 21) of the mothers were employed, and 91.3% (N = 42) reported being married or living with the father of the child. The majority of the children (65.2%, *N* = 30) were girls. All the mothers who answered the questionnaire on their socioeconomic status (*N* = 40) reported owning a color TV, 74% (*N* = 30) reported living in a house with a minimum of four rooms, 10% (*N* = 4) reported not owning a videocassette or DVD player, one woman reported not owning a fridge, and 52.5% (*N* = 21) of them reported not having a car. Fathers were, on average, 29.5 years old (SD = 6.9; range = 18–48) at the birth of their child. Forty-two percent (*N* = 19) of the fathers had not finished secondary school, 44.4% (*N* = 20) had finished secondary school, and 4.4% (*N* = 2) of them had completed higher education.

Measures

Depression Symptoms

To assess maternal and paternal depression symptoms, we used the *Edinburgh Postnatal Depression Scale* (EPDS) (Cox, Holden, & Sagovsy, 1987). The EPDS was validated in Brazil by Santos, Martins, and Pasquali (1999). The scale has also been validated for men (Matthey, Barnett, Kavanagh, & Howie, 2001). Two groups, depressed and nondepressed, were created. The depressed group was composed of participants who had a score of 11 points or more on the scale. This cutoff point of 11 was suggested by Santos et al. (1999) in their validation study. A mother's profile scale variable was created considering the EPDS scores at 3, 8, and 36 months. Three groups of mothers were created: 1. *never depressed* (51%, *N* = 21), 2. *recovery of depression over time* (10%, *N* = 4) (mothers from this group were either depressed at 3 or 8 months but not depressed at 36 months), and 3. *severe depression* (39%, *N* = 16) (mothers from this group presented symptoms of depression at 36 months and symptoms of previous depression at all times or at least at 3 or 8 months).

Father-Child Interaction

To assess father-child interaction, we used the *Taxonomy of Interactional Synchrony* (De Mendonça, Bourçois, Sinclair, & Strayer, 2015a) This coding system scheme adopts a microanalytical approach with a multidimensional focus (interpersonal distance, visual and body orientation, and play involvement). After several viewings of the videotapes, a four-point grading scale, representing different levels of synchrony, was created for each of the interactional synchrony dimensions, based on the dyadic interactional behaviors. Each dimension of interactional synchrony was then rated using this scale, with higher numbers representing greater interactional synchrony. The data was coded by one of the observers after the inter-rater reliability kappa test coefficient reached .70 for each category. The mean value of each category of the father-child interaction synchrony measures was calculated and used for subsequent analysis.

Family Relationship

To assess family relationships, we used the *Father Involvement, Marital, and Co-parental Relationship Questionnaire* (PATER). This questionnaire was developed for this study, and it is adapted from other questionnaires (Smith & Howard, 2008; Spanier, 1976). It consists of 16 five-point self-report items (0 = never; 5 = always) divided into three dimensions: father involvement, co-parental, and marital relationships. A score for each dimension was obtained by adding the items that constitutes each one of them to be used for subsequent analysis. Cronbach alpha values of father involvement, co-parental relationship, and marital relationship were 0.8, 0.8, and 0.9 for mother's perception and 0.5, 0.6, and 0.9 for father's perception, respectively.

Procedure

Participants were recruited at the university hospital and health centers in the same region of São Paulo. These medical centers are part of the public health system and are used mostly by the low-income population. Participation in the study was on a volunteer basis. Transportation fees were paid, and a snack was provided for the child at the end of the interview. Ten sessions of therapy were offered to depressed mothers following the postpartum evaluation, 3 months after the child's birthday. Few mothers participated, and no mothers in our sample participated in this intervention program.

Fathers were only invited to participate in the last visit at the child's 36 months, and 46 fathers attended the interview and participated in both studies. Three couples were eliminated from the final sample due to technical problems. Mothers completed the *Edinburgh Postnatal Depression Scale* (EPDS) on three occasions (at the child's 3rd, 8th, and 36th month), and fathers completed the EPDS at the child's 36th month. Father-child interaction was assessed at the child's 36th month during a 10-minute free play interaction at the university laboratory. The laboratory setting consisted of a group of toys, including dolls, trucks, and balls, displayed on a carpet. There was no other furniture in the observation room. Fathers were instructed to play with their children as they regularly did at home. The play session was filmed and coded by the first author.

Discussion

The understanding of parental depression in new parents that we propose is based on an integrative analysis of maternal and paternal depression. The main findings of Study 1 and Study 2 (reported above) indicate that both maternal and paternal depression accounted for some of the father-child interaction total variance. Severity of maternal depression (from the postpartum period to the child's third year) was associated with closer father-child interpersonal distance and more father-child visual synchrony at the child's third year. On the other hand, symptoms of paternal depression at the child's third year correlated positively with closer father-child interpersonal distance at the child's third year.

The results of greater father-child interactional synchrony when mothers presented PPD support the evolutionary hypothesis of PPD (Hagen, 1999), according to which the main function of PDD is to gather social support, especially from the partner (presented above). This interpretation of mothers' PPD highlights the benefits elicited by mothers' depression for the family. However, the mechanisms involved in this bargaining process remain to be understood, as well as the functions that paternal depression may eventually have within the family system.

As Hagen and Rosenström (2016) affirm, unipolar depression, even after more than a century of inquiry, remains a profound scientific mystery. The authors argue, as we do, that researchers from the Western world have viewed depression mostly as an illness, so studies investigating its potential to affect ultimately positive changes in the lives of those afflicted are very few. Hagen and Rosenström point to some interesting research findings that provide additional insight into the search for a better understanding of depression.

First, they call attention to the 2:1 female bias in depression, indicating that depression is mostly a female condition. Second, research shows that depression is closely associated with the chronic activation of the hypothalamic-pituitary-adrenal axis (Nemeroff, 1998) which is a very ancient response mechanism in living organisms that prepares the body for fight or flight (present in mammals in general). Finally, past results indicate that the most significant cause of depression is a major negative life event.

Hagen and Rosenström further argue that, given the dimorphism characteristic of humans, where women are physically weaker than men, it makes sense for women to try to influence the behavior of others (or to bargain), especially with a physically stronger male partner, by withholding benefits (not caring appropriately for offspring) despite the apparent costs to oneself (the unconscious induction of depression elicited by the emotion of sadness), instead of using an aggressive strategy (e.g., physical threats), often elicited by the emotion of anger and more often employed by powerful organisms (e.g., physically stronger males). All together, these findings reinforce the understanding of depression as a female adaptive reaction response to environmental threats. But what about fathers' depression? How can we make sense of it in the context of mothers' PPD?

Mother-child interaction and mothering have been a major area of inquiry in psychology, whereas much less attention has been given to father-child interaction and fathering (Volling & Cabrera, 2019). Thus, we know much more about mothers' functioning in the family than we know about fathers', and many questions about the functioning of fathers remain unclear. Moreover, research results on fathers are inconsistent and controversial, especially in relation to the impacts of paternal depression on father-child interaction.

Numerous studies have shown that maternal PPD has a negative impact on mother-child interaction and child development. Mothers with symptoms of postpartum depression are less contingent (Stanley et al., 2004) and interact with their children in a less affectionate way, and with less visual and vocal communication (Field, 2010), in addition to structuring the interaction less (Fonseca et al., 2010). Moreover, in a low-income Brazilian sample, the correlation between mothers' verbalization, smile, and eye contact (a pattern that is suggestive of a more consistent interactive style) was only found in non-PPD mother-child dyads (DeFelipe, 2009).

Furthermore, previous analysis in our database reinforces the negative impact of the mother's depression on the marital relationship (De Mendonça, Bussab, & Siqueira, 2013a). Past research has shown that both maternal depression and marital conflict are important risk factors for the child's social adaptation (Cummings, Keller, & Davies, 2005; Morais, Lucci, & Otta, 2013). However, it is important to note that when marital conflict was considered together with mothers' high social support and education in a multivariate analysis, a significant effect of mothers' high social support and high education (but not of marital conflict) on maternal PPD was found (De Mendonça, Bussab, Siqueira, & Lucci, 2013b), suggesting that other factors may work as protection for the mother. It is possible that the negative effects of marital conflict on maternal PPD are attenuated in the presence of other kinds of social support (other members of the family and friends) that may function as a safety net for the mother.

The impact of paternal depression on the child's development and family functioning is less understood and, as mentioned above, the results are less consistent (Paulson & Bazemore, 2010). Past research has shown that paternal depression impairs parenting (Wilson & Durbin, 2010) and has negative consequences for the child's development (Ramchandani et al., 2008; Weitzman, Rosenthal, & Liu, 2011). Moreover, Kvalevaag et al. (2013) demonstrated a small positive association between fathers' prenatal mental health and emotional difficulties of their children at 36 months.

However, studies looking at the link between paternal depression and father-infant interactions, specifically, report contradictory findings. For example, Lundy (2002) found that paternal depression symptoms were unrelated to the quality of father-infant interactions. In another study, Field, Hossain, and Malphurs (1999) report that depressed and nondepressed fathers were found to interact similarly with their infants and that depressed fathers displayed more positive behavior toward their children than depressed mothers. The few recent studies found that fathers with depression may be more withdrawn, displaying less verbal and behavioral stimulation during free play interactions with their 3-month-old infants (Sethna, Murray, Netsi, Psychogiou, & Ramchandani, 2015). In addition, Sethna, Murray, Edmondson, Iles, and Ramchandani (2018) report that white well-educated depressed fathers (compared to nondepressed fathers) engaged in fewer episodes of playful excitation, less gentle touch, and less active engagement with their 3-month-old infants. Results also indicate an association between symptoms of paternal depression and marital conflict (Franck & Buehler, 2007), in particular for affection within the relationship (reported by both men and their partners) (Ramchandani et al., 2011).

These inconsistencies in research on fathers may be due to the fact that individual and group differences in the research are still rare, even though research shows that there is a great variability in paternal care expression (Hrdy, 2014). Studies on the biological mechanisms involved in paternal care behavior show that fathers have the same potential to nurture as mothers, although they do not express it as often. For example, research indicates there are common endocrinal mechanisms in mothers and fathers. Moreover, new fathers present a similar response to infants as mothers: a comparable elevation of oxytocin levels to those in mothers; a rise in prolactin levels (the hormone associated with childcare behavior in mammals), although not as high as in mothers; and a decline in testosterone levels (Hrdy, 2014). In addition, several authors have demonstrated that lower testosterone levels are associated with greater paternal responsiveness (Alvergne, Faurie, & Raymond, 2009). Hrdy (2014) refers to it as the "paradox of facultative fathering," pointing out that human fathers have the potential to nurture, though this potential is not always expressed. In fact, in most contemporary human societies, mothers are the main caretakers while fathers can be either very present (and share childcare responsibilities) or completely absent from the child's life (note that there is also variability in maternal care behavior).

Nevertheless, the understanding of the evolution of paternal care behavior in nature may provide a framework that accounts for the variability in fathers' behavior. The literature shows that paternal care expression evolved as a system with maximum flexibility in species where it is not mandatory for infant survival, such that males and their partners can maximize reproductive success in different ways, depending on different conditions (Royle, Russell, & Wilson, 2014; Storey, Delahunty, McKay, Walsh, & Wilhelm, 2006) and, on the contrary, being more fixed (shaped less by social experience and ecological pressures) in species where it is mandatory for offspring survival. Moreover, according to Storey and Walsh (2011), when paternal care is not mandatory for offspring survival, its manifestation may be more susceptible to a variable immediate environment. In addition, research on the evolution of paternal care behavior in nature shows that paternal care is rarely present among most animal species. It occurs in less than 5% of all mammal species (Geary, 2000; Storey & Walsh, 2011).

Researchers agree that paternal care in humans must have been selected in the ancestral environment because it helped offspring survival (Hrdy, 1999, 2014). The difficulties that ancestral mothers must have faced to raise their offspring alone must have had a great impact on the evolution of a cooperative breeding pattern of parental care, involving both parents as well as other alloparents (e.g., other caregivers) in the human species. Hrdy further suggests that infant care involving other members of the social group was probably the typical infant care arrangement in the ancestral environment and a valuable strategy to promote infant survival.

Considering that paternal care in most contemporary societies (different from the ancestral period) is not mandatory for offspring survival, we argue that maternal PPD may be one of the circumstances in which an increase in paternal care is necessary to promote offspring well-being. Hagen suggests that if mothers believe that they are incurring fitness[2] costs from the current care arrangement and are unable to raise the newborn child without more external help, they must somehow convince their partners that this is the case, before fathers agree to increase their investment in the infant. According to Hagen's hypothesis, mothers' depression symptoms and the subsequent impaired infant care provide such evidence. The questions we pose are as follows: Does the increase in fathers' investment, when mothers present PPD, comes from fathers' perception of mothers' depression symptoms and impaired care alone, or is it related to other mechanisms? If so, what other mechanisms are fathers' increased investment related to?

Research shows that changing the social contract of a group can be very costly, with most group members resisting such a change without the robust evidence of its necessity (Watson & Andrews, 2002). We argue, then, that nature may

[2]The fitness of an individual organism refers to the survival and reproductive success of its kin, each relative being valued according to the probability of shared genetic information, an offspring or sibling having a value of 50 percent and a cousin 25 percent.

have provided the organisms with a mechanism to force a change in fathers' behavior when it is necessary for promoting offspring well-being. We further argue that in the context of maternal PPD, this mechanism could be the triggering of paternal depression.

The ideas of Trivers, a well-known evolutionary biologist, provide an interesting input into these questions. Trivers theorizes that the degree to which human parents invest in their offspring is intimately related to the concept of reproductive success (Trivers, 1972). Trivers' research shows the high cost that caring behavior imposes on men pointing out that the different reproductive strategies of men and women account for the level of parental investment in offspring. Trivers argues that men can increase their reproductive success by caring for offspring and/or by mating with other women, given the characteristics of their reproductive physiology (production of a great quantity of spermatozoids during the life course). Women, on the other hand, can rarely increase their reproductive success by increasing mating effort because they produce a limited number of eggs and undertake a long and demanding pregnancy and lactation. For these reasons, they have to rely principally on caring for offspring to promote their reproductive success. In fact, empirical evidence shows that men with more sexual opportunities were more depressed postpartum (Hagen & Rosenström, 2016).

Then, Trivers points out that men, but not women, can substantially increase their reproductive success by mating with multiple partners. In addition, Trivers' theory predicts an increase in paternal care investment (and a loss of mating opportunities) when it is necessary for offspring well-being (survival, growth, and social adaptation) during phylogeny and ontogeny.

Based on these ideas, we argue that it is likely that the biological drive to mate in men promotes a special openness to the outside world of the immediate environment and that paternal depression, in the context of maternal PPD, may function to bring fathers closer to the family in a moment of family need. In what follows, we will further develop our argument.

The Functions of Paternal Depression

Bringing together an evolutionary perspective of depression and paternal care, as well as a systemic approach to the family, we propose that paternal depression in the context of mothers' PPD may function to force a change in fathers' behavior by inhibiting their openness to the outside world and, thus, promoting their greater involvement with the family in the context of family adversity (e.g., maternal PPD).

Trivers suggests that, in the case of maternal depression, fathers unconsciously "calculate" that the increase in the investment in the child may also increase their reproductive success. However, it is not clear how this "calculation" is done. What are the mechanisms involved in this "calculation"? Our hypothesis is that this "calculation" involves the triggering of paternal depression. Moreover, we propose that, given the high costs of paternal investment, paternal depression evolved in the context of mothers' PPD as an unconscious mechanism with the main function of inhibiting fathers' activity outside of the family by inducing a general low mood and passivity that characterizes depressive moods. By inhibiting activity outside the family, paternal depression may inversely promote fathers' approximation to the family in a situation of family adversity, such as mothers' depression and the resulting impaired care capabilities. Thus, in the context of maternal PPD, paternal depression can also be understood as an adaptation to difficult environmental conditions.

More specifically, (1) the literature indicates an association between maternal and paternal depression during the postpartum period, and maternal depression has also been considered the main risk factor for paternal depression (Cameron, Sedov, & Tomfohr-Madsen, 2016; Goodman, 2004; Paulson & Bazemore, 2010; Wee, Skouteris, Pier, Richardson, & Milgrom, 2011); (2) our previous analysis (using both self-report and observational measures) demonstrated that paternal depression can bring fathers closer to the family; (3) then, it is possible that depression in new mothers increases the chances of fathers also becoming depressed to force them to change their behavior by inhibiting activity outside of the family and, thus, promoting their increased proximity to the family. Nevertheless, severe paternal depression will probably have negative consequences for family interaction. Furthermore, it is important to consider that fathers with a mild depression, such as the fathers in our sample, may also look for emotional bonding and more time together with their wives and children as a strategy to overcome their own depression.

Finally, we would like to reinforce that an evolutionary approach to depression and parental care and investment enlarges our comprehension of parental depression within the family as it challenges the traditional view of depression as an illness and proposes that depression may also be seen as a defense mechanism with the potential to bring benefits to the family. Nevertheless, it is important to keep in mind that the analysis of the possible adaptive function of depression does not replace nor should it be confused with the investigation of the causal conditions of the emergence of depression.

We would also like to emphasize that an evolutionary perspective adds another layer of analysis for the understanding of human behavior and development, providing a window to our history as a species. To understand that our behavior reflects, at least partially, years and years of past adaptations shaped over our evolutionary history, and that we carry the history of our species not only in our genes but also in our behavior and development, is an important step to better understanding ontogeny. Developmental psychologists have much to gain from a careful look at the evolutionary history of our species as it provides the fundamentals of what we humans are right now.

To conclude, we would like to reinforce the need for further research to test the hypothesis we set out in this chapter—that the main function of paternal depression in the context of maternal PPD is to promote fathers' proximity to the family. Research looking at maternal and paternal depression together is still rare, and more studies are needed to better understand family dynamics and the child's development when both parents are depressed. Furthermore, given that development is highly contingent upon sociocultural influences (Kärtner, Keller, Chaudhary, & Yovsi, 2012; Henrich, Heine, & Norenzayan, 2010), it is important to test this hypothesis in different countries, communities, and family structures in order to test the universality of this mechanism. Finally, we would like to end this chapter reinforcing the need to include the whole family in prevention and treatment programs for PPD.

Summary and Key Points

Unipolar depression, even after more than a century of inquiry, remains a profound scientific mystery. Researchers from the Western world have viewed depression primarily as an illness, so studies investigating its potential to work ultimately positive changes in the lives of those afflicted have been quite rare. It is also clear that the field of fathering studies is moving in the direction of integrating mothering and fathering studies. Hagen's evolutionary perspective on depression highlights the impact of maternal PPD on fathers' behavior. According to Hagen, depression has a signal function, indicating mother's need for extra support, and can be seen as a psychological functional adaptation to a situation evaluated as more costly than the mother can cope with. This interpretation of mothers' PPD allows for the understanding of depression as a female adaptive reaction response to environmental threats and highlights the benefits elicited by mothers' depression for the family.

However, the mechanisms involved in this bargaining process remain to be understood. Research results on fathers are inconsistent and controversial especially in relation to the impact of paternal depression on father-child interaction. Evolutionary biology, and especially Trivers' research, shows the high cost that caring behavior imposes on men. Trivers further argues that men (but not women) can substantially increase their reproductive success by mating with multiple partners. Thus, we argue that it is likely that this biological drive to mate promotes in men a special openness to the outside world of the immediate environment. In addition, the literature indicates an association between maternal and paternal depression during the postpartum period in which maternal depression has been considered the main risk factor for paternal depression.

We propose that fathers' depression, in the context of mothers' PPD, may function to force a change in fathers' behavior by inhibiting their openness to the outside world. By inhibiting activity outside the family, paternal depression may inversely promote fathers' approximation to the family in a situation of family adversity (e.g., mothers' depression and impaired care capabilities due to depression). Thus, paternal depression, in the context of maternal PPD, can also be understood as an adaptation to difficult environmental conditions. Nevertheless, severe paternal depression will probably have negative consequences for family interaction.

References

Ades, C. (2009). Um olhar evolucionista Para a psicologia. [An evolutionary look at psychology]. In E. Otta & M. E. Yamamoto (Eds.), *Psicologia Evolucionista* [Evolutionary Psychology] (pp. 10–21). Guanabara: Koogan.

Alvergne, A., Faurie, C., & Raymond, M. (2009). Variation in testosterone levels and male reproductive effort: Insight from a polygynous human population. *Hormones and Behavior, 56*(5), 491–497.

Cameron, E. E., Sedov, I. D., & Tomfohr-Madsen, L. M. (2016). Prevalence of paternal depression in pregnancy and the postpartum: An updated meta-analysis. *Journal of Affective Disorders, 206*, 189–203.

Cox, J. L., Holden, J. M., & Sagovsy, R. (1987). Detection of postnatal depression: Development of the 10-item Edinburgh postnatal depression scale. *British Journal of Psychiatry, 150*, 782–786. https://doi.org/10.1192/bjp.150.6.782

Cummings, E. M., Keller, P. S., & Davies, P. T. (2005). Towards a family process model of maternal and paternal depressive symptoms: Exploring multiple relations with child and family functioning. *Journal of Child Psychology and Psychiatry, 46*, 479–489.

DeFelipe, R. (2009). Análise do efeito da depressão pós-parto na interação mãe-bebê via categorias comportamentais e estilos interativos maternos. [Analysis of the effect of postpartum depression on mother-infant interaction via maternal behavioral categories and interactive styles]. Unpublished Doctoral Thesis. University of São Paulo, Brazil.

De Mendonça, J. S., Cossette, L., Lapointe, M. N., & Strayer, F. F. (2008). Vers une analyse systémique des liens d'attachement [Toward a systemic analysis of attachment bonds]. *Bulletin de psychologie, 3*, 257–266.

De Mendonça, J. S., Cossette, L., Strayer, F., & Gravel, F. (2011). Mother-child and father-child interactional synchrony in dyadic and triadic interactions. *Sex Roles, 64*, 132–142.

De Mendonça, J. S., Bussab, V., Rodrigues, A., Siqueira, J., & Cossette, L. (2012). Postpartum depression, father's involvement, and marital and co-parental relationships from mothers' and fathers' perspectives in a low-income Brazilian sample. *Family Science, 4*, 1–10. https://doi.org/10.1080/19424620.2012.783423

De Mendonça, J. S., Bussab, V. S., & Siqueira, J. (2013a). Depressão pós-parto e conflito conjugal: estudo longitudinal das associações bidirecionais em famílias de baixa renda. [Postpartum depression and marital conflict: longitudinal study of two-way associations in low-income families.]. *Psico, 44*(4), 581–589.

De Mendonça, J. S., Bussab, V., Siqueira, J. & Lucci, T. (2013b). Postpartum depression, marital conflict and attachment in a Brazilian sample. Poster presented at *6th International Attachment Conference*, Pavia, Italy.

De Mendonça, J. S., Bourçois, V., Sinclair, F., & Strayer, F. F. (2015a). *Taxonomy of interactional synchrony*. [Database Record]. PsycTESTS, American Psychological Association, U.S.A.

De Mendonça, J. S., Bussab, V. S., Lucci, T. K., & Kärtner, J. (2015b). Father-child interactional synchrony in Brazilian families with maternal depression. *Human Ethology Bulletin, 30*(1), 121–138.

De Mendonça, J. S., & Bussab, V. S. (2016). Father-child interactional synchrony as a function of paternal depression in a low-income Brazilian sample. Conference paper at *15th World Congress of the World Association for Infant Mental Health*, Prague.

De Mendonça, J. S., Bussab, V. S. R., & Kärtner, J. (2019). Interactional synchrony and child gender differences in dyadic and triadic family interactions. *Journal of Family Issues, 40*(8), 959–981.

Edhborg, M., Lundh, W., Seimyr, L., & Widström, A. M. (2003). The parent-child relationship in the context of maternal depressive mood. *Archives of women's mental health, 6*(3), 211–216.

Favez, N., Frascarolo, F., & Tissot, H. (2017). The family alliance model: A way to study and characterize early family interactions. *Frontiers in Psychology, 8*, 1441.

Field, T. (2010). Postpartum depression effects on early interaction, parenting, and safety practices: A review. *Infant Behavior and Development, 33*, 1–6.

Field, T. M., Hossain, Z., & Malphurs, J. (1999). "Depressed" fathers' interactions with their infants. *Infant Mental Health Journal, 20*(3), 322–332.

Fivaz-Depeursinge, E., & Corboz-Warnery, A. (1999). *The primary triangle: A developmental system view of mothers, fathers, and infants*. New York, NY: Basic Books.

Fonseca, V. R. J., Silva, G. A. D., & Otta, E. (2010). Relação entre depressão pós-parto e disponibilidade emocional materna. [Relationship between postpartum depression and maternal emotional availability.]. *Cadernos de Saúde Pública, 26*, 738–746.

Franck, K. L., & Buehler, C. (2007). A family process model of marital hostility, parental depressive affect, and early adolescent problem behavior: The roles of triangulation and parental warmth. *Journal of Family Psychology, 21*(4), 614.

Gray, P., & Anderson, K. (2010). *Fatherhood: Evolution and human paternal behavior*. Cambridge, MA: Harvard University Press. https://doi.org/10.1111/j.1548-1352.2010.01165.x

Geary, D. (2000). Evolution and proximate expression on human paternal investment. *Psychological Bulletin, 126*(1), 55–77. https://doi.org/10.1037/0033-2909.126.1.55

Goodman, J. H. (2004). Paternal postpartum depression, its relationship to maternal postpartum depression, and implications for family health. *Journal of Advanced Nursing, 45*, 26–35.

Hagen, E. H. (1999). The functions of postpartum depression. *Evolution and Human Behavior, 20*, 323–336. https://doi.org/10.1016/S1090-5138(99)00016-1

Hagen, E. H. (2002). Depression as bargaining: The case postpartum. *Evolution and Human Behavior, 23*, 323–336. https://doi.org/10.1016/S1090-5138(01)00102-7

Hagen, E. H. (2011). Evolutionary theories of depression: A critical review. *The Canadian Journal of Psychiatry, 56*(12), 716–726.

Hagen, E. H., & Rosenström, T. (2016). Explaining the sex difference in depression with a unified bargaining model of anger and depression. *Evolution, Medicine, and Public Health, 2016*(1), 117–132.

Hagen, E. H., & Thornhill, R. (2017). Testing the psychological pain hypothesis for postnatal depression: Reproductive success versus evidence of design. *Evolution, Medicine, and Public Health, 2017*(1), 17–23.

Henrich, J., Heine, S. J., & Norenzayan, A. (2010). The weirdest people in the world? *Behavioral and Brain Sciences, 33*, 61–83.

Hrdy, S. (1999). *Mother nature: A history of mothers, infants and natural selection*. New York, NY: Pantheon.

Hrdy, S. (2014). Born human: How the utterly dependent survive. In. Birth to and motherhood: Childrearing in human evolution (symposium). In *Center for Academic Research & training in Anthropogeny*. USA.

Kärtner, J., Keller, H., Chaudhary, N., & Yovsi, R. D. (2012). The development of mirror self-recognition in different sociocultural contexts. *Monographs of the Society for Research in Child Development, 77*(4), 1–87.

Kvalevaag, A. L., Ramchandani, P. G., Hove, O., Assmus, J., Eberhard-Gran, M., & Biringer, E. (2013). Paternal mental health and socioemotional and behavioral development in their children. *Pediatrics, 131*(2), e463–e469.

Lundy, B. L. (2002). Paternal socio-psychological factors and infant attachment: The mediating role of synchrony in father–infant interactions. *Infant Behavior and Development, 25*(2), 221–236.

Luz, F., & Bussab, V. S. (2009). Psicopatologia evolucionista [Evolutionary Psychopathology]. In E. Otta & M. E. Yamamoto (Eds.), *Psicopatologia Evolucionista* [Evolutionary Psychology] (pp. 163–175). Guanabara: Koogan.

Matthey, S., Barnett, B., Kavanagh, D., & Howie, P. (2001). Validation of the Edinburgh postnatal depression scale for men, and comparison of item endorsement with their partners. *Journal of Affective Disorders, 64*, 175–184. https://doi.org/10.1016/S0165-0327(00)00236-6

McKelvey, L. M., Burrow, N. A., Mesman, G. R., Pemberton, J. L., Bradley, R. H., & Fitzgerald, H. E. (2012). Supportive fathers lessen the effects of mothers' alcohol problems on children's externalizing behaviors. *Family Science, 3*(3–4), 189–200.

McVey, C., & Tuohy, A. (2007). Differential effects of marital relationship and social support on three subscales identified within the Edinburgh postnatal depression scale. *Journal of Reproductive and Infant Psychology, 25*(3), 203–209.

Minuchin, P. (1985). Families and individual development: Provocations from the field of family therapy. *Child Development, 56*, 289–302.

Morais, M., Lucci, T., & Otta, E. (2013). Postpartum depression and child development in the first year of life. Campinas. *Estudos de Psicologia, 30*, 1–Y1. https://doi.org/10.1590/S0103-166X2013000100002

Nemeroff, C. B. (1998). The neurobiology of depression. *Scientific American, 278*(6), 42–49.

Nesse, R. M., & Williams, G. C. (1997). Evolutionary biology in the medical curriculum: What every physician should know. *Bioscience, 47*(10), 664–666.

Nesse, R. M., & Williams, G. C. (2012). *Why we get sick: The new science of Darwinian medicine*. Vintage.

Otta, E. Bussab, V., & Morais, M. (2006). Depressão pós-parto como um fator de risco para o desenvolvimento do bebê: estudo interdisciplinar dos fatores envolvidos na gênese do quadro e em suas consequências. [Postpartum depression as a risk factor for infant development: an intedisciplinary study of the factors involved in the genesis of the condition and its consequences.] Thematic Project FAPESP, University of São Paulo.

Paulson, J. F., Dauber, S., & Leiferman, J. A. (2006). Individual and combined effects of postpartum depression in mothers and fathers on parenting behavior. *Pediatrics, 118*, 659–668. https://doi.org/10.1542/peds.2005-2948

Paulson, J. F., & Bazemore, S. D. (2010). Prenatal and postpartum depression in fathers and its association with maternal depression: A meta-analysis. *JAMA, 303*(19), 1961–1969.

Price, J., Sloman, L., Gradner, R., Gilbert, P., & Rohde, P. (1994). The social competition hypothesis of depression. *British Journal of Psychiatry, 164*, 309–315. https://doi.org/10.1192/bjp.164.3.309

Ramchandani, P. G., Stein, A., O'Connor, T. G., Heron, J. O. N., Murray, L., & Evans, J. (2008). Depression in men in the postnatal period and later child psychopathology: A population cohort study. *Journal of the American Academy of Child & Adolescent Psychiatry, 47*(4), 390–398.

Ramchandani, P. G., Psychogiou, L., Vlachos, H., Iles, J., Sethna, V., Netsi, E., et al. (2011). Paternal depression: An examination of its links with father, child and family functioning in the postnatal period. *Depression and Anxiety, 28*(6), 471–477.

Royle, N., Russell, A., & Wilson, A. (2014). The evolution of flexible parenting. *Science, 345*, 776–781. https://doi.org/10.1126/science.l253294

Santos, M. F., Martins, F. C., & Pasquali, L. (1999). Escalas de auto-avaliacão de depressão pós-parto: Estudo no Brasil. [Postpartum depression self-assessment scales: A study in Brazil.]. *Revista de Psiquiatria Clínica, 26*, 32–40.

Sethna, V., Murray, L., Netsi, E., Psychogiou, L., & Ramchandani, P. G. (2015). Paternal depression in the postnatal period and early father–infant interactions. *Parenting, 15*(1), 1–8.

Sethna, V., Murray, L., Edmondson, O., Iles, J., & Ramchandani, P. G. (2018). Depression and playfulness in fathers and young infants: A matched design comparison study. *Journal of Affective Disorders, 229*, 364–370.

Spinelli, L. H. (2009). Quando as mulheres se tornam mães: a história reprodutiva feminina numa visão evolucionista. [When women become mothers: female reproductive history in an evolutionary view]. Unpublished Doctoral Thesis. Federal University of Rio Grande do Norte, Brazil.

Sroufe, L. A. (1997). *Emotional development: The organization of emotional life in the early years*. Cambridge University Press.

Stanley, C., Murray, L., & Stein, A. (2004). The effect of postnatal depression on mother-infant interaction, infant response to the still-face perturbation, and performance on an instrumental learning task. *Development and Psychopathology, 116*, 1–18.

Storey, A., & Walsh, C. (2011). How fathers evolve: A functional analysis of fathering behavior. In A. Booth, S. McHale, & N. Landale (Eds.), *Biosocial foundations of family processes* (pp. 35–47). New York: Springer. https://doi.org/10.1007/978-1-4419-7361-0_2

Storey, A., Delahunty, K., McKay, D., Walsh, C., & Wilhelm, S. (2006). Social and hormonal bases for individual differences in the parental behavior of bird and mammals. *Canadian Journal of Experimental Psychology, 60*, 237–245. https://doi.org/10.1037/cjep2006022

Tamis-LeMonda, C. (2004). Conceptualizing fathers' role: Playmates and more. *Human Development, 47*, 220–227.

Trivers, R. L. (1972). Parental investment and sexual selection. In B. Campbell (Ed.), *Sexual selection and the descent of man* (pp. 1871–1971). Chicago: Aldine Publishing Company.

Volling, B., & Cabrera, N. (2019). Advancing research and measurement on fathering and child development: Introducing the issues and a conceptual framework. *Monographs of the Society for Research in Child Development, 84*(1), 7–160.

Watson, P. J., & Andrews, P. W. (2002). Toward a revised evolutionary adaptationist analysis of depression: The social navigation hypothesis. *Journal of Affective Disorders, 72*(1), 1–14.

Wee, K. Y., Skouteris, H., Pier, C., Richardson, B., & Milgrom, J. (2011). Correlates of ante-and postnatal depression in fathers: a systematic review. *Journal of Affective Disorders, 130*(3), 358–377.

Weitzman, M., Rosenthal, D. G., & Liu, Y. H. (2011). Paternal depressive symptoms and child behavioral or emotional problems in the United States. *Pediatrics-English Edition, 128*(6), 1126.

Smith, L., & Howard, K. (2008). Continuity of paternal support and depressive symptoms among new mothers. *Journal of Family Psychology, 22*, 763–773.

Spanier, G. B. (1976). Measuring dyadic adjustment: New scales for assessing the quality of marriage and similar dyads. *Journal of Marriage and the Family, 38*, 15–26.

Wilson, S., & Durbin, C. E. (2010). Effects of paternal depression on fathers' parenting behaviors: A meta-analytic review. *Clinical psychology review, 30*(2), 167–180.

African American Fathers and Their Young Children: Images from the Field

29

Vivian L. Gadsden and Iheoma U. Iruka

In the past 25 years, there has been a clear upsurge in research studies focused on fathers and fathering and equally widespread agreement that fathers matter to the well-being of their children, families, and communities. Whether fathers are involved with their children is only outweighed by how they are involved. In other words, the field has moved past efforts that seek support for the idea that "father presence matters" and "fathers care"—critical concepts that helped frame the early work in the field—to unpacking the multiple paths to and instantiations of both presence and care. Similarly, the field has moved from a primary focus on White middle-class fathers to investing in a more deepened understanding of the lives of and demands on fathers representing ethnic minority groups and those living in low-resourced communities. While there is still considerable work to be done, researchers, practitioners, and policymakers have come to challenge "one-size-fits-all" paradigms that attempt to explain multifaceted issues within a single narrative or a single approach. The increased attention to the issues facing African American fathers constitutes one critical dimension of the response to this challenge. In this chapter, we use the descriptor, African American, to refer to the expanse of fathers who share a common African diasporic history and who reside in the United States, either as a result of immigration or forced labor, including African Americans, Africans, Afro-Caribbeans, Afro-Latinos/Afro-Latinas, or any other group that identifies as Black and/or having ancestral heritage from Africa (see also Roopnarine, 2004).

V. L. Gadsden (✉)
Graduate School of Education, University of Pennsylvania, Philadelphia, PA, USA
e-mail: viviang@upenn.edu

I. U. Iruka
Center for Early Education Research & Evaluation, HighScope Educational Research Foundation, Ypsilanti, MI, USA

African American fathers are a distinctive subset of the U.S. population and the constellation of fathers in diverse family forms. Similar to other fathers, they represent a range of sociopolitical histories, social classes and contexts, educational backgrounds, school experiences, and cultural practices and values. They reflect different parenting knowledge, beliefs, and practices, and they draw on a range of resources (e.g., their experience and observations) to determine the best approaches to parenting and to promote the health and well-being of their children (Johnson & Young, 2016). However, given their racial history in the United States, unlike many other fathers, they have often confronted multiple barriers that are deterrents to being present in their children's lives and supporting their families (McAdoo, 1993). Whether, how, and how much African American fathers are engaged with their children depend upon a cascade of macro- and micro-systemic factors, from employment and

H. E. Fitzgerald et al. (eds.), *Handbook of Fathers and Child Development*,
https://doi.org/10.1007/978-3-030-51027-5_29

employability to their interpretation of responsibility and commitment (Cochran, 1997; Cooper, 2009; McAdoo, 1993). These factors are affected by social, economic, and educational access and prevailing opportunity structures. As several ethnographic studies have noted, they are related to issues of race and discrimination and to fathers' success in navigating at once systemic barriers, cultural expectations, and personal goals (Edin & Nelson, 2013; Hamer, 2001; Jones, 2018).

This chapter focuses on African American fathers of young children and their engagement and involvement with their young children's care, development, and learning. African American fathers, specifically young, low-income African American fathers, have been a focus of discussions across family research, practice, and policy, in large part, because of their status both as fathers and as men historically marginalized by race. Basic and intervention research continues to center on their absence or on their conceptions of fathering, while other studies, including evaluation studies, address their participation in fathering and family-focused initiatives designed to increase father involvement or promote marriage (see Avellar, Dion, Zaveri, & Hershey, 2006; Wood, Moore, Clarkwest, Killewald, & Monahan, 2012). Comparatively less empirical data and fewer evaluation studies examine the ways in which these fathers are engaged in the early cognitive and social-emotional development of their children, the effects of this engagement over time in and out of formal educational settings, or the social ecologies that shape it. This chapter presents a brief synthesis of the literature from research and on-the-ground efforts. It draws from a range of analyses to capture the complexity of the issues, lapses in the existing knowledge base, and possibilities for research as a resource for practice and policy.

In examining the experiences of both African American fathers and their children, we consider two broad issues. The first acknowledges the inconsistent designations of African American fathers, in particular the ways in which race and class are conflated to describe them. African American fathers are described throughout the literature by any number of references (e.g., urban fathers and young low-income fathers). They constitute a disproportionate share of research and policy discussions on nonresidential and noncustodial fathers that focus largely on the problems that these fathers' presence or absence creates rather than the ways their presence facilitates or guides the development of their children. Hamer (2001) suggests that these men are often targeted—with little regard for the intractability of structural barriers—as a "notorious group," an image that defines them as unable and unwilling to take responsibility for their children. The intersections of race and class and the dearth of research are duly noted in other literature as well (see National Academies of Sciences, Engineering, & Medicine, 2016, 2019). Overwhelmingly, the young African American fathers who have been highlighted in research and policy studies have been poor. Yet, the attention to these fathers, important and critical that it is, is inconsistent in acknowledging the different levels of poverty (e.g., working poor versus deep poverty), merges nonresidential and noncustodial fathering, relies often on narrow definitions of presence and absence, and ignores the diversity within and among both low-income young African American fathers and the larger population of African American fathers. As a result, the field is constrained in its ability to paint either the big picture or the small, more nuanced descriptions of African American fathers and fathering.

The second is the historical backdrop against which the experiences of African American fathers are understood or misunderstood within racial formations and systems of discrimination in the United States (see Omi & Winant, 2014). The forced formal separation of African fathers from their children and families for a significant part of the U.S. history (i.e., the enslavement period) and the resulting barriers to family reunification (Drake & Cayton, 1970; DuBois, 1935; Gans, 1965) and employment from Reconstruction to the present have persistently marginalized these men within and across communities. Several researchers have referred to this problem in relation to the instrumental and expressive roles of African American fathering (Bowman & Forman, 1997), linking the problems of work and the ability to obtain jobs (Anderson, 1990, 2008; Smeeding, Garfinkel, & Mincy, 2011). While several texts have pointed to the effects of racial discrimination on African American men (e.g., Chetty, Hendren, Jones, & Porter, 2018; Wilson, 1996, 2008), relatively few have unpacked and addressed these effects fully or sufficiently in the study of African American fathers and fathering. In addition, the literature typically does not address the diversity of African American fathers by age and ethnicity or by national origin, e.g., those born in the United States versus those who have immigrated; shifting lifestyles and statuses of these fathers, e.g., single fathers and gay fathers; and the transitions within and to American culture.

Throughout the chapter, we draw primarily on work describing what we know about low-income African American fathers, largely because so much of the literature focuses on low-income African American fathers and so little literature examines other African American fathers. However, where data exist and where they help to frame a more robust portrait of African American fathers, we draw on studies and writings related to middle-class African American fathers. We examine the experiences of African American fathers as both broad and nuanced and their fatherhood practices as being derived from individual beliefs and shared cultural contexts and familial histories in the United States. We consider contemporary and historical barriers and perceptions that put the fathers and their children at risk and denote the different forms of agency on which they draw. In other words, we attempt to consider the multiple cultural identities of African American fathers and common themes across their experiences within the different family systems, networks, and cultures of which they are a part.

This chapter is divided into four sections. The first briefly lays out broad issues in ongoing discussions on fathering, father engagement, and father caregiving. It is intended to situate the subsequent section focusing on African American fathers by offering a context for the national discussion and effort that emerged in the 1990s. The second focuses on African American fathers, examining major themes in basic and intervention studies including findings from cross-ethnic studies and studies specifically highlighting African American fathers' involvement in their young children's development. The third section draws on reports and commentaries from a subset of African American fathers participating in fathering programs and offers two profiles of low-income African American fathers to demonstrate their engagement with their children and the possibilities and tensions that lie within their experiences. We conclude with potential areas for study, practice, and policy.

Background on Father Caregiving and the Culture of Fatherhood

The attention to African American fathers is both the precursor to and the result of larger discussions on fatherhood and fathering. Such discussions were spurred by federal mandates related to families and public welfare such as the *Family Support Act* of 1988 and the *Personal Responsibility and Work Opportunity Reconciliation Act* of 1996. Once these legislative items were passed, low-income African American fathers became the focus of much of the effort associated with the legislation. However, for research, these discussions became much more. They not only opened up a more expansive dialogue on the role of fathers, fathering, and father involvement but also began to unpack the question of what constitutes father caregiving. Moreover, as society shifted its perspectives regarding the traditional roles of men and women as parents, new questions were raised regarding the role of fathers (Griswold, 1993; LaRossa, 1997; Parke, 2000).

Several studies have referred to the ways that father involvement differs from mothering (Cabrera, Fitzgerald, Bradley, & Roggman, 2014). However, considerably fewer have acknowledged the fundamental differences in how the purpose and orientations of research on fathers differ from research on mothers. We have come to know how mothers contribute to children's learning and development primarily by examining the achievement and well-being of their children, centering the child as the unit of analysis. In research on fathers, the father is the unit of analysis—i.e., understanding how he interprets and acts on his responsibilities as a parent alongside his children and how his understanding of fatherhood and fathering behaviors affects his children. This results in part from the family-related policy in the 1980s and 1990s (described in the previous paragraph). Unmarried low-income, nonresidential, and noncustodial fathers became the focal point of research and programs, and arguments centered on children needing financial support from men who ostensibly had irregular contact with their children. Attention to fathers as parents was directed to "finding" fathers, determining their capacity to contribute to their children's financial well-being, and assessing barriers (e.g., paternity establishment and incarceration) to their fulfilling this role of support.

While focused on the financial dimensions of fathering, several researchers began to address the emotional and nurturing dimensions of fathering. They brought into one conversation the relatively small database on middle-class White fathers, both residential fathers and divorced fathers living apart from their children. Little was known about low-income White, Latino, or African American fathers. Most of the attention was directed toward fathers who were typically not married to the mothers of their children and who often had children with more than one mother (see Edin & Nelson, 2013). A series of research initiatives ensued and highlighted the population of men who were parents and whose involvement with their children would be influenced by any combination of marital status, culture, race, class, parenting values and beliefs, and opportunity.

In other words, to gauge the well-being of the children, researchers, practitioners, and policymakers alike were generating two knowledge streams: one focused on whether fathers were able to provide financial support and a second focused on fathers' understanding of their role in the lives of their children, the factors that contribute to their involvement, and the factors that work against their involvement. These two streams began to converge, as is evident in the evolution of studies from 1993 to the early 2000s. However, still absent from many of these discussions, emanating from the fatherhood work, was a simultaneous focus on father and child, including the developmental effects of fathers' involvement. Fathers were slowly integrated into research on parents, parenting, and families and their effects on young children.

Fathers' interactions with and influence on children have been examined in relation to their importance as a second parent (to mothers) and in relation to infants and young children. Research on infant-parent attachment demonstrates the significant role of fathers in infant attachment (Belsky, Gilstrap, & Rovine, 1984; Lamb, Chuang, & Cabrera, 2003) and of fathers' sensitivity to their infant and young children's needs (Braungart-Rieker, Garwood, Powers, & Notaro, 1998). Father involvement is thought to be directly related to children's understanding of their social worlds and their ability to interact and make sense of their worlds. Studies such as the Fragile Fathers Study were especially astute in their recognition of birth as a critical moment for fathers to become engaged with their children. They spoke to the high likelihood that early engagement would lead to sustained involvement over time. While the findings are limited and mixed in regard to whether relationships from the early cohorts of fathers studied have been sustained and whether the fathers and the mothers married, the data are clear for the shorter-term engagement (Cabrera, Fagan, & Farrie, 2008). The studies reinforced birth and pregnancy as pivotal moments to promote father engagement and responsibility. The time before birth may be a sensitive period especially in light of studies showing racial disparities in maternal and infant mortality (Petersen et al., 2019), with some indication that paternal involvement may reduce the mortality rate for Black infants (Alio, Kornosky, Mbah, Marty, & Salihu, 2010; Alio et al., 2011; Alio, Salihu, Kornosky, Richman, & Marty, 2010). Hence, father involvement may support expectant mothers to engage in more health and pregnancy-promoting behaviors while also reducing financial and emotional stressors harmful to pregnancy.

In a study of participants in the National Early Head Start evaluation study, Shannon, Cabrera, Tamis-LeMonda, and Lamb (2009) found that fathers' residence at birth and prenatal involvement (e.g., attending doctor's visits) decreased their risk of being inaccessible to their children over the first 5 years. On the one hand, residence at birth was a stronger predictor of the timing of father inaccessibility than was prenatal involvement for European American and Latin American fathers. Prenatal involvement among African American fathers was a stronger predictor of the timing of father inaccessibility than nonresidential status at birth. However, 50% of fathers who were inaccessible at birth were inaccessible by the time the child was 3 months old. The authors note the strengths and constraints of the study, including the self-selection process of the study, inability to pinpoint all dimensions of the timing of accessibility, use of maternal reports, differential marital status of participants (which influences if not determines fathers' access to their children), and the different ways that fathers chose to stay involved.

This approach, of observing and chronicling fathers' engagement from birth, is laden with possibilities for charting the growth of men as fathers, the effects of growth, and fathers' engagement in their children's care, health, and well-being. Caregiving involves generativity—that is, psychological and emotional investment in the role of caregiver and in the children for whom one provides such care (Erikson, 1969; Erikson & Erikson, 1981). Children who receive inconsistent, neglectful, or inadequate physical and emotional caregiving are at greater risk for negative developmental outcomes (Downer, Campos, McWayne, & Gartner, 2014; McLoyd, 1990). In high-risk communities characterized by chronic long-term poverty, a nurturing and supportive parent reduces risk (Fantuzzo, McWayne, Perry, & Childs, 2004) and is the single most important source of resiliency in children (Boller et al., 2006; Luthar & Zigler, 1991; National Academies of Sciences, Engineering, & Medicine, 2019; Wakschlag & Hans, 1999).

Fathers' roles range from instrumental (i.e., ensuring children's basic needs for food and protection) to expressive (i.e., nurturing and emotional engagement, love, attachment, and security). They include culturally appropriate physical acts of affection and comfort such as touching, hugging, kissing, and cuddling; verbal expressions of care such as comforting with reassuring words and sounds; and behaviors that help to maintain communication between children and caregivers such as listening and giving timely responses to children's concerns. Paternal caregiving includes the managerial tasks that permit caregivers cooperatively and consistently to meet children's basic needs (e.g., shopping for food and clothing) but is as likely to focus on play and engagement. Just as the frequency and accessibility of fathering contribute to care (Shannon et al., 2009), the quality of caregiving and parenting can have a profound effect on children (Gadsden, Davis, Fagan, & Ray, 2001).

In addition to greater government interest in fathering from the 1990s to present, several factors have led to initiatives on fathers' roles in caregiving: e.g., the increasing numbers of mothers entering the workforce (Pleck, 1997), evolving societal expectations of fathers' roles (Johnson & Young, 2016), and changing patterns of family formation and organization (Gadsden, Wortham, & Turner III, 2003). The result of this cultural shift is that both fathers and mothers have been forced to weigh how they will negotiate their roles as parents, provide children with consistent and competent caregiving, and provide the emotional investment and support they require.

The majority of research on fathers' caregiving has focused on their presence, absence, and accessibility to their young children. Research on fathers who reside with their children suggests that they are assuming more childcare responsibilities than did their predecessors. The degree to which fathers can and do engage in caregiving activities changes over the life course and within different cultural contexts. However, the contributing factors are little understood. Differences in levels of father-child engagement may also be influenced by differences in fathers' experiences, capacities, and characteristics. Characteristics of the child (e.g., temperament and disability) may shape caregiving, whether father or mother (National Academies of Sciences, Engineering, & Medicine, 2016). Research presents contradictory findings related to fathers of children with disabilities. Some early studies report that fathers of disabled children may become more involved in childcare than fathers of children without these challenges (Tallman, 1965), while other research suggests that they may be less involved (Bristol, Gallagher, & Schopler, 1988).

Research on fathers' caregiving tends to describe the frequency of care and the tasks performed but focuses less on the quality of father care or its relationship to child outcomes. In less economically advantaged families, fathers reportedly have played a critical role in caring for young children. In a study by Hans, Ray, Bernstein, and Halpern (1995) of low-income, unmarried African American mothers, the mothers stated that, after themselves, fathers were the most frequent providers of care to very young children. A majority of mothers (53%) indicated that fathers provided solo care to toddlers at least 1 or 2 days per week. Cohen (1998) found that 43% of low-income fathers, compared to 24% of more economically advantaged fathers, care for their young children while their wives work. According to Livingston (2014), based on the U.S. Census data from the 1990–2013 Annual Social and Economic Supplement (ASEC) of the Current Population Survey (CPS), the number of stay-at-home fathers jumped from 1.1 million in 1989 to 2.2 million in 2012 primarily because of the recession, with approximately 18% of preschool children regularly cared for by theirs father during their mothers' working hours (National Responsible Fatherhood Clearinghouse, n.d.). This may be due, in part, to their limited education and poverty status. Stay-at-home fathers are twice as likely to lack a high school diploma as working fathers (22% vs. 10%), and almost half (47%) of stay-at-home fathers are living in poverty, compared with 8% of working fathers.

Several studies have offered insights into fathers' contributions to young children's cognitive and social-emotional development, and many have investigated fathering behaviors across different groups. While these studies are still relatively few, as compared to studies on mothers and children, they show some distinctive effects of father involvement. Fathers who are described as having authoritarian parenting styles (i.e., characterized by highly controlling, punitive, harsh, and intrusive behaviors and low warmth and responsiveness directed toward the child) appear to have children who display more externalizing behavior (Hart, DeWolf, Wozniak, & Burts, 1992; Parke, Cassidy, Burks, Carson, & Boyum, 1992). Isley, O'Neil, Clatfelter, and Parke (1999) found that fathers' negative interactions during a physical play task were significantly and negatively related to boys' social competence as assessed by teachers in kindergarten and first grade and by peers in kindergarten. An earlier study by MacDonald and Parke (1984) found that fathers who were more direct during play sessions had preschool-age children, particularly sons, who were less popular with peers. In a study of fathers' use of physical punishment and children's externalizing behavior among White and African American children, Deater-Deckard and his colleagues (1996) found a significantly greater association between fathers' use of physical punishment and higher levels of externalizing and aggressive behavior for European American children than for African American children. More recently, Cabrera and Mitchell (2009) found that low-income African American fathers reported moderate levels of parenting stress, were moderately engaged with their children across a range of activities, and displayed medium levels of responsiveness and low levels of negativity during interactions with their toddlers.

Fathers play roles that relate to children's social competence. Across race, ethnicity, and social class, fathers appear to spend more of their total time with children engaging in play activities than do mothers (Hossain & Roopnarine, 1994). Especially when children are young, fathers and mothers appear to have different playing styles (Lamb, 1997). Fathers are more likely than are mothers to engage in more physical and rambunctious play, such as rough-and-tumble games. This pattern of play has been reported in African American, Latino, and European American fathers. In contrast, mothers tend to engage infants with objects, as well as to read to and talk with children (Parke, 1996).

The specific contributions of fathers to children's cognitive development are less clear, although studies have focused on children's academic preparation and experiences. Studies dating back to the 1990s have shown higher levels of participation of resident fathers than nonresident fathers, though the results are at best mixed. Research shows that paternal stimulation of infants seems to be important for the development of boys' mastery motivation (Yarrow et al., 1984). Clarke-Stewart (1978) found that the intellectual skill of 15–30-month-olds was significantly related to fathers' engagement in play, positive ratings of children, the amount they interacted, and their aspirations for the child's independence. Research on parent-child interaction has shown that there are special characteristics of fathers' and mothers' child-directed speech. The earliest studies found that the structural characteristics of fathers' language (e.g., mean length of utterance, type-token ratio, the mean number of verbs per utterances, and proportion of sentence types) were similar to those used by mothers. (See Tomasello & Barton, 1994, for a review; Leech, Salo, Rowe, & Cabrera, 2013.) Studies that have focused on the pragmatic or conversational aspects of parent-child communication have documented differences in the ways that fathers and mothers communicate with their children (Hammond, Caldwell, Brooks, & Bell, 2011). One robust finding is that fathers' speech to their children is more linguistically and cognitively demanding (Bernstein, 1988; Duursma, Pan, & Raikes, 2008; Tomasello, Conti-Ramsden, & Ewert, 1990). Fathers allow fewer speaker turns than do mothers, use more rare and abstract words, respond less to children's utterances, are less adept at understanding their children, ask for fewer clarifications, and are less inclined to accept violations of discourse rules. In their vocabulary choices, fathers appear to be less attuned to their children's linguistic level than mothers. Leech and her colleagues (2013) found considerable variability in the input that fathers offer to their children on a daily basis. As they note, while there may be little difference in the quantity of conversation, fathers tend to use more conversation-eliciting utterances and clarification requests than mothers do.

There is a small body of literature examining the impact of paternal involvement in children's early schooling and academic achievement. Research on parents' roles in children's cognitive development has demonstrated the significance of parent-child interaction to improve children's school performance. In areas such as children's early reading, for example, Gadsden and Bowman (1999) suggest that fathers' participation in literate activities, the barriers they face as a result of low literacy, and their perceptions of the role they can play in their children's literacy development affect whether and how well children are prepared for school. Such factors also may influence the direct and subtle messages that fathers convey to their children about the value, achievability, and power associated not only with literacy but also with schooling and knowledge. Although mother's education historically has been used as the primary predictor of children's achievement, educational research increasingly is examining father-child interaction on children's early learning within and outside of school, particularly among low-income fathers (Lee & Rispoli, 2019; Reynolds, Howard, & Jones, 2015). What these and other studies suggest is that a father's ability to support his child's learning affects the child's engagement with books and schooling. As is true for mothers, however, fathers who have limited schooling and reading and writing abilities are constrained in their attempts to participate in many school-related activities requiring high levels of literacy (Duursma et al., 2008).

Even when fathers have limited schooling, their involvement in children's schools and school lives is a powerful predictor of children's academic achievement. Nord, Brimhall, and West (1998) found that fathers from two-parent families who were moderately or highly involved in school were significantly more likely to have children who received mostly high marks, enjoy school, and never repeat a grade. Nonresidential fathers' involvement in school also predicted the same outcome measures for children (Nord et al., 1998). In their study of 11- to 14-year-old children, Grolnick and Slowiaczek (1994) found that fathers who participate in school activities have children with a higher degree of self-perceived academic competence and greater self-regulation. Father involvement in intellectual and cultural activities at home was also related to children's perceived academic competence (Grolnick & Slowiaczek, 1994). Fagan and Iglesias (1999) found a positive association between high-level participation in a father involvement project and children's mathematics readiness change scores. Using the Early Childhood Longitudinal Study—Birth Cohort (ECLS-B), Baker (2013) found that above and beyond mothers' effects, fathers who participated in more frequent home literacy involvement (e.g., shared book reading) had children with better reading, math, and social-emotional outcomes (i.e., sustained attention and fewer negative behaviors) in preschool.

Research that examines the extent to which fathers are involved with their child's school, such as the national representative study undertaken by Nord et al. (1998) and the Head Start study by Gary, Beatty, and Weaver (1987), has generally shown that fathers are less involved than mothers in all types of school activities, including volunteering and attending class events, parent-teacher conferences, and general school meetings. Fathers with less than a high school education were also much less likely to be involved in their child's school than fathers with higher levels of education (Nord et al., 1998). However, as Nord and her colleagues (1998) suggest, while nonresidential fathers were found to be substantially less involved with the child's school than residential fathers, the involvement of nonresidential fathers was in no way trivial (see Grolnick & Slowiaczek, 1994). As children move into adolescence, fathers and mothers play a less dominant, although not unimportant, role in their children's education (Baker, 2013; Hosley & Montemayor, 1997). Some researchers (e.g., Johnson & Young, 2016) have noted the differential pathway of African American fathers' engagement, particularly as children move into adolescence, suggesting a different, more culture-focused analysis of their participation.

African American Fathers

African American or Black fathers have been studied in relation to other groups such as Latino fathers and in comparison to European American fathers. Studies have been designed not only to gauge their responses to fatherhood but also to situate their practices within dominant social expectations regarding fathering. Current discussions continue to grapple with how to represent them in the rapidly changing cultural landscape, dominant societal practices, and economic contingencies. Moreover, the history and experiences of African American fathers are different from those of Latino or other ethnic minority fathers and vice versa. Johnson and Young (2016) suggest that because the roles and expectations associated with fatherhood in American society have become increasingly diversified, contemporary depictions of African American fathers are too narrow. They cite a need for a broader conceptualization of what the role entails, which has implications for African American fathers and fathers more generally. Pointing to the internal diversity of the category, Black fathers, the authors suggest that studies of Black fathers must reconcile the ways in which Black families and communities are both affected by and implicated in the expectations of fathers not only in the Black community but also in the larger society.

We know little about middle-income African American fathers. Cazenave's (1979) study, based on interviews with postal workers, was among the first to demonstrate the importance of the provider role to African American men. While studies by Cazenave and others such as Perry and colleagues (2012) focus on resident, middle-class fathers, they address neither fathers' parenting practices specifically nor their parenting ideologies. In earlier writings (e.g., Drake & Cayton, 1970; DuBois, 1935; Gans, 1965), scholars referred to the deleterious effect that forced separation of fathers and families had on father involvement while describing the critical role that African American fathers played in Reconstruction and in response to limited employment opportunities. During this period, often with migration from rural to urban areas, African American women were able to obtain jobs when the men were not, and African American fathers often assumed childcare responsibilities of young children. Drawing on both research findings and anecdotal evidence, some authors (e.g., Childs & Dalmage, 2010; Hill, 2001) have argued that the parenting practices of middle-class African American fathers may look similar to those of White middle-class fathers, except for the ways they support their children in navigating issues of cultural and social identity in the face of contemporary threats such as discrimination and racial profiling.

The issues facing African American fathers in one context may be different from those facing African American fathers in another context, particularly around culture and cultural expectations. Cultural experiences vary across African American men. Hence, simplistic appropriations of culture do not fully provide the necessary framing to examine these fathers. However, irrespective of class and subcultural histories, African American fathers share a particular racial identity within U.S. contexts and economies, which at any point may serve as barriers to their engagement with their children and their ability to support their families and themselves (Anderson, 2008; Chetty et al., 2018; Wilson, 1996, 2008). Such structural barriers have led to explanations of African American fathering among low-income, nonresidential and noncustodial men that reinforce race-based analyses.

In the discussion that follows, we focus on low-income, nonresidential African American fathers, not as representatives of the range of African American fathers but because of limited research on African American fathers more broadly. The work on African American fathers in many cases has restricted itself to focusing on African American fathers who are low-income, absent in their children's lives, variably engaged with their children, or unable to provide financial contributions. It has separated out nonresidential and noncustodial fathers from those who live with and are financially responsible for their children. The focus on income and class, especially poverty, is appropriate and needed, given the impact of poverty on children's well-being, parents' ability to contribute to their children's health and welfare, and parents' capacities to make sound decisions regarding their parenting (Hamer, 2001; National Academies of Sciences, Engineering and Medicine, 2019; Smeeding et al., 2011).

However, despite the constraints of poverty, many young African American fathers are highly engaged with their children, and most report that they value fatherhood, want to be involved in their children's lives, but are limited by a range of factors including financial stability and inaccessibility to their children due to relationship tensions (Hamer, 2001). Several researchers have noted the nurturing contributions that many low-income African American men make to their children's well-being and their reported sensibilities and sensitivities to the importance of care (Edin & Nelson, 2013). A core of research, beginning in the 1990s, redirected the focus on fathers' financial contributions to include a critical analysis of fathers' contributions to children's emotional well-being, social environments, and care (National Center on Fathers and Families, 1995).

The focus on African American fathers' residential status, in particular, does not represent a binary of presence and absence. It is experienced along a continuum of engagement, dependent on individual factors such as a father's decision to be involved with his children and the number of children he may have with different mothers. It is also affected by societal factors such as a father's ability to obtain employment with sufficient wages to support his children and the disproportionate number of African American fathers who are incarcerated. Individually, these factors create a complex pathway to responsible fathering. Together, they create an impossible trajectory to ensuring that these fathers are engaged with their children and that they are able to overcome structural racism and intergenerational poverty and hardship that serve as barriers to their engagement, positive father-child relationships, or the fathers' sense of their own agency.

Although much has been written about Black fathers' invisibility, the 2013 report from the Centers for Disease Control (CDC) suggests that African American fathers have comparably higher levels of involvement than White fathers though lower levels of residence. Data were collected from 12,279 interviews with women and 10,403 men aged 15–44 from June 2006 through June 2010. The report is mainly limited to the data collected from the sample of 3928 men who are fathers and found that African American fathers had higher levels of engagement for children five and under. Both co-residential and non-residential fathers reported that in the 4 weeks prior to the survey, they were most likely to have bathed, dressed, diapered, or helped their children use the toilet every day; taken their children to or from activities every day; read to them; or helped with homework. These findings do not disagree with findings in other studies and draw attention to the disjuncture between the popular conceptions of African American father absence and the need for more intricate, carefully developed studies that uncover the nature, content, and potential of father involvement.

Similar to other studies, the CDC study uses a comparative framework across White, Latino, and Black fathers. In general, the White-Black comparison is relatively constricted, as it positions the practices of White middle-class fathers as the gold standard of engagement. Data suggest that studies on African American father engagement and involvement might focus more on what they do and, when focused on their presence or absence, give more attention to how their presence matters for children's academic success and social-emotional development and when and why they are absent.

For example, a major barrier to fathers' presence in their children's homes was federal welfare policies of the past which often encouraged father invisibility, if not absence, by withholding benefits from low-income mothers whose husbands or partners lived at home (Edin, Lein, & Nelson, 1998; Lerman & Sorensen, 2000; Edin & Nelson, 2013). These social and economic factors and the resulting policy mandates removed lower-income African American fathers from their children's homes and typically from communities to a greater extent than for other U.S. neighborhoods and communities. Research from the 1990s reinforces this point. Sullivan (1993) suggested that inner-city African American youth tend to acknowledge their paternity readily, although not formally, and that the African American community facilitates the informal establishment of paternity and a young father's involvement in informal child-support arrangements. Others such as Waller (2001) found that for many of the fathers, the breadwinner role was less important than their desire to provide guidance and discipline for his children. The fathers in Waller's study (part of the Fragile Families Study) emphasized the need for fathers to ensure that their children lived comfortably and that their children's needs were met, either through in-kind informal support or more formal payment arrangements. Studies by Gadsden et al. (2003) and Parents' Fair Share (Knox & Redcross, 2000; Miller & Knox, 2001) not only found a similar emphasis on the nurturing role from young urban fathers but also noted fathers' emphasis on the breadwinner role even when consistent employment was difficult to be found.

The issues around class and the residual effects of class (e.g., poor-quality schooling, limited education, unemployment, and incarceration) have centered on a specific time period, late adolescence and young adulthood, in the lives of many young fathers, a period often fraught with inconsistencies and common questions related to transitions. Studies such as the Fragile Families Study provided a rich analysis of whether and how young fathers—disproportionately African American, low-income men, and men with similar backgrounds—were and could be engaged with their children from birth and the real and perceived barriers to their engagement. Several studies describe some of the experiences of young fathers, highlighting the realities of unemployment and intergenerational father absence as barriers to overcome (Waldfogel, Craigie, & Brooks-Gunn, 2010). Despite the strengths of these studies, few have demonstrated the ways that African American fathers of young children, in particular, take on the responsibilities of parenting their children—i.e., the nature of engagement, not only whether they are engaged but also their understanding of their roles, the activities that they take on and with what outcomes, their definitions of their roles in the present and future, and the evolution and enactments of these definitions.

Unlike older children, very young children, typically, from birth to age 5, are uniquely positioned as dependents. Because of their age and relative helplessness, they rely directly on parents and other caregivers to address the fundamental needs of food and care. However, they are also reliant on parents as primary mechanisms for socialization and preparation for the expectations of their environments. As the National Academies of Sciences report, *Parenting Matters* (2016) writes:

> The impact of parents may never be greater than during the earliest years of life, when children's brains are developing rapidly and when nearly all of their experiences are created and shaped by their parents and by the positive or difficult circumstance in which the parents find themselves (p. 1).

Later in the same report, the authors note the dearth of research studies and research data on fathers, in general, to inform a discussion about the natural pathways to father involvement for young children; the different directions they have taken; or their effects on children's cognition, social-emotional development, or health and well-being.

Similar to other work on fathers, studies on African American fathers are limited by a lack of theory that links specific acts of father involvement to child developmental outcomes. Several researchers have drawn upon social ecological theory as an appropriate framework. Cabrera and her colleagues (2014) offer a theoretical framing developed out of social ecological theory that focuses on the bidirectionality between fathers and children over time, in addition to context and fathers' personality and behavior. Others have reframed it as a cultural ecological theory (Threlfall, Seay, & Kohl, 2013). While these theoretical framings have been applied to uncover what is known about African American fathers and young children, much of what is uncovered must be disaggregated from cross-ethnic studies. For example, several studies reinforce the importance of parents in stimulating children's cognitive development and social competence, in particular their language development and specific abilities in reading, writing, and other early literacies (Baker, 2013; Leech et al., 2013). Some research reports take note of the higher levels of caregiving and play activities between African American and Latino fathers (Baker, 2016). They point to African American and Latino fathers' lower levels of engagement in children's cognitive development, which they agree may be attributed in large part to the lower levels of education among the fathers studied. These and other data are compelling, but several of the studies to date are consistently small, drawn from convenience samples, and unable to inform the field about the levels of engagement or the duration and content of engagement. In addition, it may be that within-class diversity may be minimized such that middle-class White fathers are compared with working-class or middle-class African American and Latino fathers, and the studies may not weigh systematically the wealth differential between Blacks and Whites (see Chetty et al., 2018; Oliver & Shapiro, 2013), as well as the stressors African American and Latino fathers face due to their gender, race, ethnicity, and culture.

In a study of fathers' contributions to children's self-regulation among low-income ethnic minority preschoolers, Owen and her colleagues (2013) focused on 404 fathers, 182 of whom were African American, and their 30-month-old children. While they did not find a clear pattern when profiling for fathers' education, they found in follow-up tests, stratified by child ethnicity, that higher levels of father education were associated with more child-oriented fathering among African American but not Latino fathers. That is, African American fathers with more than a high school education exhibited more child-oriented fathering than among fathers with less education. The authors note that African American, child-oriented fathers held unique importance in predicting their children's emerging self-regulation in an attention conflict task, which is consistent with others highlighting the developmental importance of fathers' sensitive and challenging play. These findings are reinforced by studies of toddlers with co-residing mothers and fathers (Cabrera, Hofferth, & Chae, 2011). African American and Latino fathers reported being engaged with their infants in physical play and caregiving (Cabrera et al., 2011).

Mullins (2011) reports that African American fathers are more likely to stress the importance of behavior (i.e., behaving according to some designated rules) for children under the age of 61 months. The fathers indicated that following rules, being kind and considerate towards others, controlling temper, and obeying parents were all important behaviors in children. However, contradicting the self-reports in the CDC study, African American fathers were found to be the least likely to read to their children.

Among the criticisms of research, practice, and policy that affect African American fathers is that they have relied on a single story that does not reflect the diversity in its broadest sense—e.g., cultural histories, nationality, single-parent status, income differences, sexual orientations, or any of the intersectional identities that African American fathers similar to other fathers reflect. This is not to say that African American fathers are just like all other fathers. Instead, it cautions references that place fathers into a single nonporous category that intentionally minimizes or erases the multiplicity of identities and pathways to father involvement. The increased attention to low-income, nonresidential, noncustodial African American fathers in the past 20 years has drawn attention to African American families and the cultural practices within them.

African American Fathers: Images from Programs

A source of information for the field has been programs designed to serve fathers. Most of these programs serve young, low-income, ethnic minority men who are new fathers or fathers of young children. Many have provided support to the men to ensure that they have the employment and emotional support to establish and sustain engagement with their children. Early programs such as Parents' Fair Share and others were intended to provide consistent support, and as a result, these programs provided evaluation data that led to the expansion of research and policy initiatives on fatherhood. In many ways, they have been a major source of information about how fathers are faring and have served as a site for a range of research studies. Like many basic and intervention studies, evaluation studies have often focused on whether fathers are participating in programs and/or whether fathers report being engaged with their children. In other cases, they highlight the number of reported father-child encounters from either program staff or fathers, leaving the potential for inaccuracy on the actual level of engagement and little information on the nature of the participation, the manifestations of participation in different contexts, fathers' persistence, or programmatic preparation that measures children's short- and long-term effects. Still, these programs and the fathers in them offer powerful insights on what young fathers experience in their efforts to parent their young children.

Fathering programs are diverse in that several are supported in part by federal funds and aimed at increasing paternity, child support, and fathers' presence and involvement. In the mid-1990s when programs began to expand and since, they have served an important but not always empirically charted path. Programs ranged from small on-the-ground efforts conducted by community-based organizations to formal efforts in maternal and child health centers, Head Start and Early Head Start, that integrate or support fathers separately. The services vary not only in their focus but also in the degree to which they are able to support fathers' parenting or focus on young children. Subsequent requirements regarding marriage redirected the early purposes of these programs, resulting in national evaluations to determine their efficacy, though still offering clear directions.

Much of what we know from programs about fathers of young children has come from studies and evaluations of large, federally funded programs such as Head Start and Early Head Start. For example, in a study of Early Head Start, Raikes, Summers, and Roggman (2007) focus on Hispanic, African American, and White fathers. Similar to other studies (e.g., Cabrera et al., 2004), they found that in what is described as mature programs, Hispanic men are more likely than African American or White men to be involved. However, the odds of higher participation were approximately 3 to 1 for Hispanics and African Americans/Blacks compared to Whites. While the data showed lower average monthly visits by African American fathers, the authors note that in their interviews with African American fathers, several placed "a high value on their children's education and appeared to be motivated to be involved in order to improve their children's prospects in life" (p. 47).

In programs designed for fathering, the primary emphasis is on engaging the father in more direct contact with his child and supporting him to sustain the engagement. In our review of 20 programs, few linked fathering practices and children's well-being in anything other than references to the overall importance of fathering and parenting (Gadsden & Rethemeyer, 2003) In other words, there was little in the programs' descriptions that teased apart dimensions of the relationship between fathering behaviors and children's outcomes. This, along with child-serving evaluations of programs such as Head Start and Early Head Start that focused on the effects of African American fathers, points to the need for more purposeful efforts to chart whether and how father engagement is sustained over time and with what results for the child and father.

A second source of information about African American fathers is the fathers themselves. Two images of African American, described in several relevant studies (Gadsden, Davis, & Johnson, 2015; Gadsden & Ray, 2002; Gadsden et al., 2003), reflect the ways in which low-income fathers have engaged and understood their responsibilities as fathers of young children and how they have aimed to make sense of their role. For example, in a study of 50 young African American fathers in a program located in an urban setting, the fathers, all of whom had children under 8 years of age, ostensibly understood the importance of their involvement with their children. The dominant theme throughout their narratives is described in relation to the importance of a father "being there" for his children, followed by providing for their children. Fathers complemented this description with commentaries on their desire to construct a different, future self that reconciles past identity with present and future goals. They reported that they aimed to eliminate intergenerational father absence in their families while searching for a transformed identity. These dimensions of identity and change are reflected in our description of CJ in which he highlights "the predicament" of low-income, African American fathers and how transformative events have motivated him to break the intergenerational pattern of father absence.

Image One: CJ

> **CJ:** All the years of not having one [a father], wishing that I did….The pain in my life is what made me want to be a father to my child, because I wanted my father, you know. I prayed at night that my father would come. Just knowing the loneliness of not having a father … you don't want your child to go through that same thing
> I did like 45 days one time in the lock-up and then I thought about, you know, me. It's actually a little of both. I thought about, you know, me being locked up, which I didn't like, and I never knew my father, and I thought if I spent all my time locked up, then my son would never know his father. So it's actually, I did it half for him and half for myself.

During most of his son's early life, CJ was either in prison or living apart from his son, with relatively little time to understand his son's development or to act on the changes of his young child. During this time, CJ's son and his mother relocated to another state and then returned shortly after CJ was released from prison. CJ noted that when his son returned from out of state (when the son was five), he acted on the decision he had made in prison—i.e., getting a job to take care of his son, establishing a regular schedule for visitation and overnight stays, and becoming involved in his son's life.

From our meetings with CJ, it was clear that he and his son had a good relationship, but a relationship that was more peer-like than parent-child. CJ reported that his son likes to "hang out with him" and that they "do a variety of things. It just depends on what we wanna do that day." CJ describes their relationship as "pretty open." This dependence on the child as peer runs through many of the interviews that we have conducted. Edin and Nelson (2013) describe similar relationships between low-income African American and White fathers in their study. However, throughout our interview, CJ demonstrated his commitment to "acting" more like a parent, noting that he had little knowledge of his son's early years as he discusses his son's emergent behaviors around an incident in which he determined that his son had been dishonest. In relation to this incident and his son's behavior, CJ describes himself as taking responsibility and acting more like a parent: "I know, I feel like sometimes he just flat out lies to keep himself from getting in trouble. So that bothers us sometimes."

Here, CJ voices himself, together with his son's mother, as being concerned in a parental way that his son may be "lying." He also talks about wanting to earn more money, so that he could get his son "the things that [he] would like him to have, which is not actually the things that he has." At this point and on this topic, CJ adopts a more parental voice. He articulates a father's responsibility to be able to distinguish what a young child actually needs to have from what he wants to have. CJ is not unique. Like over half of the fathers interviewed, CJ's father was on the streets, while his mother created a safe home for him and his stepfather later provided a good role model. Nonetheless, as an adolescent and young man, CJ ended up on the streets like his father. He lived what he described as a fast life there for several years, even after his son was born. However, his son's move out of state, while he was in jail, inspired CJ to slow down and become a responsible parent, and served as an incentive to seek a new possible self.

CJ's story is not unlike the stories of other African American fathers in its focus on personal transformation and the material and emotional dimensions of fathering. The contradiction of his behavior "in the streets" is mapped against an understanding of his role as a father, an understanding garnered through his relationship with his stepfather. What is significant in CJ's commentary is an absence of focus on the age of his child and plans for his child's development. He does not voice a perspective on what it means to support his child's early development and how he might ensure seamless development through adolescence and over the life course.

Just as CJ focused on his own life and the changes that have allowed him to change and contribute to his child's early learning, PR describes his relationship with the young daughter of his girlfriend. Both CJ and PR are nonresident fathers without custody of their young children. Again, the contrasts and similarities between the two men reinforce the dangers of a single story to describe the experiences of the young fathers.

Image 2: PR

PR's father lived with his mother for the first 2 years of PR's life. After that period, he states, "he disappeared." His daughter was born when he was 19. He was arrested, incarcerated at 20, and became a father of a son (with a different mother) at 24. At age 25, he made a major decision to change and redirect his life, entering the father resource program. It was during this time that he began a relationship with still another woman who had a daughter of her own. At the time of the interview, PR was 26 and was engaged to his girlfriend, had a good job, and saw his two biological children regularly for supervised visitation. He also cared for his girlfriend's daughter at home "as if she were [his] own."

At the very beginning of the interview, PR gives information that establishes him as a young African American man who has fathered two children with two different mothers and who has been involved with the court system. When asked about daily routines in his role as a father, he responded:

> **PR:** Well, it depends if I'm off, well even if I'm not off work, that little girl will come in there and wake me up, so that I have to get up maybe I have to go in there and cook something.
> **Interviewer:** okay, what about like in the evening, when you all come back, do you all have dinner together?
> **PR:** no, see I work nights. I work from two thirty till eleven. so when I'm home, she's sleeping, so…
> **Interviewer:** so, tell me a little bit about, for example, when your daughter comes to wake you up and then you have to cook breakfast, like do the two of you have a chance to talk?
> **PR:** yeah.
> **Interviewer:** so, what are you talking about?
> **PR:** anything. I mean, the little girl is so…aw, man. it seem like she is very intelligent. like, this morning. this morning. her tooth fell out last night. and …, so I put some money under her pillow. and she woke me up at seven o'clock this morning and showed me her little, and said look what I get. I said where'd you get that from?" she said the tooth fairy gave it to me. I said when did your tooth come out? she didn't know I knew her tooth came out, because she was sleeping when I came home, so her mother showed me her tooth. so she woke me up this morning, and told me she had a little money and stuff, so and I hugged her and kissed her and stuff. she went on to daycare. we talk about everything. she's smart. she's so, she wants to know everything.
> **Interviewer:** sounds like she's very curious.
> **PR:** curious. that's the word I'm looking for. she's very curious. she asks me a question, I give her the best answer I can.

PR goes on to talk about translating the desire to end the intergenerational absence of fathers in his family, as evident in this exchange:

> **Interviewer:** …so it was actually his absence and watching your mother provide for you in [your father's] absence that you, and as you were a child, you could see what you wish you would have had.
> **PR:** exactly.
> **Interviewer:** and therefore, you want to take that wish list and sort of pass it on to your kids.
> **PR:** exactly. I think that's exactly the way I feel about it, too. that's the only way that I can, that's exactly what it is.

PR fits into two categories, biological and stepfather, or what has been described as a social father, taking on, in this case, the formal role of father to a nonbiological child. However, his apparent commitment is greater than that of a casual or social relationship. His description of his fiancée's daughter as possessing a high level of cognitive ability motivates him to support her, to capture her ability in just the right word: "Curious." What informs PR's understanding of his stepdaughter's ability, and how is he prepared to support her cognitive and social-emotional development? His real or potential contributions to his fiancée's daughter are measured not only in the amount of time he spends with her but also in the quality of that time and his capacity to indulge and stimulate her curiosity and support her in academically important ways.

Several of the messages from our interviews and the more focused case study of CJ and PR suggest that, despite the potential and real distractions of father absence, poverty, and poor schooling, these fathers, like other fathers, form significant and nurturing bonds with their children and work to negotiate the roles and expectations of parenting with the mothers of their children. They construct future images of themselves as fathers that are based on sometimes limited understanding of their chosen strategies and are constrained in part by the paucity of economic, educational, and societal supports. In some cases, including the two fathers described here, they seek to nurture and support their children in the ways that are presented visually on television and other media and in teachings from their families and the programs in which many participate. In particular, noncustodial, nonresidential African American fathers are similar to their peers from other ethnic groups and other social classes who are testing the boundaries of engaged fatherhood, trying on their new roles, and negotiating these boundaries across legal, social, and familial lines.

Summary and Key Points

Several researchers (e.g., Gordon, 2000) point to what is considered a stark disconnect between current vestiges of fatherhood and historical expectations, perceptions, and practices in African American communities. Like other fathers, African American fathers' parenting practices are informed and shaped by a range of social determinants that motivate them to take on the role of a caregiver and father or that complicate their pathways to engaged fathering. A series of social factors over time have shifted the practices, patterns, and nature of father engagement in many African American communities, challenged by the onslaught of high levels of incarceration and social problems and exacerbated by the economic downturn. Research studies on low-income African American fathers indicate relative success in assuming this role. What these studies do not provide is a systematic understanding of what transpires in the child-father experience, driven from field studies and observations. What we do know is that from birth through early childhood (Threlfall et al., 2013), the fathers from several studies reinforce the importance of being providers and nurturers, and do not see these roles as incongruous. This chapter underscores that African American fathers have a unique position in children's development. However, to ensure that policies and programs are father-centered, there is a need for research that is father-centric and relevant.

At least five issues are important in uncovering the role of African American fathers of young children. They have relevance across research, practice, and policy. The first refers to a point made early in the chapter—questioning how we study the father's role within the developmental trajectory of the child. To deepen our understanding requires a different kind of mapping, including longitudinal studies that run from birth through the third or fifth grade, matching other relevant studies that typically chart the course of children. Because fathers rather than their children are the focal point of many studies on fathers' engagement, the changes or outcomes for children are overwhelmed by the desire to see change in the father. How are fathers understanding and interpreting the developmental stages of their children? How are they contributing to children's development and school experiences? What are the relationships between fathers' care and children's self-regulation? Does father presence affect children's externalizing behaviors? In what ways does a father's level of education influence his willingness and capacity to engage with his children and maintain a relationship through schooling?

The second builds upon the findings of several studies of young children and African American fathers that reveal the fathers' willingness and capacity to be engaged. In particular, the focus on low-income African American fathers in urban settings is both warranted or necessary—not only as a research and practice issue but also as a community and social justice concern. Nowhere is there more urgency about father involvement than in inner-city African American communities. What are the settings that will allow us to capture the ways in which the commitments unfold and the challenges of and successes in parenting young children are managed over time?

Third, low-income, nonresidential and noncustodial African American fathers have been a primary focus of family-related programming and policy initiatives over the past 25 years. How have these opportunities for fathers changed, and how have fathers changed as a result of their engagement with these programs? How are economic and educational factors, including structural racism, continuing to serve as barriers? Despite this clear increase in our fundamental knowledge of father-child interaction, the field has not gone significantly further, and this failure to extract more information includes African American fathers.

The fourth centers on middle-income African American fathers and whether and how they are studied. The knowledge base on middle-class African American fathers is meager, and to study these fathers will require a different methodological and conceptual paradigm, which is likely to look like a hybrid of the intersections of race, class, and gender.

Lastly, are we using the appropriate frames to study African American fathers of young children, and why do we not know more? Several studies on African American fathers focus on adolescence, with others concerned with the ways that the fathers interpret and embrace their roles. By and large, these studies address questions of youths' identity and social racialization rather than their engagements with school, persistence, and related matters. This suggests that gauging our purposes for studying African American fathers of young children or adolescents will not only need to be more clearly fine-grained but also need to expand to be less deficit-oriented or deficit-leaning. That is, the studies need to provide a lens into what fathers and fathering look like that leads to optimal health, development, and learning for African American children. However, it also suggests that to understand the fathers of young children might require examining fathers' roles with older children as well. These are issues to be understood for African American fathers but are surely issues to be uncovered for all fathers.

References

Alio, A. P., Kornosky, J. L., Mbah, A. K., Marty, P. J., & Salihu, H. M. (2010). The impact of paternal involvement on feto-infant morbidity among Whites, Blacks and Hispanics. *Maternal and Child Health Journal, 14*(5), 735–741.

Alio, A. P., Mbah, A. K., Kornosky, J. L., Wathington, D., Marty, P. J., & Salihu, H. M. (2011). Assessing the impact of paternal involvement on racial/ethnic disparities in infant mortality rates. *Journal of Community Health, 36*(1), 63–68.

Alio, A. P., Salihu, H. M., Kornosky, J. L., Richman, A. M., & Marty, P. J. (2010). Feto-infant health and survival: Does paternal involvement matter? *Maternal and Child Health Journal, 14*(6), 931–937.

Anderson, E. (1990). *Streetwise: Race, class, and change in an urban community*. Chicago: University of Chicago Press.

Anderson, E. (2008). Against the wall: Poor, young, Black, and male. In E. Anderson (Ed.), *Against the wall: Poor, young Black, and male* (pp. 1–27). Philadelphia: University of Pennsylvania Press.

Avellar, S., Dion, M. R., Zaveri, H. H., & Hershey, A. M. (2006). *Early lessons from the building strong families project*. Washington, DC: Mathematica Policy Research.

Baker, C. E. (2013). Fathers' and mothers' home literacy involvement and children's cognitive and social emotional development: Implications for family literacy programs. *Applied Developmental Science, 17*(4), 184–197.

Baker, C. E. (2016). African American and Hispanic fathers' work characteristics and preschool children's cognitive development. *Journal of Family Issues, 37*(11), 1514–1534.

Belsky, J., Gilstrap, B., & Rovine, M. (1984). The Pennsylvania Infant and Family Development Project, I: Stability and change in mother-infant and father-infant interaction in a family setting at one, three, and nine months. *Child Development, 55*(3), 692–705.

Bernstein, R. N. (1988). Patterns of parental vocabulary selection in speech to young children. *Journal of Child Language, 15*(3), 481–492.

Boller, K., Bradley, R., Cabrera, N., Raikes, H., Pan, B., Shears, J., et al. (2006). The early head start father studies: Design, data collection, and summary of father presence in the lives of infants and toddlers. *Parenting, 6*(2–3), 117–143.

Bowman, P. J., & Forman, T. A. (1997). Instrumental and expressive family roles among African American fathers. In R. J. Taylor, J. S. Jackson, & L. M. Chatters (Eds.), *Family life in Black America* (pp. 216–247). Thousand Oaks, CA: Sage Publications, Inc.

Braungart-Rieker, J., Garwood, M. M., Powers, B. P., & Notaro, P. C. (1998). Infant affect and affect regulation during the still-face paradigm with mothers and fathers: The role of infant characteristics and parental sensitivity. *Developmental Psychology, 34*(6), 1428–1437.

Bristol, M. M., Gallagher, J. J., & Schopler, E. (1988). Mothers and fathers of young developmentally disabled and nondisabled boys: Adaptation and spousal support. *Developmental Psychology, 24*(3), 441–451.

Cabrera, N., & Mitchell, S. (2009). An exploratory study of fathers' parenting stress and toddlers' social development in low-income African American families. *Fathering, 7*(3), 201.

Cabrera, N. J., Fagan, J., & Farrie, D. (2008). Explaining the long reach of fathers' prenatal involvement on later paternal engagement. *Journal of Marriage and Family, 70*(5), 1094–1107.

Cabrera, N. J., Fitzgerald, H. E., Bradley, R. H., & Roggman, L. (2014). The ecology of father-child relationships: An expanded model. *Journal of Family Theory & Review, 6*(4), 336–354.

Cabrera, N. J., Hofferth, S. L., & Chae, S. (2011). Patterns and predictors of father–infant engagement across race/ethnic groups. *Early Childhood Research Quarterly, 26*(3), 365–375.

Cabrera, N. J., Ryan, R. M., Shannon, J. D., Brooks-Gunn, J., Vogel, C., et al. (2004). Low-income fathers' involvement in their toddlers' lives: Biological fathers from the Early Head Start Research and Evaluation Study. *Fathering, 2*(1), 5–30.

Cazenave, N. A. (1979). Middle-income Black fathers: An analysis of the provider role. *Family Coordinator*, 583–593.

CDC Health Disparities and Inequalities Report—United States. (2013). CDC health disparities and inequalities report—United States. *Morbidity and Mortality Weekly Report (MMWR), 62*(3), 1–187.

Chetty, R., Hendren, N., Jones, M. R., & Porter, S. R. (2018). *Race and economic opportunity in the United States: An intergenerational perspective* (No. w24441). National Bureau of Economic Research.

Childs, E. C., & Dalmage, H. M. (2010). Raising biracial children: The experiences of black married fathers.

In *The myth of the missing Black father* (pp. 65–79). New York: Columbia University Press.

Clarke-Stewart, K. A. (1978). And daddy makes three: The father's impact on mother and young child. *Child Development, 49*, 466–478.

Cochran, D. (1997). African American fathers: A decade review of the literature. *Families in Society: The Journal of Contemporary Human Services, 78*(4), 340–350.

Cohen, O. (1998). Parental narcissism and the disengagement of the non-custodial father after divorce. *Clinical Social Work Journal, 26*(2), 195–215.

Cooper, S. M. (2009). Associations between father-daughter relationship quality and the academic engagement of African American adolescent girls: Self-esteem as a mediator? *Journal of Black Psychology, 35*(4), 495–516.

Deater-Deckard, K., Dodge, K. A., Bates, J. E., & Pettit, G. S. (1996). Physical discipline among African American and European American mothers: Links to children's externalizing behaviors. *Developmental Psychology, 32*(6), 1065–1072.

Downer, J., Campos, R., McWayne, C., & Gartner, T. (2014). Father involvement and children's early learning: A critical review of published empirical work from the past 15 years. In W. Jeynes (Ed.), *Family factors and the educational success of children* (pp. 72–113). New York: Routledge.

Drake, S. C., & Cayton, H. R. (1970). *Black metropolis: A study of Negro life in a northern city*. Chicago: University of Chicago Press.

DuBois, W. E. B. (1935). *Black reconstruction in America: An essay toward a history of the part which Black folk played in the attempt to reconstruct democracy in America* (pp. 1860–1880). New York: Harcourt, Brace and Company.

Duursma, E., Pan, B. A., & Raikes, H. (2008). Predictors and outcomes of low-income fathers' reading with their toddlers. *Early Childhood Research Quarterly, 23*(3), 351–365.

Edin, K., Lein, L., & Nelson, T. (1998). *Low-income, non-residential fathers: Off-balance in a competitive economy, in initial analysis*. Washington, DC: US Department of Health and Human Services.

Edin, K., & Nelson, T. J. (2013). *Doing the best I can: Fatherhood in the inner city*. Oakland, CA: University of California Press.

Erikson, E., & Erikson, J. (1981). On generativity and identity: From a conversation with Erik and Joan Erikson. *Harvard Educational Review, 51*(2), 249–269.

Erikson, E. H. (1969). Adult stage: Generativity versus stagnation. In *Dialogue with Erik Erickson* (pp. 50–53). New York: Dutton.

Fagan, J., & Iglesias, A. (1999). Father involvement program effects on fathers, father figures, and their Head Start children: A quasi-experimental study. *Early Childhood Research Quarterly, 14*(2), 243–269.

Fantuzzo, J., McWayne, C., Perry, M. A., & Childs, S. (2004). Multiple dimensions of family involvement and their relations to behavioral and learning competencies for urban, low-income children. *School Psychology Review, 33*(4), 467–480.

Gadsden, V., & Ray, A. (2002). Engaging fathers: Issues and considerations for early childhood educators. *Young Children, 57*(6), 32–42.

Gadsden, V. L., & Bowman, P. (1999). African American males and the struggle toward responsible fatherhood. In V. Polite & J. Davis (Eds.), *A continuing challenge in times like these: African American males in schools and society* (pp. 166–183). New York: Teachers College Press.

Gadsden, V. L., Fagan, J., Ray, A., & Davis, J. (2001). Fathering Indicators Framework. Philadelphia, PA: National Center on Fathers and Families, University of Pennsylvania.

Gadsden, V. L., Davis, J. E., & Johnson, C. J. (2015). African American fathers and families within cultural and historical perspective. In J. L. Roopnarine (Ed.), *Fathers across cultures: The importance, roles, and diverse practices of dads* (pp. 155–182). Santa Barbara, CA: ABC-CLIO.

Gadsden, V. L., & Rethemeyer, R. K. (2003). Linking father involvement and parental incarceration: Concepts and contexts for considering "what works". In *Heading home: Offender reintegration into the family*. Lanham, MD: American Correctional Association.

Gadsden, V. L., Wortham, S. E., & Turner III, H. M. (2003). Situated identities of young, African American fathers in low-income urban settings: Perspectives on home, street, and the system. *Family Court Review, 41*(3), 381–399.

Gans, H. J. (1965). The Negro family: Reflections on the Moynihan report. *Commonwealth, 83*, 47–51.

Gary, L., Beatty, L., & Weaver, G. (1987). *Involvement of Black fathers in Head Start. (Final report submitted to the Department of Health and Human Services, ACYF, Grant No. 90-CD-0509)*. Washington, DC: Institute for Urban Affairs and Research, Howard University.

Gordon, E. W. (2000). The myths and realities of African American fatherhood. In R. D. Taylor & M. C. Wang (Eds.), *Resilience across contexts: Family, work, culture, and community* (pp. 217–232). Maliwah, NJ: Lawrence Erlbaum.

Griswold, R. L. (1993). *Fatherhood in America: A history*. New York: Basic Books.

Grolnick, W. S., & Slowiaczek, M. L. (1994). Parents' involvement in children's schooling: A multidimensional conceptualization and motivational model. *Child Development, 65*(1), 237–252.

Hamer, J. (2001). *What it means to be daddy: Fatherhood for Black men living away from their children*. New York: Columbia University Press.

Hammond, W. P., Caldwell, C. H., Brooks, C., & Bell, L. (2011). Being there in spirit, fire, and mind: Expressive roles among nonresidential African American fathers. *Research on Social Work Practice, 21*(3), 308–318.

Hans, S., Ray, A., Bernstein, V., & Halpern, R. (1995). *Care giving in the inner city*. Chicago: The University of Chicago and The Erikson Institute.

Hart, C. H., DeWolf, D. M., Wozniak, P., & Burts, D. C. (1992). Maternal and paternal disciplinary styles: Relations with preschoolers' playground behavioral orientations and peer status. *Child Development, 63*(4), 879–892.

Hill, N. E. (2001). Parenting and academic socialization as they relate to school readiness: The roles of ethnicity and family income. *Journal of Educational Psychology, 93*(4), 686.

Hosley, C. A., & Montemayor, R. (1997). Fathers and adolescents. In M. E. Lamb (Ed.), *The role of the father in child development* (pp. 162–178). New York: Wiley.

Hossain, Z., & Roopnarine, J. L. (1994). African-American fathers' involvement with infants: Relationship to their functioning style, support, education, and income. *Infant Behavior and Development, 17*(2), 175–184.

Isley, S. L., O'Neil, R., Clatfelter, D., & Parke, R. D. (1999). Parent and child expressed affect and children's social competence: Modeling direct and indirect pathways. *Developmental Psychology, 35*(2), 547.

Johnson, M. S., & Young, A. A. (2016). Diversity and meaning in the study of Black fatherhood: Toward a new paradigm. *Du Bois Review: Social Science Research on Race, 13*(1), 5–23.

Jones, N. (2018). *The chosen ones: Black men and the politics of redemption*. Oakland, CA: University of California Press.

Knox, V., & Redcross, C. (2000). *Parenting and providing: The impact of parents' fair share on paternal involvement*. New York: Manpower Demonstration Research Corp.

Lamb, M. (1997). *The development of father-infacnt relationships*. In M.E. Lamb (Eds.), The Role of the father in child development (pp.104-120), New York: John Wiley & Sons, Inc.

Lamb, M. E., Chuang, S. S., & Cabrera, N. (2003). Promoting child adjustment by fostering positive paternal involvement. In R. M. Lerner, F. Jacobs, & D. Wertlieb (Eds.), *Handbook of applied developmental science* (Vol. 1, pp. 211–232). Thousand Oaks, CA: Sage.

LaRossa, R. (1997). *The modernization of fatherhood: A social and political history*. Chicago: University of Chicago Press.

Lee, K., & Rispoli, K. (2019). Head start impact on fathers' involvement and Black children's development. *Journal of Social Work Education, 55*(4), 777–797.

Leech, K. A., Salo, V. C., Rowe, M. L., & Cabrera, N. J. (2013). Father input and child vocabulary development: the importance of Wh questions and clarification requests. In *Seminars in speech and language* (Vol. 34, No. 04, pp. 249–259). New York: Thieme Medical Publishers.

Lerman, R., & Sorensen, E. (2000). Father involvement with their nonmarital children: Patterns, determinants, and effects on their earnings. *Marriage & Family Review, 29*(2–3), 137–158.

Livingston, G. (2014). *Growing number of dads home with the kids: Biggest increase among those caring for family*. Retrieved from Pew Research Center website: http://www.pewsocialtrends.org/2014/06/05/growing-number-of-dads-home-with-the-kids/

Luthar, S. S., & Zigler, E. (1991). Vulnerability and competence: A review of research on resilience in childhood. *American Journal of Orthopsychiatry, 61*(1), 6–22.

MacDonald, K., & Parke, R. (1984). Bridging the gap: Parent-Child Play Interaction and Peer Interactice Competence. *Child Development, 55*(4), 1265–1277.

McAdoo, J. L. (1993). The roles of African American fathers: An ecological perspective. *Families in Society, 74*(1), 28–35.

McLoyd, V. C. (1990). Minority children: Introduction to the special issue. *Child Development, 61*(2), 263–266.

Miller, C., & Knox, V. (2001). *The challenge of helping low-income fathers support their children: Final lessons from parents' fair share*. New York: Manpower Demonstration Research Corporation.

Mullins, D. F. (2011). Linkages between children's behavior and nonresident father involvement: A comparison of African American, Anglo, and Latino families. *Journal of African American Studies, 15*(1), 1–21.

National Academies of Sciences, Engineering, and Medicine. (2016). *Parenting matters: Supporting parents of children ages 0–8*. Washington, DC: National Academies Press.

National Academies of Sciences, Engineering, and Medicine. (2019). *Vibrant and healthy kids: Aligning science, practice, and policy to advance health equity*. Washington, DC: The National Academies Press.

National Center on Fathers and Families. (1995). *Fathers and families core learnings*. Philadelphia: University of Pennsylvania.

National Responsible Fatherhood Clearinghouse. (n.d.). *Dad Stats*. Retrieved on December 13, 2019 from https://www.fatherhood.gov/content/dad-stats

Nord, C. W., Brimhall, D., & West, J. (1998). *Father involvement in schools*. Champaign, IL: ERIC Clearinghouse on Elementary and Early Childhood Education, University of Illinois.

Oliver, M., & Shapiro, T. (2013). *Black wealth/white wealth: A new perspective on racial inequality*. New York: Routledge.

Omi, M., & Winant, H. (2014). *Racial formation in the United States*. New York: Routledge.

Owen, M. T., Caughy, M. O., Hurst, J. R., Amos, M., Hasanizadeh, N., & Mata-Otero, A.-M. (2013). Unique contributions of fathering to emerging self-regulation in low-income ethnic minority preschoolers. *Early Child Development Care, 183*(3–4), 464–492.

Parke, R. D. (1996). *Fatherhood*. Boston: Harvard University Press.

Parke, R. D. (2000). Father involvement: A developmental psychological perspective. *Marriage & Family Review, 29*(2–3), 43–58.

Parke, R. D., Cassidy, J., Burks, V. M., Carson, J. L., & Boyum, L. (1992). Family contributions to peer relationships among young children. In R. D. Parke &

G. W. Ladd (Eds.), *Family-peer relations: Modes of linkage* (pp. 107–134). New York: Routledge.

Perry, A. R., Harmon, D. K., & Leeper, J. (2012). Resident black fathers' involvement: A comparative analysis of married and unwed, cohabitating fathers. *Journal of Family Issues, 33*(6), 695–714.

Petersen, E. E., Davis, N. L., Goodman, D., Cox, S., Syverson, C., Seed, K., et al. (2019). Racial/ethnic disparities in pregnancy-related deaths—United States, 2007–2016. *Morbidity and Mortality Weekly Report, 68*(35), 762–765.

Pleck, E. H. (1997). Paternal involvement: Levels, sources, and consequences. In M. E. Lamb (Ed.), *The role of the father in child development* (pp. 66–103). New York: Wiley.

Raikes, H. H., Summers, J. A., & Roggman, L. A. (2007). Father involvement in Early Head Start research programs. *Fathering: A Journal of Theory, Research, and Practice About Men as Fathers, 3*(1), 29–58.

Reynolds, R. E., Howard, T. C., & Jones, T. K. (2015). Is this what educators really want? Transforming the discourse on Black fathers and their participation in schools. *Race Ethnicity and Education, 18*(1), 89–107.

Roopnarine, J. L. (2004). African American and African Caribbean fathers: Level, quality, and meaning of involvement. In M. E. Lamb (Ed.), *The role of the father in child development* (p. 552). Hoboken, NJ: Wiley.

Shannon, J. D., Cabrera, N. J., Tamis-LeMonda, C., & Lamb, M. E. (2009). Who stays and who leaves? Father accessibility across children's first 5 years. *Parenting: Science and Practice, 9*(1–2), 78–100.

Smeeding, T. M., Garfinkel, I., & Mincy, R. B. (2011). *Young disadvantaged men: Fathers, families, poverty, and policy: An introduction to the issues*. Institute for Research on Poverty, Discussion Paper no. 1383-10.

Sullivan, M. L. (1993). Culture and class as determinants of out-of-wedlock childbearing and poverty during late adolescence. *Journal of Research on Adolescence, 3*(3), 295–316.

Tallman, I. (1965). Spousal role differentiation and the socialization of severely retarded children. *Journal of Marriage and the Family, 27*, 37–42.

Tamis-LeMonda, C. S., Shannon, J. D., Cabrera, N. J., & Lamb, M. E. (2004). Fathers and mothers at play with their 2-and 3-year-olds: Contributions to language and cognitive development. *Child Development, 75*(6), 1806–1820.

Threlfall, J. M., Seay, K. D., & Kohl, P. L. (2013). The parenting role of African-American fathers in the context of urban poverty. *Journal of Children and Poverty, 19*(1), 45–61.

Tomasello, M., & Barton, M. E. (1994). Learning words in nonostensive contexts. *Developmental Psychology, 30*(5), 639–650.

Tomasello, M., Conti-Ramsden, G., & Ewert, B. (1990). Young children's conversations with their mothers and fathers: Differences in breakdown and repair. *Journal of Child Language, 17*(1), 115–130.

US Department of Health and Human Services. (1996). *The personal responsibility and work opportunity reconciliation act*

Wakschlag, L. S., & Hans, S. L. (1999). Relation of maternal responsiveness during infancy to the development of behavior problems in high-risk youths. *Developmental Psychology, 35*(2), 569–579.

Waldfogel, J., Craigie, T. A., & Brooks-Gunn, J. (2010). Fragile families and child wellbeing. *The Future of Children/Center for the Future of Children, the David and Lucile Packard Foundation, 20*(2), 87–112.

Waller, M. R. (2001). High hopes: Unwed parents' expectations about marriage. *Children and Youth Services Review, 23*(6–7), 457–484.

Waller, M. R., & Swisher, R. (2014). Fathers' risk factors in fragile families: Implications for "healthy" relationships and father involvement. *Social Problems, 53*(3), 392–420.

Wilson, W. J. (1996). *When work disappears: The world of the new urban poor*. New York: Knopf.

Wilson, W. J. (2008). The economic Plight of inner-city Black males. In E. Anderson (Ed.), *Against the wall: Poor, young Black, and male* (pp. 55–70). Philadelphia: University of Pennsylvania Press.

Wood, R. G., Moore, Q., Clarkwest, A., Killewald, A., & Monahan, S. (2012). *The long-term effects of building strong families: A relationship skills education program for unmarried parents*. Washington, DC: Office of Planning, Research and Evaluation, Administration for Children and Families, U.S. Department of Health and Human Services (OPRE).

Yarrow, L. J., MacTurk, R. H., Vietze, P. M., McCarthy, M. E., Klein, R. P., & McQuiston, S. (1984). Development course of parental stimulation and its relationship to mastery motivation during infancy. *Developmental Psychology, 20*(3), 492–503.

Latino Fathers and Their Preschool Children

30

Cristina Mogro-Wilson

As the diversity of the population in the United States changes, there is an urgent need to understand the cultural and contextual factors that apply to its various ethnoracial populations. In this chapter, I focus on Latinos, the largest racial and ethnic minority group in the United States. If current immigration patterns continue, Latinos will continue to expand their proportion of the population. Latino is used to describe individuals from Latin America, usually Cuba, Mexico, Puerto Rico, South or Central America, or other Spanish culture of origin regardless of their race. Research on fathers has disproportionally involved White non-Latino fathers in contrast to minority fathers. In the past 20 years, we have begun to explore the role of the Latino father and how parental involvement and other attributes of fatherhood affect Latinos differently (Cabrera & Bradley, 2012). Over half of US Latinos are US citizens or US national at birth (66%) and 35% are foreign born (U.S Census Bureau, 2018). Of all Latinos in the United States, 62% identify as Mexican, 9% as Puerto Rican, 9% as Central American, 9% as other Hispanic, 7% as South American, and 4% as Cuban (U.S. Census Bureau, 2018). The nuanced understanding of each cultural group within Latinos as well as other defining characteristics including the length of time they have been in the United States, citizen status, socioeconomic status, and educational level makes Latino fathers an exceptionally diverse group. Due to the complexity of Latinos in the United States and the scope of this chapter, I will not cover the research contrasting within group similarities and differences.

Nearly 25% of school-aged children in the United States are Latino (U.S. Census Bureau, 2018). Most Latino children (76%) are living in two-parent households where the father is participating in parenting (Lopez & Velasco, 2010; U.S. Census Bureau, 2018). When Latino fathers are not living in the household, they are often co-parenting, or continuing to remain active in their child's lives. As the population grows, understanding the role Latino fathers play in their child's lives, how to best integrate them into our systems of care, and how culture influences their parenting is an urgent need.

Latino males in the United States are facing incredible barriers; compared to non-Latino males, they are less likely to enroll in early educational programs, complete high school or college, and have health care and insurance (Cabrera, Guzman, Turner, Malin, & Cooper, 2016; U.S. Bureau of Labor Statistics., 2017). Latino families are poorer (median household income $50,486 compared to the median income for White non-Latino of $68,145) and have the largest family size (3.87 members per family compared to 2.37 for non-Latino families)

C. Mogro-Wilson (✉)
School of Social Work, University of Connecticut, Hartford, CT, USA
e-mail: cristina.wilson@uconn.edu

H. E. Fitzgerald et al. (eds.), *Handbook of Fathers and Child Development*,
https://doi.org/10.1007/978-3-030-51027-5_30

(U.S. Census Bureau, 2018). Latinos comprise 18% of the US population, but in nine states, the percentage is higher, led by New Mexico (49%), Texas (39%), California (39%), and Arizona (31%). These differences in socioeconomic status and family size directly affect the role that Latino fathers play in their families' lives. For example, the father's education level has been found to affect how much time they spend with their children. Those fathers who attended at least some college spend more time with their child compared to noncollege-educated fathers (Yeung, Sandberg, Davis-Kean, & Hofferth, 2001).

As a large fraction of Latino fathers are also immigrants, a quick discussion of acculturation is important. Acculturation is defined as a process where one culture adopts the standards, actions, and behaviors of the dominant population, where this process is bidirectional and the majority population is affected through contact with the minority group (Alba, 2003; Gordon, 1964). The length of time spent in the United States, as well as generational status, directly affects how much of the culture of origin one adheres to. For example, first-generation Latino immigrants are less likely than men born in the United States to adhere to egalitarian gender norms that are more common in US culture, and this in turn affects father involvement (Adams, Coltrane, & Parke, 2007; Bulanda, 2004). The acculturation process is a complicated one, and while the father is acculturating at his own rate, his family (children, mother) is acculturating at differing rates. Language ability plays a large role in how fathers, and all parents, interact with various systems and affects the ease with which fathers can communicate with schools, medical providers, and other social service agencies. How acculturation affects parenting for Latino fathers is less clear; there is some evidence suggesting that as Latino immigrant fathers acculturate, they are involved less with their children (Coltrane, Parke, & Adams, 2004). This could be related to the loss of some Latino cultural values in the acculturation process such as *familismo*, or the solidarity and cohesion of the family, and an increase of focus on individuality. However, other research has supported more involvement of Latina mother's acculturation in their child's school activities (Terriquez, 2012; Turney & Kao, 2009); whether this translates to fathers is still unknown.

Bioecological Framework

To better understand families, particularly ethnic minority families, and how their roles influence a child, a cultural-ecological approach can be used. Bronfenbrenner's bioecological model is a conceptual guide allowing us to better understand how parenting, cultural values, and the environment can influence the father, child, and family (Bronfenbrenner, 1986). The bioecological model is a conceptual guide for designing research that examines multiple influences on targeted aspects of child development. It is one example of a systems approach to complex problems, particularly those where systems are nested in other systems (child, family, neighborhood, etc.). During early childhood development, at the ages between birth and five, the relationship between the child and their parents develops the building blocks for how they establish relationships prior to school entry (Bronfenbrenner, 2005). The bioecological model has the child at the center in the microsystem which is the closest to the child, their home, and family and builds out to the mesosystem which stresses the relationship between the microsystems and includes schools, religious institutions, neighborhoods, and friends. The exosystem moves further away from the individual child and includes the parents' workplace but also policies that affect the child. The macrosystem is the larger cultural norms or environment where the child lives. Finally, the chronosystem emphasizes the effects of time on a child's development; those events in a child's life will affect them as they develop over time. There is great strength in Bronfenbrenner's framework because it illustrates how systems are nested in other systems, thus encouraging investigators to develop conceptual research models that are multilevel such as that developed by Cabrera, Fitzgerald, Bradley, and Roggman (2014) to organize research on father involvement in child development.

Microsystem: The Home Environment The child and the microsystem include the family home environment which can provide learning stimulation that influences more than just a child's cognitive skills but also extends to improved behavioral competence (McWayne, Downer, Campos, & Harris, 2013). A longitudinal study of children found that when fathers engaged in play with their toddler-aged children, such as reading, singing, and storytelling, the child benefited in academic and social-emotional outcomes (Baker, 2013). This at-home communication and creating a learning environment are important for fathers to engage in during the early years of their child's development. The extended Latino family often includes uncles, aunts, and first and second cousins, and there is a large emphasis placed on their role in the development of the child and their level of involvement in parenting (Mogro-Wilson, Rojas, & Haynes, 2016). A child that is raised where there is a large Latino community presence may have extended family and community members playing a role in their development and lives.

As mentioned earlier in the chapter, Latinos have the largest family size (3.87 members per family compared to 2.37 for non-Latino families) (U.S. Census Bureau, 2018). The increase in size could of course mean more children but also more extended family such as grandparents or aunts and uncles. One of the factors that affect child development is the residential status of the father and the size of the family. Some work indicates that more children at home is related to positive parenting decreasing, partially due to the increasing demands (Crnic & Greenberg, 1990), while others have found that more children in the home minimizes the demands on the parents because there are older siblings to help remove some of the pressure (Behrman & Taubman, 1986).

Mesosystem: Religion The church, healthcare system, and school system are examples of mesosystem providers that function in integral roles in young children's lives. Particularly for young Latino children, religion often plays a large role, with Latinos reporting to be more religious than non-Latinos, 59% reporting that religion is very importance in their life (Taylor, Lopez, Martinez, & Velasco, 2012). In addition, Latinos are more likely to attend church services weekly or more often, with six in ten Latinos reporting that religion is very important in their lives (Taylor et al., 2012). Therefore, religion may play a substantial role in the lives of Latino children. Children and families may attend weekly church services and be involved in their church and religious community, and the religious value systems may influence parenting and family roles. Most notably in the early years of the child's life, or prenatally, parental coping and stress may be dealt with through religion. In cases where there is heightened stress, such as a developmental disability or health problems, this may be even more prominent. Latinos confronted with health issues of their child (e.g., asthma) often site religion playing a major role in their lives and believing that the fate of their child is in God's hands (Coffey, Cloutier, Meadows-Oliver, & Terrazos, 2012; Garro, 2011; Skinner, Correa, Skinner, & Bailey Jr., 2001).

Mesosystem: Healthcare System Fathers and families interact with many systems, including medical systems that are a large part of the early life of a child. There are often regular prenatal and first-year doctor visits and sick visits as well as visits that may occur around concerns about child development. A language barrier is the most cited reason for not seeking medical care, as few Spanish-speaking healthcare providers in the United States exist, in addition to difficulties in arranging transportation to healthcare facilities (Garro, 2011; Hinojosa et al., 2012). Latinos suffer disproportionately from obesity, asthma, HIV/AIDS, low birth weight, infant mortality, and diabetes (Office of Minority Health, 2019). In addition, Latinos report the lowest access to private insurance, Medicaid, and state health programs compared to non-Latinos of the same socioeconomic status affecting medical care and receiving appropriate medications (Garro, 2011). Mothers and fathers manage healthcare issues differently; however, there is a lack of understanding on how Latino fathers cope with health-related issues for their children. This is vitally important given the usual role of the Latino father as protector and income provider.

Mesosystem: School System The school system is a chance for families to interact and develop connections with teachers and to monitor their child's development academically and socially-emotionally. Family engagement in the school systems, both at preschool and entering kindergarten, has a large influence on Latino student outcomes (Hill & Torres, 2010; Rodríguez-Brown, 2010). For Latinos, the education of a child stems from the home, with moral and social relationships expected to serve as the foundation of education that takes place in the school setting (Auerbach, 2011). Latino fathers have often not been the focus of engagement for school outreach and are often thought of as an untapped resource (Behnke, Gonzalez, & Cox, 2010). The reported involvement of Latino fathers in a child's school has been lower than for non-Latinos; however, the systematic barriers to involvement such as cultural and linguistic issues and feeling unwelcome in the school community may be creating these issues (Hill & Torres, 2010; Hyslop, 2000). Latino fathers believe it is important to be involved in a child's education beyond just the mother's involvement (Lopez & Velasco, 2010). However, Latino fathers have noted their distrust with the school system (Quiñones & Kiyama, 2014) yet continue to monitor, advocate, and help their child succeed in school. Latino fathers utilize the home environment and the family unit to promote education, by having high expectations and goals for their family and advocating, monitoring, and finding information to help support their children in the educational environment (Quiñones & Kiyama, 2014). In addition, Latino fathers tend to promote passivity and silence toward school personnel (Quiñones, 2012), in accordance with the cultural value of *simpatía* (discussed further below) which emphasizes getting along with others particularly those in positions of authority.

Exosystem: External Environment The exosystem, or the external environment, also plays a large role in the child's development as well as influencing the father's role. Exposure to poverty at young ages, low parent education, and young fathers are negatively associated with the quality of the child's home and learning environment within the home and are often associated with less parental warmth and inconsistent discipline (Davis-Kean, 2005; McLoyd, 1998). Local and national policies that have created an anti-immigrant rhetoric create an environment where Latino parents with any immigration concerns may be less likely to address health issues, bring their child to school, and seek out social services or any other provider that may ask of them to report any personal information. In addition, the antipathy toward Latino undocumented immigrants, many of whom are fathers, subjects them to high levels of stress in relation to immigration and deportation concerns (Cervantes, Gattamorta, & Berger-Cardoso, 2019). This stress can overflow to all areas of Latino fathers' lives, adding to distrust of professionals and creating barriers to connections with the external environment.

Macrosystem: Cultural Values The macrosystem, which includes the role of cultural values, is an integral part of family life and parenting and affects how the father and child interact with all the systems. Parenting is a cultural construct, and thus, one's culture influences how one parents and how parenting is perceived by the child and the father. While there are many cultural constructs embedded into Latino families, a few of the primary ones will be discussed and their impact on parenting. The following is a discussion of how fathering is influenced by Latino culture particularly *familismo*, *respeto*, *personalismo*, *simpatía*, traditional *machismo*, and *caballerismo*. Of note is that all these cultural values change over time and are impacted by immigration status, socioeconomic status, and acculturation levels.

Familismo is the cultural value of emphasizing a duty to the family and an interconnection and cooperation among members of the family (Rodriguez et al., 2007). Fathers who value *familismo* feel a strong obligation to maintain family ties, emphasizing the importance of the family as the primary emotional support system. Latino fathers, due to this cultural value, may feel an added pressure to preserve the family unit by focusing on cooperation and agreement in parenting and relationships within the family unit. Latino families view the family unit as more expansive and utilize the role of uncles, aunts, and other extended members of the family in parenting activities. Latino fathers view the behavior of their children as a way their family is represented to the outside community; Latino fathers want to maintain respect for their family and their role as a father and want the community to see that through the behavior of their children (Mogro-Wilson et al., 2016).

Respeto is a cultural value where the importance for maintaining respect toward oneself and others during interpersonal relationships is an expected part of being a member of the family, and each member of the family is respected in the roles that they play (Livas-Dlott et al., 2010). Latino fathers have noted the importance of this cultural value in their parenting, confirming this bidirectional relationship of respect, them for their child and their child for them (Mogro-Wilson et al., 2016). Latino fathers utilize the role of respect as a way to control and monitor their children both in public and at home. For example, Latino fathers tend to not loudly discipline or spank their children in public because they respect their children and do not want to embarrass them (Mogro-Wilson et al., 2016). Respect has an influence on the father and mother relationship in their roles as co-parents suggesting that fathers who value *respeto* have better co-parenting harmonization (Yu et al., 2008).

Personalismo is a cultural value that centers on reliance, warmness, and respect in relationships and can be seen as a cornerstone for the development of the parent-child relationship (Altarriba & Santiago-Rivera, 1994; Mogro-Wilson, 2013). The parent-child relationship is a unique relationship that lies outside of the parenting style constructs; it is developed between the father and each child. The father-child relationship is different depending on the personality, gender, and other characteristics of that child as well as dependent on father characteristics. However, parenting styles tend to be more consistent within the family for all the children in a family unit. The parent-child relationship centers on trust and getting along, and the cultural value of *personalismo* further enhances these concepts. In order to develop the father-child relationship, fathers are attentive to the child's interests and abilities and engage in child directed play (Mogro-Wilson et al., 2016). For example, child-directed play tends to stem from child interests, like playing with dolls for a young girl, and not the interest of the father, which may be playing baseball instead.

Simpatía is a cultural value that emphasizes creating harmony in relationships, being empathic to others, having an easygoing attitude, and being open to conform to authority figures (including medical and school personnel) (Triandis, Marín, Lisansky, & Betancourt, 1984). This avoidance of conflict and tendency to lean toward agreeableness translates for Latino fathers as having a family system that is in agreement, where there is sharing of responsibilities and decision-making that is done collaboratively with the mother. Latino fathers who highly value *simpatía* are more likely to agree upon parenting values with the mother (Yu et al., 2008). Latino fathers often portray their warmth and love for their child through the cultural value of *simpatía*, and this value is often displayed differently depending on the gender of the child (Mogro-Wilson et al., 2016). Latino fathers may show warmth and love toward their girl children through hugs and kisses and utilize more physical play and roughhousing with their boy children (Mogro-Wilson et al., 2016).

Traditional machismo is a gender role construct where male authority and female passivity are adhered to (Guilamo-Ramos et al., 2007). Within the family, traditional *machismo* is demonstrated by the father's adherence to a firm division of gender-based family roles, where the mother is the caregiver and the father is the financial provider. However, there is evidence that traditional *machismo* is not practiced as extensively as implied by the stereotype (Cabrera & Garcia Coll, 2004). For example, both Mexican American and Puerto Rican fathers actively interact with their children, playing, showing warmth and love, and providing emotional support (Davis & Chavez, 1995; Mogro-Wilson et al., 2016). In addition, Toth and Xu (1999) found that Latino fathers spent more time with their children in direct interactions than White non-Latino fathers did. An explanation for these differences is the cultural value of *caballerismo*, which encompasses other, still gender-based, values that may help explain the differences we are seeing for Latino fathers in their caregiving roles.

Caballerismo is an expansion to the traditional *machismo* cultural value that includes positive values such as Latino fathers valuing a sense of obligation and responsibility toward their family and the need to protect the family as a unit (Torres, Solberg, & Carlstrom, 2002). *Caballerismo* differs from *familismo* in that it contains obligation and responsibility to the family unit, rather than just the observance of the family over the individual. In addition, the adherence to this cultural value for Latino fathers has been connected to outcomes that include better life satisfaction for the father, better relationships, and a sense of responsibility toward the larger community (Cruz et al., 2011; Mogro-Wilson et al., 2016). Increased Latino father involvement has also been connected to fathers who endorse values centered on *caballerismo* (Cruz et al., 2011). Latino fathers that adhere to these positive values of *caballerismo* not only feel financially responsible for their children but emotionally responsible as well. In a qualitative study, Latino fathers have described their parenting role as being involved with their child(ren) including attending parent-teacher conferences and in the day-to-day activities of their child (Mogro-Wilson et al., 2016). The responsibility and pride Latino fathers feel toward their child(ren) and family is a benefit not only to the child but to the father as well.

These cultural values affect the way fathers' parent, develop relationships with their child, and interact with other members of their families and communities. Parenting styles, discussed below, are often viewed through traditional westernized lenses of understanding parenting roles. These cultural values give context to these parenting styles and relationships. Viewing parenting practices through the cultural lens of Latino cultural values adds a layer of complexity to the understanding of how Latino fathers parent (Mogro-Wilson, 2013).

Parenting Styles Research on early childhood demonstrates that fathers have a long-lasting effect on their child's lives including behavioral control, language development, literacy, and social and emotional skills (Lamb, 2012; Malin, Cabrera, & Rowe, 2014; Martin, Ryan, & Brooks-Gunn, 2010; Towe-Goodman et al., 2014). In line with a bioecological theory, families and children do better with supportive, responsive parenting, where parents show love and care toward their children and assist their child to gain new cognitive, social, and emotional skills. Latino fathers, who portray warmth through touch (hugging and kissing) to their child, have children with better language and social-emotional relationship skills (Fagan, 2000; Martin et al., 2010). In a longitudinal study of low-income children, Coley, Lewin-Bizan, and Carrano (2011) found that fathers who showed warmth and love toward their toddler lead to improved academic outcomes in math and reading in middle school. Father warmth has also been linked to better behavior management of children. For example, Towe-Goodman and colleagues (2014) found that father warmth and responsiveness while a child was playing at 2 years old predicted children's decision-making functioning, including inhibitory control, working memory, and attention, when the child was 3 years of age.

Diana Baumrind (1997) constructed four main parenting typologies based on the idea that parenting is a combination of warmth/love and control/discipline. Authoritative parenting characterized by high levels of warmth and love and low amounts of control/discipline has long been established as the most beneficial for children in the Western world (Baumrind, 1997). The other types of parenting styles are as follows: authoritarian (low warmth, high control), permissive (high warmth, low control), and uninvolved (low warmth, low control). Research suggests that authoritative parents have children with better academic and social outcomes; however, this has been shown with non-Latinos and primarily with mothers (Baumrind, 1997; Darling & Steinberg, 1993; Mistry, Vandewater, Huston, & McLoyd, 2002). Research with fathers shows different results; those fathers who are more controlling or focused more on discipline may decrease opportunities for learning and relationship building and thus decrease positive outcomes for children (Coley et al., 2011; Mackenzie, Nicklas, Waldfogel, & Brooks-Gunn, 2013). Coley et al. (2011) found that low-income fathers who used more control and discipline had children with lower academic scores compared to fathers who reported using less control. There is building evidence suggesting that there are cultural variations of how we define and perceive warmth and control that may influence outcomes for other ethnic minority groups.

Fitting with Baumrind's authoritarian parenting style, past research has characterized Latino parenting by harsh discipline, obeying with no questioning, and lacking in warmth and intimacy toward their children (Mirandé, 1991). However, as our understanding of families and parenting has evolved, evidence now shows that Latino fathers are highly involved, value their relationship with their children, show warmth and love, and feel the importance of transmitting cultural values such as respect (Campos, 2008; Mogro-Wilson, 2008; Mogro-Wilson et al., 2016; Perez-Brena, Cookston, Fabricius, & Saenz, 2012; Taylor & Behnke, 2005). Latino fathers are playing an increased role in their child's lives as they develop from prenatal care to early childhood. These changing roles are beyond that of provider and contributor financially to the child's lives but involve more emotional and developmental support.

Latino families are often portrayed as following typical gender roles, where the mother stays at home and provides the most caregiving and fathers work outside the house and are less involved in parenting (Diaz, Miville, & Gil, 2013). However, as Latina mothers become more economically able to provide financial support to their families, the involvement of the fathers in daily caregiving is increasing, eliminating the once large gap between Latina mothers and fathers in caregiving activities (Coltrane et al., 2004; Lamb, 2012; Shwalb, Shwalb, & Lamb, 2013).

Latino Fathers During the Prenatal Period Father involvement during the prenatal period can lead to better health outcomes for children and also better father-child relationships. How Latino fathers interact with the mother during this parental time is important. Research has supported that Latino males influence health behavior such as contraceptive and condom use as well as breastfeeding (Lovera, Sanderson, Bogle, & Vela Acosta, 2010; Tschann, Flores, de Groat, Deardorff, & Wibbelsman, 2010). For Latinos, even if the mother did not intend onthe pregnancy, there is a protective factor if the father wanted the child, where the fathers support the mothers to receive early and sustained prenatal care (Sangi-Haghpeykar, Mehta, Posner, & Poindexter, 2005). During the prenatal period and beyond, relationship quality and co-parenting between mother and father are important factors that can influence the involvement of the father. Research supports the importance of supportive co-parenting relationship as aligned with more father involvement (Carlson, McLanahan, & Brooks-Gunn, 2008; Sobolewski & King, 2005). Thus, many parenting interventions are aimed at creating a favorable co-parenting relationship placing a focus on both the mother and the father (Guilamo-Ramos, Bowman, Santa Maria, Kabemba, & Geronimo, 2017).

Latino Fathers from Birth Until Age Five At birth, it is important for all fathers, including Latino fathers, to develop their ability to be sensitive and responsive to their babies. Early caregiving tasks allow for bonding and attachment between the child and the father and predict attachment when the child is a year old and then predict father sensitivity when the child is three (Brown, Mangelsdorf, & Neff, 2012). Research has partially demonstrated that depending on level of acculturation, Latino fathers are similar to non-Latino fathers in some caregiving activities. In the level of involvement with the child, Latino fathers compared to non-Latinos tend to be quite similar (Hofferth, 2003; Sotomayor-Peterson, Card, & Wilhelm, 2013; Toth & Xu, 1999). However, acculturation is also once again at play for Latino fathers. Latino fathers that are less acculturated tend not to engage in cognitive stimulation of their infant (under age of one), perhaps deeming it not developmentally appropriate (Cabrera, Shannon, West, & Brooks-Gunn, 2006; Sotomayor-Peterson et al., 2013). Thus, reading a book to an infant for a less acculturated Latino father may not seem age appropriate.

Sotomayor-Peterson and colleagues (2013) found that against stereotypical beliefs about Latino father parenting, Latino fathers were more involved and nurturing compared to non-Latino fathers, even while controlling for acculturation levels. Latino fathers were more soothing to babies, got up more during the night to respond to a baby, or stayed home while the child was sick (Sotomayor-Peterson et al., 2013). This nurturing, or responding in the moment to their young child's needs, is a way Latino fathers may be expressing the cultural value of *familismo* (Mogro-Wilson et al., 2016; Sotomayor-Peterson et al., 2013). Latino fathers spend more time on the weekends with their children than non-Latino fathers do; however, there is no difference in the time spent during the week (Yeung et al., 2001). While Latino fathers are spending similar amounts of time with their children as non-Latinos, they are taking more responsibility over their care and are assuming less control over their behavior than non-Latino fathers (Hofferth, 2003).

As children enter preschool around age three or four, or if they wait until kindergarten at around age five, parents are expected to interact with institutional settings such as schools and medical facilities. Direct participation in schools allows a father to monitor their child academically and socially, create relationships with teachers and community members, and contribute to the development of the school culture and community. Latino immigrant fathers tend to participate less in their child's school compared to US-born Latinos (Terriquez, 2012). It is important to note that school and medical settings contain institutional discrimination that limits the abilities of Latinos to completely interact (Telles & Ortiz, 2008). These institutions prioritize White, middle-class norms and expectations including the privileging of mothers in these settings over fathers (Auerbach, 2006; Lareau, 2000). However, fathers continue to voice the importance of their involvement in these systems (Mogro-Wilson et al., 2016). In addition, Latino fathers remain committed to the academic needs of their children and working at home with them (Auerbach, 2006; Lopez, 2001).

Family Interventions When Latino males become fathers, it may be a natural time in their life for change, a transformative life event. Others have spoken about this time as a teaching moment, a time when there is an event that can increase your motivation to change your behavior (McBride, Emmons, & Lipkus, 2003). Becoming a father can change how fathers perceive risk and self-image. For example, Latino males have shown a greater desire to quit smoking when they learn of their partners' pregnancy or after the birth of the child (Pollak et al., 2010, 2015). Interventions that utilize motivational interviewing with fathers may be able to use these reasons of breaking from the past and as a transitional period of change to stop any risky behaviors. The opportunity of using a commitment to fatherhood coupled with the cultural tenants that underlie Latino cultural values, such as a strong commitment to the family, may offer a chance for intervention.

However, family interventions that are truly father-centric and inclusive of the father that also include cultural sensitivity are limited. For example, research shows that only 20% of parent training involves fathers (Lundahl, Tollefson, Risser, & Lovejoy, 2008). Head Start and Early Head Start programs have added portions of their outreach to fathers either in the home or in center-based programs (https://eclkc.ohs.acf.hhs.gov/family-engagement/article/engaging-fathers). However, involvement and engagement in interventions for Latino fathers can be challenging, and there are many barriers to overcome (Mogro-Wilson et al., 2019). The "Helping Our Toddlers, Developing Our Children's Skills" 7-week training program helps families of toddlers who have challenging behaviors by teaching parents in six session how to identify features in the environment and in interactions with others that may contribute to the reinforcement or maintenance of problem behaviors (Salinas, Smith, & Armstrong, 2011). Approximately 200 families receive the training program, which occurs outside the home, and at least 29% of the participants are fathers. The program utilizes role playing, modeling, and homework for families to try at home. In one study, more than half the participants were Latino fathers and reported difficulty going to the sessions due to conflicts with work schedules, difficulty in finding childcare, and partners who did not participate (Salinas et al., 2011). There are studies on parenting interventions that report fathers not always reporting positive changes in their parenting compared to mothers; however, this could be due to the interventions not always targeting fathers (Lundahl et al., 2008). There is a need to create tailored interventions for Latino fathers that integrate the cultural values and help develop close parent-child relationships. Family-based interventions need to address issues of culture and parenting that is culturally attuned to Latino fathers to build emotional connections. Multidimensional family therapy could be one such avenue as it can encourage strong parent-child connections through a developmental and contextual system framework (Liddle, 2004; Liddle, Rowe, Dakof, Henderson, & Greenbaum, 2009).

Summary and Key Points

Latinos comprise 18% of the US population from various countries of origin, including Mexico, Central and South American, and Puerto Rico. Yet, Latino men are still facing incredible barriers, compared to non-Latino males (Cabrera et al., 2016; U.S. Bureau of Labor Statistics., 2017). The focus in the past decades has been on how mothers affect child development. However, becoming ever more prominent is the unique role fathers play in parenting and child development. Given the growth of the Latino population and that nearly 25% of school-aged children in the United States are Latino (U.S. Census Bureau, 2018), there is a need to include Latino fathers in the parenting discussion.

Bronfenbrenner's bioecological model allows for a look at parenting, cultural values, and the environment that can influence the father, child, and family (Bronfenbrenner, 1986). The bioecological model has the child at the center in the microsystem which is the closest to the child, their home, and family. Latino families may include grandparents, aunts, uncles, and community members. These extended family members may play a large role in the parenting and development of a child.

For Latino families, religion (part of the mesosystem) may play an integral part in establishing roles, responsibilities, and value systems within the family. In early life, fathers may use religion as a way to cope and deal with stressful situations such as a disability or health-related problem for their child. Also part of the mesosystem is the medical system, and for Latino fathers, integration into the medical system may be difficult as they may experience language and cultural barriers. Often, the role of the Latino father as the provider and protector causes a strain on the family when insurance and medical issues arise. Finally, Latino fathers continue to be a resource for school systems because Latino fathers want to be involved in their child's education. However, various barriers exist including language and cultural barriers that can influence Latino fathers and lead to a distrust in the school system.

Exposure to poverty is related to the child's home and learning environment and is often associated with less parental warmth and inconsistent discipline (Davis-Kean, 2005; McLoyd, 1998). Local and national policies with anti-immigrant rhetoric create a country that is less hospitable to Latino fathers. It can create an environment where Latino fathers are more hesitant to address health issues, bring their child to school, or seek out social services.

Parenting is a cultural construct, and thus, one's culture influences how one parents and how parenting is perceived by the child and father. Fathering is influenced by Latino culture particularly *familismo*, *respeto*, *personalismo*, *simpatía*, traditional *machismo*, and *caballerismo.* Fathers who value *familismo* feel a strong obligation to maintain family ties, emphasizing the importance of the family as the primary emotional support system. Latino fathers have noted *respeto* in their parenting, confirming this bidirectional relationship of respect as a way to control and monitor their children both in public and at home. The parent-child relationship centers on trust and getting along, and the cultural value of *personalismo* further enhances these concepts. In order to develop the father-child relationship, fathers are attentive to the child's intrests and abilities and engage in child directed play. Latino fathers who highly value *simpatía* are more likely to agree upon parenting values with the mother (Yu et al., 2008) and may show warmth differently depending on the gender of their child (Mogro-Wilson et al., 2016). Traditional *machismo* is demonstrated by the father's adherence to a firm division of gender-based family roles; however, there is evidence that it is not practiced as extensively. Adherence to *caballerismo* has been connected to better life satisfaction and relationships and a sense of responsibility toward the larger community (Cruz et al., 2011; Mogro-Wilson et al., 2016).

As discussed in the chapter, involvement of Latino fathers during the prenatal and early years is related to better child outcomes across various domains (Fagan, 2000; Martin et al., 2010). Latino fathers are playing an important role in their child's lives as they develop from prenatal care to early childhood. These changing roles are beyond that of provider and financial contributor to a child's life but involve emotional and developmental support. Latino fathers are involved in various child-rearing activities including reading books, soothing babies, and spending time on the weekends in child-directed activities. There is an overall lack of family-based interventions that truly involve the father and that are culturally relevant to Latino fathers in particular.

The Future of Latino Fathers Perhaps one of the most critical questions for the next decade is how to integrate the Latino father into the services we are providing to the child, to the mother, and to the family. Service providers, social workers, psychologists, health professionals, and teachers have to understand the unique role that Latino fathers play in the family. In order for Latino families to reach their full potential, the father must be involved in the child's life, to the benefit of the child, the family, and the father himself. As we move forward, service providers must continue to integrate the work that they are doing to engagne, involve, and retain the father in various parts of treatment.

The next set of critical questions for the following decade is how to move this conversation into policy change. Most of the policy change around fathers is focused on economic contributions to the family. However, Latino fathers are changing the landscape of immigration; as more men cross the border to find employment, they are away from their families and children for extended periods of time. The impact on child development and on the mental health of Latino fathers is not yet understood. Given the current political climate and changes to health insurance, medical coverage, health access, and family support and leave policies, the role of the father is often left out of the discussion. Work must be done to continue the integration of fathers into the policies being created that is accessible to Latino fathers. With the political climate affecting anti-immigration and anti-Latino sentiments, the increased policing and criminalization of Latino males will have an impact on their involvement with their children and families. As increasing numbers of Latino families become involved in the criminal justice system, the child welfare system, and other institutions, the interventions we employ to assist these families must include the father. How we create spaces that are not elaborations of systematic oppression toward Latinos that can provide services and comprehensive education and care that involve fathers frames our next set of challenges.

Finally, we must keep the voices of the Latino fathers present in the work we do to move forward child, father, and family development. The ever-changing role of the father is moving toward more egalitarian roles, with more technology integrated into parenting and relationship development. The modern Latino male will respond to the responsibilities of parenting and developing relationships with their partners and children, in ever-changing ways. In all these coming changes, we must turn to the men who know and are experiencing these parenting roles in a complex political and social environment. We must use this moment of transition into parenthood as an opportunity to change and for positive movement forward in self-development for the Latino male. Utilizing a strengths-based perspective, we have to see the Latino father as an essential component of the Latino family.

References

Adams, M., Coltrane, S., & Parke, R. D. (2007). Cross ethnic applicability of the gender based attitudes toward marriage and child rearing scales. *Sex Roles, 56*(5–6), 325–339.

Alba, R. D. (2003). *Remaking the American mainstream: Assimilation and contemporary immigration*. Cambridge, MA: Harvard University Press.

Altarriba, J., & Santiago-Rivera, A. (1994). Current perspectives on using linguistic and cultural factors in counseling the Hispanic client. *Professional Psychology: Research and Practice, 25*(4), 388–397. https://doi.org/10.1037/0735-7028.25.4.388

Auerbach, S. (2006). "If the student is good, let him fly": Moral support for college among Latino immigrant parents. *Journal of Latinos & Education, 5*(4), 275–292. https://doi.org/10.1207/s1532771xjle0504_4

Auerbach, S. (2011). Learning from Latino families. *Educational Leadership, 68*(8), 16–21.

Baker, C. E. (2013). Fathers' and mothers' home literacy involvement and children's cognitive and social emotional development: Implications for family literacy programs. *Applied Developmental Science, 17*(4), 184–197. https://doi.org/10.1080/10888691.2013.836034

Baumrind, D. (1997). The discipline encounter: Contemporary issues. *Aggression and Violent Behavior, 2*(4), 321–335. https://doi.org/10.1016/S1359-1789(97)00018-9

Behnke, A. O., Gonzalez, L. M., & Cox, R. B. (2010). Latino students in new arrival states: Factors and services to prevent youth from dropping out. *Hispanic Journal of Behavioral Sciences, 32*(3), 385–409. https://doi.org/10.1177/0739986310374025

Behrman, J. R., & Taubman, P. (1986). Birth order, schooling, and earnings. *Journal of Labor Economics, 4*(3), S121–S145. https://doi.org/10.1086/298124

Bronfenbrenner, U. (1986). Ecology of the family as a context for human development: Research perspectives. *Developmental Psychology, 22*(6), 723–742. https://doi.org/10.1037/0012-1649.22.6.723

Bronfenbrenner, U. (2005). *Making human beings human: Bioecological perspectives on human development*. Thousand Oaks, CA: Sage.

Brown, G. L., Mangelsdorf, S. C., & Neff, C. (2012). Father involvement, paternal sensitivity, and father–child attachment security in the first 3 years. *Journal of Family Psychology, 26*(3), 421–430. https://doi.org/10.1037/a0027836

Bulanda, R. E. (2004). Paternal involvement with children: The influence of gender ideologies. *Journal of Marriage & Family, 66*, 40–45.

Cabrera, N. J., & Bradley, R. H. (2012). Latino fathers and their children. *Child Development Perspectives, 6*(3), 232–238. https://doi.org/10.1111/j.1750-8606.2012.00249.x

Cabrera, N. J., Fitzgerald, H. E., Bradley, R. H., & Roggman, L. (2014). The ecology of father child relationships: An expanded model. *Journal of Family Theory & Review, 6*(4), 336–354. https://doi.org/10.1111/jftr.12054

Cabrera, N. J., & Garcia Coll, C. (2004). Latino fathers: Uncharted territory in need of much exploration. In M. E. Lamb (Ed.), *The role of the father in child development* (pp. 98–120). Hoboken, NJ: Wiley.

Cabrera, N. J., Guzman, L., Turner, K., Malin, J., & Cooper, P. M. (2016). *A national portrait of the health and education of Hispanic boys and young men*. Retrieved from https://www.childtrends.org/wp-content/uploads/2016/09/National-Portrait-of-Hispanic-Boys-Young-Men-9.15.16.pdf

Cabrera, N. J., Shannon, J. D., West, J., & Brooks-Gunn, J. (2006). Parental interactions with Latino infants: Variation by country of origin and English proficiency. *Child Development, 77*(5), 1190–1207. https://doi.org/10.1111/j.1467-8624.2006.00928.x

Campos, R. (2008). Considerations for studying father involvement in early childhood among Latino families. *Hispanic Journal of Behavioral Sciences, 30*(2), 133–160. https://doi.org/10.1177/0739986308316658

Carlson, M. J., McLanahan, S., & Brooks-Gunn, J. (2008). Coparenting and nonresident fathers' involvement with young children after a nonmarital birth. *Demography, 45*(2), 461–488.

Cervantes, R. C., Gattamorta, K. A., & Berger-Cardoso, J. (2019). Examining difference in immigration stress, acculturation stress and mental health outcomes in six Hispanic/Latino nativity and regional groups. *Journal of Immigrant and Minority Health, 21*(1), 14–20. https://doi.org/10.1007/s10903-018-0714-9

Coffey, J., Cloutier, M., Meadows-Oliver, M., & Terrazos, C. (2012). Puerto Rican families' experiences of asthma and use of the emergency department for asthma care. *Journal of Pediatric Health Care, 26*(5), 356–363. https://doi.org/10.1016/j.pedhc.2011.01.006

Coley, R. L., Lewin-Bizan, S., & Carrano, J. (2011). Does early paternal parenting promote low-income children's long-term cognitive skills? *Journal of Family Issues, 32*(11), 1522–1542. https://doi.org/10.1177/0192513X11402175

Coltrane, S., Parke, R. D., & Adams, M. (2004). Complexity of father involvement in low income Mexican American families. *Family Relations, 53*(2), 179–189. https://doi.org/10.1111/j.0022-2445.2004.00008

Crnic, K. A., & Greenberg, M. T. (1990). Minor parenting stresses with young children. *Child Development, 61*(5), 1628–1637. https://doi.org/10.1111/j.1467-8624.1990.tb02889

Cruz, R. A., King, K. M., Widaman, K. F., Leu, J., Cauce, A. M., & Conger, R. D. (2011). Cultural influences on positive father involvement in two-parent Mexican-origin families. *Journal of Family Psychology, 25*(5), 731–740. https://doi.org/10.1037/a0025128

Darling, N., & Steinberg, L. (1993). Parenting style as context: An integrative model. *Psychological Bulletin, 113*(3), 487–496. https://doi.org/10.1037/0033-2909.113.3.487

Davis, S. K., & Chavez, V. (1995). Hispanic househusbands. In A. M. Padilla (Ed.), *Hispanic psychology: Critical issues in theory and research* (pp. 257–287). Thousand Oaks, CA: SAGE.

Davis-Kean, P. (2005). The influence of parent education and family income on child achievement: The indirect role of parental expectations and the home environment. *Journal of Family Psychology, 19*(2), 294–304. https://doi.org/10.1037/0893-3200.19.2.294

Diaz, M. A., Miville, M. L., & Gil, N. (2013). Latino male gender role. In M. L. Miville (Ed.), *Multicultural gender roles: Applications for mental health and education* (pp. 97–132). Hoboken, NJ: Wiley.

Fagan, J. (2000). African American and Puerto Rican American parenting styles, paternal involvement, and head start children's social competence. *Merrill-Palmer Quarterly, 46*(4), 592–612.

Garro, A. (2011). Coping patterns in Latino families of children with asthma. *Journal of Pediatric Health Care, 25*(6), 347–354. https://doi.org/10.1016/j.pedhc.2010.04.005

Gordon, M. (1964). *Assimilation in American life: The role of race, religion and national origins*. Oxford, UK: Oxford University Press.

Guilamo-Ramos, V., Bowman, A. S., Santa Maria, D., Kabemba, F., & Geronimo, Y. (2017). Addressing a critical gap in U.S. national teen pregnancy prevention programs: The acceptability and feasibility of father-based sexual and reproductive health interventions for Latino adolescent males. *Journal of Adolescent Health, 62*(3). https://doi.org/10.1016/j.jadohealth.2017.08.015

Guilamo-Ramos, V., Dittus, P., Jaccard, J., Johansson, M., Bouris, A., & Acosta, N. (2007). Parenting practices among Dominican and Puerto Rican mothers. *Social Work, 52*(1), 17–30. https://doi.org/10.1093/sw/52.1.17

Hill, N. E., & Torres, K. (2010). Negotiating the American dream: The paradox of aspirations and achievement among Latino students and engagement between their families and schools. *Journal of Social Issues, 66*(1), 95–112. https://doi.org/10.1111/j.1540-4560.2009.01635.x

Hinojosa, M. S., Knapp, C. A., Madden, V. L., Huang, I., Sloyer, P., & Shenkman, E. A. (2012). Caring for children with life-threatening illnesses: Impact on White, African American, and Latino families. *Journal of Pediatric Nursing, 27*(5), 500–507. https://doi.org/10.1016/j.pedn.2011.06.013

Hofferth, S. L. (2003). Race/ethnic differences in father involvement in two-parent families: Culture, context, or economy? *Journal of Family Issues, 24*(2), 185–216. https://doi.org/10.1177/0192513X02250087

Hyslop, S. (2000). *Hispanic parental involvement in home literacy* (ERIC Digest, D158 ed.). (ERIC No. ED 446340). Retrieved from http://www.ericdigests.org/2001-3/hispanic.htm

Lamb, M. E. (2012). Mothers, fathers, families, and circumstances: Factors affecting children's adjustment. *Applied Developmental Science, 16*(2), 98–111. https://doi.org/10.1080/10888691.2012.667344

Lareau, A. (2000). *Home advantage: Social class and parental intervention in elementary education*. Lanham, MD: Rowman & Littlefield.

Liddle, H. A. (2004). Family-based therapies for adolescent alcohol and drug use: Research contributions and future research needs. *Addiction, 99*(s2), 76–92.

Liddle, H. A., Rowe, C. L., Dakof, G. A., Henderson, C. E., & Greenbaum, P. E. (2009). Multidimensional family therapy for early adolescent substance abusers: Twelve month outcomes of a randomized controlled trial. *Journal of Consulting and Clinical Psychology, 77*, 12–25.

Livas-Dlott, A., Fuller, B., Stein, G. L., Bridges, M., Mangual Figueroa, A., & Mireles, L. (2010). Commands, competence, and cariño: Maternal socialization practices in Mexican American families. *Developmental Psychology, 46*(3), 566–578. https://doi.org/10.1037/a0018016

Lopez, G. R. (2001). The value of hard work: Lessons on parent involvement from an (im)migrant household. *Harvard Educational Review, 71*(3), 416–437.

Lopez, M. H., & Velasco, G. (2010). *Childhood poverty among Hispanics sets record, leads nation*. Pew Hispanic Center. Retrieved from https://www.pewhispanic.org/2011/09/28/childhood-poverty-among-hispanics-sets-record-leads-nation/

Lovera, D., Sanderson, M., Bogle, M. L., & Vela Acosta, M. S. (2010). Evaluation of a breastfeeding peer support program for fathers of Hispanic participants in a Texas special supplemental nutrition program for women, infants, and children. *Journal of the American Dietetic Association, 110*(11), 1696–1702. https://doi.org/10.1016/j.jada.2010.08.001

Lundahl, B. W., Tollefson, D., Risser, H., & Lovejoy, M. C. (2008). A meta-analysis of father involvement in parent training. *Research on Social Work Practice, 18*(2), 97–106. https://doi.org/10.1177/1049731507309828

Mackenzie, M. J., Nicklas, E., Waldfogel, J., & Brooks-Gunn, J. (2013). Spanking and child development across the first decade of life. *Pediatrics, 132*(5), e1118. https://doi.org/10.1542/peds.2013-1227

Malin, J. L., Cabrera, N. J., & Rowe, M. L. (2014). Low-income minority mothers' and fathers' reading and children's interest: Longitudinal contributions to children's receptive vocabulary skills. *Early Childhood Research Quarterly, 29*(4), 425–432. https://doi.org/10.1016/j.ecresq.2014.04.010

Martin, A., Ryan, R. M., & Brooks-Gunn, J. (2010). When fathers' supportiveness matters most: Maternal and paternal parenting and children's school readiness. *Journal of Family Psychology, 24*(2), 145–155. https://doi.org/10.1037/a0018073

McBride, C. M., Emmons, K. M., & Lipkus, I. M. (2003). Understanding the potential of teachable moments: The case of smoking cessation. *Health Education Research, 18*(2), 156–170.

McLoyd, V. C. (1998). Socioeconomic disadvantage and child development. *American Psychologist, 53*(2), 185–204. https://doi.org/10.1037/0003-066X.53.2.185

McWayne, C., Downer, J., Campos, R., & Harris, R. (2013). Father involvement during early childhood and its association with children's early learning: A meta-analysis. *Early Education & Development, 24*(6), 898–922. https://doi.org/10.1080/10409289.2013.746932

Mirandé, A. (1991). Fatherhood and ethnicity. In F. W. Bozett & S. M. H. Hanson (Eds.), *Fatherhood and families in cultural context* (pp. 53–81). New York: Springer.

Mistry, R. S., Vandewater, E. A., Huston, A. C., & McLoyd, V. C. (2002). Economic well-being and children's social adjustment: The role of family process in an ethnically diverse low-income sample. *Child Development, 73*(3), 935–951.

Mogro-Wilson, C. (2008). The influence of parental warmth and control on Latino adolescent alcohol use. *Hispanic Journal of Behavioral Sciences, 30*(1), 89–105. https://doi.org/10.1177/0739986307310881

Mogro-Wilson, C. (2013). Parenting in Puerto Rican families. *Families in Society: The Journal of Contemporary Social Services, 94*(4), 235–241.

Mogro-Wilson, C., Hayes, C., Loomis, A., Drake, A., Martin-Peele, M., & Fifield, J. (2019). Supporting recruitment and retention of young African American and Hispanic fathers in community-based parenting interventions research. *Advances in Social Work, 18*(4), 1068–1084. https://doi.org/10.18060/22293

Mogro-Wilson, C., Rojas, R., & Haynes, J. (2016). A cultural understanding of the parenting practices of Puerto Rican fathers. *Social Work Research, 40*(4), 1–12. https://doi.org/10.1093/swr/svw019

Office of Minority Health. (2019). *Profile: Hispanic/Latino Americans*. Retrieved from: https://minorityhealth.hhs.gov/omh/browse.aspx?lvl=3&lvlid=64

Perez-Brena, N., Cookston, J. T., Fabricius, W. V., & Saenz, D. (2012). Patterns of father self-evaluations among Mexican and European American men and links to adolescent adjustment. *Fathering, 10*(2), 213. https://doi.org/10.3149/fth.1002.213

Pollak, K. I., Denman, S., Gordon, K. C., Lyna, P., Rocha, P., Brouwer, R., et al. (2010). Is pregnancy a teachable moment for smoking cessation among U.S. Latino expectant fathers? A pilot study. *Ethnicity & Health, 15*(1), 47–59. https://doi.org/10.1080/13557850903398293

Pollak, K. I., Lyna, P., Bilheimer, A. K., Gordon, K. C., Peterson, B. L., Gao, X., et al. (2015). Efficacy of a couple-based randomized controlled trial to help Latino fathers quit smoking during pregnancy and postpartum: The parejas trial. *Cancer Epidemiology, Biomarkers & Prevention, 24*(2), 379. https://doi.org/10.1158/1055-9965.EPI-14-0841

Quiñones, S. (2012). *Educated entremundos: Understanding how Puerto Rican diaspora teachers conceptualize and enact ser bien educado and being well-educated* (Doctoral dissertation).

Quiñones, S., & Kiyama, J. M. (2014). "Contra la corriente" (against the current): The role of Latino fathers in family-school engagement. *School Community Journal, 24*(1), 149–176.

Rodriguez, R. A., Henderson, C. E., Rowe, C. L., Burnett, K. F., Dakof, G. A., & Liddle, H. A. (2007). Acculturation and drug use among dually diagnosed Hispanic adolescents. *Journal of Ethnicity in Substance Abuse, 6*(2), 97–113. https://doi.org/10.1300/J233v06n02-07

Rodríguez-Brown, F. (2010). Latino families: Culture and schooling. In E. G. Murillo et al. (Eds.), *Handbook of Latinos and education: Theory, research, and practice* (pp. 350–360). New York: Routledge.

Salinas, A., Smith, J. C., & Armstrong, K. (2011). Engaging fathers in behavioral parent training: Listening to fathers' voices. *Journal of Pediatric Nursing, 26*(4), 304–311. https://doi.org/10.1016/j.pedn.2010.01.008

Sangi-Haghpeykar, H., Mehta, M., Posner, S., & Poindexter, A. (2005). Paternal influences on the timing of prenatal care among Hispanics. *Maternal and Child Health Journal, 9*(2), 159–163. https://doi.org/10.1007/s10995-005-3012-9

Shwalb, D., Shwalb, B., & Lamb, M. (2013). *Fathers in cultural context*. New York: Routledge.

Skinner, D. G., Correa, V., Skinner, M., & Bailey Jr., D. B. (2001). Role of religion in the lives of Latino families of young children with developmental delays. *American Journal on Mental Retardation, 106*(4), 297–313. https://doi.org/10.1352/0895-8017(2001)1062.0.CO;2

Sobolewski, J. M., & King, V. (2005). The importance of the coparental relationship for nonresident fathers' ties to children. *Journal of Marriage and Family, 67*(5), 1196–1212. https://doi.org/10.1111/j.1741-3737.2005.00210.x

Sotomayor-Peterson, M., Card, N. A., & Wilhelm, M. S. (2013). Fathers' care-giving and nurturing: The role of ethnicity and acculturation in European American and Hispano-Americans. *Interamerican Journal of Psychology, 47*(3), 449–455.

Taylor, B., & Behnke, A. (2005). Fathering across the border: Latino fathers in Mexico and the U.S. *Fathering, 3*(2), 1–25.

Taylor, P., Lopez, M. H., Martinez, J., & Velasco, G. (2012). *When labels don't fit: Hispanics and their views of identity.* Pew Research Center, Hispanic Trends. Retrieved from https://www.pewhispanic.org/2012/04/04/when-labels-dont-fit-hispanics-and-their-views-of-identity/

Telles, E., & Ortiz, V. (2008). *Generations of exclusion: Mexican Americans, assimilation, and race*. New York: Russell Sage Foundation.

Terriquez, V. (2012). Civic inequalities? Immigrant incorporation and Latina mothers' participation in their children's schools. *Sociological Perspectives, 55*(4), 663–682. https://doi.org/10.1525/sop.2012.55.4.663

Torres, J. B., Solberg, V. S., & Carlstrom, A. H. (2002). The myth of sameness among Latino men and their machismo. *American Journal of Orthopsychiatry, 72*(2), 163–181. https://doi.org/10.1037/0002-9432.72.2.163

Toth, J. F., & Xu, X. (1999). Ethnic and cultural diversity in fathers' involvement: A racial/ethnic comparison of African American, Hispanic, and white fathers. *Youth and Society, 31*, 76–99. https://doi.org/10.1177/0044118X99031001004

Towe-Goodman, N., Willoughby, M., Blair, C., Gustafsson, H. C., Mills-Koonce, W., & Cox, M. J. (2014). Fathers' sensitive parenting and the development of early executive functioning. *Journal of Family Psychology, 28*(6), 867–876. https://doi.org/10.1037/a0038128

Triandis, H. C., Marín, G., Lisansky, J., & Betancourt, H. (1984). Simpatía as a cultural script of Hispanics. *Journal of Personality and Social Psychology, 47*(6), 1363–1375. https://doi.org/10.1037/0022-3514.47.6.1363

Tschann, J. M., Flores, E., de Groat, C. L., Deardorff, J., & Wibbelsman, C. J. (2010). Condom negotiation strategies and actual condom use among Latino youth. *Journal of Adolescent Health, 47*(3), 254–262. https://doi.org/10.1016/j.jadohealth.2010.01.018

Turney, K., & Kao, G. (2009). Barriers to school involvement: Are immigrant parents disadvantaged? *The Journal of Educational Research, 102*(4), 257–271. https://doi.org/10.3200/JOER.102.4.257-271

U.S. Bureau of Labor Statistics. (2017). *Labor force characteristics by race and ethnicity*. Retrieved from https://www.bls.gov/

U.S. Census Bureau. (2018). *Current population survey, annual social and economic supplement, 2018*. Retrieved from https://www.census.gov/data/tables/2018/demo/hispanic-origin/2018-cps.html

Yeung, W., Sandberg, J., Davis-Kean, P., & Hofferth, S. (2001). Children's time with fathers in intact families. *Journal of Marriage and Family, 63*(1), 136–154.

Yu, J. J., Lucero-Liu, A., Gamble, W. C., Taylor, A. R., Christensen, D. H., & Modry-Mandell, K. (2008). Partner effects of Mexican cultural values: The couple and parenting relationships. *The Journal of Psychology, 142*(2), 169–192. https://doi.org/10.3200/JRLP.142.2.169-192

Fathering Across Military Deployment and Reintegration

33

Tova B. Walsh and Katherine L. Rosenblum

The total number of US military personnel is close to 3.5 million, and nearly 40% of US service members are parents, most of them fathers (U.S. Department of Defense, 2018). The largest percentage of the 1.65 million American children who have at least one parent serving in the military are under 6 years of age (U.S. Department of Defense, 2018). Multiple deployments are common among military personnel since 2001 (IOM, 2013), and families, including many young children, have cycled through deployments alongside service members (Bonds, Baiocchi, & McDonald, 2010). A 2013 Institute of Medicine report on "The Assessment of Readjustment Needs of Veterans, Service Members, and Their Families" highlighted the pressing need for effective support for military families with young children (http://nationalacademies.org/hmd/Reports/2013/Returning-Home-from-Iraq-and-Afghanistan.aspx).

The normative challenges faced by fathers of young children and by deploying military service members are compounded when early fatherhood and military deployment intersect. New fathers experience significant developmental demands, including developing an identity as a father, establishing a co-parenting relationship with a partner, and learning to balance their new role and responsibilities as a father with existing roles and responsibilities at home and at work (Roy, 2005). Surrounding a deployment, service members face multiple challenges, including extended separation from family members and reconnecting with family members after long separation. These challenges are reflected in elevated rates of mental health symptoms and relationship stress, child maltreatment, divorce, and suicide in military families during and following deployment (Flake, Davis, Johnson, & Middleton, 2009; Gibbs, Martin, Kupper, & Johnson, 2007; Hoge, Auchterlonie, & Milliken, 2006; Hoge et al., 2004; Lapierre, Schwegler, & LaBauve, 2007; Gibbs et al., 2007; Rentz et al., 2007; Sayer et al., 2010; Smith et al., 2008). The disruption to relationships incurred by a military deployment adds complexity in the formative period of early fatherhood, and the emotional and practical demands of early fatherhood further complicate the experiences of deployment and reunification, already a time of heightened stress and transition.

Service member-fathers of young children have reported significant levels of parenting stress and have identified unique challenges associated with their deployment, including managing separations and reunions that may involve

T. B. Walsh (✉)
Sandra Rosenbaum School of Social Work, University of Wisconsin, Madison, WI, USA
e-mail: tbwalsh@wisc.edu

K. L. Rosenblum
Departments of Psychiatry and Obstetrics & Gynecology, University of Michigan, Ann Arbor, MI, USA

H. E. Fitzgerald et al. (eds.), *Handbook of Fathers and Child Development*,
https://doi.org/10.1007/978-3-030-51027-5_33

significant periods of their child's early development, reconnecting with young children, adapting expectations between military and family life, and co-parenting across periods of extended separation (Walsh et al., 2014). A service member-father who deploys when his child is an infant and returns home to a toddler may experience reunification as requiring him to get to know an entirely different child. Early development is marked by a rapid progression of physical and cognitive changes, and consequently, the child's evolving needs may require markedly different parenting behavior from the newly returned father, in comparison to the parenting behavior that was responsive to his child's needs at the time that he deployed.

Some populations of military fathers face additional challenges in navigating and adjusting to early separations and the return to life at home and day-to-day parenting of young children. Fathers in dual military and single-parent families may not be able to rely on a partner's availability to manage the home front during their deployment. Fathers who experience psychological and/or physical injury during a deployment must contend with the impacts of their injury even as they seek to reestablish relationships and readjust to the home environment. Relative to active duty service members, fathers who serve in the National Guard and Reserve Component often face added challenges associated with geographic dispersion, including greater isolation and reduced access to services.

A growing, but still limited, body of research addresses the family impacts of deployment and supports for families surrounding a deployment. Due to the high proportion of young children in military-connected families, young children are disproportionately impacted by a father's military deployment. Separation from a primary caregiver, transitions and associated stress, heightened distress, and emotional symptoms in parents place young children at particular risk (Jensen, Martin, & Watanabe, 1996; Rosen, Teitelbaum, & Westhuis, 1993); yet few resources are available for young children and their caregivers during and following deployment. In recent years, a number of preventive interventions have been developed to support families impacted by deployment-related separations, but relatively few have focused on very young children.

This chapter will explore the experiences of fathers parenting young children across the "deployment cycle," considering what is known about fathering in the pre-deployment period, during deployment, and post-deployment as fathers and their families are reunited and readjust. Early relationship disruptions pose risks to children's social, emotional, and cognitive development (Shonkoff, Garner, & Committee on Psychosocial Aspects of Child and Family Health, 2012). Reuniting brings relief and joy; yet, it is also stressful as families begin the extended process of reestablishing relationships, roles, and routines. This chapter will describe the resilience of military fathers and their families, as well as the challenges they face across the deployment cycle. There is increasing evidence that healing and reconnection are possible and relationships can recover following disruptions (Dodge, Gonzalez, Muzik, & Rosenblum, 2018; Julian, Muzik, Kees, Valenstein, & Rosenblum, 2018).

Fathering in the Pre-deployment Period

During the pre-deployment period, service member-fathers and their families prepare for the changes ahead. In this time of transition, as fathers and their families anticipate the coming separation, they may experience anticipatory worry and heightened tension. The time between notification of deployment and departure varies, and both long and short windows are stressful. Waiting to deploy may feel like being stuck in a holding pattern (Lapp et al., 2010); yet, shorter notice limits time available to make preparations. During this time, deploying fathers grapple with concerns about family and household functioning and child and family well-being in their absence, as well as what they themselves may experience during deployment (DeVoe, Ross, & Paris, 2012;

Maguen, Turcotte, Peterson, et al., 2008; Renshaw, Rodrigues, & Jones, 2009). Specific challenges include preparing their children (and partners, if partnered) as well as themselves for physical separation, trying to figure out how to sustain emotional connections across distance, and confronting their own and their children's (and partner's) fear that they might not return. These challenges have a particular character with very young children, who do not have the cognitive capacity or verbal skills to understand the impending separation and talk about its meaning to them or ways of coping.

DeVoe et al. (2012) theorized a "parenting cycle of deployment," wherein "Looking Ahead" and "Saying Goodbye" are characteristic processes of the pre-deployment period. Looking Ahead involves considering and making efforts to ensure the needs of families will be met during the deployment, for example, making childcare and other arrangements to fill in the responsibilities usually filled by the deploying service member. Simultaneous with practical preparations, families make emotional preparations for deployment. Saying Goodbye is the culmination of preparing to be apart and involves facing the service member's actual departure.

Pre-deployment training itself may require extended time away from home, and fathers and families may experience tension as service member-fathers simultaneously make preparations on the home front and take part in deployment preparations with their unit. In this stressful context, service member-fathers may withdraw, emotionally disconnecting as a way of protecting themselves against potentially overwhelming feelings about leaving their family for deployment (Willerton, Schwarz, Wadsworth, & Oglesby, 2011). Fathers who are partnered frequently rely on their partner to support them and their children during times of adjustment across the deployment cycle (Dayton, Walsh, Muzik, Erwin, & Rosenblum, 2015; Walsh et al., 2014). Single fathers and fathers who are typically the primary caregiver in their household face heightened challenges during this period of practical and emotional preparation for deployment.

Fathering During Deployment

Despite the profound challenges of deployment separation, many military families demonstrate positive adaptation and coping across the deployment cycle (Park, 2011; Saltzman, Pynoos, Lester, Layne, & Beardslee, 2013). However, many families struggle. Over the span of an extended separation from a young child, fathers miss important events and developmental milestones as well as daily involvement in parenting. This can be a source of distress both during and after deployment (Newby, McCarroll, Ursano, Fan, Shigemura, & Tucker-Harris, 2005; Walsh et al., 2014). High levels of parenting stress make it difficult to effectively manage family roles throughout and following deployment (Lincoln, Swift, & Shorteno-Fraser, 2008), and deployment is associated with increased behavioral problems among the children of a deployed parent (Burrell, Adams, Durand, & Castro, 2006; Chartrand, Frank, White, & Shope, 2008; Esposito-Smythers et al., 2011; Lester & Flake, 2013). Specifically, in very young children, responses to deployment may include difficulty eating or sleeping, regressing to earlier behaviors, being clingy, or acting out (Pincus, House, Christensen, & Adler, 2001).

Immediately after departing for deployment, fathers may feel sadness and guilt regarding separation from their family yet also experience relief that the difficult and tense period of preparing to deploy has passed (Pincus et al., 2001; Weins & Boss, 2006). After the early weeks of deployment are complete, the emotional disorganization experienced initially is typically replaced by a sense of stability as the deployed father (and his family at home) adjusts to separation. Both the deployed father and his family at home establish new routines.

His primary focus while in theater must be on his military duties, but the deployed father may be preoccupied with child and family well-being at home (MacDermid et al., 2005; Renshaw et al., 2009). Parenting stress can impact a father's ability to carry out his duties, and it is thus imperative that deployed fathers find ways to limit or manage stress so that it does not undermine their capacity to ensure the safety of themselves and others. Sustaining connection to the child and family at home is important to fathers and families but largely dependent on the extent to which communication is logistically possible and the parent/caregiver at home is able and willing to facilitate contact between the deployed father and the child (ren) at home (Schachman, 2010; Willerton et al. 2011). Phone and online communication facilitate a sense of connection and involvement from afar, but access to such communication varies, and the age/verbal skills/attention span of the young child may further constrain opportunities to connect and communicate virtually.

While the at-home parent/caregiver bears the burden of responding to children's questions and distress, the deployed father bears the burden of relinquishing control and recognizing the new limits to his ability to be present for his children, knowledgeable of their experiences, and involved in their care. Although direct interaction with children is necessarily limited during a deployment, many deployed fathers do not disengage from their children but rather remain psychologically engaged and maintain a sense of responsibility for children's well-being (MacDermid et al., 2005). Others, however, withhold involvement as a means of self-protection, finding emotional distance necessary in order to tolerate physical separation and remain focused on military duties (Willerton et al., 2011). Some fathers report that frequent communication helps to alleviate psychological distress during separation (Schachman, 2010), while others find that it is a painful reminder of what they are missing (Willerton et al., 2011). Research suggests that regular communication is valuable for sustaining relationships, limiting risk for attachment insecurity, and promoting successful reintegration (DeVoe et al., 2012).

Both excitement and unease may mount as deployment draws to an end. Reunification is eagerly anticipated but also prompts questions and worries about when and how to explain and prepare young children for the service member-father to reenter the family, how the child will respond, and whether very young children will recognize their father after an extended separation (DeVoe et al., 2012). Informal and formal support for families can promote individual and family coping, adjustment, and well-being (Chapin, 2011; Flake et al., 2009; Maholmes, 2012; Rosenblum et al., 2015), with community support and resources more readily available to families located on an active duty base than families of fathers who serve in the National Guard and Reserve.

Fathering Post-Deployment

Reunification is often joyful; yet, it also places significant stress on families. Normative challenges upon reunification include the reestablishment of relationships, roles, and routines. These challenges are compounded when a returning service member is coping with a service-related physical injury or psychological distress, or when family members are experiencing mental health problems. It is estimated that 25–40% of service members returning from Afghanistan and Iraq experience symptoms that suggest a need for mental health treatment (Milliken, Auchterlonie, & Hoge, 2007; Seal, Bertenthal, Miner, Sen, & Marmar, 2007; Seal et al., 2009), and rates of mental health problems among military spouses are nearly as high as those among service members themselves (Eaton et al., 2008; Mansfield et al., 2010; Renshaw et al., 2009).

Traumatic brain injury (Lew, Poole, Alvarez, & Moore, 2005) and post-traumatic stress disorder (Tanielian & Jaycox, 2008) are among the most common diagnoses for returning service members, and these conditions add difficulty to the inherent challenges of returning to daily parenting and restoring parent-child and co-parenting relationships (Gorman, Fitzgerald, & Blow, 2010). Service members returning from combat deployment also are at increased risk for substance use problems (Jacobson et al., 2008), and this too can interfere with effective and sensitive parenting. The impact of deployment and reunification on young children is heavily influenced by parental stress and corresponding sensitivity to child needs (Alink et al., 2009; De Wolff,

& van IJzendoorn, 1997; Hirsh-Pasek & Burchinal, 2006; Hoffman, Marvin, Cooper, & Powell, 2006; Lincoln et al., 2008), and studies have found increased internalizing and externalizing behaviors among children of deployed parents (Chartrand et al., 2008; Flake et al., 2009). However, very little is yet known about the influence of combat-related physical and mental health injuries on parenting and relationship processes in infants, toddlers, and young children (Lieberman & Van Horn, 2013).

At the same time that service member-fathers are making their own adjustment, their children and families require support for their individual and collective processes of adjustment following reunification. For fathers of young children, the post-deployment return to civilian life poses the challenge of reconnecting with a child too young to have the cognitive capacity to understand a deployment-related separation, leaving them more vulnerable to experiencing the dysregulating effects associated with separation and loss (Bowlby, 1994). Reunification requires reestablishing connections with a child who has undergone significant developmental transitions and who, by nature of age, may not communicate directly, may exhibit challenging behaviors, and yet is dependent on parents for meeting emotional needs.

In qualitative research, returning fathers of young children describe heavy reliance on their spouse/partner for support in the post-deployment period, including support for their reengagement in daily parenting and managing their own mental health and responses to challenging child behavior (Dayton et al., 2015; Walsh et al., 2014). Readjusting from the structured lifestyle of deployment to the dynamics of home life with a young child can be difficult. In the words of one father:

> Um, you know, I'm a military guy and I, I emphasize on discipline, so that's my hard point is not realizing the age factor and they're not soldiers. (Walsh et al., 2014)

Trauma symptoms experienced by returning service member-fathers may compound the difficulty of tolerating a young child's age-typical distress, upset, or demandingness (Walsh et al., 2014).

The "post-deployment" period encompasses the short-term experience of reunion and the longer-term establishment of a new family equilibrium that accommodates the family's present reality, including the child(ren)'s current developmental stage(s) and capacities and deployment's impacts on the service member-father and other family members. Immediately upon returning home, families may experience a honeymoon period. Subsequently, reintegration may require patience, adjustment, and renegotiation as family members work to restore relationships and establish a "new normal." A level of stabilization is achieved as new routines are established, but difficulty related to enduring impacts of deployment may be maintained over an extended period, with returned service members experiencing family challenges as many as 3 years after deployment (Sayer et al., 2010). Extended family support and community support are often offered during the deployment, but the need for support continues during the extended period of reintegration.

Military fathers of young children report multiple challenges as they reengage in parenting after deployment, as well as strong motivation to be the best parents they can be (Walsh et al., 2014). Challenges identified by fathers include reconnecting with their young child after time apart, a continuing sense of loss about missed time together, adapting expectations from military to family life, and co-parenting across the deployment cycle. Fathers express the desire to increase their parenting skills and knowledge, build their capacity to provide affection and nurture to their children, learn to more effectively manage their temper, and connect with and learn from others who can relate to their experiences. In the words of one father:

> I want to be a better parent, I want to learn to be a better parent… When I came home from the Marine Corps, uh, I really had a hard time adjusting to it. And so, um, you know coming from a structured lifestyle, being told what to do, how to do it, when to do it, um, to coming home and being a full-time dad, um, and everything else, I didn't know how to adjust to it. I didn't—I didn't know what to do. And I didn't spend as much one-on-one

> time with her as I should have. I'm still learning. (Walsh et al., 2014)

Fathers recognize the impact of their military service on their attitudes toward their child and their parenting and express profound commitment to foster strength and resilience in their children (Dayton et al., 2015).

> I think when I came back from Iraq, I was scared and still am … at how easy it is for me to lose him. Um, and I'm, I'm … you know, I'm afraid for him to go out there [into the world] and put himself out there, but I encourage him… (Dayton et al., 2015)

In a study of fathers who participated in the Strong Military Families program (Rosenblum et al., 2015)—a multifamily parenting and self-care skills group that aims to strengthen protective factors and promote military family resilience in the reunification period—service member-fathers reported two primary hopes for their program participation (Dodge et al., 2018). They wanted to strengthen connection within their family and build connection with other families, and they wanted to gain insight into their own family and families in general. These findings underscore the commitment of military fathers to strengthening relationships with their children and understanding the dynamics at play within families following a deployment. Notably, fathers with PTSD feared that stressors they faced might impede their ability to sustain participation in the program, demonstrating the need for comprehensive support for multi-stressed fathers and their families surrounding a deployment.

Supports for Military-Connected Fathers, Young Children, and Families

Responsive to the need for family and community support across the deployment cycle, including support during the extended period that follows homecoming, a number of programs have been developed for fathers (and mothers) to promote adjustment in military and veteran families with young children (e.g., Gewirtz, Pinna, Hanson, & Brockberg, 2014; Lester et al., 2011). A variety of family supports are available to families on military installations, and these include both the informal supports inherent to living in proximity to a density of military families and the corresponding sense of community and camaraderie around parenting across the deployment cycle, as well as more formal supports, including, for example, full family health care, family housing, accredited and affordable day care with extended hours, programs and activity centers for children, and new parent support programs. Fewer resources for support are available to fathers and their families, including some active duty as well as National Guard and Reserve families, who live off base, in communities throughout the country. A small but increasing number of programs exist to support military families in the community, with varied emphasis on specific periods in the deployment cycle or spanning the full cycle from pre-deployment through reintegration.

In this section, we highlight several of these programs aimed at supporting family health and resilience among military and veteran fathers of young children. A consistent goal across many of these programs is to mitigate the potentially negative impacts of challenges faced by military families by strengthening protective factors such as familial and military social supports, parental well-being, and access to care. Evaluation of many of these programs has indicated high levels of satisfaction, as well as significant improvements in mental health and parenting for the service members and their parenting partners (DeVoe et al., 2012; Dodge et al., 2018; Julian, Muzik, Kees, Valenstein, & Rosenblum, 2018; Lester et al., 2011).

Two of these interventions are specifically targeted at military families with younger children: Strong Military Families (Rosenblum et al., 2015; Rosenblum & Muzik, 2014) and Strong Families Strong Forces (DeVoe et al., 2012). Both Strong Military Families and Strong Families Strong Forces share a focus on support for parenting infants, toddlers, and young children, an invitation for both the father and his parenting partner/spouse to be involved, and an emphasis on enhancing parental reflective functioning or insight regarding their own and their child's thoughts, feelings, and emotions, including those regarding deployment and reconnection.

Strong Families Strong Forces (SFSF) is an in-home intervention designed specifically for families with young children who have experienced deployment and is delivered by a trained clinician. The **intervention** is comprised of eight modules that aim to reduce **parenting** stress and parental mental health concerns and to enhance parental capacity for reflective functioning. Modules include foci such as military identity, parental/child deployment narratives, co-parenting, and parental self-awareness. Evaluation of SFSF using a waitlist control design indicates improvements in key domains including parenting stress and reflective capacity, particularly for those with mental health symptoms (DeVoe, Paris, Emmert-Aronson, Ross, & Acker, 2017).

Strong Military Families (SMF) is a resilience enhancing parenting and mental health program adapted from an existing civilian program (Muzik et al., 2015; Rosenblum et al., 2017). To increase access for families, SMF has two versions—a homebased psychoeducational materials program ("Homebased") and a multifamily therapeutic group ("Multifamily Group"). The SMF Multifamily Group includes a parent group along with a simultaneous "child team" in which children engage in child-directed play with team members. The parent group provides parent education, especially focused on the parent-child relationship, with specific attention to the experiences of military families with young children. The group context increases social support and social connectedness among participants. The SMF Homebased program consists of mailed psychoeducational materials that are parallel to the information that is provided in the Multifamily Group.

SMF is based on five key therapeutic "pillars" and is specifically tailored to military family experience, with a particular focus on families connected to the National Guard and Reserves. (1) Guard and Reserve families are often geographically dispersed and isolated; thus, *Social Support* is enhanced by creating a shared group experience, with opportunities for informal relationship building during shared mealtime and the parent group. (2) Children and parents experience significant challenges around separation and reunion associated with deployment cycles; the *Parenting Education* curriculum provides information about typical reactions of preschool-aged children and teaches strategies for sensitively responding to young children's emotional and relational needs. In the parent group, participants are introduced to key topics in parenting and child development, observe video interactions and apply concepts learned, engage in activities designed to develop and practice skills, and reflect on interactions with their own children. An integral concept is helping parents understand that while deployment poses challenges for the parent-child relationship, everyday experiences provide opportunities for nurturing, restoring balance, and repairing smaller disruptions and that this is the process by which relationships are restored and strengthened. Another core aspect of the curriculum is attention to the need for "balanced parenting," as we encourage parents as they strive to integrate being both strong and kind into their everyday interactions with their children, including "balanced" approaches to discipline. (3) *Child Routines and Parent-Child Interaction* are supported by a curriculum that emphasizes creating safe, predictable routines, acknowledging "goodbyes" when parents leave for their class, developmentally appropriate play-based activities, and observation of and support for reunions when parents return from their group. These brief separations and reunions provide an opportunity for real-time practice, negotiating feelings about separations and return, and helping parents identify and respond to their children's needs for support. Parents are encouraged to anticipate, observe, and reflect upon these separations and reunions, as well as identify ways they might want to "try something new" to address their children's feelings during separation/reunion at the next session. (4) Service members and spouses report high levels of parenting stress and PTSD. The *Self-Care/Stress-Reduction* curriculum addresses parents' needs for strategies for reducing their own levels of stress. Each parent group session includes hands-on practice of evidence-based stress-reduction "skills" including guided breathing, relaxation, or mindfulness. This has the added benefit of helping parents prepare for reuniting with their children in a calmer, more relaxed state. (5) Individual meetings with parents are held midway through the 10-week intervention to provide opportunities for *Connecting Families to Care*, including individualized referrals to relevant community resources, including mental health treatment when indicated.

Prior evaluation suggests that participation in SMF is associated with high levels of satisfaction and improvements in parenting behavior, reflective functioning, and parent mental health (DeVoe et al., 2012; Julian et al., 2018; Julian, Muzik, Kees, Valenstein, & Rosenblum, 2018). For example, fathers noted that participation in SMF increased feelings of hope and motivation, and reduced feelings of isolation, in regard to military family experience. As described by one father (Dodge et al., 2018):

> "I think it was hopeful. You know, it was kind of, it made me feel like I was less of a person being all by themselves trying to accomplish this monumental task of bringing a kid up but. It showed me commonalities that I shared with the other parents and stuff like that…"

In addition to the programs focused more exclusively on the experiences of military families with young children, two other interventions target military families with children in a broader age range, extending beyond the infant and preschool age period. These include Families OverComing Under Stress (FOCUS), a resilience-enhancing program for military families with children aged 3 to 17 (Lester et al., 2011), and ADAPT, a group-based Web-enhanced parenting program for military families with children ages 4 to 12 (Gewirtz, DeGarmo, & Zamir, 2017). FOCUS supports families in developing a narrative about their experience of deployment and, in addition, provides psychoeducation and coping strategies including an emphasis on emotion regulation, communication, problem-solving, goal setting, and managing trauma and stress reminders. Components of the program are designed for service members, spouses, and children and are delivered in person on installation or via technology (Lester et al., 2011). The After Deployment, Adaptive Parenting Tools (ADAPT) intervention is a 14-week group-based, Web-enhanced parenting program for military families with children ages 4 to 12 (Gewirtz et al., 2017). It is adapted from the Parent Management Training Oregon Model. Evaluation of ADAPT indicates that participation in the program is associated with improvements in parenting self-efficacy, child behavior, and parent mental health.

In addition to intervention programs to promote resilience in military families with young children, resources have been developed and distributed for military families by national organizations such as Zero to Three (www.zerotothree.org), including resources (e.g., books, apps, and materials) for parents to support "Families on the Homefront" and for early childhood providers working with military and veteran families with very young children.

While each of the programs described in this chapter address critical issues facing service member-fathers of young children, there continues to be a need to increase the reach and impact of supports, particularly for fathers with young children who are geographically dispersed and may not have access to resources housed on military installations (IOM, 2013). The promising data in regard to the efficacy of existing programs suggests that future work should focus on implementation strategies that expand the reach and impact of such programming to best serve the thousands of military families with young children living across the United States and around the globe.

Summary and Key Points

Men who are both military service members and fathers of young children face a complex set of demands before, during, and after deployment. Research demonstrates the profound commitment of service member-fathers to both their military and family roles and responsibilities and illuminates both the resilience of many military fathers and families and the scope of the challenges they face. The specific challenges faced by service member-fathers of young children at each stage of the deployment cycle and the limitations of existing resources for meeting the needs of fathers and families, particularly those who do not live on military installations, underscore the need for expanded services designed to meet the needs of military families with young children across the deployment cycle. There remains a need for continued research to consider the distinct experiences and support needs of diverse service member-fathers of young children and their families (e.g., single fathers, fathers in dual military partnerships, fathers who deploy when children are infants, toddlers, or preschoolers). Services that are responsive to the distinct experiences and needs of service member-fathers of young children have the potential to strengthen father well-being, parenting, father-child and co-parenting relationships, and child and family well-being.

References

Alink, L. R. A., Mesman, J., van Zeijl, J., Stolk, M. N., Juffer, F., Bakermans-Kranenburg, M. J., et al. (2009). Maternal sensitivity moderates the relation between negative discipline and aggression in early childhood. *Social Development, 18*(1), 99–120.

Bonds, T. M., Baiocchi, D., & McDonald, L. L. (2010). *Army deployments to OIF and OEF*. Santa Monica, CA: RAND Corporation. https://www.rand.org/pubs/documented_briefings/DB587.html

Burrell, L. M., Adams, G. A., Durand, D. B., & Castro, C. A. (2006). The impact of military lifestyle demands on Well-being, army, and family outcomes. *Armed Forces & Society, 33*(1), 43–58.

Bowlby, J. (1994). Pathological mourning and childhood mourning. In R.V. Frankiel (Ed.), *Essential papers on object loss* (pp. 185–221). New York: New York University Press.

Chartrand, M. M., Frank, D. A., White, L. F., & Shope, T. R. (2008). Effect of parents' wartime deployment on the behavior of young children in military families. *Archives of Pediatrics & Adolescent Medicine, 162*(11), 1009–1014.

Chapin, M. G. (2011). Family resilience and the fortunes of war. *Social Work in Health Care, 50*(7), 527–542.

Dayton, C. J., Walsh, T. B., Muzik, M., Erwin, M., & Rosenblum, K. L. (2015). Strong, safe, and secure: Negotiating early fathering and military service across the deployment cycle. *Infant Mental Health Journal, 35*(5), 509–520.

DeVoe, E. R., Paris, R., Emmert-Aronson, B., Ross, A., & Acker, M. (2017). A randomized clinical trial of postdeployment parenting intervention for service members and their families with young children. *Psychological Trauma: Theory, Research, Practice, and Policy, 9*, 25–34.

DeVoe, E. R., Ross, A., & Paris, R. (2012). The parenting cycle of deployment. *Military Medicine, 177*(2), 184–190.

De Wolff, M., & van IJzendoorn, M. H. (1997). Sensitivity and attachment: A meta-analysis on parental antecedents of infant attachment. *Child Development, 68*, 571–591.

Dodge, J., Gonzalez, M. M., Muzik, M., & Rosenblum, K. (2018). Fathers' perspectives on strengthening military families: A mixed method evaluation of a 10-week resilience building program. *Clinical Social Work Journal, 46*, 145–155.

Eaton, K. M., Hoge, C. W., Messer, S. C., Whitt, A. A., Cabrera, O. A., McGurk, D., et al. (2008). Prevalence of mental health problems, treatment need, and barriers to care among primary care-seeking spouses of military service members involved in Iraq and Afghanistan deployments. *Military Medicine, 173*(11), 1051–1056.

Esposito-Smythers, C., Wolff, J., Lemmon, K. M., Bodzy, M., Swenson, R. R., & Spirito, A. (2011). Military youth and the deployment cycle: Emotional health consequences and recommendations for intervention. *Journal of Family Psychology, 25*(4), 497.

Flake, E. M., Davis, B. E., Johnson, P. L., & Middleton, L. S. (2009). The psychosocial effects of deployment on military children. *Journal of Developmental and Behavioral Pediatrics, 30*(4), 271–178.

Gewirtz, A. H., DeGarmo, D. S., & Zamir, O. (2017). After deployment, adaptive parenting tools: 1-year outcomes of an evidence-based parenting program for military families following deployment. *Prevention Science, 19*, 589–599.

Gewirtz, A. H., Pinna, K. L., Hanson, S. K., & Brockberg, D. (2014). Promoting parenting to support reintegrating military families: After deployment, adaptive parenting tools. *Psychological Services, 11*(1), 31–40.

Gibbs, D. A., Martin, S. L., Kupper, L. L., & Johnson, R. E. (2007). Child maltreatment in enlisted soldiers' families during combat-related deployments. *JAMA, 298*(5), 528–535.

Gorman, L. A., Fitzgerald, H. E., & Blow, A. J. (2010). Parental combat injury and early child development: A conceptual model for differentiating effects of visible and invisible injuries. *Psychiatric Quarterly, 81*, 1–21.

Hirsh-Pasek, K., & Burchinal, M. (2006). Mother and caregiver sensitivity over time: Predicting language and academic outcomes with variable- and person-centered approaches. *Merrill-Palmer Quarterly, 52*(3), 449–485.

Hoffman, K. T., Marvin, R. S., Cooper, G., & Powell, B. (2006). Changing toddlers' and preschoolers' attachment classifications: The circle of security intervention. *Journal of Consulting and Clinical Psychology, 74*, 1017–1026.

Hoge, C. W., Auchterlonie, J. L., & Milliken, C. S. (2006). Mental health problems, use of mental health services, and attrition from military service after returning from deployment to Iraq or Afghanistan. *JAMA, 295*(9), 1023–1032.

Hoge, C. W., Castro, C. A., Messer, S. C., McGurk, D., Cotting, D. I., & Koffman, R. L. (2004). Combat duty in Iraq and Afghanistan, mental health problems, and barriers to care. *New England Journal of Medicine, 2004*(351), 13–22.

IOM (Institute of Medicine). (2013). *Returning home from Iraq and Afghanistan: Assessment of readjustment needs of veterans, service members, and their families*. Washington, DC: The National Academies Press. http://nationalacademies.org/hmd/Reports/2013/Returning-Home-from-Iraq-and-Afghanistan.aspx

Jacobson, I. G., Ryan, M. A. K., Hooper, T. L., Smith, T. C., Amoroso, P. J., Boyko, E. J., et al. (2008). Alcohol use and alcohol-related problems before and after military combat deployment. *Journal of American Medical Association, 300*, 663–675.

Julian, M., Muzik, M., Kees, M., Valenstein, M., Dexter, C., & Rosenblum, K. (2018). Intervention effects on reflectivity explain change in positive parenting in military families with young children. *Journal of Family Psychology, 32*, 804–815.

Julian, M., Muzik, M., Kees, M., Valenstein, M., & Rosenblum, K. L. (2018). Strong military families intervention enhances parenting reflectivity and representations in families with young children. *Infant Mental Health Journal, 39*(1), 106–118.

Jensen, P. S., Martin, D., & Watanabe, H. (1996). Children's response to parental separation during Operation Desert Storm. *Journal of the American Academy of Child & Adolescent Psychiatry, 35*(4), 433–441.

Lapierre, C. B., Schwegler, A. F., & LaBauve, B. J. (2007). Posttraumatic stress and depression symptoms in soldiers returning from combat operations in Iraq and Afghanistan. *Journal of Traumatic Stress, 20*(6), 933–943.

Lapp, C. A., Taft, L. B., Tollefson, T., Hoepner, A., Moore, K., & Divyak, K. (2010). Stress and coping on the home front: Guard and reserve spouses searching for a new normal. *Journal of Family Nursing, 16*(1), 45–67.

Lester, P., Mogil, C., Saltzman, W., Woodward, K., Nash, W., Leskin, G., et al. (2011). Families overcoming under stress: Implementing family-centered prevention for military families facing wartime deployments and combat operational stress. *Military Medicine, 176*, 19–25.

Lester, P., & Flake, L. C. E. (2013). How wartime military service affects children and families. *The Future of Children, 23*(2), 121–141.

Lew, H. L., Poole, J. H., Alvarez, S., & Moore, W. (2005). Soldiers with occult traumatic brain injury. *American Journal of Physical Medicine & Rehabilitation, 84*(6), 393–8.53.

Lieberman, A. F., & Van Horn, P. (2013). Infants and young children in military families: A conceptual model for intervention. *Clinical Child and Family Psychology Review, 16*(3), 282–293.

Lincoln, A., Swift, E., & Shorteno-Fraser, M. (2008). Psychological adjustment and treatment of children and families with parents deployed in military combat. *Journal of Clinical Psychology, 2008., 64*(8), 984–992.

MacDermid, S., Schwarz, R., Faber, A., Adkins, J., Mishkind, M., & Weiss, H. (2005). Military fathers on the front lines. In W. Marsiglio, K. Roy, & G. L. Fox (Eds.), *Situated fathering: A focus on physical and social spaces*. Oxford, UK: Rowman & Littlefield Publishers.

Maguen, S., Turcotte, D. M., Peterson, A. L., et al. (2008). Description of risk and resilience factors among military medical personnel before deployment to Iraq. *Military Medicine, 173*(1), 1–9.25.

Mansfield, A. J., Kaufman, J. S., Marshall, S. W., Gaynes, B. N., Morrissey, J. P., & Engel, C. C. (2010). Deployment and the use of mental health services among U.S. Army wives. *New England Journal of Medicine, 362*, 101–109.

Milliken, C. S., Auchterlonie, J. L., & Hoge, C. W. (2007). Longitudinal assessment of mental health problems among active and reserve component soldiers returning from the Iraq war. *JAMA, 298*(18), 2141–2148.

Muzik, M., Rosenblum, K. L., Alfafara, E. A., Schuster, M. M., Miller, N. M., Waddell, R. M., et al. (2015). Mom power: Preliminary outcomes of a group intervention to improve mental health and parenting among high-risk mothers. *Archives of Women's Mental Health, 18*(3), 507–521.

Maholmes, V. (2012). Adjustment of children and youth in military families: Toward developmental understandings. *Child Development Perspectives, 6*(4), 430–435.

Newby, J. H., McCarroll, J. E., Ursano, R. J., Fan, Z., Shigemura, J., & Tucker-Harris, Y. (2005). Positive and Negative Consequences of a Military Deployment. *Military Medicine, 170*(10), 815–819.

Park, N. (2011). Military children and families: Strengths and challenges during peace and war. *American Psychologist, 66*(1), 65–72.

Pincus, S. H., House, R., Christensen, J., & Adler, L. E. (2001). The emotional cycle of deployment: A military family perspective. *US Army Medical Department Journal, 4*(5), 15–23.

Renshaw, K. D., Rodrigues, C. S., & Jones, D. H. (2009). Combat exposure, psychological symptoms, and marital satisfaction in National Guard soldiers who served in operation Iraqi freedom from 2005 to 2006. *Anxiety, Stress & Coping, 22*(1), 101–115.

Rentz, E. D., Marshall, S. W., Loomis, D., Casteel, C., Martin, S. L., & Gibbs, D. A. (2007). Effect of deployment on the occurrence of child maltreatment in military and nonmilitary families. *American Journal of Epidemiology, 165*(10), 1199–1206.

Rosenblum, K. L., & Muzik, M. (2014). STRoNG military families: A multifamily group intervention for military families with young children. *Psychiatric Services, 65*, 399–400.

Rosenblum, K. L., Muzik, M., Morelen, D. M., Alfafara, E. A., Miller, N. M., Waddell, R. M., et al. (2017). A community-based randomized controlled trial of mom power parenting intervention for mothers with interpersonal trauma histories and their young children. *Archives of Women's Mental Health, 20*(5), 673–686.

Rosenblum, K. L., Muzik, M., Waddell, R., Thompson, S., Rosenberg, L., Masini, G., et al. (2015). Strong military families program: A multifamily group approach to strengthening family resilience. *ZERO TO THREE, 36*(2), 8–14.

Roy, K. M. (2005). Transitions on the margins of work and family life for low-income African-American fathers. *Journal of Family and Economic Issues, 26*(1), 77–100.

Rosen, L. N., Teitelbaum, J. M., & Westhuis, D. J. (1993). Children's reactions to the Desert Storm deployment: Initial findings from a survey of Army families. *Military Medicine, 158*(7), 465–469.

Saltzman, W. R., Pynoos, R. S., Lester, P., Layne, C. M., & Beardslee, W. R. (2013). Enhancing family resilience through family narrative coconstruction. *Clinical Child and Family Psychology Review, 16*(3), 294–310.

Sayer, N. A., Noorbaloochi, S., Frazier, P., Carlson, K., Gravely, A., & Murdoch, M. (2010). Reintegration problems and treatment interests among Iraq and Afghanistan combat veterans receiving VA medical care. *Psychiatric Services, 61*(6), 589–597.

Schachman, K. A. (2010). Online fathering: The experience of first-time fatherhood in combat-deployed troops. *Nursing Research, 59*(1), 11–17.

Seal, K. H., Bertenthal, D., Miner, C. R., Sen, S., & Marmar, C. (2007). Bringing the war Back home: Mental health disorders among 103 788 US veterans returning from Iraq and Afghanistan seen at Department of Veterans Affairs Facilities. *Archives of Internal Medicine, 167*(5), 476–482.

Seal, K. H., Metzler, T. J., Gima, K. S., Bertenthal, D., Maguen, S., & Marmar, C. R. (2009). Trends and risk factors for mental health diagnoses among Iraq and Afghanistan veterans using Department of Veterans Affairs Health Care, 2002–2008. *American Journal of Public Health, 99*(9), 1651–1658.

Shonkoff, J. P., Garner, A. S., & Committee on Psychosocial Aspects of Child and Family Health, Committee on Early Childhood, Adoption, and Dependent Care, Section on Developmental and Behavioral Pediatrics. (2012). The lifelong effects of early childhood adversity and toxic stress. *Pediatrics, 129*, e232–e246.

Smith, T. C., Ryan, M. A., Wingard, D. L., Slymen, D. J., Sallis, J. F., & Kritz-Silverstein, D. (2008). New onset and persistent symptoms of post-traumatic stress disorder self reported after deployment and combat exposures: Prospective population based US military cohort study. *BMJ, 336*(7640), 366–371.

Tanielian, T., & Jaycox, L. (2008). *Invisible wounds of war: Psychological and cognitive injuries, their consequences, and services to assist recovery*. Santa Monica, CA: RAND Corporation.

U.S. Department of Defense. (2018). *Demographics Report: Profile of the Military Community.* Retrieved 16 January 2020 from http://download.militaryonesource.mil/12038/MOS/Reports/2018-demographics-report.pdf

Weins, T. W., & Boss, P. (2006). Maintaining family resiliency before, during and after military separation. In C. A. Castro, A. B. Adler, & C. A. Britt (Eds.), *Military life: The psychology of serving in peace and combat* (pp. 13–38). Bridgeport, CT: Praeger Security International.

Walsh, T. B., Dayton, C. J., Erwin, M. S., Muzik, M., Busuito, A., & Rosenblum, K. L. (2014). Fathering after military deployment: Parenting challenges and goals of fathers of young children. *Health & Social Work, 39*(1), 35–44.

Willerton, E., Schwarz, R. L., Wadsworth, S. M. M., & Oglesby, M. S. (2011). Military fathers' perspectives on involvement. *Journal of Family Psychology, 25*(4), 521–530.

Part V

Father's and Children's Mental Health

Overview to Part V: Fathers and Children's Mental Health

34

Kai von Klitzing

In the second part of the twentieth century, an enhanced understanding that deviations from normative human behavior and mental illness have to be viewed not as misconduct but as an expression of biological, psychological, and social imbalance evolved. In the context of this understanding, the modern concept of mental health emerged and was increasingly understood in parallel to the concept of somatic health. This lead to a de-stigmatization of psychiatric disorders and symptoms that is not completed in Western industrialized countries nor in other parts of the world. Furthermore, an awareness developed that mental health problems are embedded in relational contexts and that psychological problems in one individual can only be understood in the context of relationships with others, including family, members of the community, and individuals in broader society. In this context emerged an understanding that mental disorders have to be diagnosed and treated with a developmentally sensitive approach, especially with respect to relationships between very young children and their immediate caregivers. Mental health in infancy is predictive for mental health during the whole life cycle and is imbedded in the relationships of infants to their closest attachment figures (Lyons-Ruth et al., 2017). Therefore, mental problems of caregivers have been identified as the most evident risk factors for mental health problems of their young offspring.

In this light researchers and clinicians who work on health issues of young children usually have a close look at the mental health status of children's caregivers. For example, maternal postpartum depression has been identified as the most prominent risk factor for depressive disorders of their children (Murray et al., 2011). For years, clinical work with young children as well as developmental research nearly exclusively focused on the mother as the primary caregiver. In research, fathers were not included because adding a third person and his relationship to the infant made analyses more complicated. In clinical practice fathers are often not involved because clinicians would have to change much of their practice (e.g., different times of consultation, other clinical approaches, etc.) in order to include them. A further problem in clinical work beyond the absent father is the violent father. As we very often work with families with low social economic status we are frequently confronted with high levels of violence in social disadvantaged neighborhoods. Mostly we see fathers as the obvious perpetrators. Violence in families and conflictual relationships often spring from men who feel narcissistically wounded and do not know how to regulate their impulses. The attitude that the violent father is the typical indicator of a precarious and maltreating environment is wide

K. von Klitzing (✉)
Department of Child and Adolescent Psychiatry, University of Leipzig, Leipzig, Germany
e-mail: Kai.vonklitzing@uniklinik-leipzig.de

H. E. Fitzgerald et al. (eds.), *Handbook of Fathers and Child Development*,
https://doi.org/10.1007/978-3-030-51027-5_34

spread. For example, Lieberman and van Horn (2005) titled their seminal book on psychotherapy with young stressed and traumatized children and their parents *Don't hit my Mommy* and thereby positioned the violent father into the center of the clinical problem. It is the aim of this clinical section to approach the significance of the father for the mental development of his young offspring in an open and innovative manner, no matter whether it is about the loving and caring father, the absent father, or the violent father.

In their chapter Godleski and Eiden focus on the transgenerational transmission of antisocial behavior showing the interweaving of genetic and environmental factors. Especially boys seem to absorb antisocial behavior of their fathers, with biological and psychological pathways for this absorption. Many studies show that fathers' antisocial behavior increases risk for children's externalizing behavior problems, especially for boys. In addition to significant genetic risk, two primary environmental risk processes may be partner conflict and fathers' harsh parenting or father-to-child hostility. As the risk seems mitigated by limiting child exposure to antisocial fathers, the authors suggest that treatment for antisocial behavior may have cascading positive effects for both fathers and children.

McMahon reports a number of epidemiological and longitudinal studies documenting the effects of substance abuse on fatherhood and parenting practices. Substance use remains one of the more common threats to family processes known to promote the social and psychological well-being of fathers, mothers, and children. Substantial empirical evidence points to a vicious circle: substance use affects the production and parenting of children by men and the production and parenting of children affects substance use by men. The author designed a conceptual model of nested familial influences likely to be operative in the lives of infants, toddlers, and preschool children living in family systems affected by paternal addiction including factors like child temperament, children's representations of substance use, family process, and parental psychopathology.

In view of the fact that father's behavior and mental health status is of major predictive significance for child development outcomes, it is obvious that sufficient therapeutic efforts should involve fathers regardless of the problematic nature of their behavior. Von Klitzing and White report empirical evidence that psychotherapeutic treatments of young children have better outcomes if fathers are involved in the therapeutic work. Research still has a long way to go, since, as a rule, studies examine the effect of fathers in what are inherently mother-focused interventions, though exceptions to this rule are emerging in the literature. In their chapter, the authors also describe different psychotherapeutic tools for father involvement and outline tiers at which to pitch father-focused interventions (for a broad overview see Baradon, 2019). They believe that it is important to tailor therapeutic techniques to the role of fathers in child development and study their effects using appropriate designs to capture therapeutic processes.

Based on the rationale that father involvement in therapeutic practice is difficult but important in order to improve the effectiveness of most intervention strategies, three chapters focus on intervention programs that are tailored towards the needs of fathers with the aim to improve father involvement. Pruett and Pruett present a specific preventive intervention program, the California Supporting Father Involvement, which has been studied in different trials within diverse settings. The program is designed for parents of very young children (2–3 years of age) with the expectation that strengthening family relationships early will lead to less child abuse and better relationships throughout family life. Fletcher presents the SMS4Dads program, a text-based perinatal support program for fathers that has been developed and tested in Australia. This program aims to: (1) scaffold fathers as they navigate psychosocial vulnerabilities across the transition to fatherhood, (2) build capacity in fathers to offer support to the mother while developing their co-parenting partnership and form a secure attachment with their infant, and (3) pay particular attention to the fathers' identity in accessing and engaging in support. DeGarmo delineates the Fathering Through Change (FTC) program which is tailored to the needs of divorced and separating fathers, with a major focus on the relevance of the fathering role and its impact on children. The FTC intervention program uses a number of instructional processes, including video sequences, web-based interactivity, web-based social connectivity and networking, and email and phone text instructional prompting. From the experience with these father-oriented programs, the authors draw general conclusions for principles of father involvement, for example that it is important to work with fathers and not on fathers. Furthermore, practical recommendations are extracted from the authors' experiences, for example, to offer hours of service that are flexible enough to accommodate the fathers' work responsibilities, to contact fathers directly and not via mothers, or to look at service intake procedures through the eyes of an anxious young father.

In his concluding chapter, Bradley starts from a cultural historic overview of father research. He comes to the conclusion that there is more respect for the roles played by fathers in children's lives and in family life more broadly and that there is also greater appreciation for the dynamic interplay of the personal and contextual factors that determine how men enact the roles that fathers play in the lives of children. He advocates for a stepping up of efforts to guide meaningful and actionable research on fatherhood taking into account advances in technology, the evolving roles of men and women in the workforce, diverse family constellations, and progress of neurobiological sciences. He concludes that fatherhood is not only essential for family life and child development but also for many men's identity.

References

Baradon, T. (Ed.). (2019). *Working with fathers in psychoanalytic parent-infant psychotherapy*. New York: Routledge. https://doi.org/10.4324/9781315106830

Lieberman, A. F., & van Horn, P. (2005). *Don't hit my mommy!: A manual for child-parent psychotherapy with young witnesses of family violence*. Washington, DC: Zero to Three.

Lyons-Ruth, K., Todd Manly, J., von Klitzing, K., Tamminen, T., Emde, R., Fitzgerald, H., et al. (2017). The worldwide burden of infant mental health and emotional disorder: Report of the task force of the World Association for Infant Mentahal Health. *Infant Mental Health Journal, 38*(6), 695–705. https://doi.org/10.1002/imhj.21674

Murray, L., Arteche, A., Fearon, P., Halligan, S., Goodyer, I., & Cooper, P. (2011). Maternal postnatal depression and the development of depression in offspring up to 16 years of age. *Journal of the American Academy of Child & Adolescent Psychiatry, 50*(5), 460–470. https://doi.org/10.1016/j.jaac.2011.02.001

Fathers' Antisocial Behavior and Early Childhood

35

Stephanie Godleski and Rina D. Eiden

An antisocial personality disorder (ASPD) diagnosis requires a consistent pattern of behavior that indicates a disregard for or violation of rights of others. Symptoms include significant impairments in self-functioning with self-esteem and goal setting based on personal gain or power and absence of conscience; impairments in interpersonal functioning characterized by lack of empathy or capacity for mutual intimacy, that is based on exploitation, coercion, or intimidation; lack of inhibition; and being manipulative, deceitful, callous, or hostile in interactions with others. These antisocial behaviors may occur along a continuum of severity that may or may not meet criteria for ASPD. The history and evolution of antisocial personality disorder in western psychology has been well described by the National Collaborating Centre for Mental Health (NCCMH, 2010) and recent reviews (e.g., Black, 2015). Antisocial personality disorder is temporally preceded by conduct disorder in childhood, although not all conduct-disordered children continue to display ASPD in adulthood. Indeed, the DSM-5 definition of ASPD diagnosis requires evidence of conduct problems (i.e., serious, repetitive disruptive behaviors such as aggression and defiance) by age 15 years. Antisocial behaviors are also more common among men and have greater continuity over time among men compared to women (Black, 2015; NCCMH, 2010; Paris, 2003). Thus, antisocial behavior among fathers may have particular significance for long-lasting effects on parenting and developmental outcomes in children given greater prevalence and greater continuity over time.

S. Godleski (✉)
College of Liberal Arts, Department of Psychology, Rochester Institute of Technology, Rochester, NY, USA
e-mail: saggsh@rit.edu

R. D. Eiden
Department of Psychology, Consortium for Combating Substance Abuse, Pennsylvania State University, State College, PA, USA

Prevalence and Comorbidity

There are few epidemiological studies on prevalence of high antisocial behavior or ASPD among fathers, making it difficult to ascertain the extent of the problem. However, there are some epidemiological studies on prevalence of ASPD among men and women using nationally representative samples. These rates vary by country and methods used to ascertain the incidence of antisocial behavior and ASPD (Black, 2015; NCCMH, 2010). In the USA, the rates of ASPD have varied from 2 to 8% among men and about 0.5–0.8% among women (Compton, Conway, Stinson, Colliver, & Grant, 2005; Grant et al., 2004; Kendler, Davis, & Kessler, 1997; Robins & Price, 1991; Swanson, Bland, & Newman, 1994). However, rates of adult antisocial behavior have

H. E. Fitzgerald et al. (eds.), *Handbook of Fathers and Child Development*,
https://doi.org/10.1007/978-3-030-51027-5_35

been much higher. For instance, data from the National Epidemiologic Survey on Alcohol and Related Conditions-III indicated an adult antisocial behavior rate of 20%, with highest prevalence among Caucasian and Native American males who were younger and unmarried with high school or below education and low income (Goldstein et al., 2017). In Europe, rates of ASPD have varied from 1 to 1.3% among men and 0 to 0.2% among women (Coid et al., 2006; Torgersen et al., 2008). In addition, there are a number of studies that have used more select samples or examined comorbidity with other paternal psychopathology that may offer some evidence regarding prevalence among fathers in contrast to men in general. For instance, using data from two consecutive birth cohorts of twins born in England and Wales, Jaffee and colleagues (Jaffee, Moffitt, Caspi, & Taylor, 2003) noted that of 1116 participants, 171 fathers (15%) scored at or above the 85th percentile on a measure of antisocial behavior symptoms and 97% of these fathers met DSM-IV criteria of ASPD. Similarly, in a sample of Finnish twins, 51 fathers of 478 families (11%) met DSM-IV criterion (three or more symptoms) for antisocial personality disorder. These rates are much higher than prevalence rates for men (who may or may not be fathers) based on nationally representative samples, perhaps indicating that these samples may be more selective for higher levels of antisocial behavior compared to nationally representative samples.

Antisocial behavior is also highly comorbid with other psychopathology, such as other personality and mood disorders, anxiety, and substance abuse (e.g., Goldstein et al., 2017; Tielbeek et al., 2018; Werner, Few, & Bucholz, 2015). Indeed, one recent report noted substantial correlations between antisocial behavior with lifetime cannabis use and number of cigarettes smoked per day and a small but significant genetic correlation between antisocial behavior and these substance use behaviors (Tielbeek et al., 2018). Results from national surveys have further noted that adults with ASPD were seven to 17 times more likely to also meet criteria for alcohol, drug, and nicotine dependence compared to those without ASPD (Lenzenweger, Lane, Loranger, & Kessler, 2007). Thus, studies of fathers' antisocial behavior and ASPD on early childhood development need to consider the role of comorbid conditions as potentially exacerbating risks associated with fathers' antisocial behaviors on family processes and child outcomes.

Theoretical Framework

Although there is no specific unifying theory for the etiology and generational transmission of antisocial behavior, a behavioral genetics perspective or biosocial model is frequently used to frame these processes. Genetically informed research has demonstrated that there is a significant heritable component to antisocial behavior, as well as comorbid and phenotypically similar behaviors such as impulsivity (for review, see Baker, Bezdijian, & Raine, 2006; Ferguson, 2010). Indeed, there may be similar etiological pathways for the development of an externalizing behavior factor (Krueger et al., 2002), which would help to explain the generational transmission and comorbidity of similar, albeit heterogeneous, psychopathological patterns, such as emotional and behavioral dysregulation, substance problems, and antisocial behavior. The risk may be particularly exacerbated in the context of and in interaction with adverse environmental influences, such as through social learning (e.g., low parenting quality; Smith & Farrington, 2004) or stress (e.g., neighborhood violence; Fitzgerald, McKelvey, Schiffman, & Montanez, 2006). For example, Dodge (2009) proposed a developmental model of the development of conduct disorder to antisocial behavior/ASPD that includes a discussion of gene by environment interaction effects. When children have extended and frequent exposure with a father who exhibits antisocial behavior, such as when they live in the same home, the risk for transmission of externalizing and antisocial behavior may be elevated (Jaffee et al., 2003). Further, from a developmental psychopathology and developmental cascade perspective, the developmental timing of environmental influences may also play an important role. Early experiences during the first few years of life with paternal antisocial behavior and comorbid and associated risks, such as substance problems (Eiden, Edwards, & Leonard, 2007), ineffective or harsh parenting (e.g., Coley, Carrano, & Lewin-Bizan, 2011), socioeconomic status (Tuvblad & Beaver, 2013), as well as partner conflict (Loukas, Fitzgerald, Zucker, & Von Eye, 2001) could have a lasting and cascading influence throughout development (Dodge, 2009; Rutter, 1997).

Genetic Associations and Environmental Risk

There are few behavior genetic studies examining associations between fathers' antisocial behavior and early childhood outcomes. However, studies of older age groups indicate that antisocial behavior has strong intergenerational continuity with family history of antisocial behavior being one of the strongest risk factors for child's externalizing behavior problems (e.g., Frick et al., 1992; Salvatore et al., 2015). Results from behavior genetic studies with older age groups regarding heritability of antisocial behavior have been mixed, and estimates have varied from none for child aggression (Plomin & Foch, 1981) to 71% heritability for antisocial behaviors (Slutske, 2001). Meta-analytic reviews and more recent studies have reported heritability estimates in the range of 38% to 56% (Ferguson, 2010; Rhee & Waldman, 2002; Torgersen et al., 2008). These variations may be due to differences in the nature of the sample and degree of sample risk (clinic vs. community samples), sex of the participants (males having higher risk), and differences in measurement of antisocial behavior and ASPD. There have also been discussions of variations in family risk profiles based on subgroups of child externalizing problems such as those with a diagnosis of conduct disorder or less severe conduct problems that reflect negative, non-compliant behaviors (e.g., Frick et al., 1992). Among clinic referred school-aged boys, those with a diagnosis of conduct disorder (severe conduct problems) were more likely to have parents with ASPD and substance use problems compared to those with milder conduct problems. However, the family history risk does not seem to be limited to externalizing disorders alone. Results from the National Comorbidity Study (Kendler et al., 1997) indicate linkages between parent ASPD and child externalizing as well as internalizing disorders.

Although there is clearly a strong genetic component to intergenerational transmission of antisocial behaviors, studies of father presence vs. absence described below provide support for environmental mechanisms as well (e.g., Blazei, Iacono, & McGue, 2008). In addition, studies using comprehensive assessments of both fathers and mothers indicate that associations between family process variables such as parenting and the parent-intimate partner relationship continue to be significant even when accounting for the role of fathers' antisocial behavior (e.g., Bornovalova, Blazei, Malone, McGue, & Iacono, 2013). As noted by these authors, it is possible that passive gene-environment associations (i.e., association between parent genotype and environments they create for their children) may also account for these relationships by transmission of genetic liability for both couple discord and externalizing disorders as genetic predispositions could contribute to the manifestation of antisocial disorder as well as the kind of developmental environment that parents may create for their children (Scarr & McCartney, 1983). Further, evocative and active gene-environment associations could also potentially account for the transmission of antisocial behavior and associated harsh parenting as a child's genetic propensity for externalizing behaviors may pull for more negative parenting behaviors as well as increase the likelihood of engaging in higher levels of parent-child conflict (Bornovalova et al., 2013). In addition, children may actively choose environmental contexts that fit better with their genetic predispositions, such as spending time with peers who are more similar to them (Scarr & McCartney, 1983). In a study using a novel, genetically informative design, Harold and colleagues (Harold, Elam, Lewis, Rice, & Thapar, 2012) included families with 4- to 10-year-old children, who conceived children through in vitro fertilization (IVF). They examined theoretical pathways from parents' antisocial behavior to child antisocial behavior via parent to child hostility and through associations between antisocial behavior and partner conflict among genetically related and genetically unrelated families. Results indicated that for both genetically related and genetically unrelated families, the association between father and child antisocial behavior was mediated via father to child hostility, thus supporting hostile parenting as a significant environmental mechanism. Fathers' antisocial behavior was also associated with higher partner conflict, which in turn was predictive of child antisocial behavior via father to child hostility – supporting a spillover mechanism from interparental relationship to parenting (Harold et al., 2012).

Additional support for socialization practices as explanatory environmental mechanism for transmission of father to child antisocial problems was provided by a large sample study of 5-year-old twins and their parents (Jaffee et al., 2003). Results from behavior genetic analyses indicated that fathers' presence in the home was protective against child conduct problems only when fathers had low levels of antisocial behavior. Among fathers with high antisocial behavior, more time spent in the home was associated with higher child conduct problems, supporting a combined effect of genetic and environmental risk. In contrast, in a study of intergenerational transmission of severe antisocial behavior (criminal offenses) across three generations, there were both within and between generation continuities that were not completely mediated by parenting (Smith & Farrington, 2004). Having two antisocial parents and being male conferred additional risk. In addition, higher parent-partner conflict was a predictor of child problems across two generations – again supporting spillover effects. Results from these studies on older children support both genetic risk and environmental mechanisms. Indeed, meta-analytic reviews have noted that about 16% of the variance may be explained by shared environmental and about 43% by individual-specific environmental mechanisms (Rhee & Waldman, 2002).

Importance of Early Experiences

Although there is limited research on the impact of fathers' antisocial behavior during the early child period, this developmental period is critical for investigating the impact of parents and for understanding child development in several key cognitive and social domains (Gentile & Sesma, 2003; Thompson, 2006). Importantly, early experiences can set the stage for success or difficulty with later developmental tasks, such as negotiating peer relationships and academic demands. Cognitively, children are increasing in their memory and language abilities during the early childhood period (Bauer, 2006; Tomasello, 2006) as well as their abilities to focus and pay attention (DeMarie-Dreblow & Miller, 1988; Nelson, Thomas, & de Haan, 2006). Socially, children are undergoing important changes in their social perspectives and social relationships, such as developing critical attachment relationships and understanding that others may have different thoughts or beliefs than one's own (Bowlby, 1973; Astington, 1993). Preschool-aged children are learning scripts, social knowledge structures, and schemas for behaviors (Fivush, 2002; Gentile & Sesma, 2003), such as routines or everyday interactions that have been acquired through experience (Burks, Laird, Dodge, Pettit, & Bates, 1999; Murphy & Medin, 1985). Children are learning and developing the ability to consciously self-regulate their own thoughts, behaviors, and emotions (Aber & Jones, 1997; Moore, Evans, Brooks-Gunn, & Roth, 2001; Moore & Symons, 2005). In addition, development often proceeds with some degree of continuity, and early experience is often thought to have an important influence on later development (Sroufe, 1997), and thus the influences of a father's antisocial behavior, even as early as the period from birth to preschool age, could have an enduring impact on a child's developmental pathways toward adjustment or maladjustment prior to the middle childhood and adolescent developmental periods. Further, children who exhibit behavioral problems earlier in life are often at greater risk of continued, and potentially exacerbating, behavioral problems throughout development (Caspi, 2000;

Moffitt, 1993; NICHD Early Child Care Research Network, 2004; Smith & Farrington, 2004).

Impact on Early Development

Past research has demonstrated the increased risk for social-emotional maladjustment for children of antisocial fathers (e.g., Lahey, Waldman, & McBurnett, 1999; Smith & Farrington, 2004). However, as noted earlier, much of the research has focused on the impact of fathers' antisocial behavior on children during middle childhood, adolescence, and adulthood (e.g., Bornovalova et al., 2013; Capaldi & Patterson, 1991).

Much of the research on early childhood outcomes among children of antisocial fathers has been with samples of fathers who were heavy drinking or met criteria for alcohol abuse or dependence (e.g., Eiden et al., 2016; Loukas, Zucker, Fitzgerald, & Krull, 2003). Results from these studies that consider the role of antisocial behavior in the context of fathers' alcohol problems have varied, depending on child age and the specific outcome of interest. For instance, fathers' lifetime antisocial behavior was not associated with infant-father attachment security at 12 months of infant age (Eiden, Edwards, & Leonard, 2002) or stability of attachment security from 12 to 18 months of child age (Edwards, Eiden, & Leonard, 2004), with parent reports of internalizing (e.g., depression, anxiety, withdrawn behavior) or externalizing (aggression, attention problems) behavior problems at toddler age (Edwards, Leonard, & Eiden, 2001), with aspects of child self-regulation such as internalization of rules of conduct at preschool age (Eiden, Edwards, & Leonard, 2006), or with parent reports of laxness or over-reactive discipline styles across early childhood (18 months to 5 years; Edwards, Homish, Eiden, Grohman, & Leonard, 2009).

In contrast, fathers' antisocial behavior scores were significantly correlated with fathers' observed parenting behavior during father-infant interactions at 12 months of infant age (Eiden, Chavez, & Leonard, 1999) and at toddler age (2 years; Eiden et al., 2007). Higher fathers' lifetime antisocial scores were associated with lower warmth and sensitivity and higher harshness during observations of laboratory-based play interactions, supporting results from studies of older children indicating father to child hostility as a primary mediator of father to child antisocial behavior associations (Harold et al., 2012). Similarly, fathers' lifetime antisocial behavior was associated with higher paternal aggravation toward their child from infancy to early school age (Eiden, Molnar, Colder, Edwards, & Leonard, 2009) and higher externalizing behavior problems at 3 years of child age (Eiden, Colder, Edwards, & Leonard, 2009). In a prospective study of preschool children of alcoholics, Jansen and colleagues (Jansen, Fitzgerald, Ham, & Zucker, 1995) demonstrated that parents of boys falling within the clinical range of problem behavior on the Child Behavior Checklist (Achenbach, 1991) had higher levels of antisocial behavior, with fathers reporting significantly higher levels of antisocial behavior than mothers. Results from this study also indicated that continuity of externalizing problems from under control at preschool age to disruptive behaviors at school entry was stronger with increasing age among boys with antisocial fathers (Loukas et al., 2003). However, in many of these described analyses, fathers' antisocial behavior did not account for unique variance in fathers' parenting behaviors or child outcomes when analytic models included fathers' alcohol problems, depression, and other family risk factors (Eiden et al., 1999; Eiden, Colder, et al., 2009; Eiden, Molnar, et al., 2009; Eiden et al., 2007).

A family risk factor that has been especially implicated in children's emotional and social development is parent-intimate partner conflict (e.g., Davies & Cummings, 1994). Indeed, fathers' lifetime antisocial behavior did account for unique variance in intimate partner conflict in early childhood even in the context of alcohol problems (e.g., Finger et al., 2010), and high intimate partner conflict had a spillover effect on parenting in early childhood, with subsequent effects on child outcomes such as social competence at early school age (Finger, Eiden, Edwards, Leonard, & Kachadourian, 2010). One conclusion from these results is that similar to studies of older children, fathers' antisocial behavior that often occurs in the context of other paternal and family risk factors may impact developmental outcomes in early childhood indirectly via the couple relationship and the impact of the intimate partner relationship on parenting. An important issue to consider is that these analyses included community recruited families of fathers with alcohol problems who had generally lower levels of antisocial behavior than fathers who may be in treatment for substance abuse. A second issue of note is that the measure of antisocial behavior in these analyses was a measure of lifetime antisocial behavior that may have happened during adolescence or young adulthood for the fathers and not current antisocial behavior or current diagnosis of ASPD. Fathers' antisocial behavior may have more direct implications for child outcomes when these behaviors occur after the child's birth and are current and not lifetime. However, others have noted that externalizing behaviors tend to be fairly stable past the preschool years, and fathers' with lifetime antisocial behavior are more likely to continue to have interpersonal problems and display higher hostility compared to fathers with low lifetime antisocial behavior (Broidy et al., 2003; Caspi, 2000; Caspi, Moffitt, Newman, & Silva, 1998; Moffitt & Caspi, 2001).

As noted earlier, much of the literature on father's antisocial behavior and early childhood outcomes has been on samples of fathers with alcohol use disorders, with a few exceptions. In a longitudinal study of children and families in low-income neighborhoods in Boston, Chicago, and San Antonio (Coley et al., 2011), fathers' antisocial behavior predicted growth in children's externalizing and internalizing behavior problems from the preschool period to early school age, with links stronger among resident-father families. Further, Coley et al. (2011) demonstrated an interactive effect of fathers' antisocial behavior and harsh discipline on children's internalizing behavior problems. High levels of harsh discipline exacerbated the association between fathers' antisocial behavior and higher internalizing behavior problems among children, whereas low levels of harsh discipline were protective against effects of fathers' antisocial behavior. These effects again support parenting as a primary mechanism for linkages between fathers' antisocial behavior and child behavior problems.

In addition to the role of fathers' antisocial behavior on family functioning and parenting as primary mechanisms of risk for poor child outcomes, dosage is important to consider. As discussed previously, the effects of fathers' antisocial behavior on child psychopathology are thought to be particularly strong when the dosage of exposure is highest, such as when the father lives in the same home (Blazei et al., 2008; Coley et al., 2011; Jaffee et al., 2003). For instance, results from a community sample of adolescent twins and their parents indicated that the association between fathers' antisocialilty and child's externalizing behavior problems was moderated by fathers' presence in the household (Blazei et al., 2008; Jaffee et al., 2003). The association between father and child antisocial/externalizing behaviors was stronger when fathers had been present in the home for a longer period of time (as measured by the proportion of the child's life that the fathers had been living with the children) perhaps reflecting socialization influences and indicating a significant role of the environment as well. However, others have reported that antisocial fathers were less involved in child rearing activities even when they were in the home, thus highlighting the importance of measuring father involvement in studies of fathers' antisocial behavior (Bornovalova et al., 2013). Similarly, risk is highest when there is cumulative or synergistic risk exposure, such as when there are high levels of neighborhood violence (Fitzgerald et al., 2006). More specifically, Fitzgerald et al. (2006) found an interactive effect of exposure to high levels of neighborhood violence with father's antisocial behavior predicting higher levels of emotion dysregulation for 3-year-old children. Indeed, Thornberry's (1987) interactional model suggests the pervasive social and contextual impact of parent antisocial behavior on other systems, leading to associated and comorbid risk such as poverty, stress, instability, comorbid substance use, partner and family conflict, and maladaptive parenting practices (e.g., Coley et al., 2011; Jaffee et al., 2003; Thornberry & Krohn, 2005). For example, Loukas et al. (2001) found an indirect path from father's antisocial behavior via family and parent-child conflict on children of alcoholics' externalizing behavior. Therefore, although there is genetic risk for antisocial behavior, additive and exacerbated risk from the caregiving or environmental context is also critical (Harold et al., 2012; Jaffee et al., 2003).

Future Research

Although there has been significant investigation in the area of fathers' antisocial behavior, understanding the impact during early development and the subsequent potential cascade of risk into later development is less well understood. In particular and as reviewed previously, past research has suggested the importance of early experiences. As such, parsing out the developmental timing or exposure to risk and protective factors within the context of fathers' antisocial behavior will be an important area for future work. In particular, it may be informative to investigate promotive or protective factors, such as a high-quality relationship with another caregiver (e.g., attachment security with non-antisocial mother in the context of fathers' antisocial behavior), as well as the dosage of exposure to fathers' antisocial behavior and associated risk factors (e.g., Jaffee et al., 2003) beginning in infancy. Emphasizing and focusing on early development is especially critical given that fathers' antisocial behavior predicts child dysregulation and problem behavior, which are then precursors to more serious adult outcomes (i.e., poorer academic achievement, substance problems).

Future research would also benefit from incorporating the larger systems and transactional factors at play in children's development over time. In particular, it may be interesting to investigate risk factors within the context of neighborhood influences, such as community violence (Fitzgerald et al., 2006). Further, even when an antisocial father does not live within the home with the child, there could be indirect influences via other caregivers, such as negative perceptions of children's behavior as being consistent with the father's antisociality. These negative perceptions may be particularly salient for boys compared to girls. This is an important area for future study. Additionally, much of the work conducted longitudinally that incorporates the impact of father's antisocial behavior on early child development has done so under the circumstances of father alcohol problems. Although antisocial behavior and alcohol use are often comorbid, future research could examine the interactive or additive effects of antisocial behavior with other comorbid conditions or risk factors, to enhance our understanding of the role of paternal alcohol problems as well as other comorbid risks versus antisocial behavior. Similarly, an additional important area for future research is to continue the examination of indirect, mediating, or moderating factors (Eiden et al., 2007; Coley et al., 2011) that may impact the relation between fathers' antisocial behavior and early child development. There is ample evidence that harsh discipline may exacerbate the impact of fathers' antisocial behavior; however, the sex constellation of the parent-child dyad could also play an important role in the transmission of risk (e.g., Thornberry et al., 2003). Indeed parents may respond differently to their children based on their sex, and different vulnerabilities may be present for boys and girls (Golding & Fitzgerald, 2017). It has been suggested that boys may be particularly biologically predisposed to violence and antisocial behavior (i.e., lower heart rate leading to greater sensation seeking; Golding & Fitzgerald, 2019) and that boys may be especially vulnerable to early experiences with stress, such as inadequate caregiving (Schore, 2017; Thornberry et al., 2003).

Methodologically and statistically, future research can emphasize obtaining fathers' self-reports of their behavior to reduce confounds introduced by maternal reports of fathers' antisocial behavior (e.g., Tremblay et al., 2004). Observational paradigms of parent-child interactions with all significant caregivers (e.g., Eiden et al., 2016), family dynamics, and dosage of exposure to both risk and protective factors can be incorporated. In addition, across many studies, parent antisocial behavior is included as a covariate instead of as a direct hypothesized predictor (e.g., Ramchandani et al., 2013). Studies that specifically focus on fathers' antisocial behavior in the context of other risk factors may be more informative.

Implications for Preventive Interventions

Intervening early in childhood development, perhaps even during pregnancy when motivation for change could be heightened, is crucial for preventing the potential cascade of risk to children's externalizing behavior problems as well as subsequent social-emotional maladjustment in adulthood, such as substance use problems (e.g., Tremblay & Côté, 2019). With emphasis on understanding the myriad of interacting risk and protective factors, preventative interventions may target the child-, family-, and community-level influences that may make the intergenerational transmission of antisocial behavior more likely. For instance, potential genetic risk may be mitigated by targeting fathers' antisocial behaviors and the cascading impact as well as comorbid risk of this antisocial behavior in order to mitigate potential environmental exposure and socialization experiences.

Further, by taking into account developmental timing and cascade of influence, such interventions can focus on establishing and maintaining secure attachment relationships (Eiden et al., 2002; Edwards et al., 2004) during early development as well as improving parent's ability to provide coordinated and high-quality caregiving. Given the direct impact of fathers' antisocial behavior on parent-partner conflict, which is then associated with child emotional and behavioral adjustment (e.g., Finger, Eiden, et al., 2010; Loukas et al., 2001), preventing the spillover of parent-intimate partner discord and conflict to the parent-child relationship (e.g., Harold et al., 2012) could be another area to target. In particular, co-parenting may be an additional intervention area, as both parenting practices and family conflict have been demonstrated to be indirect pathways from fathers' antisocial behavior to child externalizing and internalizing behavior problems (Coley et al., 2011; Finger, Eiden, et al., 2010; Loukas et al., 2001). Co-parenting is not exclusive to parents who cohabitate, as emphasizing interparental adaptive communication and consistent, positive care for children may be important protective factors across many family circumstances and compositions (e.g., Cowan, Cowan, Kline Pruett, & Pruett, 2007).

Summary and Key Points

In conclusion, the literature on fathers' antisocial behavior on early childhood outcomes is fairly limited. The majority of this literature is focused on fathers' antisocial behavior in the context of fathers' substance abuse. However, there are some consistent themes that have emerged from these studies in combination with studies on older children. First, fathers' antisocial behavior increases risk for children's externalizing behavior problems, especially for boys (e.g., Golding & Fitzgerald, 2019; Tremblay & Côté, 2019). Second, in addition to significant genetic risk, two primary environmental risk processes may be partner conflict and fathers' harsh parenting or father to child hostility. Risk may be mitigated by limiting child exposure to antisocial fathers, suggesting that treatment for antisocial behavior may have cascading positive effects for both fathers and children.

References

Aber, J. L., & Jones, S. J. (1997). Indicators of positive development in early childhood: Improving concepts and measures. In R. M. Hauser, B. V. Brown, & W. R. Prosser (Eds.), *Indicators of children's Well-being*. New York, NY: Sage Foundation.

Achenbach, T. M. (1991). *Manual for the child behavior checklist/4–18 and 1991*. Burlington, VT: University of Vermont, Department of Psychiatry.

Astington, J. W. (1993). *The child's discovery of the mind*. Cambridge MA: Harvard University Press.

Baker, L. A., Bezdijian, S., & Raine, A. (2006). Behavioral genetics: The science of antisocial behavior. *Law and Contemporary Problems, 69*(1–2), 7–46.

Bauer, P. (2006). Event memory. In D. Kuhn & R. S. Siegler (Eds.), *Handbook of child psychology (6th edition): Cognition, perception, and language*. New York, NY: Wiley.

Black, D. W. (2015). The natural history of antisocial personality disorder. *Canadian Journal of Psychiatry. Revue Canadienne de Psychiatrie, 60*(7), 309–314.

Blazei, R. W., Iacono, W. G., & McGue, M. (2008). Father-child transmission of antisocial behavior: The moderating role of father's presence in the home. *Journal of the American Academy of Child and Adolescent Psychiatry, 47*(4), 406–415.

Bornovalova, M. A., Blazei, R., Malone, S. H., McGue, M., & Iacono, W. G. (2013). Disentangling the relative contribution of parental antisociality and family discord to child disruptive disorders. *Personal Disord, 4*(3), 239–246.

Bowlby, J. (1973). *Attachment and loss: Vol. 2 separation*. New York, NY: Basic Books.

Broidy, L. M., Nagin, D. S., Tremblay, R. E., Bates, J. E., Brame, B., Dodge, K. A., et al. (2003). Developmental trajectories of childhood disruptive behaviors and adolescent delinquency: A six-site, cross-national study. *Developmental Psychology, 39*(2), 222–245.

Burks, V. S., Laird, R. D., Dodge, K. A., Pettit, G. S., & Bates, J. E. (1999). Knowledge structures, social information processing, and children's aggressive behavior. *Social Development, 8*, 220–236.

Capaldi, D. M., & Patterson, G. R. (1991). Relation of parental transitions to boys' adjustment problems: I. a linear hypothesis: II. *Mothers at risk for transitions and unskilled parenting. Developmental Psychology, 27*(3), 489–504.

Caspi, A. (2000). The child is the father of the man: Personality continuities from childhood to adulthood. *Journal of Personality and Social Psychology, 78*(1), 158–172.

Caspi, A., Moffitt, T. E., Newman, D. L., & Silva, P. A. (1998). Behavioral observations at age 3 years predict adult psychiatric disorders: Longitudinal evidence from a birth cohort. In M. E. Hertzig & E. A. Farber (Eds.), *Annual progress in child psychiatry and child development* (pp. 319–331). Philadelphia, PA: Brunner/Mazel.

Coid, J., Yang, M., Roberts, A., Ullrich, S., Moran, P., Bebbington, P., et al. (2006). Violence and psychiatric morbidity in the national household population of Britain: Public health implications. *The British Journal of Psychiatry, 189*(1), 12–19. https://doi.org/10.1192/bjp.189.1.12

Coley, R. L., Carrano, J., & Lewin-Bizan, S. (2011). Unpacking links between fathers' antisocial behaviors and children's behavior problems: Direct, indirect, and interactive effects. *Journal of Abnormal Child Psychology, 39*(6), 791–804. https://doi.org/10.1007/s10802-011-9496-4

Compton, W. M., Conway, K. P., Stinson, F. S., Colliver, J. D., & Grant, B. F. (2005). Prevalence, correlates, and comorbidity of DSM-IV antisocial personality syndromes and alcohol and specific drug use disorders in the United States: Results from the National Epidemiologic Survey on alcohol and related conditions. *The Journal of Clinical Psychiatry, 66*(6), 677–685. https://doi.org/10.4088/JCP.v66n0602

Cowan, C. P., Cowan, P. A., Kline Pruett, M. A. R. S. H. A., & Pruett, K. (2007). An approach to preventing coparenting conflict and divorce in low-income families: Strengthening couple relationships and fostering fathers' involvement. *Family Process, 46*(1), 109–121.

Davies, P. T., & Cummings, E. M. (1994). Marital conflict and child adjustment: An emotional security hypothesis. *Psychological Bulletin, 116*(3), 387–411. https://doi.org/10.1037/0033-2909.116.3.387

DeMarie-Dreblow, D., & Miller, P. H. (1988). The development of children's strategies for selective attention: Evidence for a transitional period. *Child Development, 59*, 1504–1513.

Dodge, K. A. (2009). Mechanisms of gene-environment interaction effects in the development of conduct disorder. *Perspectives on Psychological Science, 4*(4), 408–414. https://doi.org/10.1111/j.1745-6924.2009.01147.x

Edwards, E. P., Eiden, R. D., & Leonard, K. E. (2004). Impact of fathers' alcoholism and associated risk factors on parent-infant attachment stability from 12 to 18 months. *Infant Mental Health Journal, 25*(6), 556–579.

Edwards, E. P., Homish, G. G., Eiden, R. D., Grohman, K. K., & Leonard, K. E. (2009). Longitudinal prediction of early childhood discipline styles among heavy drinking parents. *Addictive Behaviors, 34*(1), 100–106.

Edwards, E. P., Leonard, K. E., & Eiden, R. D. (2001). Temperament and behavioral problems among infants in alcoholic families. *Infant Mental Health Journal, 22*(3), 374–392.

Eiden, R. D., Chavez, F., & Leonard, K. E. (1999). Parent-infant interactions among families with alcoholic fathers. *Development and Psychopathology, 11*, 745–762.

Eiden, R. D., Colder, C., Edwards, E. P., & Leonard, K. E. (2009). A longitudinal study of social competence among children of alcoholic and nonalcoholic parents: Role of parental psychopathology, parental warmth, and self-regulation. *Psychology of Addictive Behaviors, 23*(1), 36–46.

Eiden, R. D., Edwards, E. P., & Leonard, K. E. (2002). Mother-infant and father-infant attachment among alcoholic families. *Development and Psychopathology, 14*(2), 253–278.

Eiden, R. D., Edwards, E. P., & Leonard, K. E. (2006). Children's internalization of rules of conduct: Role of parenting in alcoholic families. *Psychology of Addictive Behaviors, 20*(3), 305–315.

Eiden, R. D., Edwards, E. P., & Leonard, K. E. (2007). A conceptual model for the development of externalizing behavior problems among kindergarten children of alcoholic families: Role of parenting and children's self-regulation. *Developmental Psychology, 43*(5), 1187–1201.

Eiden, R. D., Lessard, J., Colder, C. R., Livingston, J., Casey, M., & Leonard, K. E. (2016). Developmental cascade model for adolescent substance use from infancy to late adolescence. *Developmental Psychology, 52*(10), 1619–1633.

Eiden, R. D., Molnar, D. S., Colder, C., Edwards, E. P., & Leonard, K. E. (2009). A conceptual model predicting internalizing problems in middle childhood among children of alcoholic and nonalcoholic fathers: The role of marital aggression. *Journal of Studies on Alcohol and Drugs, 70*(5), 741–750.

Ferguson, C. J. (2010). Genetic contributions to antisocial personality and behavior: A meta-analytic review from an evolutionary perspective. *The Journal of Social Psychology, 150*(2), 160–180.

Finger, B., Eiden, R. D., Edwards, E. P., Leonard, K. E., & Kachadourian, L. (2010). Marital aggression and child peer competence: A comparison of three conceptual models. *Personal Relationships, 17*(3), 357–376.

Finger, B., Kachadourian, L. K., Molnar, D. S., Eiden, R. D., Edwards, E. P., & Leonard, K. E. (2010). Alcoholism, associated risk factors, and harsh parenting among fathers: Examining the role of marital aggression. *Addictive Behaviors, 35*(6), 541–548.

Fitzgerald, H. E., McKelvey, L. M., Schiffman, R. F., & Montanez, M. (2006). Exposure of low-income families and their children to neighborhood violence and paternal antisocial behavior. *Parenting: Science & Practice, 6*(2 & 3), 243–258.

Fivush, R. (2002). Scripts, schemas, and memory of trauma. In N. L. Stein, P. J. Bauer, & M. Rabinowitz (Eds.), *Representation, memory, and development: Essays in honor of Jean Mandler*. Mahwah, NJ: Erlbaum.

Frick, P. J., Lahey, B. B., Loeber, R., Stouthamer-Loeber, M., Christ, M. G., & Hanson, K. (1992). Familial risk factors to oppositional defiant disorder and conduct behavior: Parental psychopathology and maternal parenting. *Journal of Abnormal Child Psychology, 27*, 383–392.

Gentile, D. A., & Sesma, A. (2003). Developmental approaches to understanding media effects on individuals. In D. A. Gentile (Ed.), *Media violence and children*. Westport, CT: Praeger.

Golding, P., & Fitzgerald, H. E. (2017). Psychology of boys at risk: Indicators from 0-5. *Infant Mental Health Journal, 38*, 5–14. https://doi.org/10.1002/imhj.21621

Golding, P., & Fitzgerald, H. E. (2019). The early biopsychosocial development of boys and the origins of violence in males. *Infant Mental Health Journal, 40*, 5–22. https://doi.org/10.1002/imhj.21753

Goldstein, R. B., Chou, S. P., Saha, T. D., Smith, S. M., Jung, J., Zhang, H., et al. (2017). The epidemiology of antisocial behavioral syndromes in adulthood: Results from the National Epidemiologic Survey on alcohol and related conditions-III. *Journal of Clinical Psychiatry, 78*(1), 90–98. https://doi.org/10.4088/JCP.15m10358

Grant, B. F., Hasin, D. S., Stinson, F. S., Dawson, D. A., Chou, S. P., Ruan, W. J., et al. (2004). Prevalence, correlates, and disability of personality disorders in the United States: Results from the National Epidemiologic Survey on alcohol and related conditions. *The Journal of Clinical Psychiatry, 65*(7), 948–958. https://doi.org/10.4088/JCP.v65n0711

Harold, G. T., Elam, K. K., Lewis, G., Rice, F., & Thapar, A. (2012). Interparental conflict, parent psychopathology, hostile parenting, and child antisocial behavior: Examining the role of maternal versus paternal influences using a novel genetically sensitive research design. *Development and Psychopathology, 24*(4), 1283–1295. https://doi.org/10.1017/S0954579412000703

Jaffee, S. R., Moffitt, T. E., Caspi, A., & Taylor, A. (2003). Life with (or without) father: The benefits of living with two biological parents depend on the father's antisocial behavior. *Child Development, 74*(1), 109–126.

Jansen, R., Fitzgerald, H. E., Ham, H. P., & Zucker, R. A. (1995). Pathways into risk: Temperament and behavior problems in three- to five-year-old sons of alcoholics. *Alcoholism: Clinical & Experimental Research, 19*(2), 501–509.

Kendler, K. S., Davis, C. G., & Kessler, R. C. (1997). The familial aggregation of common psychiatric and substance use disorders in the National Comorbidity Survey: A family history study. *British Journal of Psychiatry, 170*, 541–548.

Krueger, R. F., Hicks, B. M., Patrick, C. J., Carlson, S. R., Iacono, W. G., & McGue, M. (2002). Etiologic connections among substance dependence, antisocial behavior, and personality: Modeling the externalizing spectrum. *Journal of Abnormal Psychology, 111*(3), 411–424.

Lahey, B. B., Waldman, I. D., & McBurnett, K. (1999). Annotation: The development of antisocial behavior: An integrative causal model. *The Journal of Child Psychology and Psychiatry and Allied Disciplines, 40*(5), 669–682.

Lenzenweger, M. F., Lane, M. C., Loranger, A. W., & Kessler, R. C. (2007). DSM-IV personality disorders in the National Comorbidity Survey Replication. *Biological Psychiatry, 62*(6), 553–564. https://doi.org/10.1016/j.biopsych.2006.09.019

Loukas, A., Fitzgerald, H. E., Zucker, R. A., & Von Eye, A. (2001). Parental alcoholism and co-occurring antisocial behavior: Prospective relationships to externalizing behavior problems in their young sons. *Journal of Abnormal Child Psychology, 29*(2), 91–106.

Loukas, A., Zucker, R. A., Fitzgerald, H. E., & Krull, J. L. (2003). Developmental trajectories of disruptive behavior problems among sons of alcoholics: Effects of parent psychopathology, family conflict, and child undercontrol. *Journal of Abnormal Psychology, 112*(1), 119–131.

Moffitt, T. E. (1993). Adolescence-limited and life-course-persistent antisocial behavior: A developmental taxonomy. *Psychological Review, 100*(4), 674–701.

Moffitt, T. E., & Caspi, A. (2001). Childhood predictors differentiate life-course persistent and adolescence-limited antisocial pathways among males and females. *Development and Psychopathology, 13*(2), 355–375.

Moore, C., & Symons, D. (2005). Attachment, theory of mind, and delay of gratification. In B. D. Homer & C. S. Tamis-LeMonda (Eds.), *The development of social cognition and communication*. Mahwah, NJ: Lawrence Erlbaum Associates, Publishers.

Moore, K. A., Evans, V. J., Brooks-Gunn, J., & Roth, J. (2001). What are good child outcomes? In A. Thornton (Ed.), *The Well-being of children and families: Research & data needs*. Ann Arbor, MI: University of Michigan Press.

Murphy, G. L., & Medin, D. L. (1985). The role of theories in conceptual coherence. *Psychological Review, 92*, 289–316.

National Collaborating Centre for Mental Health (UK). (2010). Antisocial personality disorder. In *Antisocial personality disorder: Treatment, management and prevention*. British Psychological Society.

Nelson, C. A., Thomas, K. M., & de Haan, M. (2006). Neural bases of cognitive development. In D. Kuhn & R. S. Siegler (Eds.), *Handbook of child psychology (6th edition): Cognition, perception, and language*. New York, NY: Wiley.

NICHD Early Child Care Research Network. (2004). Trajectories of physical aggression from toddlerhood to middle childhood: Predictors, correlates, and outcomes. *Monographs of the Society for Research in Child Development, 69*(4), vii–1.

Paris, J. (2003). Personality disorders over time: Precursors, course and outcome. *Journal of Personality Disorders, 17*(6), 479–488. https://doi.org/10.1521/pedi.17.6.479.25360

Plomin, R., & Foch, T. T. (1981). Bobo clown aggression in childhood: Environment, not genes. *Journal of Research in Personality, 15*(3), 331–342.

Ramchandani, P. G., Domoney, J., Sethna, V., Psychogiou, L., Vlachos, H., & Murray, L. (2013). Do early father-infant interactions predict the onset of externalising behaviours in young children? Findings from a longitudinal cohort study. *Journal of Child Psychology and Psychiatry and Allied Disciplines, 54*(1), 56–64.

Rhee, S. H., & Waldman, I. D. (2002). Genetic and environmental influences on antisocial behavior: A meta-analysis of twin and adoption studies. *Psychological Bulletin, 128*(3), 490–529. https://doi.org/10.1037/0033-2909.128.3.490

Robins, L. N., & Price, R. K. (1991). Adult disorders predicted by childhood conduct problems: Results from the NIMH epidemiologic catchment area project. *Psychiatry: Interpersonal and Biological Processes, 54*(2), 116–132.

Rutter, M. (1997). Nature-nurture integration. *American Psychologist, 52*(4), 390–398.

Salvatore, J. E., Meyers, J. L., Yan, J., Aliev, F., Lansford, J. E., Pettit, G. S., et al. (2015). Intergenerational continuity in parents' and adolescents' externalizing problems: The role of life events and their interaction with GABRA2. *Journal of Abnormal Psychology, 124*(3), 709–728. https://doi.org/10.1037/abn0000066

Scarr, S., & McCartney, K. (1983). How people make their own environments: A theory of genotype→ environment effects. *Child Development, 54*(2), 424–435.

Schore, A. N. (2017). All our sons: The developmental neurobiology and neuroendocrinology of boys at risk. *Infant Mental Health Journal, 38*, 15–52. https://doi.org/10.1002/imhj.21616

Slutske, W. S. (2001). The genetics of antisocial behavior. *Current Psychiatry Reports, 3*(2), 158–162. https://doi.org/10.1007/s11920-001-0014-1

Smith, C. A., & Farrington, D. P. (2004). Continuities in antisocial behavior and parenting across three generations. *Journal of Child Psychology and Psychiatry, 45*(2), 230–247.

Sroufe, L. A. (1997). Psychopathology as an outcome of development. *Development and Psychopathology, 9*, 251–286.

Swanson, M. C., Bland, R. C., & Newman, S. C. (1994). Antisocial personality disorders. *Acta Psychiatrica Scandinavica, 89*(376, Suppl), 63–70. https://doi.org/10.1111/j.1600-0447.1994.tb05792.x

Thompson, R. A. (2006). The development of the person: Social understanding, relationships, conscience, self. In N. Eisenberg (Ed.), *Handbook of child psychology (6th edition): Social, emotional, and personality development*. New York, NY: Wiley.

Thornberry, T. P. (1987). Toward an interactional theory of delinquency. *Criminology, 25*, 863–891.

Thornberry, T. P., Freeman-Gallant, A., Lizotte, A. J., Krohn, M. D., & Smith, C. A. (2003). Linked lives: The intergenerational transmission of antisocial behavior. *Journal of Abnormal Child Psychology, 31*(2), 171–184. https://doi.org/10.1023/A:1022574208366.

Thornberry, T. P., & Krohn, M. D. (2005). Applying interactional theory to the explanation of continuity and change in antisocial behavior. *Integrated Developmental and Life-course Theories of Offending, 14*, 183–209.

Tielbeek, J. J., Vink, J. M., Polderman, T. J. C., Popma, A., Posthuma, D., & Verweij, K. J. H. (2018). Genetic correlation of antisocial behaviour with alcohol, nicotine, and cannabis use. *Drug and Alcohol Dependence, 187*, 296–299. https://doi.org/10.1016/j.drugalcdep.2018.03.020

Tomasello, M. (2006). Acquiring linguistic constructions. In D. Kuhn & R. S. Siegler (Eds.), *Handbook of child psychology (6th edition): Cognition, perception, and language*. New York, NY: Wiley.

Torgersen, S., Czajkowski, N., Jacobson, K., Reichborn-Kjennerud, T., Røysamb, E., Neale, M. C., et al. (2008). Dimensional representations of DSM-IV cluster B personality disorders in a population-based sample of Norwegian twins: A multivariate study.

Psychological Medicine, 38(11), 1617–1625. https://doi.org/10.1017/S0033291708002924

Tremblay, R. E., Nagin, D. S., Séguin, J. R., Zoccolillo, M., Zelazo, P. D., Boivin, M., Perusse, D., & Japel, C. (2004). Physical aggression during early childhood:Trajectories and predictors. *Pediatrics, 114*(1), e43–e50. https://doi.org/10.1542/peds.114.1.e43.

Tremblay, R. E., & Côté, S. M. (2019). Sex differences in the development of physical aggression: An intergenerational perspective and implications for preventive interventions. *Infant Mental Health Journal, 40*(1), 129–140.

Terence P. Thornberry, Adrienne Freeman-Gallant, Alan J. Lizotte, Marvin D. Krohn, Carolyn A. Smith, Journal of Abnormal Child Psychology 31 (2):171-184

Tuvblad, C., & Beaver, K. M. (2013). Genetic and environmental influences on antisocial behavior. *J Crim Justice, 41*(5), 273–276. https://doi.org/10.1016/j.jcrimjus.2013.07.007

Werner, K. B., Few, L. R., & Bucholz, K. K. (2015). Epidemiology, comorbidity, and behavioral genetics of antisocial personality disorder and psychopathy. *Psychiatric Annals, 45*(4), 195–199. https://doi.org/10.3928/00485713-20150401-08

Fatherhood, Substance Use, and Early Child Development

36

Thomas J. McMahon

Although the gender gap in the use of some substances may be slowly closing in postindustrial cultures (Grant et al., 2017; Hasin et al., 2015), epidemiologic data indicate that, with very few exceptions, men use more alcohol, nicotine, marijuana, and other drugs than women across the life span (Schulenberg et al., 2018). As they move through adolescence, girls tend to begin using substances sooner than boys, but boys generally use substances more consistently with more negative consequences (Miech et al., 2019). During the transition to adulthood, young men continue to use substances more frequently than young women with greater risk for a substance use disorder (Schulenberg et al., 2018), and they remain much more likely to be misusing alcohol, nicotine, marijuana, and other drugs during early to middle adulthood when a majority of men first become a parent (Grant et al., 2017; Grant et al., 2015, 2016; Martinez, Chandra, Abma, Jones, & Mosher, 2006).

As definitions of socially responsible fathering have changed in response to social, economic, and political influences occurring across technologically oriented cultures (Gavanas, 2002), the epidemiologic data raise important questions about the prevalence, dynamics, and consequences of substance use in the lives of men as they become fathers (McMahon & Rounsaville, 2002). Despite evidence that substance use is one of the more pressing health problems in the lives of men, substance use is often not clearly acknowledged in the conceptualization of public policy, research, and service delivery designed to promote more effective fathering (McMahon & Rounsaville, 2002). Consequently, this chapter will outline what is presently known about substance use and fathering during the process of family formation, broadly defined here as a variable process that begins with the selection of a sexual partner and ends when a first child begins elementary school.

The discussion will be presented in five sections. The first section will focus on the epidemiology of substance use and fathering when examined from several different perspectives; the second will outline two somewhat different positions on the relationship between substance use and fathering derived from developmental theory and research. The third section will summarize what is known about the potential impact of

Support for preparation of this chapter was provided by the National Institute on Drug Abuse (R01 DA017294).
Correspondence concerning this chapter should be addressed to Thomas McMahon, Ph.D., Yale University School of Medicine, Connecticut Mental Health Center, West Haven Mental Health Clinic, 270 Center Street, West Haven, Connecticut 06516. Electronic mail may be sent to thomas.mcmahon@yale.edu.

T. J. McMahon (✉)
Yale University School of Medicine, Connecticut Mental Health Center, New Haven, CT, USA
e-mail: thomas.mcmahon@yale.edu

H. E. Fitzgerald et al. (eds.), *Handbook of Fathers and Child Development*,
https://doi.org/10.1007/978-3-030-51027-5_36

substance use at each step in the process of family formation, and the next will outline what is known about the consequences of paternal addiction for children from conception through the preschool years. The final section will integrate the existing literature into a conceptual model that outlines the process by which paternal addiction influences early child development. Each section will present the results of representative research and conclude with a summary statement. The chapter will then end with a summary of key findings and a call for policymakers, researchers, and providers to use the expanding literature on substance use and fathering to inform the systematic development of preventive and clinical interventions designed to minimize the harm associated with paternal addiction.

Throughout this selective review of the research, five general themes will be emphasized. First, there will be recognition that the period from conception to enrollment in elementary school is a time of profound change, not just for children, but for fathers and mothers. Second, there will be acknowledgment that fatherhood is an important developmental transition in the lives of men with the potential to have both positive and negative effects on the well-being of fathers, mothers, and children. Third, substance use by men will consistently be presented as a threat to the development of men, women, and children during this time in the life cycle of a family. Fourth, there will be an emphasis on the idea that pathways to fatherhood, with or without substance use, are best understood as a developmental process that unfolds over time in a specific social ecology. Finally, there will be an emphasis on the idea that there is undoubtedly a reciprocal relationship between substance use and fathering such that, for better or worse, each influences the other as men become fathers.

Epidemiology of Substance Use and Fathering

Epidemiologic data on the prevalence of substance use by fathers are limited seemingly because of measurement issues within large-scale surveys of different populations of men. Most demographic surveys examining patterns of pair-bonding, procreation, and parenting, like the Fragile Families and Child Wellbeing Study (Reichman, Teitler, Garfinkel, & McLanahan, 2001), do not usually include detailed measures of substance use. Likewise, most epidemiologic surveys of substance use, like the National Survey on Drug Use and Health (Substance Abuse and Mental Health Services Administration, 2019) and the National Epidemiologic Survey on Alcohol and Related Conditions (Chen, Slater, Castle, & Grant, 2016), do not usually include detailed measures of relationship and parenting status. Consequently, information concerning fathering and substance use generally comes from secondary analysis of data collected for other reasons where there are significant limitations on the quality of the information imposed by either measurement of the substance use or measurement of parenting status. It is also important to note that the available data on substance use during the transition from adolescence to early adulthood when men are most likely to be producing children come primarily from older, longitudinal investigations done in North America, Europe, Australia, and New Zealand (Degenhardt, Stockings, Patton, Hall, & Lynskey, 2016). Much of the available data come from nations where per capita income is high, attitudes toward substance use are relatively liberal, attitudes toward fathering have changed in response to social and economic pressures, and the social costs associated with substance use are high (Degenhardt et al., 2016; Gavanas, 2002). Much less is known about substance use and fathering in other cultural settings.

Substance Use by Men in the General Population

Epidemiologic data drawn from the National Epidemiologic Survey on Alcohol and Related Conditions (Chou et al., 2016; Grant et al., 2015, 2016; Hasin et al., 2016) suggest that, over the past year, more than 75% of men in the general population have used alcohol and approximately

17% confirm an alcohol use disorder. Similarly, approximately 23% of men confirm a nicotine use disorder, and approximately 5% confirm a drug use disorder involving something other than alcohol or nicotine. After nicotine and alcohol, cannabis is, by far, the drug most frequently misused. Across the life span, rates of use and misuse are consistently highest in men 18 to 29 and then 30 to 44 years of age. Taken together, these data suggest that misuse of nicotine, alcohol, marijuana, and other drugs is most prevalent during early to middle adulthood when more than 75% of men father at least one child (Martinez et al., 2006).

Substance Use by Fathers in the General Population

Because rates of substance use may vary with the parenting status of men, surveys of substance use by men who report being a parent compared with men who report not being a parent also help define the prevalence of the problem. Using data from the longitudinal component of the Monitoring the Future Study, Merline, O'Malley, Schulenberg, Bachman, and Johnston (2004) found that, when compared with men without any children, fathers living with at least one of their children were less likely to be smoking cigarettes, drinking alcohol heavily, or using other drugs at approximately 35 years of age. Approximately 25% of men living with at least some of their children versus 27% of men with no children reported smoking cigarettes in the past 30 days, 29% versus 36% reported using alcohol excessively during the previous 2 weeks, and approximately 10% versus 16.5% reported using marijuana over the previous 30 days. However, when compared with men without any children and men living with at least one of their children, men not living with any of their children were most likely to be using substances. Approximately 42% of fathers not living with any of their children reported smoking cigarettes in the past 30 days, 41% reported using alcohol excessively during the previous 2 weeks, and approximately 20% reported using marijuana during the previous 30 days. Generally, data from representative samples of middle-age men drawn from the general population consistently indicate that fathers living with at least some of their children report the lowest rates of substance use followed by men without any children and fathers not living with any of their children.

Parenting Status of Men Entering Substance Use Treatment

Noting that there is very little information about the parenting status of men entering substance use treatment, McMahon, Winkel, Luthar, and Rounsaville (2005) surveyed a local cohort of men and women seeking medication-assisted treatment for an opioid use disorder over a 12-month period. Using data provided by 362 men and 162 women, they found that women (80%) were more likely than men (54%) to be the parent of at least one biological child. However, because the men dramatically outnumbered the women, men with at least one biological child (37%) represented the largest group within the cohort followed by men without any biological children (32%), women with at least one biological child (25%), and women without any biological children (6%).

When compared with the mothers in the cohort, the fathers were significantly older when they first became a parent, and they were more likely to have been using opioids when their first child was born. There were, however, no significant differences in (a) the number of children, (b) the number of minor children, (c) age of the youngest child, or (d) age of the oldest child. As expected, mothers (45%) were more likely than fathers (20%) to be living with at least one of their biological children. However, because the men outnumbered the women, nonresident fathers (48%) defined, by far, the largest group of parents seeking treatment followed by nonresident mothers (22%), resident mothers (18%), and resident fathers (12%). Unfortunately, the study did not document the presence of men with other types of parenting relationships with children. When considered with the results of a limited number of similar surveys (e.g., U.S. Department of Health & Human Services, 1994), these data suggest that there is a substantial, but poorly documented, population of fathers, principally nonresident fathers, seeking treatment for a substance use disorder.

Children Affected by Parental Substance Use

When questions about exposure to paternal substance use are examined from the perspective of minor children, epidemiologic data drawn from the National Survey on Drug Use and Health (Huang, Cerbone, & Gfroerer, 1998; Lipari & Van Horn, 2017; Substance Abuse and Mental Health Services Administration, 2009) suggest that approximately 8.7 million children or more than 12% of all minor children reside in a household with at least one adult with an alcohol or illicit drug use disorder. Although the estimates vary somewhat in response to operational definitions, this general rate of exposure has proven relatively consistent over time. Given the focus of this volume, it is important to note that most recent estimates suggest that approximately 13% of children birth to 2 years of age and approximately 12% of children 3 to 5 years of age are living with a parent struggling with an addiction to alcohol or illicit drugs. Some estimates (Substance Abuse and Mental Health Services Administration, 2009) suggest that, when compared to school-age children and teens, children less than 5 years of age may be more likely to be living with an affected parent.

Moreover, these data (Huang et al., 1998; Lipari & Van Horn, 2017; Substance Abuse and Mental Health Services Administration, 2009) indicate that approximately 80% of the children living with a parent struggling with an alcohol or illicit drug use disorder reside in a two-parent household, approximately 16% reside in a household headed by a single mother, and approximately 4% reside in a household headed by a single father. Although they represent a small number of children, children living in a household headed by a single father are at greatest risk for exposure to a parent misusing alcohol or an illicit drug. Repeated analysis of data drawn from this national survey consistently indicates that misuse of alcohol by the affected parent exceeds, by far, the misuse of illicit drugs and concurrent misuse of alcohol and an illicit drug. A majority (59%) of the affected children live with a father struggling with an addiction to alcohol or an illicit drug. Many (35%) live with a mother struggling with an addiction, and relatively few (6%) live with two parents struggling with an addiction.

Conclusion

Although these epidemiologic data help define the scope of the problem, they are not exhaustive. Despite the limitations, McMahon and Giannini (2003) concluded that the existing data consistently indicate that there is a sizable population of children in technologically oriented cultures living in the same household as a father misusing a licit or illicit substance. They also concluded that there appears to be an even larger, but poorly documented, population of children separated from a father misusing a substance. Given the focus of this volume, it is important to note that infants and toddlers may be more likely to be living in the same household as a father misusing primarily alcohol, while older children and adolescents may be more likely to be living away from a father misusing alcohol, nicotine, or other drugs.

Substance Use and Family Formation: A Developmental Perspective

Acknowledging that use of alcohol, nicotine, and marijuana is normative from middle adolescence through the transition to early adulthood, developmental researchers working from several different perspectives have documented empirical links between substance use and family process in the lives of men. Generally, this literature indicates that greater involvement in family life during early to middle adulthood is consistently associated with less substance use. Within this literature, there have, however, been persistent questions about whether this relationship represents a *selection* versus a *socialization* process into positive parenting roles. That is, there have been questions about whether empirical links between family formation and substance use are best explained by (a) a common developmental pathway that begins during childhood and extends into adulthood or (b) the direct influence of family formation on substance use during the transition from adolescence to early adulthood.

Common Developmental Pathways

Although some policy statements imply socially responsible fathering is a choice men make, developmental researchers (e.g., Belsky, 1997, 2000; Belsky, Steinberg, & Draper, 1991) have begun to outline ways genetic, psychological, interpersonal, and social factors influence the reproductive and parenting behavior of men as they move from childhood through adolescence into early to middle adulthood. Similarly, developmental researchers (e.g., Tarter & Vanyukov, 1994; Zucker, 2006) have, for many years, been outlining ways the same constellation of genetic, psychological, interpersonal, and social factors influence risk for the misuse of substances by men as development unfolds over time. Broadly, biopsychosocial influences that put boys on developmental pathways away from problematic use of substances as an adult seem to also put them on pathways to fatherhood within more stable sexual partnerships where there is more social and economic support for family formation. Likewise, biopsychosocial influences that put boys on developmental pathways toward problematic use of substances as an adult seem to also put them on pathways to fatherhood within less stable sexual partnerships where there is less social and economic support for family formation.

Consistent with this concept of common developmental pathways, researchers have used epidemiologic and longitudinal data to show that boys with early use of alcohol and illicit drugs are also at risk for early first sexual intercourse, more sexual partners, and an early unplanned pregnancy in the context of an unstable sexual partnership with limited social support and limited financial resources. For example, Lowry et al. (1994) and Santelli, Brener, Lowry, Bhatt, and Zabin (1998) used data from the Youth Risk Behavior Survey to show that use of alcohol and illicit drugs by boys during adolescence was consistently associated with sexual behavior involving risk for an unplanned pregnancy. Likewise, Capaldi, Crosby, and Stoolmiller (1996) examined data from the Oregon Youth Study and found that early initiation of sexual intercourse by boys was clearly associated with early, frequent, and persistent use of substances during adolescence. Using data from the Rochester Youth Development Study, Krohn, Lizotte, and Perez (1997) found that, among boys at risk for delinquency, early use of alcohol and other drugs was associated with risk for early fatherhood, failure to complete high school, and an early move to independent living. Moreover, transitions into adult roles during adolescence were associated with risk for continued use of alcohol and illicit drugs during early adulthood. Finally, Oesterle, Hawkins, and Hill (2011) defined three pathways through early adulthood for men involving pursuit of post-secondary education, employment, marital status, and fatherhood. When compared with married fathers working full-time and married men with post-secondary education working full-time who delayed having children, unmarried men with less education were more likely to be a father, less likely to be working full-time, and more likely to report problematic use of alcohol, nicotine, and marijuana that began early in adolescence.

Developmental Transitions

As developmental theory has become increasingly sophisticated, the concept of developmental pathways has been complemented by the concepts of *developmental transitions* and *turning points* in development. When discussing continuity and discontinuity in substance use during adolescence, Schulenberg, Maggs, and O'Malley (2003) defined developmental transitions as common, critical, proximal points in development. From their perspective, developmental transitions may be characterized as either *global*, like the transition from adolescence to early adulthood, or *specific*, like the transition to parenthood. When there is continuity in development, developmental transitions serve as an opportunity for an individual to demonstrate continued movement toward positive or negative adaptation. Developmental transitions, like the transition to parenthood, may also serve as turning points where, for a variety of reasons, movement along a developmental pathway may be altered significantly. That is, they may represent a turning toward adaptation in a pathway toward maladaption or a turning toward maladaption in a pathway to adaptation. Therefore, although genetic influences, quality of early family environments, and social context may put boys on broad developmental pathways, more proximal events in lives of young men, like a new sexual partnership or the birth of a first child, may serve as turning points in development.

Substance Use During Transitions into Sexual Partnerships

Consistent with the concept of developmental transitions, Bachman and his associates (Bachman et al., 2002; Bachman, Wadsworth, O'Malley, Johnston, & Schulenberg, 1997) used data from the Monitoring the Future Study to demonstrate that transitions into a committed sexual partnership, like engagement to marry, cohabitation, and marriage, were generally associated with less use of alcohol, nicotine, and illicit drugs by men. Although the focus here is on family formation, it is important to note that Bachman et al. (1997, 2002) also found that separation from a sexual partner was consistently associated with an increase in the use of alcohol by men. Several years later, Staff et al. (2010) used data from the same study to show that use of alcohol, cigarette, marijuana, and cocaine continued to decline with a transition into marriage or cohabitation during early adulthood. Consistent with the concept of turning points in developmental pathways, Lee, Chassin, and MacKinnon (2015) showed that, although there was a general decline in problematic use of alcohol by men following marriage, the potential influence of marriage on alcohol consumption proved most dramatic for men with more serious problems with alcohol prior to the marriage. They concluded that the transition into marriage for men demonstrating less problematic prior use of alcohol seemed to represent continuity in a low-risk developmental trajectory, but the transition for men demonstrating more problematic prior use of alcohol seemed to represent a turning point in a high-risk developmental trajectory.

Unfortunately, some of the relationships between transitions into committed sexual partnerships and substance use outlined by Bachman et al. (1997, 2002) have not proven consistent across investigations. Generally, the existing data most consistently document a relationship between the transition into marriage and a decline in the use and misuse of alcohol by men. For example, Duncan, Wilkerson, and England (2006) examined data drawn from the National Longitudinal Survey of Youth and found that marriage, but not cohabitation, was associated with less problematic use of alcohol and less frequent use of marijuana. Duncan et al. did not find any evidence that a transition into either marriage or cohabitation had any effect on the use of cigarettes. Staff, Greene, Maggs, and Schoon (2014) used data collected from men participating in the National Child Development Study in Great Britain to show that, when compared with men who were not involved in a marital or cohabitating relationship, men who were involved in such a relationship demonstrated less use of alcohol.

Substance Use During Transitions into Fatherhood

Women, much more clearly than men, consistently decrease their substance use during the transition to parenthood. For men, changes in substance use during the transition to parenthood, although generally evident, appear to vary depending on marital status, timing of parenthood, and residential status of the father-child dyad. Following the birth of a child, the stage of parenting may also influence the degree to which changes in substance use persist.

Combining data from three epidemiologic surveys done in Australia, Borschmann et al. (2019) recently found that, although much less dramatic than differences among women, fatherhood was associated with less use of alcohol by men and lower rates of an alcohol use disorder, particularly among men with children less than 12 months of age. Kendler, Lonn, Salvatore, Sundquist, and Sundquist (2016) recently noted a similar pattern among married couples in Sweden. Using data from the Monitoring the Future Study, Bachman et al. (1997, 2002) also showed that the transition to fatherhood was associated with less use of alcohol, nicotine, and illicit drugs. However, the changes in substance use were generally accounted for by a marriage that predated the transition to parenthood. Similarly, Pampel, Mollborn, and Lawrence (2014) used data from the National Longitudinal Study of Adolescent Health to show that the potential impact of fatherhood on the use of tobacco seemed to be dependent on marital status. When compared with men not married without children, married men and married men with children were less likely to be smoking cigarettes, but unmarried men with children were more likely to be smoking cigarettes. Ironically, Verges et al. (2012) used longitudinal data from the National Epidemiologic Survey on Alcohol and Related Conditions to show that the transition to parenthood, but not the transition to marriage, was associated with less risk for both the persistence of an alcohol use disorder and the emergence of an alcohol use disorder. They also noted that the potential impact of parenthood on the persistence of an alcohol use disorder seemed to be more pronounced among older men.

Working with longitudinal data from a sample that included boys at risk for an alcohol use disorder because of a positive family history, Little, Handley, Leuthe, and Chassin (2009) found that men who became parents during early adulthood demonstrated a decrease in alcohol consumption during early adulthood, while men who became parents during adolescence demonstrated an increase in alcohol consumption during early adulthood. Krohn et al. (1997) also noted that an early transition to parenthood was associated with more frequent use of alcohol and illicit drugs during early adulthood. Using longitudinal data from the Christchurch Health and Development Study, Fergusson, Boden, and Horwood (2012) found that, when compared with men 18 to 30 years of age who were not a father, men who were fathers directly involved in the care of children demonstrated less risk for an alcohol or illicit drug use disorder during early adulthood. The finding did not, however, prove true for fathers who were not directly involved in the care of children. Consistent with this, Staff et al. (2010) noted that fathers living with their children were less likely to be using alcohol, marijuana, or cocaine when compared with fathers not living with their children. Given the focus of this volume, it is important to note that Staff et al. (2014) showed that, when compared with men not living with a minor child, men living with a biological, adopted, or stepchild less than 5 years of age most clearly reported less use of alcohol. Men living with a child 5 to 16 years of age also reported less use of alcohol, but men living with a child 16 to 21 years of age reported more use of alcohol.

Personality, Developmental Pathways, and Developmental Transitions

When considering the relationship between substance use and family process, it is important to acknowledge that the existing literature suggests that the consolidation of personality traits during the transition to early adulthood may be an important factor in developmental pathways to fatherhood. Although debate about the exact nature of the relationships continues, personality traits involving conscientiousness, emotionality, and behavioral control have been linked with both substance use and family process. For example, Lee, Ellingson, and Sher (2015) showed that there was moderate to high correlation of problematic use of alcohol and personality traits across early to middle adulthood. They also found that more behavioral control and more conscientiousness at 21 years of age were associated with a greater probability of marriage and parenthood at 25 years of age which were associated with less problematic use of alcohol at 29 years of age. Both personality traits at 29 years of age were also associated with less problematic use of alcohol at 34 years of age. Negative emotionality did not seem to be related to either family transitions or problematic use of alcohol.

Similarly, Pears, Capaldi, and Owen (2007) found that poor behavioral control in boys during middle adolescence was associated with (a) misuse of alcohol and illicit drugs during late adolescence and (b) poor discipline practices during early adulthood when the boys were the father of a 21-month-old child. Likewise, Bailey et al. (2013) found that vulnerability to negative emotion mediated the relationship between illicit drug use during early adulthood and subsequent compromise of parenting behavior with children 2 to 8 years of age. Unlike other researchers (e.g., Lee, Ellingson, & Sher, 2015; Pears et al., 2007), they did not find a significant influence for behavioral control over time.

Using data collected from a cohort of male and female college students, Littlefield, Sher, and Wood (2009, 2010) showed that more conscientiousness at 21 years of age was associated with less problematic use of alcohol and greater probability of marriage and parenthood from 21 to 35 years of age which was associated with a decline in problematic use of alcohol during the same period. In one statistical model (Littlefield et al., 2010) but not the other (Littlefield et al., 2009), less negative emotionality at 21 years of age appeared to be associated with selection into family transitions. Impulsivity did not appear to be related to selection into family transitions. However, they also found that a decrease in negative emotionality, a decrease in impulsivity, and an increase in conscientiousness were each independently associated with a decrease in problematic use of alcohol during this phase of life after allowance for the potential influence of the family transitions.

Conclusion

When considered together, variable and individual-based research designs suggest that, as proposed by Belsky et al. (1991), there are at least two broad developmental pathways that link substance use and family formation as boys move through adolescence into early adulthood. For many boys, biological, psychological, and social advantage that accumulates over childhood and adolescence puts them on developmental pathways to time-limited substance use that resolves as they begin the process of family formation with adequate social and economic resources. Marriage, more so than any other step in the process of family formation, appears to be most clearly associated with a decline in substance use. For other boys, biological, psychological, and social disadvantage that accumulates over childhood and adolescence puts them on developmental pathways to early substance use that persists as they begin the process of family formation without adequate social and economic resources. Early parenthood in the context of unstable sexual partnerships with little involvement in childcare appears to be most clearly associated with persistent substance use. Regardless which developmental pathway young men seem to be on, the consolidation of specific personality traits during the transition from adolescence to early adulthood appears to be a critical influence in the direction they move, and for some young men, specific transitions into relationships as a partner and a parent may represent turning points in a developmental trajectory with unexpected movement toward either more or less substance use.

Substance Use and the Process of Family Formation

Given the prevalence of substance use by men within the general population, it is not surprising that the misuse of substances, particularly alcohol and illicit drugs, appears to be a potential influence on the process of family formation. When considered in total, the existing literature, albeit somewhat limited and inconsistent, suggests that there is a relationship between the misuse of substances and the production and parenting of children by men. It is important to note that most of the research examining the reciprocal relationship between substance use and family process during this phase of life has been done primarily with Euro-American, heterosexual couples living together while the male partner was misusing alcohol. Much less is known about substance use and family process in other contexts.

Substance Use and the Selection of Sexual Partners

Substance use appears to play an important role in the selection of sexual partners and the persistence of those sexual partnerships. Research consistently indicates that, when compared with other men, heterosexual men misusing alcohol or illicit drugs appear to be more likely to select a female sexual partner who has personality, psychiatric, or substance use problems. For example, Leonard and Eiden (1999) noted a significant degree of consistency in the use of alcohol within dyads planning to marry. They also noted that men's use of alcohol may contribute to increases in women's use of alcohol during the transition into marriage. Leonard and Mudar (2004) replicated that finding and noted that spousal influence may, over time, become bidirectional. Ostermann, Sloan, and Taylor (2005) also noted consistency in the use of alcohol within a nationally representative sample of married couples.

Moreover, Eiden, Leonard, Hoyle, and Chavez (2004) found that, when compared with other couples with infant children, approximately 25% of mothers living with a father experiencing problems with alcohol also reported problems involving the use of alcohol. Floyd, Cranford, Daugherty, Fitzgerald, and Zucker (2006) noted a similar pattern among mothers of preschool children living with a father misusing alcohol. Edwards, Eiden, and Leonard (2006) reported that, when compared with other mothers, mothers of preschool children living with a father experiencing problems with alcohol also reported more depression.

Longitudinal research examining links between substance use and family process also suggests that early substance use continuing into the transition to adulthood is generally associated with less stable sexual partnerships that are less likely to serve as the foundation for supportive family environments. For example, McMahon, Winkel, and Rounsaville (2008) found that, when compared with fathers with no history of an alcohol or drug use disorder, men with an opioid use disorder were more likely to have cohabitated with a series of sexual partners and less likely to have been involved in a marriage. Moreover, Hall, Fals-Stewart, and Fincham (2008) found that, even when they do marry, men with an alcohol use disorder are more likely to report being involved in extramarital sexual activity with risk for an unplanned pregnancy. Collins, Ellickson, and Klein (2007) showed that more frequent use of alcohol to intoxication was associated with greater risk for divorce during early adulthood, and Ostermann et al. (2005) showed that risk for divorce may be greatest across the life span when use of alcohol by spouses is discrepant.

Substance Use and Preparation for Conception

Generally, surveys of the general population (Martinez et al., 2006) indicate that fathers report that, from their perspective, pregnancy is most often not planned. This makes it difficult for men to change their substance use when preparing to conceive a child. Moreover, research (e.g., Shawe et al., 2019) suggests that even when preparing for conception many men continue using alcohol, nicotine, and other drugs. Lack of preparation for pregnancy is important because research (e.g., Gundersen et al., 2015; Jensen et al., 2014) suggests that substance use may affect the quality of sperm. Although the results have been inconsistent across investigations, systematic reviews of this literature (e.g., Sharma, Harlev, Agarwal, & Esteves, 2016) indicate that heavy, persistent use of alcohol, cigarettes, and illicit drugs may affect the quantity, mobility, and morphology of sperm in ways that can influence conception.

Substance Use During Pregnancy

Although very few men curtail their substance use in preparation for conception, the research on ways pregnancy influences their substance use has been somewhat inconsistent. Bachman et al. (1997) noted a decrease in the frequency of substance use associated with pregnancy, but much of the change appeared to be associated with a previous transition into a marriage. Several years later, Staff et al. (2010) again examined data from the Monitoring the Future Study and found that frequency of alcohol consumption declined for men when a sexual partner was pregnant, but pregnancy did not seem to affect the use of cigarettes, marijuana, or cocaine. Bailey, Hill, Hawkins, Catalano, and Abbott (2008) showed that use of cigarettes by men declined during pregnancy, but use of alcohol and marijuana did not. It is important to note that, when men continue using substances during pregnancy, women appear to also be more likely to continue using substances, particularly the same substance. For example, Perreira and Cortes (2006) examined data from the Fragile Families and Child Wellbeing Study and noted that men's use of alcohol, nicotine, and illicit drugs correlated strongly with women's use of alcohol, nicotine, and illicit drugs during pregnancy with some specificity in the correlation. That is, when men reported smoking cigarettes during a pregnancy, women were more likely to also report smoking cigarettes during the pregnancy. When men reported using alcohol during a pregnancy, women were more likely to also report using alcohol during the pregnancy.

Substance Use, Sexual Partnerships, and Co-parenting Relationships

Within the substance abuse literature, there is fairly consistent evidence that the quality of sexual partnerships and co-parenting relationships is poorer when men are misusing alcohol and illicit drugs, particularly when men are misusing something and women are not. When couples remain together following the birth of a child, researchers (Finger, Eiden, Edwards, Leonard, & Kachadourian, 2010; Finger et al., 2010; Keller, Cummings, & Davies, 2005; Keller, Cummings, Davies, & Mitchell, 2008; Kachadourian, Eiden, & Leonard, 2009) have consistently shown that, when compared with other couples, couples where father is misusing alcohol or illicit drugs consistently report (a) less marital satisfaction, (b) more marital conflict, (c) less resolution of marital conflict, (d) more verbal aggression, and (e) more physical aggression through the time the child enters kindergarten. Moreover, research done by Homish and Leonard (2007) showed that there was even less satisfaction and more conflict within a marriage when the spouses of men misusing alcohol were also not misusing alcohol or an illicit drug. Consistent with this general trend, McMahon and his colleagues (McMahon et al., 2008; Moore, Easton, & McMahon, 2011) found that there was less negotiation and more aggression in the co-parenting relationships of fathers receiving medication-assisted treatment for opioid addiction when they were compared with fathers with no history of addiction. Risk for psychological, physical, and sexual aggression seemed to be bidirectional, and the risk proved to be surprisingly robust despite the fact that the fathers struggling with drug addiction were much less likely than the other fathers to be living with the mother of their youngest child. That is, risk for aggressive behavior present when the couple was involved in a sexual partnership seemed to persist after the sexual relationship ended.

Substance Use and Parenting Behavior

Systematic reviews of the literature (e.g., McMahon, 2013) suggest that problematic use of alcohol and illicit drugs is generally associated with less positive and more negative parenting behavior by fathers from infancy through adolescence. For example, Eiden and her colleagues (Eiden, Chavez, & Leonard, 1999; Eiden, Edwards, & Leonard, 2007; Eiden, Leonard, et al., 2004; Kachadourian et al., 2009) showed that, when compared with other fathers, fathers misusing alcohol demonstrated less verbal interaction, less positive emotion, and less emotional sensitivity during parent-child interactions with children when the children were 12 to 36 months of age. However, they (Eiden et al., 1999; Finger, Kachadourian, et al., 2010) also found that, although the fathers misusing alcohol reported more frustration and demonstrated more negative emotion during interaction with their 12-month-old children, they did not consistently demonstrate more negative parenting behavior with their children through entry into kindergarten. Within a sample of parents with 3-year-old children at risk for externalizing difficulty, Harvey, Stoessel, and Herbert (2011) found that the misuse of alcohol and illicit drugs by fathers was associated with self-report of more lax parenting behavior, but not self-report of more emotionally reactive parenting behavior nor observer rating of less emotionally responsive or more emotionally reactive parenting behavior. Finally, Eiden, Edwards, and Leonard (2002) showed that, although a surprising number of children were able to establish a secure attachment with a father misusing alcohol, the differences in positive and negative parenting behavior evident in fathers misusing alcohol contributed to significantly fewer children establishing a secure attachment with their father during this phase of development.

Substance Use and Family Environments

Although researchers typically focus on the quality of parenting and co-parenting behavior as a proximal influence on the sense of well-being as parents for men and women, some scholars (e.g., McHale, Kuersten, & Lauretti, 1996) have argued that quality of the general family environment may also contribute to the psychological well-being of both fathers and mothers. After allowance for the quality of parenting behavior, quality of the general family environment may also contribute directly to the cognitive, emotional, and behavioral adjustment of young children. After a systematic review of the limited literature on the topic, McMahon (2013) concluded that the existing, but limited, research shows that, when fathers are present in the home, paternal addiction appears to be associated with family environments characterized by (a) more family conflict, (b) less family cohesion, (c) less consistency in daily routines, (d) more financial stress, and (e) fewer family rituals. Paternal addiction also seems to be associated with (a) more difficulty establishing family rules, (b) poorer communication, (c) more difficulty with emotional expression, (d) less emotional support for everyone, and (e) less instrumental support for everyone. Given the focus of this volume, it is important to highlight the fact that researchers (Fitzgerald et al., 1993; Noll, Zucker, Fitzgerald, & Curtis, 1992; Sanford, Bingham, & Zucker, 1999; Whipple, Fitzgerald, & Zucker, 1995) have also shown that paternal addiction to alcohol has been associated with family environments characterized by less emotional, cognitive, and social stimulation for young children.

Conclusion

Research done over more than 30 years consistently indicates that moderate to severe substance use by men is associated with compromise of family process known to support the production and parenting of children. Most of this research has focused on the potential impact of problems involving the use of alcohol. Significantly less is known about the potential impact of problems involving the use of nicotine and illicit drugs. Despite the gaps in the existing literature, there is sufficient evidence to conclude that the misuse of substances by men is consistently associated with risk for difficulty at every step in the process of family formation.

Paternal Addiction: Consequences for Children

When compared with children whose father has no history of addiction, children whose father is struggling with addiction are much more likely to develop emotional and behavioral difficulty as they move from infancy through childhood and adolescence into early adulthood. Reviews of the existing research (e.g., McMahon, 2013) indicate that, although the risks associated with paternal addiction to nicotine are less clear, children at risk because of paternal addiction to alcohol or illicit drugs are clearly more likely to develop externalizing difficulty characterized by overactive, oppositional, defiant, impulsive, and aggressive behavior. Much of the same research indicates that, although the comparative difference may not be as robust, children at risk because of paternal addiction to alcohol or illicit drugs are also more likely to develop internalizing difficulty characterized by anxiety, depression, and somatic preoccupation. Although the data are limited and inconsistent, this research raises questions about whether children with a father misusing alcohol or illicit drugs are also at risk for relatively poorer intellectual development and relatively poorer academic achievement. Without dispute, this research very clearly indicates that children affected by paternal addiction are much more likely to (a) begin using substances early, (b) use more frequently, (c) use more per occasion, and (d) more quickly develop serious problems.

Consequences for Infants, Toddlers, and Preschool Children

Although limited, research done with infants, toddlers, and preschool children living with a father misusing principally alcohol consistently indicates that risk for emotional-behavioral difficulty emerges very early. Even when there are not clear indications of clinically significant problems, children with a father misusing alcohol and illicit drugs demonstrate a relative disadvantage when compared with other children. For example, Eiden, Leonard, and Morrisey (2001) showed that, when compared with boys the same age living with a father not misusing alcohol or illicit drugs, 18- to 24-month-old boys living with a father misusing alcohol presented with less behavioral compliance when interacting with their father and their mother. Eiden, Edwards, and Leonard (2004) later showed that boys living with a father misusing alcohol also demonstrated less behavioral inhibition at 24 and 36 months of age; and Edwards, Eiden, and Leonard (2006) found that, at 18, 24, and 36 months of age, children living with a father misusing alcohol demonstrated more internalizing and more externalizing difficulty than other children. There was also a general trend for children living with a father misusing alcohol to demonstrate higher rates of clinically significant emotional and behavioral difficulty.

Across a series of investigations done using both parent and observer ratings, Zucker, Fitzgerald, and their colleagues (Jansen, Fitzgerald, Ham, & Zucker, 1995; Martel et al., 2009; Wong et al., 2006; Wong, Zucker, Puttler, & Fitzgerald, 1999) also found that, when compared with other children, 3- to 5-year-old boys and girls living with a father misusing alcohol, particularly a father with antisocial personality traits misusing alcohol, demonstrated more difficult temperament characterized by (a) less attentional capacity, (b) less behavioral inhibition, (c) less adaptability, (d) more activity, and (e) more emotional reactivity. They (Jansen et al., 1995; Puttler, Zucker, Fitzgerald, & Bingham, 1998) also documented higher levels of externalizing and internalizing difficulty in the children living with a father misusing alcohol. Moreover, although Leonard and Eiden et al. (2002) did not find any significant differences in cognitive or motor development when infants and toddlers living with a father who was misusing alcohol were compared with other infants and toddlers, Zucker, Fitzgerald, and their colleagues (Poon, Ellis, Fitzgerald, & Zucker, 2000; Puttler et al., 1998) found significant differences in cognitive development at 3 to 8 years of age in a comparative study of children affected by paternal addiction. They also documented significant differences in academic achievement at 6 to 8 years of age. Finally, Zucker, Kincaid, Fitzgerald, and Bingham (1995) showed that 3- to 5-year-old boys living with a father misusing alcohol were more likely than other boys to correctly identify alcoholic beverages and they were likely to attribute the use of alcoholic beverages to men, suggesting that very early in life the boys were developing cognitive representations of alcohol consumption that may reflect environmental risk for early experimentation with alcohol during adolescence.

Conclusion

Research done with children of all ages clearly indicates that parental addiction, including paternal addiction, is clearly associated with risk for compromise of normative child development. Limited research done with infants, toddlers, and preschool children suggests that, although development may still fall within a normative range, relative disadvantages emerge early in the life of these children, primarily in the form of (a) difficult temperament as an infant, (b) difficulty with emotional and behavioral control as a toddler, and (c) early externalizing difficulty as a preschool child. Most of the difficulty seems to be in the emotional-behavioral domain. If they incur disadvantages in cognitive and academic domains, those differences may not be evident until children make the transition into elementary school.

Paternal Addiction: A Conceptual Model of Family Process and Child Development

Paternal substance use clearly represents risk for poor developmental outcomes in children during their formative years. However, because of complex relationships involving any marker of risk and other potential influences in the lives of children, paternal substance use appears to represent a global risk in the lives of children that confers both genetic and environmental risk for poor developmental outcomes that undoubtedly gets attenuated and exacerbated in multiple ways over time. At this time, there appears to be agreement (Tarter & Vanyukov, 1994; Fitzgerald, Davies, & Zucker, 2002; Zucker, 2006) that family process interacts in complex ways with genetic vulnerability to influence developmental outcomes for children. Although not exhaustive, Fig. 36.1 outlines a conceptual model of nested familial influences likely to be operative in the lives of infants, toddlers, and preschool children living in family systems affected by paternal addiction. As research designs examining mediation and moderation of threats to normative development present in the lives of children have become increasingly sophisticated, prospective research done with children at risk has begun to clarify ways paternal substance use influences developmental outcomes in children from conception through the preschool years. Generally, this research suggests that, during these initial phases of life, paternal substance use seems to represent a more distal influence that impacts the biopsychosocial development of children through proximal mechanisms involving genetic transmission of difficult temperament and compromise of family environments.

Distal Risks: Parental Addiction, Psychopathology, and Personality Difficulty

Within the limited literature on the dynamics of substance use and family formation, researchers have found support for many of the mechanisms of potential influence outlined in Fig. 36.1. During this phase of the family life cycle, paternal substance use may, consistent with the conceptual model outlined by Kraemer, Stice, Kazdin, Offord, and Kupfer (2001), best be understood as an overlapping or concurrent threat to normative child development through association with comorbid personality and psychiatric disturbance. That is, risk for disruption of family process may not necessarily be limited to just the substance use; personality difficulty and psychiatric disturbance common among men misusing

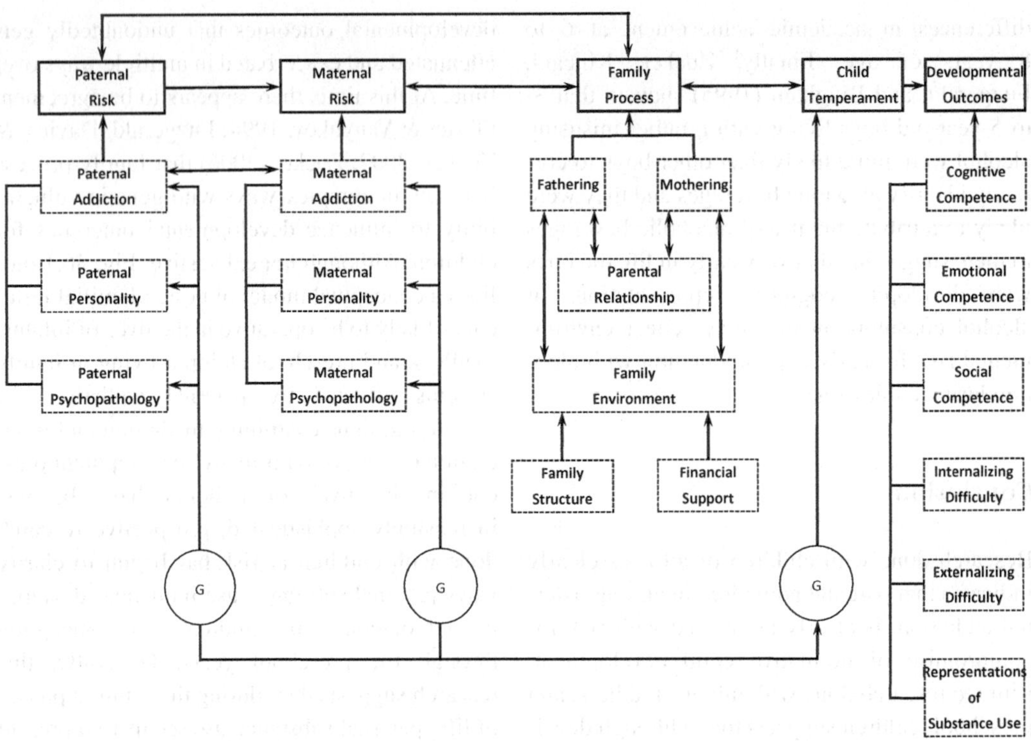

Fig. 36.1 Conceptual Model of Paternal Addiction, Family Process, and Child Development During Family Formation

substances may also be contributing. Consistent with this, Eiden and her colleagues (Eiden et al., 1999; Eiden & Leonard, 2000) illustrated how difference in positive and negative parenting behavior associated with the misuse of alcohol by men may more clearly be related to comorbid depression. They (Edwards, Eiden, Colder, & Leonard, 2006) also found that risk for internalizing difficulty in toddlers associated with paternal addiction may be more clearly linked with comorbid depression. Moreover, Poon et al. (2000) and Johnson, Cohen, Kasen, and Brook (2004) showed that combinations of paternal substance use, personality, and psychiatric problems may affect genetic liability and family process in an additive manner. Similarly, research mentioned above suggests that paternal addiction may be a proxy for substance use, personality, or psychiatric problems in the mother or some combination of substance use, personality, and psychiatric problems in both parents. Repeatedly, researchers (e.g., Eiden, Edwards, & Leonard, 2004) have shown that the presence or absence of maternal psychopathology and substance use may mitigate or exacerbate the potential impact of paternal addiction, and they (Poon et al., 2000; Hussong et al., 2007; Osborne & Berger, 2009) have shown that risk for children appears to be greatest when both parents are experiencing serious difficulty.

Genetic Liability: Difficult Child Temperament

Research mentioned above suggests that, during early childhood, a positive family history of substance use, personality, and psychiatric difficulty appears, as noted in Fig. 36.1, to confer genetic liability for difficult temperament which represents early risk for the development of substance use and related problems across generations. Work done by Eiden and her colleagues (Edwards, Eiden, & Leonard, 2006) and Zucker, Fitzgerald, and their colleagues (Jansen et al., 1995; Martel et al., 2009; Wong et al., 2006; Wong et al., 1999) suggests links between paternal addiction and infant temperament characterized by extreme emotionality, and behavioral disinhibition seems to represent early risk for externalizing and internalizing difficulty during childhood and adolescence. Substance use and comorbid personality and psychiatric difficulty in fathers, with or without similar difficulty in mothers, appear to contribute to the attenuation or exacerbation of risk associated with temperamental differences, primarily through the impact of the addiction and related problems on different dimensions of family process represented in Fig. 36.1 as (a) general family environment, (b) quality of the parental relationship, (c) the parenting behavior of mothers and fathers, and (d) the quality of the parent-child relationships.

Proximal Influences: Family and Marital Environments

Substantial support for potential mechanisms of influence outlined in Fig. 36.1 comes from the limited literature on family process and early child development in the context of paternal addiction to alcohol. For example, Loukas, Fitzgerald, Zucker, and von Eye (2001) examined data drawn for the Michigan Longitudinal Study and showed that, even after allowance for parent-child conflict during the preschool years, general family conflict contributed to mediation of links between addiction to alcohol and antisocial behavior in fathers and risk for externalizing behavior in boys during early elementary school. Loukas, Zucker, Fitzgerald, and Krull (2003) then found that conflictual family environments more frequently associated with paternal addiction were linked with more disruptive behavior during the preschool years and a slower rate of decline in disruptive behavior from 3 to 6 to 12 years of age. Subsequently, Jester et al. (2005) showed that high-risk developmental pathways from early childhood into adolescence more likely among children affected by paternal addiction were predicted by quality of the family environment during the preschool years.

Similarly, quality of parental relationship appears to be an important influence in family process occurring in the context of paternal addiction. For example, Kachadourian et al. (2009) showed that less satisfaction with their marital relationship mediated the link between paternal addiction to alcohol and less emotionally responsive parenting behavior in mothers with preschool children. Likewise, Finger, Kachadourian, et al. (2010) found prospective links between misuse of alcohol, depression, and antisocial behavior in fathers when children were 12 to 24 months of age and marital aggression when children were 36 months of age and negative parenting behavior in fathers when children were 60 months of age. Similarly, Keller et al. (2008) outlined a family process illustrating how concurrent misuse of alcohol by fathers and mothers when children were enrolled in kindergarten was associated with serious marital conflict which was associated with less positive and more negative parenting by both mothers and fathers which was then associated with more internalizing difficulty and more externalizing difficulty in children.

Proximal Influences: Parenting Behavior

The existing literature on paternal addiction generally supports the idea that the parenting behavior of fathers and mothers which impacts the quality of parent-child relationships is undoubtedly the most proximal influence in comprehensive models of risk during this phase of life. Consistent with this, Eiden et al. (2002) demonstrated that risk for insecure father-child attachment associated with paternal addiction was, as expected, accounted for by less emotionally sensitive parenting behavior among the fathers misusing alcohol. Subsequently, Eiden, Edwards, and Leonard (2004, 2006) noted that difficulty internalizing parental rules of conduct and difficulty with inhibitory control over behavior that may be more common among 24- to 36-month-old children with a father misusing substances seemed to be associated with compromise of positive parenting behavior in both mothers and fathers. Similarly, Wong et al. (1999) illustrated how negative parenting behavior by fathers and mothers partially explained links between difficult child temperament during the preschool years and externalizing behavior during early elementary school within family systems affected by paternal addiction. Furthermore, Finger, Eiden, et al. (2010) found that compromise of social competence in children during enrollment in kindergarten associated with exposure to the marital aggression more common among couples affected by paternal addiction was largely explained by the impact of the marital relationship on the positive parenting behavior of mothers and fathers.

Mitigating, Exacerbating, and Reciprocal Influences

Paternal substance use represents global risk for relatively poorer developmental outcomes, but the psychosocial adjustment of children tends to be variable. Many children do not demonstrate signs or symptoms of serious emotional, behavioral, cognitive, or academic difficulty, particularly during early childhood before the relative disadvantages incurred by children affected by parental addiction have had a cumulative effect on child development. On a limited basis, researchers (Brook et al., 2002; Brook et al., 2002) have begun to explore ways protective and vulnerability factors may interact across different levels of social organization to modify the risk incurred by children affected by paternal substance use. Given the focus of this volume, it is important to note that Eiden et al. (2002) showed that risk for internalizing and externalizing difficulty associated with exposure to paternal addiction may be moderated by a secure attachment with a mother as children move from 12 to 36 months of age. Because of clear bias for researchers to focus on disruption of parenting and the maladjustment of children, McMahon (2013) highlighted the fact that virtually nothing is known about ways positive parenting behavior occurring despite the presence of problematic use of substances may promote normative development in young children. Although not represented in Fig. 36.1, researchers (Andreas, O'Farrell, & Fals-Stewart, 2006, Andreas & O'Farrell, 2009; Andreas & O'Farrell, 2007; Rounsaville, O'Farrell, Andreas, Murphy, & Murphy, 2014) have demonstrated that abstinence following substance use treatment for fathers may attenuate exposure to conflictual family environments and attenuate risk for internalizing and externalizing difficulty in children, including preschool children. However, very little is known about ways comorbid personality and psychiatric difficulty common among men struggling with addiction may continue to influence family process after fathers are no longer misusing substances.

Finally, risk to children associated with paternal addiction may also vary with characteristics of the child. When considering quality of parent-child interaction within family systems affected by paternal addiction, Eiden, Leonard, et al. (2004) found that fathers seemed to interact more positively with daughters versus sons at 12 months of age and paternal addiction did not appear to contribute to compromise of positive parenting behavior in mothers or fathers until the infants were 24 months of age. Although researchers interested in parenting (e.g., Bornstein, 2019) have suggested reciprocal mechanisms of influence in parent-child interactions, Eiden, Leonard, Hoyle, and Chaves found no evidence that the behavior of toddlers evoked parental behavior in the context of paternal addiction to alcohol. Prospective links suggested that parental behavior, more clearly maternal behavior, was influencing child behavior much more than child behavior was influencing parental behavior when children were 12 to 24 months of age.

Conclusion

Although neither exhaustive nor definitive, this conceptual model of family formation in the context of paternal addiction illustrates how the principles of developmental psychopathology (Cicchetti, 2006) can be used to organize the existing literature and clarify ways misuse of alcohol, nicotine, and illicit drugs by men affects the psychosocial adjustment of fathers, mothers, and children during this phase of life. When grounded in a systematic review of the existing literature, conceptual models like this can inform (a) research designed to address gaps in the knowledge base, (b) clinical intervention designed to address family issues among parenting receiving substance use treatment, and (c) targeted prevention designed to promote normative development among children affected by paternal addiction.

Summary and Key Findings

Fatherhood is an important developmental transition in the lives of most men that has, over the previous 20 years, been redefined by an array of social, economic, and political changes. Amid calls by policymakers for programs to promote socially responsible fathering, substance use remains one of the more common threats to family process known to promote the social and psychological well-being of fathers, mothers, and children. Although the existing literature is, in many instances, limited or inconsistent, there is substantial empirical evidence that substance use affects the production and parenting of children by men and the production and parenting of children affects substance use by men.

There are six key findings supported by this comprehensive review of this literature. First, epidemiologic data collected in several different ways indicate that (a) there is a sizable population of children living in the same household as a father misusing substances and (b) there is a sizable, but poorly documented, population of children separated from a father misusing substances. Infants, toddlers, and preschool children may be more likely than older children and teens to be living in the same household as a father misusing primarily alcohol. Second, despite implications that socially responsible fathering is a choice for men to make, developmental research suggests that, consistent with a life history perspective on procreation, there appears to be a complex set of biopsychosocial influences that put boys on broad developmental pathways toward fatherhood in the context of more stable sexual partnerships, minimal substance use, and more social and economic support for family formation versus fatherhood in the context of less stable sexual partnerships, more substance use, and less social and economic support for family formation. Consolidation of personality traits associated with individual differences in substance use and sexuality may exert substantial influence on the general direction development takes. Third, as boys move through adolescence into early adulthood, transitions into sexual partnerships and parenthood may represent turning points where the direction of a developmental trajectory may change for better or worse.

Fourth, substance use by men appears to be a threat to successful family formation from selection of a sexual partner through the parenting of children into the preschool years. Next, substance use by men also appears to represent a threat to normative child development during this phase of life. Risk for externalizing and, to a lesser extent, internalizing difficulty linked with early, problematic use of substances during adolescence emerges early in childhood among children affected by paternal addiction. Finally, risk for intergenerational transmission of substance use and related difficulty during this phase of life appears to be best characterized as the early expression of genetic liability in the form of difficult temperament attenuated or exacerbated by family process. Positive versus negative parenting behavior occurring within complex reciprocal interactions between children and both fathers and mothers may, over time, appear to be the critical, proximal influence on the psychosocial adjustment of children living in family systems affected by paternal addiction.

To close, McMahon and Rounsaville (2002) argued, almost 20 years ago, that the potential impact of substance use on fathering and fathering on substance use needed to be more clearly acknowledged in the conceptualization of public policy, service delivery, and research as fathering emerged as one of the more prominent social issues of the new millennium. At that time, research (e.g., Eiden et al., 1999; Eiden & Leonard, 1996; Fitzgerald et al., 1993; Jansen et al., 1995; Puttler et al., 1998) on ways paternal addiction to alcohol might influence family process and child development during this phase of life was just beginning. As the literature on substance use and fathering during family formation continues to expand, policymakers, researchers, and providers need, as McMahon and Rounsaville suggested, to use this literature to inform the development of creative preventive and clinical interventions designed to minimize the harm associated with paternal addiction for fathers, mothers, and children.

References

Andreas, J. B., & O'Farrell, T. J. (2007). Longitudinal associations between fathers' heavy drinking patterns and children's psychosocial adjustment. *Journal of Abnormal Child Psychology, 35*, 1–16.

Andreas, J. B., & O'Farrell, T. J. (2009). Alcoholics Anonymous attendance following 12-step treatment participation as a link between alcohol-dependent fathers' treatment involvement and their children's externalizing problems. *Journal of Substance Abuse Treatment, 36*, 87–100.

Andreas, J. B., O'Farrell, T. J., & Fals-Stewart, W. (2006). Does individual treatment for alcoholic fathers benefit their children? A longitudinal assessment. *Journal of Consulting and Clinical Psychology, 74*, 191–198.

Bachman, J. G., O'Malley, P. M., Schulenberg, J. E., Johnston, L. D., Bryant, A. L., & Merline, A. C. (2002). *The decline of substance use in young adulthood: Changes in social activities, roles, and beliefs*. Mahwah, NJ: Lawrence Erlbaum Associates.

Bachman, J. G., Wadsworth, K. N., O'Malley, P. M., Johnston, L. D., & Schulenberg, J. E. (1997). *Smoking, drinking, and drug use in young adulthood: The impacts of new freedoms and new responsibilities*. Mahwah, NJ: Lawrence Erlbaum Associates.

Bailey, J. A., Hill, K. G., Guttmannova, K., Oesterle, S., Hawkins, J. D., Catalano, R. F., et al. (2013). The association between parent early adult drug use disorder and later observed parenting practices and child behavior problems: Testing alternate models. *Developmental Psychology, 49*, 887–899.

Bailey, J. A., Hill, K. G., Hawkins, J. D., Catalano, R. F., & Abbott, R. D. (2008). Men's and women's patterns of substance use around pregnancy. *Birth, 35*, 50–59.

Belsky, J. (1997). Attachment, mating, and parenting: An evolutionary interpretation. *Human Nature, 8*, 361–381.

Belsky, J. (2000). Conditional and alternative reproductive strategies: Individual differences in susceptibility to rearing experiences. In J. L. Rodgers, D. C. Rowe, & W. B. Miller (Eds.), *Genetic influences on human fertility and sexuality: Theoretical and empirical contributions from the biological and behavioral sciences* (pp. 127–146). Boston, MA: Clair Academic Publishing.

Belsky, J., Steinberg, L., & Draper, P. (1991). Childhood experience, interpersonal development, and reproductive strategy: An evolutionary theory of socialization. *Child Development, 62*, 647–670.

Bornstein, M. H. (2019). *Parenting infants. Handbook of parenting, vol. I: Children and parenting* (3rd ed.pp. 3–55). New York, NY: Routledge.

Borschmann, R., Becker, D., Spry, E., Youssef, G. J., Olsson, C. A., Hutchinson, D. M., et al. (2019). Alcohol and parenthood: An integrative analysis of the effects of transition to parenthood in three Australasian cohorts. *Drug and Alcohol Dependence, 197*, 326–334.

Brook, D. W., Brook, J. S., Richter, L., Whiteman, M., Arencibia-Mireles, O., & Masci, J. R. (2002). Marijuana use among the adolescent children of high-risk drug-abusing fathers. *American Journal on Addictions, 11*, 95–110.

Brook, D. W., Brook, J. S., Whiteman, M., Arencibia-Mireles, O., Pressman, M. A., & Rubenstone, E. (2002). Coping in adolescent children of HIV-positive and HIV-negative substance-abusing fathers. *Journal of Genetic Psychology, 163*, 5–23.

Capaldi, D. M., Crosby, L., Stoolmiller, M. (1996). Predicting the timing of first sexual intercourse for at-risk adolescent males. *Child Development, 67*, 344–359.

Chen, C. M., Slater, M. E., Castle, I. -J. P., & Grant, B. F. (2016). U.S. alcohol epidemiologic data reference manual: Vol. 10. Main findings from the 2012–2013 National Epidemiologic Survey on Alcohol and Related Conditions-III (NESARC-III) (NIH Publication No. 16-AA-8020). Bethesda, MD: National Institute on Alcohol Abuse and Alcoholism.

Chou, S. P., Goldstein, R. B., Smith, S. M., Huang, B., Ruan, W. J., Zhang, H., et al. (2016). The epidemiology of DSM-5 nicotine use disorder: Results from the National Epidemiologic Survey on alcohol and related conditions-III. *Journal of Clinical Psychiatry, 77*, 1404–1412.

Cicchetti, D. (2006). Development and psychopathology. In D. Cicchetti & D. J. Cohen (Eds.), *Developmental psychopathology, Vol. 1: Theory and method* (2nd ed., pp. 1–23). New York, NY: John Wiley & Sons.

Collins, R. L., Ellickson, P. L., & Klein, D. J. (2007). The role of substance use in young adult divorce. *Addiction, 102*, 786–794.

Degenhardt, L., Stockings, E., Patton, G., Hall, W. D., & Lynskey, M. (2016). The increasing global health priority of substance use in young people. *Lancet Psychiatry, 3*, 251–264.

Duncan, G. J., Wilkerson, B., & England, P. (2006). Cleaning up their act: The effects of marriage and cohabitation on licit and illicit drug use. *Demography, 43*, 691–710.

Edwards, E., Eiden, R., & Leonard, K. E. (2006). Behavior problems in 18- to 36-month-old children of alcoholic fathers: Secure mother–infant attachment as a protective factor. *Development and Psychopathology, 18*, 395–407.

Edwards, E. P., Eiden, R. D., Colder, C. R., & Leonard, K. E. (2006). The development of aggression in 18 to 48-month-old children of alcoholic parents. *Journal of Abnormal Child Psychology, 34*, 409–423.

Eiden, R. D., Chavez, F., & Leonard, K. E. (1999). Parent-infant interactions among families with alcoholic fathers. *Development and Psychopathology, 11*, 745–762.

Eiden, R. D., Edwards, E. P., & Leonard, K. E. (2002). Mother-infant and father-infant attachment among alcoholic families. *Development and Psychopathology, 14*, 253–278.

Eiden, R. D., Edwards, E. P., & Leonard, K. E. (2004). Predictors of effortful control among children of alcoholic and nonalcoholic fathers. *Journal of Studies on Alcohol, 65*, 309–319.

Eiden, R. D., Edwards, E. P., & Leonard, K. E. (2006). Children's internalization of rules of conduct: Role of parenting in alcoholic families. *Psychology of Addictive Behaviors, 20*, 305–315.

Eiden, R. D., Edwards, E. P., & Leonard, K. E. (2007). A conceptual model for the development of externalizing behavior problems among kindergarten children of alcoholic families: Role of parenting and children's self-regulation. *Developmental Psychology, 43*, 1187–1201.

Eiden, R. D., & Leonard, K. E. (1996). Paternal alcohol use and the mother-infant relationship. *Development and Psychopathology, 8*, 307–323.

Eiden, R. D., & Leonard, K. E. (2000). Paternal alcoholism, parental psychopathology, and aggravation with infants. *Journal of Substance Abuse, 11*, 17–29.

Eiden, R. D., Leonard, K. E., & Morrisey, S. (2001). Paternal alcoholism and toddler noncompliance. *Alcoholism: Clinical and Experimental Research, 25*, 1621–1633.

Eiden, R. D., Leonard, K. E., Hoyle, R. H., & Chavez, F. (2004). A transactional model of parent-infant interactions in alcoholic families. *Psychology of Addictive Behaviors, 18*, 350–361.

Fergusson, D. M., Boden, J. M., & Horwood, L. J. (2012). Transition to parenthood and substance use disorders: Findings from a 30-year longitudinal study. *Drug and Alcohol Dependence, 125*, 295–300.

Finger, B., Eiden, R. D., Edwards, E. P., Leonard, K. E., & Kachadourian, L. (2010). Marital aggression and child peer competence: A comparison of three conceptual models. *Personal Relationships, 17*, 357–376.

Finger, B., Kachadourian, L. K., Molnar, D. S., Eiden, R. D., Edwards, E. P., & Leonard, K. E. (2010). Alcoholism, associated risk factors, and harsh parenting among fathers: Examining the role of marital aggression. *Addictive Behaviors, 35*, 541–548.

Fitzgerald, H. E., Davies, W. H., & Zucker, R. A. (2002). Growing up in an alcoholic family: Structuring pathways for risk aggregation and theory-driven intervention. In R. J. McMahon & R. D. Peters (Eds.), *The effects of parental dysfunction on children* (pp. 127–146). New York, NY: Kluwer Academic/Plenum Publishers.

Fitzgerald, H. E., Sullivan, L. A., Ham, H. P., Zucker, R. A., Bruckel, S., & Schneider, A. M. (1993). Predictors of behavioral problems in three-year-old sons of alcoholics: Early evidence for onset of risk. *Child Development, 64*, 110–123.

Floyd, F. J., Cranford, J. A., Daugherty, M. K., Fitzgerald, H. E., & Zucker, R. A. (2006). Marital interaction in alcoholic and nonalcoholic couples: Alcoholic subtype variations and wives' alcoholism status. *Journal of Abnormal Psychology, 115*, 121–130.

Gavanas, A. (2002). The fatherhood responsibility movement: The centrality of marriage, work and male sexuality in reconstructions of masculinity and fatherhood. In B. Hobson (Ed.), *Making men into fathers: Men, masculinities, and the social politics of fatherhood* (pp. 213–242). Cambridge, England: Cambridge University Press.

Grant, B. F., Chou, S. P., Saha, T. D., Pickering, R. P., Kerridge, B. T., Ruan, W. J., et al. (2017). Prevalence of 12-month alcohol use, high-risk drinking, and DSM-IV alcohol use disorder in the United States, 2001-2002 to 2012-2013: Results from the National Epidemiologic Survey on alcohol and related conditions. *JAMA Psychiatry, 74*, 911–923.

Grant, B. F., Goldstein, R. B., Saha, T. D., Chou, S. P., Jung, J., Zhang, H., et al. (2015). The epidemiology of DSM-5 alcohol use disorder: Results from the National Epidemiologic Survey on alcohol and related conditions-III. *JAMA Psychiatry, 72*, 757–766.

Grant, B. F., Saha, T. D., Ruan, W. J., Goldstein, R. B., Chou, S. P., Jung, J., et al. (2016). Epidemiology of DSM-5 drug use disorder: Results from the National Epidemiologic Survey on alcohol and related conditions-III. *JAMA Psychiatry, 73*, 39–47.

Gundersen, T. D., Jørgensen, N., Andersson, A., Bang, A. K., Nordkap, L., Skakkebæk, N. E., et al. (2015). Association between use of marijuana and male reproductive hormones and semen quality: A study among 1,215 healthy young men. *American Journal of Epidemiology, 182*, 473–481.

Hall, J. H., Fals-Stewart, W., & Fincham, F. D. (2008). Risky sexual behavior among married alcoholic men. *Journal of Family Psychology, 22*, 287–292.

Harvey, E., Stoessel, B., & Herbert, S. (2011). Psychopathology and parenting practices of parents of preschool children with behavior problems. *Parenting, 11*, 239–263.

Hasin, D. S., Kerridge, B. T., Saha, T. D., Huang, B., Pickering, R., Smith, S. M., et al. (2016). Prevalence and correlates of DSM-5 cannabis use disorder, 2012-2013: Findings from the National Epidemiologic

Survey on alcohol and related conditions-III. *American Journal of Psychiatry, 173*, 588–599.

Hasin, D. S., Saha, T. D., Kerridge, B. T., Goldstein, R. B., Chou, S. P., Zhang, H., et al. (2015). Prevalence of marijuana use disorders in the United States between 2001-2002 and 2012-2013. *JAMA Psychiatry, 72*, 1235–1242.

Homish, G. G., & Leonard, K. E. (2007). The drinking partnership and marital satisfaction: The longitudinal influence of discrepant drinking. *Journal of Consulting and Clinical Psychology, 75*, 43–51.

Huang, L. X., Cerbone, F. G., & Gfroerer, J. C. (1998). Children at risk because of parental substance abuse. In *Substance Abuse and Mental Health Services Administration, Office of Applied Studies, Analysis of substance abuse and treatment need issues* (pp. 5–18). Rockville, MD: U.S. Department of Health & Human Services.

Hussong, A. M., Wirth, R. J., Edwards, M. C., Curran, P. J., Chassin, L. A., & Zucker, R. A. (2007). Externalizing symptoms among children of alcoholic parents: Entry points for an antisocial pathway to alcoholism. *Journal of Abnormal Psychology, 116*, 529–542.

Jansen, R. E., Fitzgerald, H. E., Ham, H. P., & Zucker, R. A. (1995). Pathways into risk: Temperament and behavior problems in three to five-year-old sons of alcoholics. *Alcoholism: Clinical and Experimental Research, 19*, 501–509.

Jensen, T. K., Gottschau, M., Madsen, J. O. B., Andersson, A., Lassen, T. H., Skakkebæk, N. E., et al. (2014). Habitual alcohol consumption associated with reduced semen quality and changes in reproductive hormones: A cross-sectional study among 1,221 young Danish men. *BMJ Open, 4*, e005462.

Jester, J. M., Nigg, J. T., Adams, K. M., Fitzgerald, H. E., Puttler, L. I., Wong, M. M., et al. (2005). Inattention/hyperactivity and aggression from early childhood to adolescence: Heterogeneity of trajectories and differential influence of family environment characteristics. *Development and Psychopathology, 17*, 99–125.

Johnson, J. G., Cohen, P., Kasen, S., & Brook, J. S. (2004). Paternal psychiatric symptoms and maladaptive paternal behavior in the home during the child rearing years. *Journal of Child and Family Studies, 13*, 421–437.

Kachadourian, L. K., Eiden, R. D., & Leonard, K. E. (2009). Paternal alcoholism, negative parenting, and the mediating role of marital satisfaction. *Addictive Behaviors, 34*, 918–927.

Keller, P., Cummings, E., Davies, P., & Mitchell, P. (2008). Longitudinal relations between parental drinking problems, family functioning, and child adjustment. *Development and Psychopathology, 20*, 195–212.

Keller, P. S., Cummings, E. M., & Davies, P. T. (2005). The role of marital discord and parenting in relations between parental problem drinking and child adjustment. *Journal of Child Psychology and Psychiatry and Allied Disciplines, 46*, 943–951.

Kendler, K., Lonn, S. L., Salvatore, J., Sundquist, J., & Sundquist, K. (2016). Effect of marriage on risk for onset of alcohol use disorder: A longitudinal and co-relative analysis in a Swedish national sample. *American Journal of Psychiatry, 173*, 911–918.

Kraemer, H. C., Stice, E., Kazdin, A., Offord, D., & Kupfer, D. (2001). How do risk factors work together? Mediators, moderators, and independent, overlapping, and proxy risk factors. *American Journal of Psychiatry, 158*, 848–856.

Krohn, M., Lizotte, A., & Perez, C. (1997). The interrelationship between substance use and precocious transitions to adult statuses. *Journal of Health and Social Behavior, 38*, 87–103.

Lee, M. R., Chassin, L., & MacKinnon, D. P. (2015). Role transitions and young adult maturing out of heavy drinking: Evidence for larger effects of marriage among more severe premarriage problem drinkers. *Alcohol: Clinical and Experimental Research, 39*, 1064–1074.

Lee, M. R., Ellingson, J. M., & Sher, K. J. (2015). Integrating social contextual and intrapersonal mechanisms of "maturing out": Joint influences of familial role transitions and personality maturation on problem drinking reductions. *Alcohol: Clinical and Experimental Research, 39*, 1775–1787.

Leonard, K. E., & Eiden, R. D. (1999). Husbands and wives drinking: Unilateral or bilateral influences among newlyweds in a general population sample. *Journal of Studies on Alcohol, Suppl., 13*, 130–138.

Leonard, K. E., & Mudar, P. (2004). Husbands influence on wives' drinking: Testing a relationship motivation model in the early years of marriage. *Psychology of Addictive Behaviors, 18*, 340–349.

Lipari, R. N., & Van Horn, S. L. (2017, August). *Children living with parents who have a substance use disorder*. Rockville, MD: Substance Abuse and Mental Health Services Administration, Center for Behavioral Health Statistics and Quality.

Little, M., Handley, E., Leuthe, E., & Chassin, L. (2009). The impact of parenthood on alcohol consumption trajectories: Variations as a function of timing of parenthood, familial alcoholism, and gender. *Development and Psychopathology, 21*, 661–682.

Littlefield, A. K., Sher, K. J., & Wood, P. K. (2009). Is "maturing out" of problematic alcohol involvement related to personality change? *Journal of Abnormal Psychology, 118*, 360–374.

Littlefield, A. K., Sher, K. J., & Wood, P. K. (2010). Do changes in drinking motives mediate the relation between personality change and "maturing out" of problem drinking? *Journal of Abnormal Psychology, 119*, 93–105.

Loukas, A., Fitzgerald, H. E., Zucker, R. A., & von Eye, A. (2001). Parental alcoholism and co-occurring antisocial behavior: Prospective relationships to externalizing behavior problems in their young sons. *Journal of Abnormal Child Psychology, 29*, 91–106.

Loukas, A., Zucker, R. A., Fitzgerald, H. E., & Krull, J. L. (2003). Developmental trajectories of disruptive behavior problems among sons of alcoholics: Effects of parent psychopathology, family conflict, and child undercontrol. *Journal of Abnormal Psychology, 112*, 119–131.

Lowry, R., Holtzman, D., Truman, B. I., Kann, L., Collins, J. L., & Kolbe, L. J. (1994). Substance use and HIV-related sexual behaviors among US high school students: Are they related? *American Journal of Public Health, 84*, 1116–1120.

Martel, M. M., Pierce, L., Nigg, J. T., Jester, J. M., Adams, K., Puttler, L. I., et al. (2009). Temperament pathways to childhood disruptive behavior and adolescent substance abuse: Testing a cascade model. *Journal of Abnormal Child Psychology, 37*, 363–373.

Martinez, G. M., Chandra, A., Abma, J. C., Jones, J., & Mosher, W. D. (2006). Fertility, contraception, and fatherhood: Data on men and women from cycle 6 (2002) of the National Survey of family growth. *Vital and Health Statistics, 23*(26).

McHale, J. P., Kuersten, R., & Lauretti, A. (1996). New directions in the study of family-level dynamics during infancy and early childhood. In J. P. McHale & P. A. Cowan (Eds.), *Understanding how family-level dynamics affect children's development: Studies of two-parent families* (pp. 5–26). San Francisco, CA: Jossey-Bass.

McMahon, T. J. (2013). Substance-abusing fathers: A developmental perspective. In N. E. Suchman, M. Pajulo, & L. C. Mayes (Eds.), *Parenting and substance addiction: Developmental approaches to intervention* (pp. 156–182). New York, NY: Oxford University Press.

McMahon, T. J., & Giannini, F. D. (2003). Substance-abusing fathers in family court: Moving from popular stereotypes to therapeutic jurisprudence. *Family Court Review, 41*, 337–353.

McMahon, T. J., & Rounsaville, B. J. (2002). Substance abuse and fathering: Adding poppa to the research agenda. *Addiction, 97*, 1109–1115.

McMahon, T. J., Winkel, J. D., Luthar, S. S., & Rounsaville, B. J. (2005). Looking for poppa: Parenting responsibilities of men versus women seeking drug abuse treatment. *American Journal of Drug and Alcohol Abuse, 31*, 79–91.

McMahon, T. J., Winkel, J. D., & Rounsaville, B. J. (2008). Drug-abuse and responsible fathering: A comparative study of men enrolled in methadone maintenance treatment. *Addiction, 103*, 269–283.

Merline, A. C., O'Malley, P. M., Schulenberg, J. E., Bachman, J. G., & Johnston, L. D. (2004). Substance use among adults 35 years of age: Prevalence, adulthood predictors, and impact of adolescent substance use. *American Journal of Public Health, 94*, 96–102.

Miech, R. A., Johnston, L. D., O'Malley, P. M., Bachman, J. G., Schulenberg, J. E., & Patrick, M. E. (2019). *Monitoring the future national survey results on drug use, 1975-2018: Vol. I, Secondary school students*. Ann Arbor, MI: University of Michigan, National Center for Health Statistics.

Moore, B. C., Easton, C. J., & McMahon, T. J. (2011). Drug abuse and intimate partner violence: A comparative study of opioid-dependent fathers. *American Journal of Orthopsychiatry, 81*, 218–227.

Noll, R. B., Zucker, R. A., Fitzgerald, H. E., & Curtis, W. J. (1992). Cognitive and motoric functioning of sons of alcoholic fathers and controls: The early childhood years. *Developmental Psychology, 28*, 665–675.

Oesterle, S., Hawkins, J. D., & Hill, K. G. (2011). Men's and women's pathways to adulthood and associated substance misuse. *Journal of Studies on Alcohol and Drugs, 72*, 763–773.

Osborne, C., & Berger, L. M. (2009). Parental substance abuse and child well-being: A consideration of parents' gender and coresidence. *Journal of Family Issues, 30*, 341–370.

Ostermann, J., Sloan, F. A., & Taylor, D. H. (2005). Heavy alcohol use and marital dissolution in the USA. *Social Science and Medicine, 61*, 2304–2316.

Pampel, F. C., Mollborn, S., & Lawrence, E. M. (2014). Life course transitions in early adulthood and SES disparities in tobacco use. *Social Science Research, 43*, 45–59.

Pears, K., Capaldi, D. M., & Owen, L. D. (2007). Substance use risk across three generations: The roles of parent discipline practices and inhibitory control. *Psychology of Addictive Behaviors, 21*, 373–386.

Perreira, K. M., & Cortes, K. E. (2006). Race/ethnicity and nativity differences in alcohol and tobacco use during pregnancy. *American Journal of Public Health, 96*, 1629–1636.

Poon, E., Ellis, D. A., Fitzgerald, H. E., & Zucker, R. A. (2000). Intellectual, cognitive and academic performance among sons of alcoholics during the early elementary school years: Differences related to subtypes of familial alcoholism. *Alcoholism: Clinical and Experimental Research, 24*, 1020–1027.

Puttler, L. I., Zucker, R. A., Fitzgerald, H. E., & Bingham, C. R. (1998). Behavioral outcomes among children of alcoholics during the early and middle childhood years: Familial subtype variations. *Alcoholism: Clinical and Experimental Research, 22*, 1962–1972.

Reichman, N. E., Teitler, J. O., Garfinkel, I., & McLanahan, S. S. (2001). Fragile families: Sample and design. *Children and Youth Services Review, 23*, 303–326.

Rounsaville, D., O'Farrell, T. J., Andreas, J. B., Murphy, C. M., & Murphy, M. M. (2014). Children's exposure to parental conflict after father's treatment for alcoholism. *Addictive Behaviors, 39*, 1168–1171.

Sanford, K., Bingham, C. R., & Zucker, R. A. (1999). Validity issues with the family environment scale: Psychometric resolution and research application with alcoholic families. *Psychological Assessment, 11*, 315–325.

Santelli, J. S., Brener, N. D., Lowry, R., Bhatt, A., & Zabin, L. S. (1998). Multiple sexual partners among U. S. adolescents and young adults. *Family Planning Perspectives, 30*, 271–275.

Schulenberg, J. E., Johnston, L. D., O'Malley, P. M., Bachman, J. G., Miech, R. A., & Patrick, M. E. (2018). *Monitoring the Future national survey results on drug use, 1975-2017: Vol. II, College students and adults ages 19-55*. Ann Arbor, MI: University of Michigan, Institute for Social Research.

Schulenberg, J. E., Maggs, J. L., & O'Malley, P. M. (2003). How and why the understanding of developmental continuity and discontinuity is important: The sample case of long-term consequences of adolescent substance use. In J. T. Mortimer & M. J. Shanahan (Eds.), *Handbook of the life course* (pp. 413–436). New York, NY: Plenum Press.

Sharma, R., Harlev, A., Agarwal, A., & Esteves, S. C. (2016). Cigarette smoking and semen quality: A new meta-analysis examining the effect of the 2010 World Health Organization laboratory methods for the examination of human semen. *European Urology, 70*, 635–645.

Shawe, J., Patel, D., Joy, M., Howden, B., Barrett, G., & Stephenson, J. (2019). Preparation for fatherhood: A survey of men's preconception health knowledge and behaviour in England. *PLoS One, 14*, e0213897.

Staff, J., Greene, K. M., Maggs, J. L., & Schoon, I. (2014). Family transitions and drinking in adulthood. *Addiction, 109*, 227–236.

Staff, J., Schulenberg, J. E., Maslowsky, J., Bachman, J. G., O'Malley, P. M., Maggs, J. L., et al. (2010). Substance use changes and social role transitions: Proximal developmental effects on ongoing trajectories from late adolescence through early adulthood. *Development and Psychopathology, 22*, 917–932.

Substance Abuse and Mental Health Services Administration. (2019). *Key substance use and mental health indicators in the United States: Results from the 2018 National Survey on Drug Use and Health* (HHS publication no. PEP19 5068). Rockville, MD: Substance Abuse and Mental Health Services Administration, Center for Behavioral Health Statistics and Quality.

Substance Abuse and Mental Health Services Administration, Office of Applied Studies. (2009). *Children living with substance-dependent or substance-abusing parents: 2002 to 2007*. Rockville, MD: Author.

Tarter, R. E., & Vanyukov, M. (1994). Alcoholism: A developmental disorder. *Journal of Consulting and Clinical Psychology, 62*, 1096–1107.

U.S. Department of Health and Human Services, Office of the Assistant Secretary for Planning and Evaluation. (1994, July). *Substance abuse among women and parents*. Washington, DC: Author.

Verges, A., Jackson, K. M., Bucholz, K. K., Grant, J. D., Trull, T. J., Wood, P. K., et al. (2012). Deconstructing the age-prevalence curve of alcohol dependence: Why "maturing out" is only a small piece of the puzzle. *Journal of Abnormal Psychology, 121*, 511–523.

Whipple, E. E., Fitzgerald, H. E., & Zucker, R. A. (1995). Parent-child interactions in alcoholic families: Implications for psychological child maltreatment. *American Journal of Orthopsychiatry, 65*, 153–159.

Wong, M. M., Nigg, J. T., Puttler, L. I., Fitzgerald, H. E., Jester, J. M., Glass, J. M., et al. (2006). Behavioral control and resiliency in the onset of alcohol and illicit drug use: A prospective study from preschool to adolescence. *Child Development, 77*, 1016–1033.

Wong, M. M., Zucker, R. A., Puttler, L. I., & Fitzgerald, H. E. (1999). Heterogeneity of risk aggregation for alcohol problems between early and middle childhood: Nesting structure variations. *Development and Psychopathology, 11*, 727–744.

Zucker, R. A. (2006). Alcohol use and alcohol use disorders: A developmental-biopsychosocial systems formulation covering the life course. In D. Cicchetti & D. J. Cohen (Eds.), *Developmental psychopathology: Vol. 3. Risk, disorder and adaptation* (2nd ed., pp. 620–656). Hoboken, NJ: John Wiley & Sons.

Zucker, R. A., Kincaid, S. B., Fitzgerald, H. E., & Bingham, C. R. (1995). Alcohol schema acquisition in preschoolers: Differences between children of alcoholics and children of non-alcoholics. *Journal of Clinical and Experimental Research, 19*, 1011–1017.

Fathers in Child Psychotherapy

37

Kai von Klitzing and Lars O. White

"Someone once described the joy and anxiety of parenthood as the equivalent of having your heart outside of your body all the time, walking around."

—A father and US president

In many ways, this quote from Barack Obama not only captures the chimera of parenthood but also, more specifically, fatherhood. Echoing and extending this view, in an autobiographical account of the birth of his first son and his first steps as a father, Bevington (2019) elegantly recounts numerous feelings and situations that might be considered prototypical of fatherhood. His account stretches from feeling amazed and overwhelmed as his child entered the world, to feeling inadequate for being "just a small part of this huge soft engine" (p. 10) and merely attending to "the practical stuff to support mother and baby" (p. 9), all the way to the pride at witnessing his child's "first steps outwards, away from [the parents] into the world" (p. 12) coupled with the fear of "not being there" to protect his child (p. 8). As already implied by the length of the previous sentence, his account suggests a great many "father roles", as opposed to a single all-encompassing role.

At a theoretical level, fatherhood and motherhood share much in common which can be captured by multiple dimensions, such as warmth, sensitivity, availability, and responsibility (Lamb, 2010). At the same time, however, much theory casts fathers in a unique role for the child, as their "primary playmates" as well as the main limit setters who promote separation within the early mother-infant bond (Paquette, 2004b). In so doing, the father is arguably instrumental in ushering the child into the triadic and symbolic universe that allows for representing others with interpersonal and internal worlds of their own (von Klitzing, 2019). As part and parcel of paternally aided separation from the mother, children encounter a world which can become "their oyster", brimming with exciting things to explore but, in turn, demanding a father to meet the child's need for protection. The father excludes, but he simultaneously facilitates reinclusion into a wider world (Paquette, 2004b). But as the Obama quote above and many other contemporary sources remind us, we are witnessing upheavals in traditional gender roles, perhaps more so today than ever before, and hence many of these points apply to the "father as a principle" (Bürgin, 1998), as opposed to the actual father, which can also be taken on alternately by either parent, including, of course, each parent in homosexual partnerships.

As varied as Bevington's (2019) recollections and theory suggest is the role of the father in child development (see Lamb, 2010), and thus, one might also venture, in child psychotherapy. Certainly, this impression is confirmed by some

K. von Klitzing (✉) · L. O. White
Department of Child and Adolescent Psychiatry, University of Leipzig, Leipzig, Germany
e-mail: Kai.vonklitzing@uniklinik-leipzig.de

H. E. Fitzgerald et al. (eds.), *Handbook of Fathers and Child Development*,
https://doi.org/10.1007/978-3-030-51027-5_37

of the clinical literature on the topic (e.g. Baradon, 2019a). However, in this case, the clinical literature far exceeds the body of systematic empirical research studies in terms of the elaborateness and specificity accorded to the role of fathers in child psychotherapy. Thus, based on empirical research, the role of the father in child psychotherapy remains opaque, raising many basic questions, for example, about the father's status as a moderator or mediator of child treatment outcomes, with a rich clinical literature offering many exciting (but so far untested) hypotheses.

In other words, as will become clear below, empirical research supports *that* fathers may exert an important influence on child mental health and (to a lesser extent) on outcomes of child psychotherapy, but *how* they do so in the latter case still largely remains the remit of the clinician. Closely linked to this is a variant of the same question that has haunted much of developmental research on fathers over the last decades (Pleck, 2010): Is the father's role in child psychotherapy unique and essential or merely that of a "second parent" or, more provocatively, a "second mother"? In an effort to do justice to the researcher and the clinician in us, we will attempt to straddle these domains, first proffering an empirical account and then, in an admittedly more speculative vein, delving into the complexities of clinical work with fathers, before closing by reflecting on this clinical work from a research perspective. This chapter thus aims to not only throw the importance of fathers for achieving success in child psychotherapy into relief but also accentuate the richness and often untapped potential of father work in child psychotherapy. In so doing, it is our hope to help kindle a dialogue between research and practice, a bridge that allows both sides to learn from each other.

The Empirical Account

Fathers in Interventions for Externalizing Problems

The vast majority of research to date on the effects of fathers in child psychotherapy derives from parent training programs (Phares, Rojas, Thurston, & Hankinson, 2010). Given that these programs typically target disruptive behaviour disorders (DBDs), it may come as no surprise that research in this area has primarily focused on fathers of children suffering from DBDs from preschool-age onwards (Lundahl, Tollefson, Risser, & Lovejoy, 2007), with a dearth of work on father involvement in interventions for other externalizing problems, such as attention deficit hyperactivity disorder (Fabiano, 2007) or internalizing problems (Bögels & Phares, 2008). Lundahl et al.'s (2007) meta-analysis suggests that joint involvement of fathers and mothers in parent training for child DBDs resulted in superior outcomes with moderate effect sizes (ES) on child and parenting behaviours relative to mother-only parent training which merely yielded negligible to small ES. Interestingly, when fathers were involved, it was mothers who tended to observe greater treatment gains (large ES) compared to fathers (moderate ES), both in relation to child behaviour and their own parenting behaviours, thus helping to rule out a mere respondent bias (e.g. whereby fathers may have portrayed effects more positively when involved).

As far as father-directed parent training is concerned, preliminary data from Head Start programs suggest that fathers from ethnic minorities in the United States showed larger improvements in parenting behaviour than fathers in a control group (Helfenbaum-Kun & Ortiz, 2007). Yet, despite initially promising turnout of fathers, large attrition rates were documented in this study with fathers attending less than 70% of the sessions, raising the question whether targeting both parents simultaneously may yield better retention rates. Indeed, the oft-noted pattern of lacking father participation (Panter-Brick et al., 2014) has prompted researchers to tailor studies and treatments more strongly to fathers' preferences (e.g. countering beliefs about gender roles) (Sicouri et al., 2018). A more recent adaptation of father-directed parent training, the "Fathers Supporting Success in Preschoolers" (FSSP) program, emphasized skills promotion during shared book reading, obtaining far better attendance rates of fathers (Chacko, Fabiano,

Doctoroff, & Fortson, 2018). Among 126 predominantly male Head Start Latino children with an average age of 4 years, Chacko et al. (2018) thus demonstrated superiority in reducing father-reported child behaviour problems, self- and observer-rated negative parenting (e.g. critical statements), and improvements in self- and observer-rated positive parenting behaviours (e.g. positive affect). However, follow-up data on maintenance of FSSP effects are currently still lacking.

In a similar vein – ever since Webster-Stratton's (1985) pioneering work showing superior maintenance of treatment gains when fathers were involved – the question has arisen whether father involvement in parent training might primarily exert salutary effects at follow-up, by serving to stabilize treatment effects. Reasons for this may involve the achievement of greater inter-parental congruence, lower conflict, and more cooperation between parents, if interventions target both parental parties. Yet, Lundahl et al.'s (2007) meta-analysis comparing joint mother-father to mother-only training failed to support the conclusion that father involvement results in more maintenance of treatment gains at follow-up. However, this result should be considered tentative, given that only very few studies contributed to the mother-only follow-up ES. Moreover, a frequently cited pre-post study by Bagner and Eyberg (2003) on the involvement of fathers in parent-child interaction therapy (PCIT) – a behavioural intervention mainly targeting DBDs combining parent training, behavioural, and play therapy elements (Eyberg, Boggs, & Algina, 1995) – also yielded equivocal results; though, this result was and still often is taken as evidence that maintenance of PCIT treatment gains is conditional upon involving fathers (Bagner & Eyberg, 2003). To be sure, the 4-month follow-up comparison of an involved-father group ($n = 23$; defined as participation in at least one treatment session), to an absent-father group ($n = 15$), yielded a group by time interaction on maternal reports of child behaviour problems, with a greater rate of relapse in the absent-father group. However, upon closer inspection, it was the *absent-father group* which initially showed greater treatment gains, so that after relapsing a similar level of behaviour problems were attained as compared to the involved father group at follow-up. In addition, the study was plagued by an exceedingly high dropout rate across all conditions in the order of 33–44%, without using intent-to-treat analyses to control results accordingly, additionally making the results difficult to interpret.

Conversely, more recent work hints at the possibility that father-adapted parenting interventions may potentially result in more sustained treatment gains. For example, targeting a recruited sample of middle- to high-income families of preschool- to school-age children with clinical-level behaviour problems, Frank, Keown, and Sanders (2015) supplemented father-relevant content (e.g. discussing the importance of father involvement and father-identified parenting challenges, such as balancing the pressures of work and family) to the Group Triple P parenting intervention, focusing on positive parenting strategies. Compared to the waitlist, their adapted Group Triple P not only coincided with a low attrition rate but also gave rise to a sustained reduction of behaviour problems among their offspring at 6-month follow-up.

Fathers in Interventions for Internalizing Problems

In contrast to treatments for externalizing problems, evaluation of father involvement in psychotherapy targeting child internalizing problems is still in its infancy and has focused almost exclusively on school-age children (Bögels & Phares, 2008). Though early efforts already involved some form of parent work, this was often equated with mother involvement, and even in the few cases where fathers and mothers were successfully mobilized to attend group therapy, no data were reported on potential additional benefits of father involvement (e.g. Manassis et al., 2002). However, a recent meta-analytic review identifying five studies with school-age children compared child-only cognitive behaviour therapy (ICBT) with CBT for children plus both parents

(PCBT) detecting comparable treatment gains on anxiety symptoms for both approaches (Carnes, Matthewson, & Boer, 2019), thus not supporting clear guidelines as to the uniform involvement of fathers. That said, research on older children also indicates that short- and long-term treatment success for child anxiety may be specifically impeded by fathers' anxiety and depressive symptoms, somatization, and rejection of the child (Crawford & Manassis, 2001; Liber et al., 2008; Rapee, 2000) and that fathers' own anxiety may recede following family treatment targeting their anxious child (Bögels & Siqueland, 2006). This is in line with recent longitudinal findings showing cross-lagged effects of child anxiety on paternal mental health (Andreas et al., 2018).

Studies on recent adaptations of CBT for preschool anxiety disorders (reviewed by Barrett, Games, Fisak, Stallard, & Phillips, 2019), though typically parent-focused, rarely report rates of father involvement or results separately for both parents. In one recent exception on a preliminary pre-post study of an 8-session parent-only CBT, fathers were involved in 11 of 26 cases (van der Sluis, van der Bruggen, Brechman-Toussaint, Thissen, & Bögels, 2012). While the authors aggregated reports from both parents on child outcomes, they reported that mothers, but not fathers, perceived significant improvement in their own anxiety-reducing parenting behaviours (e.g. positive, reinforcement, providing reassurance). Similarly, in an RCT of 16-session CBT ($n = 21$) versus waitlist ($n = 22$) among 5- to 7-year-olds with separation anxiety disorder, Schneider et al. (2011) did not report rates of father involvement, but showed that mothers, fathers, and children alike rated separation anxiety to be reduced following treatment and 4-week follow-up, with additional improvements in distress and quality of life reported by both parents, alike.

The Role of Fathers in Attachment and Prevention Approaches

Compared to parent training, evidence for the importance of father involvement in other types of interventions is currently limited and/or only of indirect clinical relevance. For example, within the largest meta-analysis of attachment interventions to date (e.g. video-feedback), the few intervention studies involving fathers yielded larger effects on parental sensitivity as compared to mother-only interventions (Bakermans-Kranenburg, van Ijzendoorn, & Juffer, 2003). However, this result must be weighed against several factors. First, this result was based on a comparison of effects between three studies ($N = 81$) that included fathers and 78 studies ($N = 7555$) that did not. Furthermore, effects in these studies were apparently attributable to increases primarily in paternal sensitivity, which seemingly came at the cost of maternal sensitivity which was substantially lower in these studies. Finally, and perhaps most importantly, attachment interventions mainly demonstrate salutary effects on attachment insecurity, rather than attachment disorganization (Bakermans-Kranenburg et al., 2003). Indeed, recent meta-analyses suggest that direct effects of attachment insecurity on externalizing and internalizing symptoms are weak (though significant) and at least in the case of externalizing symptoms primarily emerge in clinical samples, mainly driven by attachment disorganization (Fearon, Bakermans-Kranenburg, Van Ijzendoorn, Lapsley, & Roisman, 2010; Groh, Roisman, van Ijzendoorn, Bakermans-Kranenburg, & Fearon, 2012).

A particularly noteworthy group-based parenting couple intervention approach known as Supporting Father Involvement (SFI) has received impressive support across ample recent large-scale RCTs (reviewed by Cowan, Cowan, Pruett, & Pruett, 2018). Among others, SFI targets the psychological state of each parent individually as well as their functioning as a couple, both in terms of their romantic partnership and as co-parents. Besides its replicated positive effects in preventing the emergence of behavioural problems among at-risk children, the couple approach was specifically also able to maintain satisfaction in the parental partnership as compared to a father-only intervention group, thus addressing an important risk factor for child behaviour problems and paving the way to sustained treatment gains.

Critical Evaluation of the Empirical Research

The widely received view in this line of research is that evidence has accrued over the last decades to include fathers' yields important benefits for child psychotherapy, and therefore, researchers and clinicians are well-advised to do so (Bögels & Phares, 2008; Cowan & Cowan, 2019a; Panter-Brick et al., 2014). While we generally adhere to this view, such broad summary statements always run the risk of glossing over important ambiguities of the evidence base. Thus, empirical findings remain equivocal concerning the value of father involvement (1) in psychotherapy for young children, (2) in the maintenance of treatment gains, (3) for effects on internalizing problems, and, more generally, (4) for psychotherapy formats besides parent training. A number of other criticisms of the evidence base were voiced over 10 years ago by Tiano and McNeil (2005) including the lack of statistical power, comparisons between maternal and paternal data, and the omission of parent-specific attendance rates, which still largely apply today. Certainly, an uncritical wholesale application of intervention approaches to fathers originally formulated with "mothers in mind" cannot be recommended, given the high level of dropout documented by some studies. Conversely, tailoring interventions to fathers' needs and interests seems to yield more promising results (e.g. Chacko et al., 2018; Frank et al., 2015).

More important than these gaps in our view is the pressing need to elaborate on the theoretical mechanisms underlying the presumed benefits of father involvement in child psychotherapy and develop *and* assess interventions in accordance with these theoretical principles. To this end, Kazdin (2007) has spelt out the criteria for evaluating treatment moderators, mediators, and mechanisms. While a mediator accounts for the relationship between intervention and outcomes and may hint at an underlying therapeutic mechanism of therapeutic change, a moderator "refers to some characteristic that influences the direction or magnitude of the relation between intervention and outcome" (Kazdin, 2007, p. 3). Crucially, it is often tacitly assumed that father involvement is a moderator of treatment success. "All we need to do is to get fathers on board and all will be well!" goes the battle cry. Thus, researchers and clinicians alike often seem to be most strongly concerned with identifying the right techniques to involve fathers and then use the same intervention approach as with mothers or minimal variants thereof.

However, it might be worth pointing out that research to date does not enable us to disentangle to what extent we are dealing with a moderator or mediator of treatment outcome in Kazdin's (2007) sense. Thus, in the aforementioned studies, father involvement was never assigned randomly. Either post hoc comparisons were made between treatments in which fathers were involved versus uninvolved (based on grouping cases together following treatment completion) or between completely different studies (meta-analyses) which can vary dramatically in terms of various characteristics, from recruitment procedures, intervention aspects, and so on. In other words, successful father-involvement may characterize a certain species of father (or mother, or family, etc.) or, conversely, may reflect a different, more successful treatment trajectory. At this point, we simply do not know. However, if the father involvement merely is a proxy for favourable preconditions for intervention, this warrants a qualitatively different approach than just bringing the father on board. Rather, clinicians and researchers would then be called on to develop alternative father interventions and/or initially work with families and fathers to identify and address the reasons for the lack of father involvement in order to create the preconditions for treatment success.

Echoing Kazdin (2007), the field currently lacks theoretical rigor in defining the specific contribution of fathers to child development and child psychopathology and, in turn, using this knowledge as a point of departure for elaborating intervention techniques for fathers. By way of example, paternal challenging behaviour, rough-and-tumble play, paternal activation relationship, and triadic capacity have emerged as fundamental components of child development to which fathers make a substantial and unique contribution (see below). For example, research has recently demonstrated that paternal (but not maternal) challenging behaviour may carry important protective effects for child anxiety (Majdandžić, de Vente, Colonnesi, & Bögels, 2018; Majdandžić, Möller, de Vente, Bögels, & van den Boom, 2014). However, very few if any of these concepts have found their way into the aforementioned intervention approaches or even entered into the clinical researcher's vocabulary. For these reasons, we now turn to the second part of this chapter which focuses on precisely these theory-driven mechanisms, thought to underlie the influence of fathers in child psychotherapy.

A Three-Tiered Model for Targeting the Father in Child Psychotherapy

Based on developmental theory and research (Bögels & Phares, 2008; Paquette, 2004b) as well as clinical case studies (see Baradon, 2019a) about the partly unique role of the father in child development, we propose three levels at which fathers (often inevitably) influence child psychotherapy, whether they are directly involved in child psychotherapy or not. We believe that the key question is whether the clinician can keep in mind and make effective use of these levels or, conversely, whether therapy directly or indirectly comes under the detrimental influence of unresolved paternal interpersonal or internal conflicts. In our view, the principal ways at which fathers influence child development (von Klitzing, 2019) and, by extension, child psychotherapy can usefully be classified into (1) the "real father" or the direct effects of fathers on children via parenting, play, and so on; (2) the father as part of the mother-father-child triad which also includes the indirect effects of the father via the relationship with the mother; and (3) the child's and the mother's internalized father representation. We will cover each of these levels in turn below and provide clinical examples and a brief case vignette illustrating how the clinician can address each level. At the outset, we would like to point out that due to the dearth of empirical research on *how* fathers promote the success of child psychotherapy, this section necessarily remains speculative insofar as we extrapolate from the known effects of fathers on child development and psychopathology to how therapeutic interventions might capitalize on these effects in the context of child psychotherapy.

An Episode of Father-Child Play

To set the scene, we begin with a brief example of a typical father-child interaction. This observation was captured on video within a longitudinal study focusing on early triadic interaction (Klitzing & Burgin, 2005; von Klitzing, Simoni, Amsler, & Bürgin, 1999). At the time, the mother was pregnant again with her second child. In line with the Lausanne triadic play paradigm (Corboz-Warnery, Fivaz-Depeursinge, Bettens, & Favez, 1993), the parents were instructed to play in a set sequence with their 18-month-old son.

First, the mother played with the boy. They used a toy cup and toy pitcher, and the mother tried to scaffold her son towards engaging in pretend play. "Look, you can use the pitcher and pour lemonade into the cup. Then, you can drink lemonade. Yum, this tastes so good." The boy seemed confused by these statements as there was no real lemonade either in the pitcher or in the cup. He repeatedly responded with, "Nothing, nothing." He even went over to his father several times who was sitting close by, observing the scene, and said, "Nothing to drink!", while shaking his head and shrugging his shoulders to convey the absence of content both verbally and gesturally. The mother was very patient and attuned, adjusting her behaviour almost perfectly to the needs of her son. She seemed to sense that the onset of pretend play would reflect promising developmental progress for the boy but that he was having difficulties to enter into this new symbolic space. Again and again, she tried to explain to her son, "We can just pretend that there is lemonade in the pitcher". Then, the parents decided to take turns. The mother withdrew into the pas-

sive role of the observer and transferred the active role of a player to the father. Initially, the child seemed somewhat frustrated about the mother's withdrawal but then cautiously glanced at the father, as if to suggest that he perceived him as an intruder.

The father behaved in a completely different way. First, he built a tower with toy bricks and appeared unresponsive to the boy's emotional state. The father simply did not seem to care much about either the previous play or the boy's problems with pretend play, instead of following his own agenda. In turn, the boy was not really interested in his father's play. Instead, he offered the cup to the father, hoping that the father could pour some real lemonade into it. Responding to this offer, the father now took the cup, and lifting it to his mouth, he shouted, "tut, tut, tut", as if the cup were a microphone. Surprisingly, his son immediately moved into a state of excitement and joy, exclaiming, "More! More! More!" An episode of joyful cooperative play ensued, involving singing and shouting and using the toy cup as a pretend microphone.

In this episode, the father's unresponsiveness to the boy's insecure emotional state thus served as a "door opener" to a universe of symbolic play between father and son. But how exactly did the father achieve this? At the risk of overgeneralizing from a single episode as well as overstating the difference between mothers and fathers, we contend that such father-child play interactions markedly contrast with typical mother-child interactions (see Fonagy, Gergely, Jurist, & Target, 2002). Drawing on some of the theories outlined below, the interaction could be described as follows (see Fig. 37.1): In the first step, an internal mental state coupled with an expectancy is expressed by the child, as he hands the father the cup. The father picks up on this internal state and the related expectancy, but rather than directly responding and complying with the child's expectancy, he decouples himself from it, pursues his own agenda, and creates challenging alternatives in his mind. In opting for the cup as a microphone, he violates the child's expectancy, switching to an even higher level of "decontextualized" symbolic play where the play object (referent) and what it symbolizes show little or no outward resemblance (see Smith, 2010). Thus, he playfully and somewhat intrusively gives the child a gentle push to yet a higher developmental level and surprises the child with an entirely different intentionally mismatched bid. In this style of interaction, fathers thus convey a "yes, you can" message which simultaneously poses a stark contrast between internal states of self and other, in terms of "what's mine" and "what's yours", challenging the child to adapt to or compete with the father's bid.

The Real Father

As suggested by the observation above, much developmental theory and research now indicate that fathers impact child development for better *and* for worse by virtue of direct interactions with their children. In what follows, we will provide insight into those roles and how they might go awry, presenting potential targets for parent work in child psychotherapy. We will draw on two case vignettes to illustrate how interventions can harness this father role to bring about change at the level of the child.

Theory and Evidence for the Real Father

Early on, Lamb (1975) portrayed fathers as connecting children to the outside world. Others broadened this paternal function to engaging children in exciting activities and play, much like in the example above, sometimes even scaffolding children "to hear and do some things mothers would avoid as dangerous" (Murphy, 1997, p. 9). In what is now considered a watershed paper, Paquette (2004b) casts fathers in the role of "primary playmates", relating to the child in the "activation relationship", in contrast to the maternal role of the "primary caregiver" relating to the child within the "attachment relationship". As opposed to the attachment-related maternal provision of comfort under duress, the activative role of the father "satisfies the child's need to be stim-

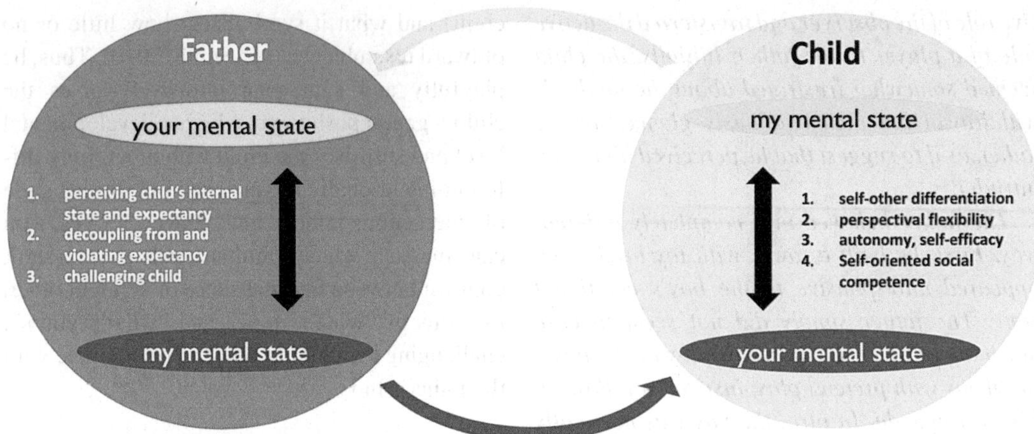

Fig. 37.1 Mental processes underlying father-child interaction during activation play

ulated, to overcome limits and to learn to take chances in contexts in which the child is confident of being protected from potential dangers" (Paquette, 2004b, p. 202). Akin to the observation described above, the activation relationship often involves mild to moderate levels of disruption and intrusiveness. As part and parcel of this activative function, when confronted with potential dangers, as is often the case in rough and tumble play (RTP), the child is also exposed to a more directive, rule-bound style of interaction in which obedience to parental authority is required to ensure safety. Accordingly, RTP typically involves subordinate and dominant roles while preserving the affectional bond and affording the child a practice ground to regulate aggression and learn to decode others' affective states in an emotionally charged situation (Paquette, 2004b).

In a similar vein, but building on attachment theory, scholars have proposed that the caregiver function of safe haven to which children return in times of distress typifies mothers, whereas the caregiver function of a secure base from which children explore in times of safety typifies fathers (Cowan & Cowan, 2019b; Grossmann et al., 2002; Kerns, Mathews, Koehn, Williams, & Siener-Ciesla, 2015). However, unlike Paquette's view (2004b) which conceives of fathers as activators, the attachment perspective appears to suggest that fathers are primarily *passive* supporters of autonomy in the context of safety, avoiding disruptiveness and primarily posing sensitive and non-intrusive challenges to the child (e.g. Grossmann et al., 2002). Conversely, not unlike the observation reported above, others stress precisely this mistimed, disruptive, directive, competitive, and moderately intrusive nature of father-child interaction, occurring, of course, against the backdrop of a positive, supportive, and encouraging relationship (Volling & Cabrera, 2019). In turn, the latter may promote the child's perception of the father as a separate entity with a mind of his own (as in the example above), eventually imbuing children with a greater sense of autonomy and self-efficacy.

Various overlapping facets of the father-typical activative function emerge across recent research. In early development, for example, father-infant face-to-face interactions with high levels of synchrony were characterized by sudden, highly intense bouts of positive arousal, thus contrasting with the well-calibrated medium to low levels of arousal and gradually emerging positive effect in synchronous mother-infant interactions (Feldman, 2003). Across later development scholars have operationalized the activative function in terms of encouragement of risk-taking (Paquette & Bigras, 2010), sensitive-challenging behaviour (Grossmann et al., 2002), dominance and quality of rough and tumble play (Flanders et al., 2010; Fletcher, StGeorge, & Freeman, 2013), and challenging parenting behaviour (Majdandžić, de Vente, & Bögels, 2016). These parenting behaviours have proven quite stable across the first years (Majdandžić et al., 2016) and appear distinguishable from infant attachment security (Paquette & Bigras, 2010; Volling, Stevenson, Safyer, Gonzalez, & Lee, 2019), though interesting links to infant attachment disorganization (high risk for overactivated, reckless infants; Paquette & Bigras, 2010) and narrative attachment measures in middle childhood and adolescence have arisen (Grossmann et al., 2002). Moreover, as suggested by the latter findings, suboptimal levels of activative parenting of fathers are linked to psychosocial maladjustment, including less externalizing and internalizing problems (Bögels & van Melick, 2004; Flanders, Leo, Paquette, Pihl, & Séguin, 2009; Majdandžić et al., 2014; Majdandžić et al., 2018).

Much debate revolves around the question whether these activative patterns truly typify fathers as opposed to mothers and, even if they do, how much importance to accord to them. This issue is particularly pressing if we choose to foreground this function in our intervention efforts. Notably, some researchers claim that "differences between mothers and fathers seem much less important than similarities" (Lamb, 2010, p. 10). Thus, regardless of whether expressed by mothers or fathers, parental dimensions, such as warmth, closeness, comfort, and acceptance, exert positive effects, while controlling behaviour and negative affect expression exert negative effects on child psychosocial adjustment and achievement (Lamb, 2010; Volling & Cabrera, 2019). More closely related to the postulated activative function, fathers only engage in more play with children on a relative scale, but because mothers, on average, spend more time with children, they actually engage in more play in absolute terms, thus partly debunking the claim of the father as the primary playmate (Pleck, 2010). Going a step further, a number of researchers have taken issue with Paquette's (2004b) claims, arguing that mothers and fathers even share most qualitative aspects of play in common (e.g. amount of affection, type of play) (Roggman, 2004). Pleck (2010) – based, among others, on a meta-analysis of parental gender differences in language use reporting small effect sizes throughout (e.g. mothers use more supportive but less directive and informative speech than fathers; Leaper, Anderson, & Sanders, 1998) – thus claims that gender differences in parenting have been exaggerated and fathers do not account for *unique* variance (in the sense of the variance that is nonsubstitutable by others) in child outcomes.

While we acknowledge that the difference between mothers and fathers may be better characterized as one of degree rather than of kind, we believe there are good reasons not to downplay this difference. As statisticians remind us, even small effects can amount to important differences over time and account for much variance if they derive from stable traits (Abelson, 1985). Moreover, it is noteworthy that none of the recent large-scale meta-analyses showing highly robust small-to-moderate effects of infant attachment patterns on social competence, internalizing, or externalizing behaviours, detected a significant effect of father-infant attachment patterns on these outcomes (Fearon et al., 2010; Groh et al., 2012; Groh et al., 2014), even though paternal sensitivity robustly predicts father-infant attachment security (Lucassen et al., 2011). In other words, the undeniable effects of fathers on child development do not seem to solely or even *primarily* occur via a common route mediating many effects of mothers on child development. For treatment, this implies that clinicians might be well-advised to, at least, also focus intervention efforts with fathers at other levels.

While the activation-attachment dichotomy in some regards might offer a crucial point of departure, we agree with its critics that it is important to resist the temptation to caricature fathers (and mothers) in *only* these terms, a risk that was indeed immediately acknowledged by Paquette (2004a) himself. Furthermore, recent research testifies to the considerable overlap in the activative function of fathers and mothers. For example, during a teaching task both mothers and fathers were observed to engage in so-called "activation parenting" not only involving cognitive stimulation, sensitivity, and positive affect but also coupled with moderate intrusiveness (Volling et al., 2019). Nevertheless, the activative function appears to be slightly more characteristic of father-child than mother-child interactions (Feldman, 2003; Kerns et al., 2015; Volling et al., 2019), though some results are more equivocal (Majdandžić et al., 2016; Paquette & Bigras, 2010). Yet, even if activation occurs at similar rates in mothers and fathers, the intensity of these behaviours in fathers, both in terms of intrusiveness and positive affect, seems to exceed that of mothers and gives rise to more positive affect expression of their children (Karberg, Cabrera, Malin, & Kuhns, 2019).

Finally, it is crucial not to ignore the possibility that mothers may adopt the activative function, potentially in an effort to buffer against or compensate for a limited activative function or an absent father (Majdandžić et al., 2018). Here, it is particularly noteworthy that first hints have emerged that the consequences of activative parenting may differ somewhat when originating from mothers as opposed to fathers. For example, when fathers promote autonomy, this appears to protect their child against anxiety, but when mothers do so, this is merely indicative of lower maternal anxiety (Bögels & van Melick, 2004). Indeed, more recent work has repeatedly supported the specific protective function of parental challenging behaviour when it originates from fathers, but not from mothers (Majdandžić et al., 2014), though some compensation between parents may be possible (Majdandžić et al., 2018).

Intervening at the Level of the Real Father

The research reviewed above, we contend, warrants an interventional focus on the activation relationship during father-related work in child psychotherapy. While this should not occur to the exclusion of other parenting functions that fathers share in common with mothers, a plethora of effective interventions already exist to successfully address these shared parenting functions (partly reviewed above). Therefore, when it comes to these shared functions, the most important task for the clinician may indeed be to bring the father on board, so that he can also benefit from the intervention. Conversely, in the case of the father-child activation relationship interventions may need to "beat a new path" altogether.

To begin with, we feel that the two words of warning are in order. First, recent work has linked paternal risk encouragement to higher rates of physical injury in children (StGeorge, Fletcher, Freeman, Paquette, & Dumont, 2015). Therefore, simply encouraging fathers to take up activative behaviour without attending to the cognitive and emotional states underlying their inhibition to express this behaviour may entail considerable risks. Indeed, such an approach would ignore the complex psychological negotiation process with the child that respects their developmental boundaries and allows fathers to pitch the level of intrusion and challenge at the "right" level, i.e. not too low to make it boring, but not too high to make it overwhelming, as illustrated by Baradon's (2019b) and Perez's (2019) case vignettes outlined below.

Second, clinicians should carefully weigh the advantages against the potential risks of bringing the father on board (Jones, 2019). Thus, if it has been confirmed that the father subjected the mother or the child to physical or sexual abuse, these may be warning signs that involvement of the father may not be desirable or possible. That said, reports of what the father has or has not done can be contradictory, and the risk is to all too readily give up on the often arduous task of involving the father and fully rely on what is sometimes a highly skewed view of the father through the mother's eyes. Undertaking a concerted effort to meet the father in person jointly with the mother or separately can thus pay dividends, also in terms of informing ensuing intervention efforts (Salomonsson, Baradon, & von Klitzing, 2019).

With these caveats in mind, we discuss two brief vignettes as examples of how to intervene at the level of the real father in parent-child psychotherapy. A crucial "port of entry" may be addressing the father's own caregiving history to make links on the intergenerational effects these might be having on his parenting, akin to intervention approaches targeting parental "ghosts in the nursery" (Lieberman, Ghosh Ippen, & Van Horn, 2015) which Barrows (2004) elegantly extended to fathers. To this end, Joyce (2019) describes a father included in parent-infant therapy that was originally premised on tackling the mother's postnatal depression and treating their 6-month-old fussy son who would not stop crying. Early on in treatment, it emerged, however, that the mother felt the father to lack parenting competence and that "the early death of his father meant ... that he had no sense of how to be a father [himself]" (Joyce, 2019, p. 31). Rated as dismissing on the Adult Attachment Interview, the father shrugged off the loss of both of his father at age 5 and his mother at age 11, believing that he was too young for it to bear any significance, instead of emphasizing how important it is to "pull up your socks, get on with life, and be happy [and not to] dwell on things so much" (Joyce, 2019, p. 30). It is telling that the parents reported adhering to Gina Ford's parenting book on early child-care, so that the therapist was confronted with "rule-bound parents creating a rule-bound baby" (Joyce, 2019, p. 33).

However, after scheduling individual sessions with the father, he was able to discuss the pain related to the losses in his childhood. With the help of the therapist, the father eventually came to realize that his son was being coerced into pseudo-autonomy, "pushing him to keep achieving, driving forward, not relaxing" (Joyce, 2019, p. 36), much like the precocity or pseudo-maturity the father had acquired himself as a child in response to the loss of his own father. Towards the end of treatment, the mother asserted that their son was responsive to when the father did not return from work at the usual time. In turn, the father made the analogy that "if a six-month-old could register and show his feelings about his dad's presence and absence, then in all likelihood a five- or six-year-old would certainly have noticed when his dad died and was absent forever" (Joyce, 2019, p. 36).

Whether or not this intervention enabled the father to more optimally express an activative parenting function is difficult to know without any observations before and after therapy. However, in light of the documented links between paternal attachment insecurity and some aspects of the activation function (Feldman, 2003), this certainly seems possible. What seems like a safer guess is that the intervention might well have helped the parental couple to relax the constraints of their "rule-bound life" which may have kept the activative function – with its creative and somewhat rule-breaking elements – at bay. At any rate, by the end of treatment, the father was clearly more attuned to the needs of his son, presumably owing in part to working through his own childhood losses and giving them meaning in the father-infant relationship. If not directly stimulating the father-child activation relationship, this intervention appears to have created favourable preconditions for its emergence.

In a second relevant vignette, Baradon (2019b) reports on parent-infant psychotherapy with a father with a history of abuse and facing a precarious situation as a destitute illegal immigrant who had passively withdrawn from the relationship to his 8-month-old daughter. During one of the joint mother-father-infant sessions, the therapist encouraged the father to respond to the daughter who was showing signs of distress. Drawing his daughter's attention to a toy train, he proceeded to gradually roll it towards her. The therapist commented on what his daughter might be thinking (Was it driving too fast? Where was it headed?), thus alerting him to his daughter's internal states, upon which he "started monitoring [his daughter's] responses and moving the train accordingly" (Baradon, 2019b, p. 88). After she had calmed down and was relaxing on dad's lap, the therapist interpreted the father's choice of the train as a toy: Perhaps, this was "symbolic of his arrival in the United Kingdom with no one to help him make safe connections to his new country, and his wish to provide a safe emotional environment to his daughter" (Baradon, 2019b, p. 88), which seemed to touch the father very deeply.

In both vignettes, the therapists leveraged the fathers' respective biographies to target their inhibited parenting function (see Barrows, 2004). As pointed out in the discussion of these cases (Salomonsson, Baradon, & von Klitzing, 2019), in openly addressing these issues the therapist presumably conveyed an empathic attitude towards the paternal difficulties, thus also serving to mitigate the negative transference that can readily develop towards a therapist who may be perceived as yet another "know-it-all mind-reader" with no inkling of the father's plight. Moreover, Baradon (2019b) gives us insight into the work that can be conducted in father-child play interactions scaffolding the father to attend closely to the child's signals during play. As acknowledged many times above, proponents of the father-child activation relationship stress that activation must occur in the context of an attuned father-child bond.

Father in the Parent-Child Triad

Given that the field of early child development is steeped in a "bastion of dyadic, mother-infant relationship models and interventions" (McHale, 2007, p. 372), it may seem audacious to stress the importance of pitching father-related interventions at the level of the parent-child triad. However, as will become abundantly clear below, we believe that neglecting this level may fundamentally put intervention efforts in many families at risk. As in the previous section, we first begin with a short clinical vignette to illustrate what it is we mean by the father in the parent-child triad.

Seven-year-old Melanie was enrolled in psychoanalytic focal psychotherapy in the context of one of our clinical trials on depression and anxiety in preschool- and young school-age children (Göttken & von Klitzing, 2014; Göttken, White, Klein, & von Klitzing, 2014). *She suffered from eating problems, depressive mood, suicidal ideation, anxiety, and sleeping problems. The parental partnership was highly conflictual. Whereas Melanie's mother was very concerned about her symptoms, her father who was exceedingly absorbed by his newly established business downplayed the girls suffering. The initial parent interview – usually conducted with both parents – was attended by the mother on her own. The female therapist formulated the focus of short-term therapy after the first two sessions with the child: "Melanie has problems in regulating her aggression. She worries that her mother cannot tolerate her aggressive feelings, and she fears that her father cannot help as he shows no interest in her. Therefore, she turns her aggression inwards onto herself and becomes depressed and suicidal." A central technique of focal therapy consists of zeroing in on and repeatedly verbalizing this focus in a child-and-parent appropriate way during suitable moments (e.g. during child-play). Furthermore, the therapist insisted that the father should attend the regularly scheduled parent sessions which are part of the child therapy. Finally, the father somewhat reluctantly consented to this. From now on, he not only attended the parent sessions but also, surprisingly, brought Melanie to the child sessions each time. In so doing, he created a space for some time and activity together with his daughter, something Melanie apparently relished.*

In the 12th child session, Melanie drew her family as animals. She drew her mother as a fox and herself as a mooncalf. After some hesitation, she drew her father as an elephant, but from behind so that one could only see his bottom. The ensuing dialogue between her and the therapist revolved around the girl's aggressive feelings when being together with her family. The therapist interpreted that Melanie was trying her best to stymy her aggression so as to protect her mother, also in drawing the elephant facing away. Then, the therapeutic conversation fell upon the conflicts that apparently were part of her parents' marital relationship. Melanie asked herself whether Mom still loves Dad and Dad still loves Mom. On the one hand, the thought that feelings of love and attraction between her parents still existed raised some concerns of being excluded in her. On the other hand, she felt relief that she was not solely responsible for her mother's happiness. At the end of this session, she altered the drawing of her father by adding a nose, eyes, and a mouth on the elephant so that the elephant was now visible from the front. The therapist understood this as an indication that the father was more involved in her life, that it was now possible to see that he was male, not an undefined creature, and that he might as such be of interest or even attractive for her mother (and also for herself). Apparently, this provided some consolation to the troubled girl.

In psychotherapy with children, we typically encounter mothers as our primary "port of entry" for parent work. They provide an important ingredient for the therapeutic process, while fathers often "blend into the woodwork" or even completely drop out. The case of Melanie shows how important it is to fight for the engagement of fathers. Not only that the father could help in practical things (like bringing the child to therapy), but the participation of fathers can also have meanings for the internal world of the child in treatment. Thus, through encouraging autonomy in challenging situations, the father representation can help manage problematic feelings, such as aggression, in a well-regulated way. In Melanie's case, aggression is understandable, for example, in light of constantly squabbling parents, a disappointingly absent father or an overprotective and overly anxious mother. In picking up on this, her therapist not only conveys that aggression is tolerable and "survivable" (i.e. does not necessarily result in further rejection or retaliation; Winnicott, 1971), but carries meaning which, if verbalized, rather than being turned inwards, can generate positive outcomes, such as more father involvement (see next section on the internalized father).

As the father emerged onto the scene and the father and daughter began to show greater interest in each other, the concept of the "father being with the mother" inevitably gained prominence. While the emergence of this concept reflects a necessary developmental step which can cause anxieties of exclusion in its own right, it can also alleviate feelings of responsibility for her mother's well-being and guilt harboured towards the mother or father due to wishes for an exclusive relationship with either party – feelings which required working through in the case of Melanie. These processes lie at the heart of what we mean by the family as a triad.

Theory and Evidence on the Role of the Father in the Triad

As can be gleaned from the case of Melanie, the triadic focus involves attending to patterns of exclusion, disengagement, interference, or undermining of any one member of the parent-child triad. A number of methods have been devised to tap into these capacities from infancy onwards (see McHale, 2007). Notably, the Lausanne Triadic Play (LTP; Corboz-Warnery et al., 1993) task, already referred to above, uses a standardized series of free play situations involving so-called "two-plus-ones", where each member of the triad alternately assumes a passive role, while the other two are interacting followed by a "three-together", where all members are active and need to jointly coordinate their play. Much work using the LTP has focused on young infants' capacity for "coordination", as indexed, for example, by rapid back-and-forth gaze shifts between both parents and affective signals directed at both parents simultaneously ("triangular bids"). These and similar capacities of infants have proven stable across time and interaction contexts, are predicted by marital distress, and protect against ample domains of later psychosocial maladjustment of the child (see McHale, 2007 and von Klitzing, 2019 for reviews).

Here, we lay our focus on the paternal contribution to this matrix, in the form of the parental triadic competence, which refers to the ability of mothers and fathers to contemplate family relationships "without excluding themselves or their partners from the relationship to the infant" (von Klitzing, Simoni, & Bürgin, 1999, p. 76). Operationalizing this capacity in a prenatal interview with both parents, von Klitzing and colleagues (von Klitzing, Simoni, & Bürgin, 1999) found that parental triadic competence predicted postnatal triadic capacities in the LTP at age 4 months as well as in a triadic stressful separation-reunion procedure modelled on the Strange Situation (Ainsworth, Blehar, Waters, & Wall, 1978) at 1 year. Crucial for the present purposes, in a follow-up analysis, von Klitzing, Simoni, Amsler, and Bürgin (1999) could trace the effect on the LTP primarily to the prenatal paternal as opposed to the maternal triadic competence.

These findings raise questions similar to the ones encountered at the level of the real father, i.e. whether the father is merely an interchangeable part of the triad or has a distinct role in the family triad. In short, some theorists primarily view the father as a third that is external to the mother-infant bond (Target & Fonagy, 2002). As such, the father acts as a vehicle to prevent the child from directly incorporating the mother representation in the sense of a false or alien self, instead of helping to "represent the relationship [to the mother] as a relationship" (Target & Fonagy, 2002, p. 60), thereby expediting mentalizing capacities. Intriguingly, some empirical work indeed demonstrates that triadic functioning of the family predicts later theory of mind of the child (Favez et al., 2012). From this view, the father as the third helps turn the mother in the child's mind into a thinking entity with goals and desires of her own that lead her outside the relationship to the child (Fonagy & Target, 1995). Notably, Target and Fonagy et al. (2002) consider mothers to perform a parallel function for the father-child relationship, thus suggesting that the essence of the father's role as a third is basically interchangeable.

This contrasts markedly with views that are in keeping with the attachment-activation dichotomy, whereby the mother's role typically involves "state-matching" and "homeostatic attunement," while the father's role involves "state-changing" and "disruptive attunement" (Herzog, 1991/1998). Although these functions can sometimes be observed simultaneously or rapid succession in a single parent – somewhat analogous to the notion of contingent marked mirroring of caregivers (Fonagy et al., 2002) – Herzog (1991/1998) contends that this is not the norm. Rather, he postulated a "division of labour" whereby disruptive attunement (primarily emanating from the father) is advantageous only inasmuch as it occurs in the context of ongoing homeostatic attunement (primarily emanating from the mother). Moreover, disruptive attunement often occurs in the context of play, whereas homeostatic attunement may be most vital in times of distress. This model therefore casts the father in a distinct role within the triad.

Primarily, the distinctiveness of the father's role in the triad derives from the function of separating the child from the mother which may also be secondary to his activation function (Paquette, 2004b). Accordingly, some theorists have posited that the symbiotic origin of the mother-child relationship may place the father in a better position to facilitate such separation (Mahler & Gosliner, 1955), partly also by sustaining an exclusive relationship with the mother that sets clear generational boundaries and creates symbolic distance between the mother and the child (see von Klitzing, 2019). Yet, potentially a key task for the father is to initially accept the central place of the nurturing mother-infant relationship (Bevington, 2019) and serve "as a repository for the infant's experience of the 'bad', depriving mother" (Davids, 2002, p. 85). With increasing maturity, the need for such splitting is thought to diminish (Kernberg, Weiner, & Bardenstein, 2000), enabling the infant to become aware of the real qualities of both parents and develop a more differentiated relationship to both mother and father. Drawing on Herzog (1991/1998), this maturational process may, however, crucially depend on the actual presence of the father who continually survives the infant's projections as long as the representational capacities have not yet been fully consolidated.

In sum, the evidence to date robustly supports the importance of that parent-child triad for well-adjusted child development. Yet, at present, research does not warrant conclusive inferences on the interchangeable or unique contribution of the father to the triad and the developing triadic competence of the infant. Preliminary evidence, however, dovetails with a somewhat unique role, which may involve a separating function that scaffolds the child's nascent triadic competence (Herzog, 1991/1998; von Klitzing, Simoni, Amsler, & Bürgin, 1999).

Intervening at the Triadic Level

To illustrate the power of intervening at the level of the triad, we offer another example from parent-infant psychotherapy where all partners of the triad are present. Perez (2019) reports on a family where the mother was diagnosed with borderline personality disorder and is described as a gatekeeper, derogating and curtailing all interactions between her 2½-month-old son and his father, who has become increasingly withdrawn, mirroring the busy father he had experienced in his own childhood. A few months into treatment, an episode is described where the father calls the therapist to confess that their son had to be taken to the emergency unit, because he fell off the sofa and hurt his head. While the doctor reassured the father and the mother that their son was healthy, the father divulges his excessive feelings of guilt to the therapist, fearing that he might have caused their son lasting damage through his incompetent care. In the following session, all his anxieties about the role as the father come to the fore as he reports being at a loss about how to play with his son, especially as the mother was reproaching him for playing in a too lively and energetic manner. Perez (2019) speculates that for the mother seeing her child engaged in this type of play may have posed too great a threat because it conveyed a sense of separateness from her son and exclusion from the father-child bond.

The "port of entry" selected by Perez was to awaken the father's concern for the infant who was increasingly entering into an "autistic-like state". Thus, during a session where the mother was absorbed in her own anxieties and low mood while their son was looking out of the window with "a dazed, absent look on his face", Perez (2019) "wondered out loud whether [their son] felt that it was all too much and was trying to escape, if only with his eyes and his mind" (p. 47). Repeated situations where Perez voiced such concerns when the child was at the risk of being forgotten slowly set in motion a willingness of the father to overcome his fears and become more involved, even at the expense of now being the primary target of the mother's retaliatory impulses. At the end of the case report, the father, full of pride, recounts an episode where he successfully saved his son from an injury during play, also seeking recognition of this from Perez.

This case brings to the fore many of the themes encountered in the previous sections and illustrates the inherent interrelatedness of the various levels. Thus, although Perez's intervention targeted the triad, it served to simultaneously address the conflicted activative function of the father. Here, the father has at least temporary access to the activative function, even though it is continually reined in by a gatekeeping mother who devalues his livelihood. Accordingly, the therapist did not opt for individual sessions with the father, but, rather, drew on a joint parent-child setting as a means to intervene on behalf of the child in order to give the father a "gentle push" (almost modelling the activation function herself). The therapist in recognizing the need for the father and in harnessing the concern for his child against his passive withdrawal addresses the internal conflict of the father, also allowing him to brace the ensuing conflict and stand up to his domineering wife. In turn, the father after thus gaining confidence in his role also successfully embraces a protective role that might have previously been distorted by his internal conflict between taking initiative with his son and fearing the rupture this might cause with his wife.

The Represented Father

In this brief final section, we turn from the direct influence of the actual father, per se, to the representation of the father and the parental relationship in the minds of the mother and the child. At the theoretical and empirical levels, this section primarily involves a shift of emphasis to the subjective level of the mother and the child which includes the cognitive-affective mechanisms whereby the real and the triadic levels of fathering influence child development. At the clinical level, this shift of emphasis entails a range of child- and parent-focused interventions, often informed by the transference relationship to the therapist. This was already hinted at in the aforementioned case of Melanie: the father's lack of interest not only in Melanie but also in therapy (after all, he did not attend the initial interview), thus implicitly conveyed to the therapist the same derogating message that Melanie was exposed to day by day, whereby feelings of disappointment and anger may be unimportant and unacceptable and, if expressed, may lead to yet more rejection. The therapist, by not succumbing to this logic, but instead tackling the lack of father involvement head-on, may well have offered a corrective experience to everyone, including Melanie. Analogously, some theorists propose that the father is critical for scaffolding development of capacities of healthy regulation and expression of aggression, for example, in RTP (Paquette, 2004b).

Theory and Evidence for the Represented Father

As noted by theorists of various stripes, representations of caregivers do not simply replicate reality, but, rather, encompass the individual's subjective construal and elaboration of the history of past interactions, how they might unfold in the future, and the product of emotion regulation processes (Bretherton, 2005; Clyman, 2003; Main, Kaplan, & Cassidy, 1985; Sandler & Rosenblatt, 1962; Stern, 1985). The representation of the caregiver becomes a part of the individual that guides new interactions and relationships, a part which is present even in the caregiver's absence and is thought to account for continuity across time and context. Though behavioural and physiological evidence for the existence of such representations has accrued from infancy onwards (Johnson, Dweck, & Chen, 2007; White, Wu, Borelli, Mayes, & Crowley, 2013), as a rule, this work has not focused on the specific contributions of fathers.

In a notable exception, Verschueren and Marcoen (1999) adapted a widely used story-stem technique with 4- to 6-year-olds, such that children separately completed stories focused on the mother and the father. Interestingly, children's portrayals of a positive and open father-child interaction better accounted for the child's anxious/withdrawn behaviour than analogous mother-child portrayals. By contrast, the latter better accounted for the child's positiveness of self than analogous father-child portrayals. Using a similar story-stem technique, Page and Bretherton (2003) found that positive father representations predicted better teacher-rated socialization, but only for boys, with girls surprisingly showing a reverse pattern. Potentially, the activative paternal function may indirectly exert its protective influence on anxiety and social behaviour (for boys) via such internal father representations of the child. However, this research has applied the same attachment-related criteria to the coding of both mothers and father representations, without factoring in their putatively distinct qualities.

Kerns et al. (2015) have recently begun to tease out the distinctiveness of mother and father representations using the Friends and Family Interview (N = 107), among older children and adolescents (10–14 years). While mothers more strongly performed a safe-haven function than fathers, fathers more strongly performed a secure-base function than mothers. Moreover, both the secure base and the safe haven were correlates of academic and peer competence, indicating their predictive value beyond the parent-child matrix and thus validating that the researchers were indeed tapping into the representational level.

While intriguing, it remains unclear whether similarly distinct mother and father functions also operate among younger children. Furthermore, whether or not the safe haven and secure base functions *independently* predicted social or academic competence was not assessed in this study. In following up this research, it may help to bear in mind that social competencies promoted by the father-child activation relationship may primarily involve self-efficacy and learning to stand up for yourself (Paquette, 2004b). Crucially, this type of self-oriented social competence is both empirically theoretically distinct from "other-oriented" social competence involving cooperation and collaboration towards a common goal (Perren, Forrester-Knauss, & Alsaker, 2012; Rose-Krasnor & Denham, 2009).

Besides the effect of the father in the child's mind, theories have also speculated on the importance of the "father in the mother's mind". This not only enables children to engage with the actual father but also helps them endow the mother with a mind and relationships of her own, facilitating self-other differentiation processes (see von Klitzing, 2019). To this end, Winnicott's (1975) famous phrase "There is no such thing as a baby" (p. 99) was elegantly expanded by Green (2004) to "there is no such thing as a mother-infant relationship" (p. 101) in order to underscore the importance of the mother's internalized father. However, very little direct evidence exists to date to corroborate these theoretical positions. Perhaps, most relevant in this regard is the finding that higher prenatal maternal triadic competence predicts better quality of the postnatal father-child dyadic interactions (von Klitzing, Simoni, Amsler, & Bürgin, 1999). In other words, a stronger father-child bond appears to hinge on the capacity of the mother to contemplate this bond as a salient entity before birth. In other words, maternal triadic competence may inversely relate to maternal gatekeeping, in line with the idea that mothers may facilitate or limit the father's access to the infant (Winnicott, 1964).

In a similar vein, scholars draw attention to the child's growing awareness of the couple relationship between mother and father. Within a small-scale observational research study, Herzog (1991/1998) reports on several play interviews where children from about age 2 showed a sense of the parental couple together, portraying them as fighting and making up with the help of the child. Analogous patterns have also emerged from more systematic research, showing that 4- to 7-year-old offspring of divorced parents sometimes portray wished-for reunions in their play (Bretherton & Page, 2004). From these data, we can surmise that young children represent not only the father but also his relationship to the mother.

Intervening at the Level of the Father Representation

Though evidence for the relevance of representations of the father is still somewhat preliminary, the effects may well be ubiquitous in the sense of providing an important mechanism whereby the real father and the father as part of the triad exert influence on child development. Given that representational models are imposed on new relationships, they naturally also come to influence how the therapist is perceived in what is termed the transference relationship. Indeed, a distinct feature of psychodynamic approaches is their extensive use of the transference relationship which may reflect a key ingredient in explaining therapeutic success in psychodynamic psychotherapy (see Høglend, 2014 for evidence).

To illustrate these points, we draw on the case of 5-year-old Julian who has also featured in previous publications of our focal short-term psychodynamic psychotherapy model for children. Here, we focus on how Julian transferred the excluded role of the father onto the (female) therapist. He did so partly in an effort to maintain the symbiotic tie to his mother, who had separated from Julian's father soon after birth and, in many ways, had elevated Julian to the role of a substitute partner. Feeling excluded from the mother-child relationship, the father had largely withdrawn. Among others, Julian suffered from intense social phobia and separation anxiety, as expressed by severe tantrums ensuing on a daily basis before leaving for daycare. The therapist interpreted these symptoms as an expression of his anxiety that in daycare, his special role as substitute partner would be challenged by other children (whom he reported hating) and he would merely be "one among many".

In accordance with this, Julian initially also rejected the therapist, especially in the presence of the mother who, in her turn, also seemed to relish in telling the therapist just how reluctant Julian was to attend therapy. During the initial sessions, Julian ordered the therapist around, condemning her to the position of an audience member, and depriving her of a sense of individuality. Fittingly, he disavowed any feelings of vulnerability and neediness, among others, because these posed a threat to his role as a partner substitute for his mother.

These themes picked up the therapeutic focus which the therapist repeatedly verbalized in a developmentally sensitive way towards Julian as well as the mother and the father. As therapy progressed, Julian increasingly engaged in collaborative play with the therapist, relating to her as a person with a mind of her own. He now openly acknowledged his enjoyment of therapy, even directly expressing affection towards the therapist. Ultimately, he also came to embrace his vulnerability which seemed to coincide with feelings of relief that he could be a child and was not solely responsible for the well-being of his mother. By the end of therapy, his social phobia and separation anxiety had subsided, and he was even able to attend class trips and spend the weekend at his father's place.

Among others, Julian's case illustrates how the relationship with the therapist can come under the influence of the father representation the child and the mother carry forwards into therapy. It was crucial for the therapist to acknowledge her initial role as the excluded father in the countertransference in order to survive the attacks of the child and mother, rather than withdraw into the same passive role the father had adopted. In turn, this allowed her to take on the role of a separating third which Julian and his mother eventually came to embrace.

Summary and Key Points

This chapter attempted to accomplish two main aims: First, we sought to provide a state-of-the-art review of the evidence base on the role of fathers in child psychotherapy. From this review, we concluded that the field has yielded some promising evidence, suggesting the potential of including fathers in our intervention efforts. At the same time, however, research still has a long way to go, since, as a rule, studies examine the effect of fathers in what are inherently mother-focused interventions, though exceptions to this rule are emerging in the literature (e.g. Cowan et al., 2018).

For this reason, this chapter also pursued its second aim of outlining different tiers at which to pitch father-focused interventions and providing concrete examples from practitioners with years of experience. On this basis, we believe it is now time to tailor therapeutic techniques to the role of fathers in child development and study their effects using appropriate designs to capture therapeutic processes (Kazdin, 2007). To be sure, in some cases, fathers and their effects on children may call for a similar toolbox already in use with mothers, but in some documented cases, these efforts have already proven to be in vain. What kind of therapeutic techniques to use under these circumstances, surprisingly, is still largely uncharted territory. At this juncture, we drew on what can largely be considered modern psychodynamic work, in part, because this therapeutic orientation has been very vocal about the specific role of fathers in development and has a long tradition of publishing case reports which we found helpful in illustrating specific techniques. In so doing, we did not intend to downplay the important work of other orientations in the field, but felt that other chapters in this volume would close this gap. Moreover, as stimulating as the second section may have been, it is now time to put some of these proposals to test in empirical research on child psychotherapy. We believe this to be a crucial ingredient in moving this field from the realm of speculation to one that can inform disseminatable clinical guidelines and policies for intervening with fathers.

In closing, we would like to return to the introductory quote by Barack Obama. Obama made this comment in a speech penned by himself for the ceremony of the Sandy Hook Elementary School shooting in 2012, which he described as the most challenging time of his presidency in his autobiography. It goes without saying that these sorts of traumatic events have the power to destabilize the parenting function. Such circumstances may also interfere with the joys of fatherhood, in particular, which, almost by definition, require tolerating a certain level of anxiety in order to meet the child's needs for activation, challenges, autonomy, encouragement of exploration, and so on. As we enter into the thick of the role of fathers in child psychotherapy, it is thus wise to remain humble and remind ourselves just how challenging it might prove to effect changes at this level.

References

Abelson, R. P. (1985). A variance explanation paradox: When a little is a lot. *Psychological Bulletin, 97*(1), 129–133.

Ainsworth, M. D. S., Blehar, M. C., Waters, E., & Wall, S. (1978). *Patterns of attachment: A psychological study of the strange situation*. Hillsdale, NJ: Erlbaum.

Andreas, A., White, L. O., Sierau, S., Perren, S., von Klitzing, K., & Klein, A. M. (2018). Like mother like daughter, like father like son? Intergenerational transmission of internalizing symptoms at early school age: A longitudinal study. *European Child & Adolescent Psychiatry, 27*, 985–995. https://doi.org/10.1007/s00787-017-1103-y

Bagner, D. M., & Eyberg, S. M. (2003). Father involvement in Parent training: When does it matter? *Journal of Clinical Child & Adolescent Psychology, 32*(4), 599–605. https://doi.org/10.1207/S15374424JCCP3204_13

Bakermans-Kranenburg, M. J., van Ijzendoorn, M. H., & Juffer, F. (2003). Less is more: Meta-analyses of sensitivity and attachment interventions in early childhood. *Psychological Bulletin, 129*(2), 195–215.

Baradon, T. (2019a). *Working with fathers in psychoanalytic parent-infant psychotherapy*. Oxon, UK: Routledge.

Baradon, T. (2019b). Working with the triad. In T. Baradon (Ed.), *Working with fathers in psychoanalytic parent-infant psychotherapy* (pp. 85–93). Oxon, UK: Routledge.

Barrett, P., Games, N., Fisak, B., Stallard, P., & Phillips, L. (2019). The treatment of anxiety disorders in preschool-aged children. In B. Fisak & P. M. Barrett (Eds.), *Anxiety in preschool children: Assessment, treatment, and prevention* (p. 99). New York: Routledge.

Barrows, P. (2004). Fathers and families: Locating the ghost in the nursery. *Infant Mental Health Journal, 25*(5), 408–423. https://doi.org/10.1002/imhj.20016

Bevington, D. (2019). A journey into fatherhood: The art of failing gracefully. In T. Baradon (Ed.), *Working with fathers in psychoanalytic parent-infant psychotherapy* (pp. 1–13). Oxon, UK: Routledge.

Bögels, S. M., & Phares, V. (2008). Fathers' role in the etiology, prevention and treatment of child anxiety: A review and new model. *Clinical Psychology Review, 28*(4), 539–558. https://doi.org/10.1016/j.cpr.2007.07.011

Bögels, S. M., & Siqueland, L. (2006). Family cognitive behavioral therapy for children and adolescents with clinical anxiety disorders. *Journal of the American Academy of Child & Adolescent Psychiatry, 45*(2), 134–141. https://doi.org/10.1097/01.chi.0000190467.01072.ee

Bögels, S. M., & van Melick, M. (2004). The relationship between child-report, parent self-report, and partner report of perceived parental rearing behaviors and anxiety in children and parents. *Personality and Individual Differences, 37*(8), 1583–1596. https://doi.org/10.1016/j.paid.2004.02.014

Bretherton, I. (2005). In pursuit of the internal working model construct and its relevance to attachment relationships. In K. Grossmann, K. Grossmann, & E. Waters (Eds.), *Attachment from infancy to adulthood: The major longitudinal studies* (pp. 13–47). New York: Guilford.

Bretherton, I., & Page, T. F. (2004). Shared or conflicting working models? Relationships in postdivorce families seen through the eyes of mothers and their preschool children. *Development and Psychopathology, 16*(03), 551–575.

Bürgin, D. (1998). Vater als Person und Vater als Prinzip. In D. Bürgin (Ed.), *Triangulierung–Der Übergang zur Elternschaft* (pp. 179–214). Stuttgart, Germany: Schattauer.

Carnes, A., Matthewson, M., & Boer, O. (2019). The contribution of parents in childhood anxiety treatment: A meta-analytic review. *Clinical Psychologist*. https://doi.org/10.1111/cp.12179

Chacko, A., Fabiano, G. A., Doctoroff, G. L., & Fortson, B. (2018). Engaging fathers in effective parenting for preschool children using shared book reading: A randomized controlled trial. *Journal of Clinical Child & Adolescent Psychology, 47*(1), 79–93. https://doi.org/10.1080/15374416.2016.1266648

Clyman, R. B. (2003). Portrayals in maltreated children's play narratives: Representations or emotion regulation. In R. N. Emde, D. P. Wolf, & D. Oppenheim (Eds.), *Revealing the inner worlds of young children. The MacArthur story stem battery and parent-child narratives* (pp. 201–221). Oxford: Oxford University Press.

Corboz-Warnery, A., Fivaz-Depeursinge, E., Bettens, C. G., & Favez, N. (1993). Systemic analysis of father-mother-baby interactions: The Lausanne triadic play. *Infant Mental Health Journal, 14*(4), 298–316. https://doi.org/10.1002/1097-0355

Cowan, C. P., & Cowan, P. A. (2019a). Enhancing parenting effectiveness, Fathers' involvement, couple relationship quality, and Children's development: Breaking down silos in family policy making and service delivery. *Journal of Family Theory & Review, 11*(1), 92–111.

Cowan, P. A., & Cowan, C. P. (2019b). Introduction: Bringing dads back into the family. *Attachment & Human Development, 21*(5), 419–425. https://doi.org/10.1080/14616734.2019.1582594

Cowan, P. A., Cowan, C. P., Pruett, M. K., & Pruett, K. D. (2018). Supporting father involvement: A father inclusive couples group approach to parenting interventions. In H. Steele & M. Steele (Eds.), *Handbook of attachment-based interventions* (pp. 466–491). New York: Guilford.

Crawford, A. M., & Manassis, K. (2001). Familial predictors of treatment outcome in childhood anxiety disorders. *Journal of the American Academy of Child & Adolescent Psychiatry, 40*(10), 1182–1189. https://doi.org/10.1097/00004583-200110000-00012

Davids, M. F. (2002). Fathers in the internal world: from boy to man to father. In S. Budd (Series Ed.) & J. Trowell & A. Etchegoyen (Vol. Eds.), *New library of psychoanalysis. The importance of fathers - a psychoanalytic re-evaluation*. Hove: Brunner-Routledge.

Eyberg, S. M., Boggs, S. R., & Algina, J. (1995). Parent-child interaction therapy: A psychosocial model for the treatment of young children with conduct problem behavior and their families. *Psychopharmacology Bulletin, 31*(1), 83–91.

Fabiano, G. A. (2007). Father participation in behavioral parent training for ADHD: Review and recommendations for increasing inclusion and engagement. *Journal of Family Psychology, 21*(4), 683–693. https://doi.org/10.1037/0893-3200.21.4.683

Favez, N., Lopes, F., Bernard, M., Frascarolo, F., Lavanchy Scaiola, C., Corboz-Warnery, A., et al. (2012). The development of family Alliance from pregnancy to toddlerhood and child outcomes at 5 years. *Family Process, 51*(4), 542–556. https://doi.org/10.1111/j.1545-5300.2012.01419.x

Fearon, R. P., Bakermans-Kranenburg, M. J., Van Ijzendoorn, M. H., Lapsley, A.-M., & Roisman, G. I. (2010). The significance of insecure attachment and disorganization in the development of Children's externalizing behavior: A meta-analytic study. *Child Development, 81*(2), 435–456. https://doi.org/10.1111/j.1467-8624.2009.01405.x

Feldman, R. (2003). Infant–mother and infant–father synchrony: The coregulation of positive arousal. *Infant Mental Health Journal, 24*(1), 1–23. https://doi.org/10.1002/imhj.10041

Flanders, J. L., Leo, V., Paquette, D., Pihl, R. O., & Séguin, J. R. (2009). Rough-and-tumble play and the regulation of aggression: An observational study of father–child play dyads. *Aggressive Behavior, 35*(4), 285–295. https://doi.org/10.1002/ab.20309

Flanders, J. L., Simard, M., Paquette, D., Parent, S., Vitaro, F., Pihl, R. O., et al. (2010). Rough-and-tumble play and the development of physical aggression and emotion regulation: A five-year follow-up study. *Journal of Family Violence, 25*(4), 357–367. https://doi.org/10.1007/s10896-009-9297-5

Fletcher, R., StGeorge, J., & Freeman, E. (2013). Rough and tumble play quality: Theoretical foundations for a new measure of father–child interaction. *Early Child Development and Care, 183*(6), 746–759. https://doi.org/10.1080/03004430.2012.723439

Fonagy, P., Gergely, G., Jurist, E. L., & Target, M. (2002). *Affect regulation, mentalization, and the development of the self.* London: Karnac.

Fonagy, P., & Target, M. (1995). Understanding the violent patient: The use of the body and the role of the father. *The International Journal of Psychoanalysis, 76*(3), 487–501.

Frank, T. J., Keown, L. J., & Sanders, M. R. (2015). Enhancing father engagement and Interparental teamwork in an evidence-based parenting intervention: A randomized-controlled trial of outcomes and processes. *Behavior Therapy, 46*(6), 749–763. https://doi.org/10.1016/j.beth.2015.05.008

Göttken, T., & von Klitzing, K. (2014). *Manual for short-term psychoanalytic child therapy (PaCT)*. London: Karnac Books.

Göttken, T., White, L. O., Klein, A. M., & von Klitzing, K. (2014). Short-term psychoanalytic child therapy for anxious children: A pilot study. *Psychotherapy, 51*(1), 148–158. https://doi.org/10.1037/a0036026

Green, A. (2004). Thirdness and psychoanalytic concepts. *The Psychoanalytic Quarterly, 73*, 99–135.

Groh, A. M., Fearon, R. P., Bakermans-Kranenburg, M. J., van Ijzendoorn, M. H., Steele, R. D., & Roisman, G. I. (2014). The significance of attachment security for children's social competence with peers: A meta-analytic study. *Attachment & Human Development, 16*(2), 103–136. https://doi.org/10.1080/14616734.2014.883636

Groh, A. M., Roisman, G. I., van Ijzendoorn, M. H., Bakermans-Kranenburg, M. J., & Fearon, R. P. (2012). The significance of insecure and disorganized attachment for children's internalizing symptoms: A meta-analytic study. *Child Development, 83*(2), 591–610. https://doi.org/10.1111/j.1467-8624.2011.01711.x

Grossmann, K., Grossmann, K. E., Fremmer-Bombik, E., Kindler, H., Scheuerer-Englisch, H., & Zimmermann, P. (2002). The uniqueness of the child–father attachment relationship: fathers' sensitive and challenging play as a pivotal variable in a 16-year longitudinal study. *Social Development, 11*(3), 301–337. https://doi.org/10.1111/1467-9507.00202

Helfenbaum-Kun, E. D., & Ortiz, C. (2007). Parent-training groups for fathers of head start children: A pilot study of their feasibility and impact on child behavior and intra-familial relationships. *Child & Family Behavior Therapy, 29*(2), 47–64. https://doi.org/10.1300/J019v29n02_04

Herzog, J. M. (1991/1998). Early interaction and representation: The father's role in early and later triads, the father as expediter from dyad to triad. [initially presented as a paper in Basel, Switzerland in 1991]. In D. Bürgin (Ed.), *Triangulierung–Der Übergang zur Elternschaft* (pp. 162–178). Stuttgart, Germany: Schattauer.

Høglend, P. (2014). Exploration of the patient-therapist relationship in psychotherapy. *American Journal of Psychiatry, 171*(10), 1056–1066. https://doi.org/10.1176/appi.ajp.2014.14010121

Johnson, S. C., Dweck, C. S., & Chen, F. S. (2007). Evidence for infants' internal working models of attachment. *Psychological Science, 18*, 501–502. https://doi.org/10.1111/j.1467-9280.2007.01929.x

Jones, A. (2019). When working therapeutically with a baby's father is not possible. In T. Baradon (Ed.), *Working with fathers in psychoanalytic parent-infant psychotherapy* (pp. 50–63). Oxon, UK: Routledge.

Joyce, A. (2019). "The door in the back of my head": A father's failure to mourn the deaths of his parents. In T. Baradon (Ed.), *Working with fathers in psychoanalytic parent-infant psychotherapy* (pp. 28–38). Oxon, UK: Routledge.

Karberg, E., Cabrera, N. J., Malin, J., & Kuhns, C. (2019). Longitudinal contributions of maternal and paternal intrusive behaviors to children's sociability and sustained attention at prekindergarten. *Monographs of the Society for Research in Child Development, 84*(1), 79–93.

Kazdin, A. E. (2007). Mediators and mechanisms of change in psychotherapy research. *Annual Review of Clinical Psychology, 3*(1), 1–27. https://doi.org/10.1146/annurev.clinpsy.3.022806.091432

Kernberg, P. F., Weiner, A. S., & Bardenstein, K. (2000). *Personality disorders in children and adolescents*. New York: Basic Books.

Kerns, K. A., Mathews, B. L., Koehn, A. J., Williams, C. T., & Siener-Ciesla, S. (2015). Assessing both safe haven and secure base support in parent–child relationships. *Attachment & Human Development, 17*(4), 337–353. https://doi.org/10.1080/14616734.2015.1042487

Lamb, M. E. (1975). Fathers: Forgotten contributors to child development. *Human Development, 18*(4), 245–266. Retrieved from https://www.karger.com/DOI/10.1159/000271493. https://doi.org/10.1159/000271493

Lamb, M. E. (2010). How do fathers influence children's development? Let me count the ways. In M. E. Lamb (Ed.), *The role of the father in child development* (5th ed., pp. 1–26). Hoboken: John Wiley & Sons Inc.

Leaper, C., Anderson, K. J., & Sanders, P. (1998). Moderators of gender effects on parents' talk to their children: A meta-analysis. *Developmental Psychology, 34*(1), 3–27. https://doi.org/10.1037/0012-1649.34.1.3

Liber, J. M., van Widenfelt, B. M., Goedhart, A. W., Utens, E. M. W. J., van der Leeden, A. J. M., Markus, M. T., et al. (2008). Parenting and parental anxiety and depression as predictors of treatment outcome for childhood anxiety disorders: Has the role of fathers been underestimated? *Journal of Clinical Child & Adolescent Psychology, 37*(4), 747–758. https://doi.org/10.1080/15374410802359692

Lieberman, A. F., Ghosh Ippen, C., & Van Horn, P. (2015). *"Don't hit my mommy!": A manual for child-parent psychotherapy with young children exposed to violence and other trauma*. Washington, DC: Zero to Three.

Lucassen, N., Tharner, A., Van IJzendoorn, M. H., Bakermans-Kranenburg, M. J., Volling, B. L., Verhulst, F. C., et al. (2011). The association between paternal sensitivity and infant–father attachment security: A meta-analysis of three decades of research. *Journal of Family Psychology, 25*(6), 986.

Lundahl, B. W., Tollefson, D., Risser, H., & Lovejoy, M. C. (2007). A meta-analysis of father involvement in parent training. *Research on Social Work Practice, 18*(2), 97–106. https://doi.org/10.1177/1049731507309828

Mahler, M. S., & Gosliner, B. J. (1955). On symbiotic child psychosis. *The Psychoanalytic Study of the Child, 10*(1), 195–212. https://doi.org/10.1080/00797308.1955.11822556

Main, M., Kaplan, N., & Cassidy, J. (1985). Security in infancy, childhood, and adulthood: A move to the level of representation. *Monographs of the Society for Research in Child Development, 50*(1/2), 66–104.

Majdandžić, M., de Vente, W., & Bögels, S. M. (2016). Challenging parenting behavior from infancy to toddlerhood: Etiology, measurement, and differences between fathers and mothers. *Infancy, 21*(4), 423–452. https://doi.org/10.1111/infa.12125

Majdandžić, M., de Vente, W., Colonnesi, C., & Bögels, S. M. (2018). Fathers' challenging parenting behavior predicts less subsequent anxiety symptoms in early childhood. *Behaviour Research and Therapy, 109*, 18–28. Retrieved from. https://doi.org/10.1016/j.brat.2018.07.007

Majdandžić, M., Möller, E. L., de Vente, W., Bögels, S. M., & van den Boom, D. C. (2014). Fathers' challenging parenting behavior prevents social anxiety development in their 4-year-old children: A longitudinal observational study. *Journal of Abnormal Child Psychology, 42*(2), 301–310. https://doi.org/10.1007/s10802-013-9774-4

Manassis, K., Mendlowitz, S. L., Scapillato, D., Avery, D., Fiksenbaum, L., Freire, M., . . . Owens, M. (2002). Group and individual cognitive-behavioral therapy for childhood anxiety disorders: A randomized trial. Journal of the American Academy of Child & Adolescent Psychiatry, 41(12), 1423–1430. doi:https://doi.org/10.1097/00004583-200212000-00013

McHale, J. P. (2007). When infants grow up in multiperson relationship systems. *Infant Mental Health Journal, 28*(4), 370–392. https://doi.org/10.1002/imhj.20142

Murphy, L. B. (1997). Fathers. *Zero to Three, 18*(1), 9.

Page, T., & Bretherton, I. (2003). Representations of attachment to father in the narratives of preschool girls in post-divorce families: Implications for family relationships and social development. *Child and Adolescent Social Work Journal, 20*(2), 99–122. https://doi.org/10.1023/A:1022864614244

Panter-Brick, C., Burgess, A., Eggerman, M., McAllister, F., Pruett, K., & Leckman, J. F. (2014). Practitioner review: Engaging fathers – Recommendations for a game change in parenting interventions based on a systematic review of the global evidence. *Journal of Child Psychology and Psychiatry, 55*(11), 1187–1212. https://doi.org/10.1111/jcpp.12280

Paquette, D. (2004a). Dichotomizing paternal and maternal functions as a means to better understand their primary contributions. *Human Development, 47*(4), 237–238. https://doi.org/10.1159/000078726

Paquette, D. (2004b). Theorizing the father-child relationship: Mechanisms and developmental outcomes. *Human Development, 47*(4), 193–219. https://doi.org/10.1159/000078723

Paquette, D., & Bigras, M. (2010). The risky situation: A procedure for assessing the father–child activation relationship. *Early Child Development and Care, 180*(1–2), 33–50. https://doi.org/10.1080/03004430903414687

Perez, A. (2019). Waking daddy up: Restoring a father's place in a borderline personality couple. In T. Baradon (Ed.), *Working with fathers in psychoanalytic parent-infant psychotherapy* (pp. 39–49). Oxon, UK: Routledge.

Perren, S., Forrester-Knauss, C., & Alsaker, F. D. (2012). Self-and other-oriented social skills: Differential associations with children's mental health and bullying roles. *Journal for Educational Research Online/Journal für Bildungsforschung Online, 4*(1), 99–123.

Phares, V., Rojas, A., Thurston, I. B., & Hankinson, J. C. (2010). Including fathers in clinical interventions for children and adolescents. In M. E. Lamb (Ed.), *The role of the father in child development* (5th ed., pp. 459–485). Hoboken, NJ: John Wiley & Sons Inc.

Pleck, J. H. (2010). Fatherhood and masculinity. In M. E. Lamb (Ed.), *The role of the father in child development* (5th ed., pp. 27–57). Hoboken, NJ: John Wiley & Sons Inc.

Rapee, R. M. (2000). Group treatment of children with anxiety disorders: Outcome and predictors of treatment response. *Australian Journal of Psychology, 52*(3), 125–129. https://doi.org/10.1080/00049530008255379

Roggman, L. A. (2004). Do fathers just want to have fun? *Human Development, 47*(4), 228–236. https://doi.org/10.1159/000078725

Rose-Krasnor, L., & Denham, S. A. (2009). Social-emotional competence in early childhood. In K. H. Rubin, W. M. Bukowski, & B. Laursen (Eds.), *Handbook of peer interactions, relationships and groups* (pp. 162–179). New York: Guildford.

Salomonsson, B., Baradon, T., & von Klitzing, K. (2019). Three themes about father in parent-infant psychotherapy. In T. Baradon (Ed.), *Working with fathers in psychoanalytic parent-infant psychotherapy* (Vol. 154–168). Oxon, UK: Roultledge

Sandler, J., & Rosenblatt, B. (1962). The concept of the representational world. *The Psychoanalytic Study of the Child, 17*(1), 128–145.

Schneider, S., Blatter-Meunier, J., Herren, C., Adornetto, C., In-Albon, T., & Lavallee, K. (2011). Disorder-specific cognitive-behavioral therapy for separation anxiety disorder in young children: A randomized waiting-list-controlled trial. *Psychotherapy and Psychosomatics, 80*(4), 206–215. https://doi.org/10.1159/000323444

Sicouri, G., Tully, L., Collins, D., Burn, M., Sargeant, K., Frick, P., . . . Dadds, M. (2018). Toward father-friendly parenting interventions: A qualitative study. Australian and New Zealand Journal of Family Therapy, 39(2), 218–231. doi:https://doi.org/10.1002/anzf.1307

Smith, P. K. (2010). *Children and play*. John Wiley & Sons. New York.

Stern, D. N. (1985). *The interpersonal world of the infant: A view from psychoanalysis and developmental psychology*. New York: Basic Books.

StGeorge, J., Fletcher, R., Freeman, E., Paquette, D., & Dumont, C. (2015). Father–child interactions and children's risk of injury. *Early Child Development and Care, 185*(9), 1409–1421. https://doi.org/10.1080/03004430.2014.1000888

Target, M., & Fonagy, P. (2002). Fathers in moder psychoanalysis and in society: The role of the father in child development. In J. Trowell & A. Etchegoyen (Eds.), *The importance of fathers – A psychoanalytic re-evaluation* (pp. 45–66). Hove, UK: Brunner-Routledge.

Tiano, J. D., & McNeil, C. B. (2005). The inclusion of fathers in behavioral Parent training: A critical evaluation. *Child & Family Behavior Therapy, 27*(4), 1–28. https://doi.org/10.1300/J019v27n04_01

van der Sluis, C. M., van der Bruggen, C. O., Brechman-Toussaint, M. L., Thissen, M. A. P., & Bögels, S. M. (2012). Parent-directed cognitive behavioral therapy for young anxious children: A pilot study. *Behavior Therapy, 43*(3), 583–592. https://doi.org/10.1016/j.beth.2011.10.002

Verschueren, K., & Marcoen, A. (1999). Representation of self and socioemotional competence in kindergartners: Differential and combined effects of attachment to mother and to father. *Child Development, 70*(1), 183–201. https://doi.org/10.1111/1467-8624.00014

Volling, B. L., & Cabrera, N. J. (2019). Advancing research and measurement on fathering and Children's development. *Monographs of the Society for Research in Child Development, 84*(1), 7–160. Retrieved from https://doi.org/10.1111/mono.12404

Volling, B. L., Stevenson, M. M., Safyer, P., Gonzalez, R., & Lee, J. Y. (2019). IV. In search of the father–infant activation relationship: A person-centered approach. In B. L. Volling & N. J. Cabrera (Eds.), *Monographs of the Society for Research in child development: Advancing research and measurement on fathering and children's development* (Vol. 84, pp. 50–63). New York: John Wiley & Sons.

von Klitzing, K. & Burgin, D. (2005). Parental capacities fro triadic relationships during pregnancy: Early predictors of children's behavioral and representational functioning at preschool age. *Infant Mental Health Journal, 26*(1), 19–39.

von Klitzing, K. (2019). The role of father in early child development. In T. Baradon (Ed.), *Working with fathers in psychoanalytic parent-infant psychotherapy* (pp. 14–27). Oxon, UK: Routledge.

von Klitzing, K., Simoni, H., Amsler, F., & Bürgin, D. (1999). The role of the father in early family interactions. *Infant Mental Health Journal, 20*(3), 222–237. https://doi.org/10.1002/1097-0355

von Klitzing, K., Simoni, H., & Bürgin, D. (1999). Child development and early triadic relationships. *The International Journal of Psychoanalysis, 80*(1), 71–89. https://doi.org/10.1516/0020757991598576

Webster-Stratton, C. (1985). The effects of father involvement in parent training for conduct problem children. *Journal of Child Psychology and Psychiatry, 26*(5), 801–810. https://doi.org/10.1111/j.1469-7610.1985.tb00593.x

White, L. O., Wu, J., Borelli, J. L., Mayes, L. C., & Crowley, M. J. (2013). Play it again: Neural responses to Reunion with excluders predicted by attachment patterns. *Developmental Science, 16*(6), 850–863. https://doi.org/10.1111/desc.12035

Winnicott, D. W. (1964) What about father? *In The child, the family and the outside world* (pp. 113–118). New York: Da Capo Press.

Winnicott, D.W. (1971). *Playing and Reality*. London: Tavistock Publications.

Engaging Fathers of Young Children in Low-Income Families to Improve Child and Family Outcomes: A Preventive Intervention Perspective

38

Kyle Dean Pruett and Marsha Kline Pruett

This volume bears witness to efforts by leading behavioral scientists, clinicians, researchers, and policy makers to advance our understanding fathers' roles – biological and nonbiological – on young and very young children's well-being and development. Its publication is timely, coming as it does on the heels of many countries' interest and recent investment in paternal engagement programs, driven by their concern about the myriad vulnerabilities that many children and families are known to suffer when fathers are absent (Panter-Brick et al., 2014).

Several recent summaries of the effects of those early investments, however, detail how difficult it has proven to use traditional matricentric-centric approaches to evaluate child-father interactions sufficient to generating positive change. Panter-Brick et al. (2014) reviewed 1172 global publications that reported "fathering effects" on child development and were able to distill just 36 reports that met sufficiently rigorous standards to support the conclusion that positive paternal engagement improves child outcomes. Phares (1996) found that in the few journal articles purporting to measure "fathering effects," when paternal-generated variables were included, they were nearly always significant. Einstein summarized this dilemma: "When you always do what you always did, you will always get what you always got."

Fabiano and Caserta (2018) found that despite 40 years of science supporting contributions made by fathers to child well-being, research literature continues to lag far behind in the investigation of cause and effect of paternal impact on child development. This chapter presents the context for, the design and implementation of, and lessons learned from a unique RCT paternal engagement intervention design that demonstrated reductions of risk factors for abuse and neglect in a large number of diverse vulnerable families with infants and toddlers.

Although we may not yet have a robust inventory of proven interventions at hand, we are increasingly well-informed about the nature and mechanisms of positive paternal engagement from infancy to preK. Emotional and behavioral regulation, coping, and stress management are all areas of infant and toddler development impacted by paternal engagement. Karberg, Cabrera, Malin, and Kuhns (Volling et al., 2019) compared maternal and paternal intrusiveness in interactions with their 24-month-old Early Head Start low-income, minority children and found that while mothers and fathers did not differ in the frequency of their intrusive interactive episodes, fathers tended to be more intensely intrusive, while staying within the context of more positive

K. D. Pruett (✉)
Yale Study Center, Northampton, MA, USA
e-mail: kyle.pruett@yale.edu

M. K. Pruett
School for Social Work, Smith College, Northampton, MA, USA

H. E. Fitzgerald et al. (eds.), *Handbook of Fathers and Child Development*,
https://doi.org/10.1007/978-3-030-51027-5_38

shared affect with their child. Children were found to demonstrate more positive affect during intrusive exchanges with fathers than with mothers. These findings might suggest that father's more intense intrusiveness is generally well tolerated by toddlers, who themselves are exploring the boundaries of aggression and autonomy. The positive affect may evidence that the shared pleasure in that interaction experienced with father may be more characteristic of that dyad.

Baptista, Sousa, Soares, and Martins (2018) deepened our understanding of some of these differences by extending observations of behavioral regulation from the dyadic parent-child plane of interaction to the coparenting domain and its influence on young children's behavioral regulation. Coding videotapes of 70 preschoolers engaged in the "Head-Shoulders-Knees-and-Toes" task (standing children singing a simple tune guiding them to repeat the cycle of touching their head, then shoulders, then knees, and then toes in unison) found that paternal sensitivity during the task correlated significantly with the reported amount of cooperation in coparenting. Their strong recommendation for programs designed to promote child self-regulation was to employ strategies focused on both individual and coparenting skill building, not simply mother-child dyads.

Play has been a primary focus of father-focused research for decades, given the observation that fathers spend a higher percentage of their interactive time with their children in play than do mothers. The intense emotions that often accompany play are identified by fathers as reasons that they and their children enjoy it. Fathers are also aware that such play offers a laboratory for learning how to regulate those very emotions. Bocknek et al. (2017), with a large population of Early Head Start families, measured the relationship between father's active play (measured at 36-month birthday-related assessment) and subsequent cognitive-social and emotional regulation at kindergarten entry. Regular, active physical play between fathers and young children was associated with improved developmental outcomes, especially moderate doses of such play. Too little or too much active physical play, however, worsens such outcomes, particularly among children with more reactive temperaments. Interestingly, children with highly emotional reactive temperaments benefited especially from this type of play with fathers. Reading or mealtime engagement was not associated with improved emotional regulation, suggesting that there is a unique dynamic inherent in this type of play.

One of the least researched, but more salient to mental health outcome topics, has been the paternal-child emotional regulation paradigm of anxiety, especially in infants and toddlers. While it is well known that negative infant affectivity predisposes to childhood anxiety, most of the attention and attribution has focused on maternal risk or resilience variables, with varying degrees of understanding about causality, suggesting that there are more pieces to the puzzle.

Metz, Colonnesi, Majdandžić, and Bögels (2018) suggest that a key puzzle piece may well be the nature of the coparenting relationship. In their longitudinal study of 116 couples, they coded cooperative, mutual, neutral, and competitive coparenting behaviors during a clothes-changing task at 4 months, with follow-up evaluation of child anxiety symptoms at 30 months. While both parents endorsed that infant negative affectivity predicted childhood anxiety, the association was moderated by each parent's divergent cooperative coparenting. The association strengthened when mothers were cooperative and fathers stayed neutral and weakened when fathers were cooperative while mothers stayed neutral. When fathers "stepped up" and became more cooperative, mothers took a "step back," leaving room for the father-child relationship to thrive (less gatekeeping). The authors conclude that this dynamic may reduce the odds of their at-risk child developing anxiety.

Building on the importance to the Zero to Three field of understanding the power of coparenting relationships in positive and negative child outcomes, Favez, Tissot, Frascarolo, Stiefel, and Despland (2016) studied the degree to which feeling competent about parental roles in mothers and fathers influenced coparenting and child engagement in triadic interactions during the first

24 months of life, *after* marital satisfaction and postpartum depression were controlled for (the usual suspects). Using the Lausanne Trialogue Play assessment, 69 triads were assessed for coparenting support and conflict and child engagement. Questionnaires evaluating parental sense of competence, beliefs about parental roles, marital satisfaction, and postpartum depression (in mothers and fathers) were done at 3, 9, and 18 months. Paternal beliefs about the importance of father's and mother's roles were main predictors of child engagement at 18 months, and discrepancies between mothers and fathers in beliefs about the importance of the mother's role is the main predictor of coparenting conflict at 18 months. They also found that maternal competence is positively linked with coparenting support, especially at 18 months. A useful thing to have when raising a toddler.

The bulk of research connecting positive child outcomes from efforts to positively engage fathers has centered on at-risk populations in or near urban centers (Panter-Brick et al., 2014). A recent controlled study in Vietnam focused on couples raising their infants in rural or semirural communes (Rempel, Rempel, Khuc, & Vui, 2017). The study tested the thesis that fathers could be taught and encouraged to develop positive relationships with their children, even when few of them had enjoyed mutually satisfying relationships with their own fathers during childhood. Mothers and fathers in the intervention and the control completed pre-birth and 1-month, 4-month, and 9-month post-birth questionnaires. Intervention fathers received direct counseling, and mothers joined them for periodic group discussions. Intervention fathers were reported both by themselves and their partners to feel more attached to their infants, right from birth. The 9-month follow-up developmental assessment revealed that their infants demonstrated higher levels of motor, language, and personal/social development than controls. The authors concluded that fathers can be taught, supported, and encouraged to interact more sensitively, responsively, and effectively with their newborns and that such increased interaction can lay the foundation for enhanced infant and toddler development.

On this foundation of recent research regarding contributions fathers can make when they are included, supported, and explicitly expected to participate in their infant and toddler's lives, we ground our discussion of the large RCT that is the central contribution of this chapter.

California Supporting Father Involvement (SFI)

The Supporting Father Involvement (SFI) program was launched in 2003 by the California Department of Social Services, Office of Child Abuse Prevention, as the first coparenting-focused, father involvement program evaluated with a longitudinal randomized clinical trial (RCT) research methodology (Cowan, Cowan, Pruett, Pruett, & Wong, 2009; Epstein et al., 2015). The program was based on prevention theory in that it was steered toward parents of very young children (2.3 years of age) with the expectation that strengthening family relationships early would lead to less child abuse and better relationships throughout family life, possibly lowering risk to subsequent births in the family.

While child well-being is the focus and purpose of the program, it targets the parents' relationship as the locus in which to create change to directly benefit their children. The opening expectation was that both parents must be involved for the intervention to have maximum effect (eventually corroborated by data). Thus, the intervention was based on an ecological model (Belsky, 1984; Bronfenbrenner, 1979) and a family systems' approach (Cowan & Cowan, 2000; Heinicke, 2002) that articulated five key family domains: (1) individual well-being and mental health, primarily depression and anxiety; (2) parenting quality and stress; (3) coparenting/couple communication, problem-solving about conflicts, and relationship satisfaction; (4) three-generational transmission of parenting attitudes and behaviors; and (5) balance between stress and social support outside of the family, particularly from work inside and outside the home. Risk and protective factors in each of the domains are associated with fathers' level of positive involvement in intact families (Cookston, 1999; Pruett, Pruett, Cowan, & Cowan, 2017a), as well as in divorced families (Maccoby, Depner, & Mnookin, 1990; Pruett, McIntosh, & Kelly, 2014), and negative events in each of the domains are known to increase risks for abuse and neglect of children (Rosenberg & Wilcox, 2006).

SFI was conceptualized as a preventive intervention for community high-risk samples, intended to increase partnership parenting and father involvement before expected downturns of partner satisfaction after becoming parents (Hirschberger, Srivastava, Marsh, Cowan, & Cowan, 2009; Twenge, Campbell, & Foster, 2003) and parent stresses result in poorer coparenting and parenting, fathers' withdrawal or absence, and negative child outcomes.

SFI begins with a detailed couple interview that introduces the five domains with which parents will be working in the intervention groups, shaping a collaborative approach to motivating change in attitudes and behaviors (Miller & Rollnick, 2009; Pruett et al., 2019). For the RCT, participating parents were randomly invited to take part in one of three conditions: (1) a 16-week, 32-hour primarily fathers' group; (2) a 16-week, 32-hour couples' group; or (3) one-time informational meeting (3 hours) which served as a low-dose control condition. The fathers' groups typically have eight to ten participants, while the couples' groups include four to eight couples. The curricula differ only in who attends (fathers or both coparents) and how change is targeted (through the partners or primarily through one parent). Twice in each version of the curriculum, fathers and mothers meet separately with one of the co-leaders. "His" group meeting includes time with the fathers' youngest children, while "her" meeting focuses on issues of sharing child care with partners. Themes from the five risk/protective domains are woven together in the curriculum over the course of the groups. Each session includes a combination of didactic material, hands-on exercises, videos, and discussion in various formats (large group, small group, couples/pairs, individuals) to elicit maximum engagement and foster participants' growth.

The groups are led by clinically trained male-female Group Leader pairs, at least one having a master's degree. An SFI Case Manager refers families to other community services as needed (housing, health, food, legal, employment, etc.) and supports the family's retention in the program through regular contact. Additional program components include onsite child care and family meals before the group. The curriculum, adapted by Drs. Kline Pruett and Ebling from previous iterations of the intervention model (Cowan & Cowan, 2000, 2005), focuses on strengthening key family relationships in racially and ethnically diverse low-income families.

The first SFI study phase included 279 Mexican-American and European-American low-income couples residing in 4 California counties with a youngest child ranging in age from 0 to 7 (average 2.3 years). Participants in this first iteration (but not later ones) were all biological parents of the youngest child. This first randomized clinical trial SFI study followed families across 18 months – prior to and during a brief waiting period before the intervention's beginning and then 11 months after conclusion. While the control group fathers and mothers showed no positive changes and some negative changes at the 18-month follow-up assessment, both intervention groups reported (1) increases in fathers' involvement in care of their children, (2) reductions in parenting stress, (3) no increase in children's behavior problems (whereas control condition children showed worsening), and (4) no decline in the couple relationship – a positive finding in the context of 50 studies worldwide which show that without intervention, marital satisfaction follows a downward trajectory (Twenge et al., 2003). See Cowan et al. (2009) for complete results and Pruett, Cowan, Cowan, and Pruett (2009) for a description of lessons learned. Results were similar across Hispanic and Caucasian, married and unmarried, and higher and lower SES families.

The intervention was equally effective regardless of parental levels of depression, conflict, and couple satisfaction when entering the program. The number and range of positive outcomes, combined with careful program methodology and assessment, led SFI to be designated as an evidence-based practice by the California Evidence-Based Clearinghouse.

Extending SFI Results in California: Community and Child Welfare Samples

Following the positive results of the first SFI study, the same research team sought to establish whether the outcomes could be replicated with a more diverse participant population. Therefore, a second SFI trial (Cowan, Cowan, Pruett, Pruett, & Gillette, 2014) was conducted in the original four California sites with the addition of a new site comprised of an African-American family sample. Other variations in SFI II involved extending the age range of the youngest child from 0–7 to 0–11 and including any fathering figures (stepparent, siblings, grandparents). Most families continued to opt for the program as married couples, especially when their youngest child was a toddler (average age 2.5 years).

The most significant change in the design of Study II included eliminating the control group and RCT design. Because results from the first study showed that participants in the control group experienced no positive and many negative changes in their relationships as couples or in their children's behavior (Cowan et al., 2009), ethical concerns drove the decision to eliminate the control group. When sites were also allowed to choose whether to implement fathers' or couples' groups, the vast majority chose couples' groups. They had been more successful in the previous study, and partners reported that they enjoyed the chance to work together for their children and themselves. In the initial study, Group Leaders observed participants as delving deeper into issues when both partners were involved; fathers' groups produced positive changes in individual and parental domains but did not affect the couple domain, and the Group Leaders reported that families – especially mothers – preferred the couples' group option. This preference was borne out by participant attendance: couples' groups attendance averaged 80%, while fathers' groups attendance averaged 70%. SFI researchers chose to use a "benchmarking" strategy (Hunsley & Lee, 2007) by comparing the results from the Study II replication, which offered the same curriculum and program to a more inclusive population, with the already published data from the original SFI I (Cowan et al., 2009). The researchers conceptualized SFI II as an opportunity to gather systematic practice-based evidence through a community-based application of the SFI approach.

In SFI II, 236 low-income parents participated in an SFI couples' group with participant couples in all 3 ethnic groups (European-American, Mexican-American, African-American) showing positive changes in measures of parent-child relationships, couple relationship quality, and children's problem behaviors. A pre-post assessment of the couples' groups found (1) stable relationship satisfaction, (2) statistically significant increases in father involvement and (3) increases in household income [average 4K], (4) declines in parents' reports of violent problem-solving, (5) lower parenting stress, and (6) decreases in their children's aggressive behavior. Couples in most difficulty at Baseline showed the greatest benefits. The SFI intervention for low-income families produced effects ranging from the 0.20s to mid-0.40s, with only the impact of parent participation on children's socially withdrawn behavior reaching a very high level ($d = 1.88$). Cohen (1988) tentatively described effect sizes as small (0.20), medium (0.50), and large (0.80). Compared with other interventions with low-income couples, the effect sizes described here are above average (Hawkins, Blanchard, Baldwin, & Fawcett, 2008). The significant rise in household income was notable, but without a control group, we could not determine whether increased income could be attributed causally to participation. Also, in our intervention study sample, we had predicted and found a direct intervention effect on the change from Pre to Post 1 couple conflict ($\beta = 0.14$, $t = 3.05$, $p < 0.001$, equivalent to small to medium effect size of $d = 0.4$).

In addition to individual- and family-level effects, systems-level results confirmed that both

Studies I and II showed positive changes in the community agencies responsible for implementing SFI in terms of their father friendliness and family focus across various organizational measures such as staffing, policies, reputation in the community, and so on (Vann & Nelson-Hooks, 2000). These changes were sustained at the 18-month follow-up and held for 3 years beyond.

SFI II demonstrated that replicating the SFI intervention with a more diverse sample (inclusion of African-American families and nonbiological fathering figures) produced positive results comparable to – or better than – those obtained in SFI I, increasing the evidence base of SFI (Cowan et al., 2014). The results of both studies support the combined focus on couple relationships, parenting, and coparenting to produce positive outcomes for the entire family.

Father involvement itself increased significantly in this replication of SFI – somewhat less than it had in the benchmark study – while parenting stress declined in the current study as much as it had in the earlier benchmark findings. Satisfaction with the couple relationship remained stable in the current study as it had earlier, whereas the decline in violent problem-solving for current parents was significantly greater than for parents in the benchmark couples' groups. The stability in children's problem behavior in both current and benchmark families contrasted with the increase in children's problem behavior for the benchmark controls.

In SFI III, we accepted couples referred from the Child Welfare System (CWS) who were not currently at risk for harming their partner or child. While we were cautious about using a couples' systems approach when intimate partner violence or child abuse had been previously identified (Stith, McCollum, Amanor-Boadu, & Smith, 2011), studies indicate that working with couples conjointly is efficacious and appropriate in many situations (Karakurt, Whiting, van Esch, Bolen, & Calabrese, 2016), e.g., when situational violence, rather than coercive control, is involved (Hardesty, Crossman, Khaw, & Raffaelli, 2016). With ongoing monitoring for safety, SFI III supported direct couples work on communication issues, negative attributions, and self-control of aggression. It also provided opportunities to reduce harsh parenting and strengthen commitments by the coparents to curb aggressive or neglectful tendencies. Notably, the group approach used in SFI III enabled couples to draw strength from the community created by participants sharing their experiences.

SFI III began with 239 heterosexual pairs, most of whom were romantic partners and half of whom were Hispanic (mostly Mexican-American). After 18 months, 162 coparents remained in the program and study. Including only randomized couples' groups and a waitlist control in structural equation modeling, analyses showed that couple conflict was associated, both contemporaneously and over time, with anxious/harsh parenting, which in turn was associated with children's externalizing and internalizing problem behaviors at 18 months postintervention. The intervention reduced couple conflict at Post 1 (2 months after the groups ended) statistically more in the couples' groups than among the randomly assigned waitlist-control parents, which was then associated with parenting and child outcomes. Thus, the mechanism operating in SFI was decreasing couple conflict, an effect which spilled over to both the couple relationship and parenting quality at Post 2 (18 months after the program began), with benefits for the child primarily in terms of externalizing behaviors.

Child welfare-referred parents and community sample parents benefitted equally. Interestingly, when parents' conflict decreased from participation in the intervention, the improvement was connected to parenting behavior and child benefits. Among controls, positive changes in the couple did not become linked with parenting and child outcomes. The intervention helped parents systemically by linking their behavior toward each other to their behavior toward the child. Father involvement and income growth in the family were both again linked to the intervention.

Of particular interest to the early childhood research community were these findings from the child welfare SFI III study: overall, there were very few differences in intervention effects for parents of younger (0–2) and older (3–12) children. Couple violence decreases for parents of both ages (though not in controls). When SFI works, it works for parents when the youngest child is 0–2 and also when the parents' youngest child is 3–12 years old. There were no special intervention effects for parents of younger children. This is of interest given the frequently made argument that special interventions are required with populations of parents with infants, toddlers, or preschoolers. SFI suggests that a comprehensive coparenting intervention is effective for children across the first twelve years of life, if not beyond.

Father involvement increased significantly in this replication of SFI – somewhat less than it had in the benchmark study – while parenting stress declined in the current study as much as it had in the earlier benchmark findings. Satisfaction with the couple relationship remained stable in the current study as it had earlier, whereas the decline in violent problem-solving for current parents was significantly greater than for parents in the benchmark couples' groups. The stability in children's problem behavior in both current and benchmark families contrasted with the increase in children's problem behavior for the benchmark controls. Finally, statistically significant increases in annual income of these families seemed to reflect the more secure base from which they could now carry on the business of raising children, making an income, which often now included the ability of both partners to work, usually part-time.

In this replication of the Supporting Father Involvement couples' group intervention, participant couples in all three ethnic groups, who were at risk because of their low incomes, showed positive changes in questionnaire measures of parent-child relationship quality, couple relationship quality, children's problem behaviors, and family income. One of 11 measures in the current replication of the SFI couples' group intervention failed to replicate the positive results obtained in the earlier benchmark RCT (an increase in men's psychological involvement as "father"). Of the remaining ten measures completed by the current couples, one revealed a significant change that was not statistically different from the benchmark results (authoritarian parenting ideas), and one showed a positive change that was smaller than that reported by benchmark couples (father involvement). The central finding was that six of the measures showed positive Baseline to Post 2 changes that were equal to those of the benchmark intervention participants (declines in parenting stress, stability in couple relationship satisfaction, children's aggression, hyperactivity, social isolation, and psychological symptoms) and two showed significantly more positive changes than those of couples in the benchmark intervention (decline in couples' violent problem-solving and their children's aggression).

Populations for Which SFI Worked and for Which It Did Not

In Study I's 11 randomized designs ($n = 289$ couples), fathers and mothers who participated in the one-time informational meeting control experience revealed no positive changes and some negative changes over 18 months – as individuals, couples, and parents. They also described increases in acting out, aggressive or shy, withdrawn, depressed behaviors in their children. Partners who participated in the 16-week fathers-only groups reported increased father involvement, no increase in the children's problematic behaviors, but, as in the control condition, declining satisfaction as a couple. By contrast, parents who participated in a couples' group reported all the positive changes of those in the fathers-only groups, as well as reductions in parenting stress, and no declines in their satisfaction as couples over 18 months. Trial 2 ($n = 236$ couples) focused predominantly on couples' groups, yielding equivalent findings and several even more positive results. Over both trials, the intervention was equally effective for fathers and mothers and for parents with initially higher or lower levels of income, conflict, depressive symptoms, and couple satisfaction. Moreover, the program was equally successful for European-American, Mexican-American, and African-American families.

As seen in this summary, there are inherent biases present in that in all cohorts two partners had to agree to participate. They were screened and referred out of the intervention for services for serious domestic violence, mental illness, and substance abuse. Recruiting methods were biased to the extent that the communities sourced for 800 families were intentionally broad: agencies (health and educational), community gatherings and festivals, radio and newspaper announcements, word of mouth, and walk-ins – obviously a large naturalistic epidemiologic sampling of adults willing to participate with their coparenting partner in the program.

Ways in which the studies have not been biased: In the first two trials, participants were not referred because of identified family distress nor did they constitute a special, well-functioning subgroup of the low-income population. In the third trial of this intervention, the Office of Child Abuse Prevention asked us to extend the intervention to higher-risk couples who had come to the attention of the Child Welfare System because of domestic violence, child abuse, or neglect. Across the first two trials, results of which have been published (Cowan et al., 2009, 2014).

There were no statistically significant retention differences between fathers and mothers, CWS-referred and community couples, or immediate and waitlist-control conditions.

None of the measures indicated baseline differences in level of risk or distress between those who dropped out and those who completed the 18-month follow-up. Overall, the retention rate for this low-income, relatively high-risk sample over 18 months was 68%, not much different from the 71% and 74% retention rate of our two earlier intervention studies of low-income parents (Cowan et al., 2009, 2014).[1] There were no statistically significant differences in the retention of fathers or mothers in the community or CWS-referred samples as a function of age, marital status, ethnicity, being born in the USA, having a high school diploma, or involvement in paid work during the previous 2 weeks.

To summarize the primary outcomes or variables in all SFI studies: reduced relationship/parental conflict, improved parenting quality, such as reduced harsh parenting, reduced internal and externalizing behaviors in their children at follow-up. Secondary variables: improved parental well-being with reductions in depression and anxiety and increases in relationship satisfaction, decreased stress, increased father involvement (both observed and psychological), higher income, lower substance use, and improved parent-child relationship.

As thorough as we tried to be across the wide range of families and variables with which we worked, we also look forward to future analysis of additional data with sufficient diversity that we can move beyond testing for family structural and ethnic differences to elucidate the contributions of fathering and mothering figures versus parents and gender differences that might emerge in those analyses. We have learned that father involvement, worthy goal that it is, is one thing and coparenting is another. Elucidated this difference would help interventionist improve their aim. Attendant to these successes, we attempted to validate SFI's effectiveness for other populations, outside of the USA.

SFI Replication in Alberta, Canada

In 2011, the Norlien (now called Palix) Foundation brought SFI to Canada and implemented the program at three family resource centers, with a scaled-back evaluation component. SFI Alberta focused on offering program components that make replication effective (Durlak & DuPre, 2008), including sufficient funding, coordination with other agencies, provider skill proficiency, training, and technical assistance. The goal of preventive science is expansion of the evidence base of "what works" by identifying commonalities of success across interventions (Schorr & Farrow, 2011). The SFI Alberta program entailed the same 32-hour group intervention (either for fathers or couples with clinically trained co-leaders), case management, and efforts to enhance father friendliness in the social ser-

[1]Thanks to Phil Cowan for the data analysis for this observation

vice agencies in which SFI was embedded. The Canada sample was assessed using a longitudinal design of 12 months.

The study of the SFI intervention with 106 Caucasian couples with middle- and working-class incomes couples in Alberta, Canada (Pruett, Pruett, Cowan, & Cowan, 2017b), used a pre-post quasi-experimental design. The parents had higher conflict levels and mothers were more depressed than the CA couples. Twelve months after entering the Canadian study, SFI participants changed positively on 9 of 11 measures used in prior SFI studies, including fathers' involvement in care of the children, parenting stress, and coparenting and parenting quality. Also, parents reported that their children's behavior problems held steady over time.

Further Replication in the UK

A further study of the efficacy of the SFI curriculum in the UK, renamed "Parents as Partners" (Casey et al., 2017), found similarly positive results for low-income parents from varied ethnic backgrounds. A pre-post design to evaluate changes in the first 100 participating couples revealed statistically significant reductions in the parents' reports of anxiety and depression, parenting stress, violent problem-solving, and behavior problems in their children. As in our second US study, UK participants in most distress as they entered the study showed the most gains after participating in a couples' group.

Summary and Key Points: Policies Which Engage Fathers Positively

SFI has shown us that paternal engagement, in combination with maternal inclusion, is a robust and effective agent of change in lowering risk to children of abuse or neglect (see page 11). Such engagement, however, is not a given in most interventions, especially when everything from intake procedures to parent information forms and to artwork on the walls of children's clinics has traditionally been designed around the understandable desire to support strong mother-child relationships whenever we have the chance. Father-friendly practice, however, requires conscious effort if it is to be anything beyond the ineffective simply asking the mother if the "father is involved."

It has been the author's experience when engaging with programs that want to increase paternal engagement, the conversation often begins with the refrain, "We want to include them, but they just won't come." Suggestions based on our research and clinical experience (Pruett et al., 2009) to increase father friendliness: (1) look at your intake procedures and clinic spaces through the eyes of an anxious young father, to see what you can change to make him feel he is doing the right thing for his child by coming in the front door to your program; (2) are your hours of service flexible enough to accommodate his work, part-time work, or welfare-to-work responsibilities?; (3) do you offer services that are especially important to him, job training, legal assistance, etc.?; (4) are there any men on the staff – paid or volunteer – that might make him feel welcomed in a place that is not just for mothers and their children?

Finally, suggestions for policies to promote effective and positive paternal engagement that reflects in improved outcomes for, and protection of, children at risk:

1. *Intervene early*. We need to intervene early with fathers and fathering partners who are still connected emotionally to their children and the children's mother. The influential Fragile Families Study (McLanahan, 2009) underlined how crucial early engagement is in pregnancy in the absence of marriage, but the presence of a strong wish to be involved in the life and well-being of the child, and "give this kid the chance I never had to know my father."
2. *Invite fathers directly* (not through mothers) and invite them to work on the father-child relationship. This is less intimidating than inviting them into a group that focuses solely on the couple relationship. Invitations from community leaders and past participants in

SFI or other father-engagement programs are especially productive.
3. *Work on the coparenting and couple relationship* within existing child-focused interventions, since children fare better when their parenting figures have positive interactions with each other and are collaborative in their approach to their children rather than in conflict.
4. *Extend the definition* of the coparenting couple to include same-sex fathers and other instances of actively coparenting fathering figures such as grandparents, parent-grandparent pairs, aunts/uncles, siblings, and close friends.
5. *Avoid being prescriptive*, implying that the intervenors have "the answers" about how to parent effectively. Support parents in their work together to become the kinds of parents and partners that they want to be.

The senior author chaired a plenary session on "Father Engagement with Infants and Toddlers" at the annual meeting of *Zero to Three* two decades ago in which two fathers of infants and toddlers testified to the barriers they faced being taken seriously as nurturing influences in their children's lives by professionals whom they knew to be talented clinicians. A senior clinician spoke of her "hesitation" in reaching out directly to men because of her extensive experience treating domestic violence having become "habituated to seeing men as more problem than solution, turning a blind eye to what they might mean to their children and their well-being." Their narratives and conversation led to a standing ovation from a deeply appreciative audience that sensed the urgency of needed change. Time has helped, but it hasn't eliminated those barriers; hence, SFI.

References

Baptista, J., Sousa, D., Soares, I., & Martins, C. (2018). Fathers' sensitive guidance moderates the association between coparenting and behavioral regulation in preschoolers. *International Journal of Behavioral Development, 42*(6), 574–580.

Belsky, J. (1984). The determinants of parenting: A process model. *Child Development, 55*(1), 83–96.

Bocknek, E. L., Dayton, C., Raveau, H. A., Richardson, P., Brophy-Herb, H. E., & Fitzgerald, H. E. (2017). Routine active playtime with fathers is associated with self-regulation in early childhood. *Merrill-Palmer Quarterly, 63*(1), 105–134.

Bronfenbrenner, U. (1979). *The ecology of human development: Experiments by nature and design.* Cambridge, MA: Harvard University Press.

Casey, P., Cowan, P. A., Cowan, C. P., Draper, L., Mwamba, N., & Hewison, D. (2017). Parents as partners: A U.K. trial of a U.S. couples-based parenting intervention for at-risk low-income families. *Family Process, 56*(3), 589–606.

Cohen, J. E. (1988). *Statistical power analysis for the behavioral sciences.* Hillsdale, NJ: Lawrence Erlbaum Associates, Inc..

Cookston, J. T. (1999). Parental supervision and family structure: Effects on adolescent problem behaviors. *Journal of Divorce & Remarriage, 32*(1–2), 107–122.

Cowan, C. P., & Cowan, P. A. (2000). *When partners become parents: The big life change for couples.* Mahwah, NJ: Lawrence Erlbaum Associates, Inc..

Cowan, C. P., & Cowan, P. A. (2005). Two central roles for couple relationships: Breaking negative intergenerational patterns and enhancing children's adaptation. *Sexual and Relationship Therapy, 20*(3), 275–288.

Cowan, P. A., Cowan, C. P., Pruett, M. K., Pruett, K., & Gillette, P. (2014). Evaluation a couples group to enhance father involvement in low-income families using a benchmark comparison. *Family Relations, 63*(3), 356–370.

Cowan, P. A., Cowan, C. P., Pruett, M. K., Pruett, K., & Wong, J. J. (2009). Promoting fathers' engagement with children: Preventive interventions for low-income families. *Journal of Marriage and Family, 71*(3), 663–679.

Durlak, J. A., & DuPre, E. P. (2008). Implementation matters: A review of research on the influence of implementation on program outcomes and the factors affecting implementation. *American Journal of Community Psychology, 41*(3–4), 327–350.

Epstein, K., Pruett, M. K., Cowan, P., Cowan, C., Pradhan, L., Mah, E., et al. (2015). More than one way to get there: Pathways of change in coparenting conflict after a preventive intervention. *Family Process, 54*(4), 610–618.

Fabiano, G. A., & Caserta, A. (2018). Future directions in father inclusion, engagement, retention, and positive outcomes in child and adolescent research. *Journal of Clinical Child & Adolescent Psychology, 47*(5), 847–862.

Favez, N., Tissot, H., Frascarolo, F., Stiefel, F., & Despland, J. N. (2016). Sense of competence and beliefs about parental roles in mothers and fathers as predictors of coparenting and child engagement in mother–father–infant triadic interactions. *Infant and Child Development, 25*(4), 283–301.

Hardesty, J. L., Crossman, K. A., Khaw, L., & Raffaelli, M. (2016). Marital violence and coparenting quality after separation. *Journal of Family Psychology, 30*(3), 320–330.

Hawkins, A. J., Blanchard, V. L., Baldwin, S. A., & Fawcett, E. B. (2008). Does marriage and relationship education work? A meta-analytic study. *Journal of Consulting and Clinical Psychology, 76*(5), 723–734. https://doi.org/10.1037/a0012584

Heinicke, C. M. (2002). *The transition to parenting*. Mahwah, NJ: Lawrence Erlbaum Associates, Inc..

Hirschberger, G., Srivastava, S., Marsh, P., Cowan, C. P., & Cowan, P. A. (2009). Attachment, marital satisfaction, and divorce during the first fifteen years of parenthood. *Personal Relationships, 16*(3), 401–420.

Hunsley, J., & Lee, C. M. (2007). Research-informed benchmarks for psychological treatments: Efficacy studies, effectiveness studies, and beyond. *Professional Psychology: Research and Practice, 38*(1), 21–33.

Karakurt, G., Whiting, K., van Esch, C., Bolen, S. D., & Calabrese, J. R. (2016). Couples therapy for intimate partner violence: A systematic review and meta-analysis. *Journal of Marital and Family Therapy, 42*(4), 567–583.

Maccoby, E. E., Depner, C. E., & Mnookin, R. H. (1990). Coparenting in the second year after divorce. *Journal of Marriage and the Family, 52*(1), 141–155.

McLanahan, S. (2009). Fragile families and the reproduction of poverty. *The Annals of the American Academy of Political and Social Science, 621*(1), 111–131.

Metz, M., Colonnesi, C., Majdandžić, M., & Bögels, S. M. (2018). When father steps forward and mother steps back: The moderating role of simultaneity in parents' coparenting behaviors in the development of anxiety in 4-to 30-month-olds. *Infancy, 23*(1), 103–123.

Miller, W. R., & Rollnick, S. (2009). Ten things that motivational interviewing is not. *Behavioural and Cognitive Psychotherapy, 37*(2), 129–140.

Panter-Brick, C., Burgess, A., Eggerman, M., McAllister, F., Pruett, K., & Leckman, J. F. (2014). Practitioner review: Engaging fathers – recommendations for a game change in parenting interventions based on a systematic review of the global evidence. *Journal of Child Psychology and Psychiatry, 55*(11), 1187–1212.

Phares, V. (1996). Conducting nonsexist research, prevention, and treatment with fathers and mothers: A call for a change. *Psychology of Women Quarterly, 20*(1), 55–77.

Pruett, M. K., Cowan, C. P., Cowan, P. A., & Pruett, K. (2009). Lessons learned from the Supporting Father Involvement study: A cross-cultural preventive intervention for low-income families with young children. *Journal of Social Service Research, 35*(2), 163–179.

Pruett, M. K., McIntosh, J. E., & Kelly, J. B. (2014). Parental separation and overnight care of young children, part 1: Consensus through theoretical and empirical integration. *Family Court Review, 52*(2), 240–255.

Pruett, M. K., Nakash, O., Welton, E., Cowan, C. P., Cowan, P. A., & Gillette, P. (2019). Using an initial clinical interview to assess the coparenting relationship: Preliminary examples from the Supporting Father Involvement Program. *Smith College Studies in Social Work, 89*(1), 38–65.

Pruett, M. K., Pruett, K. D., Cowan, C. P., & Cowan, P. A. (2017a). Enhancing father involvement in low-income families: A couples group approach to preventive intervention. *Child Development, 88*(2), 398–407.

Pruett, M. K., Pruett, K. D., Cowan, C. P., & Cowan, P. A. (2017b). Enhancing paternal engagement in a coparenting paradigm. *Child Development Perspectives, 11*(4), 245–250.

Rempel, L. A., Rempel, J. K., Khuc, T. N., & Vui, L. T. (2017). Influence of father–infant relationship on infant development: A father-involvement intervention in Vietnam. *Developmental Psychology, 53*(10), 1844–1858.

Rosenberg, J., & Wilcox, W. B. (2006). *The importance of fathers in the healthy development of children: Fathers and their impact on children's well-being*. U.S. Children's Bureau, Office on Child Abuse and Neglect. Retrieved from https://www.childwelfare.gov/pubpdfs/fatherhood.pdf

Schorr, L. B., & Farrow, F. (2011). *Expanding the evidence universe: Doing better by knowing more*. Washington, DC: Center for the Study of Social Policy.

Stith, S. M., McCollum, E. E., Amanor-Boadu, Y., & Smith, D. (2011). Systemic perspectives on intimate partner violence treatment. *Journal of Marital and Family Therapy, 38*(1), 220–240.

Twenge, J., Campbell, W., & Foster, C. (2003). Parenthood and marital satisfaction: A meta-analytic review. *Journal of Marriage and Family, 65*(3), 574–583.

Vann, N., & Nelson-Hooks, J. (2000). *Father-friendliness organizational self-assessment and planning tool*. Retrieved May, 8, 2007.

Volling, B. L., Cabrera, N. J., Feinberg, M. E., Jones, D. E., McDaniel, B. T., Liu, S., et al. (2019). Advancing research and measurement on fathering and children's development. *Monographs of the Society for Research in Child Development, 84*(1), 7–160.

Connection, IT and Identity: SMS4dads as Health Promotion for New Fathers

39

Richard Fletcher, Jacqui A. Macdonald, and Jennifer Mary StGeorge

Men's psychological functioning in the transition to fatherhood is now understood as a public health issue which may pose a risk to the wellbeing of the mother and to the cognitive, social and emotional development of their offspring (Ramchandani & Iles, 2014).

The potential benefits of providing support to fathers across the perinatal period are clear. However, fathers are less likely than mothers to access or have access to organised, institutional support for adjustment to their parenting role (Bremberg, 2016; Panter-Brick et al., 2014). They are also less likely than mothers to access, or have access to, informal social supports for parenting (Baldwin, Malone, Sandall, & Bick, 2018; Fletcher, Matthey, & Marley, 2006). Currently, interventions or services that aim to assist men making this transition are add-ons to maternal programmes or developed out of generalised family models rather than being father-specific prompting calls to develop frameworks that more effectively recognise and include fathers (Dennis & Letourneau, 2007; Panter-Brick et al., 2014). In responding to this call, we make a case for considering fathers' identity in the design of support that is tailored to fathers' preferences and needs and addresses paternal, and therefore family, psychosocial wellbeing. We take particular note of the changed communication environment, where the internet and mobile phones have created ways of delivering information and support outside of traditional face-to-face modalities.

In this chapter, we outline a model that aims to (1) scaffold fathers as they navigate psychosocial vulnerabilities across the transition to fatherhood, (2) build capacity in fathers to offer support to the mother while developing their co-parenting partnership and form a secure attachment with their infant and (3) pay particular attention to the fathers' identity in accessing and engaging in support. We illustrate the application of this model through a case study of SMS4dads, a text-based perinatal support programme for fathers that has been developed and tested in the Australian context (Fletcher, Kay-Lambkin, et al., 2017; Fletcher, May, et al., 2017). Our model posits that the method of delivering information and support as well as the scripting and online resourcing can be attuned to fathers' identity to interact with mechanisms internalised within the individual in a way that creates a tailored, father-specific support during

R. Fletcher (✉)
Fathers and Families Research Program – Faculty of Health and Medicine, The University of Newcastle, Callaghan, NSW, Australia
e-mail: richard.fletcher@newcastle.edu.au

J. A. Macdonald
School of Psychology, Deakin University, Burwood, VIC, Australia

J. M. StGeorge
Family Action Centre, Faculty of Medicine & Health, University of Newcastle, Callaghan, NSW, Australia

H. E. Fitzgerald et al. (eds.), *Handbook of Fathers and Child Development*,
https://doi.org/10.1007/978-3-030-51027-5_39

the inherent psychological upheaval of a major life adjustment (Fletcher, Knight, Macdonald, & StGeorge, 2019).

Identity Theory in the Design of Fatherhood Support

Identity theory has been useful for framing research of fathers, particularly examinations of fathers' involvement with their children and relationship with their partner. Applied to fathers, the theory suggests that male parents incorporate 'being a father' into a hierarchy of identities, each informed by societies' expectations of behaviours. For example, expectations of fathers include providing care or finances. When integrating this identity, the new father will then ascribe particular meanings to the identity (e.g. good fathers play with their children) (Pasley, Petren, & Fish, 2014). Paternal identity salience and centrality, which indicate the level of importance the father assigns to the parenting identity, have been found to be associated with positive parental engagement, involvement and caregiving in a range of samples including fathers of disabled children and divorced, married, incarcerated and expectant fathers (Adamsons & Pasley, 2016; Dyer, 2005; Fox, Nordquist, Billen, & Savoca, 2015). However, findings are mixed. Studies have used varying definitions and measures of fathers' identity such that meaning, salience or centrality may differ in their effects on behaviours and interactions with children and partners for different sub-groups of fathers and different fathering roles (Pasley et al., 2014).

In this chapter, we take it as axiomatic that a father's ideas and feelings about his identity as a father will influence his interactions with his partner and his infant. We describe how the existing links, evident in the literature, between men's sense of connection to others, their notions of fatherhood and the possible consequences for their own and their families' wellbeing form a basis for designing support services to fathers. In describing the SMS4dads case study, we also pay particular attention to the value of overtly 'normalising' fathering experiences and emotions and to 'reflected appraisals', a key concept of identity theory that refers to an individual's perceptions of others' evaluations of their identities (Maurer, Pleck, & Rane, 2001). At the interpersonal level, mothers' views on how the father should or does carry out his role may strongly influence fathers' caring behaviours. In addition, social policy initiatives such as parental leave for fathers, which affirm fatherhood, have been found to influence paternal involvement in caring for infants over time (Dermott & Miller, 2015). In the case study presented here, we identify identity-affirming processes that occur at a social level through the father-only promotion of SMS4dads and at an interpersonal level through the targeted content and tone of the text messages.

How Connection and Identity Are Linked to Health for Fathers

Transitions are periods of disequilibrium (Cowan, 1991). They are balancing acts between loss and gain, decline and growth and risk and possibility (Parke, 1988; Schlossberg, 1981), and the passage into fatherhood is no exception (Palkovitz & Palm, 2009). Not surprisingly, transitions, while often leading to positive change, are nevertheless associated with elevated susceptibility to physical and psychological risk (Draper, 2003; Saxbe, Rossin-Slater, & Goldenberg, 2018). In the transition to fatherhood across high-income societies, at least 1 in 10 men will experience symptoms of psychological distress, depression, anxiety or generalised stress (Paulson & Bazemore, 2010; Philpott, Leahy-Warren, FitzGerald, & Savage, 2017). More than half of new fathers report they are poorly affected by sleep problems (Wynter et al., 2019). After the first child is born, intimate partner relationship quality is consistently reported to decline (Doss, Rhoades, Stanley, & Markman, 2009; Kohn et al., 2012), fathers gain more weight than childless men of the same age (Umberson, Liu, Mirowsky, & Reczek, 2011) and they experience increased financial stress (Da Costa et al., 2019), while some feel incompetent to be a carer (Hildingsson, Haines, Johansson,

Rubertsson, & Fenwick, 2014) and one in five becomes socially isolated from peers and supports (Baldwin et al., 2018; Ipsos-Mori, 2019). Risk for these mental and physical health problems is higher when access to support is limited and a sense of social connection diminishes.

Identity clarity and role expectations are each argued to be psychologically protective (Greenaway, Cruwys, Haslam, & Jetten, 2016). Identity facilitates belonging, group membership, co-operation and the potential for support and is therefore associated with physical and psychological wellbeing (Greenaway et al., 2016). Role expectations reduce ambiguity and the likelihood of conflicting objectives and present clear parameters for role success. However, clarity is often not a feature of the contemporary transition to fatherhood (Genesoni & Tallandini, 2009; Hodkinson & Brooks, 2018). While it is usual to feel unsure of oneself while developing mastery of parenting tasks, it is now commonplace for fathers to question broadly what it means to be a 'good father'. Baldwin et al. (2018) found that men often worried about not 'getting it right' (p. 2128). There is now ample evidence that a generational shift in gender-oriented expectations and a widening of the father role have increased ambiguity and reduced role clarity (Cabrera, Tamis-LeMonda, Bradley, Hofferth, & Lamb, 2000; Genesoni & Tallandini, 2009). 'I've been struggling in a way to try and find what... what is my role with this child?' is a father's comment in one interview that illustrates the confusion that can accompany adjustment to parenting (Baldwin et al., 2018, p. 2161). A contemporary emphasis on fathers engaging in more nurturing responsibilities, in shared household tasks and in emotional bonding with their infants is not always congruent with men's preconception notions of a father identity (Genesoni & Tallandini, 2009; Crespi & Ruspini, 2015). Nor are modern expectations congruent with the fathering role modelled to many men by their own fathers (Baldwin et al., 2018; Dermott & Miller, 2015). It is therefore difficult for fathers to know what is 'normal' and common for stress to arise from this lack of knowledge (Philpott et al., 2017).

Identities are reinforced by connections with peers who share social roles or by role models and individuals in authority who guide engagement in role tasks. These connections elevate the salience of expectations and affirm competence and belonging. For men, these connections are often lacking concerning fatherhood. In Baldwin et al.'s (2018) meta-synthesis, 20 findings identified fathers' lack of support as characterised by feelings of drifting away from friends, by peers not understanding the new identity or providing support and by marginalisation by health professionals who regularly failed to acknowledge or involve fathers in their consultations with the new family. These findings are reinforced by a study of 1680 fathers in the United Kingdom, Australia, the United States and Canada, which found that 20% of fathers reported a decrease in the number of close friends in the 12 months following the birth of their first child (Ipsos-Mori, 2019). Of young fathers 18–35 years, 40% reported feeling isolated after becoming a parent (Ipsos-Mori, 2019). This lack of support is likely to inhibit men's progress in defining for themselves the importance of new roles as caregiver, breadwinner or co-parent.

Fatherhood as a Catalyst for Change

We have focused to this point on factors that might prevent a clear sense of role identity across the transition to fatherhood and the related associations with psychological distress and relationship quality decline. This serves to highlight the need for intervention. The flip side to the heightened risk narrative is the opportunity for growth and behavioural change. Saxbe et al. (2018) present the transition to parenthood, for both fathers and mothers, as a period of sensitivity underpinned by a 'third window of neuroplasticity' during which there are both psychological and biological propulsions towards positive behaviours. The psychological motivation to be 'a good father' is consistently apparent in the literature (Baldwin et al., 2018), and in the United States, the United Kingdom and Australia, the transition to fatherhood has been recognised as a possible turning point for young men whose experience of parenting has been problematic and who lack economic and social resources (Faulkner, Hammond, Nisbet, & Fletcher, 2018; Ferguson & Gates, 2015; Roy & Dyson, 2010). The motivation accompanying fatherhood extends from being 'hands-on' in the care of the infant (Baldwin et al., 2018) to caring for the self because the new role brings with it responsibilities to be healthy and reliable to enable provision of care (Garfield, Isacco, & Bartlo, 2010). Across the transition to parenthood, among those for whom family identity is more salient than competing identities, a father may be far less inclined to smoke, for example (Haslam, Jetten, Postmes, & Haslam, 2009). This suggests that reinforcing and supporting the development of a man's 'father identity' may strengthen his intrinsic motivation to engage in behaviours that indicate he is performing the role well. The transition to parenthood is described as an opportunity for 'teachable moments' when the 'newborn engenders in both parents an overwhelming need to protect it from harm' (Winickoff et al., 2010, p. 522). Canadian researchers have promoted fathers' protective role in programmes to reduce men's cigarette smoking 'When I found out I was going to be a father, change was in the air. After the baby's born, change is there. It's not in the air anymore. I've found myself starting to re-think my smoking' (Oliffe, Bottorff, & Sarbit, 2010). Studying healthy eating intentions, Bassett-Gunter et al. (2013) also found that fathers, compared to non-fathers, had significantly greater intentions to eat healthily. However, fathers in the first 6 months postpartum perceived their control over intentions to be lower than fathers with older children. These findings suggest that while motivation might be high for positive behaviours after the birth of child, the demands of the period may prevent the enactment of the desired behaviours, warranting support to help new fathers attain their goals.

Support for the New Father Identity

Normalising a father's experiences is one way to clarify the breadth and parameters of the contemporary father role. Identity serves to situate an individual within a group where the stronger the identity salience, the greater the sense of belongingness and 'normalcy' (Stryker & Burke, 2000). Among fathers in high-income countries, there are certain experiences that are commonplace: the 2 am frustration with an unsettled child, the fear of not being a good enough dad, the sadness over changes in intimacy with a partner, the wishing for a night off, the enormous feeling of responsibility and more. These are the simple things that a disconnected father, lacking support, might not recognise as 'normal' aspects of infant care. Lack of clear parameters around normality within roles increases stress and anxiety and limits a sense of mastery (Elloy & Smith, 2003). In these circumstances, it may provide temporary relief from stress to prioritise and give salience to the roles in which clarity of expectation exists (Rothbard, 2001; Winkel & Clayton, 2010). Imagine a father unsure of whether his infant's behaviours are typical, unsure of how to manage the change in intimacy with his partner and unclear about when to step into caregiving tasks and whether the way he is showing care is 'right'. In contrast, he may have a workplace where role expectations are established and understood, his competence is recognised by colleagues and his economic value to the organisation is clear.

In transitions, the hierarchy of existing identities is reorganised to incorporate new identities (Burke & Stets, 2009). Thus, in a context of unclear expectations and low support, two responses may be identified in the transition to fatherhood. In the first response, the father selects the psychologically protective route of prioritising the salient identity where the benefits of the accompanying role, such as belongingness, a sense of autonomy and recognised value, are maintained (Hirsh & Kang, 2016). In this scenario, the father may prioritise career and narrowly conceptualise fatherhood around the provider component of the role. The second response is one where the father prioritises the new parenting identity, but his transition may be marked by strain and uncertainty. Rather than the new identity fulfilling psychological needs, without support and role clarity, it may highlight role deficits, prolong the disequilibrium of transition and increase risk for mental health problems (Hirsh & Kang, 2016).

There are consequences for the members of the family in each of these scenarios. When a father prioritises the role of 'breadwinner' or 'provider', for example, he is less likely to be involved in his infant's care and provide the warm, sensitive, challenging interactions that are clearly established as beneficial to children's development (Daniel, Madigan, & Jenkins, 2016; Grossmann et al., 2002; StGeorge, Wroe, & Cashin, 2018). Furthermore, his role as co-parent and partner to a new mother may be compromised, as his ability to co-parent with the mother (avoiding undermining and criticism) will impact on her health and on the wellbeing of their children (Cutrona, Russell, & Gardner, 2005; Morse, Buist, & Durkin, 2000). Equally, when struggling to clarify his roles as caregiver, provider or co-parent, fathers' anxiety, stress or depression will negatively influence on both their partners' mental health and their infant's wellbeing (Dennis & Letourneau, 2007; Fletcher, Freeman, & Matthey, 2011).

In seeking to support men as they transition into fatherhood, therefore, the goal is to foster fathering identities that enhance father-infant connection and father-partner support and co-operation in raising their child. Specifically, the aim is to nurture the development of the new caregiving and infant-oriented identity while protecting the salience and centrality of the partner-couple identity and acknowledging the provider/breadwinner role where relevant. Identity theory does not posit a finite number of identities that an individual can incorporate. Evidence even suggests that a wider variety of identities may be protective against mental health risk if the identities combine to meet basic psychological needs. These needs include belonging, maintaining self-esteem, exerting some control over one's outcomes and the sense of living a meaningful life (Cruwys et al., 2013). By contrast, mental health risk increases when these psychological needs are no longer met because of identity loss (Cruwys et al., 2013). It is not uncommon for postpartum fathers to feel loss with regard to their intimate partner relationship (Darwin et al., 2017), but under the right conditions, particularly when opportunities are encouraged for communication, a deeper and richer partnership evolves (Fägerskiöld, 2008). Central to the development of SMS4dads was the hypothesis that m-health support for new fathers would be most effective if it promoted the salience of both the father and partner identities through caring for the infant, partner and self.

The SMS4dads Programme

The Conception of the SMS4dads Programme

The conception and development of SMS4dads arose from two decades of researchers working in collaboration with health, education and welfare services who were attempting to include fathers in their practice. A number of initiatives instigated by government and nongovernment services reported some success, and across the sectors, a gradual shift could be seen to include fathers (Fletcher & Silberberg, 2006; Fletcher, St George, May, Hartman, & King, 2015). Professionals from a variety of disciplines began to recognise that fathers are not simply mother substitutes, and government departments and nongovernment organisations initiated programmes for fathers as a separate group for service delivery (Fletcher, 2008). At the same time, perinatal health services, who were aware of maternal depression (Department of Health WA. 2007), were beginning to recognize that fathers' mental health was also an important issue in the early years of family formation (Fletcher et al., 2006).

Attempting to Reach Fathers Through Email

As part of the impetus to involve fathers in perinatal services, fathers attending antenatal classes were recruited to the New Fathers Information Project comprising email messages offering information, links to online resources and participation in a confidential email discussion group with other fathers attending antenatal classes. The study, a randomised controlled trial ($N = 307$), aimed to test the impact on father-infant attachment of email-based information and peer group support (Fletcher, 2008). The measurements of father-infant attachment from antenatal to postnatal failed to demonstrate a significant difference between intervention and control.

However, the experience gained through this project provided guidance for the design of SMS4dads. First, clinicians' agreement with the purpose of the study did not translate into effective recruitment actions. Second, although previous research had suggested that peer discussion was of high value (Friedewald, Fletcher, & Fairbairn, 2005), very few fathers participated in the email discussion with peers. Third, the study highlighted the information preferences for fathers-to-be and new fathers. Participants were offered seven topics to receive emailed information: father-baby games, fathers helping breastfeeding, father-infant bonding, fathering a fussy baby, sex after the birth, postnatal depression and work-family balance. The most frequently requested topics were *father-baby bonding* (85) and *father-baby games* (77), while the least popular were *fathers helping breastfeeding* (17) and *sex after the birth* (17).

SMS4dads: A Phone-Optimised Web-Based Programme

The SMS4dads programme consists of a set of 296 brief (160 characters or less) text messages delivered to participants' mobile phones at varying days and times approximately three times per week. Fathers may enrol from when their partner is 16 weeks' gestation and can receive messages until the infant is 6 months of age. Fathers enter the expected date of birth at enrolment so that the messages are keyed to foetal and infant development. Message content addresses various aspects of new fathers' roles: his relationship with his baby, his relationship with and support of the baby's mother and his own self-care. All messages begin with '4dad' and are tailored to a father's perspective. Most are written in the 'voice' of the baby. Every 3 weeks, one of the messages will remind participants that they can exit by texting 'stop', and almost one in three messages includes a link to a not-for-profit parenting website for further information. Examples are given in Table 39.1.

In addition to the messages, every 3 weeks, an interactive Mood Tracker text asked participants to indicate their current mood by selecting one of five one-click options ('awesome', 'cool', 'OK', 'shaky' or 'bad'). Indications of high distress triggered an escalation process from a national helpline for perinatal mental health support. An important feature of the pro-

Table 39.1 Text messages

Week	Message	Content area
−19	4dad: At 20 weeks, my eyelids and eyebrows are forming and I can even blink! Not much to see yet but lots to look forward to dad	Father-infant
−17	4dad: Breastfeeding. Great for baby, good for mum and easy on the wallet. If mum wants to breastfeed, then let her know you also want this for your family [LINK]	Father-partner
−6	4dad: Walking together is good for health and good for relationships [txt STOP to OptOut]	Father self-care
+1	4dad: I am going to triple my weight in the first year of life. Don't let this happen to you too dad [LINK]	Father self-care
+8	4dad: Notice something your partner is doing well and tell her about it. It is important for her to hear this now	Father-partner
+17	4dad: I love a book with pictures of faces that have big eyes. They can be animals, people or even machines. I am interested in all sorts of faces now dad	Father-infant

gramme is its ability to communicate with fathers irrespective of location (the studies have enrolled participants from across Australia) for the cost of a text message, suggesting it is a relatively inexpensive method of supporting fathers. The process of developing the text messages and the programme features are reported elsewhere (Fletcher et al., 2016; Fletcher, Kay-Lambkin, et al., 2017; Fletcher, May, et al., 2017).

Approval and Impact of SMS4dads

Reviews of eHealth programmes have reported dropout rates of between 2% and 83%, even for brief online programmes (Melville, Casey, & Kavanagh, 2010) leading some researchers to recommend that, due to the lack of sustained participation, computerised programmes be not supported as front-line services (Twomey et al., 2014). Overall attrition rates from the programmes of SMS4dads to date range from 10% to 21% (see Table 39.2). In SMS4dads programmes, participants are repeatedly reminded 'to opt out text STOP' providing a specific opportunity to exit approximately every 3 weeks over a period of up to 70 weeks. The pattern of dropping out appears to be similar across various implementations of the programme and indicates considerable commitment. Those who do text back 'STOP' have usually received messages for some time. In the SMS4dads feasibility, for example, the average time from enrolment to dropout was 11 weeks by which time they would have received approximately 33 messages (Fletcher, Kay-Lambkin, et al., 2017 , Fletcher, May, et al., 2017).

Two of the SMS4dads studies have included evaluations by fathers. At the conclusion of the SMS4dads feasibility messages, 101/520 fathers completed an online survey. Responses indicated high approval of the programme: 92.9% found the messages helpful, 83.3% said they felt less isolated as a result of the programme, 65.4% found the messages helped their relationship with their infant and 80.9% found the messages helped their relationship with their partner (Fletcher, Kay-Lambkin, et al., 2017, Fletcher, May, et al., 2017). In a subsequent study of 244 fathers, similar approval rates were reported. Fathers completed surveys at four points during the 13-month study: T1, third trimester; T2, 6–8 weeks post birth; T3, 12–14 weeks post birth; and T4, final survey at 24 weeks. The overall rating, approve or strongly approve for four evaluation questions, was 97% (see Table 39.3).

The sustained engagement of the fathers, over more than 12 months for many, and the positive evaluations reported by participants suggest that the SMS4dads programme may provide a model of relatively low-cost support to fathers with the potential to improve the wellbeing of all family members.

Table 39.2 Attrition rates for programmes

Programme	Population	Enrolled	Attrition (%)
SMS4dads feasibility[1]	National	520	78 (15)
SMS4dads RCT[2]	National	788	165 (21)
SMS4dads defence health [3]	Members/relatives defence health	53	10 (19)
SMS4PP QLD [4]	Partners of mothers with severe mental illness	67	7 (10)
SMS4dadsSA [5]	South Australian fathers	254	42 (17)
SMS4dads aboriginal [6]	Young aboriginal fathers from regional areas	20	1 (0.05)

1. Fletcher, Kay-Lambkin, et al. (2017) and Fletcher, May, et al. (2017)
2. SMS4dads RCT Report to beyondblue
3. SMS4dads Defence Health Final Report
4. SMS4Perinatal Parents Final Report
5. SMS4dadsSA Final Report
6. Faulkner et al. (2018)

Table 39.3 Total responses to survey at four times during enrolment in sms4dads

Survey question	Very/ somewhat helpful
Have the texts been helpful in becoming a new dad? (1 = very helpful to 4 = not helpful at all)	210/214 (98%)
Over the last month, you have been sent texts about your own self-care and wellbeing. How did they go with you? (1 = very helpful to 4 = not helpful at all)	206/214 (96%)
Over the last month, you have been sent texts about your new baby. How did they go with you? (1 = very helpful to 4 = not helpful at all)	210/214 (98%)
Over the last month, you have been sent texts about your relationship with your partner. How did they go with you? (1 = very helpful to 4 = not helpful at all)	205/214 (96%)

Contributing to Fathers' Identity Through SMS4dads

The initial formulation of SMS4dads was situated within theories of health communication (Fleisher et al., 2008) with a focus on tailoring information and eHealth delivery (De Nooijer, Lechner, & de Vries, 2002; Fletcher et al., 2011; Kreuter & Wray, 2003). However, it is important to understand the mechanisms operating within programmes that keep participants engaged and that produce the targeted outcomes (Hall & Bierman, 2015). Reproducing or scaling up of interventions is dependent not only on systematic documentation of implementation but also on a deep understanding of the pathways or mechanisms by which the effects are produced (Astbury & Leeuw, 2010; Moore et al., 2015). Therefore, we wondered if the programme mechanisms that led to its positive reception were more intrinsically linked to a combination of identity theory and transition concepts; if so, could they be explicated through close analysis of interviews with participants (Fletcher et al., 2019)?

Forty fathers who had completed the programme were interviewed in a semi-structured format. Their responses were analysed to draw out the effective features of the programme as seen by this group. In the following section, we draw on this interview material to tease out the possible content and structural features of SMS4dads that supports fathers' identity formation.

Programme Content

The branding of SMS4dads underlines the salience of the fathering role and the legitimacy of fathers' involvement in the direct care of their infant. Over the perinatal period, fathers will encounter or become aware of multiple services aiming to assist new 'parents'; however, in reality, the high dropout rate of fathers in these programmes suggests that targeting services 'for parents' does not fully engage many fathers. By positioning itself as 'for dads', the programme title points to differentiation within the generalised parenting role and suggests that there are diverse or unique responsibilities and experiences for men. Among the many services that parents encounter, there are few for new fathers, and thus the programme title conveys a sense of importance about this role. Men experienced this focus as 'taking into account the dad', as 'having their own thing', that 'reflected your own experience', where 'you felt you were valued'.

> They were kind of like my little thing, I got a message. Just having some helpful advice, I was just going over some previous messages before. So it helped, like a personal support network maybe, I don't know, it's not really a support network but you know.

Three target domains of information were embedded in the messages: the father-infant relationship, the father-partner relationship and father self-care. These centred on areas where, at a point postconception, men conceivably enter a process of reshaping their behavioural patterns and priorities. The first two domains explicitly reflect the new roles undertaken by men when they become fathers: one role encompassing the expectations, practices and responsibilities of bonding and caregiving and other roles being that of partner to a new mother and co-parent. Addressing the domains of father-infant and father-partner relationships in the SMS4dads programme is an attempt to redress the generally imbalanced representation of the fathering role, at least in the perinatal period, as being only a support for mother through labour and breastfeeding (Litton Fox, Bruce, & Combs-Orme, 2000). These two domains represent the most pressing and potentially complex relational domains of a new father's life. Separating fatherhood activities or practices into these distinctive roles serves to better describe each and draws attention to the potential challenges within and between them. To this extent, the SMS4dads programme underscores the importance of the fatherhood status.

An explicit focus on the father-infant relationship begins with the video promotion of the programme and was shared with fathers through messages about bonding and child development, phrased in terms of either information or action points and often written in the first person, as if from the baby. This focus on infant bonding, play and development accords with men's interests and concerns as documented in research on new fathers (e.g. Baldwin et al., 2018), in the New Fathers Information Project described above (Fletcher, 2008) and in developmental phases of the programme (Fletcher, Kay-Lambkin, et al., 2017; Fletcher, May, et al., 2017). The information in the messages pragmatically guides behaviours and provides implications of father-child interaction in ways that gave many men a more nuanced knowledge base and strengthened their bond with their child. Through learning to focus on the child, the range of parenting behaviours within the fathering role was expanded at the same time as men's emotional and relational investment (their identity commitment) increased.

> The message I really probably remember the most was interaction with the baby and facial expressions and talking to the baby. Just sitting there telling him about your day. Getting him used to your voice there. Probably the ones I took the most out of from the SMSs. Some of them had links with videos in regards to those as well.

Similarly, the explicit focus on the domain of partner relationship in the messages signalled to men the emergence of a family system where specific roles, rules and boundaries were to be negotiated. The message content enhanced this process by providing useful tips and examples of actions or behaviour that endorsed the value of men's support to the mother, such as, 'Notice something your partner is doing well and tell her about it. It is important for her to hear this now', thus giving men confidence in this new role as intimate partner to a new mother: 'when I got that message, I just understood what the issue was [with her and I] and I just gave it time'.

Messages also highlighted the new interactional role of co-parent. Fathers' role as a partner in parenting was promoted by message content that directly addressed this interaction and which more broadly stimulated conversations about their new child, which in turn promoted cohesion. For example, after a difficult night with their infant, one father said that it was 'a really good message for both of us to hear, so I think it does help having something come to me that I can then take to her and to re-assure her as well'. At the same time, message content strengthened their relationship through the increased understanding and interaction that the messages encouraged, bringing 'something else which is really positive'.

Message Structure and Tone

A second element in SMS4dads that potentially contributes to identify formation was the structure and tone of the communication. Messages were created as brief information statements with links to webpages of highly relevant, evidence-based, government and not-for-profit sources. Pilot study results confirmed that fathers preferred direct messages that were specific advice and prompts (Fletcher, Kay-Lambkin, et al., 2017; Fletcher, May, et al., 2017). While the scheduling of the messages was synchronised to the baby's birth date (see below), the delivery time of the messages varied through the week, and fathers preferred this format (Fletcher, Kay-Lambkin, et al., 2017; Fletcher, May, et al., 2017). The tone was designed to be engaging, using humour, the first person 'baby's voice' and an encouraging, nonjudgemental tone. Together, these strategies appeared to contribute to men's confidence in parenting their child and in helping them orient to their new fathering roles. Speaking about receiving messages before the birth of his first child, one father explained how this worked:

> I think messages that really resonated with me, and made me think more about, 'what I've got myself into', is when you've said, one of the messages says, like 'how will you make time for me, dad?' So it's putting me in that role before I'm actually in that role.

The voice of the baby messages appeared to provide an external appraisal of his new fathering role and support for commitment to this role. These messages seemed to create a virtual conversation between baby and father where the father was urged to engage with the 'person', that is, the infant who is addressing him, and where directions and instructions would be acceptable as they were enhancing his father role 'When other people tell me what to do that doesn't really work for me but when the message came from my baby asking me to read to her, well what could I do?' Messages in the baby's voice strengthened both the father's understanding of the baby's mind and his bond with the infant, thus enhancing his affective commitment to the role.

A further component to the SMS4dads aimed at promoting positive outcomes in general, and identity support in particular was the purposeful 'function' embedded in the message. While message content was constructed to convey information in the three target domains of father-infant, father-partner and self-care, each message was also assigned a function. These were explicitly embedded in the content and timing of the messages and included (1) evidence-based information synchronised to specific gestational and postpartum needs, (2) normalisation of paternal experiences, (3) prompts to interact and reflect and (4) the provision of a safety net (through the Mood Tracker).

The most important design feature was *synchronisation* of all messages to the antenatal and postnatal journey, based on the baby's expected date of delivery. Many of the challenges new fathers and mothers face, which are known to lead to parental stress, are well understood. Sensory and motor development, feeding, crying and sleeping capabilities and behaviours that evolve through the perinatal period can be mapped chronologically with some precision. The messages therefore arrived in a highly personalised format tailored to the father's likely experiences. Men's negative reactions to receiving mistimed messages that did not fit their situation reinforced the importance for fathers of this 'just in time' information. Fathers recognised the messages as a high-quality resource, 'something I could trust in'. Relevant information would 'pop up at the right time', when fathers might have had 'questions that need answers' or needed a signal, 'Hey, now's the time to start thinking about this'.

> You get overloaded. The hospital give you information, there are plenty of people that refer you to a website. So I suppose it was quite good that this referred you specifically to an article, in a brief and also timely, it came in at the right time, and said 'here's something that you should read about this thing that's going on right now'. I didn't have to go in and LOOK for something.

Normalisation of experience was a second explicit design feature embedded in the message content. A proportion of the messages were constructed to inform fathers about typical occurrences throughout the perinatal period, for example, difficulties in breastfeeding, crying, sleeping or mood. With the intention of normalising men's experiences, as in health behaviour change theory, these types of messages conveyed to an extent the likelihood and prevalence of the issues (McEachan, Conner, Taylor, & Lawton, 2011). The normalisation messages gave a positive frame to men's experiences, helping them realise that 'the things that I'm going through are not, I suppose, unique or isolated just to me'. 'So just of planting those ideas that OK, that could be why the child's crying, it's not to do with me being a bad parent or anything like that. You know, this is what a normal kid does. It gave me some insight into that I guess'.

A third purposeful function embedded in a proportion of the messages was *prompts to act*: reminders, prompts, questions or instructions to act or reflect. These were intended to activate fathers' interactions with his baby or partner, 'I definitely tried things after seeing messages'. A fourth intended function for messages specifically about self-care was to prompt men to reflect on their own mood and wellbeing. The messages were experienced as a 'check-up', 'check in' or 'pick me up', giving 'a bit of hope' and providing resources during a difficult time, presenting the information in an objective yet supportive way.

> Because you know some of the messages there have spoke about, you know, exercise and even alcohol intake, just being smart and being aware that, you know, you have a responsibility at the end of the day, so yeah, they would have. Look, they're really good check-ins, and I enjoyed that one in particular about exercise, you know, do it right, look after myself first and then I'm able to help someone else.

Mechanisms of Support for Identity

In our analysis of exit interviews ($N = 40$) (Fletcher et al., 2019), we found that some of these design features interacted with basic psychological processes related to transition and social cognitive theory: change in knowledge, feelings of confidence, ability to cope, role orientation and feeling connected (Meleis, Sawyer, Im, Messias, & Schumacher, 2000). The interaction of these features and psychological processes created mechanisms for changes in fathers' understanding of their role, their relationship quality and a reduction of feelings of isolation, as documented in programme outcomes (Fletcher, Kay-Lambkin, et al., 2017; Fletcher, May, et al., 2017; Fletcher, May, Attia, Garfield, & Skinner, 2018). In this way, the identity support provided by the SMS4dads programme helped fathers value and celebrate their new fatherhood status; begin to define and distinguish their roles as father, partner and co-parent; and strengthen their affective commitment or investment in these roles. Examples of how these design features and psychological processes interacted to create mechanisms of change are given in Table 39.3. Below, we demonstrate how these changes may contribute to identity development (Table 39.4).

Enhancing the Salience of Fatherhood

The mechanisms that appeared to most clearly emphasise the salience or centrality of fatherhood were interactions between synced evidence-based messages, normalising messages and safety-net messages, with the psychological processes of knowledge construction, coping and connection. The information in the synced evidence-based messages interacted with men's recognition of their new role. Men described that the information alerted them to their specific influence and responsibilities, for one father, because 'I massively underestimated my role in the key period of his development'. In the same way, the gravitas and permanence of fatherhood was underlined when normalising messages helped fathers cope with the changes: 'after a hard night', for example, because 'if you know that there's other people that have the same sort of issue, it's easier for you to deal with it'. Safety-net messages that enhanced fathers' coping skills similarly signalled the importance of the transition and the value of self. The texts 'really helped, particularly with the mental side of everything'. Together, the interactions between these core design features and normative psychological processes created positive outcomes for fathers and indicated that the messages specifically affirmed and buttressed the value and centrality of fatherhood.

The infant's 'voice' in the text messages appeared to be a key factor in supporting a developing father identity. Applying the notion of 'reflected appraisals', the men were encouraged to see themselves through their infants' eyes or mind, 'it was just nice to be called Dad in a mes-

Table 39.4 Structural features and psychological processes in SMS4dads

Structural features	Psychological processes				
	1. Increase in knowledge	2. Feelings of confidence	3. Ability to cope	4. Role orientation	5. Feeling connected
1. Synced info	So having that information ready is really a good strategy	Can interact in ways that are appropriate	So the timing worked really well... It helps when you get a bit stressed	Because the article and stuff and the link went through how that was beneficial, you feel like you're contributing	Again, it was just a text message but you're checking in on me and you're saying things that actually are happening to me as I'm getting the text messages
2. Normalising	Once or twice one would come in just as she was having a bit of a worse off time, and it was just helpful to remember that it's fairly natural thing for them to go through	Just having the little reminders that it's not actually anything we were doing specifically, but it's just how this whole process works. It definitely helps restore your confidence when you've had a hit	So it sort of like calmed me a little bit, from the perspective of not freaking out or whatever or not – you know, not being too concerned about something that really wasn't a concern; it was just normal	Just of planting those ideas that OK, that could be why the child's crying; it's not to do with me being a bad parent or anything like that	I suppose it sort of reinforces in me that she is doing a good job and what she's doing is perfectly normal and she is going to experience these rough times as well
3. Prompts to interact	Some of those messages that were a bit instructive about different interactions or things to try. I definitely tried things after seeing messages	I think they definitely gave me some other ideas… made me feel more confident	It's a prompt for me to raise something that maybe I would have left until things had gotten sort of to the point where it would have been harder	That's what triggered something in me to say, 'you know what, I really need to be a little bit more active in that area'	Every time I got it, she was like, 'what was the message today?' and then we'd have a joke about the video camera being in the corner of the room
4.Safety net	…click on to the links and go through the articles. But I often find it's better that way because … (people say) 'if you're not doing it the way I did you're doing it wrong'	And you get these coming through and you go, well even if it's not a friend, at least it's something that's reminding me that I'm doing a good job	It felt like somebody just walked into my office, put their hand on my shoulder and said, 'are you okay?' and that's golden	'Look after myself first and then I'm able to help someone else'	A 'sort of mate tapping you on the shoulder'

Sourced from Fletcher et al. (2019)

sage'. Texts documented the importance of the father to the infant, for example, 'I will learn to love your face and I will try to copy things that you do with your face from a very early age'. They also described what the infant could see when looking up at the father, 'My favourite view will be your face gazing at me. It will be easier when you come just close enough 15–20 cm'. There is no claim to suspension of disbelief. Rather, the men acknowledged the origin of the texts to be from 'experts', which increased their trust in the information and allowed them to focus on the content and meaning.

> Knowing that it's from an actual research organisation and geared towards dads it added an element of trust that what they were sending me was something that I could trust in, that the information would be evidence-based and backed, and appropriate.

Much of the literature on fathers and reflected appraisal has focused on how men come to see themselves as parents based on a partner's appraisal (Maurer & Pleck, 2006). Here we have shifted the perspective, giving the father a lens through which to appraise himself as hugely significant to his infant's security and development from the viewpoint of the infant itself.

Scoping Multiple and Potentially Competing Roles

Because the messages were synchronised to infant development over the perinatal period, men gained knowledge about infant behaviours and needs and how to interact with them. The messages also helped fathers understand the infant's mind, because 'you don't know what they are thinking'. One father explained how the prompt to interact with the baby sharpened his realisation that he is important, that he is 'actively doing something for the baby, and that was good'. Even when men felt they were 'pretty aware', the messages 'keep you on your toes', prompting action when 'you know you haven't been doing it as much as should have'. In this way, the father was called on to take responsibility for the wellbeing of his infant and, at the same time, is recognised for his contribution to the health and wellbeing of his infant. Both the simulated baby dialogue and the suggested actions encouraged fathers to seek time alone with their infant, a hallmark of high-level father involvement (Craig, 2006) and clear demonstration of his new understandings of the paternal role.

Similarly, texts with prompts to action that opened lines of communication between partners helped fathers better understand the expectations of this new co-parenting role. Texts sparked positive conversations between partners about sleep, crying or shared household labour. By acting on these messages, fathers could show their partners that they were supportive, 'involved' and 'actually be more present and helpful'. The messages also prompted fathers to take up 'difficult conversations' with their partner, to discuss struggles and to ameliorate or avoid conflict.

> She found they're good, yeah, she found they're good. I think, you know, if she finds them good, but she might have read something similar or different and, you know, it's just good that I suppose I'm being active as well and, you know, we're all on the same page basically, which is great.

Strengthening Commitment

The messages that prompted men to support their partner or discuss their infant functioned to increase men's sense of connection with both, as demonstrated in the highly positive ratings of these factors across evaluations (Fletcher et al., 2018; Fletcher, Kay-Lambkin, et al., 2017; Fletcher, May, et al., 2017). Men acknowledged that they now had to consider the family system, 'you know you're in it together, you know what's going on, where you're up to, but the reminder to check in with them and look after them [is very important]'. This sense of togetherness and responsibility appears to be a key component of the emotional and relational investment that characterises affective or socio-emotional commitment within identity theory (Burke & Reitzes, 1991). Likewise, SMS4dads provided for men another socio-emotional connection that buttressed their new status as father. The attribution of a persona to the messages appeared to create a sense of anticipation that kept men balanced and in the loop, 'Put it this way: if I wasn't receiving the message, I'd miss them', because 'you're the only one who's texted me saying how are things going'.

Summary and Key Points

The way that men carry out their fathering role, starting before the birth, has a profound influence on the long-term development of their children and on their partner's wellbeing. We know this, yet we have not been effective in finding ways to engage with men as they make this transition. Our interventions and services for family members lag behind the society-wide changes in how men and women see themselves as parents, changes in the conception of fathering which include caring for infants alongside the traditional provider roles. A new framework, looking beyond what has worked in supporting mothers, is needed, one which values fathers both for the way that they parent and for the way that they partner in their parenting with the mother. In this chapter, we have suggested that a father's identity, the way he conceptualises and enacts the various aspects of his role as father, is key to designing effective support. This is not a new idea, but in the modern information technology context, specifically the ubiquity of mobile phone use, new avenues for supporting his identity are available. We use the text-based SMS4dads programme to suggest key processes in support as they relate to the fathers' identity.

The SMS4dads programme, which begins before birth, is intentionally father-only, sends brief messages directly to the father every few days and does not require downloading or logging on. The programme design takes account of widely acknowledged, contradictory aspects of new fathers' role in high-income countries. These include the necessity to take up the fathering role in the absence of intergenerational models of how to be a father; the expectation to be 'involved' with the pregnancy and baby contradicted by work pressure, mother-focused services and limited parental leave; the enormous range of parenting information available online without the means to find trustworthy, relevant advice; and the reduction of social contact at a time when knowing how other fathers are managing the same challenges would be helpful. Fathers enrolling in the programme (>1300) report high approval ratings of the programme overall, appreciation of the texts in regard to the effect on their fathering in the relationships with their infant and partner and their confidence in the fathering role.

The constructs from identity theory, such as normalisation, role salience and reflected appraisal, may help explain the mechanisms at play in the satisfaction of participating fathers and suggest a way to design effective supports for new fathers. The key features of the programme which support the fathers' positive identity are valuing the identity of father as caregiver for his infant; valuing fathers' support for, and co-parenting with, the mother; and strengthening his identity by connection with other men.

Valuing the Identity of Father as Caregiver for his Infant

The badging of the programme, as being specifically for fathers, calls attention to the value placed on this role by the existence of the programme. The fathers' identity as carer is supported in the texts which are tailored to the interactions that fathers typically encounter throughout the pregnancy and early months. The emphasis on infant care reinforces the value attributed to his caring role, and strategies, 'tips', are offered for enacting the role. The 'voice' of the baby, used in most messages, offers a positive appraisal which fathers comment had a powerful effect on their commitment to the role of nurturing fathers and to interacting with their infants. These texts scaffold his attention on the baby's development and encourage and applaud his interactions. They create a virtual conversation between baby and father where the father is urged to engage with the 'person', that is, the infant who is addressing him, before birth and in the preverbal months after the birth.

Valuing Fathers' Support for, and Co-parenting with, the Mother

The messages suggesting that he offer verbal encouragement to the mother, in bearing or in caring for their infant, build the father's identity as a partner with a different but valuable role in the parenting team. Fathers say that the texts are a conversation starter, a way to engage with the task of parenting more as a partner and less as a helper.

Strengthening His Identity by Connection with Other Men

Knowing that other fathers in the same situation are receiving the same messages can create a 'virtual' community, one which can help normalise the emotional turmoil arising from stressful situations which are very common in learning to parent a new baby. The trustworthiness of the programme, in an online environment where information is not easily verified, offers a low-stress source of support.

References

Adamsons, K., & Pasley, K. (2016). Parents' fathering identity standards and later father involvement. *Journal of Family Issues, 37*(2), 221–244.

Astbury, B., & Leeuw, F. L. (2010). Unpacking black boxes: Mechanisms and theory building in evaluation. *American Journal of Evaluation, 31*(3), 363–381.

Baldwin, S., Malone, M., Sandall, J., & Bick, D. (2018). Mental health and wellbeing during the transition to fatherhood: A systematic review of first time fathers' experiences. *JBI Database of Systematic Reviews and Implementation Reports, 16*(11), 2118.

Bassett-Gunter, R. L., Levy-Milne, R., Naylor, P. J., Downs, D. S., Benoit, C., Warburton, D. E., et al. (2013). Oh baby! Motivation for healthy eating during parenthood transitions: A longitudinal examination with a theory of planned behavior perspective. *International Journal of Behavioral Nutrition and Physical Activity, 10*(1), 88.

Bremberg, S. (2016). Supporting fathers is essential in the child health field. *Acta Paediatrica, 105*(9), 992–993.

Burke, P. J., & Reitzes, D. C. (1991). An identity theory approach to commitment. *Social Psychology Quarterly*, 239–251.

Burke, P. J., & Stets, J. E. (2009). *Identity theory*. Oxford University Press.

Cabrera, N., Tamis-LeMonda, C. S., Bradley, R. H., Hofferth, S., & Lamb, M. E. (2000). Fatherhood in the twenty-first century. *Child Development, 71*(1), 127–136.

Cowan, P. A. (1991). Individual and family life transitions: A proposal for a new definition. In P. A. Cowan & M. Hetherington (Eds.), Family Transitions (pp. 3–30). Hillsdale, NJ: Lawrence Erlbaum Associates

Craig, L. (2006). Does father care mean fathers share? A comparison of how mothers and fathers in intact families spend time with children. *Gender & Society, 20*(2), 259–281.

Crespi, I., & Ruspini, E. (2015). Transition to fatherhood: New perspectives in the global context of changing men's identities. *International Review of Sociology, 25*(3), 353–358.

Cruwys, T., Dingle, G. A., Haslam, C., Haslam, S. A., Jetten, J., & Morton, T. A. (2013). Social group memberships protect against future depression, alleviate depression symptoms and prevent depression relapse. *Social Science & Medicine, 98*, 179–186.

Cutrona, C. E., Russell, D. W., & Gardner, K. A. (2005). The relationship enhancement model of social support. In T. A. Revenson, K. Kayser, & G. Bodenmann (Eds.), *Decade of behavior. Couples coping with stress: Emerging perspectives on dyadic coping* (pp. 73–95). Washington, DC: American Psychological Association.

Da Costa, D., Danieli, C., Abrahamowicz, M., Dasgupta, K., Sewitch, M., Lowensteyn, I., et al. (2019). A prospective study of postnatal depressive symptoms and associated risk factors in first-time fathers. *Journal of Affective Disorders, 249*, 371–377.

Daniel, E., Madigan, S., & Jenkins, J. (2016). Paternal and maternal warmth and the development of prosociality among preschoolers. *Journal of Family Psychology, 30*(1), 114.

Darwin, Z., Galdas, P., Hinchliff, S., Littlewood, E., McMillan, D., McGowan, L., et al. (2017). Fathers' views and experiences of their own mental health during pregnancy and the first postnatal year: A qualitative interview study of men participating in the UK Born and Bred in Yorkshire (BaBY) cohort. *BMC Pregnancy and Childbirth, 17*(1), 45.

De Nooijer, J., Lechner, L., & de Vries, H. (2002). Tailored versus general information on early detection of cancer: A comparison of the reactions of Dutch adults and the impact on attitudes and behaviors. *Health Education Research, 17*(2), 239–252.

Dennis, C. L., & Letourneau, N. (2007). Global and relationship-specific perceptions of support and the development of postpartum depressive symptomatology. *Social Psychiatry and Psychiatric Epidemiology, 42*(5), 389–395.

Department of Health WA. State Perinatal Reference Group and the Western Australian Perinatal Mental Health Unit (2007). State Perinatal Mental Health

Initiative: Report 2003–2007. Perth: Department of Health WA.

Dermott, E., & Miller, T. (2015). More than the sum of its parts? Contemporary fatherhood policy, practice and discourse. *Families, Relationships and Societies, 4*(2), 183–195.

Doss, B. D., Rhoades, G. K., Stanley, S. M., & Markman, H. J. (2009). The effect of the transition to parenthood on relationship quality: An 8-year prospective study. *Journal of Personality and Social Psychology, 96*(3), 601.

Draper, J. (2003). Men's passage to fatherhood: An analysis of the contemporary relevance of transition theory. *Nursing Inquiry, 10*(1), 66–78.

Dyer, W. M. (2005). Prison, fathers, and identity: A theory of how incarceration affects men's paternal identity. *Fathering, 3*(3).

Elloy, D. F., & Smith, C. R. (2003). Patterns of stress, work-family conflict, role conflict, role ambiguity and overload among dual-career and single-career couples: An Australian study. *Cross Cultural Management: An International Journal, 10*(1), 55–66.

Fägerskiöld, A. (2008). A change in life as experienced by first-time fathers. *Scandinavian Journal of Caring Sciences, 22*(1), 64–71.

Faulkner, D., Hammond, C., Nisbet, L., & Fletcher, R. (2018). How do young aboriginal fathers in Australia 'stay on track'?–Perspectives on the support networks of aboriginal fathers. *Journal of Family Studies*, 1–14.

Ferguson, H., & Gates, P. (2015). Early intervention and holistic, relationship-based practice with fathers: evidence from the work of the Family Nurse Partnership. *Child & Family Social Work, 20*(1), 96–105.

Fleisher, L., Buzaglo, J., Collins, M., Millard, J., Miller, S. M., Egleston, B. L., et al. (2008). Using health communication best practices to develop a web-based provider–patient communication aid: The CONNECT™ study. *Patient Education and Counseling, 71*(3), 378–387.

Fletcher, R., Knight, T., Macdonald, J. A., & StGeorge, J. (2019). Process evaluation of text-based support for fathers during the transition to fatherhood (SMS4dads): Mechanisms of impact. *BMC Psychology, 7*(1), 1–11.

Fletcher, R. J., Matthey, S., & Marley, C. G. (2006). Addressing depression and anxiety among new fathers. *Medical Journal of Australia, 185*(8), 461–463.

Fletcher, R. (2008). *The assessment and support of new fathers: Father-infant attachment as a basis for psychosocial assessment and support*. Berlin, Germany: Verlag.

Fletcher, R., Freeman, E., & Matthey, S. (2011). The impact of Behavioural parent training on fathers' parenting: A meta-analysis of the triple P-positive parenting program. *Fathering, 9*(3).

Fletcher, R., Kay-Lambkin, F., May, C., Oldmeadow, C., Attia, J., & Leigh, L. (2017). Supporting men through their transition to fatherhood with messages delivered to their smartphones: A feasibility study of SMS4dads. *BMC Public Health, 17*(1), 953.

Fletcher, R., May, C., Attia, J., Garfield, C. F., & Skinner, G. (2018). Text-based program addressing the mental health of soon-to-be and new fathers (SMS4dads): Protocol for a randomized controlled trial. *JMIR research protocols, 7*(2), e37.

Fletcher, R., May, C., Kay Lambkin, F., Gemmill, A. W., Cann, W., Nicholson, C. R., et al. (2017). SMS4dads: Providing information and support to new fathers through mobile phones–a pilot study. *Advances in Mental Health, 15*(2), 121–131.

Fletcher, R., May, C., Wroe, J., Hall, P., Cooke, D., Rawlinson, C., et al. (2016). Development of a set of mobile phone text messages designed for new fathers. *Journal of Reproductive and Infant Psychology, 34*(5), 525–534.

Fletcher, R., & Silberberg, S. (2006). Involvement of fathers in primary school activities. *Australian Journal of Education, 50*(1), 29–39.

Fletcher, R., St George, J., May, C., Hartman, D., & King, A. (2015). Father-inclusive practice in a family center: An Australian perspective. *Zero to Three, 35*(5), 60–67.

Fox, G. L., Nordquist, V. M., Billen, R. M., & Savoca, E. F. (2015). Father involvement and early intervention: Effects of empowerment and father role identity. *Family Relations, 64*(4), 461–475.

Friedewald, M., Fletcher, R., & Fairbairn, H. (2005). All-male discussion forums for expectant fathers: Evaluation of a model. *The Journal of Perinatal Education, 14*(2), 8.

Garfield, C. F., Isacco, A., & Bartlo, W. D. (2010). Men's health and fatherhood in the urban Midwestern United States. *International Journal of Men's Health, 9*(3).

Genesoni, L., & Tallandini, M. A. (2009). Men's psychological transition to fatherhood: an analysis of the literature, 1989–2008. *Birth, 36*(4), 305–318.

Greenaway, K. H., Cruwys, T., Haslam, S. A., & Jetten, J. (2016). Social identities promote well-being because they satisfy global psychological needs. *European Journal of Social Psychology, 46*(3), 294–307.

Grossmann, K., Grossmann, K. E., Fremmer-Bombik, E., Kindler, H., Scheuerer-Englisch, H., & Zimmermann, A. P. (2002). The uniqueness of the child–father attachment relationship: Fathers' sensitive and challenging play as a pivotal variable in a 16-year longitudinal study. *Social Development, 11*(3), 301–337.

Hall, C. M., & Bierman, K. L. (2015). Technology-assisted interventions for parents of young children: Emerging practices, current research, and future directions. *Early Childhood Research Quarterly, 33*, 21–32.

Haslam, S. A., Jetten, J., Postmes, T., & Haslam, C. (2009). Social identity, health and well-being: An emerging agenda for applied psychology. *Applied Psychology, 58*(1), 1–23.

Hildingsson, I., Haines, H., Johansson, M., Rubertsson, C., & Fenwick, J. (2014). Childbirth fear in Swedish fathers is associated with parental stress as well as poor physical and mental health. *Midwifery, 30*(2), 248–254.

Hirsh, J. B., & Kang, S. K. (2016). Mechanisms of identity conflict: Uncertainty, anxiety, and the behavioral inhibition system. *Personality and Social Psychology Review, 20*(3), 223–244.

Hodkinson, P., & Brooks, R. (2018). Interchangeable parents? The roles and identities of primary and equal carer fathers of young children. Current Sociology, 0011392118807530.

Ipsos-Mori. (2019). *Fatherhood and social connections report*. Australia: Ipsos Public Affairs for Movember.

Kohn, J. L., Rholes, S. W., Simpson, J. A., Martin III, A. M., Tran, S., & Wilson, C. L. (2012). Changes in marital satisfaction across the transition to parenthood: The role of adult attachment orientations. *Personality and Social Psychology Bulletin, 38*(11), 1506–1522.

Kreuter, M. W., & Wray, R. J. (2003). Tailored and targeted health communication: Strategies for enhancing information relevance. *American Journal of Health Behavior, 27*(1), S227–S232.

Litton Fox, G., Bruce, C., & Combs-Orme, T. (2000). Parenting expectations and concerns of fathers and mothers of newborn infants. *Family Relations, 49*(2), 123–131.

Maurer, T. W., & Pleck, J. H. (2006). Fathers' caregiving and breadwinning: A gender congruence analysis. *Psychology of Men & Masculinity, 7*(2), 101.

Maurer, T. W., Pleck, J. H., & Rane, T. R. (2001). Parental identity and reflected-appraisals: Measurement and gender dynamics. *Journal of Marriage and Family, 63*(2), 309–321.

McEachan, R. R. C., Conner, M., Taylor, N. J., & Lawton, R. J. (2011). Prospective prediction of health-related behaviours with the theory of planned behaviour: A meta-analysis. *Health Psychology Review, 5*(2), 97–144.

Meleis, A. I., Sawyer, L. M., Im, E. O., Messias, D. K. H., & Schumacher, K. (2000). Experiencing transitions: An emerging middle-range theory. *Advances in Nursing Science, 23*(1), 12–28.

Melville, K. M., Casey, L. M., & Kavanagh, D. J. (2010). Dropout from internet-based treatment for psychological disorders. *British Journal of Clinical Psychology, 49*(4), 455–471.

Moore, G. F., Audrey, S., Barker, M., Bond, L., Bonell, C., Hardeman, W., et al. (2015). Process evaluation of complex interventions: Medical Research Council guidance. *BMJ, 350*, h1258.

Morse, C. A., Buist, A., & Durkin, S. (2000). First-time parenthood: Influences on pre-and postnatal adjustment in fathers and mothers. *Journal of Psychosomatic Obstetrics and Gynecology, 21*(2), 109–120.

Oliffe, J. L., Bottorff, J. L., & Sarbit, G. (2010). The right time, the right reasons: Dads talk about reducing and quitting smoking. *Okanagan, British Columbia, Canada: Institute for Healthy Living and Chronic Disease Prevention, University of British Columbia.*

Palkovitz, R., & Palm, G. (2009). Transitions within fathering. *Fathering, 7*(1).

Panter-Brick, C., Burgess, A., Eggerman, M., McAllister, F., Pruett, K., & Leckman, J. F. (2014). Practitioner review: Engaging fathers–recommendations for a game change in parenting interventions based on a systematic review of the global evidence. *Journal of Child Psychology and Psychiatry, 55*(11), 1187–1212.

Parke, R. D. (1988). Families in life-span perspective: A multilevel developmental approach. In E. M. Hetherington, R. M. Lerner, & M. Perlmutter (Eds.), *Child development in life-span perspective* (pp. 159–190). Hillsdale, NJ, US: Lawrence Erlbaum Associates, Inc.

Pasley, K., Petren, R. E., & Fish, J. N. (2014). Use of identity theory to inform fathering scholarship. *Journal of Family Theory & Review, 6*(4), 298–318.

Paulson, J. F., & Bazemore, S. D. (2010). Prenatal and postpartum depression in fathers and its association with maternal depression: A meta-analysis. *JAMA, 303*(19), 1961–1969.

Philpott, L. F., Leahy-Warren, P., FitzGerald, S., & Savage, E. (2017). Stress in fathers in the perinatal period: A systematic review. *Midwifery, 55*, 113–127.

Ramchandani, P., & Iles, J. (2014). Commentary: Getting fathers into parenting programmes–a reflection on Panter-Brick et al. (2014). *Journal of Child Psychology and Psychiatry, 55*(11), 1213–1214.

Rothbard, N. P. (2001). Enriching or depleting? The dynamics of engagement in work and family roles. *Administrative Science Quarterly, 46*(4), 655–684.

Roy, K. M., & Dyson, O. (2010). Making daddies into fathers: Community-based fatherhood programs and the construction of masculinities for low-income African American men. *American Journal of Community Psychology, 45*(1-2), 139–154.

Schlossberg, N. K. (1981). A model for analyzing human adaptation to transition. *The Counseling Psychologist, 9*(2), 2–18.

Saxbe, D., Rossin-Slater, M., & Goldenberg, D. (2018). The transition to parenthood as a critical window for adult health. *American Psychologist, 73*(9), 1190.

StGeorge, J. M., Wroe, J. K., & Cashin, M. E. (2018). The concept and measurement of fathers' stimulating play: A review. *Attachment & Human Development, 20*(6), 634–658.

Stryker, S., & Burke, P. J. (2000). The past, present, and future of an identity theory. *Social Psychology Quarterly*, 284–297.

Twomey, C., O'Reilly, G., Byrne, M., Bury, M., White, A., Kissane, S., et al. (2014). A randomized controlled trial of the computerized CBT programme, MoodGYM, for public mental health service users waiting for interventions. *British Journal of Clinical Psychology, 53*(4), 433–450.

Umberson, D., Liu, H., Mirowsky, J., & Reczek, C. (2011). Parenthood and trajectories of change in body weight over the life course. *Social Science & Medicine, 73*(9), 1323–1331.

Winickoff, J. P., Healey, E. A., Regan, S., Park, E. R., Cole, C., Friebely, J., et al. (2010). Using the postpartum hospital stay to address mothers' and fathers' smoking: The NEWS study. *Pediatrics, 125*(3), 518–525.

Winkel, D. E., & Clayton, R. W. (2010). Transitioning between work and family roles as a function of boundary flexibility and role salience. *Journal of Vocational Behavior, 76*(2), 336–343.

Wynter, K., Francis, L., Fletcher, R., McBride, N., Dowse, E., Wilson, N., ... & Macdonald, J. (2019). *Sleep, mental health and wellbeing among fathers of infants up to 1 year postpartum: A scoping review.* https://doi.org/10.31219/osf.io/wukp7

Designing and Tailoring Preventive Interventions for Fathers' Parenting

40

David S. DeGarmo

This chapter focuses on effective parent training interventions for fathers of young children and how research can inform the tailoring of cognitive and behavioral treatments to be more salient for fathers and, therefore, more efficacious. A key element of tailoring interventions for fathers is adapting interventions based on sound theoretically grounded principles that are specifically relevant to the fathering role and fathering behaviors. In general, the primary theoretical perspectives discussed throughout this chapter are attachment theory for fathers of infants, social interaction learning theory for children ages three and above, and identity theory for fathers of children across the life course. This chapter is organized in sections that first reviews evidence-based non-tailored and father-tailored parent training programs. Next, recommendations for practice and implementation science are reviewed from a treatment and from a methodological perspective. Finally, data are presented from a recently tailored program for single and separating fathers using principles of father-focused adaptation of an effective parent training program.

D. S. DeGarmo (✉)
Department of Counseling Psychology and Human Services, Prevention Science Institute, University of Oregon, Eugene, OR, USA
e-mail: degarmo@uoregon.edu

The Need for Effective Parent Training with Fathers

Children's problem behaviors remain a costly burden both nationally and globally (Salmanian, Mohammadi, Keshavarzi, & Brand, 2018) with effective parent training one cost-effective strategy for addressing developmental behavioral psychopathology as a public health concern. Children's externalizing and internalizing disorders including conduct disorder (CD), oppositional defiant disorder (ODD), attention-deficit disorder (ADD), anxiety, and depression, are the leading reasons for referral of children to mental health agencies (Weber, Kamp-Becker, Christiansen, & Mingebach, 2019). Meta-analyses have shown that conduct disorder is associated with the long-term outcomes relating to criminality, mental health problems, substance use disorders, antisocial personality disorder, early pregnancy, and failure to complete high school (Erskine et al., 2016).

The worldwide prevalence of externalizing disorders in children and adolescents is estimated to be roughly 6% (Polanczyk, Salum, Sugaya, Caye, & Rohde, 2015). Prevalence is even higher in the contemporary USA, with initial national data reporting that one in every four to five youth will meet criteria for a mental health disorder across their lifetime (Merikangas et al., 2010). Prevalence of disorders with severe impairment was estimated to be 22.2% (11.2% with mood

H. E. Fitzgerald et al. (eds.), *Handbook of Fathers and Child Development*,
https://doi.org/10.1007/978-3-030-51027-5_40

disorders, 8.3% with anxiety disorders, and 9.6% behavior disorders). Onset of these disorders occurs early and lasts through adolescence with mediation age of onset earliest for anxiety (age 6), externalizing behavior (median age 11), mood disorders (median age 13), and substance use (median age 15) (Merikangas et al., 2010).

Among the complex biological and environmental factors contributing to the etiology of child and adolescent conduct problems, *parenting behaviors* are the key socializing agent predicting the development of problem behaviors, in particular, *harsh coercive parenting* and *inconsistent discipline*, with *prosocial positive parenting behavior* serving as a protective factor (Duncombe, Havighurst, Holland, & Frankling, 2012). Fathers' coercive parenting is uniquely problematic. Relative to mothers' developmental studies have shown that coercive fathering explains greater variance in children's problem behaviors (DeGarmo, Nordahl, & Fabiano, 2016). As a protective factor, it is also well established that independent of mothers' influence, quality fathering behaviors of both residential and nonresidential fathers matter in the healthy development of their children (Asmussen & Weizel, 2010; Flouri, 2005). Quality father involvement and effective parenting is associated with better academic outcomes and reduced internalizing and externalizing behaviors across development (Jeynes, 2015; Leidy, Schofield, & Parke, 2013).

Together, these data above underscore the need for early intervention and effective preventive intervention and treatment targeting parenting practices and behaviors during early childhood. Indeed, there is long-standing evidence from meta-analyses that behavioral parent training shows positive effects not only on children's short-term outcomes (Furlong et al., 2013; Lee, Niew, Yang, Chen, & Lin, 2012; Lundahl, Risser, & Lovejoy, 2006); but higher-order meta-analyses also show that parent training has beneficial maintenance, emergent, and crossover effects for parents (Weber et al., 2019). Short-term effects on child behavior problems tend to be more consistent, with long-term effects of child adjustment exhibiting considerable heterogeneity as do longer-term effects on parent well-being.

Moreover, non-tailored parent training implemented with mothers and fathers consistently shows that for two-parent families, participation of fathers in treatment has greater benefits for relative gains and maintenance compared to families in which fathers do not participate (Bagner, 2013; Cowan, Cowan, & Knox, 2010; Sicouri et al., 2018). Unfortunately, at the same time reviews show rapid increase in efforts to engage fathers in psychosocial parenting education or behavioral parent training, and evidence still suggests that relative to mother-child and mother-focused programs, rigorously evaluated father-focused parenting interventions remain few in number and participation of fathers remains notoriously low (DeGarmo et al., 2016; Lee, Knauer, Lee, MacEachern, & Garfield, 2018; Panter-Brick et al., 2014).

In general, roughly one in five fathers when offered participate in parent training programs. A recent systematic review found that at least 25% of parents in need of behavioral parent training (BPT) do not enroll or engage in treatment when offered, and of those who do initially engage, 26% prematurely drop out, leaving fewer than half of the parents who had been identified as likely to benefit from BPT actually receiving appropriate treatment (Chacko et al., 2016). In addition, fathers are uniquely more challenging to engage in BPT (DeGarmo et al., 2016). In the Triple P meta-analysis, Fletcher, Freeman, and Mathey (2011) report that overall only 20% of fathers participated in 28 total evaluations, with only 50% of the studies reporting data on factors associated with father participation.

From a prevalence perspective, an Australian sample of 1001 fathers showed that only 15% of fathers participated in parenting interventions or treatment for children as young as 2 years of age (Tully et al., 2017). Although participation was higher for fathers of children with problem behaviors, fathers of children with higher externalizing reported more participation barriers relative to fathers of children with low levels of externalizing. The top four practical barriers included costs of service, conflicts with work commitments, time to participate in general, and convenience of location of services. Similarly, a comprehensive survey of social service practitioners in the UK found that among two-parent families attending structured parenting courses, 21% of fathers participated (Scourfield, Cheung, & Macdonald, 2014). From a systemic point of view on implementation effectiveness and sustainability of effective programs for fathers, it is essential that parent training programs are compelling not only to fathers but to all stakeholders and decision-makers including fathers and other primary caregivers, mothers, program directors, policymakers, and funders (Panter-Brick et al., 2014).

Non-tailored Parenting Intervention and Fathers

This section presents non-tailored parenting intervention programs defined as well-established behavioral parent training programs based on universal parenting principles. That is, cumulative clinical intervention programs are considered here that have utilized randomized controlled designs testing theory-driven parenting training interventions that were applied as manualized but "off the shelf" for both mothers and fathers.

Infancy Interventions for Fathers

For infancy (i.e., birth to 2), fathering interventions have been dominated by attachment theory (Cabrera, Shannon, & Tamis-LeMonda, 2007; Lamb & Lewis, 2013). Attachment theory focuses on parental sensitivity and responsiveness to the infant's signals as the key dimension of prosocial positive parenting that contributes to children's secure attachment and healthy emotional adjustment. Fathers' sensitivity has been less studied (Lamb & Lewis, 2013). Nevertheless, research on fathers' behavior during early childhood reveals that they can be equally sensitive as mothers and that their skillful parenting contributes to child adjustment (Tamis-LeMonda, Shannon, Cabrera, & Lamb, 2004). The negative impact of unskilled parenting for early child development, unfortunately, is better understood. Disruptions in fathers' sensitive and responsive parenting and their intrusive, detached, or harsh parenting predict poor child attachment (Lucassen et al., 2011) and poor child outcomes (Ramchandani et al., 2013).

Attachment-based interventions have been developed almost exclusively for mothers (Bakermans-Kranenburg, van IJzendoorn, & Juffer, 2005). Relatively fewer exist for fathers. Evidence-based father programs include infant massage, didactic parent training groups, direct observation, strength-based video feedback, and modeling care of infants (Magill-Evans, Harrison, Rempel, & Slater, 2006). For example, based on the Steps Toward Effective Enjoyable Parenting (STEEP) program, Doherty, Erickson, and LaRossa (2006) developed an 8-week pre- and postnatal psychoeducational and behavioral program for couples transitioning to parenthood. The goal was to increase fathers' knowledge and skill and commitment to the fatherhood role. Couple components focused on co-parenting and contextual factors associated with fathers such as work and cultural expectations. The randomized trial of 165 couples demonstrated the program was successful in promoting increased father involvement and quality father-baby interactions. Employing similar theoretical perspectives, Shapiro, Gottman, and Fink (2020) recently tested a couple-focused intervention designed to promote father involvement in childcare and strengthen the couple relationships. A randomized trial of 136 couples showed that fathers in the Bringing Baby Home intervention reported increased father involvement relative to controls, greater satisfaction with the division of parenting labor, and feeling more appreciated by partners. Both husbands and wives reported greater satisfaction when fathers were more involved in parenting tasks.

In a recent randomized trial evaluating skin-to-skin contact (SSC) program (Chen, Gau, Liu, & Lee, 2017), 83 young Taiwanese fathers were allocated to either SSC or to a control condition. The SSC program involved 15-minute touch sessions for the first 3 days postpartum. Fathers in the SSC program reported significantly higher attachment on the Father-Child Attachment Scale. Another recent example is the Fathers Club intervention for new fathers (Rempel, Rempel, Khuc, & Vui, 2017). Employing communes in Vietnam, Fathers Clubs were developed to provide opportunities for ongoing peer support and validation. Fathers Club meetings provide fathers with opportunities to discuss their positive and negative experiences, discuss concerns, and ask questions about being actively involved fathers. One primary activity included group participation in friendly competitions between father groups and invited community members (e.g., family and friends). The competitions were designed to increase social learning of the program content and to increase community awareness. More tailored attachment approaches with fathers are presented further below.

Early Childhood Interventions for Fathers

For early childhood (i.e., ages 2–3 to adolescence), the predominant evidence-based programs for early childhood reporting findings on fathers include but are not limited to Parent-Child Interaction Therapy (PCIT), Triple P, Incredible Years (IY), and Parent Management Training-Oregon Model (PMTO). In general, meta-analytic approaches report moderate to medium effect sizes for the benefits of parent training on fathers' effective parenting practices, while small sample clinical trials often report large effects for fathers. Reviews indicate that the active engagement of fathers in parenting interventions can be a key factor promoting maintenance and long-term success of maternal, child, and family outcomes (Lechowicz et al., 2019; Lundahl et al., 2008).

In a meta-analysis of 28 randomized control trials, Fletcher et al. (2011) reported positive overall benefits of participating in Triple P on the Parenting Scale, a validated 30-item scale of parenting practices, measuring dimensions of *laxness-permissiveness*, *overreactivity-harshness*, and *verbosity,* obtaining an overall effect size (ES) of 0.77 [95% CI, 0.71–0.84]. However, when comparing mothers with fathers separately, the ES for mothers was 0.77 [95% CI, 0.65–0.87] and was 0.51 [95% CI, 0.37–0.63] for fathers. In a small wait-listed control trial of the IY program of 36 Portuguese families where fathers were willing to participate with co-parents, Homem, Gaspar, Seabra-Santos, Canavarro, and Azevedo (2014) reported significant 6-month pre-post improvements in fathers' reported parenting practices on the Parenting Scale with a partial η^2 of 0.25 a large effect size ($d = 1.15$).

In a rigorously designed comparative effectiveness study of the IY program, Webster-Stratton, Reid, and Hammond (2004) compared 159 families with children aged 4–8 years with problem behaviors. Families were randomly assigned to six parent training conditions: a wait-listed control (WL), parent training only (PT), child training only (CT), (PT + TT), (CT + TT), and (PT + CT + TT) conditions. The intervention was effective in reducing fathers' negative parenting behaviors in only conditions including PT ($d = 0.51$, 0.91, and 0.77 for PT, PT + TT, and PT + CT + TT, respectively). The effects of PT on mothers' negative parenting were comparable to the reductions in fathers' negative parenting (d ranged from 0.74 to 0.84 across PT conditions).

In a nonrandomized comparison of families participating in the intensive PCIT program, Bagner and Eyberg (2003) compared 107 families in which fathers participated, families with non-participating fathers (uninvolved but present), versus absent-father families. All PCIT groups of families reported improvements in child behavior and parenting stress. At immediate post-test, absent-father families showed better gains compared to participating father families. However, follow-up data showed that families with participating fathers maintained treatment gains on child behavior problems, while absent-father families reported significant declines. These data support the notion that father participation is important for the maintenance and support of sustaining beneficial treatment effects. More recently, in a study of 44 families with children presenting with conduct disorder and developmental delay participating in PCIT, Bagner (2013) showed that families in which fathers participated in treatment exhibited lower levels of externalizing behavior problems compared to children from single-mother families or families in which fathers did not participate. The PCIT program would better address the impact of father participation with the use of randomized designs to better address potential selection effects accounting for differences in father participation effects.

In the Marital and Parenting in Stepfamilies (MAPS) study, PMTO has demonstrated reduced marital conflict (Bullard et al., 2010) and medium effect sizes for observed co-parenting latent constructs of parenting practices measured with observed parent-child interactions (i.e., *problem solving, coercive discipline, monitoring, skill encouragement, and positive involvement*) (Forgatch, DeGarmo, & Beldavs, 2005; $d = 0.80$, partial $\eta^2 = 0.14$). Counter to reviews of self-reported parenting reviews, larger effect sizes on observed effective parenting practices were higher for stepfathers relative to biological mothers (DeGarmo & Forgatch, 2007; $d = 0.54$ and 0.46 for fathers and mothers, respectively). It is possible that effect sizes could be larger for more marginalized fathers or at-risk father populations for which few evidence-based programs exist such as stepfathers, nonresidential fathers, or single fathers (DeGarmo et al., 2016). Other evidence-based parent training programs that focus on co-parenting alliances, parenting as a united front, and parenting as a team include the Supporting Father Involvement for socially disadvantaged fathers (Cowan, Cowan, Pruett, & Pruett, 2007) and Dads for Life for divorcing couples (Cookston, Braver, Griffin, De Lusé, & Miles, 2007).

Tailored Evidence-Based Parenting Intervention and Fathers

This section provides a few exemplars of tailored father-focused interventions during infancy and early childhood. Tailoring of fathering intervention should be based on theoretical models of paternal engagement and functions of fathering roles (Doherty, Kouneski, & Erickson, 1998; Pleck, 1997). In general, empirical data and theory suggest that father-centric programming that promotes fathers' identification with the parenting role and raise fathers' awareness of their developmental impact on children may be more effective in tailoring programs for fathers (DeGarmo et al., 2016; Frank, Keown, Dittman, & Sanders, 2015).

Additionally, Panter-Brick et al. (2014) caution that engaging fathers in gender-equitable role definitions needs to be sensitive to cultural and contextual characteristics of participants. For example, although historically fathers are becoming more involved in their children's lives, fathers still identify with "breadwinning" (Mauer & Pleck, 2006), and "caregiving" is still primarily defined as woman's work, which means that many fathers need to cognitively redefine tasks that are nontraditional for men as still somehow being masculine (Doucet, 2004). Psychoeducational and behavioral treatments need to reframe men's perspectives as being partners not as helpers to mothers; couples err by neglecting to give parenting the same weight as other domestic chores.

Within a broader ecological model, tailoring needs to be culturally sensitive as well. *Cultural adaptation* refers to the systematic modification of an evidence-based intervention to consider language, behavioral traditions, and context that are compatible with and relevant to a focal population's shared values and beliefs (Parra-Cardona et al., 2017). One early example of cultural tailoring for fathers was the Parent Empowerment Project (PEP: Parra-Cordona et al., 2006). Contextually, teen fathers face greater financial difficulties and greater educational barriers and are at higher risk for relationship instability relative to more on-time fathers (Parra-Cardona, Wampler, & Sharp, 2006). Furthermore, Mexican origin teens in the contemporary USA are at high risk for teen pregnancy, with few programs focusing on inclusion or experiences of the adolescent father. The Parent Empowerment Project (PEP) was a state-funded teen parent program implemented in Latinx communities for high-risk families. Qualitative analyses indicated that fathers participating in the PEP obtained a higher sense of parenting efficacy and skill for caring for infants and reported a greater commitment to the fathering role (Parra-Cordona et al., 2006). The goals of the parenting program were to increase adolescent fathers' understanding of their own issues about becoming a father as a reflection of his experiences as a son, to offer resources to cope with issues between himself and the child's mother, to increase comfort in childcare for infants, and to teach adolescent fathers fundamental parenting and childcare skills.

A recent single-subject design for a father of a 3-year-old child with autism tested an Applied Behavioral Analysis intervention based on fatherhood theories of paternal engagement. In-home father coaching sessions included weekly sessions targeting four responsive strategies. These included follow-in comments, follow-in directives, symbolic object play, and rough-tumble play. The father-focused intervention was associated with competency in three of the four targeted strategies (follow-in comments, follow-in directives, and rough-and-tumble/physical play). Child use of single words increased over baseline and beginning use of multiword utterances were also observed (Flippin, 2018).

Another engagement-based tailoring is the Coaching Our Acting-Out Children: Heightening Essential Skills program (COACHES: Fabiano, 2007; Fabiano et al., 2009). The approach behind the COACHES program development was to first identify activities that often have high levels of father involvement such as sports activities and little leagues for young children. COACHES integrated the salient activity of sports activities into an evidence-based parent training program. For the first hour, children practice soccer skills while the fathers meet in a large group and review effective parenting strategies. During the second hour, fathers coach their children in a soccer little league game, and they are asked to practice the parenting strategies (e.g., catching the child being good) within the context of the sport. In an initial randomized trial of 75 families randomly assigned to COACHES versus a wait-list control condition, fathers who attended COACHES attended more parent training sessions and were more likely to complete homework assignments. Moreover, fathers and their children in the COACHES condition were less likely to drop out and were more satisfied with treatment process, and at posttreatment fathers rated their children as more improved relative to a traditional parent training approach ($d = 0.49$; Fabiano et al., 2009). In another independent evaluation of 55 randomized families testing father-only participation in COACHES and parent training relative to a wait-list control, similarly, medium effects were obtained for reductions in fathers' negative talk ($d = 0.57$) and for increases in father praise ($d = 0.54$).

A more recent father-focused intervention from the same research group focused on another salient father-child activity for young children, reading books together (Chacko, Fabiano, Doctoroff, & Fortson, 2018). Testing the Fathers Supporting Success in Preschoolers: A Community Parent Education Program (FSSP), 126 families were randomized to either FSSP or wait-list controls. Random-effects regression models revealed significant improvements for reductions in father-reported coercive discipline ($d = 0.82$), increases in reported positive parenting behaviors ($d = 0.91$), and medium effects for reductions in observed negative parenting ($d = 0.53$) and improvements in observed positive parenting ($d = 0.63$). Participating fathers in the FSSP were not recruited to work on parenting or to reduce child behavior problems, but rather were recruited to learn skills to support their children's school readiness. Chacko et al. (2018) argue that these strength-based procedures reduce stigma and contributed to the high rates of father engagement in intervention components (79% average attendance by FSSP fathers).

Finally, identity theory shows promise for tailoring motivational and social learning components of father interventions. Identity theories have garnered much theoretical attention in an effort to explain variation in father involvement. At the same time, however, very little empirical attention has been paid to these theories for intervention development. Fathering identity theories simply posit that the more a father identifies with the father role and the more important or central it is to his self-conception, the more involved he will be with his children (Ihinger-Tallman, Pasley, & Buehler, 1995; Madden-Derdich & Leonard, 2000).

Identity theory emphasizes both how behavioral interactions shape meanings and definitions of self and conversely how identities provide behavioral guidance. Because of their desire to stay involved with their children, effective programs targeting father identities may benefit from father-oriented components increasing men's awareness of the fathering role and how it impacts child development and fills child-centered needs (Brotherson, Dollahite, & Hawkins, 2005). Using causal modeling, DeGarmo (2010) demonstrated that increases in fathering identity predicted growth in the quality of observed father involvement for residential and nonresidential fathers. That is, fathers' identification with the fathering role was more predictive of fathering behaviors, than were the effects of father involvement on changes in fathering identity. Fathering identity was measured as identity salience, the forced-choice ranking of importance of the fathering role, relative to other role domains. Identity salience also predicted well as longitudinal reductions in father health problems and substance use (DeGarmo, Reid, Leve, Chamberlain, & Knutson, 2010).

Identity theory also posits that positive behavioral and interactional feedback can reinforce and strengthen positive and more desirable definitions of self-identity and fathering roles, a plausible putative mechanism for increasing fathers' commitment to parenting roles (Høivik et al., 2015). DeGarmo, Jones, and Rains (2019) recently tested a within-group pilot study of a strength-based video feedback program designed to improve fathers' sense of efficacy in the parenting role. Trained therapists treated eleven divorced fathers with three to five home-visit, video feedback sessions over 12 months. Data showed reductions in harsh discipline and inept parenting and evidence of improvements in efficacy and father involvement. Changes in fathering identity were significantly associated with changes in parental efficacy ($r = 0.47$), harsh parenting ($r = 0.64$), and inept parenting ($r = 0.42$).

Recommendations for Promoting Father Engagement in Parent Training

Given that fathers independently and jointly impact healthy child development and that fathers are at risk for lack of engagement in parenting interventions, directly below are bulleted and explicated recommendations for researchers and practitioners based on studies reviewed above.

Employ a Generative Fathering Perspective to Raise Awareness of Fathers' Impact on Their Child and Avoid a Deficit Model

Reviews consistently show that a primary factor for overcoming fathers' lack of engagement in parent training is avoiding internalized negative attitudes toward fathers. Programs that employ a deficit model emphasizing fathering flaws needing corrective action are averse to fathers and a threat to their participation (Lechowicz et al., 2019; Panter-Brick et al., 2014). Moreover, negative attitudes by service providers and beliefs on whether father involvement in treatment is beneficial are an external and relational barrier for father engagement in services or treatments (Pfitzner, Humphreys, & Hegarty, 2017).

Rather, strength-based and generative fathering perspectives are needed to raise awareness of fathers' developmental impact on their children. For social services, it is essential to build rapport and trust and emphasize that services or treatments are a partnership working with fathers rather than working on fathers (Pfitzner et al., 2017). Clinical strategies from programs involving maltreating and abusive fathers have shown that fathers are more responsive to interventions raising awareness of father impacts on their children and focusing on the welfare and needs of the children as a focal point for addressing harmful interactions with spouses and children (Rosenberg & Wilcox, 2006; Scott & Crooks, 2007). For example, in a recent pilot evaluation of the *Dads Matter* program, a perinatal home visitation program for new parents at risk for abuse and neglect,

Guterman, Bellamy, and Banman (2018) designed an enhanced home visitation program for new parents. Large effect sizes were obtained with d ranging from −0.75 to −0.90 for self-report of child neglect, physical assault, and psychological aggression toward child. The program also directly impacted fathers' attitudes regarding the values of their contributions to their children's well-being ($d = 0.42$).

Employ Father-Friendly Treatment Implementation Strategies

Father engagement in evidence-based programs is hampered by interpersonal and service-based barriers to participation (DeGarmo et al., 2016). Identified barriers include scheduling conflicts and timing, transportation and childcare, fatigue, motivation, stigma, and geographic location. Alternate modalities of intervention implementation may be more acceptable for fathers' contextual factors and may provide greater reach for participation. Web and mobile connectivity to deliver parenting education is sensible and logical given the technology habits of today's parents, the "digital natives," immersed in digital media (Oblinger, Oblinger, & Lippincott, 2005).

Implementation through mobile and smartphone technology can also provide greater efficiency and timeliness to capture real-time, ongoing data on a large scale to better understand and perhaps to provide more immediate support, feedback, and engagement in parent training (Chacko et al., 2016).

Reviews consistently report that the use of male facilitators and, more importantly, peer and contextually relatable facilitators is also key for successful engagement (DeGarmo et al., 2016; Lechowicz et al., 2019). In two-parent families, the use of male-female facilitators for demonstrating manualized co-parenting practices and for providing meaningful role-play opportunities is important for effective uptake of parent training.

Raising Awareness, Advertising, and Providing Better Outreach

Beyond views of program purveyors, reviews of participation barriers from fathers' perspectives indicate that in general there is a lack of knowledge and experience of available parenting programs (Frank et al., 2015; Siccouri et al., 2018). The father-infant Fathers Club discussed above (Rempel et al., 2017), for example, employed a specific strategy for increasing community awareness. It is key that effective programs are also designed for portability and sustainability. For many father programs, local advocacy is needed for successful adoption by service agencies.

Engage and Support Both Parents and Other Primary Caregivers

For two-parent families, evidence remains mixed on whether father-only groups are more effective than mixed-parent groups. First, preference data suggest that fathers prefer father-only groups (Frank et al., 2015). Indeed, tailored programs focusing on individual father development of fathering skills within the family exhibit beneficial effects for fathers. The Re:Membering Fatherhood Program was designed for fathers motivated to improve their individual fathering experience (Gearing, Colvin, Popova, & Regehr, 2008). However, several sets of empirical data suggest that mixed gender mother-father groups are more effective than father-only groups for at-risk families (Cowan et al., 2010). Moreover, experimental evidence for two-parent families suggests that father-only parent training groups do not generalize benefits within the family to untreated mothers (Fabiano et al., 2012).

There are several related factors that are likely driving the effectiveness of two-parent engagement relative to father-only treatments. These include increased interparental consistency and the promotion of a united front in the implementation of parenting practices, addressing coercive parenting practices of both parents, and reducing co-parenting conflict (DeGarmo & Forgatch, 2007; Sicouri et al., 2018). The evidence reviewed in the first sections of this report also suggests that more effective parent training involves the family as a system and consideration of shared parenting values.

Experimental Strategies for Tailoring Father Programs

This section focuses on experimental approaches for identifying causal mechanism for increasing father engagement in parent training and for identifying "tailoring variables" to enhance compliance. These include the use of preference trials, comparative effectiveness studies, and sequential multiple assignment randomized trials (SMART studies).

Preference Trials

Using a mixed method survey approach with a community sample of 160 fathers, Frank et al. (2015) examined father preferences for participation in parent training programs. Consistent with a strength-based focus on child well-being, the highest-rated preferences include building a positive parent-child relationship, increasing children's socioemotional and behavioral skills, and programs that include the importance of fathers' contribution to child development. From an implementation point of view, fathers' preferred delivery methods include father-only groups, individually tailored programs, and less intensive options such as seminars, video-based content, and self-directed web-based series (Frank et al., 2015). In a larger community sample of 1001 Australian fathers, Tully et al. (2017) report that fathers reported understanding what is involved in the program and knowing that a facilitator is well-trained as the two leading factors affecting the decision to participate.

More formal and rigorous testing of preferences involves experimental tests of preferences among participants. Preferences represent what individuals would want in intervention programs if they were given the choice. Lack of consideration of choice/preference can lead to higher rates of noncompliance and greater rates of attrition (Brown et al., 2009). In a meta-analysis of 35 treatment studies, Swift, Callahan, and Vollmer (2011) found that clients who were matched to their preferred therapy conditions were less likely to drop out of therapy prematurely (odds ratio [OR] 0.59, $p < 0.001$) and showed greater improvements in treatment outcomes ($d = 0.31$, $p < 0.001$). In a recent doubly randomized PMTO preference trial (Gewirtz, Lee, August, & He, 2018; He, Gewirtz, Lee, Morrell, & August, 2016), 129 families referred to community mental health clinics for child conduct problems were randomized to either choice or no-choice conditions. In the stage 2 randomization, parents were offered choices between (or were randomized to) home- or clinic-based, individual, and group versions of PMTO or services as usual within the mental health clinics. Families assigned to the no-choice condition were significantly more likely to drop out of treatment than those in the choice condition ($OR = 3.12$; 95% confidence interval [1.18–8.29]). In the choice condition, in-home treatment was the preferred modality, and across conditions, families were more likely to drop out of group and clinic modalities. Moreover, assignment to the choice condition was associated with greater teacher-reported reductions in some child problem behaviors at 6 months post-treatment termination and with improved observed parenting practices among those in the choice group who selected PMTO, compared with those who selected treatment as usual. A larger empirical database is needed to causally determine preferences that are associated with greater father engagement.

Comparative Effectiveness Studies

Comparative effectiveness designs can directly inform how previously validated programs can be modified to determine if more cost-effective, brief, or alternative delivery methods will be as efficacious as standing evidence-based treatments. Advantages of intensive individual- or group-based parent training include greater coverage of content, direct monitoring and feedback, normalization and support through participation in group interventions, and troubleshooting. Some disadvantages of intensive behavioral interventions, however, are costs, the need to train staff and maintain fidelity, scheduling that is inconvenient to families and staff, location of services, and stigma for families. These factors can be particularly relevant for fathers (Tully et al., 2017; DeGarmo & Jones, 2019).

As a result, service providers often struggle with striking an adequate balance between implementation resources and intensity of parenting training or services; that is, if a program is too brief and too cost-effective, it may not be effective enough for successful learning and uptake by clients. As suggested above, one strategy is increasing the use of online and digital parent training. As such, with the growing number of interactive modular interventions being developed and adopted, evaluation of evidence for the effectiveness is imperative using randomized comparative effectiveness.

For example, two recent meta-analyses suggest online programs have potential for effectiveness. Using studies with direct comparison of in-person BPT versus digital online BPT, Baumel and colleagues found that reduced professional support compared with full-contact conditions was not inferior and showed slight improvement in comparison with usual care (Cohen's $d = 0.34$; Baumel, Pawar, Kane, & Correll, 2016). For children younger than age 9 years, digital parent training programs have obtained Cohen's d ranging from 0.41 to 0.80 (Baumel et al., 2016), and for adolescents, Cohen's d has ranged from 0.17 to 0.20 (Baumel, Pawar, Mathur, Kane, & Correll, 2017).

Adaptive Interventions and SMART Designs

Adaptive intervention strategies, also referred to as *dynamic treatment regimens*, are sequential individualized, multiple component interventions in which the intensity or type of treatment is varied after treatment begins in response to the evolving needs and monitored progress of study participants (Almirall & Chronis-Tuscano, 2016). Response to intervention designs are based on the idea that with early evaluation of data, adaptations and design characteristics can be altered to improve effectiveness either in terms of responsiveness or in terms of implementation efficiency. Because response to interventions is evaluated during the course of the study, adaptive designs are often *accelerated* designs.

The primary rationale for response to intervention studies is identifying and addressing slow responding and nonresponding individuals within a given intervention program. Many fathers may remain symptomatic at the end of multiyear traditional randomized control trial (RCT). Through carefully executed sequencing and multiple randomization, one can accelerate the pace at which inferences are made about program effectiveness, thus providing information on optimal intervention strategies in a shorter time frame than would be the case in traditional RCTs. Data-informed decisions might be made to vary dosage or delivery modalities, or to further tailor options to the needs of fathers by providing indicated or high-intensity treatments, as opposed to fixed allocated treatments or universal approaches only. Adaptive designs are characterized by several key design and planning elements: decision points, decision rules, tailoring variables, and intervention options. The aim of decision points and decision rules is to guide researchers or clinicians on when and which intervention options to use at each stage of the adaptive intervention. Decisions are based on readily available information relating to the characteristics or ongoing performance of the participant.

Specifically, in an adaptive intervention, the intervention options are based on participant scores on a *tailoring variable*. Tailoring variables are person-level data used to make decisions about alterations in further randomization. A tailoring variable can be (a) an important precursor to an intended outcome, (b) an important moderator of intervention uptake, or (c) an important moderator of intervention effectiveness. Thus, a tailoring variable may not be directly related to the criterion outcome, but simply to engagement in or adherence to the intervention. For many adaptive designs, the focus of the research is to tailor interventions that promote greater engagement or to enhance full uptake of an intervention. The tailoring variable is then associated with identifying nonresponders and slow responders. A nonresponder may be defined simply as a person who does not attend intervention sessions or a person who attends but does not complete all the required components of treatment. These tailoring variables can be readily assessed with implementation process variables such as attendance and compliance and simply require cut scores to determine those classified as responders versus nonresponders. For example, fathers who are not responding to initial sessions of parent training may be further randomized to receive motivational interviewing. With the accelerated experimental design, outcome data would determine if motivational interviewing is effective or not in providing greater gains for fathers who are initially nonresponders. Thus, an adaptive design is an ideal candidate for better improving fathers' participation in evidence-based parent training.

The SMART—the sequential multiple assignment randomized trial—is a specific type of adaptive design. The focus of a SMART is to better understand what sequence of interventions is more effective. For example, Pelham et al. (2016) conducted a SMART adaptive intervention to treat young children (ages 5–12) with attention-deficit/hyperactivity disorder (ADHD). A sample of 146 children was randomized to start with low amounts of either behavioral parent training (BPT) or extended-release ADHD medication. After 8 weeks, nonresponders to BPT or medication were re-randomized to secondary interventions that either increased the intensity of BPT or dosage of medication. The group beginning with BPT showed significantly fewer disciplinary referrals and lower rates of problem behaviors observed in the classrooms at school. Adding medication as a secondary treatment was more beneficial to the BPT group than it was for adding it to the initial medication group. Parents who initially began BPT had better attendance than those receiving BPT after medication. Thus, sequencing and beginning treatment with BPT produced better overall outcomes than starting with medication.

Adaptive designs can determine what programs are more effective for fathers; what types of interventions lead to better retention, participation, and compliance; and what programs are equally effective using an accelerated timeline. To date, adaptive designs have not been designed or tested to demonstrate what factors improve father participation in parent training. Tailoring variables can be piloted and determined a priori, or they can be determined by evaluation of moderators after data is collected in a given SMART trial.

The SIL Model and Fathering Through Change (FTC)

To illustrate a recently tailored intervention, this last section provides data from a recently adapted PMTO model designed to address the specific needs of single fathers. The evidence-based program was tailored to be father-centric, to focus on and enhance the father-child relationship, and was delivered in a modality to provide greater access and coverage of single fathers by employing interactive and standardized online parent training (DeGarmo & Jones, 2019). The study was predicated on the social interaction learning (SIL) model. The SIL model focuses on how the family social environment shapes and establishes overlearned patterns of behavior that can generalize across social settings for a developing child. Parenting practices are the key agent of child socialization. Parent-child social interaction patterns are the behavioral mechanism that reinforces a child's likelihood of engaging in future prosocial or antisocial behaviors. Relatedly, the coercion model more specifically focuses on how antisociality and harsh, punitive, and ineffective discipline are associated with growth in children's aggression and comorbid problem behaviors. For example, unskilled and antisocial parents may use hitting, yelling, and harsh punishment to discipline a child to stop an aversive child behavior. Coercive discipline works in the short run; however, in the long run, a child can learn that coercion among family members can be used to terminate aversive behaviors of other family members. A child may then learn to apply aggression and coercion in relationships with peers and other adults. From the SIL perspective, treatment and prevention of coercive process entails teaching parents how to rearrange and manage consequences to decrease aggressive behavior and to increase more prosocial behaviors through effective parenting practices (Patterson, 2005). This work involving fathers and the role of family structure transitions laid the theoretical foundation for Fathering Through Change (FTC).

The Fathering Through Change (FTC) Program

The FTC was funded by a phase 2 small business innovation research grant (R44 HD075499) and was adapted from the evidence-based BPT program PMTO. Based on separate focus group data from key stakeholders, including fathers, judges, and court administrators, the FTC was tailored to the needs of divorced and separating fathers, with a major focus on the relevance of the fathering role and its impact on children. Several focus groups were conducted in both phase 1 and phase 2 of the study prior to intervention development. Father-identified challenges included reduced contact with children, conflict with the ex-spouse over parenting, and lack of opportunities for peer support. One theme was the lack of an "instructional manual" for parenting on your own. Desired content for a fathering program included themes on how to strengthen their relationship with their children, how to deal with stress and emotions, and specific help with discipline; one father stated this as "How to find a good balance between being a 'Disneyland dad' and being a firm one." Integrating these preferences and further translation and tailoring of PMTO for FTC involved formal consultation with several PMTO-certified trainers and consultation with the director of the Association of Families and Conciliation Courts. When completed, the FTC was designed to improve parenting skills, strengthen the father-child relationship, and reduce stress in the lives of fathers. In turn, these targeted outcomes were intended to decrease child adjustment problems during and after the separation and divorce process.

The FTC intervention program uses a number of instructional processes, including video sequences, web-based interactivity, web-based social connectivity and networking, and email and phone text instructional prompting. Each of these modalities was also identified as desirable in focus groups and was tested for acceptability and usability before conducting phase 2 of the study. The FTC modules use several instructional methods, including explicit instruction, modeling, and practice. The theory of instruction (Engelmann & Carnine, 1991) relies on clear presentation of conceptual material, skill-based material presented through instructional pacing, use of positive and negative examples, and cumulative review of previously taught materials. The program also includes an electronic journal to tailor progress, note challenges and successes, and provide evaluation with checks for fidelity.

The FTC program curriculum includes ten content modules. The first 6 weeks include sequentially ordered core cumulative program content that is *precedent* ordered, meaning fathers are required to complete one assigned module per week in order to proceed to new content. The first 6 weeks include the modules *Introduction to the Program, Give Effective Directions, Teach Through Encouragement, Recognize and Regulate Emotions,* and *Use Discipline That Works*. Week 6 consists of review and refinement designed to review and troubleshoot. Weeks 7 through 10 include *Solve Problems, Protect Children From Conflict, Active Communication,* and *Strengthen Your Relationship*.

The efficacy study was a 12-week, two-arm, randomized controlled trial design. Fathers were randomly assigned to the FTC online parent training or to the wait-list control condition (see Fig. 40.1). The final study sample included 426 participating fathers; 225 were randomly assigned

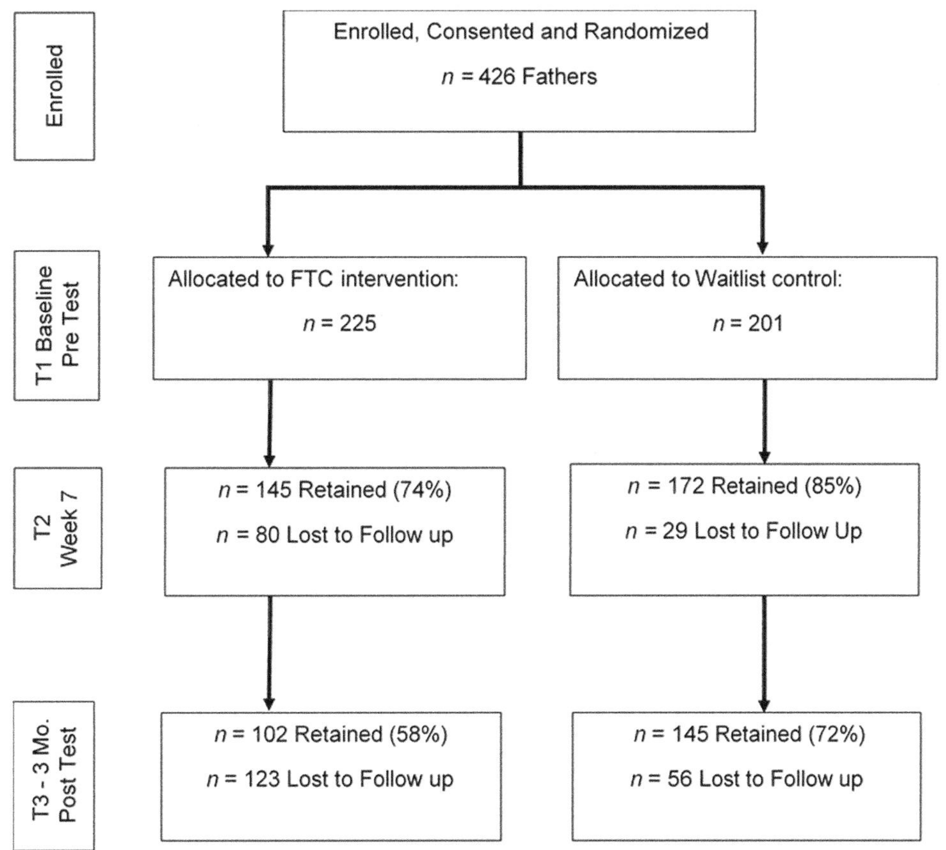

Fig. 40.1 CONSORT flow chart for study fathers

to the FTC intervention condition and 201 to the wait-list control condition. Among the fathers, 74% were legally married prior to separation, 61% had joint legal custody, 14% had full legal custody, 6% reported that the co-parent had legal custody, and 19% reported custody had not yet been finalized. The average age of the fathers was 37.24 and average age of the focal child was 7.88 years. Boys comprised 56% of the sample of focal children.

Initial evaluation data were reported in DeGarmo and Jones (2019) with the primary targeted outcome being self-reported parenting practices. The intent to treat analyses showed that the FTC obtained a small direct effect on father-reported pre-post changes in child adjustment problems ($d = 0.20$) measured with a latent variable specified with the Eyberg Child Behavior Inventory T scales (Burns & Patterson, 2000) and the Prosocial Subscale of the Strengths and Difficulties Questionnaire (Ford, Hutchings, Bywater, Goodman, & Goodman, 2009). A medium effect on pre-post changes in fathers' coercive parenting ($d = 0.61$) was detected using a latent variable of coercive parenting, prosocial, and inept subscales of the Parenting Practices Interview (Webster-Stratton, Reid, & Hammond, 2001). To illustrate effectiveness of the intervention uptake, Fig. 40.2 displays boxplots and fitted group mean trajectories with 95% confidence intervals for the FTC knowledge test. The knowledge test was a measure designed to objectively assess uptake of the intervention content. The knowledge test was comprised of 15 true or false items on intervention components and thus ranged from 0 to 15. The knowledge test was assessed in both conditions at pre- and post-intervention and at follow-up. The control group is the left panel and the FTC is on the right.

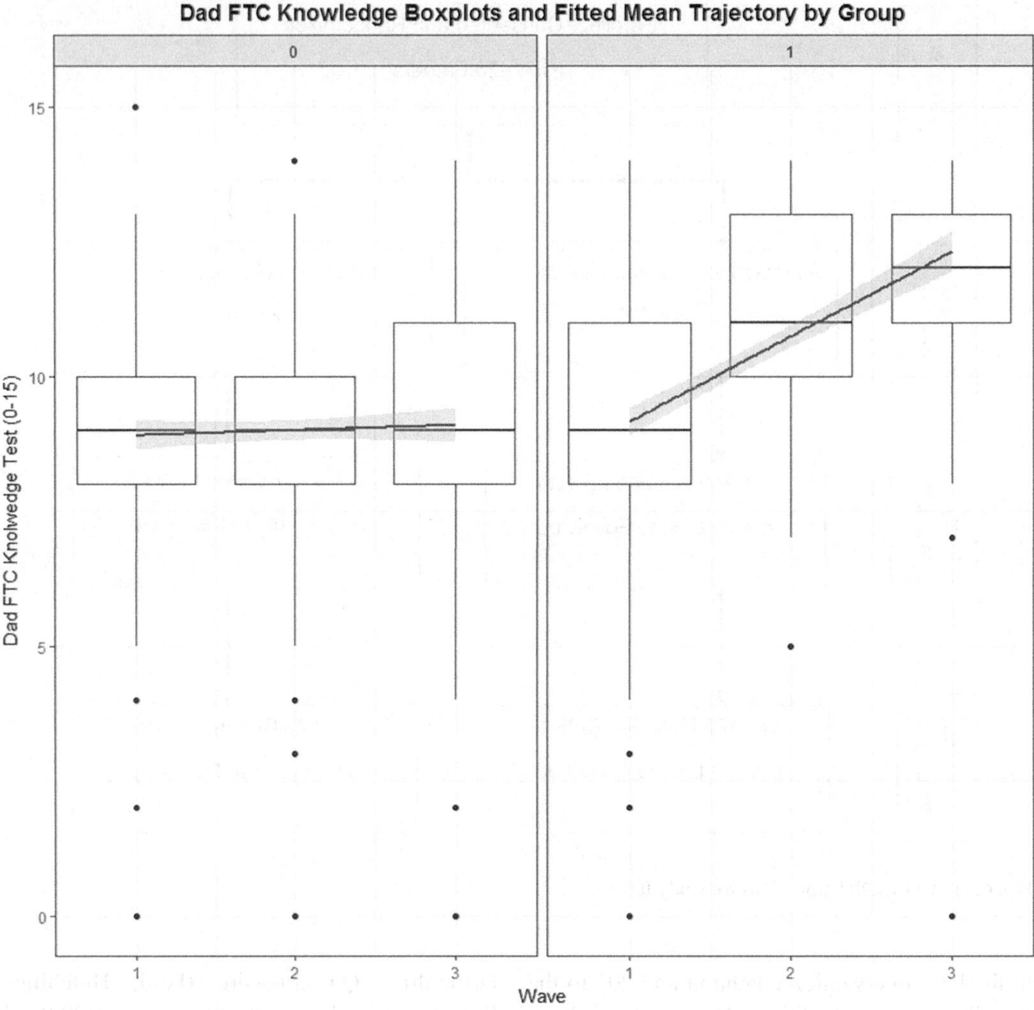

Fig. 40.2 Boxplots and fitted mean trajectories by group across time for FTC knowledge test of intervention content

As shown in the CONSORT flow, there were differential rates of attrition by group condition, with 85% of controls retained at T2 compared with 64% of the FTC condition and 72% of controls at T3 compared with 45% of FTC condition. Among 54 baseline demographic variables and key outcome study scales, attrition analyses indicated only one significant difference observed between those retained and those lost to follow-up, fewer than expected by chance false discovery. Fathers lost to follow-up were lower in reported education compared with those retained (T2 $M = 4.46$ and 4.11, $n = 317$ and 104, respectively, $t = 2.19$*; T3 $M = 4.54$ and 4.14, $n = 247$ and 174, respectively, $t = 2.83$**).

Because differential rates of attrition were observed between randomized conditions, intervention effects could be overestimated if higher functioning fathers were retained in the treatment condition. Therefore, complier average causal effect (CACE) models were specified to estimate the intervention effects adjusting for compliers and noncompliers in the intervention group and estimated "would-be" compliers in the control group. CACE uses mixture models, or estimated categorical profiles, to provide unbiased estimates of intervention effect by estimating the unknown compliance status of the control condition as missing data. This unbiased estimate provides a better understanding of how a program

Table 40.1 Y standardized indirect effects and confidence intervals for intent to treat and complier average causal effect model

Indirect path	Indirect effect	95th percent *CI*
FTC ITT → −.61*** → Change father coercive → .49*** → Change child problems	−0.30***	[−0.53, −0.14][1]
FTC CACE → −.80*** → Change father coercive → .45** → Change child problems	−0.36*	[−0.60, −0.12]

Data from DeGarmo and Jones (2019)
Note. [1]Bias-corrected bootstrapped confidence intervals with 1000 draws
***$p < 0.001$
**$p < 0.01$
*$p < 0.05$

works by estimating what would happen to the control group had they been offered the intervention by directly comparing characteristics of participants in the intervention group that complied with treatment (observed compliance) with estimates of would-be compliers or noncompliers in the control condition (estimated compliance), based on their study and group-matched characteristics. Findings are shown in Table 40.1.

CACE models indicated intervention effects were robust compared with findings from the ITT models. These models address fathers who were retained but did not engage. Unfortunately, threats to internal validity remained because of potential dropouts of the study. However, attrition analyses of all outcome and baseline demographics revealed only one difference for fathers' education, which was controlled for in the analyses.

In summary, the FTC was illustrated here as an example of adapting an evidence-based parent training program and tailoring it to the needs and preferences of fathers. The efficacy evaluation supported the notion that online interactive interventions can be acceptable and efficacious for fathers. The differential attrition also suggests that adaptive designs could be employed to better understand factors that will promote father retention and participation rates. Preference trials may also lend themselves to improving father participation and effectiveness.

Summary and Key Points

This chapter focused on parent training evidence for fathers of young children, mainly the periods of perinatal infancy and early childhood. Despite several decades of developing, testing, replicating, and disseminating effective behavioral parent training and psychosocial education, worldwide evidence suggests that children's social emotional and behavioral adjustment remains a public health concern. At the same time, cumulative data also show that effective parent training demonstrates short- and long-term benefits for children and for parents' well-being.

Unfortunately, when offered, fathers' participation remains low. In addition, it remains extremely surprising that very few theory-driven and rigorously evaluated father-focused parenting programs exist. This is still the case despite the increase in father time in childcare (Sullivan, Coltrane, McAnnally, & Altintas, 2009) and the explosion of archival and prospective research conducted on father involvement as a result of federal fatherhood initiatives (Lamb, 2004). Public policy and fatherhood research has come a long way in accepting changing cultural values and empirical data that residential and nonresidential fathers matter in the healthy development of children. What remains to be accomplished is better inclusion of fathers in social, behavioral, genetic, and epidemiological studies of child and family development. More importantly, because fathers are at risk for low participation and yet, independently contribute to child development, more father-inclusive, father-friendly, and father-focused parent training programs are needed as stand-alone or in unison with couples' parent training. In addition to qualitative studies, more rigorous experimental designs are needed to inform the field on how to better engage fathers and how to tailor programs to be more father-inclusive. Directly, below are final summary points based on the data reviewed above.

- Evidence still shows that compared to mothering, relatively few parent training interventions are tailored to fathers or multifarious father populations.
- Engaging fathers in evidence-based programs leads to better maintenance and outcomes for mothers, fathers, and children.
- Although preference data suggest fathers prefer father groups, benefits of conducting father-only groups remain mixed.
- When offered to couples, roughly one in five fathers participates in parent training.
- Traditional and cultural contexts regarding breadwinning identities need to be incorporated to promote fathers as co-equal co-parenting partners.
- Social services and parent training need to focus on working *with* fathers and not *on* fathers.
- Tailoring father-focused programs need to avoid deficit models and focus on generative fathering and strength-based approaches, particularly raising awareness of fathers' impact on their children.
- Programs need to consider fathers' associated breadwinner and employment identities in tailoring more flexible, accessible, and more time-sensitive programs.
- In addition to qualitative studies, rigorous experimental designs are needed to test factors predicting engagement of fathers. These include comparative effectiveness, preference trials, and SMART trials, each of which is in their nascency regarding studies of father engagement and compliance.

References

Almirall, D., & Chronis-Tuscano, A. (2016). Adaptive Interventions in child and adolescent mental health. *Journal of Clinical Child & Adolescent Psychology, 45*(4), 383–395. https://doi.org/10.1080/15374416.2016.1152555

Asmussen, K., & Weizel, K. (2010). *Evaluating the evidence: Fathers, families and children*. National Academy for Parenting Research, King's College.

Bagner, D. M. (2013). Father's role in parent training for children with developmental delay. *Journal of Family Psychology, 27*(4), 650–657. https://doi.org/10.1037/a0033465

Bagner, D. M., & Eyberg, S. M. (2003). Father involvement in parent training: When does it matter? *Journal of Clinical Child & Adolescent Psychology, 32*, 337–342. https://doi.org/10.1207/S15374424JCCP3204_13

Bakermans-Kranenburg, M. J., van IJzendoorn, M. H., & Juffer, F. (2005). Disorganized infant attachment and preventive interventions: A review and meta-analysis. *Infant Mental Health Journal, 26*(3), 191–216. https://doi.org/10.1002/imhj.20046

Baumel, A., Pawar, A., Kane, J. M., & Correll, C. U. (2016). Digital parent training for children with disruptive behaviors: Systematic review and meta-analysis of randomized trials. *Journal of Child and Adolescent Psychopharmacology, 26*(8), 740–749. https://doi.org/10.1089/cap.2016.0048

Baumel, A., Pawar, A., Mathur, N., Kane, J. M., & Correll, C. U. (2017). Technology-assisted parent training programs for children and adolescents with disruptive behaviors: A systematic review. *Journal of Clinical Psychiatry, 78*(8), e957–e969. https://doi.org/10.4088/JCP.16r11063

Brotherson, S. E., Dollahite, D. C., & Hawkins, A. J. (2005). Generative fathering and the dynamics of connection between fathers and their children. *Fathering, 3*(1), 1–28.

Brown, C. H., Ten Have, T. R., Jo, B., Dagne, G., Wyman, P. A., Muthén, B., et al. (2009). Adaptive designs for randomized trials in public health. *Annual Review of Public Health, 30*, 1–25. https://doi.org/10.1146/annurev.publhealth.031308.100223

Bullard, L., Wachlarowicz, M., DeLeeuw, J., Snyder, J., Low, S., Forgatch, M. S., et al. (2010). Effects of the Oregon Model of Parent Management Training (PMTO) on marital adjustment in new stepfamilies: A randomized trial. *Journal of Family Psychology, 24*(4), 485–496. https://doi.org/10.1037/a0020267

Burns, G., & Patterson, D. R. (2000). Factor structure of the Eyberg Child Behavior Inventory: A parent rating scale of oppositional defiant behavior toward adults, inattentive behavior, and conduct problem behavior. *Journal of Clinical Child Psychology, 29*, 569–577. https://doi.org/10.1207/S15374424JCCP2904_9

Cabrera, N. J., Shannon, J. D., & Tamis-LeMonda, C. (2007). Fathers' influence on their children's cognitive and emotional development: From toddlers to pre-K.

Applied Developmental Science, 11, 208–213. https://doi.org/10.1080/10888690701762100

Chacko, A., Fabiano, G. A., Doctoroff, G. L., & Fortson, B. (2018). Engaging fathers in effective parenting for preschool children using shared book reading: A randomized controlled trial. *Journal of Clinical Child & Adolescent Psychology, 47*(1), 79–93. https://doi.org/10.1080/15374416.2016.1266648

Chacko, A., Jensen, S., Lowry, L., Cornwell, M., Chimklis, A., Chan, E., et al. (2016). Engagement in behavioral parent training: Review of the literature and implications for practice. *Clinical Child & Family Psychology Review, 19*(3), 204–215. https://doi.org/10.1007/s10567-016-0205-2

Chen, E. M., Gau, M. L., Liu, C. Y., & Lee, T. Y. (2017). Effects of father-neonate skin-to-skin contact on attachment: A randomized controlled trial. *Nursing Research and Practice, 2017*, 8612024. https://doi.org/10.1155/2017/8612024

Cookston, J. T., Braver, S. L., Griffin, W. A., De Lusé, S. R., & Miles, J. C. (2007). Effects for the Dads for Life intervention on interparental conflict and co-parenting in the two years after divorce. *Family Process, 46*(1), 123–137. https://doi.org/10.1111/j.1545-5300.2006.00196.x

Cowan, C. P., Cowan, P. A., Pruett, M. K., & Pruett, K. (2007). An approach to preventing coparenting conflict and divorce in low-income families: Strengthening couple relationships and fostering fathers' involvement. *Family Process, 46*(1), 109–121. https://doi.org/10.1111/j.1545-5300.2006.00195.x

Cowan, P. A., Cowan, C. P., & Knox, V. (2010). Marriage and fatherhood programs. *The Future of Children, 20*(2), 205–230. https://doi.org/10.1353/foc.2010.0000

DeGarmo, D. S. (2010). A time varying evaluation of identity theory and father involvement for full custody, shared custody, and no custody divorced fathers. *Fathering, 8*(2), 181–202. https://doi.org/10.3149/fth.1802.181

DeGarmo, D. S., & Forgatch, M. S. (2007). Efficacy of parent training for stepfathers: From playful spectator and polite stranger to effective stepfathering. *Parenting: Science and Practice, 7*(4), 1–25. https://doi.org/10.1080/15295190701665631

DeGarmo, D. S., Jones, J., & Rains, L. A. (2019). A pilot study evaluation of Marte Meo for divorced fathers. *Journal of Family Therapy, 41*(2), 232–250. https://doi.org/10.1111/1467-6427.12221

DeGarmo, D. S., & Jones, J. A. (2019). Fathering Through Change (FTC) intervention for single fathers: Preventing coercive parenting and child problem behaviors. *Development and Psychopathology, 31*(5), 1801–1811. https://doi.org/10.1017/S0954579419001019

DeGarmo, D. S., Nordahl, K. B., & Fabiano, G. A. (2016). Fathers and coercion dynamics in families. In T. Dishion & J. Snyder (Eds.), *Oxford Handbook of Coercive Dynamics in Close Relationships: Implications for Development, Psychopathology and Intervention Science* (pp. 114–128). Oxford, NY: Oxford University Press.

DeGarmo, D. S., Reid, J. B., Leve, L. D., Chamberlain, P., & Knutson, J. F. (2010). Patterns and predictors of growth in divorced fathers' health status and substance use. *American Journal of Men's Health, 4*(1), 60–70. https://doi.org/10.1177/1557988308329454

Doherty, W. J., Erickson, M. F., & LaRossa, R. (2006). An intervention to increase father involvement and skills with infants during the transition to parenthood. *Journal of Family Psychology, 20*(3), 438–447. https://doi.org/10.1037/0893-3200.20.3.438

Doherty, W. J., Kouneski, E. F., & Erickson, M. F. (1998). Responsible fathering: An overview and conceptual framework. *Journal of Marriage and the Family, 60*, 277–292. https://doi.org/10.2307/353848

Doucet, A. (2004). "It's almost like I have a job, but I don't get paid": Fathers at home reconfiguring work, care, and masculinity. *Fathering, 2*(3), 277–303.

Duncombe, M. E., Havighurst, S. S., Holland, K. A., & Frankling, E. J. (2012). The contribution of parenting practices and parent emotion factors in children at risk for disruptive behavior disorders. *Child Psychiatry & Human Development, 43*(5), 715–733. https://doi.org/10.1007/s10578-012-0290-5

Engelmann, S., & Carnine, D. (1991). *Theory of instruction: Principles and applications*. Eugene, OR: ADI Press.

Erskine, H. E., Norman, R. E., Ferrari, A. J., Chan, G. C., Copeland, W. E., Whiteford, H. A., et al. (2016). Long-term outcomes of attention-deficit/hyperactivity disorder and conduct disorder: A systematic review and meta-analysis. *Journal of the American Academy of Child & Adolescent Psychiatry, 55*(10), 841–850. https://doi.org/10.1016/j.jaac.2016.06.016

Fabiano, G. A. (2007). Father participation in behavioral parent training for ADHD: Review and recommendations for increasing inclusion and engagement. *Journal of Family Psychology, 21*(4), 683–693. https://doi.org/10.1037/0893-3200.21.4.683

Fabiano, G. A., Chacko, A., Pelham, W. E., Robb, J., Walker, K. S., Wymbs, F., et al. (2009). A comparison of behavioral parent training programs for fathers of children with attention-deficit/hyperactivity disorder. *Behavior Therapy, 40*(2), 190–204. https://doi.org/10.1016/j.beth.2008.05.002

Fabiano, G. A., Pelham, W. E., Cunningham, C. E., Yu, J., Gangloff, B., Buck, M., et al. (2012). A waitlist-controlled trial of behavioral parent training for fathers of children with ADHD. *Journal of Clinical Child & Adolescent Psychology, 41*(3), 337–345. https://doi.org/10.1080/15374416.2012.654464

Fletcher, R., Freeman, E., & Mathey, S. (2011). The impact of behavioral parent training on fathers' parenting: A meta-analysis of the Triple P-Positive Parenting Program. *Fathering, 9*(3), 291–312. https://doi.org/10.3149/fth.0903.291

Flippin, M. (2018). Using father-mediated intervention to increase responsive parental behaviors and child communication in children with autism spectrum disorder:

A pilot study. *Journal of Clinical and Translational Science, 2*(S1), 50–50. https://doi.org/10.1017/cts.2018.192

Flouri, E. (2005). *Fathering and child outcomes*. Chichester, UK: Wiley.

Ford, T., Hutchings, J., Bywater, T., Goodman, A., & Goodman, R. (2009). Strengths and difficulties questionnaire added value scores: Evaluating effectiveness in child mental health interventions. *The British Journal of Psychiatry, 194*, 552–558. https://doi.org/10.1192/bjp.bp.108.052373

Forgatch, M. S., DeGarmo, D. S., & Beldavs, Z. G. (2005). An efficacious theory-based intervention for stepfamilies. *Behavior Therapy, 36*(4), 357–365. https://doi.org/10.1016/S0005-7894(05)80117-0

Frank, T. J., Keown, L. J., Dittman, C. K., & Sanders, M. R. (2015). Using father preference data to increase father engagement in evidence-based parenting programs. *Journal of Child and Family Studies, 24*(4), 937–947. https://doi.org/10.1007/s10826-014-9904-9

Furlong, M., McGilloway, S., Bywater, T., Hutchings, J., Smith, S. M., & Donnelly, M. (2013). Cochrane Review: Behavioural and cognitive-behavioural group-based parenting programmes for early-onset conduct problems in children aged 3 to 12 years (Review). *Evidence-Based Child Health: A Cochrane Review Journal, 8*(2), 318–692. https://doi.org/10.1002/ebch.1905

Gearing, R. E., Colvin, G., Popova, S., & Regehr, C. (2008). Re:Membering fatherhood: Evaluating the impact of a group intervention on fathering. *Journal for Specialists in Group Work, 33*(1), 22–42. https://doi.org/10.1080/01933920701798539

Gewirtz, A. H., Lee, S. S., August, G. J., & He, Y. (2018). Does giving parents their choice of interventions for child behavior problems improve child outcomes? *Prevention Science, 19*, 589–599. https://doi.org/10.1007/s11121-018-0865-x

Guterman, N. B., Bellamy, J. L., & Banman, A. (2018). Promoting father involvement in early home visiting services for vulnerable families: Findings from a pilot study of "dads matter". *Child Abuse and Neglect: The International Journal, 76*, 261–272. https://doi.org/10.1016/j.chiabu.2017.10.017

He, Y., Gewirtz, A., Lee, S., Morrell, N., & August, G. (2016). A randomized preference trial to inform personalization of a parent training program implemented in community mental health clinics. *Translational Behavioral Medicine, 6*(1), 73–80. https://doi.org/10.1007/s13142-015-0366-4

Høivik, M. S., Lydersen, S., Drugli, M. B., Onsøien, R., Hansen, M. B., & Nielsen, T. S. B. (2015). Video feedback compared to treatment as usual in families with parent-child interactions problems: A randomized controlled trial. *Child and Adolescent Psychiatry and Mental Health, 9*(1), 3. https://doi.org/10.1186/s13034-015-0036-9

Homem, T. C., Gaspar, M. F., Seabra-Santos, M. J., Canavarro, M. C., & Azevedo, A. (2014). A pilot study with the incredible years parenting training: Does it work for fathers of preschoolers with oppositional behavior symptoms? *Fathering: A Journal of Theory, Research, and Practice about Men as Fathers, 12*(3), 262–282. https://doi.org/10.3149/fth.1203.262

Ihinger-Tallman, M., Pasley, K., & Buehler, C. (1995). Developing a middle-range theory of father involvement postdivorce. In W. Marsiglio (Ed.), *Fatherhood: Contemporary theory, research, and social policy* (pp. 57–77). Thousand Oaks, CA: Sage.

Jeynes, W. H. (2015). A meta-analysis: The relationship between father involvement and student academic achievement. *Urban Education, 50*(4), 387–423. https://doi.org/10.1177/0042085914525789

Lamb, M. E. (2004). *The role of the father in child development* (4th ed.). Hoboken, NJ: Wiley.

Lamb, M. E., & Lewis, C. (2013). Father-child relationships. In C. N. Cabrera & S. Tamis-LeMonda (Eds.), *Handbook of father involvement* (pp. 135–150). London: Routledge.

Lechowicz, M. E., Jiang, Y., Tully, L. A., Burn, M. T., Collins, D. A. J., Hawes, D. J., et al. (2019). Enhancing father engagement in parenting programs: Translating research into practice recommendations. *Australian Psychologist, 54*(2), 83–89. https://doi.org/10.1111/ap.12361

Lee, J. Y., Knauer, H. A., Lee, S. J., MacEachern, M. P., & Garfield, C. F. (2018). Father-inclusive perinatal parent education programs: A systematic review. *Pediatrics, 142*(1), 1–18. https://doi.org/10.1542/peds.2018-0437

Lee, P. C., Niew, W. I., Yang, H. J., Chen, V. C., & Lin, K. C. (2012). A meta-analysis of behavioral parent training for children with attention deficit hyperactivity disorder. *Research in Developmental Disabilities, 33*(6), 2040–2049. https://doi.org/10.1016/j.ridd.2012.05.011

Leidy, M. S., Schofield, T. J., & Parke, R. D. (2013). Fathers' contributions to children's social development. In N. J. Cabrera & C. S. Tamis-Lemonda (Eds.), *Handbook of father involvement: Multidisciplinary perspectives* (2nd ed., pp. 151–167). New York: Routledge.

Lucassen, N., Tharner, A., Van Ijzendoorn, M. H., Bakermans-Kranenburg, M. J., Volling, B. L., Verhulst, F. C., et al. (2011). The association between paternal sensitivity and infant-father attachment security: A meta-analysis of three decades of research. *Journal of Family Psychology, 25*(6), 986–992. https://doi.org/10.1037/a0025855

Lundahl, B., Risser, H. J., & Lovejoy, M. C. (2006). A meta-analysis of parent training: Moderators and follow-up effects. *Clinical Psychology Review, 26*(1), 86–104. https://doi.org/10.1016/j.cpr.2005.07.004

Lundahl, B. W., Tollefson, D., Risser, H., & Lovejoy, M. C. (2008). A Meta-Analysis of Father Involvement in Parent Training. *Research in Social Work Practice, 18*(2), 97–106. https://doi.org/10.1177/1049731507309828

Madden-Derdich, D. A., & Leonard, S. A. (2000). Parental role identity and fathers' involvement in coparental interaction after divorce: Fathers' perspectives. *Family Relations, 49*, 311–318.

Magill-Evans, J., Harrison, M. J., Rempel, G., & Slater, L. (2006). Interventions with fathers of young children: Systematic literature review. *Journal of Advanced Nursing, 55*(2), 248–264. https://doi.org/10.1111/j.1365-2648.2006.03896.x

Mauer, T. W., & Pleck, J. H. (2006). Fathers' caregiving and breadwinning: A gender congruence analysis. *Psychology of Men and Masculinity, 7*(2), 101–112. https://doi.org/10.1037/1524-9220.7.2.101

Merikangas, K. R., He, J.-P., Burstein, M., Swanson, S. A., Avenevoli, S., Cui, L., et al. (2010). Lifetime prevalence of mental disorders in U.S. adolescents: Results from the National Comorbidity Survey Replication–Adolescent Supplement (NCS-A). *Journal of the American Academy of Child and Adolescent Psychiatry, 49*(10), 980–989. https://doi.org/10.1016/j.jaac.2010.05.017

Oblinger, D., Oblinger, J. L., & Lippincott, J. K. (2005). *Educating the net generation*. Boulder, CO: EDUCAUSE. https://digitalcommons.brockport.edu/bookshelf/272

Panter-Brick, C., Burgess, A., Eggerman, M., McAllister, F., Pruett, K., & Leckman, J. F. (2014). Practitioner review: Engaging fathers-recommendations for a game change in parenting interventions based on a systematic review of the global evidence. *Journal of Child Psychology and Psychiatry, 55*(11), 1187–1212. https://doi.org/10.1111/jcpp.12280

Parra-Cardona, J. R., Bybee, D., Sullivan, C. M., Rodríguez, M. M. D., Dates, B., Tams, L., et al. (2017). Examining the impact of differential cultural adaptation with Latina/o immigrants exposed to adapted parent training interventions. *Journal of Consulting and Clinical Psychology, 85*(1), 58–71. https://doi.org/10.1037/ccp0000160

Parra-Cardona, J. R., Wampler, R. S., & Sharp, E. A. (2006). "Wanting to be a good father": Experiences of adolescent fathers of Mexican descent in a teen fathers program. *Journal of Marital and Family Therapy, 32*(2), 215–231. https://doi.org/10.1111/j.1752-0606.2006.tb01601.x

Patterson, G. R. (2005). The next generation of PMTO models. *The Behavior Therapist, 28*(2), 25–32.

Pelham, W. E., Fabiano, G. A., Waxmonsky, J. G., Greiner, A. R., Gnagy, E. M., Coxe, S., et al. (2016). Treatment sequencing for childhood ADHD: A multiple-randomization study of adaptive medication and behavioral interventions. *Journal of Clinical Child & Adolescent Psychology, 45*, 396–415. https://doi.org/10.1080/15374416.2015.1105138

Pfitzner, N., Humphreys, C., & Hegarty, K. (2017). Research review: Engaging men: A multi-level model to support father engagement. *Child & Family Social Work, 22*(1), 537–547. https://doi.org/10.1111/cfs.12250

Pleck, J. (1997). Paternal involvement: Levels, sources, and consequences. In M. E. Lamb (Ed.), *The role of fathers in child development* (3rd ed., pp. 66–103). Hoboken, NJ: Wiley.

Polanczyk, G. V., Salum, G. A., Sugaya, L. S., Caye, A., & Rohde, L. A. (2015). Annual research review: A meta-analysis of the worldwide prevalence of mental disorders in children and adolescents. *Journal of Child Psychology and Psychiatry, 56*(3), 345–365. https://doi.org/10.1111/jcpp.12381

Ramchandani, P. G., Domoney, J., Sethna, V., Psychogiou, L., Vlachos, H., & Murray, L. (2013). Do early father–infant interactions predict the onset of externalising behaviours in young children? Findings from a longitudinal cohort study. *Journal of Child Psychology and Psychiatry, 54*(1), 56–64. https://doi.org/10.1111/j.1469-7610.2012.02583.x

Rempel, L. A., Rempel, J. K., Khuc, T. N., & Vui, L. T. (2017). Influence of father-infant relationship on infant development: A father-involvement intervention in Vietnam. *Developmental Psychology, 53*(10), 1844–1858. https://doi.org/10.1037/dev0000390

Rosenberg, J., & Wilcox, W. B. (2006). *The importance of fathers in the healthy development of children: Child abuse and neglect user manual series*. Washington, DC: Department of Health and Human Services, Children's Bureau.

Salmanian, M., Mohammadi, M. R., Keshavarzi, Z., & Brand, S. (2018). An update on the global prevalence of conduct disorder (2011–2017): Study protocol for a systematic review and meta-analysis. *Journal of Forensic and Legal Medicine, 59*, 1–3. https://doi.org/10.1016/j.jflm.2018.07.008

Scott, K. L., & Crooks, C. V. (2007). Preliminary evaluation of an intervention program for maltreating fathers. *Brief Treatment and Crisis Intervention, 7*(3), 224–238.

Scourfield, J., Cheung, S. Y., & Macdonald, G. (2014). Working with fathers to improve children's well-being: Results of a survey exploring service provision and intervention approach in the UK. *Children and Youth Services Review, 43*, 40–50. https://doi.org/10.1016/j.childyouth.2014.04.009

Shapiro, A. F., Gottman, J. M., & Fink, B. C. (2020). Father's involvement when bringing baby home: Efficacy testing of a couple-focused transition to parenthood intervention for promoting father involvement. *Psychological Reports, 123*(3), 806–824. https://doi.org/10.1177/0033294119829436

Sicouri, G., Tully, L., Collins, D., Burn, M., Sargeant, K., Frick, P., … Dadds, M. (2018). Toward father-friendly parenting interventions: A qualitative study. *Australian and New Zealand Journal of Family Therapy, 39*(2), 218–231. https://doi.org/10.1002/anzf.1307

Sullivan, O., Coltrane, S., McAnnally, L., & Altintas, E. (2009). Father-friendly policies and time-use data in a cross-national context: Potential and prospects for future research. *Annals of the Academy of Political and Social Science, 624*, 214–233. https://doi.org/10.1177/0002716209335138

Swift, J. K., Callahan, J. L., & Vollmer, B. M. (2011). Preferences. *Journal of Clinical Psychology, 67*(2), 155–165. https://doi.org/10.1002/jclp.20759

Tamis-LeMonda, C. S., Shannon, J. D., Cabrera, N. J., & Lamb, M. E. (2004). Fathers and mothers at play with their 2- and 3-year-olds: Contributions to language and cognitive development. *Child Development, 75*, 1806–1820. https://doi.org/10.1111/j.1467-8624.2004.00818.x

Tully, L. A., Piotrowska, P. J., Collins, D. A. J., Mairet, K. S., Black, N., Kimonis, E. R., et al. (2017). Optimising child outcomes from parenting interventions: Fathers' experiences, preferences and barriers to participation. *BMC Public Health, 17*(1), 550. https://doi.org/10.1186/s12889-017-4426-1

Weber, L., Kamp-Becker, I., Christiansen, H., & Mingebach, T. (2019). Treatment of child externalizing behavior problems: A comprehensive review and meta-meta-analysis on effects of parent-based interventions on parental characteristics. *European Child & Adolescent Psychiatry, 28*(8), 1025–1036. https://doi.org/10.1007/s00787-018-1175-3

Webster-Stratton, C., Reid, M. J., & Hammond, M. (2001). Preventing conduct problems, promoting social competence: A parent and teacher training partnership in head start. *Journal of Clinical Child & Adolescent Psychology, 30*(3), 283–302. https://doi.org/10.1207/S15374424JCCP3003_2

Webster-Stratton, C., Reid, M. J., & Hammond, M. (2004). Treating children with early-onset conduct problems: Intervention outcomes for parent, child, and teacher training. *Journal of Clinical Child & Adolescent Psychology, 33*(1), 105–124. https://doi.org/10.1207/S15374424JCCP3301_11

Fathers and Their Very Young Children: Future Directions

41

Robert H. Bradley

To plan well for the future often requires a careful look at the past and what it may offer by way of guidance. That practice would seem useful in planning research on fathers. As other scholars have argued, past research on fathers has too often been framed using a maternal template and too often has looked at fathers as simply being present or absent in a child's life or as a "bread-winner" (Cabrera, Fitzgerald, Bradley, & Roggman, 2014). Furthermore, prior research has too often focused on the quantity of paternal actions taken in behalf of children rather than at the quality of those actions and their purpose vis-à-vis children's well-being (Palkovitz & Hull, 2018). This broad comment is offered not so much as a criticism but as a cautionary tale. Future research on fathers will be stronger and more actionable if it adopts a more comprehensive view of how fathers fit into the lives of children. Future research on fathers will also be stronger if it looks beyond how much time fathers spend with their children or the father's economic contribution to overall family resources. A more meaningful understanding of fathers will emerge if more incisive attention is given to various attributes of paternal involvement as they potentially have impact on particular aspects of child well-being at particular points in the child's life course.

R. H. Bradley (✉)
Center for Child and Family Success, Arizona State University, Tempe, AZ, USA
e-mail: robert.bradley@asu.edu

A more meaningful understanding of paternal involvement will emerge if there is attention to what the father also derives from his involvement – there is an ongoing dialectic in the father-child relationship, with paternal identity at the center of all encounters and paternal well-being as well as child well-being always in process.

It behooves those who study fathers to recognize that (1) fathers can play many roles in children's lives, roles that change through time; (2) roles that fathers play in children's lives derive from the needs children have both in and through time; (3) roles that fathers play derive from cultural values regarding what fathers should do to facilitate a child's development of the skills needed in that culture; (4) roles that fathers play depend on the broader affordances present in the environment; (5) there is interplay between the roles played by fathers and the roles played by other family members and caregivers for the child; and (6) there is interplay between the roles played by fathers in a child's life and the other roles enacted by fathers as part of their larger role in the family and in society. The proliferation of information on parenting (fathering in particular) on the Internet attests to the diverse roles played by fathers and the connection of those roles to the complex, dynamic environment we live in. The number of websites devoted to parenting is growing exponentially, with websites often citing research findings. That said, current research on fathers does not always provide the kind of

H. E. Fitzgerald et al. (eds.), *Handbook of Fathers and Child Development*,
https://doi.org/10.1007/978-3-030-51027-5_41

precise guidance needed for fathers to optimally carry out their role as parent. Thus, websites currently rely on research done with mothers even as they offer information to fathers on how to parent. In effect, websites essentially are begging for more detailed and authoritative information on fathers, so that they can provide information that is judged by viewers as more authoritative and more complete – ergo, more actionable.

To some extent, research on fathers prior to 1975 was all too much driven conceptions of maternal and paternal roles that emerged as a consequence of industrialization and the two world wars that occurred in the first half of the twentieth century (Lamb, 1975). It was a time when many fathers worked away from home for 40 or more hours a week, families were becoming smaller, and there was a decreasing prevalence of multigenerational households where care of children was shared by the adults present in the household (Cherlin, 2014).

During the late nineteenth century, when the first phase of father research was undertaken, the majority of mothers were "stay-at-home moms" and provided most child care. Research on parenting was driven by notions pertaining to the centrality of maternal care for children. Most research was also conducted in Western democracies, where most children resided in two-parent homes, homes that did not include extended family members. But these "affordances" belie the broader historical and geographic realities connected with parenting generally and fathering in particular. There have been massive changes in daily life for humans over the eons of human history (McGaughey, 2002). Initially, humans were hunters and gatherers who lived in small groups of closely connected kith and kin. They had few tools and they needed to develop a relatively small repertoire of skills to survive. Over time humans developed more tools and were less reliant on hunting and gathering to survive. Humans gathered into larger collectives; and they constructed more defined roles for various members of the collective, roles directly associated with particular goals that served the broader community as well as personal survival. As a consequence, humans needed to develop more skills, and their roles in caregiving became more specific and sometimes more hierarchically organized. Community/cultural norms and mores pertaining to child rearing began to emerge as well – albeit the specifics varied depending on where one lived (geography) and what was needed to manage daily life. Cherlin (2014) speaks to the particular impacts of industrialization and how it impacted family in the nineteenth and early twentieth centuries, beginning in Western countries and then spreading throughout the globe. All of these changes had a bearing on the role fathers needed to play in children's lives. Just as fathers' roles evolved to fit the changing affordances of the past, so those roles will continue to evolve as daily life continues to change.

As the human use of tools evolved, so did human brains. To some extent, the use of new tools changed not only what humans did and how they did it, but it also changed human perceptions of who we are and how we got here. The connection between advances in tool use and human perceptions of what it means to be human is by no means simple; but those advances came with changes in how parents provided care for their children – and, more specifically, what it means to be a father. The current advances in human tools are almost certain to do the same. One simply has to wonder about the impact artificial intelligence, robots, the Internet, social media, and "aps for everything" on the human brain and how these technological devices will shape parenting beliefs and practices. It seems almost certain that more parents will have more detailed knowledge about children and about parenting practices. It also seems almost certain the parents' social networks will be broader; thus, the social influences on parenting more dispersed. It also seems almost certain that parents will utilize advanced technologies to manage various aspects of parenting (e.g., monitoring, educating, communicating, how time is spent in joint activities). All of these "actions" on the part of parents will help shape cortical and subcortical connections in the brain and help determine brain function (Hagmann et al., 2008).

Past adaptations made to address technological, climatic, political, and social change offer hints as to what one might expect by way of future change in parental roles. However, the pace and ubiquity of the change happening now makes it difficult to fully anticipate what may be needed by children in the next generation and what parents will have by way of supports to meet those needs. To make the picture even murkier, one has to also consider the needs of the parents themselves. The full impact of advances in robotics, smart technologies, and the interface of humans with those technologies is hard to predict; but, for sure, the human "social world" is changing rapidly (Kurzweil, 2005). History suggests that human adaptations to major changes in life's circumstances can be difficult to predict in the short run. This is not surprising given that human environments are complex and involve dynamic interplay between numerous component parts. According to dynamic systems theory, the interplay of component elements in complex systems may undergo major readjustments during and immediately after periods of "chaos" or flux (Lewis, 2000). In some cases, systems revert to old modes of interaction among system members/components, while, in other cases, brand new structures are implemented. In the latter case, it can take a show for new values and new ways of doing things to become stable. Thus, future research on fathers needs to carefully track how various groups of fathers (i.e., those living in varied micro- and macro-system conditions) are starting to respond, with careful attention to factors that may move them in particular directions (e.g., technological advances and social/organizational circumstances that might directly impact parenting behavior).

Up to this point, most research on parenting has been guided by the "now" (i.e., the circumstances present a particular moment in time). Given that it takes a while for information to be disseminated, digested, and organized into an actionable form, even information on relatively recent research can be somewhat "dated." Even good research findings can be a bit behind the curve of change. Scholars have questioned the applicability of key findings from past research to the new "now," given changes that have occurred since a particular study was mounted. The accelerating pace of technological and social change means findings from research anchored to conditions in even the fairly recent past could have limited applicability to the "now." In effect, we may be getting increasingly behind the curve of change. Accordingly, future research on fathers may need to be more future-oriented, with efforts made to anticipate what is coming – even granting some uncertainties with such guesses. If, as theorists that deal with fathering (Cabrera et al., 2014; Palkovitz & Hull, 2018) contend, context matters, then the ways of doing future research may need to quickly assess emerging contexts before launching new research on fathers. This likely means finding multiple ways of doing qualitative data gathering that set the frame for the new research. Simply digging through scientific journals to guide research may undermine the real value of future research. It doesn't mean ignoring what is in journals, but it means combining the techniques (and frameworks) that were used in the past with ideas informed by thoughtful qualitative data gathering so that the new science is actually reflective of the "now." Advances in technology can help in such efforts. To some extent, this more open approach carries risks; but taking such risks may increase confidence that relevant findings will emerge. Editors and reviewers of articles submitted for publication will also need to make this shift.

In this chapter, an effort will be made to consider potentially productive areas for future research on fathers, beginning with a consideration of the primary roles played by fathers in children's lives and historical changes in human life generally. Attention will then be given to issues related to (1) the use of media and other technologies, (2) involvement of both mothers and fathers in the workforce, (3) coparenting, (4) the father-daughter and father-son relationships, (5) engagement in science and math in a technologically advancing world, and (6) children with special needs. The last major topic will be paternal identity. The chapter will end with a brief summary of key points pertaining to future research on fathers.

The Role of Fathers

Despite huge variation in macro-level conditions for families around the world, fathers generally have four key roles to play in children's lives: (1) provision of resources, (2) nurturance and support, (3) life skills development, and (4) maintenance and management of the family/community systems. These broad roles or functions in children's lives will almost certainly remain; but the ways of achieving those functions (i.e., the forms they take) will adapt to fit the circumstances of daily life (Epstein, Bishop, Ryan, Miller, & Keitner, 1993). That said, productive research on fathers will need to consider that the timing and duration of particular forms of paternal behavior will tend to vary as a consequence of child needs and contextual circumstances (Cabrera et al., 2014). During infancy, children are highly dependent on caregivers to meet basic needs, so fathers (like other family members) more likely spend time feeding a child, clothing the child, putting a child to sleep, and responding to the child's fears and frustrations. As children gain skills and become somewhat more independent, caregivers will gravitate more to functioning as playmates, teaching children simple life skills and skills needed for school, while at the same time being available for transportation and managing the child's engagement in key activities. Then, as children move through middle childhood and adolescence, fathers will likely spend more time helping them learn advanced skills, being present and helping with lessons and team activities, connecting children to key institutions and social networks, and monitoring offspring activities. These shifts in developmental needs and opportunities, notwithstanding, fathers (like other caregivers) will need to continue providing social and emotional support and affording children protection – but even for these roles, the forms could change somewhat (Joussemet, Landry, & Koestner, 2008). As an example, though children generally require at least a modest level of in-person encounters with caregivers to help them feel secure and motivated for self-actualization (Kenrick, Neuberg, Griskevicius, Becker, & Schaller, 2010), face timing a 3-year-old might go a long way to fulling some of the nurturance and support role a father needs to enact. Being there "in the flesh" may not be required all the time. Likewise, sitting with a 5-year-old child watching a well-constructed "YouTube" video or an episode from the Disney Channel that deals with a key notion about management of emotions might function to fulfill a life skills development role. Maybe even just encouraging the child to watch the episode on Disney Channel could work.

Embarking on productive lines of research on fathering will be both exciting and challenging given the rapid pace of change in human life. Part of the challenge derives from the fact that the field of father research is itself "quite fractionated," according to Palkovitz and Hull (2018). They offer a new resource theory of fathering which explicates a multiplicity of factors assumed to impact both paternal patterns of behavior and the impact those behaviors have on children. Palkovitz and Hull contend that to be maximally useful, research on these elements needs to be guided by a "father-centric view" and a recognition that the father-child relationship is unique among caregiver-child relationships. To some extent, Cabrera et al. (2014) had a similar motive in offering their expanded model, a model that addresses the ecology of father-child relationships. Others have also offered ideas on how to better integrate research on fathers (Lamb & Lewis, 2010; Pleck, 2010). None of these frameworks purports that children must have heavily involved fathers to develop adequately (i.e., that fathers are "essential"), but each presents a case for the importance of paternal involvement. Notably, each makes clear that future research will have to delve deeper into the whats, whens, hows, and for how long fathers do certain things and how it matters for children's development. Each also makes clear that context will have to be given greater attention if generalizable and actionable findings are to emerge. De facto, this is a "tall order" as details about the relations involved remain sketchy, as does theoretical guidance for how to consider them. It is a tall order for another reason as well; specifically, it is unlikely that there are adequate measures for capturing some of the behavioral, developmental, and contextual constructs that are critical for some new lines of inquiry.

Seeking the Roots of Modern Paternal Behavior

When it comes to caring for children, human males seem a bit odd compared to males from most mammalian species. In only about 5% of mammalian species do fathers take on a direct caregiving role (Geary, 2000). Gettler (2016) describes the interesting case of men in forager societies who spent significant amounts of time taking care of children while mothers are away foraging. This might be taken as an indication that evolution has prepared human males to take on social roles with respect to offspring to a greater extent than males from most mammalian species and that the exact role a father takes likely reflects the broader needs of the family (perhaps even broader social community). That does not mean that human fathers provide high levels of care in most families; but there are more instances of human fathers providing significant care for offspring than is true for most mammalian species (Abraham et al., 2014; Bureau of Labor Statistics, 2017; Hrdy, 1999; Samman, Presler-Marshall, & Jones, 2016). Moreover, fathers are spending an increasing amount of time caring for children than was true even 50 years ago Livingston & Parker, 2019). Part of the reason that human fathers tend to play a greater caregiving role likely devolves from the evolutionary underpinnings for social engagement instantiated in primates generally (Abraham et al., 2014; Hare, 2011; Plavacan, 2012). Studies of several primate species (marmosets, monkeys, tamarins, chimpanzees) reveal that they possess biological systems that facilitate paternal care and that they enact behaviors that foster or maintain bonds with offspring (Murray, Stanton, Lonsdorf, Wroblewski, & Pusey, 2016; Nunes, Fite, Patera, & French, 2001; Storey & Ziegler, 2016; Ziegler, Prudom, & Zahed, 2009). Even so, the level of diversity observed in human male care of offspring is atypical even among primates.

Over the past two decades, scholars have given increased attention to neurological and physiological factors connected with parenting (a topic that is the focus of Chap. 13). As with most studies of parenting, the vast majority were conducted with mothers, but more and more have been devoted to fathers as well. Studies using magnetic resonance imaging have shown that paternal neural responses are similar – albeit not identical – to maternal neural responses to infant behaviors (Abraham et al., 2014; Nunes-Costa, Figueriredo, & Maya-Albiol, 2016; Swain, Dayton, Kim, Tolman, & Volling, 2014). There is evidence that when fathers provide extensive care to infants, they manifest higher levels of oxytocin, a hormone that promotes caregiving (Saturn, 2014). There is evidence that the paternal brain is sensitive to child care experiences and that there is a link between fathers' neural responses and their thinking during caregiving experiences (Abraham et al., 2014; Kim et al., 2015). In a fairly recent review, Nunes-Costa et al. (2016) provide an overview of studies that address neuronal, neurochemical, hormonal, and genetic connections with paternal behavior, research that includes animal as well as human samples. They concluded that "brain image research with men suggests that networks of hypothalamic-midbrain-limbic, paralimbic-cortical circuit … that are activated in fathers' brains are highly specialized for baby stimuli, similar to those observed in women, and changes as the parent-infant relationship develops (p. 801)." However, Nunes et al. also make quite clear that extant research is quite limited and that it does not offer precise information on the genes involved in most paternal care or the timing of certain hormonal processes. They also point to the fact that some studies of the few studies extant have contradictory findings. Almost nothing is known about how certain neural or physiological processes are activated beyond infancy and the extent to which key neurochemical processes may be activated if fathers do not start playing a major caregiving role until early or middle childhood. It may be that activation is more likely in cases where fathers spend more time taking care of a child (e.g., when fathers are given dual custody after divorce, major shifts in maternal work activities, maternal death or critical illness, movement from a residence where care is provided by other kith and kin). These are areas where there is need for substantial additional research.

One of the real challenges that faces scholars who wish to study the neurological underpinnings of paternal behavior is that multiple areas of the brain come into play in the process of parenting. Abraham et al. (2014) discuss two major components of the caregiving network based on MRI research. One component is emotional processing which involves structures for processing distress, vigilance, and reward (e.g., the amygdala and ventral tegmental areas). The second component is mentalizing which includes cognitive processes connected with perspective taking, empathy, and theory of mind (e.g., ventromedial prefrontal cortex and superior temporal sulcus). These components connect to oxytocin levels that support parental care and parent-child synchrony in complex ways; but even these brain regions do not fully determine parental behavior. Other biological systems (i.e., the heart) can also become involved. The good news, according to Saturn (2014), is that these multiple systems allow fathers' brains to adapt to different parenting roles, depending on the needs of the child, the family, and the broader social network. The bad news, however, is that it can make neurophysiological studies of fathering quite challenging. One of the important conclusions drawn by Abraham et al. (2014) is "the central role of actual caregiving behavior as an important pathway to the parental brain (p. 9795)." As it happens, most of the research on paternal brains to date has been done on fathers in relatively stable, two-parent households – households that make recruitment easier and there is likely to be less chaos. The investment of fathers in child care in less stable, more challenged circumstances could be quite different; thus, the impacts could be quite different as well. In effect, studies of the paternal brain, while they are pointing to potentially actionable strategies for fathers, are in a nascent stage. The challenges of future studies on the paternal brain, notwithstanding, it would be interesting to look at how different brain regions or aspects of brain function may connect to particular forms of paternal behavior and their relation to particular domains of child functioning (e.g., social development, executive function, emotion regulation; see Chaps. 15, 16, 18, 19, 20, 21, 22, and 23). It is also critical to do research on fathers who have a history of stress or who are currently facing stress.

Imagining the World to Come

It's hard to imagine the time when you couldn't just orient your head toward your smartphone or digital assistant and say, "Siri (a.k.a., Alexa, Google, whatever), could you tell me….?" The invasion of technology into parenting space has been extraordinary in the twenty-first century. But advances in technology are just one of many changes that have occurred in human life over the past two centuries or so that would seem to have major implications for enacting the role of father. Thus, it is worth considering how key aspects of life today may bear upon both the factors that help determine how fathers engage in the four broad roles of caregiving needed to assure child well-being and the actual form those behaviors need to take to maximize offspring well-being. The breadth of change is too vast to fully consider in this chapter, but several changes would seem particularly noteworthy as regards their likely relevance for future research on fathers.

Media and Electronic Devices

Perhaps nothing has done more to change daily life than advances in technology, particularly digital technology. Technological change is pervasive and has resulted in numerous improvements in most arenas of life, including parenting. Recent surveys show that parents use TVs, computers, smartphones, electronic musical devices, and other forms of technology for a variety of caregiving purposes, with many parents mentioning that media allowed for enjoyable joint time with their children and greater opportunities to help their children learn (Center on Media and Human Development, Northwestern University, 2014; Nikken, 2019). The use of baby monitors has increased greatly over the past two decades, but with limited evidence that such they reduce injuries or increase overall well-being in children. Parents have also increased their use of digital monitoring of adolescents (Pew Research Center, 2016a, 2016b). Such monitoring has changed aspects of parent-adolescent communication and reduced parental concerns about certain types of risky behavior; but, the evidence for overall effectiveness of using such aps and devices remains unclear (Nouwen, JafariNaimi, & Zaman, 2017). There is even some evidence that parents can become overly reliant on certain types of devices when trying to protect their children from potential harm (Bonafide et al., 2018). In effect, as has been the case with most "advances" in human life, the "good news" is often accompanied by "bad news" and uncertainties as regards the actual value of the "advances." In surveys on parents' and children's use of digital technologies, the parents that used technology more often to manage parenting tasks expressed less confidence as parents and reported that their children had more problems and said that the use of media often led to conflicts between parents and children (Center on Media and Human Development, Northwestern University, 2014; Nikken, 2019). Conflicts were particularly likely when children identified themselves as being addicted to the use of a particular technology (Common Sense Media, 2016). There is even research suggesting that parents sometimes overvalue digital and media technologies when used to help protect children or assist their development (Bonafide et al., 2018). Overall, there were mixed feelings about having so many media devices in the home, with a greater proportion of parents saying that it had made parenting harder rather than easier.

More than 95% of American households have access to TV (Nielsen, 2017). As the use of media grew throughout the twentieth century, so did warnings about their effects on children. More than 75% of adults have home Internet connections as well, with the percentage being highest for adults of most likely to have young children in the household (Pew Research Center, 2018). Moreover, even adults who do not have a home Internet connection often have a smartphone which allows access to social media and websites (Pew Research Center, 2018). Research suggests that parents spend a great deal of time online, both in activities related to the parenting and activities with little or no association to their parenting (Dworkin, Connell, & Doty, 2013).

Critical to understanding how fathers are implicated in children's media experiences is determining how often children engage with TV, smartphones, computers, and other technologies. It is not easy to estimate with high confidence just how much time young children spend watching TV, watching YouTube programs, listening to electronic music, playing with smartphones, etc. However, the most recent data indicate that Sesame Street was viewed 5 billion times in 2017 and Chu Chu was watched 19 billion times (Madrigal, 2018). Programs for children have long been produced by the Public Broadcasting Network and many private firms. The most popular channel is Disney Junior Disney Junior, which had an estimated ten million viewers ages 2–8 in 2016, with Sprout and Nick Jr. also estimated to have millions as well (Futon Critic, 2017). Young children's access to smartphones and other mobile devices has also dramatically increased in the last 5 years, with evidence that by age 2 more than 70% of children use them routinely (Kabali et al., 2015). The amount of time young children spend in front of TV, watching YouTube, and engaged with smartphones and other electronic devices has given rise to concerns about negative impacts on the brain and reduced social competence (Stein, 2018). It has also given rise to concerns about cardiorespiratory fitness in children (Pfledderer, Burns, & Brusseau, 2019; Tandon et al., 2014).

The American Academy of Pediatrics (2016) has offered recommendations for how much time children should spend watching TV and using electronic devices, amounts of time that are much lower than the average current usage. AAP also recommends that parents spend more time with children in activities that are enjoyable and educational. Health and human service professionals and professional organizations familiar with children's use of media have likewise offered advice for reduction in use and parental actions that can offset some of the potential negative effects (Bozzola et al., 2018; McCarthy et al., 2018). Clearly, the diversity of media and electronic devices present in today's world offer a plethora of opportunities for fathers to support the well-being of children but a plethora of challenges as well. All this said, much remains unclear about what parents are doing to manage young children's use of media and how that is affecting children's well-being. Particularly unclear is what fathers are doing with respect to their children's use of media and how it connects to all four major roles fathers play in young children's lives.

Given the rapid growth of blogs and websites, there is need to know more about how fathers use media to support their own confidence as a parent. There is an increasing number of websites and Internet-based support groups designed to help parents (Niela-Vilen, Axelin, Salantera, & Melender, 2014). Such media outlets may be especially helpful for fathers rearing children with significant medical problems or disabilities (Kim Wyatt, Xueping, & Gaylord, 2016). However, very little is known about paternal use of these sites, whether they are optimally designed to support fathers' needs, or how much they are accomplishing by way of support (Fletcher & StGeorge, 2011).

Workforce Participation

There has been a substantial rise of women (especially mothers) in the workforce since World War II (U.S. Bureau of Labor Statistics, 2019). It is part of a worldwide shift in adult employment (Ortiz-Ospina, Tzvetkova, & Roser, 2018; Kreyenfeld, 2015). Today in more than 30% of two-parent households, women earn more than their partner (Parker & Stepler, 2017). Although mothers nowadays, on average, are spending more time in paid work, they are also spending more time in child care compared to mothers of 50 years ago – granted stay-at-home mothers are spending more time in child care than working mothers (Livingston & Bialik, 2018). Partly as a consequence, fathers are spending more time in child care nowadays too, albeit fathers do not spend as much time in child care activities as do mothers when both are employed (Livingston & Bialik, 2018). The father care-to-mother care ratio improves when mothers contribute a greater share of the household income (Raley, Bianchi, & Yang, 2012). Moreover, there is a general movement to convergence in mother and father roles as both parents try to balance the requirements of work and family (Pew Research Center, 2013). Both mothers and fathers are experiencing increased stress in trying to manage both work and child care (Pew Research Center, 2015a, 2015b). This stress, along with doubts that working parents do not have enough discretionary time to spend with children, has led to worries that maternal employment may have a negative effect on children's well-being and doubts as to whether increased child care by fathers offsets the losses (Goldberg, Prause, Lucas-Thompson, & Himsel, 2008; Hill, Waldfogel, Brooks-Gunn, & Han, 2005; Hsin & Felfe, 2014). Thus far, research does not offer precise answers. Future research needs to focus on work-family balance for fathers and to examine how father actions in behalf of children in families where both parents work connect to various aspects of children's development.

Coincident with the increasing number of women in the workforce, there has been shift in attitudes toward women as primary caregivers and men as "breadwinners" (Cunningham, 2008; Donnelly et al., 2016). It is movement toward more egalitarian gender roles. Like many changes, it is worldwide – granted the movement is stronger in some countries and it has links to parental socioeconomic status (Bosoni, 2014; Cunningham, 2008; Marks, Bun, & McHale, 2009; Olah, Kotowska, & Richter, 2018; Sweeting, Bhaskar, Benzeval, Popham, & Hunt, 2013). The shift involves viewing women as having more authority (Domingo et al., 2015). For women, gaining more authority in family decisions also derives from the increasing number of divorces that have occurred in the past half century and the increasing number of blended families now present in most advanced societies (Belch & Willis, 2002). Thus far, research does not make very clear where fathers fit into the new equation.

Not only has the composition of the workforce changed dramatically since World War 2 (with women constituting a much larger proportion of those employed), but the nature of work has also changed. Technological advances have been the primary driving factor in changing the nature of work (National Academies of Sciences, Engineering, and Medicine, 2017). A smaller proportion of workers are engaged in manual labor and factory jobs that involve limited sets of routinized activities (Pew Research Center, 2016a, 2016b). More jobs are knowledge-intensive and involve the use of computers and other forms of information technology. There are also more jobs in the service sector. Many current jobs now require high levels of social skill and more flexible responses to individualized production and service delivery. There is rapid evolution of how workers use technology to accomplish job tasks, and there tends to be less supervision of particular job tasks than in the past, leaving much online decision-making to the individual who executes the task (National Academies of Sciences, Engineering, & Medicine, 2017; Pew Research Center, 2016a, 2016b). There is also greater use of crowdsourcing platforms to divide and organize how work gets done. This changes not only the nature of work but the nature of relationships among those involved in the work. Not only technology changed the kinds of tasks performed by workers, but it has also led to a great deal more contingent work, with workers changing jobs more often, more workers who are self-employed, and more workers that have more than one job at a time (National Academies of Sciences, Engineering, and Medicine, 2017).

What do the changing patterns of employment mean for parents? It can give them more independence; but it can also lead to more uncertainty and stress. It likely changes the ideas fathers have about parenting and the methods they use to enact parenting tasks. Years ago, Kohn (1963) promulgated the notion that those in lower-level occupations tended to value obedience in their children, whereas those in higher-level occupations tended to value autonomy and critical thinking. In effect, the nature of work tends to embed itself in the values and practices of parenting. Kohn's ideas have generally received support, but their exact applicability to the current modes of paternal parenting remains poorly researched (Sherman & Harris, 2012). Particularly valuable would be research on how the nature of paternal work influences paternal efforts to support autonomy, to instill the idea of flexibility in thinking, and to work with others toward common goals. Related to this is more careful examination of how the nature of paternal work connects to paternal decisions about providing care for children and in the quality of coparenting exhibited by fathers.

Coparenting

Given the shift in maternal employment and the impact maternal employment has for child care, an important area of future research on fathers will be on documenting not just the time spent on particular caregiving tasks but the quality and manner by which certain tasks are accomplished (Hsin & Felfe, 2014; Milkie, Nomaguchi, & Denny, 2015). An important related area for future research is coparenting. Future research can aim to more fully characterize coparenting and also consider factors that may influence paternal coparenting behavior.

Although there appears to be growing convergence in mother and father roles pertaining to child care, research on coparenting remains limited. Findings from past research may no longer fully apply to the current generation of parents. Research on how coparenting is implicated in fathers' lives may be challenging given that parents' ability to coordinate with one another is likely to reflect many different contextual factors (McDaniel, Teti, & Feinberg, 2018). Additional research on coparenting would seem especially relevant given that prior research has demonstrated a connection between coparenting, mother-father relationships, parent-child relationships, and child maladaptive behavior (Barnett, Deng, Mills-Koonce, Willoughby, & Cox, 2008; Bonds & Gondoli, 2007; Feinberg & Kan, 2008; Holland & McElwain, 2013; McHale & Coates, 2014; Palkovitz, Fagan, & Hull, 2013; Parkes, Green, & Mitchell, 2019; Peltz, Rogge, & Sturge-Apple, 2018). Research on coparenting during times of instability (e.g., following divorce) would seem particularly relevant given the relatively high rates of divorce and cohabitation throughout most of the world at present (OECD, 2018). Coparenting can be particularly complicated for fathers who have remarried or who have begun cohabiting after separating from a child's mother, an issue that is highly relevant given the number of children not living in blended families and stepfamilies (American Academy of Child & Adolescent Psychiatry, 2015; U.S. Census Bureau, 2014; Pew Research Center, 2015a, 2015b; Wallerstein & Lewis, 2007). Research on coparenting would also seem highly relevant given that high-quality coparenting is less likely when there is chaos in the household (Whitsell, Teti, Crosby, & Kim, 2015). The need for such research seems all the more important given studies showing how parental conflict can have serious consequences for children's well-being under such conditions (Lamela & Figueriredo, 2016). Further research on coparenting seems particularly relevant in light of studies showing that child problems, like a difficult temperament, can undermine coparenting (Davis, Shoppe-Sullivan, Mangelsdorf, & Brown, 2009) and research showing that coparenting is associated with father's sense of parenting competence (Latham, Mark, & Oliver, 2018). This said, the role coparenting plays in child well-being beyond quality of parent-child relationships remains unclear, with evidence pointing to the parent-child relationship and time spent with parents as perhaps more influential on children (Nielsen, 2017).

Father-Child Relationship

One of the major shifts that has occurred since World War 2 is the declining percentage of children living with both biological parents (Pew Research Center, 2015a, 2015b). This often means that biological fathers do not live in the same home as their children, making it difficult to communicate effectively and take part in the children's ongoing activities. It is a problem that pertains to all subgroups of families but is more prevalent in low-income and minority households (Pew Research Center, 2015a, 2015b). Accordingly, scholars and practitioners have raised concerns about the difficulties posed for father-child relationships and how fathers can function as mature and effective models for their children. Major concerns have been raised about the father-son relationship and the challenges nonresidential status can pose for fathers who wish to provide meaningful guidance to sons at critical points in development (Burns & Caldwell, 2016; Caldwell et al., 2004, 2014). Not living with one's child also makes it more difficult for fathers to develop the kinds of skills and sense of satisfaction with parenthood that is optimal for both father and child (Qian, De Loney, & Caldwell, 2018). There have been some studies on nonresident fathers and their efforts to form satisfying relationships with their sons (and daughters) and their efforts to communicate with both the child's mother and the offspring themselves; but the research lacks details on most processes, including coparenting.

Another major shift in family life pertains to fertility. Average family size has changed dramatically over the past two centuries, with fewer households containing large numbers of children (Levni & Kopf, 2017). Having two or fewer children has become increasingly common (INED, 2013; OECD, 2016; Statistics Canada, 2018; United States Census Bureau, 2018). This change, together with the changing attitudes toward gender and evolving ideas on what constitutes desirable parenting practices, makes another area of research on fathers of particular value: the father-child relationship (Allendorf, 2012). More specifically, in smaller families, parents tend to be less authoritarian (Wagner, Schubert, & Schubert, 1985); and in society at large there has been general move toward promoting autonomy for children (National Academies of Sciences,

Engineering, and Medicine, 2016; Zimmer-Gembeck & Collins, 2003). Cornerstone to the evolving ideas about parenting is the idea of maintaining close relationships with offspring (National Academies of Sciences, Engineering, and Medicine, 2016), relationships which help fulfill the parent's own basic need for connectedness (Joussemet et al., 2008).

There is a growing literature on how fathers' involvement with children affects the father-child relationship and how the quality of the father-child relationship affects child well-being. Research suggests that when children feel close to their fathers and communicate productively with their fathers, children feel greater self-esteem and manifest stronger autonomy (Brotherson, Yamamoto, & Ackck, 2003; StGeorge & Freeman, 2017; Videon, 2005). However, the research is spotty, and findings suggest possible differences by age and gender, depending on the area of well-being (Corwyn & Bradley, 2016; McMunn et al., 2017). Moreover, most of the studies are cross-sectional and involve measures completed by a single respondent.

One of the major shifts in thinking about parent-child relationships that has occurred over the past 50 years is that fathers play an important role in girls' lives as well as boys' lives. A correlated shift in thinking is that time spent with daughters can have a significant bearing on the daughter's well-being – in past times most of the focus was on how time spent with sons helped make sons more responsible and productive (Videon, 2005). The idea that the father-daughter relationship is valuable is becoming ever more instantiated in the public mindset (e.g., dad-daughter dance routines now often incorporated into end of year dance recitals). In some respects, this evolution encourages more studies of the father-daughter relationship as well as more studies of how fathers engage boys and girls differently over the course of childhood. Several studies have shown that fathers' early involvement in girls' lives is associated with better self-esteem during adolescence and marital satisfaction during adulthood, including some studies done in non-Western countries (Algood, Beckert, & Peterson, 2012; Ali & Daoud, 2016; Flouri & Buchanan, 2002; Morman & Floyd, 2002; Perkins, 2001). However, the total canon of studies is small; and some involve cross-sectional recollections of both the father-child relationship early in the life course and later perceptions of self-esteem or life satisfaction. There are very few studies conducted on paternal behavior early in the life course (either directly observed or reported by the father when the child is young) and children's concurrent or downstream development. A more careful examination of the early father-daughter relationship would appear particularly useful given studies showing that fathers tend to engage daughters and sons differently early in the life course (Marks et al., 2009). For example, Mascaro, Renscher, Hackett, Mehl, and Rilling (2017) found that fathers were more attentively engaged with daughters than sons during normal everyday activities. Fathers were also more likely to sing to their daughters, to use both more analytical and emotion-focused language with their daughters. Finally, fathers had a stronger neural response to their daughters' happy facial expressions. By contrast, fathers were more likely to engage sons in rough and tumble play. In a separate study, Ahnert et al. (2017) found that although the quantity of fathers' play with girls and boys did not differ, the quality did, with fathers displaying greater quality with boys – the opposite was true with mothers. In all cases, higher-quality play was associated with less internalizing problems. Thus, more studies of play might be useful. It might be particularly useful to conduct more research on rough and tumble play given evidence that it appears to facilitate social competence in both boys and girls (Stgeorge & Freeman, 2017). It also appears to have some impact on emotional skills and self-regulation; but details are lacking on the exact nature of those relations and whether they affect both sons and daughters in the same way (StGeorge & Freeman, 2017).

Arenas of Child Life Needing Greater Attention

The Expanding Focus on Science and Math

More of the work in modern life involves science, math, and computer technologies. Consequently, another area where potentially fruitful studies of fathers pertains to offspring interest in science and math (STEM). Despite widespread interest in motivating children to seek STEM careers, there remains a gender gap in the pursuit of such careers (Reinking & Martin, 2018). The decision not to pursue a career in science or engineering does not derive from an innate gender difference in quantitative reasoning (Hutchison, Lyons, & Ansari, 2019; Kersey, Braham, Scumitta, Libertus, & Cantlon, 2018; Lindberg, Hyde, Petersen, & Linn, 2010), with the possible exception of the tails of the distribution (i.e., more males seem to score very low or very high; Halpern et al., 2007). Rather, girls' lower interest in math and science appears to derive from gendered socialization, stereotypes about women in science, peer affiliations, and the lack of female role models (Reinking & Martin, 2018). It is clear that these processes begin early, as parents' actions in early childhood foster less interest in science and math on the part of girls (Casey et al., 2018; Pruden & Levine, 2017; Tomasetto, Mirisola, Galdi, & Cadinu, 2015). Although fathers tend to spend more time in physical play with offspring than mothers, research does not make clear how often fathers spend time with children using blocks, legos, and other construction materials that may lend themselves to greater knowledge and interest pertaining to STEM (Schoppe-Sullivan, Kotila, Jia, Lang, & Bower, 2013; Whitebread et al., 2017). A recent survey indicated that both mothers and fathers felt less competent in their ability to help young children learn science than other subjects (Silander et al., 2018). Not only are there many more toys available for teaching science concepts than in the past, but there are also more media options to help children learn science as well. For example, the Corporation for Public Broadcasting has initiated programs to support the development of STEM concepts (e.g., The Cat in the Hat Knows a Lot About That! and Ready Jet Go!). Given that more fathers than mothers have occupations in science and engineering and occupations that involve use of math (e.g., accounting; AICPA, 2017), it would be useful to conduct research to determine how often fathers engage children in activities that include use of mathematics, scientific concepts, engineering constructs, and the like. It would also seem useful to determine such involvement was connected to girls' interest in science and math. In one of the few studies of this sort completed, Thomson, Casey, Lombardi, and Nguyen (2020) found that fathers' spatial concept support during play at age 4.5 was related to daughters' math achievement in first grade controlling for a host of other contextual factors. This finding seems quite meaningful in light of earlier findings showing that parents tend to use more spatial language with boys than girls (Pruden & Levine, 2017). It is also interesting in light of recent research showing that subtle language cues had a bearing on young girls' engagement in science (e.g., saying let's do some science today rather than let's be scientists today) (Rhodes, Leslie, Yee, & Saunders, 2019).

Children with Special Needs

Recently, the Committee on Psychosocial Aspects of Child and Family Health of the American Academy of Pediatrics issued a report on paternal involvement. It was done because research shows that paternal involvement affects children's health status and may also affect the quality of maternal care (Yogman et al., 2016). Paternal involvement is particularly critical in an area where advances in health care have increased the population of children with severe medical complications, disabilities, and mental health problems (Centers for Disease Control and Prevention, 2018; Cohen et al., 2011; GBD 2017 Child & Adolescent Health Collaborators, 2019; Kuo, Houtrow, & Council on Children with Disabilities, 2016; National Cancer Institute, 2019; Perrin, Anderson, & van Cleave, 2014;

Rice et al., 2012; United Nations Children's Fund, 2018; World Bank, 2019; Xu, Strathearn, Liu, Yan, & Bao, 2018). Children with serious health conditions often present significant challenges to practitioners and other care providers, with parents at the center (Carroll, Mollen, Aldridge, Hexem, & Feudtner, 2012; Cohen et al., 2011; Glass et al., 2015; Kuo, Lyle, Casey, & Stille, 2017; Mahone & Denckla, 2017; National Cancer Institute, 2019; Perrin et al., 2014; Robison & Hudson, 2014).

Research on how living with a child with a disability, a serious mental health problem, or serious medical condition affects parenting and family life is growing (Ha, Hong, Seltzer, & Greenberg, 2008). However, there is limited information on how fathers are affected or how their behavior affects the quality of care children or children's outcomes. Fathers often exhibit high levels of anxiety (even loss of identity) during the early stages of their relationship with a medically fragile child (Burrell, Ives, & Freudtner, 2017; Smith, Cheater, & Bekker, 2012; Swallow, Macfadyen, Sanatacroce, & Lambert, 2012). For some parents, there is a sense of chronic sorrow (Smith et al., 2012). For some fathers, the early disruption in what life means is followed by gradual acceptance of the child and what the child needs by way of care and overall support (Burrell et al., 2017). Adjustment can be incredibly difficult if the child has dim prospects for survival (Carroll et al., 2012). Fathers often report having a stronger bond with the child after learning about the child's disability (Carpenter & Towers, 2008); but fathers who have children with special needs tend to report higher levels of daily hassles, more parenting stress, and lower life satisfaction as well (Darling, Senatore, & Strachan, 2011). Fathers are often frustrated at being left out of decisions made concerning the child by practitioners (CAF, 2005; West, 2000). Overall, fathers of children with special needs exhibit signs of burden, with some turning to alcohol or drugs; but the characterization of fathers' reactions to caring for such children remains sketchy (Greenberg, 2002; Ha et al., 2008; Seltzer, Greenberg, Floyd, Pettee, & Hong, 2001).

Fathers (like mothers) often have to make major adjustments to address a disabled or chronically ill child's needs (Heiman, 2002; Long & Marsland, 2011). During this process, fathers' sense that they can control the situation is hampered by lack of support by employers and worries about the expenses connected with the child's condition (Hovey, 2005; Neil-Urban & Jones, 2002). Sometimes the experience actually increases family closeness (Fawcett, Baggaley, Wu, Whyte, & Martinson, 2005; Heaton, Noyes, & Sloper, 2005; Long & Marsland, 2011; Smith et al., 2012; Sullivan-Bolyai, Rosenberg, & Bayard, 2006); but, the stresses of dealing with a child with special needs often have a negative spillover on family relationships (Goble, 2004; Hartley, Papp, & Bolt, 2018; Smith et al., 2012; Sobsey, 2002). The stresses can be particularly daunting for low-income families and families with low social support (National Academies of Sciences, Engineering, & Medicine, 2015). Even so, some fathers of children with health problems report that their lives have strengthened and that they themselves have grown in significant ways (Goble, 2004; Hovey, 2005; Knafl & Zoeller, 2000; Smith et al., 2012). Studies show that parents more likely feel resilient when family members communicate well and offer continuous support to one another (Ha, Greenberg, & Seltzer, 2011; Heiman, 2002). More research is needed on the kinds of supports fathers need to cope well and on what fathers need to provide partners so the partner copes well.

Given the diversity of health and psychological problems present in young children, it is not surprising that little is known about the nature of father involvement with such children or how father involvement affects the long-term well-being of children that have most health and developmental problems (Wade et al., 2006). Analysis of data from the Early Childhood Longitudinal Study showed that fathers of infants with disabilities were a little less likely to be involved in the physical care of the infant than fathers of infants without disabilities; they were also less likely to provide cognitive stimulation. On the other hand, they were not any less warm or nurturing (U.S. Department of Health and Human

Services, Administration on Children and Families, 2010, February). Bronte-Tinkew, Carrano, Horowitz, and Kinukawa (2008) found that fathers' provision of cognitive stimulation was particularly helpful to children with disabilities. Likewise, Yogman and colleagues (1995) found that paternal time spent in playing with children born low birthweight was associated with higher child IQ at age 3. Fathers of children with chronic diseases are typically less involved in child care than is the case with mothers; however, when fathers are highly involved, it appears to facilitate adherence to recommended treatment protocols for the child (Wysocki & Gavin, 2004). A meta-analysis indicated that using a positive parenting style was generally beneficial to young children with disabilities, but most of the studies primarily involved assessment of maternal parenting style. So, it is difficult to ascertain how paternal parenting style may be implicated in the development of children with disabilities (Dyches, Smith, Korth, Roper, & Mandleco, 2012). As technologies and practices for addressing children with special needs advance, detailed research on how living with such children affects fathers will be important so that services can more effectively engage fathers and provide the range of supports needed to improve the lives of the children, other family members, and fathers themselves. More research on how paternal behavior affects children with various types of medical problems and disabilities will be important as well.

Paternal Identity: Kaleidoscopic Transformations of a Life with Children

One wonders what goes through the mind of daddy chimp when seeing baby chimp for the first time or when walking with his child in search of food (Krupenye, Kano, Hirata, Call, & Tomasello, 2016; Lonsdorf, Ross, & Matsuzawa, 2010). Does daddy chimp have a sense of himself as a father and does that affect what he does with the child? The human neocortex is larger than the neocortex of chimps, and there is a longer prometaphase-metaphase in human apical progenitors (Mora-Bermudez et al., 2016); but what exactly does this mean for humans' gradual development of a sense of identity?

Much has been written about the concept of identity and how it influences one's perceptions and behavior – albeit there are disagreements on how to best think about identity and what it means for human functioning (Akhtar & Samuel, 1996; Klein, 2014). Erik Erikson (1968) is considered the "father" of modern treatments of the concept of identity. He essentially argues that identity functions as an organizing principle in people's lives but that it is not a static quality. Erickson argued that identity evolves over the course of life, changing as one encounters new experiences and acquires additional information about oneself in relation to others, the demands of daily living, and the overall affordances of the settings in which one lives. As individuals encounter new experiences, they take on challenges that can help or hinder the development of identity. Research suggests that people gradually attain a reasonably well-defined identity by age 30 (Kroger, Martinussen, & Marcia, 2010). However, progress toward a well-defined identity is often nonlinear, and the pace of progress can affect commitment processes like caring for a child and the sense that one is empowered when doing so (Fox, Nordquist, Billen, & Savoca, 2015; Kroger et al., 2010).

Part of the struggle in understanding and measuring paternal identity derives from the fact that paternal identity is but one of multiple identities that fathers have. Paternal identity is one component out of many that, in the aggregate, offer the father a unified sense of coherence. This unified sense of coherence allows fathers to make key commitments and helps enable fathers to accomplish key tasks (Tsang, Hui, & Law, 2012). According to Fonagy, Gergely, and Jurist (2002), having a strong sense of oneself as a father should enable a father to engage in productive self-reflection; and it should increase the father's capacity to understand the behavior of the child and to usefully consider both his own mental state and the mental state of the child during encounters.

Because paternal identity is but one of multiple identities a father has, its capacity to direct how a father thinks, feels, and behaves in the role of parent depends on its centrality to the father's overall identity (Henley & Pasley, 2005). The more central paternal identity is to a father, the greater the role clarity and the greater the investment the father is likely to make in the child (Strauss & Goldberg, 1999). The more central paternal identity is to a father, the more likely the father will form a strong bond with the child – albeit there remains little research on this particular process (de Cock et al., 2015). Relatedly, the more central paternal identity is to a father, the greater the satisfaction the father will take when enacting the role of parent (Henley & Pasley, 2005). This said, much remains unknown about men's commitment to the role of fathering (i.e., father identity) – including what happens if the child results from an unplanned pregnancy (Nelson & O'Brien, 2012). Even as the changing world of work and the evolving notions about gender move men to take on a greater share of child caregiving, the role of fathers – compared to mothers – remains less well defined and the nature of paternal involvement more discretionary (De Graaf, Hoogenboom, De Roos, & Bucz, 2018; Gaertner, Spinrad, Eisenberg, & Greving, 2007). Not surprisingly, there are indications that men's identity as a parent may be slower to emerge than women's identity. For example, Luz, George, Vieux, and Spitz (2017) found that postnatal bonding to an infant was stronger than prenatal for both mothers and fathers, but the difference between prenatal and postnatal attachment was greater for fathers. It remains for future research to help clarify these processes and the factors connected to adoption of paternal identity as central to a father's identity.

Paternal identity is part of personal identity. It is experienced by fathers as "core" or "unique" to themselves in ways that group – and status – identities are not (Hitlin, 2003). In this regard, findings from two studies about how aspects of identity affect paternal behavior are revealing. Specifically, Rane and McBride (2000) found that a father's level of involvement with a child was related to the centrality of his identification as a nurturer of his child than to his identification with the idea of being a father (Adamasons & Pasley, 2016). Likewise, Maurer, Pleck, and Rane (2003) found no association between a father's identification with himself as being a father (a status identity) and the amount of caregiving he provided. Personal identification with a particular role one needs to play for one's child reflects a father's values and not just role obligations – it is "who I am" not just what I should be doing (Hitlin, 2003).

The more central to one's personal identity a particular parenting role is, the more likely actions related to that role will be enacted. All this said, there is very little research on these processes and the factors that promote or hinder them. One factor that provides a challenge to many fathers is work obligations; and many express that they are stressed in trying to provide care for their children while at the same time managing work obligations (Pew Research Center, 2015a, 2015b; Harrington, Fraone, & Lee, 2017). The struggle to find a comfortable work-life balance is worldwide, with research showing that only four in ten adults report little difficulty in combining work and family (OECD, 2016). Although both mothers and fathers say that the work-life balance is difficult, a recent report by the Pew Research Center (2013) found that a higher proportion of fathers indicated that they had too little time to spend with their children, and a recent study by Vandello (2013) found that more fathers desired greater work flexibility. Future research on contextual factors (like work) that affect paternal identity and parenting behavior might do well to utilize ideas from self-determination theory (SDT) as a guide (Bouchard, Lee, Asgary, & Pelletier, 2007). Specifically, SDT recognizes that enacting behaviors is jointly determined by internal drives to satisfy basic human needs and pressures external to the self. Thus, future research on paternal behavior would do well to somehow account for external forces that foster or hinder behaviors that promote child well-being and the extent to which those behaviors help satisfy the three basic human needs for competence, autonomy, and connectedness. According to theory, the more everything is aligned, the more likely positive paternal behavior will be enacted.

Becoming a father can make a man reflect (and sometimes alter) his values, a process that can continue from prior to a child's birth to late in the life course. As part of that process, the father engages in a process of self-categorization, a process that is highly contextualized and highly individualized (Deaux & Martin, 2003). Unfortunately, there is almost no research on this process. Some qualitative studies report that fathers frequently shift their orientation (part of their sense of identity) from a focus on "me" to a focus on "we." Likewise, fathers report that that shifted their attention from addressing their personal needs to addressing the needs of the child (Daly, Ashbourne, & Brown, 2012). However, the qualitative studies suggest that such shifts can be quite gradual and the movement from "me" to "we" or from my needs to their needs can be partial and idiosyncratic (Daly et al., 2012). The speed and extensity of the transition depends on where one is in the life course – a transition might be easier for a father who is nearing 30, gainfully employed, and in a meaningful relationship with the child's mother (Eliason, Mortimer, & Vuolo, 2015). Although these propositions seem reasonable, few studies on such issues have been conducted.

According to identity theory, the more a father identifies with the being a father, the more satisfaction he is likely to derive from enacting the various component roles he attaches to the personal identity (Fox & Bruce, 2001). Assuming he enacts those dispositions regularly, the more likely it is to have an impact on a child's well-being. A recent study done in the United Kingdom found that when fathers felt more fulfillment when being with their child and a greater sense of security in their role as parent, the child manifested fewer behavior problems at ages 9 and 11 (Opondo, . Redshaw, Savage-McGlynn, & Quigley, 2016). However, family systems are complex, and life can be messy. According to social relationship theory, contradictory processes are quite common (Kuczynski & Parkin, 2009). Thus, observing strong, clear paths of connection with respect to paternal identity should not be expected. According to the models presented by Cabrera et al. (2014) and Palkovitz and Hull (2018), many factors invade the space of fathering and the effects it is likely to have on a child, including the characteristics of the child himself/herself. Dynamic systems theory makes clear that aspects of a system that would generally organize themselves around one set of attractors can be disrupted and reorganize themselves around a different set of attractors (Lewis, 2000). Moreover, in different cultures or settings, elements may tend to organize themselves differently. Thus, research on paternal identity, how it develops, and how it functions for children perhaps should not be tightly tied to any one theory about identity, motivation, or self-actualization. It should perhaps not only be more father-centric, as suggested by Palkovitz and Hull, but place- and time-centric as well. For this reason, qualitative and person-centered studies should be part of the complement of studies on fathers and their children. In the real, rapidly changing world of child rearing, there are likely to be some kaleidoscopic transformations in how a father's life with his child moves through time. Even a father's relationship with a given child, his perception of that relationship, and the child's response to his behavior are likely to change if a second child is born (Volling, 2012) and life begins again.

Summary and Key Points

Research on fathers is rapidly evolving, guided by frameworks that address the factors that influence paternal behavior and processes by which fathers influence child well-being. There is more respect for the roles played by fathers in children's lives and in family life more broadly. There is also greater appreciation for the dynamic interplay of the personal and contextual factors that determine how men enact the roles that fathers play in the lives of children. Likewise, there is greater appreciation of how being a father helps shape a man's personal identity and how the centrality of paternal identity helps shape the care fathers provide children. Thus, research on fathers has moved beyond the boundaries originally considered significant by economists, social scientists, religious leaders, and policy makers. To advance what is needed to guide meaningful, actionable research on fathers for the futures requires consideration of the following key points:

- Advances in technology are penetrating into almost every aspect of human life. New technologies are affecting how fathers think and the actions they take for their children.
- The roles of both men and women in the workforce are rapidly evolving. There is more use of advanced technologies and greater need for critical thinking and flexibility in approaches to tasks. There is also more need for autonomous (sometimes coordinated) actions in carrying out work tasks. Changes in the workplace are bringing about changes in how parents think and how they perform the tasks of parenting.
- Households have become smaller; and more fathers do not live with their biological offspring on a daily basis. These changes in household composition are affecting paternal behavior and parent-child relationships.
- Fatherhood remains central to many men's identity. Brain science is making clearer how experiences with children (from prior to birth) can affect both the structural and functional characteristics of men's brains. The changes that occur in the brain affect a father's identity, his emotional responses, his motivations, and his behavior.

References

Abraham, E., Hendler, T., Shapira-Lichter, I., Kanat-Maymon, Y., Zagoory-Sharon, O., & Feldman, R. (2014). Father's brain is sensitive to childcare experiences. *Proceedings of the National Academy of Sciences USA, 111*, 9792–9797.

Adamasons, K., & Pasley, K. (2016). Parents' fathering identity standards and later father involvement. *Journal of Family Issues, 37*, 221–244.

Ahnert, L., Teufl, L., Ruiz, N., Piskernik, B., Supper, B., Remiorz, S., et al. (2017). Father-child play during the preschool years and child internalizing behaviors: Between robustness and vulnerability. *Infant Mental Health Journal, 38*, 243–256.

AICPA. (2017). *2017 CPA firm gender survey*. Available at: https://www.aicpa.org/content/dam/aicpa/career/womenintheprofession/downloadabledocuments/wiec-2017-cpa-firm-gender-survey-brochure.pdf

Akhtar, S., & Samuel, S. (1996). The concept of identity developmental origins, phenomenology, clinical relevance and measurement. *Harvard Review of Psychiatry, 3*, 254–267.

Algood, S., Beckert, T., & Peterson, C. (2012). The role of father involvement in the perceived psychological well-being of young adult daughters: A retrospective study. *North American Journal of Psychiatry, 14*, 95–110.

Ali, A., & Daoud, F. (2016). Early father-daughter relationship and demographic determinants of spousal marital satisfaction. *Psychology Research and Behavior Management, 9*, 61–70.

Allendorf, K. (2012). Like daughter, like son? Fertility decline and the transformation of gender systems in the family. *Demographic Research, 27*, 429–454.

American Academy of Child and Adolescent Psychiatry. (2015, December). *Stepfamily problems*. Available at: https://www.aacap.org/AACAP/Families_and_Youth/Facts_for_Families/FFF-Guide/Stepfamily-Problems-027.aspx

American Academy of Pediatrics. (2016). *Healthy digital media use habits for babies, toddlers, and preschoolers*. Available at: https://www.healthychildren.org/English/family-life/Media/Pages/Healthy-Digital-Media-Use-Habits-for-Babies-Toddlers-Preschoolers.aspx

Barnett, M. A., Deng, M., Mills-Koonce, W. R., Willoughby, M., & Cox, M. (2008). Interdependence of parenting of mothers and fathers of infants. *Journal of Family Psychology, 22*, 561–573.

Belch, M. A., & Willis, L. A. (2002). Family decision at the turn of the century: Has the changing structure of households impacted the family decision-making process? *Journal of Consumer Behavior, 2*, 111–124.

Bonafide, C., Lacalio, A., Ferro, D., Orenstein, M., Jamison, D., Lavanchy, C., et al. (2018). Accuracy of pulse oximetry-based home baby monitors. *JAMA, 320*, 717–719.

Bonds, D., & Gondoli, D. M. (2007). Examining the process by which marital adjustment affects maternal warmth: The role of coparenting support as a mediator. *Journal of Family Psychology, 21*, 288–296.

Bosoni, M. L. (2014). "Breadwinners" or "involved fathers?" men, fathers and work in Italy. *Journal of Comparative Family Studies, 45*, 293–315.

Bouchard, G., Lee, C. M., Asgary, V., & Pelletier, L. (2007). Fathers' motivation of involvement with their children: A self-determination theory perspective. *Fathering, 5*, 25–41.

Bozzola, E., Spina, G., Ruggiero, M., Memo, L., Agostiniani, R., Bossola, M., et al. (2018). Media devices in pre-school children: The recommendations of the Italian Pediatric Society. *Italian Journal of Pediatrics, 44*, 69.

Bronte-Tinkew, J., Carrano, J., Horowitz, A., & Kinukawa, A. (2008). Involvement among resident fathers and links to infant cognitive outcomes. *Journal of Family Issues, 29*, 1211–1244.

Brotherson, S. E., Yamamoto, T., & Acock, A. A. (2003). Connection and communication in father-chid relationships and adolescent child well-being. *Fathering, 1*, 191–214.

Bureau of Labor Statistics, U.S. Department of Labor. (2017). *Average hours per day spent caring for and helping household children as their main activity*. Available at: https://www.bls.gov/charts/american-time-use/activity-by-parent.htm

Burns, J. C., & Caldwell, C. H. (2016). Breaking the ice! Predictors about communication between nonresident African American fathers and sons about sex. *Journal of the American Association of Nurse Practitioners, 28*, 84–90.

Burrell, A., Ives, J., & Freudtner, G. (2017). The experiences of fathers who have offspring with autism spectrum disorder. *Journal of Autism and Developmental Disorders, 47*, 1135–1147.

Cabrera, N. J., Fitzgerald, H. E., Bradley, R. H., & Roggman, L. (2014). Father's influences on their children: An expanded model. *Journal of Family Theory and Review, 6*, 336–354.

CAF (Contact A Family). (2005). *Fathers factsheet*. London: Contact a Family. Available at: http://www.cafamily.org.uk/fathers.html

Caldwell, C., Wright, J., Zimmerman, M., Walsemann, K., Williams, D., & Isichei, P. (2004). Enhancing adolescent health behaviors through strengthening non-resident father-son relationships: Model for intervention with African-American families. *Health Education Research, 19*, 644–656.

Caldwell, C. H., Antonakos, C. L., Assari, S., Kruger, D., Loney, E. H., & Njai, R. (2014). Pathways to prevention: Improving nonresident African American fathers' parenting skills and behaviors to reduce sons' aggression. *Child Development, 85*, 308–325.

Carpenter, B., & Towers, C. (2008). Recognising fathers: The needs of fathers of children with disabilities. *Support for Learning, 23*, 118–125.

Carroll, K. W., Mollen, C. J., Aldridge, S., Hexem, K. R., & Feudtner, C. (2012). Influences on decision making identified by parents of children receiving pediatric palliative care. *AJOB Primary Research, 3*(1), 1–7.

Casey, B. M., Lombardi, C. M., Thomson, D., Nguyen, H. N., Paz, M., Theriault, C. A., et al. (2018). Maternal support of children's early numerical concept learning predicts preschool and first-grade math achievement. *Child Development, 89*, 156–173.

Center on Media and Human Development, Northwestern University. (2014, June). *Parenting in the age of digital technology*. Available at: https://cmhd.northwestern.edu/wp-content/uploads/2015/06/ParentingAgeDigitalTechnology.REVISED.FINAL_.2014.pdf

Centers for Disease Control and Prevention. (2018). *Health, United States, 2017 – data finder*. Available at: https://www.cdc.gov/nchs/hus/contents2017.htm?search=,Child_and_adolescent

Cherlin, A. J. (2014). *Labor's love lost*. New York: Russell Sage Foundation.

Cohen, E., Kuo, D. Z., Agrawal, R., Berry, J. G., Bhagat, S. K., Simon, T. D., et al. (2011). Children with medical complexity: An emerging population for clinical and research initiatives. *Pediatrics, 127*, 529–538.

Common Sense Media. (2016). *Technology addiction: Concern, controversy, and finding balance*. Available at: https://www.commonsensemedia.org/research/technology-addiction-concern-controversy-and-finding-balance

Corwyn, R. F., & Bradley, R. H. (2016). Fathers' autonomy support and social competence of sons and daughters. *Merrill-Palmer Quarterly, 62*, 359–387.

Cunningham, M. (2008). Changing attitudes toward the male breadwinner, female homemaker family model: Influences of women's employment and education over the lifecourse. *Social Forces, 87*, 299–323.

Daly, K. J., Ashbourne, L., & Brown, J. L. (2012). A reorientation of worldview: Children's influence on fathers. *Journal of Family Issues, 34*, 1401–1424.

Darling, C. A., Senatore, N., & Strachan, J. (2011). Fathers of children with disabilities: Stress and life satisfaction. *Stress and Health, 28*, 269–278.

Davis, E. F., Shoppe-Sullivan, S. J., Mangelsdorf, S. C., & Brown, G. L. (2009). The role of infant temperament in stability and change in coparenting across the first year of life. *Parenting: Science and Practice, 9*, 143–159.

de Cock, E. S., Henrichs, J., Vreeswijk, C. M., Maas, A. J., Rijk, C. H., & van Bakel, H. J. (2015). Continuous feelings of love: The parental bond from pregnancy to toddlerhood. *Journal of Family Psychology, 30*, 125–134.

De Graaf, J. V., Hoogenboom, M., De Roos, S., & Bucz, F. (2018). Socio-demographic correlates of fathers' and mothers' parenting behaviors. *Journal of Child and Family Studies, 27*, 2315–2327.

Deaux, K., & Martin, D. (2003). Interpersonal networks and social categories: Specifying levels of context in identity processes. *Social Psychology Quarterly, 66*, 101–117.

Domingo, P., Holmes, R., O'Neil, T., Jones, N., Bird, K., Larson, A., et al. (2015). *Women's voice and leadership in decision-making: Assessing the evidence*. London: ODI.

Donnelly, K., Twenge, J. M., Clark, M. A., Shaikh, S. K., Beiler-May, A., & Carter, N. T. (2016). Attitudes towards women's work and family roles in the United States, 1976-2013. *Psychology of Women Quarterly, 40*, 41–54.

Dworkin, J., Connell, J., & Doty, J. (2013). A literature of parents' online behavior. *Cyberpsychology: Journal of Psychosocial Research on Cyberspace, 7*(2), 2.

Dyches, T. T., Smith, T. B., Korth, B. B., Roper, S. O., & Mandleco, B. (2012). Positive parenting of children with developmental disabilities: A meta-analysis. *Research in Developmental Disabilities, 33*, 2213–2230.

Eliason, S. R., Mortimer, J. T., & Vuolo, M. (2015). The transition to adulthood: Life course structures and subjective perceptions. *Social Psychology Quarterly, 78*, 205–227.

Epstein, N. B., Bishop, D., Ryan, C., Miller, I., & Keitner, G. (1993). The McMaster model view of healthy family functioning. In F. Walsh (Ed.), *Normal family processes* (pp. 138–160). New York: Guilford Press.

Erikson, E. H. (1968). *Identity: Youth and crisis*. New York: Norton.

Fawcett, T. N., Baggaley, S. E., Wu, C., Whyte, D. A., & Martinson, I. M. (2005). Parental responses to health care services for children with chronic conditions and their families: A comparison between Hong Kong and Scotland. *Journal of Child Health Care, 9*, 8–19.

Feinberg, M., & Kan, M. (2008). Establishing family foundations: Intervention effects on coparenting, parent/infant well-being, and parent-child relations. *Journal of Family Psychology, 22*, 253–263.

Fletcher, R., & StGeorge, J. (2011). Heading into fatherhood-nervously: Support for fathering from online dads. *Qualitative Health Research, 21*, 1101–1114.

Flouri, E., & Buchanan, A. (2002). What predicts good relationships with parents in adolescence and partners in adult life? Findings from the 1958 British cohort study. *Journal of Family Psychology, 16*, 186–198.

Fonagy, P., Gergely, G., & Jurist, E. L. (2002). *Target M: Affect regulation, mentalization, and the development of the self*. New York: Other Press.

Fox, G., & Bruce, C. (2001). Conditional fatherhood: Identity theory and parental investment theory as alternative sources of explanation of fathering. *Journal of Marriage and Family, 63*, 394–403.

Fox, G. L., Nordquist, V. M., Billen, R. M., & Savoca, E. F. (2015). Father involvement and early intervention: Effects of empowerment and father role identity. *Family Relations, 64*, 461–475.

Futon Critic. (2017, March). *Ratings*. Available at: http://www.thefutoncritic.com/ratings/2017/03/28/24-hour-disney-junior-channel-celebrates-4-years-at-number-1-turbocharged-by-mickey-and-the-roadster-racers-745410/20170328disney01/

Gaertner, B., Spinrad, T., Eisenberg, N., & Greving, K. (2007). Parental childrearing attitudes as correlates of father involvement during infancy. *Journal of Marriage and Family, 69*, 962–976.

GBD 2017 Child and Adolescent Health Collaborators. (2019). Diseases, injuries, and risk factors in child and adolescent health, 1990 to 2017. Findings from the global burden of diseases, injuries, and risk factors 2017 study. *JAMA Pediatrics, 173*, E1–E17. Available at: https://jamanetwork.com/

Geary, D. C. (2000). Evolution and proximate expression of human paternal investment. *Psychological Bulletin, 126*, 55–77.

Gettler, L. T. (2016). Becoming DADS: Considering the role of cultural context and developmental plasticity for paternal socioendocrinology. *Current Anthropology, 57*(Supplement 13), S38–S55.

Glass, H. C., Costarino, T., Stayer, S. A., Brett, C., Cladis, F., & Davis, P. J. (2015). Outcomes for extremely premature infants. *Anesthesia and Analgesia, 120*, 1337–1351.

Goble, L. A. (2004). The impact of a child's chronic illness on fathers. *Issues in Comprehensive Pediatric Nursing, 27*, 153–162.

Goldberg, W. A., Prause, J., Lucas-Thompson, R., & Himsel, A. (2008). Maternal employment and children's achievement in context: A meta-analysis of four decades of research. *Psychological Bulletin, 134*, 77–108.

Greenberg, J. S. (2002). The role of fathers in the lives of their sons and daughters with mental illness. In B. J. Kramer & E. H. Thompson (Eds.), *Men as caregivers: Theory, research, and service implications* (pp. 269–293). New York: Springer Publications.

Ha, J., Greenberg, J. S., & Seltzer, M. M. (2011). Parenting a child with a disability: The role of social support for African American parents. *Families in Society, 92*, 405–411.

Ha, J., Hong, J., Seltzer, M. M., & Greenberg, J. S. (2008). Age and gender differences in the well-being of midlife and aging parents with children with mental health or developmental problems: Report of a national study. *Journal of Health and Social Behavior, 49*, 301–316.

Hagmann, P., Cammoun, L., Gigandet, X., Meuli, R., Honey, X., Wedeen, V., et al. (2008). Mapping the structural core of human cerebral cortex. *PLoS Biology, 6*(7), e159.

Halpern, D. F., Benbow, C. P., Geary, D. C., Gur, R. C., Hyde, J. S., & Gernsbacher, M. A. (2007). The science of sex differences in science and mathematics. *Psychological Science in the Public Interest, 8*, 1–51.

Hare, B. (2011). From hominoid to hominid mind: What changed and why? *Annual Review of Anthropology, 40*, 293–309.

Harrington, B., Fraone, J. S., & Lee, J. (2017). *The new dad: The career-caregiving conflict*. Center for Work and Family – Report, Boston College. Available at: http://www.thenewdad.org/yahoo_site_admin/assets/docs/BCCWF_The_New_Dad_2017.163104025.pdf

Hartley, S. L., Papp, L. M., & Bolt, D. (2018). Spillover of marital interactions with parenting stress in families of children with autism spectrum disorder. *Journal of Clinical Child and Adolescent Psychology, 47*(Supplement 1), S88–S99.

Heaton, J., Noyes, J., & Sloper, P. (2005). Families' experience of caring for technology-dependent children: A temporal perspective. *Health & Social Care in the Community, 13*, 441–450.

Heiman, T. (2002). Parents of children with disabilities: Resilience, coping, and future expectations. *Journal of Developmental and Physical Disabilities, 14*, 159–171.

Henley, K., & Pasley, K. (2005). Conditions affecting the association between father identity and father involvement. *Fathering, 3*, 59–80.

Hill, J., Waldfogel, J., Brooks-Gunn, J., & Han, W.-J. (2005). Maternal employment and child development: A fresh look using newer methods. *Developmental Psychology, 41*, 833–850.

Hitlin, S. (2003). Values as the core of personal identity: Drawing links between two theories of self. *Social Psychology Quarterly, 66*, 118–137.

Holland, A., & McElwain, N. (2013). Maternal and paternal perceptions of coparenting as a link between marital quality and the parent–toddler relationship. *Journal of Family Psychology, 27*, 117–126.

Hovey, J. K. (2005). Fathers parenting chronically ill children: Concerns and coping strategies. *Issues in Comprehensive Pediatric Nursing, 28*, 83–95.

Hrdy, S. B. (1999). *Mother nature: A history of mothers, infants, and natural selection*. New York: Pantheon Books.

Hsin, A., & Felfe, C. (2014). When does time matter? Maternal employment, children's time with parents, and child development. *Demography, 51*, 1867–1894.

Hutchison, J., Lyons, I., & Ansari, D. (2019). More similar than different: Gender differences in children's basic numerical skills are the exception not the rule. *Child Development, 90*, e66–e79.

INED. (2013). *Developed countries data base*. Available at: http://ined.fr/en/pop_figures/developed_countries_database/

Joussemet, M., Landry, R., & Koestner, R. (2008). A self-determination theory perspective on parenting. *Canadian Psychology, 49*, 194–200.

Kabali, H., Irigoyen, M., Nunez-Davis, R., Budacki, J., Mohanty, S., Leister, K., et al. (2015). Exposure and use of mobile media devices by young children. *Pediatrics, 136*, 1044–1050.

Kenrick, D. T., Neuberg, S. L., Griskevicius, V., Becker, D. V., & Schaller, M. (2010). Goal-driven cognition and functional behavior: The fundamental-motives framework. *Current Directions in Psychological Science, 19*, 63–67.

Kersey, A., Braham, E., Scumitta, K., Libertus, M., & Cantlon, J. (2018). No intrinsic gender differences in children's earliest numerical abilities. *NPJ Science of Learning, 2018*(3), 12.

Kim, P., Rigo, P., Leckman, J. F., Mayes, L. C., Cole, P. M., Feldman, R., et al. (2015). A prospective study of perceived infant outcomes at 18-24 months: Neural and psychological correlates of parental thoughts and actions assessed during the first month postpartum. *Frontiers in Psychology, 6*, 1772.

Kim, H. N, Wyatt, T. H., Li, X., & Gaylord, M. (2016). Use of social media by fathers of premature infants. *Journal of Perinatal & Neonatal Nursing, 34*, 359–366.

Klein, S. B. (2014). Sameness and the self: Philosophical and psychological considerations. *Frontiers in Psychology, 5*, 29.

Knafl, K., & Zoeller, L. (2000). Childhood chronic illness: A comparison of mothers' and fathers' experiences. *Journal of Family Nursing, 6*, 287–330.

Kohn, M. (1963). Social class and parent–child relationships: An interpretation. *The American Journal of Sociology, 68*, 471–480.

Kreyenfeld, M. (2015). Maternal and paternal employment across the life course. In R. Scott & S. Kosslyn (Eds.), *Emerging trends in the social and behavioral sciences* (pp. 1–15). Hoboken, NJ: Wiley.

Kroger, J., Martinussen, M., & Marcia, J. E. (2010). Identity change during adolescence and young adulthood: A meta-analysis. *Journal of Adolescence, 33*, 683–698.

Krupenye, C., Kano, F., Hirata, S., Call, J., & Tomasello, M. (2016). Great apes anticipate that other individuals will act according to false beliefs. *Science, 354*(6308), 110–114.

Kuczynski, L., & Parkin, C. M. (2009). Pursuing a dialectical perspective on transaction: Social relational theory of micro family processes. In A. Sameroff (Ed.), *The transactional model of development: How children and contexts shape each other* (pp. 247–268). Washington, DC: American Psychological Association.

Kuo, D. Z., Houtrow, A. J., & Council on Children with Disabilities. (2016). Recognition and management of medical complexity. *Pediatrics, 138*(6), e20163021.

Kuo, D. Z., Lyle, R. E., Casey, P. M., & Stille, C. J. (2017). Care system redesign for preterm children after discharge from the NICU. *Pediatrics, 139*(4), e2016162969.

Kurzweil, R. (2005). *The singularity is near: When humans transcend biology*. London: Penguin.

Lamb, M., & Lewis, C. (2010). The development and significance of father-child relationships in two-parent families. In M. Lamb (Ed.), *The role of the father in child development* (5th ed., pp. 94–153). Hoboken, NJ: Wiley.

Lamb, M. E. (1975). Fathers: Forgotten contributors to child development. *Human Development, 18*, 245–266.

Lamela, D., & Figueriredo, B. (2016). Coparenting after marital dissolution and children's mental health: A systematic review. *Jornal de Pediatria, 92*, 331–342.

Latham, R. M., Mark, K. M., & Oliver, B. R. (2018). Coparenting and children's disruptive behavior: Interacting processes for parenting sense of competence. *Journal of Family Psychology, 32*, 151–156.

Levni, E., & Kopf, D. (2017, October). *The decline of the large US family, in charts*. https://qz.com/1099800/average-size-of-a-us-family-from-1850-to-the-present/

Lewis, M. D. (2000). The promise of dynamic systems approaches for an integrated account of human development. *Child Development, 71*, 36–43.

Lindberg, S. M., Hyde, J. S., Petersen, J. L., & Linn, M. C. (2010). New trends in gender and mathematics performance: A meta-analysis. *Psychological Bulletin, 136*, 1123–1135.

Livingston, G., & Parker, K. (2019, June 12). 8 facts about American dads. In Pew Research Center, FACTANK. Available at: https://www.pewresearch.org/fact-tank/2019/06/12/fathers-day-facts/

Livingston, G., & Bialik, K. (2018, May). *7 facts about U.S. moms*. Pew Research Center, FACTANK. Available at: https://www.pewresearch.org/fact-tank/2018/05/10/facts-about-u-s-mothers/

Long, K., & Marsland, A. (2011). Family adjustment to childhood cancer: A systematic review. *Clinical Child and Family Psychology Review, 14*, 57–88.

Lonsdorf, E. H., Ross, S. R., & Matsuzawa, T. (2010). *The mind of the chimpanzee: Ecological and experimental perspectives*. Chicago: University of Chicago Press.

Luz, R., George, A., Vieux, R., & Spitz, E. (2017). Antenatal determinants of parental attachment and parenting alliance: How do mothers and fathers differ? *Infant Mental Health Journal, 38*, 183–197.

Madrigal, A. (2018, November). Raised by YouTube. *The Atlantic*. Available at: https://www.theatlantic.com/magazine/archive/2018/11/raised-by-youtube/570838/

Mahone, E., & Denckla, M. (2017). Attention-deficit/hyperactivity disorder: A historical neuropsychological perspective. *Journal of the International Neuropsychological Society, 23*, 916–929.

Marks, J., Bun, L. B., & McHale, S. M. (2009). Family patterns of gender role attitudes. *Sex Roles, 61*, 221–234.

Mascaro, J., Renscher, K., Hackett, P., Mehl, M., & Rilling, J. (2017). Child gender influence paternal behavior, language, and brain function. *Behavioral Neuroscience, 131*, 262–273.

Maurer, T. W., Pleck, J. H., & Rane, T. E. (2003). Methodological considerations in measuring paternal identity. *Fathering, 1*, 117–130.

McCarthy, J., Bauer, B., Sood, A., Limburg, P. J., Goodin, T., & Malleret, T. (2018). *Wellness in the age of the smartphone*. Available from the Global Wellness Institute at: https://www.globalwellnessinstitute.org/global-wellness-institute-blog/2018/4/10/new-report-wellness-in-the-age-of-the-smartphone

McDaniel, B. T., Teti, D. M., & Feinberg, M. E. (2018). Predicting coparenting quality in daily life in mothers and fathers. *Journal of Family Psychology, 32*, 904–914.

McGaughey, W. (2002). World civilization identified with five epochs of history. *Comparative Civilizations Review, 46*, 3.

McHale, J. P., & Coates, E. E. (2014). Observed coparenting and triadic dynamics in African American fragile families at 3 months postpartum. *Infant Mental Health Journal, 35*, 435–451.

McMunn, A., Martin, P., Kelly, Y., & Sacker, A. (2017). Fathers' involvement: Correlates and consequences for child socioemotional behavior in the United Kingdom. *Journal of Family Issues, 38*, 1109–1131.

Milkie, M. A., Nomaguchi, K. M., & Denny, K. E. (2015). Does the amount of time mothers spend with children or adolescents matter? *Journal of Marriage and Family, 77*, 355–372.

Mora-Bermudez, F., Badsha, F., Kanton, S., Camp, J. G., Vernot, B., Kohler, K., et al. (2016). Differences and similarities between human and chimpanzee neural progenitors during cerebral cortex development. *eLife, 5*, e18683.

Morman, M. T., & Floyd, K. (2002). A "changing culture of fatherhood": Effects on affectionate communication, closeness, and satisfaction in men's relationships with their fathers and their sons. *Western Journal of Communication, 66*, 395–411.

Murray, C., Stanton, M., Lonsdorf, E., Wroblewski, E., & Pusey, A. (2016). Chimpanzee fathers bias their behavior towards their offspring. *Royal Society Open Science, 3*, 160441.

National Academies of Sciences, Engineering, and Medicine. (2015). *Mental disorders and disabilities among low-income children*. Washington, DC: The National Academies Press.

National Academies of Sciences, Engineering, and Medicine. (2016). *Parenting matters: Supporting parents of children ages 0–8*. Washington, DC: The National Academies Press.

National Academies of Sciences, Engineering, and Medicine. (2017). *Information technology and the U.S. workforce. Where are we and where do we go from here?* Washington, DC: National Academies Press.

National Cancer Institute. (2019). *Cancer in children and adolescents*. Available at: https://www.cancer.gov/types/childhood-cancers/child-adolescent-cancers-fact-sheet

Neil-Urban, S., & Jones, J. (2002). Father-to-father support: Fathers of children with cancer share their experience. *Journal of Pediatric Oncology Nursing, 19*, 97–103.

Nelson, J. A., & O'Brien, M. (2012). Does unplanned pregnancy have long-term implications for mother-child relationships? *Journal of Family Issues, 33*, 506–526.

Niela-Vilen, H., Axelin, A., Salantera, S., & Melender, H. (2014). Internet-based peer support for parents: Systematic integrative review. *International Journal of Nursing Studies, 51*, 1524–1537.

Nielsen, L. (2017). Re-examining the research on parental conflict, coparenting, and custody arrangements. *Psychology, Public Policy, and Law, 23*, 211–231.

Nikken, P. (2019). Parents' instrumental use of media in childrearing: Relationships with confidence in parenting, and health and conduct problems in children. *Journal of Child and Family Studies, 28*, 531–546.

Nouwen, M., JafariNaimi, N., & Zaman, B. (2017). Parental controls: Reimagining technologies for parent-child interaction. In *Proceedings of 15th European conference on computer-supported cooperative work – exploratory papers*. Reports of the European Society for Socially Embedded Technologies (ISSN 2510-2591)

Nunes, S., Fite, J. E., Patera, K. J., & French, J. A. (2001). Interactions among paternal behavior, steroid hormones, and parental experience in male marmosets (Callithrix kuhlii). *Hormones and Behavior, 39*, 70–82.

Nunes-Costa, R., Figueriredo, B., & Maya-Albiol, L. (2016). The state of art of biological processes in paternal care. *Psychology/Psicologia Reflexao e Critica, 27*, 794–805.

OECD. (2016). *OECE Family Database, SF1.1: Family size and household composition*. Available at: http://www.oecd.org/els/family/SF_1_1_Family_size_and_composition.pdf

OECD. (2018). *OECD Family Database, SR3.1: Marriage and divorce rates*. Available at: http://www.oecd.org/social/family/SF_3_1_Marriage_and_divorce_rates.pdf

Olah, L. S., Kotowska, I. E., & Richter, R. (2018). Thc new roles of men and women and implications for families and societies. In G. Doblhammer & J. Guma (Eds.), *A demographic perspective on gender, family and health in Europe* (pp. 41–64). Cham, Switzerland: Springer.

Opondo, C., Redshaw, M., Savage-McGlynn, E., & Quigley, M. A. (2016). Father involvement in early child-rearing and behavioural outcomes in their pre-adolescent children: Evidence from the ALSPACK UK birth cohort. *BMJ Open, 6*, e012034.

Ortiz-Ospina, E., Tzvetkova, S., & Roser, M. (2018). *Female labor supply*. Our World Data. Available at: https://ourworldindata.org/female-labor-supply

Palkovitz, R., Fagan, J., & Hull, J. (2013). Coparenting and children's well-being. In N. J. Cabrera & C. S. Tamis-LeMonda (Eds.), *Handbook of father involvement: Multidisciplinary perspectives* (pp. 202–219). New York: Routledge/Taylor & Francis Group.

Palkovitz, R., & Hull, J. (2018). Toward a resource theory of fathering. *Journal of Family Theory and Review, 10*, 181–198.

Parker, K., & Stepler, R. (2017, September). *Americans see men as the financial providers, even as women's contributions grow*. Pew Research Center, FACTANK. Available at: https://www.pewresearch.org/2017/09/20/americans-see-men-as-the-financial-providers-even-as.women's contributions grow/

Parkes, A., Green, M., & Mitchell, K. (2019). Coparenting and parenting pathways from the couple relationship to children's behavior problems. *Journal of Family Psychology, 33*, 215–225.

Peltz, J. S., Rogge, R. D., & Sturge-Apple, M. L. (2018). Transactions within the family: Coparenting mediates associations between parents' relationship satisfaction and the parent-child relationship. *Journal of Family Psychology, 32*, 553–564.

Perkins, R. (2001). The father-daughter relationship: Familial interactions that impact a daughter's style of life. *College Studies Journal, 35*, 616–627.

Perrin, J. M., Anderson, L. E., & van Cleave, J. (2014). The rise in chronic conditions among infants, children, and youth can be met with continued health system innovations. *Health Affairs, 33*, 2099–2105.

Pew Research Center. (2013, March). *Modern parenthood: Roles of moms and dads converge as they balance work and family*. Available at: https://www.pewsocialtrends.org/2013/03/14/modern-parenthood-roles-of-moms-and-dads-converge-as-they-balance-work-and-family

Pew Research Center. (2015a, November). *Raising kids and running a household: How working parents share the load*. Available at: https://www.pewresearch.org/wp-content/uploads/sites/3/2015/11/2015-11-04_working-parents_FINAL.pdf

Pew Research Center. (2015b, December). *Parenting in America: Outlook, worries, aspirations are strongly linked to financial situation*. Available at: https://www.pewresearch.org/wp-content/uploads/sites/3/2015/12/2015-12-17_parenting-in-america_FINAL.pdf

Pew Research Center. (2016a, January). *Parents, teens and digital monitoring*. Available at: https://www.pewinternet.org/2016/01/07/parents-teens-and-digital-monitoring/

Pew Research Center. (2016b, October). *The state of American jobs: How the economic landscape is reshaping work and society and the way people think about the skills and training they need to get ahead*. Available at: https://www.pewsocialtrends.org/2016/10/06/the-state-of-American-jobs

Pew Research Center. (2018, February). *Internet/broadband connection*. Available at: https://www.pewinternet.org/fact-sheet/internet-broadband/

Pfledderer, C., Burns, R., & Brusseau, T. (2019). Association between access to electronic devices in the home environment and cardiorespiratory fitness in children. *Children, 6*, 8.

Plavacan, J. M. (2012). Social behavior of early hominins. *International Journal of Primatology, 33*, 1247–1250.

Pleck, J. H. (2010). Paternal involvement. In M. E. Lamb (Ed.), *The role of the father in child development* (5th ed., pp. 58–93). Hoboken, NJ: Wiley.

Pruden, S. M., & Levine, S. C. (2017). Parents' spatial language mediates a sex difference in preschoolers' spatial-language use. *Psychological Science, 28*, 1583–1596.

Qian, Y., De Loney, E. H., & Caldwell, C. H. (2018). Moderating effects of residential history on the effects of a fatherhood program on parenting skills satisfaction among nonresident African American fathers. *Healthcare, 6*, 13.

Raley, S., Bianchi, S., & Yang, W. (2012). When do fathers care? Mothers' economic contribution and fathers' involvement in child care. *American Journal of Sociology, 117*, 1422–1459.

Rane, T. R., & McBride, B. A. (2000). Identity theory as a guide to understanding fathers' involvement with their children. *Journal of Family Issues, 21*, 347–366.

Reinking, A., & Martin, B. (2018). The gender gap in STEM fields: Theories, movements, and ideas to engage girls in STEM. *Journal of New Approaches in Educational Research, 7*, 148–153.

Rhodes, M., Leslie, S. J., Yee, K., & Saunders, K. (2019). Subtle linguistic cues increase girls' engagement in science. *Psychological Science, 30*, 455–466.

Rice, C. E., Rosanoff, M., Dawson, G., Durkin, M. S., Croen, L. A., Singer, A., et al. (2012). Evaluating changes in the prevalence of autism spectrum disorders (ASDs). *Public Health Reviews, 34*, 1–22.

Robison, L. L., & Hudson, M. M. (2014). Survivors of childhood and adolescent cancer: Life- long risks and responsibilities. *National Review of Cancer, 14*, 61–70.

Samman, E., Presler-Marshall, E., & Jones, N. (2016). *Women's work, mothers, children and the global childcare crisis*. Available at: https://www.odi.org/publications/10349-women-s-work-mothers-children-and-global-childcare-crisis

Saturn, S. (2014). Flexibility of the father's brain. *Proceedings of the National Academy of Sciences of the United States of America, 11*(27), 9671–9672.

Schoppe-Sullivan, S. J., Kotila, L., Jia, R., Lang, S. N., & Bower, D. J. (2013). Comparisons of levels and predictors of mothers' and fathers' engagement with their preschool aged children. *Early Child Development and Care, 183*, 498–514.

Seltzer, M. M., Greenberg, J. S., Floyd, F. J., Pettee, Y., & Hong, J. (2001). Life course impacts of parenting a child with a disability. *American Journal of Mental Retardation, 106*, 265–286.

Sherman, J., & Harris, E. (2012). Social class and parenting: Classic debates and new understandings. *Social Compass, 6*, 60–71.

Silander, M., Grindal, T., Hupert, N., Garcia, E., Anderson, K., Vahey, P., et al. (2018). *What parents talk about when they talk about learning: A national survey about young children and science*. New York/Menlo Park, CA: Education Development Center, Inc./SRI International. Available at: https://www.sri.com/sites/default/files/publications/edc_sri_what_parents_talk_about.pdf

Smith, J., Cheater, F., & Bekker, H. (2012). Parents' experiences of living with a child with a long-term condition: A rapid structured review of the literature. *Health Expectations, 18*, 452–474.

Sobsey, D. (2002). Marital stability and marital satisfaction in families of children with disabilities: Chicken or egg? *Developmental Disabilities Bulletin, 32*, 62–83.

Statistics Canada. (2018). *The shift to smaller households over the past century*. https://www150.statcan.gc.ca/n1/pub/11-630-x/11-630-x2015008-eng.htm

Stein, S. (2018, March). An age-by-age guide to kids and smartphones. *Today's Parent*. Available at: https://www.todaysparent.com/family/.../an-age-by-age-guide-to-kids-and-smartphone...

Stgeorge, J., & Freeman, E. (2017). Measurement of father-child rough-and-tumble play and its relation to child behavior. *Infant Mental Health Journal, 38*, 709–725.

Storey, A. E., & Ziegler, T. E. (2016). Primate paternal care: Interactions with biology and social experience. *Hormones and Behavior, 77*, 260–271.

Strauss, R., & Goldberg, W. A. (1999). Self and possible selves during the transition to fatherhood. *Journal of Family Psychology, 13*, 244–264.

Sullivan-Bolyai, S., Rosenberg, R., & Bayard, M. (2006). Fathers' reflections on parenting young children with type 1 diabetes. *American Journal of Maternal and Child Nursing, 31*, 24–31.

Swain, J. E., Dayton, C. J., Kim, P., Tolman, R. M., & Volling, B. L. (2014). Progress on the paternal brain: Theory, animal models, human brain research, and mental health implications. *Infant Mental Health Journal, 35*, 394–408.

Swallow, V., Macfadyen, A., Sanatacroce, S., & Lambert, H. (2012). Fathers' contributions to the management of their child's long-term medical condition: A narrative review of the literature. *Health Expectations, 15*, 157–175.

Sweeting, H., Bhaskar, A., Benzeval, M., Popham, F., & Hunt, K. (2013). Changing gender roles and attitudes and their implications for well-being around the new millennium. *Social Psychiatry and Psychiatric Epidemiology, 49*, 791–809.

Tandon, P., Grow, H. M., Couch, S., Glanz, K., Sallis, J. F., Frank, L. D., et al. (2014). Physical and social home environment in relation to children's overall and home-based physical activity and sedentary time. *Preventive Medicine, 66*, 39–44.

Thomson, D., Casey, B. M., Lombardi, C. M., & Nguyen, H. N. (2020). Quality of fathers' spatial concept support during block building predicts their daughters' early math skill – but not their sons'. *Early Childhood Research Quarterly, 50*, 51–64.

Tomasetto, C., Mirisola, A., Galdi, S., & Cadinu, M. (2015). Parents' math–gender stereotypes, children's self-perception of ability, and children's appraisal of parents' evaluations in 6-year-olds. *Contemporary Educational Psychology, 42*, 186–198.

Tsang, S. K., Hui, E. K., & Law, B. C. (2012). Positive identity as a positive youth development construct: A conceptual view. *The Scientific World Journal, 2012*, 529691.

U.S. Bureau of Labor Statistics. (2019). *Civilian labor force participation rate: Women [LNS11300002]*. Retrieved from FRED, Federal Reserve Bank of St. Louis: https://fred.stlouisfed.org/series/LNS11300002

U.S. Census Bureau. (2014, April). *Adopted children and stepchildren: 2010. Population characteristics*. Available at: https://www.census.gov/prod/2014pubs/p20-572.pdf

U.S. Department of Health and Human Services, Administration on Children and Families. (2010, February). *Responsible fatherhood spotlight, father involvement – children with disabilities*. Available at: http://dhhs.nv.gov/uploadedFiles/dhhsnvgov/content/Programs/IDEA/ProjectASSIST/2010Feb-Father%20Involvement-ChildrenwithDisabilitiesUSDeptofHHSA.pdf

United Nations Children's Fund. (2018). *Levels and trends in child mortality, report 2018*. Available at: https://childmortality.org/wp-content/uploads/2018/12/UN-IGME-Child-Mortality-Report-2018.pdf

United States Census Bureau. (2018). *Historical household tables*. Table HH-4. Households by size: 1960-present. Available at: https://www.census.gov/

data/tables/time-series/demo/families/households.html

Vandello, J. (2013). When equal isn't really equal: The masculine dilemma of seeking work flexibility. *Journal of Social Issues, 69*, 301–321.

Videon, T. M. (2005). Parent-child relations and children's psychological well-being. Do dads matter? *Journal of Family Issues, 26*, 55–78.

Volling, B. L. (2012). Family transitions following the birth of a sibling: An empirical review of changes in the firstborn's adjustment. *Psychological Bulletin, 138*, 497–528.

Wade, S. L., Taylor, H. G., Walz, N. C., Salisbury, S., Stancin, T., Bernard, L. A., et al. (2006). Parent-child interactions during the initial weeks following brain injury in young children. *Rehabilitation Psychology, 53*, 180–190.

Wagner, M. E., Schubert, H. J. P., & Schubert, D. S. P. (1985). Family size effects: A review. *Journal of Genetic Psychology, 146*, 65–78.

Wallerstein, J., & Lewis, J. M. (2007). Disparate parenting and step-parenting with siblings in the post-divorce family. Report from a 10-year longitudinal study. *Journal of Family Studies, 13*, 224–235.

West, S. (2000). *Just a shadow: A review of support of fathers of children with disabilities*. Birmingham, UK: Handsel Trust.

Whitebread, D., Neale, D., Jensen, H., Liu, C., Solis, S. L., Hopkins, E., et al. (2017). *The role of play in children's development: A review of the evidence*. Billund, Denmark: The LEGO Foundation.

Whitsell, C. J., Teti, D. M., Crosby, B., & Kim, B. (2015). Household chaos, sociodemographic risk, coparenting, and parent-infant relations during the infants' first year. *Journal of Family Psychology, 29*, 211–220.

World Bank. (2019). *Infant mortality rates for the United States* (SPDYNIMRTINUSA). Available at: https://fred.stlouisfed.org/series/SPDYNIMRTINUSA

Wysocki, T., & Gavin, L. (2004). Psychometric properties of a new measure of fathers' involvement in the management of pediatric chronic diseases. *Journal of Pediatric Psychology, 29*, 231–240.

Xu, G., Strathearn, L., Liu, B., Yan, B., & Bao, W. (2018). Twenty-year trends in diagnosed attention-deficit/hyperactivity disorder among US children and adolescents, 1997-2016. *JAMA Network Open, 1*(4), e181471.

Yogman, M., Garfield, C. F., & The Committee on Psychosocial Aspects of Child and Family Health. (2016). Fathers' roles in the care and development of their children: The role of pediatricians. *Pediatrics, 138*(1), e20161128.

Yogman, M. W., Kindlon, D. & Earls, F. (1995). Father involvement and cognitive/behavioral outcomes of preterm infants. *Journal of the American Academy of Child and Adolescent Medicine, 34*, 58–66.

Ziegler, T. E., Prudom, S. L., & Zahed, S. R. (2009). Variations in male parenting and physiology in the common marmoset. *American Journal of Human Biology, 21*, 739–744.

Zimmer-Gembeck, K. J., & Collins, W. A. (2003). Autonomy development during adolescence. In G. R. Adams & M. Berzonskyi (Eds.), *Blackwell handbook of adolescence* (pp. 175–294). Oxford, UK: Blackwell Publishers.

Index

H. E. Fitzgerald et al. (eds.), *Handbook of Fathers and Child Development*,
https://doi.org/10.1007/978-3-030-51027-5

B

D

F

J

K

L

N

O

P